Gastrointestinal Hormones

Comprehensive Endocrinology

Editor-in-Chief: Luciano Martini

Endocrine Rhythms. *Dorothy T. Krieger, Editor. 1979.*

Endocrine Control of Sexual Behavior. *Carlos Beyer, Editor. 1979.*

The Adrenal Gland. *Vivian H. T. James, Editor. 1979.*

The Thyroid Gland. *Michel De Visscher, Editor. 1980.*

Gastrointestinal Hormones, *George B. Jerzy Glass, Editor. 1980.*

The Endocrine Functions of the Brain. *Marcella Motta, Editor. 1980.*

Volumes in Preparation

The Testis. *Henry Burger and David de Kretser, Editors.*

Calcium Metabolism. *John A. Parsons, Editor.*

Fertility Control. *G. Benagiano and E. Diczfalusy, Editors.*

Pediatric Endocrinology. *Robert Collu et al., Editors.*

The Ovary

The Pituitary

Diabetes

Gastrointestinal Hormones

Editor

George B. Jerzy Glass, M.D.
Dr. hon. c. Univ. Nancy and Med Acad. Krakow

Professor of Medicine and Director
Gastroenterology Research Laboratory
New York Medical College;
Consultant in Gastroenterology
Memorial Hospital for Cancer and
Allied Diseases
New York, New York

Raven Press ■ New York

Raven Press, 1140 Avenue of the Americas, New York, New York 10036

Made in the United States of America

The material contained in this volume was submitted as previously unpublished material, except in the instances in which credit has been given to the source from which some of the illustrative material was derived.

Great care has been taken to maintain the accuracy of the information contained in the volume. However, Raven Press cannot be held responsible for errors or for any consequences arising from the use of the information contained herein.

Library of Congress Cataloging in Publication Data

Main entry under title:

Gastrointestinal hormones.

    (Comprehensive endocrinology)
    Includes bibliographical references and index.
    1. Gastrointestinal hormones. I. Glass,
George B. Jerzy. II. Series. [DNLM: 1. Gastro-
intestinal hormones. WK170 G2547]
QP572.G35G36   612'.33   77–85517
ISBN 0–89004–395–7

Preface

This volume deals with one of the most explosive and important fields of modern endocrinology and gastroenterology, namely the physiology, origin, chemistry, and pharmacological and clinical aspects of the gastrointestinal hormones. The extensive contributions of analytical and synthetic peptide chemistry, immunocytochemistry, hormonal radioimmunoassay, and basic and clinical pharmacology, as well as the recent discovery of the tight interrelationships with neurosciences have opened to researchers and clinicians a new, highly promising territory for further exploration. This territory is reminiscent of a subtropical forest full of proud and established trees, jungle-like bushes interwoven with each other, beautiful flowers not yet classified in the Linnaean code, and also of frail and weak new growths struggling for survival. In this new territory the steps of the explorer are both risky and highly rewarding, but certainly full of excitement.

Unlike some of the other publications in this field, this volume is not the result of any national or international symposium on gastrointestinal hormones. It represents the collection of commissioned monographic reviews generously offered by some 40 internationally recognized gut hormone researchers and their collaborators, all of whom have significantly contributed to this new knowledge.

Sections in the volume focus on the cellular and neural origin of the gastrointestinal hormones, their morphology and functional classification, immunocytochemical methods for their study and the problems and pitfalls inherent therein, and information concerning their cellular synthesis and release. Isolation, characterization, structure-activity relationships, and biological functions are described for individual hormones and hormonal peptides: secretin, gastrin, cholecystokinin, gastric inhibitory polypeptide, motilin, vasoactive intestinal peptide, pancreatic polypeptide, gut glucagon-like immunoreactants, peptides of the amphibian skin active on the gut, including substance P, cerulein, and bombesin-like peptides, and also chymodenin and urogastrone. In addition, hormonal peptides acting both on the brain and the gut, such as somatostatin, enkephalins and endorphins, as well as their actions on the gastrointestinal tract and their radioimmunoassays, if available, are also discussed.

The volume also covers the synthesis of most of the gastrointestinal hormones, their heterogeneity, and the gastrointestinal hormone-receptor interactions in the pancreas and in the gastrointestinal tract. Effects of gastrointestinal hormones on growth of gastrointestinal tract, on gastric, pancreatic, biliary, and intestinal secretions, on the motor functions of the gastrointestinal tract and gastrointestinal sphincters, are presented and some of the gastrointestinal hormonal tumors are described. A large section is devoted to radioimmunoassays of gastrointestinal hormones, the problems and pitfalls of this technique, as well as methods for the assays of gastrin, secretin, vasoactive polypeptide, motilin, cholecystokinin, GIP, gut glucagon-like immunoreactants, somatostatin, and intraluminal secretin and gastrin.

The text concludes with a section on candidate hormones, which includes a description of some of the peptides, the final separation and characterization of which is yet to be achieved. These include villikinin and some of the substances that stimulate acid secretion (intestinal phase hormone, enterooxyntin) and those that inhibit gastric secretion and are derived from duodenal bulb (bulbogastrone) and stomach (gastrones and antral chalone). A brief description is presented of some of the work in progress in the Department of Chemistry II, Karolinska Institutet, Stockholm, on purification of five other candidate hormones obtained from porcine intestinal tissue; these may represent separate entities endowed with some interesting activities or some portions or fragments of the known peptide chains. A new chemical assay for natural peptides applicable to the isolation of candidate hormones is also presented.

The rapid flux and growth of information in the field of gastrointestinal peptides has made obsolete some of the traditional and basic concepts of anatomy, histology, physiology, and clinical sciences. This is reflected in this volume by the not infrequent divergence of views on particular topics. The complexity of hormonal interactions and plurality of hormonal effects on various organs and their functions causes some overlaps in many of the chapters, requiring frequent cross referencing. This gives the reader an additional exposure to concepts from various positions, which will be invaluable in gaining an in-depth understanding of the subject.

The editor hopes that this volume, which includes much of the information difficult to collect from other scattered sources, will be of interest and help to clinical and research endocrinologists and gastroenterologists, as well as to general internists. The researchers and teachers in basic sciences will also find here much of the information on the areas pertinent to those clinical fields.

G.B.J.G.

Acknowledgments

I am most grateful to all the authors who have by their generous collaboration contributed to this volume and thus shared with others this rich source of data. To this aim they had to accept not only my invitation, but also some of my, at times, perhaps unreasonable demands imposed on their knowledge, self discipline, and cooperative spirit.

My sincere appreciation goes also to the Raven Press and its management as well as publishing and editorial staff, who provided high standards in producing this volume. My special thanks go here to Dr. Alan Edelson and Dr. Diana Schneider for their good will and cooperation, to Berta Steiner Rosenberg for her continuous and knowledgeable support in production of this volume, to Terry Kornak for enthusiastic and careful copyediting of the text, and to Sally Fields for providing the volume with an expert and highly esthetic promotional treatment.

My deep gratitude goes also to my wife, Antonina, for her unfailing assistance, support, and patience shown me during the long time spent in organizing and editing this volume, as well as to Catherine Argiro, my office assistant for her diversified and reliable help in the preparation of this volume. I thank here also my former secretary, Maria Rivera, for her correspondence with the authors and diligent processing and retyping of some of the revised manuscripts.

George B. Jerzy Glass, M.D.

Contents

**Synthesis, Heterogeneity, and Receptor Interactions
of the Gastrointestinal Hormones and Peptides**

Candidate Peptide Hormones and Chalons

Contributors

Joel W. Adelson, M.D., Ph.D.
Institute of Medical Science
San Francisco, California 94115

Akira Arimura, M.D., Ph.D.
Department of Medicine
Tulane University
School of Medicine and
Endocrine and Peptide Laboratories
Veterans Administration Hospital
New Orleans, Louisiana 70112

Richard H. Bell, Jr., M.D.
Department of Surgery
University of California Medical Center
San Diego, California 92103

Giulio Bertaccini, M.D.
Institute of Pharmacology
University of Parma
Parma, Italy

S. R. Bloom, M.A., M.B., F.R.C.P.
Departments of Histochemistry and
  Medicine
Royal Postgraduate Medical School
London, W2OH5 England

Miklos Bodanszky, D.Sc.
Department of Chemistry
Case Western Reserve University
Cleveland, Ohio 44106

J. C. Brown, Ph.D., D.Sc.
Department of Physiology
University of British Columbia
Vancouver, British Columbia
Canada V6T 1W5

R. Buffa
Institute of Pathologic Anatomy and
  Histopathology
Histochemistry and Ultrastructure Center
University of Pavia
Pavia, Italy

P. Calderon-Attas, Ph.D.
Department of Biochemistry and Nutrition
Medical School
Universite Libre de Bruxelles
B-1000 Brussels, Belgium

C. Capella
Institute of Pathologic Anatomy and
  Histopathology
Histochemistry and Ultrastructure Center
University of Pavia
Pavia, Italy

Ruth Chang
Institutes of Medical Sciences
San Francisco, California 94115

Ta-Min Chang, Ph.D.
The Isaac Gordon Center for Digestive
  Disease and Nutrition
The Genesee Hospital and
University of Rochester
School of Medicine and Dentistry
Rochester, New York 14642

J. F. P. Chayvialle, M.D.
INSERM U 45
Hôpital E. Herriot
69374 Lyon Cedex 2 France

William Y. Chey, M.D.
The Isaac Gordon Center for Digestive
  Disease and Nutrition
The Genesee Hospital and
University of Rochester School of Medicine
  and Dentistry
Rochester, New York 55901

J. Christophe, M.D., Ph.D.
Department of Biochemistry and Nutrition
Medical School
Universite Libre de Bruxelles
B-1000 Brussels, Belgium

Sidney Cohen, M.D.
University of Pennsylvania
School of Medicine
Philadelphia, Pennsylvania 19140

David H. Coy, Ph.D.
Department of Medicine
Tulane University School of Medicine
New Orleans, Louisiana 70112

Benny Crepps, B. S.
Department of Physiology
University of North Carolina
School of Medicine
Chapel Hill, North Carolina 27514

Cora Creutzfeldt, M.D.
Division of Endocrinology and Metabolism
Department of Medicine
University of Goettingen
Goettingen, German Federal Republic

Werner Creutzfeldt, M.D.
Division of Endocrinology and Metabolism
Department of Medicine
University of Goettingen
Goettingen, German Federal Republic

Wolfram Domschke, M.D.
Department of Medicine
University of Erlangen-Nurnberg
Erlangen, German Federal Republic

M. Deschodt-Lanckman, Ph.D.
Department of Biochemistry and Nutrition
Medical School
Université Libre de Bruxelles
B-1000 Brussels, Belgium

Vittorio Erspamer, M.D.
Institute of Medical Pharmacology I
University of Rome Medical School
1–00100 Rome, Italy

R. Fiocca
Institute of Pathologic Anatomy and
   Histopathology
Histochemistry and Ultrastructure Center
University of Pavia
Pavia, Italy

Robert S. Fisher, M.D.
Temple University Medical School
Philadelphia, Pennsylvania 19140

B. Frigerio, M.D.
Institute of Pathologic Anatomy and
   Histopathology
Histochemistry and Ultrastructure Center
University of Pavia
Pavia, Italy

J. L. Frost, B.Sc.
Department of Physiology
University of British Columbia
Vancouver, British Columbia
Canada V6T 1W5

Charles B. Glaser
Institute of Medical Sciences
San Francisco, California 94115

George B. Jerzy Glass, M.D.
Gastroenterology Research Laboratory
Department of Medicine
New York Medical College
New York, New York 10029

Vay Liang Go, M.D.
Gastroenterology Unit
Mayo Clinic
Rochester, Minnesota 55901

H. Gregory, Ph.D.
Imperial Chemical Industries, Limited
Pharmaceuticals Division
Mereside, Alderley Park
Macclesfield, Cheshire, England

Roger C. L. Guillemin, M.D., Ph.D.
Neuroendocrinology Laboratory
Salk Institute
La Jolla, California 92037

L. E. Hanssen
Research Laboratory of Gastroenterology
Department of Internal Medicine
Ullevål Hospital
Oslo, Norway

Paul V. B. Hyde, M.D., F.R.C.S.
Department of Surgery
University of California Medical Center
San Diego, California 92103

Leonard R. Johnson, Ph.D.
Department of Physiology
University of Texas Medical School
Houston, Texas 77025

Eszter P. Kokas, M.D.
Department of Physiology
University of North Carolina
   School of Medicine
Chapel Hill, North Carolina 27514

Stanislaw J. Konturek, M.D.
Institute of Physiology
Medical Academy
31531 Krakow, Poland

Louis D. Kosta, M.D.
Department of Surgery
University of California Medical Center
San Diego, California 92103

S. Kwauk, B.Sc.
Department of Physiology
University of British Columbia
Vancouver, British Columbia,
Canada V6T 1W5

Joseph Z. Kwei, B. S.
Department of Chemistry
Case Western Reserve University
Cleveland, Ohio 44106

M. Lambert, Ph.D.
Department of Biochemistry and Nutrition
Medical School
Universite Libre de Bruxelles
B-1000 Brussels, Belgium

Miguel J. M. Lewin
Unité de Recherches de Gastroenterologie
Hôpital Bichat
75877 Paris Cedex 18 France

Lars-Inge Larsson, B.M., D.M.Sc.
Institute of Medical Biochemistry
University of Aarhus
DK-8000 Aarhus C, Denmark

Tsung Min Lin, M.D.
The Lilly Research Laboratories
Indianapolis, Indiana 46206

T. J. McDonald, M.D., F.R.C.P.
Department of Medicine
University of Western Ontario
London, Ontario N6A 5A5 Canada

C. H. S. McIntosh, Ph.D.
Department of Physiology
University of British Columbia
Vancouver, British Columbia
Canada V6T 1W5

Pietro Melchiorri, M.D.
Institute of Pharmacology
University of Rome
Rome 0.100 Italy

Chester A. Meyers, Ph.D.
Department of Medicine
Tulane University School of Medicine
New Orleans, Louisiana 70112

Laurence J. Miller, M.D.
Department of Gastroenterology
Mayo Medical School
Mayo Clinic
Rochester, Minnesota 55901

Alister J. Moody, M.D.
Novo Research Institute
Novo Alle
Bagsvaerd, Denmark

Viktor Mutt, Ph.D.
Department of Biochemistry II
Karolinska Institute
Stockholm, S-104-01, Sweden

J. Myren, M.D.
Research Laboratory of Gastroenterology
Department of Internal Medicine
Ulleval Hospital
Oslo, Norway

Mary Elizabeth Nelbach
Institutes of Medical Sciences
San Francisco, California 94115

Goran Nilsson, M.D.
Department of Physiology
Faculty of Veterinarian Medicine
Swedish University of Agricultural
* Sciences and*
Department of Experimental Surgery
Serafimerlasarettet
Uppsala, Sweden

Marshall J. Orloff, M.D.
Department of Surgery
University of California Medical Center
San Diego, California 92103

S. C. Otte, B.Sc.
Department of Physiology
University of British Columbia
Vancouver, British Columbia
Canada V6T 1W5

Chung Owyang, M.D.
Gastroenterology Research Unit
University of Michigan
Ann Arbor, Michigan 48109

Danielle Pansu, M.D.
Ecole Pratique des Hatues Etudes and
INSERM U 45
Hôpital E. Herriot
69374 Lyon Cedex 2 France

John J. Pisano, Ph.D.
Section of Physiological Chemistry
Laboratory of Chemistry
National Heart, Lung, and Blood Institute
Bethesda, Maryland 20205

J. M. Polak, M.D., M.R.C.Path.
Departments of Histochemistry and
Medicine
Royal Postgraduate Medical School
London, England

Lucien Pradayrol, Ph.D.
INSERM U151
C.H.U. Rangueil
F-31054 Toulouse Cedex France

Jens F. Rehfeld, D.M.Sc.
Institute of Medical Biochemistry
University of Aarhus
Aarhus, Denmark

A. Ribet, M.D.
INSERM U 51
C.H.U. Rangueil
F-31052 Toulouse Cedex France

P. Robberecht, M.D., Ph.D.
Department of Biochemistry and Nutrition
Medical School
Universite Libre de Bruxelles
B-1000 Brussels, Belgium

Grace L. Rosenquist, Ph.D.
Department of Animal Physiology
University of California
Davis, California 95616

Hans Ruppin, M.D.
Department of Medicine
University of Erlangen-Nurnberg
Erlangen, West Germany

Sami I Said, M.D.
Veterans Administration Medical Center
University of Texas
Health Science Center
Dallas, Texas 75216

E. Solcia, M.D.
Institute of Pathologic Anatomy and
Histopathology
Histochemistry and Ultrastructure Center
University of Pavia
Pavia, Italy

Fl. Stadil, M.D.
Department of Surgical
Gastroenterology D
Herlev University Hospital
Herlev 2730, Denmark

Eugene Straus, M.D.
Veterans Administration Hospital
Bronx, New York 10468

Finn Sundby, Ph.D.†
Novo Research Institute
Novo Alle
Bagsvaerd, Denmark

M. Svoboda, Ph.D.
Department of Biochemistry and Nutrition
Medical School
Universite Libre de Bruxelles
B-1000 Brussels, Belgium

Kazuhiko Tatemoto, Ph.D.
Department of Biochemistry II
Medical Nobel Institute
Karolinska Institute
S-104 01 Stockholm 60, Sweden

Norman S. Track, Ph.D.
Department of Surgery and Clinical
Biochemistry
University of Toronto
Mount Sinai Hospital
Toronto, Ontario, Canada

L. Usellini
Institute of Pathologic Anatomy and
Histopathology
Histochemistry and Ultrastructure Center
University of Pavia
Pavia, Italy

A. Vandermeers, Ph.D.
Department of Biochemistry and Nutrition
Medical School
Universite Libre de Bruxelles
B-1000 Brussels, Belgium

M. C. Vandermeers-Piret, Ph.D.
Department of Biochemistry and Nutrition
Medical School
Universite Libre de Bruxelles
B-1000 Brussels, Belgium

Monique Vagne, M.D.
INSERM U 45
Hôpital E. Herriot
69374 Lyon Cedex 2 France

John H. Walsh, M.D.
Department of Medicine
University of California
Los Angeles, California 90024

Rosalyn S. Yalow, Ph.D.
Veterans Administration Hospital
Bronx, New York 10468

Gregory B. Yates
Institutes of Medical Sciences
San Francisco, California 94115

Cellular Origin of
Gastrointestinal Hormonal Peptides

Gastrointestinal Hormones, edited by
George B. Jerzy Glass.
Raven Press, New York © 1980.

Chapter 1

Morphological and Functional Classification of Endocrine Cells and Related Growths in the Gastrointestinal Tract

E. Solcia, C. Capella, R. Buffa, B. Frigerio, L. Usellini, and R. Fiocca

Institute of Pathologic Anatomy and Histopathology, Histochemistry and Ultrastructure Center, University of Pavia, Pavia, Italy

GENERAL CYTOLOGY

Endocrine-like cells are scattered in the epithelium lining the gastric glands, intestinal crypts, and villi. They lie directly on the basal lamina. In the pyloric and intestinal mucosa most of them reach the lumen in a narrow, specialized area showing tufts of microvilli, coated vesicles, and a centriole. Most likely, this area acts as a receptor surface facing luminal contents. As a rule, granules are concentrated in the basal part of the cytoplasm, whereas the Golgi complex is located in the supranuclear portion of the cell. This pattern suggests some functional polarity of the cell (Fig. 1). In the fundic mucosa endocrine-like cells lack luminal contacts and show less evident polarity (31).

Secretory granules are released at the basal surface of the cell or along the lower part of its lateral surface (22), where involved cells may form interstitial spaces and canaliculi (Fig. 2). In the upper (juxtaluminal) part of the cell these spaces are closed by junctional complexes with neighboring epithelial cells. Granule release at the luminal surface has never been observed. Smooth vesicles are often found just below the luminal surface of the cell or in the supranuclear

1

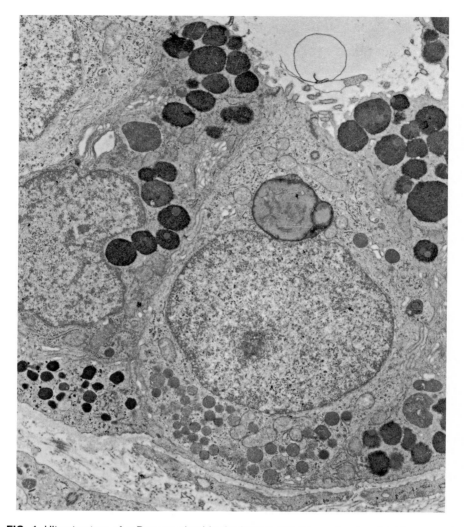

FIG. 1. Ultrastructure of a Brunner gland in the human duodenum showing, besides several mucous cells, a somatostatin D cell with infranuclear granules and a luminal process. Note part of an EC$_2$ cell in the left lower corner. ×10,000.

cytoplasm between the Golgi complex and the luminal endings. Although the exact functional meaning of these vesicles is unknown at present, their involvement in a transport system, possibly of secretory products from the Golgi to the luminal surface, is being considered. Secretion of peptide hormones such as gastrin or somatostatin from the pyloric mucosa to the gastric lumen has been reported recently (38). It seems interesting that luminal release of somatostatin has not been found in the oxyntic mucosa, where somatostatin cells lack

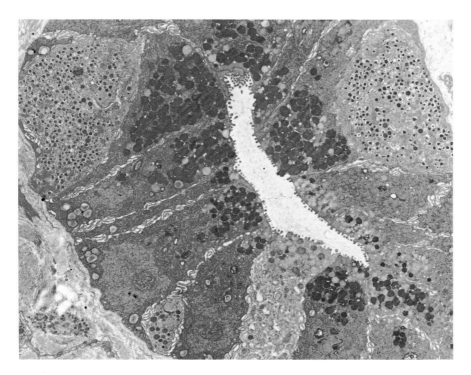

FIG. 2. Two gastrin G cells (upper left and right corners) and a small part of a D cell (below) dispersed among mucous-neck cells of a cat pyloric gland. Note extensive development of intercellular intraepithelial spaces, kept open by extrusions and infoldings of cell surface. ×3,000.

luminal contacts (37). (See also Chapter 15 by Meyers and Coy, pp. 363–385, *this volume.*)

Before entering blood capillaries that run in the lamina propria of the mucosa, active peptides and amines released by endocrine-like cells may interact with some of their targets, including nerve endings, smooth muscle fibers (with special reference to those of the villi and muscularis mucosae), and blood vessel walls. The inhibitory action of somatostatin (from D cells) on hormone release by neighboring gastrin, glucagon, and cholecystokinin (CCK) cells may be a good example of such local or "paracrine" effects of gut endocrine-like cells (28).

Although some active substances might display both blood-mediated (truly endocrine) and local (paracrine) effects, the products of several cells [such as gastrin, glucagon, secretin, CCK, and gastroinhibitory peptide (GIP)] seem to display mainly endocrine effects, whereas those of other cells [somatostatin, 5-hydroxytryptophan (5-HT), substance P, and VIP-like peptides] appear to have mainly paracrine functions. Thus, on physiological grounds, endocrine-like cells of the gut should be differentiated into paracrine cells, closely fulfilling

TABLE 1. *Classification of endocrine-like cells scattered in human gastroenteropancreatic tissues*

| | | | Stomach | | Intestine | | |
| | | | | | Small | | |
Cell	Product	Pancreas	Oxyntic, cardial	Antral	Upper	Lower	Large
P	Neuropeptides?	+[a]	+	+	+		r
D₁	Peptides?	f	+	+	+	+	+
EC	5-HT, peptides	+	+	+	+	+	+
D	Somatostatin	+	+	+	+	f	r
PP(F)	Pancreatic polypeptide	+			r	+[b]	+[b]
B	Insulin	+		+			
A	Glucagon	+	+[a]	f			
X	Unknown		+				
ECL	Unknown (H, 5-HT)		+				
G	Gastrin			+	f		
S	Secretin				+	f	
I(CCK)	Cholecystokinin				+	f	
K	GIP				+	f	
N	Neurotensin				r	+	r
L	GLI				f	+	+

[a] In human fetus or newborn, not present or only exceptionally in adults.
[b] Cells reproducing only in part the histochemistry and ultrastructure of pancreatic PP cells.
f, Few; r, rare. H, histamine; 5-HT, 5-hydroxytryptamine.

the concepts of Feyrter (12), and truly endocrine cells. Unfortunately, pertinent information is incomplete. The nature of the active products of some cells is still unknown, or rather hypothetical (see Table 1), and substances not identified as yet might be produced by cells whose function has not been clarified.

The endocrine-like cells described in the lungs, trachea, esophagus, bile ducts, prostate, and urethra display general morphological patterns similar to those of gut endocrine-like cells (8). All these cells belong to the so-called "diffuse," or "dispersed" endocrine system (DES). Truly endocrine functions have so far been identified only in the gut. The endocrine-like cells occurring in the other tissues are more likely to be interpreted as paracrine cells.

CLASSIFICATION

The first attempt to classify endocrine cells of the gut was made by Solcia, Forssmann, and Pearse during the 1969 Wiesbaden Symposium, where seven cell types were considered. The Wiesbaden classification was revised during the Bologna meeting in 1973. Two more cell types were added to the gut endocrine cells and these were tentatively compared with pancreatic endocrine cells (32). As many as 15 gastroenteropancreatic endocrine cells were considered in the Lausanne 1977 classification developed by agreement of 18 specialists (33).

This classification, rearranged and slightly improved, is reported in Table 1. It is based on ultrastructural and immunohistochemical studies interpreted in the light of available biochemical data. The products of ultrastructurally identified cells have been ascertained either by direct cytochemical techniques or by the consecutive thin-semithin section technique. This consists of electron microscopic study of a thin section of a cell stained histochemically in a consecutive semithin section.

It should be pointed out that most cytological work done so far in the field of gut endocrinology has been based on the widely held concept: "one hormone, one cell." There is increasing evidence, however, that this concept suffers from some limitations. First, instead of producing just a single peptide hormone, endocrine cells produce a family of biologically and chemically related peptides, which have to be considered in histochemical studies. Secondly, a peptide and an amine are sometimes produced by the same cell. In this case, it appears that the peptide represents a safer point of reference for cell identification and classification than the amine that is often found in ultrastructurally different cells, which produce different peptide hormones and enter different physiological reactions. For instance, 5-HT has been found in EC cells producing substance P, enkephalin, and possibly, motilin, and also in insulin B cells of guinea pig, in glucagon A cells of the pig, and in calcitonin C cells of the horse, sheep, and goat (31). As a consequence, EC like cells, so far defined by their 5-HT content, are better reclassified on the basis of the peptide they store.

When immunoreactivities with apparently unrelated peptides are detected in the same cell, one has to consider the possibility (a) of different peptides forming a portion of a bigger precursor molecule, (b) of cross-reacting sequences present in the yet unknown molecular species of a known hormone, and (c) of a mixed endocrine cell. The ultrastructural evidence suggests that the latter phenomenon occurs seldom in nonpathologic gut (11) and more frequently in the pancreas (20).

The production of two unrelated active peptides by the same cell seems possible (7,23). This may cause difficulties in attempts to introduce "functional" classifications of cells based on the hormones they produce. It seems pertinent to recall, however, that the function of a cell is not defined merely by the nature of its secretory products, but that its response to physiological stimuli and the way it releases active substances are also important.

Thus, although in many instances the "one hormone-one cell" concept still works as a basis for cell classification, this rule is not without exceptions and must be followed with caution.

DESCRIPTION OF CELL TYPES[1]

P Cells

Pulmonary-type, or P cells, are small cells with very small (from 100 to 140 nm of mean diameter), round granules, often with a thin halo surrounding

---

[1] For more detailed references and pertinent illustrations, see refs. 30 and 33.

a moderately electron-dense core. Some vesicular granules may also be present; well-developed reticulum and Golgi, small mitochondria, and numerous microfilaments are regularly found (8). The P cells are distributed in various tissues, with special reference to the upper gut and lung; however, in normal tissues they are never numerous at any site. In the human gut they are more frequently found in the duodenal and gastric mucosae.

D_1 Cells

All the small cells with round granules of mean diameter from 140 to 190 nm and showing a solid core of moderate osmiophilia with closely applied membrane or a very thin halo have been considered in Table 1 as D_1 cells. This is certainly a heterogeneous population of cells, among which slight ultrastructural differences have been observed.

The function of P and D_1 cells remains partly uncertain. The granules of some P cells closely resemble the neurosecretory granules of nerve endings in the external zone of hypothalamic median eminence; besides monoamines, some sort of neuropeptide might well be stored in such cells. A fraction of D_1 cells might be involved in the production of bombesin-like peptide(s) (36); if so, their hyperplasia in chronic atrophic gastritis might contribute to the hypergastrinemia of this condition. A relationship of some "D_1 cells" of the human duodenum and jejunum with intestinal gastrin-immunoreactive cells (5) as well as with the cells occurring in some pancreatic and duodenal gastrinomas seems possible (10). A relationship of some D_1 cell variant with the part of the cells reacting with anti-VIP sera as well as with the cells occurring in VIP-producing tumors of the pancreas (Fig. 3) also seems possible (10).

EC Cells

Argentaffin, or enterochromaffin (EC), cells (Figs. 1 and 4a) are cells with highly osmiophilic, argentaffin, and heavily argyrophil granules of pleomorphic shape storing 5-HT.

A fraction of intestinal EC cells (EC_1 cells) has been shown to store substance P (27). Other EC cells of the upper small intestine (EC_2 cells) have been found to react with some (but not all) anti-motilin sera (19). An EC cell fraction of some animal species (EC_3 cells) has been found to react with anti-enkephalin sera (1). EC cells, including human gastric EC cells, possibly storing other peptides have been called EC_n cells (33).

As producers and releasers of 5-HT, substance P, motilin, and enkephalin, EC cells seem well qualified modulators of gastrointestinal motility. Increased numbers of EC cells have been reported in intestinal tracts near to strictures or obstructions (31). Gut hypermotility is a well known component of the so-called "carcinoid syndrome" associated with argentaffin EC cell carcinoids. An obvious increase of EC cells is also found in connection with chronic inflam-

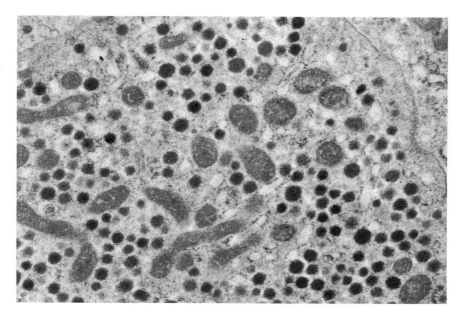

FIG. 3. Pancreatic vipoma showing small granules with osmiophilic core surrounded by a thin clear space. ×25,000.

matory diseases, with special reference to chronic gastritis, cholecystitis, appendicitis, and celiac disease (30).

D Cells

D cells (Figs. 1 and 2) show rather large (260–370 nm), poorly osmiophilic granules with closely attached membrane that are nonreactive with Grimelius' silver and easily stained with Davenport's silver. They store somatostatin (Fig. 5b) (26,29).

PP(F) Cells

PP(F) cells with irregular granules of highly variable, generally poor density, known for a long time to occur in the dog pancreas, have now been shown to store pancreatic polypeptide (PP) (25). Ultrastructurally equivalent cells have been found in all mammals so far investigated, although with some difficulty due to wide changes in the granular structure from one species to another (10). With electron immunoperoxidase or the thin-semithin section technique, PP immunoreactive cells of the human islets have been identified as cells with rather small granules that are difficult to distinguish from D_1 cells (14,25). The intense argyrophilia and occasional angularity of granules in PP(F) cells

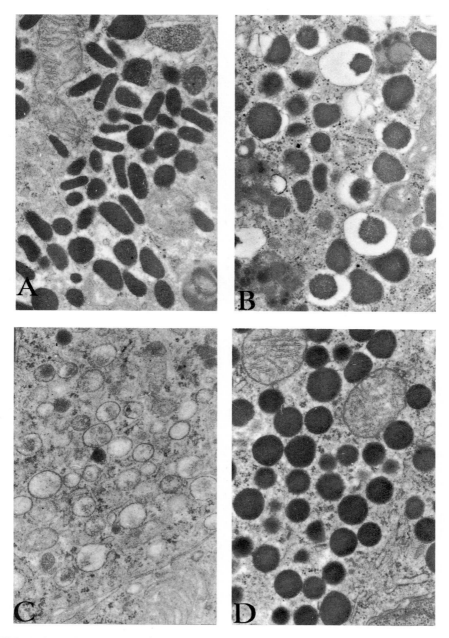

FIG. 4 a,b,c,d. Human gastrointestinal mucosa. Granules of EC_1 (**a:** jejunum), ECL (**b:** fundus), G (**c:** pylorus), and I cells (**d:** jejunum). ×25,000.

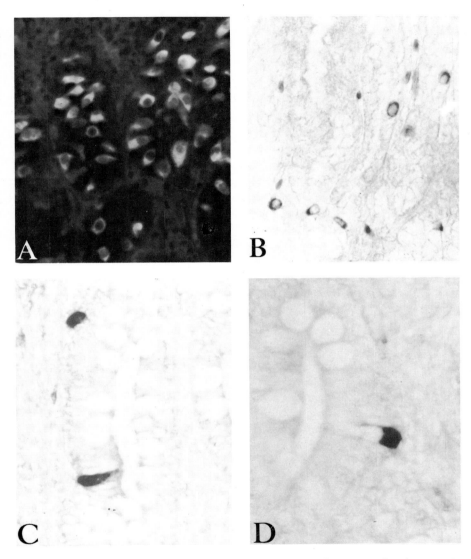

FIG. 5 a,b,c,d. Human pyloric mucosa showing gastrin (**a:** immunofluorescence) and somatostatin cells (**b:** immunoperoxidase). Dog duodenal mucosa showing secretin (**c**) and CCK cells (**d**) stained with immunoperoxidase PAP technique. **a–b:** ×300; **c:** ×600; **d:** ×800.

might be a distinguishing feature (10,14). PP(F) cells undergo hyperplastic, often micronodular, changes in chronic pancreatitis and other pathological conditions (15).

We have found very few (in the guinea pig) to relatively numerous (in the dog) PP-immunoreactive cells and ultrastructurally identified F-like cells in the pyloric mucosa. Cells storing PP-like peptide(s)—possibly differing from authentic PP—are present in the lower human intestine (6). Many of the latter cells also react with anti-glucagon and anti-glicentin sera.

A Cells

The presence of glucagon-producing A cells in the oxyntic mucosa of the dog, cat, and monkey is now established (2,17,31,35). Few A cells occur in the human fetal stomach; however, in our experience they are not a regular component of a non-diseased human adult stomach (8). Cells reacting with antiglucagon and antiglicentin sera, but only in part resembling A cells ultrastructurally (A-like or AL cells), are present in the chicken proventriculus, and, rarely, in the oxyntic mucosa of some mammals. The presence of very few, if any, A cells in the human upper small intestine is still uncertain because of the difficulty of distinguishing such cells from K cells.

B Cells

Insulin-producing B cells occur exclusively in the pancreas.

X Cells

X cells with medium-sized (approximately 250 nm), round, dense granules of closely adherent membrane and fairly Grimelius-reactive core are present, although relatively few, in the human oxyntic mucosa. They are much more numerous in other species such as dog, rat, pig, and rabbit (31); in the latter species they may also appear in the pyloric mucosa. The function of X cells remains obscure.

ECL Cells

ECL cells (Fig. 4b) in man show vesicular to relatively compact granules with coarsely granular, heavily argyrophil core (39). In small rodents these cells store histamine. Most granules of cat and rabbit ECL cells—and occasionally granules of human ECL cells—store an amine with reducing power, likely 5-HT. ECL cells are known to be stimulated by gastrin (18). In all species so far investigated ECL cells have been found exclusively or nearly exclusively in the oxyntic mucosa.

G Cells.

G cells (gastrin cells) (Figs. 4c and 5a) show vesicular to fairly dense granules of variable size (200–400 nm), slight argyrophilia, and floccular content (31,39). G cells are very numerous in the pyloric mucosa of all species investigated.

They are very scarce in adult duodenum, but are numerous and ultrastructurally pleomorphic in fetal duodenum.

S Cells

S cells (secretin cells) of several species are characterized by relatively small (approximately 200 nm), fairly irregular granules with a thin clear space interposed between the osmiophilic core and the membrane (31). S cells are slightly Grimelius-reactive; their identification with secretin immunoreactive cells is now confirmed immunocytochemically (24). S cells are scattered in the duodeno-jejunal mucosa and are less numerous in human than in dog or pig intestine (Fig. 5c).

I (CCK) Cells

I cells (Fig. 3d) show medium-sized (approximately 250 nm) round to slightly irregular, dense, argyrophobe granules (9,31). They are fairly well represented in the duodenal and jejunal mucosa, and occur only occasionally in the ileum. Their identity with the CCK cell (Fig. 5d) is now confirmed immunocytochemically (3).

K Cells

Granules of human K cells are large (approximately 350 nm), round to quite irregular, often with an osmiophilic, argyrophobe body immersed in a dense, heavily argyrophil matrix (9). Although much better represented in the duodeno-jejunal mucosa, they may also occur in the ileum. The origin of GIP from K cells is now confirmed immunocytochemically (4).

N Cells

The storage of neurotensin in some large (approximately 300 nm) granule cells scattered in the lower small intestine is now ascertained (13). In man these cells (N cells) display round, homogeneous granules with slight to moderate argyrophilia of the core.

L Cells

Granules of human L cells are smaller (approximately 250 nm) than those of dog L cells (17,31). In the lower small intestine most of them display a thin Grimelius-reactive, peripheral rim. In the colon most granules lack the argyrophil halo and are often of smaller size than those of L cells in the ileum. The presence of GLI (glucagon-like immunoreactivity, enteroglucagon, glicentin) in L cells is now confirmed (13,17).

TABLE 2. *Classification of endocrine-like tumors of the gut*

A. Endocrine tumors of the gut
  1. Gastrinomas
  2. Others?
B. Argentaffin EC cell carcinoids
  1. EC_1 cell tumor (substance P)
  2. Gastric EC cell carcinoid
  3. Others
C. Nonargentaffin carcinoids
  1. Esophagus
  2. Stomach
      (a) Gastric type: ECL cell tumor, others
      (b) Intestinal type, with intestinal endocrine cells
  3. Duodenum
  4. Jejunum, ileum, appendix, cecum
  5. Hindgut
      (a) L(GLI) cell type
      (b) others

As a whole, 14 endocrine cell types are recognized in the gastrointestinal mucosa, up to seven of which are also found in the pancreas.

CLASSIFICATION OF GUT ENDOCRINE-LIKE GROWTHS

A detailed cytological and functional classification of endocrine-like or DES tumors of the gut, based on the classification of related cells reported in Table 1, would certainly be helpful in many respects. Only a few of such tumors so far have been carefully studied, however, from the histochemical and ultrastructural points of view. This, together with the frequent occurrence of mixed tumors made up of different cell types and poorly differentiated, cytologically ambiguous tumors, makes a purely cytological classification hardly feasible and, practically, of little help at present. Thus, for the time being, it seems convenient to retain the time-honored term *carcinoid tumor* for the tumors of paracrine cells and endocrine-like cells of unknown function, and to use the term *gut endocrine tumor* for tumors composed of G, A, S, I, and K cells. Of these only G cell tumors have been described so far. A "functional" endocrine syndrome seems to appear earlier, frequently in association with the latter tumors than with carcinoids. Carcinoids are usually differentiated into argentaffin (EC cell) carcinoids—easily identified on the basis of conventional histological patterns and a few simple histochemical tests—and into nonargentaffin carcinoids (30). The present status of classification is outlined in Table 2.

At present, only two kinds of tumors appear to be well characterized from the cytological point of view, i.e., argentaffin EC cell carcinoids and gastrinomas. Both of them represent distinct pathological entities with clear-cut morphological and functional profiles. The remaining tumors , most of which are to be referred to as nonargentaffin carcinoids, are more easily classified according to the site of origin and the type of epithelium, either orthotopic or metaplastic, from which they are derived. Tumors with multiple cell types should be classified according to the prevalent cell or the associated functional syndrome.

The site of origin of endocrine-like tumors proved to be of major prognostic significance (16). Ninety-nine percent of patients with appendiceal carcinoids attained 5-year survival, despite the fact that signs of local infiltration have been observed rather often. The specific anatomy of the appendix, and the feasibility of an early and easy removal of most of these tumors, may account for this benign behavior. Patients with rectal carcinoids also have relatively good prognoses, with 5-year survival rates of 83%. Here again, factors influencing early detection and excision may account in part for these figures. Patients with carcinoid and endocrine tumors of the stomach, small intestine, and colon have poorer prognoses, with 5-year survival rates slightly above 50%. The last figures approach those for non-B cell tumors of the pancreas, among which gastrinomas (Fig. 6) and vipomas (Fig. 3) seem to have the worst prognosis.

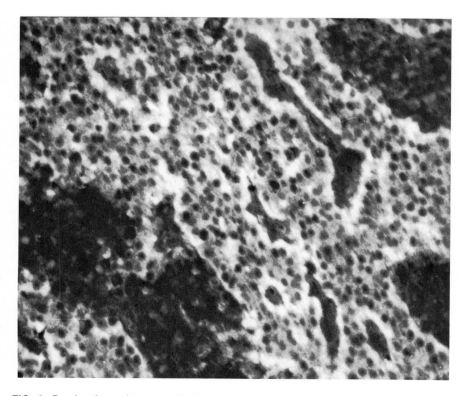

FIG. 6. Duodenal gastrinoma stained with immunofluorescence using anti-human gastrin I serum absorbed with pure porcine CCK to prevent staining of CCK cells. ×250.

Sixty-two percent of pancreatic gastrinomas and 38% of duodenal gastrinomas have been considered to be malignant (21). Conversely, only 15% of pancreatic insulinomas proved malignant (34). Thus, the functional and cytological identification of tumor cells may also be of major prognostic value.

CONCLUSIONS

It appears from the above that morphology contributed substantially to the expansion of the field of gut endocrinology. The identification of new cell types (mainly due to electron microscopy) and the localization of new hormone products (essentially by means of histochemical techniques) made a parallel progress. These two techniques have recently merged in the field of electron cytochemistry, thanks to the development of cytochemical methods at the ultrastructural level and of the thin-semithin section procedure that allowed study of consecutive sections of the same cell alternatively with histochemical and ultrastructural techniques.

Up to 14 endocrine cell types have been identified ultrastructurally and/or histochemically in the gastroenteric mucosa. Of these, gastrin (G), somatostatin (D), glucagon (A), secretin (S), and (I) (CCK) cells have been confirmed cytochemically and seem to be considered as fully established cell types. PP, GIP, neurotensin, and GLI cells have also been identified cytochemically. EC cells, although well known ultrastructurally and recognized as 5-HT producers, are still under investigation as a source of substance P, enkephalin, and motilin peptides. P, D_1, X, and ECL cells, although ultrastructurally defined, are functionally unknown, and most of their secretory products are still to be identified.

A precise cytological classification of endocrine-like tumors of the gut is hardly feasible at present. For practical purposes it seems preferable to distinguish carcinoids, either argentaffin or nonargentaffin, from true endocrine tumors of the gut (essentially gastrinomas). Nonargentaffin carcinoids will encompass a cytologically heterogeneous group of tumors, easily subdivided on simple topographical grounds.

PROJECTIONS FOR THE FUTURE

Among the most obvious goals for the future, the following morphological researches in the field of gut endocrinology can be outlined:

Complete cytochemical identification of cell products, to be exactly localized at the ultrastructural level. Problems, such as the production of several peptides by the same cell, the ultrastructural aspect of cells producing different molecular species of hormones, and the cytochemical and structural changes of cells during developmental and tumor growths, are to be carefully investigated. Consideration is to be given to these problems also from the point of view of cell classification.

Clarification of cell function with the help of cell biology approaches and experiments providing adequate cell stimulation or suppression. This is essential to an understanding of the real meaning of the various types of endocrine cells and their products as well as their role in pathology.

Morphometric evaluation of endocrine cells under basal, stimulated, or pathological conditions. Precise criteria for the identification of endocrine cell hyperplasia and hypertrophy and their correlation with clinical signs of endocrine hyperfunction are to be expected from these studies.

Clinical and pathological studies of a large number of endocrine tumors characterized fully histologically, ultrastructurally, and cytochemically. This work will provide a sound basis for establishing diagnostic and prognostic criteria and an accurate classification of these tumors.

REFERENCES

1. Alumets, J., Hakanson, R., Sundler, F., and Chang, K.-J. (1978): Leu-enkephalin-like material in nerves and enterochromaffin cells in the gut. An immunohistochemical study. *Histochemistry,* 56:187–196.
2. Baetens, D., Rufener, C., Srikant, C., Dobbs, R., Unger, R., and Orci, L. (1976): Identification of glucagon-producing cells (A cells) in dog gastric mucosa. *J. Cell Biol.,* 69:455–464.
3. Buchan, A. M. J., Polak, J. M., Solcia, E., Capella, C., Hudston, D., and Pearse, A. G. E. (1978): Electron immunocytochemical evidence for the human intestinal I cell as the source of CCK. *Gut,* 19:403–407.
4. Buchan, A. M. J., Polak, J. M., Solcia, E., Capella, C., and Pearse, A. G. E. (1978): Electron immunocytochemical evidence for the K cell localization of GIP in man. *Histochemistry,* 56:37–44.
5. Buchan, A. M. J., Polak, J. M., Solcia, E., and Pearse, A. G. E. (1979): The localization of intestinal gastrin in a distinct endocrine cell type. *Nature,* 277:138–140.
6. Buffa, R., Capella, C., Fontana, P., Usellini, L., and Solcia, E. (1978): Types of endocrine cells in the human colon and rectum. *Cell Tissue Res.,* 192:227–240.
7. Buffa, R., Chayvialle, J. A., Fontana, P., Usellini, L., Capella, C., and Solcia, E. (1979): Parafollicular cells of rabbit thyroid store both calcitonin and somatostatin and resemble ultrastructurally gut D cells. *Histochemistry,* 62:281–288.
8. Capella, C., Hage, E., Solcia, E., and Usellini, L. (1978): Ultrastructural similarity of endocrine-like cells of the human lung and some related cells of the gut. *Cell Tissue Res.,* 186:25–37.
9. Capella, C., Solcia, E., Frigerio, B., and Buffa, R. (1976): Endocrine cells of the human intestine. An ultrastructural study. In: *Endocrine Gut and Pancreas,* edited by T. Fujita, pp. 43–59. Elsevier, Amsterdam.
10. Capella, C., Solcia, E., Frigerio, B., Buffa, R., Usellini, L., and Fontana, P. (1977): The endocrine cells of the pancreas and related tumours. Ultrastructural study and classification. *Virchows Arch. (Pathol. Anat.),* 373:327–352.
11. Capella, C., Vassallo, G., and Solcia, E. (1971): Light and electron microscopic identification of the histamine-storing argyrophil (ECL) cell in murine stomach and of its equivalent in other mammals. *Z. Zellforsch.,* 118:68–84.
12. Feyrter, F. (1953): Über die peripheren endokrinen (parakrinen) Drüsen des Menschen, edited by W. Maudrich, pp. 1–231. Wien-Düsseldorf.
13. Frigerio, B., Ravazzola, M., Buffa, R., Capella, C., Solcia, E., and Orci, L. (1977): Histochemical and ultrastructural identification of neurotensin cells in the dog ileum. *Histochemistry,* 54:123–131.

14. Gepts, W., Baetens, D., and De Mey, J. (1978): The PP cell. In: *Gut Hormones,* edited by S. R. Bloom, pp. 229–233. Churchill Livingstone, Edinburgh.
15. Gepts, W., De May, J., and Marichal-Pipeleers, M. (1977): Hyperplasia of "pancreatic polypeptide" cells in the pancreas of juvenile diabetes. *Diabetologia,* 13:27–34.
16. Godwin, J. B. (1975): Carcinoid tumors. An analysis of 2837 cases. *Cancer,* 36:560–569.
17. Grimelius, L., Capella, C., Buffa, R., Polak, J. M., Pearse, A. G. E., and Solcia, E. (1976): Cytochemical and ultrastructural differentiation of enteroglucagon and pancreatic-type glucagon cells of the gastrointestinal tract. *Virchows Arch. (Cell Pathol.),* 20:217–228.
18. Hakanson, R., Larsson, L.-I., Liedberg, G., and Sundler, F. (1976): The histamine-storing enterochromaffin-like cells of the rat stomach. In: *Chromaffin, Enterochromaffin and Related Cells,* edited by R. E. Coupland and T. Fujita, pp. 243–263. Elsevier, Amsterdam.
19. Heitz, P. U., Kasper, M., Krey, G., Polak, J. M., and Pearse, A. G. E. (1978): Immunoelectron cytochemical localization of motilin in human duodenal enterochromaffin cells. *Gastroenterology,* 74:713–717.
20. Herman, L., Sato, T., and Fitzgerald, P. J. (1964): The pancreas. In: *Electron Microscopy Anatomy,* edited by S. M. Kurtz, pp. 59–95. Academic Press, New York.
21. Hofmann, J. W., Fox, P. S., and Milwaukee, S. D. W. (1973): Duodenal wall tumors and the Zollinger-Ellison syndrome. *Arch. Surg.,* 107:334–338.
22. Kobayashi, S., and Sasagawa, T. (1976): Morphological aspects of the secretion of gastro-enteric hormones. In: *Endocrine Gut and Pancreas,* edited by T. Fujita, pp. 255–271. Elsevier, Amsterdam.
23. Larsson, L.-I. (1978): Distribution of ACTH-like immunoreactivity in rat brain and gastrointestinal tract. *Histochemistry,* 55:225–233.
24. Larsson, L.-I., Sundler, F., Alumets, J., Hakanson, R., Schaffalitzky de Muckedell, O. B., and Fahrenkrug, J. (1977): Distribution, ontogeny and ultrastructure of the mammalian secretin cell. *Cell Tissue Res.,* 181:361–368.
25. Larsson, L.-I., Sundler, F., and Hakanson, R. (1976): Pancreatic polypeptide. A postulated new hormone: Identification of its cellular storage site by light and electron microscopic immunocytochemistry. *Diabetologia,* 12:211–226.
26. Orci, L., Baetens, D., Ravazzola, M., Malaisse-Lagae, F., Amherdt, M., and Rufener, C. (1976): Somatostatin in the pancreas and the gastrointestinal tract. In: *Endocrine Gut and Pancreas,* edited by T. Fujita, pp. 73–88. Elsevier, Amsterdam.
27. Pearse, A. G. E., and Polak, J. M. (1975): Immunocytochemical localization of substance P in mammalian intestine. *Histochemistry,* 41:373–375.
28. Pearse, A. G. E., Polak, J. M., and Bloom, S. R. (1977): The newer gut hormones. Cellular sources, physiology, pathology and clinical aspects. *Gastroenterology,* 72:746–761.
29. Polak, J. M., Pearse, A. G. E., Grimelius, L., Bloom, S. R., and Arimura, A. (1975): Growth-hormone release-inhibiting hormone in gastrointestinal and pancreatic D cells. *Lancet,* i:1220–1222.
30. Solcia, E., Capella, C., Buffa, R., Usellini, L., Frigerio, B., and Fontana, P. (1979): Endocrine cells of the gastrointestinal tract and related tumors. In: *Pathobiology Annual,* edited by H. L. Ioachim, pp. 163–204. Raven Press, New York.
31. Solcia, E., Capella, C., Vassallo, G., and Buffa, R. (1975): Endocrine cells of the gastric mucosa. *Int. Rev. Cytol.,* 42:223–286.
32. Solcia, E., Pearse, A. G. E., Grube, D., Kobayashi, S., Bussolati, G., Creutzfeldt, W., and Gepts, W. (1973): Revised Wiesbaden classification of gut endocrine cells. *Rendic. Gastroenterol.,* 5:13–16.
33. Solcia, E., Polak, J. M., Pearse, A. G. E., Forssmann, W. G., Larsson, L., Sundler, F., Lechago, J., Grimelius, L., Fujita, T., Creutzfeldt, W., Gepts, W., Falkmer, S., Lefranc, G., Heitz, Ph., Hage, E., Buchan, A. M. J., Bloom, S. R., and Grossman, M. I. (1978): Lausanne 1977 classification of gastroenteropancreatic endocrine cells. In: *Gut Hormones,* edited by S. R. Bloom, pp. 40–48. Churchill Livingstone, Edinburgh.
34. Stefanini, P., Carboni, M., Patrassi, N., and Basoli, A. (1974): Beta-islet cell tumors of the pancreas: results of a study on 1,067 cases. *Surgery,* 75:597–605.
35. Sundler, F., Alumets, J., Holst, J., Larsson, L.-I., and Hakanson, R. (1976): Ultrastructural identification of cells storing pancreatic-type glucagon in dog stomach. *Histochemistry,* 50:33–37.
36. Timson, C. M., Polak, J. M., Wharton, J., Ghatei, M. A., Bloom, S. R., Usellini, L., Capella,

C., Solcia, E., Brown, M. R., and Pearse, A. G. E. (1979): Bombesin-like immunoreactivity in the avian gut and its localisation. *Histochemistry,* 61:213–221.

37. Uvnas-Wallenstem, K. (1978): Personal communication to E. S.
38. Uvnäs-Wallensten, K., Efendic, S., and Luft, R. (1977): Vagal release of somatostatin into the antral lumen of cats. *Acta Physiol. Scand.,* 99:126–128.
39. Vassallo, G., Capella, C., and Solcia, E. (1971): Endocrine cells of the human gastric mucosa. *Z. Zellforsch.,* 118:49–67.

Gastrointestinal Hormones, edited by
George B. Jerzy Glass.
Raven Press, New York © 1980.

Chapter 2

Neural and Cellular Origin of Gastrointestinal Hormonal Peptides in Health and Disease

J. M. Polak and S. R. Bloom

Departments of Histochemistry and Medicine, Royal Postgraduate Medical School, London, England

INTRODUCTION

History

When Bayliss and Starling, inspired by the current trend toward organotherapy and the idea of "chemical messengers," discovered the first hormone, secretin

(4), Pavlov's well accepted theory of neural control of gut function was swept away at a single stroke. The concept of control of bodily functions by various chemical messengers capable of acting on distant organs, all included under the generic term *hormones,* acquired greater importance in the early part of the 20th century. Therefore, little attention was paid to Feyrter's original observations (25) of yet another controlling system, the diffuse endocrine system, capable of "local" (paracrine) modulation of the activity of different organs. All three of these theories of nervous, hormonal, and local regulation of gut function now are known to be valid and are contained in the modern concept of neuroendocrine control by conventional neural mechanisms and by hormone-like peptides secreted by both nerves and endocrine cells.

Technology

Knowledge of the distribution and cellular localization of these hormonal peptides has been made possible by the availability of pure or synthetic peptides and the use of two immunological methods, radioimmunoassay (RIA) and immunocytochemistry (ICC) (53). RIA provides information as to the precise quantities and molecular forms of the peptide in tissue and its concentration in local fluids and/or the peripheral circulation. ICC localizes the peptide in a histological tissue section and shows whether it is produced by the neural elements or by the endocrine cells of the gut mucosa. Details of these two techniques are given in chapters 32–38 on radioimmunoassay (pp. 751–874) and in Chapter 3 by L. I. Larsson (pp. 53–70, *this volume*).

MORPHOLOGICAL CHARACTERISTICS OF THE GUT ENDOCRINE CELLS RESPONSIBLE FOR THE PRODUCTION OF HORMONES ACTING VIA THE CIRCULATION

There are at present eight peptides commonly thought to act via the circulation. They are listed in Table 1.

The endocrine cells of the gut were recognized more than 100 years ago by Heidenhain (30). In 1897 Kultschitzky (38) associated their acidophil granules with products of resorption. These cells were therefore subsequently called Kultschitzky's cells. They appeared to be poorly stained by conventional techniques such as hematoxylin and eosin or toluidine blue. This led Feyrter to call them "clear cells" (25). He grouped them all together under the heading of the "diffuse endocrine system," attributing to them a mainly paracrine (local) function (25). The cells are scattered in the gut epithelium among the nonendocrine cells. Their amine handling properties make them members of Pearse's APUD system (46).

The gut endocrine cells have long been visualized by specialized histological staining methods including silver impregnation and lead hematoxylin. ICC, however, using specific antibodies to gut peptides, has proved the most reliable

TABLE 1. *Anatomical distribution of the gut endocrine (APUD) cells responsible for the production of hormones acting via the circulation*

Peptide	Proposed (functional or ultrastructural) name	Location	Possible action
Gastrin	AG and IG cells	Antrum, upper small intestine	Stimulation of gastric acid Trophic effect on gastric mucosa
Pancreatic polypeptide	PP cells	Pancreas	Inhibition of pancreatic enzymes and gallbladder contraction
Secretin	S cells	Duodenum and jejunum	Stimulation of pancreatic bicarbonate
Cholecystokinin-pancreazymin	CCK-I cells	Small intestine	Stimulation of pancreatic enzymes and gallbladder contraction
Motilin	M and MEC cells	Small intestine	Stimulation of upper gastrointestinal motor activity
Gastric inhibitory peptide	GIP-K cells	Small intestine	Insulinotropic effects
Neurotensin	N cells	Ileum	Inhibition of gastric motor function
Enteroglucagon	EG cells	Ileum and colon	Trophic effects on enterocyte

and informative technique available today. These endocrine cells are generally pear-shaped, with the apex reaching the gut lumen and ending in a tuft of microvilli (Fujita's open type) (27) (Fig. 1). Some cells are not in contact with the gut lumen. These are located mainly in the basal parts of the glands and are often covered by other, nonendocrine cells (Fujita's closed type) (27) (Fig. 2). Enterochromaffin-like cells (ECL), fundic somatostatin cells, and occasionally one type of motilin cell (see below) belong to this group. The presence of ultrastructurally distinguishable electron-dense secretory granules is one of the main features that characterizes the endocrine cells. An additional characteristic made noticeable by the wide use of ICC has recently been observed; this is a basal extension of the elongated APUD cell with a "finger-like" process that often terminates in a bulbous swelling on another cell, either endocrine or exocrine. This feature is particularly noticeable in the enteroglucagon cells of the large intestine, the bombesin cells of the chicken proventriculus (Fig. 3), and in the somatostatin cells, especially of the fundic mucosa. In many cells, also, ultrastructural studies show the presence of microfilaments. These are again especially noticeable in one type of motilin cell. Some workers have suggested that they take part in intracellular movements (41). A full account of the morphology of the gut endocrine cells is given by E. Solcia et al. in Chapter 1 (pp. 1–17).

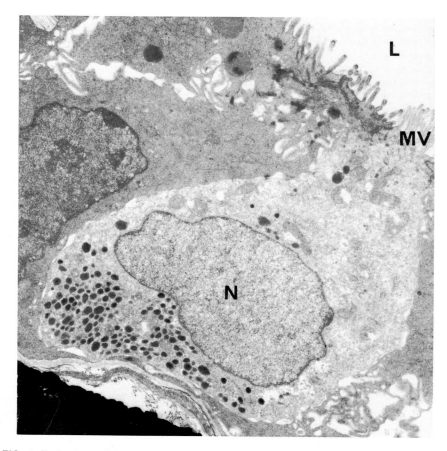

FIG. 1. Endocrine cell ("open" type) of the duodenal mucosa. L, Lumen; MV, microvilli; N, nuclei. ×10,000.

Pearse (45) suggested, on cytochemical grounds, that APUD cells and nerves had a common embryological origin in the neuroectoderm. Fujita and Kobayashi (27) noted that the APUD cells are morphologically similar to nerve cells by virtue of having an apical receptor pole with microvilli, as well as secretory (neurosecretory) granules. These observations, together with the recent discovery of peptides in both cells and nerves (47), the presence of neuroendocrine cells in the gut wall outside the mucosa (34,35,59) and the close morphological relationship between autonomic nerves and endocrine cells, particularly in the pancreas, have led Fujita (27) to support fully and further expand Pearse's original hypothesis. Further to these general morphological properties, two other features have recently emerged: (a) One resulted from the realization that a single peptide

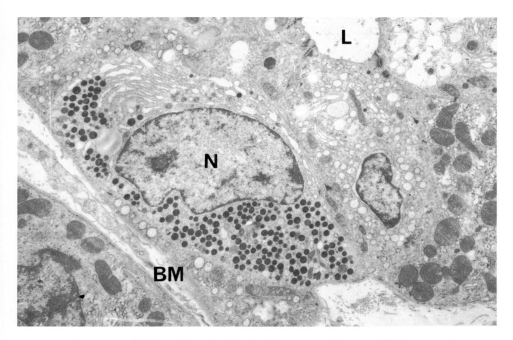

FIG. 2. Endocrine cell ("closed" type) of the fundic mucosa. L, Lumen; BM, basement membrane; N, nucleus. ×7,500.

may exist in several molecular forms. (b) The other arose as a result of further studies of the comparative morphology of secretory granules in different species.

A. Multiple Molecular Forms

It is now well established that most of the gut peptide hormones are present in tissue and in the circulation in more than one molecular form. (See Chapter 19 by F. Rehfeld, pp. 443–449, *this volume.*)

Gastrin is one of the best known examples. It has long been recognized that the antral G cells, typified by large electronlucent granules, are associated with the production of gastrin (68). We now know that antral gastrin is predominantly the small form of the G-17 molecule. It has recently been shown that the cell responsible for the production of intestinal gastrin, which is mainly the larger form, G-34, is a cell that contains much smaller and denser secretory granules than those found in the antral G cells (14) (Fig. 4). A single peptide is thus present in the tissue in at least two molecular forms that are produced and stored in two ultrastructurally distinguishable types of cell. Cholecystokinin (CCK), a peptide closely related to the gastrins, is also present in the small intestine. CCK cells constitute a totally separate cell population with larger

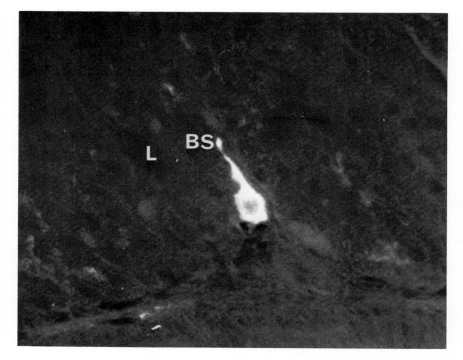

FIG. 3. Bombesin cell of the chicken proventriculus. L, Lumen; BS, bulbous swelling. ×630.

secretory granules (13), identified as type I in the ultrastructural classification (67) (Fig. 5).

In tissue and in circulation, motilin is present in two molecular forms (7). Some enterochromaffin (EC) cells of the small intestine apparently store the larger molecular form, whereas the smaller form appears to be stored in nonenterochromaffin cells containing smaller secretory granules (58) (Fig. 6). These were previously included among the D1 cells of the electron microscopic (EM) classification (67).

A glucagon-like immunoreactivity or enteroglucagon has been localized to cells of the large intestine in many species (57,60). Pure enteroglucagon has recently been extracted from porcine intestine, renamed glicentin, and suggested to be a 100-amino acid peptide, probably containing the entire sequence of pancreatic glucagon (? proglucagon) (44). (See Chapter 12 by F. Sundby and A. J. Moody, pp. 307–313, *this volume.*) The cells storing pancreatic glucagon are the well accepted A cells of the pancreas (71) containing large granules with a characteristic limiting membrane and argyrophilic halo, whereas the intestinal cells, storing the larger molecular form (glicentin or proglucagon), are characterized by the presence of similarly large granules that lack the classic argyrophilic halo of the A cells (29).

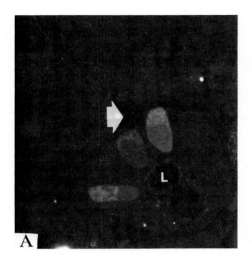

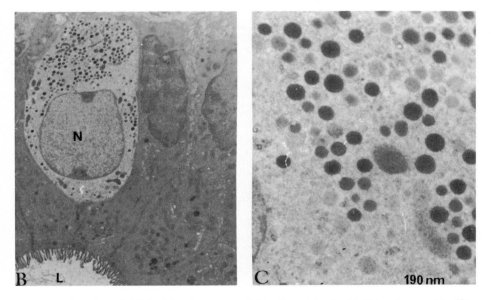

FIG. 4.a: Gastrin cell (I.G.) of the human small intestine stained with N-terminal gastrin (G-17) antibodies. Section 800-nm thick, ×500. **b:** Serial 60 nm EM section showing numerous small, round, and dense secretory granules. ×6,000. **c:** Same as **(b)**. ×30,000. L, Lumen; N, nucleus.

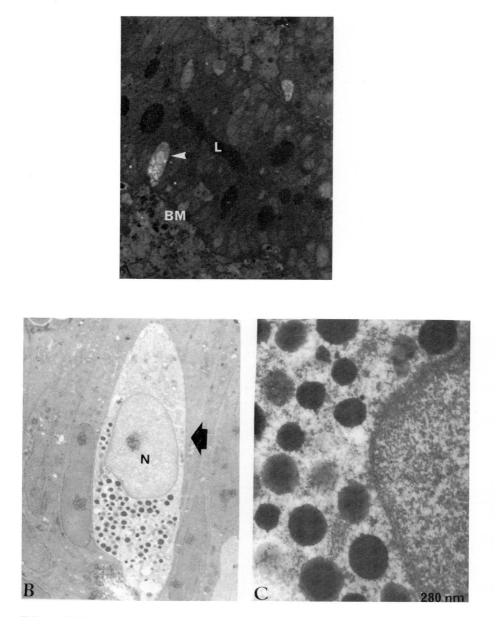

FIG. 5.a: CCK cell of the human small intestinal mucosa (800 nm section) stained with specific antibodies to CCK. ×500. **b:** 60-nm serial section stained with uranyl acetate. Note the larger size of their secretory granules when compared with Fig. 4 **b–c.** ×6,000. **c:** Same as **(b)**. ×30,000. L, Lumen; BM, basement membrane; N, nucleus.

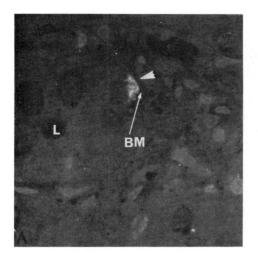

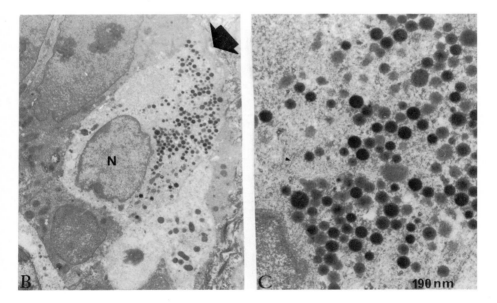

FIG. 6. Nonenterochromaffin cell of the small intestine mucosa stained in **(a)** with C-terminal directed motilin antibodies. ×500. **b** and **c:** Conventional EM showing the presence of small, round secretory granules. **b:** ×6,000. **c:** ×28,000. L, Lumen; N, nucleus; BM, basement membrane.

B. Variations in Appearance of Secretory Granules

The original observations on the morphology of gut endocrine cells have recently been expanded. Extensive combined ultrastructural and immunocyto-chemical studies have been carried out on the morphological and ultrastructural appearances of gut endocrine cells and have revealed considerable species varia-tions in the appearance of their secretory granules. This is especially noticeable in the secretin- and enteroglucagon-producing cells. In the intestine of mammals, such as the pig and the dog, the small (S) and large (L) granuled endocrine cells were associated with the production of secretin and enteroglucagon, respec-tively (16). Combined ICC and ultrastructural studies (thin-semithin method) have now shown that the reverse is true in the human gut mucosa, with secretin-containing cells having relatively large granules (260 ± 26 nm) (Fig. 7) [other mammals 170 nm (range 94–148 nm)] and enteroglucagon cells small (200 ± 36 nm) granules [other mammals (266 nm, range 130–496 nm)].

In this chapter we do not discuss in detail the individual circulating hormones listed above, as they are covered in Chapters 5 through 17 *(this volume)* but will concentrate on the hormone-like peptides with local influence on the gut.

BRAIN AND GUT PEPTIDES

As early as in 1931, substance P was shown to be a peptide present in both the brain and the gut (23). Since 1975, when somatostatin, originally extracted from the hypothalamus, was found to be present in large quantities in the gut (2), the number of peptides found to be common to these two locations has increased rapidly. Today the list comprises substance P, somatostatin, gastrin, CCK, VIP, bombesin, neurotensin, and enkephalin. All these peptides have been successfully extracted from both the brain and the gut and on many occa-sions their physicochemical identities in both locations have been established by permeation chromatography. ICC has greatly aided in establishing their tissue distribution. It has thus been recognized for some time that these neuropep-tides are present in both nervous (central and peripheral) and in endocrine tissue. Sharp distinctions cannot be drawn, as the peptides show a wide variety of cellular and neural localizations (66).

GENERAL CHARACTERISTICS OF THE "NEUROPEPTIDES"

Unlike the hormones acting via the circulation, the neuropeptides that act either locally, in a paracrine manner, or as neurotransmitters or neuromodula-tors, have a very short half-life. Once they are released, they are rapidly destroyed, possibly by the actions of proteolytic enzymes. They have a very widespread distribution and a corresponding versatility of pharmacological actions. They are found not only in the gut but also in most other peripheral tissues, such as lung (74,75), genitourinary tract (5), skin, nasal, buccal, and other mucosae, salivary glands (63), and so forth.

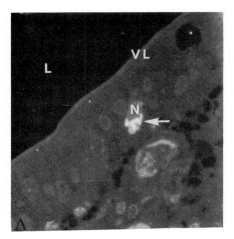

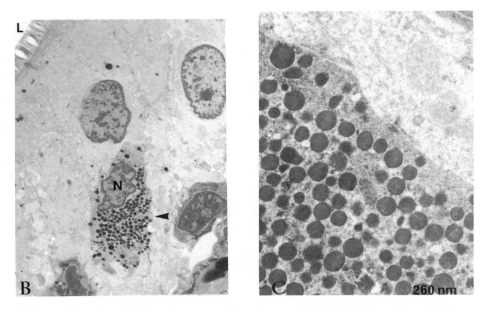

FIG. 7.a: Secretin cell of the human small intestine. ×500. **b:** Serial EM section ×3,000. **c:** Detail of secretory granules of this cell. ×28,000. V.L., Villi; L, lumen; N, nucleus.

PEPTIDERGIC AUTONOMIC INNERVATION

Despite the early description by Dogiel (21) of three types of neurons in the myenteric plexus of the gut, the challenge to Langley's (39) division of the autonomic nervous system into two components, sympathetic and parasympathetic, did not come until much later. In 1970 Baumgarten et al. (3) described a third type of autonomic nerve fiber, distinguishable at the ultrastructural level by the presence of neurosecretory granules that appeared larger and denser than those seen in the adrenergic and cholinergic types of fiber. The authors termed their newly described nerve fibers "p-type" because of the resemblance of their secretory granules to those seen in the central nervous system neurons that are responsible for the production of vasopressin and oxytocin. The complexity and variety of autonomic nerve fibers was later emphasized in 1976 by Cook and Burnstock, who described at least eight different types of neurosecretory granules in the autonomic innervation of the guinea pig gut (18). It has now become clear from neurophysiological and morphological studies that there exists, as part of the autonomic nervous system, an important and powerful noncholinergic, nonadrenergic component often referred to as purinergic (15).

INDIVIDUAL NEUROPEPTIDES

In this section we discuss the peripheral distribution of the following neuropeptides: substance P, somatostatin, enkephalins, bombesin, and VIP. A brief mention of their pharmacological actions will also be given but the details can be found in other chapters of this volume. Also, reference to the peripheral distribution of neurotensin and of the gastrin family of peptides is omitted, as these are discussed in other chapters.

Substance P

Substance P was the first neuropeptide to be found in a dual localization in the brain and the gut (23). Abdominal vagal nerve stimulation releases a substance, unaffected by atropine and thus different from acetylcholine, that exerts powerful contractile effects on an isolated guinea pig ileal smooth muscle preparation. This substance has been shown to be an 11-amino acid peptide known as substance P. Its actions are numerous and varied. (See Table 2).

Distribution

Substance P is found throughout the gut, from the esophagus to the colon, mostly in fine nerve fibers in all areas of the gut wall, including the two muscle layers, the two myenteric plexuses, the mucosa, and the submucosa. The intrinsic origin of these nerve fibers from the myenteric plexus, suggested before (48),

TABLE 2. *Reported pharmacological actions of substance P*

Gut
  Muscle contraction
  Gallbladder contraction
  ↑ Pancreatic exocrine secretion
  ↑ Saliva secretion

Nervous system
  Sensory
  Axon reflex (skin)
  Analgesia
  Behavior

Cardiovascular system
  Vasodilation
  ↑ Blood flow
  Bradychardia

Respiratory system
  Bronchoconstriction
  ↑ Glycoprotein-mucus
  ↑ Respiration (frequency)
  ↑ Nasal secretion

Endocrine system
  Anterior pituitary
    (↑ GH, LH/FSH, Prolatin)
  Pancreas
    (↑ Glucagon, ↓ insulin, ↑ glucose)
  ↓ Gastrin

Urogenital tract
  Vas deferens
  Uterus and fallopian tube   Smooth muscle contraction
  Ureter
  Bladder

Data from ref. 66.

has been fully confirmed by the use of separate Auerbach and Meissner tissue explant techniques (Fig. 8) and extrinsic gut denervation procedures (Fig. 9) (33). Apart from its localization in the gut, an important net of substance P fine nerve fibers is seen in the lung (Fig. 10) (75), urogenital tract (Fig. 11) (especially vagina and ureter), skin (Fig. 12), and tongue.

Somatostatin

Somatostatin is a 14-amino acid peptide, originally extracted from the hypothalamus during the search for the factor that inhibited the release of growth hormone (11). It was later discovered that somatostatin is also a potent inhibitor of the release of thyroid-stimulating hormone and that it can block completely the release of numerous gut hormones.

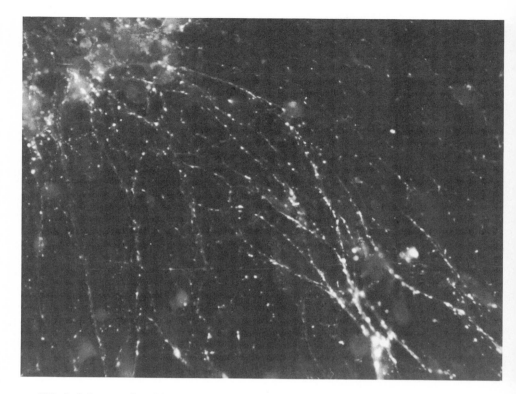

FIG. 8. Substance P cell bodies and nerve fibers after 8 days of explanting the Auerbach's plexus of the guinea pig *taenia coli.* ×344.

Distribution

Somatostatin is found in the gastrointestinal tract in quantities even larger than in the brain. The principal locations are the antrum and the pancreas, although some can be found throughout the gut, including the colon and the rectum. The physicochemical properties of gastrointestinal somatostatin are almost indistinguishable from those of the brain peptide, and pure preparations of gut somatostatin display biological actions similar to those of pure synthetic somatostatin (6). Somatostatin is produced by the D cells of the gut and pancreas (62). Immunocytochemical staining shows that the somatostatin cells are provided with cytoplasmic processes that connect them to other endocrine or exocrine cells and end in a bulbous swelling like a nerve terminal (Fig. 13). These processes are particularly noticeable in the fundus and pancreatic islets, where somatostatin cells, unlike those of the antrum and pancreatic ducts, are rarely connected with the lumen. These and other features suggest a possible local or paracrine role for somatostatin. The occasional presence of somatostatin in the peripheral circulation may merely indicate an overflow phenomenon.

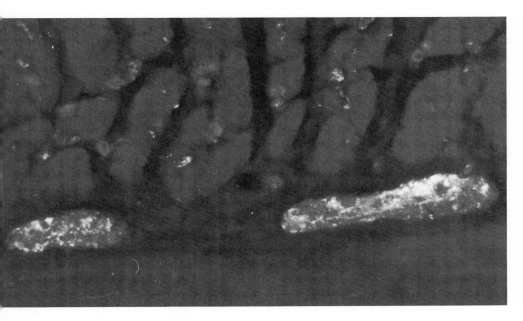

FIG. 9. Substance P nerve fibers in Auerbach's plexus of the guinea pig *taenia coli* 3 weeks after extrinsic autonomic denervation. ×254.

Pathology

Duodenal Ulceration

Information provided by quantitative ICC in the antra from patients with duodenal ulceration suggested a relative decrease of the somatostatin content (56). This led to the postulate that a somatostatin deficiency may result in unrestrained acid secretion and thus be one of the numerous factors contributing to the development of duodenal ulceration (56). This suggestion has been recently strengthened by a reduced somatostatin content in the antral tissue of patients with duodenal ulceration found by RIA (17).

Apudomas

Two pancreatic endocrine tumors were reported to produce somatostatin (28,40). The patients had gallstones, diabetes, and reduced acid secretion. In the same year our group reported the finding of somatostatin in a number of glucagonomas, vipomas, gastrinomas, and insulinomas (9,10), which could explain the relatively refractory response to somatostatin treatment in some cases of Apudomas. Our findings have been confirmed recently by various groups

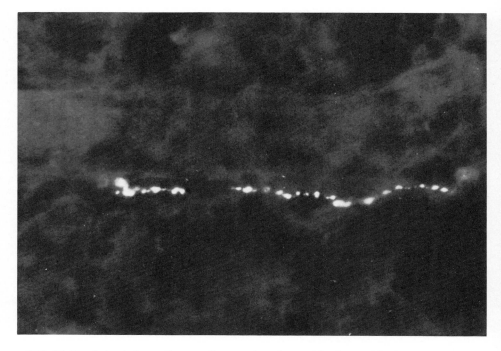

FIG. 10. Beaded substance P nerve fiber running along a blood vessel in the outer third of the guinea pig lung. ×630.

(1,26). Studies have included experimental insulinomas, in which the presence of somatostatin has also been shown (19).

Persistent Neonatal Hypoglycemia with Nesidioblastosis

We have recently shown a significant decrease in somatostatin levels in children with persistent neonatal hypoglycemia and hyperinsulinemia and the pathological features of nesidioblastosis (54). This somatostatin failure may be one of the factors leading to the excessive insulin release. These findings have been supported by the successful treatment with somatostatin of two children with nesidioblastosis (31,69).

Enkephalins

Methionine and leucine enkephalin are two pentapeptides that differ in only one amino acid at the C-terminal end. Methionine enkephalin (met-enkephalin) is included in a larger group of chemically related peptides known as endorphins

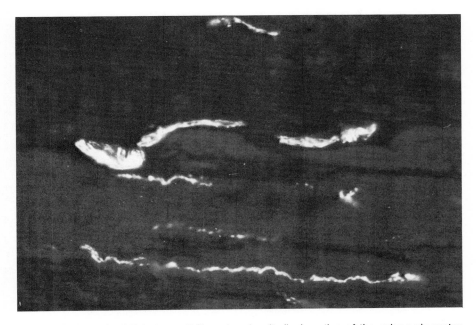

FIG. 11. Rich mesh of Substance P fibers in a longitudinal section of the guinea pig ureter. ×346.

(endogenous morphine). Their name, indicating that they are endogenous opiates, was coined after the surprising discovery of morphine receptors in the brain. The enkephalins powerfully modulate intestinal functions. Their actions include reduction of intestinal motility and secretion, relaxation of gallbladder tone, and contraction of the sphincter of Oddi, as well as suppression of pancreatic bicarbonate or enzyme secretion after endogenous or exogenous stimulation (36,37).

Distribution

The enkephalins are present throughout the gastrointestinal tract but are particularly concentrated in the upper parts. ICC shows that the enkephalins are localized mostly in the innervation of the gut, their cell bodies being found intrinsically in the gut wall. Their intrinsic gut wall origin is further supported by the finding of positive immunostaining in extrinsically denervated pieces of gut and in tissue explants of myenteric plexus (33). In addition, the enkephalins are often found in sympathetic ganglia (65) and in normal (65) and tumorous adrenal medulla (70). More information on this subject may be found in Chapter 15 by C. A. Myers and D. H. Coy, pp. 363–385, and in Chapter 28 by S. Konturek, pp. 693–716, *this volume.*

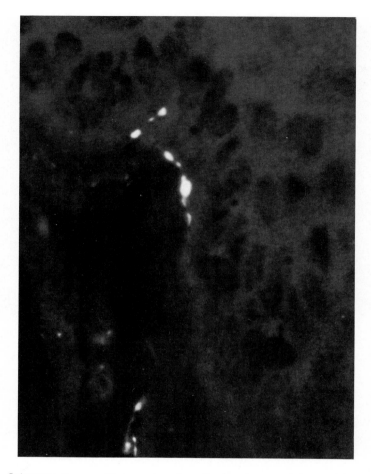

FIG. 12. Substance P nerve fiber running along the basal parts of the cat skin (foot pad) and extending into the epidermis. ×604.

Bombesin

Bombesin is a 14-amino acid peptide originally extracted from the skin of the discoglossid frog *Bombina bombina* after the systematic search for active peptides in more than 500 amphibian species (22). Like many other amphibian

FIG. 13.a: Dog fundic mucosa double stained with antibodies to glucagon and somatostatin. Observe the "finger-like" process of the somatostatin cell (SM) in close contact with parietal cells. ×500. PG, pancreatic glucagon cells; L, lumen; FL, "finger-like" process; SM, somatostatin cell; P, parietal cell. **b:** Same tissue, conventional EM. Observe the elongated somatostatin process in close contact with an A (pancreatic glucagon) cell of the fundic mucosa. ×12,500.

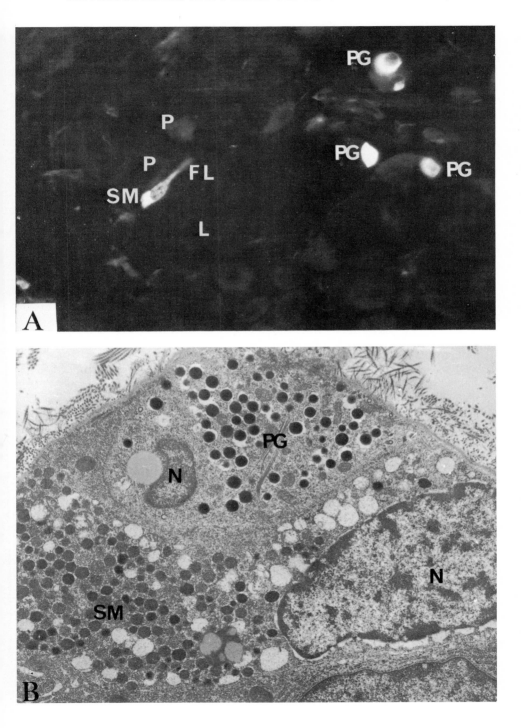

TABLE 3. *Reported pharmacological actions of bombesin*

Stomach
  pH independent gastrin release
  Stimulation of gastric acid secretion (either directly or gastrin mediated)

Pancreas
  (a) Exocrine
    In vitro: Enzyme secretion
      Calcium efflux (direct, cholinergic-independent)
    In vivo: Enzyme secretion
      (indirect, cholinergic-dependent ?CCK or others)
  (b) Endocrine: release of
    Insulin
    Glucagon
    PP (cholinergic dependent)

Smooth muscle
  Gallbladder contraction
  Bronchoconstriction

Vascular
  Stimulation of the renin-angiotensin system
  Erythropoietin release

Brain
  Hyperglycemia
  Thermoregulation

skin peptides, bombesin displays a wide spectrum of pharmacological actions in the mammal (43) (See Table 3).

Distribution

Bombesin is found in the gut (61), brain (61), and lung (61,74), where it may be present either in the innervation (61) or in endocrine (APUD) cells (72). For more information see Chapters 14 by V. Erspamer, pp. 343–361 and 29 by P. Melchiorri, pp. 717–725, *this volume.*

Vasoactive Intestinal Polypeptide (VIP)

VIP was originally extracted from porcine intestine as a powerful vasoactive substance. It was later found to be a highly basic, 28-amino acid peptide with close sequence similarity to glucagon, GIP, and secretin (64).

Distribution

VIP is the "neuropeptide" with the widest distribution within and outside the gut. Large quantities of extractable VIP, with the physicochemical properties identical to those of natural and synthetic porcine VIP, are found in the brain (12), pituitary (73), gut (12), salivary glands (63) (Fig. 14), tongue, genitourinary

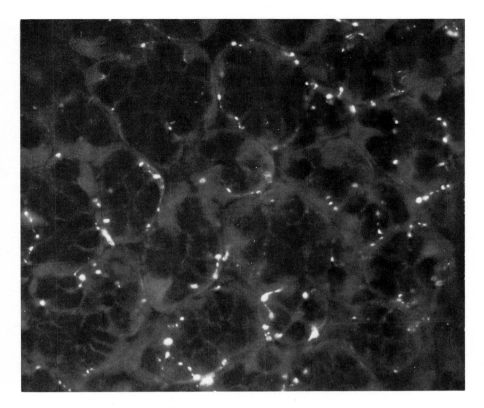

FIG. 14. VIP nerve fibers of the rat sublingual gland. ×378.

tract (5), nasal mucosa (Fig. 15), and pancreas (51). ICC localizes VIP mainly to fine nerve fibers containing neurosecretory granules that, when analyzed at the ultrastructural level, seem to correspond to the nonadrenergic, noncholinergic "p" (peptidergic) secretory granules described by Baumgarten (3). In the gut, VIP nerve fibers are seen throughout the entire length and width (Fig. 16). Their cell bodies are intrinsic to the gut wall (33) and localized in Meissner's plexus (Fig. 17). Nerve fibers originating at this level innervate the mucosa and submucosa, the two muscle layers, the blood vessels, and the Auerbach's plexus. VIP is also well represented in the pancreas (Table 4), where it appears to innervate both the exocrine and endocrine pancreas (Fig. 18) (51). Numerous immunoreactive ganglion cells are also seen within the pancreas.

Actions

VIP is a powerful vasodilator, smooth muscle relaxant, and modulator of intestinal secretion. These actions correspond well to the anatomical localization

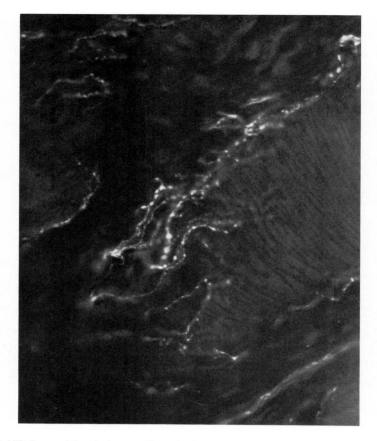

FIG. 15. VIP fine and beaded nerve fibers in the cat nasal mucosa. Observe a tight mesh around an artery. ×600.

of the VIP nerves in structures involved in secretion (e.g., gut mucosa and endometrium) and vasodilation (e.g., around blood vessels). The extensive smooth muscle VIP innervation supports the idea that VIP is a modulator of smooth muscle activity. Its actions may be mediated by cyclic AMP, which has been shown to be increased by VIP in several systems (for details, see Chapter 10 by S. Said, pp. 245–273 *this volume*). A number of atropine-resistant, nerve-mediated gastrointestinal responses such as antral muscle relaxation and pancreatic alkaline bicarbonate secretion can now be mimicked by intravascular infusion of VIP in small quantities (24, 32).

Pathology

Tumors

VIP has been shown to be the agent responsible for the Verner-Morrison syndrome of watery diarrhea, hypokalemia, and achlorhydria (WDHA) (8). This syndrome is always associated with an endocrine tumor (APUDOMA) often found in the pancreas, producing and secreting large quantities of VIP. Of these VIPomas, 25% are extrapancreatic and present all the morphological features of ganglioneuroblastomas (Fig. 19). (For further details see Chapter 31 by C. Owyang and V. L. Go, pp. 741–748, *this volume.*)

Non-tumors

An interesting recently discovered example of VIP involvement in nontumor pathology is found in the bowel of patients suffering from Crohn's disease, where the VIP-containing nerves are highly immunoreactive and appear hyperplastic, thickened, and disorganized. (Fig. 20 a,b) (50). These features are found not only at the level of the stricture but also in the nongranulomatous areas. These VIP abnormalities are seen in all the layers of the gut wall and are also found in the younger group of patients (teenagers). The VIP content of colonic extracts is also significantly elevated (Table 5). An increase in the number of ganglion cells and nerves in Crohn's disease was recognized as early as in 1955 (20). The extent of this increase was not suspected until the application of ICC methods for neuropeptides. It should now be possible to investigate the possible neurally mediated malfunctions in this disease.

CONCLUSIONS

In the light of these various new findings, one fact is immediately obvious. Our old preconceived idea that the endocrine cells produce and secrete "true" hormones, and nerves release neurotransmitters, must be changed to accommodate the recent discovery of an increasing number of peptides with a dual localization in both neural and endocrine elements, comprising what is now widely known as the diffuse neuroendocrine system. A number of conclusions may therefore be drawn.

Common Embryological Origin of Neuroendocrine Cells

In 1966 Pearse (45) postulated a common embryological origin for the cells of the diffuse neuroendocrine system in the neural crest. He later suggested that the common origin was neuroectodermal and proposed that the endocrine system was an outpouch of the brain. On this premise, it was likely that further similarities between the nervous and the endocrine systems would be found.

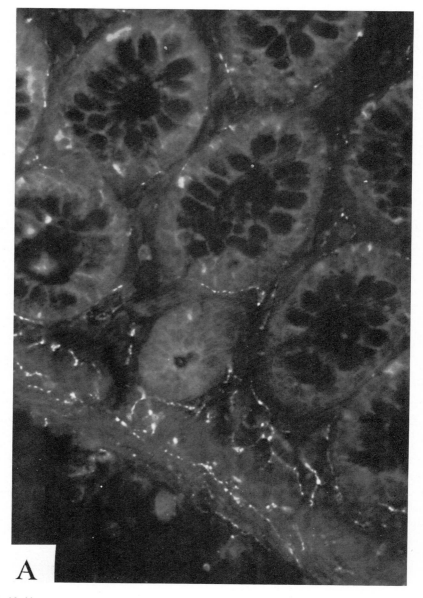

FIG. 16. Human gut. **a:** VIP nerve fibers in the mucosa. × 300. **b:** VIP nerves in the gut wall (muscle). ×300.

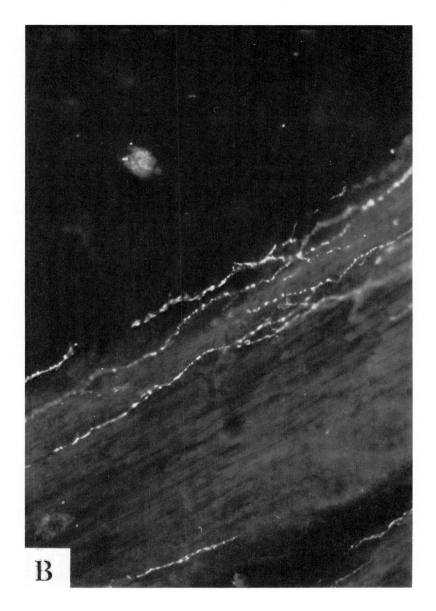

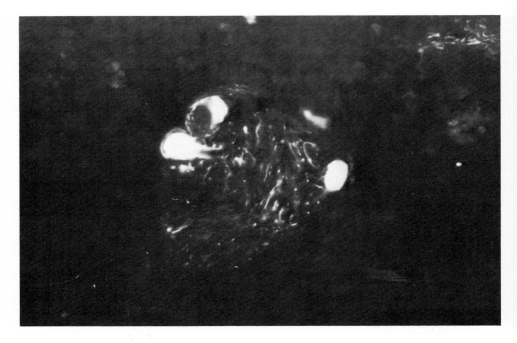

FIG. 17. Immunoreactive VIP cell bodies and fibers in the myenteric plexus. ×315.

Pavlov Theory versus Theory of Bayliss and Starling

Strict divisions cannot be made between peptides localized in cells and those localized in nerves; it is thus no longer valid to view the endocrine and the nervous systems as two separate entities. The discovery of the diffuse neuroendocrine system has reconciled the two opposing views of control of gut function. Pavlov's theory of nervous control and Bayliss and Starling's theory of control by chemical messengers may now be combined. A hormonal peptide may act in at least three separate ways. First, it can be produced by a neuron, transported down an axon, and released from a synapse by axonal depolarization, whence it has a local action and is rapidly destroyed. Second, a hormonal peptide

TABLE 4. *VIP content in human and rat pancreas (whole tissue and isolated islets) estimated by RIA of tissue extracts*

Tissue	pmole/g wet weight	± SEM
Whole human pancreas	49 ± 15	$n = 7$
Whole rat pancreas	27 ± 7	$n = 7$
Isolated rat islets	304 ± 30	$n = 5$

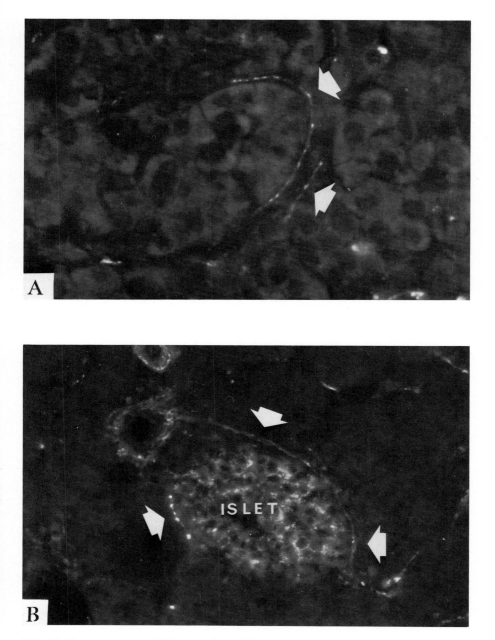

FIG. 18. Human pancreas. VIP innervation of **(a)** pancreatic islet and **(b)** exocrine pancreas. **a:** ×250. **b:** ×300.

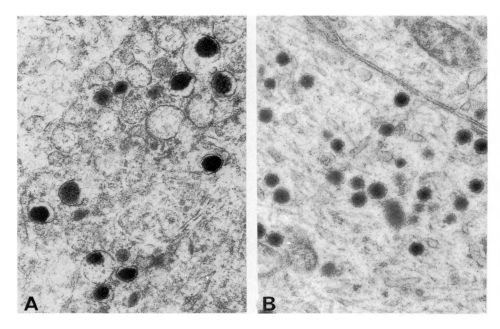

FIG. 19. VIPoma with the classic morphological features of ganglioneuroblastoma, showing two different types of secretory granules: **(a)** amine granules; **(b)** VIP granules. ×30,000.

may be stored in an endocrine cell but is released only locally and influences the surrounding tissues only as far as it can diffuse (local hormone or paracrine system). Third, the peptide may be released into the bloodstream to act at a distance in the classic hormonal manner.

Peptidergic Component of the Autonomic Nervous System

In 1970 full recognition of a new division of the autonomic nervous system came from the clear description of Baumgarten and associates (3), who observed neurosecretory (peptidergic) granules as quite distinct from the classic profiles of the adrenergic and cholinergic components. Some of the neuropeptides that we have described [e.g., VIP (52) and substance P (48)], appear to be stored in these large and highly electron-dense secretory granules of autonomic nervous system (Baumgarten's "p-type"). The rapid advances seen in the last decade (see Chapter 1 by E. Solcia et al., pp. 1–17, *this volume,* on the classification of the endocrine cells of the gut) can now be predicted with respect to the peptidergic innervation of the gut that has just come to light (55).

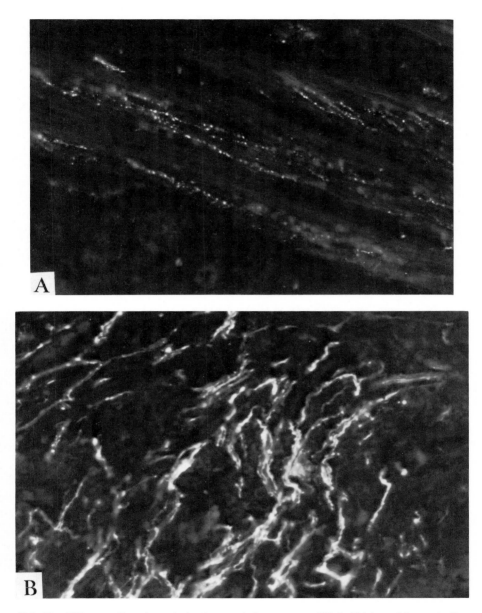

FIG. 20.a: VIP nerve fibers in control gut, muscularis mucosa. ×450. **b:** Thickened, hyperplastic, and disorganized VIP nerve fibers of the gut wall. ×450.

TABLE 5. *Increased VIP content in Crohn's disease*

Gut wall	VIP pmole/g wet weight	± SEM
Control	119 ± 8	$n = 5$
Crohn's	271 ± 39	$n = 5$

PROJECTIONS FOR THE FUTURE

The concept of endocrine cells and nerves as a single integrated neurohormonal system is clear and logical. However, there are many facets to its organization. Peptides released by paracrine cells may reach such concentrations that they overflow into the bloodstream and are thus carried to distant sites that may be receptive. Equally, a peptide released from synapses into the pituitary portal circulation may also act as a "classic" hormone.

The classic idea of an "inhibitory" (sympathetic) and "excitatory" (parasympathetic) role for the autonomic nervous system will have to be modified to account for the extensive and powerful components of this system secreting peptides with a consequent array of agonistic and antagonistic effects. Many atropine-resistant responses of the gastrointestinal tract after nerve stimulation can now be explained by the release of these neuropeptides acting as neurotransmitters or neuromodulators. The complexity of many gastrointestinal functions and their controlling factors are beginning to fall into place and we may now look forward to profitable years of further insight into gut functions in health and disease.

ACKNOWLEDGMENTS

This work was carried out with the generous support from the Medical Research Council, Cancer Research Campaign, Council for Tobacco Research (U.S.A.), and Janssen Pharmaceutical (U.K.).

REFERENCES

1. Alumets, J., Ekelund, G., Hakanson, R., Ljungberg, O., Ljungqvist, U., Sundler, F., and Tibblin, S. (1978): Jejunal endocrine tumour composed of somatostatin and gastrin cells and associated with duodenal ulcer disease. *Virchows Archiv. (Pathol. Anat.),* 17–22.
2. Arimura, A., Sato, H., Dupont, A., Nishi, N., and Schally, A. V. (1975): Somatostatin: Abundance of immunoreactive hormone in rat stomach and pancreas. *Science,* 189:1007–1009.
3. Baumgarten, H. G., Holstein, A. F., and Owman, C. H. (1970): Auerbach's plexus of mammals and man—electron microscopical identification of three different types of neuronal processes in myenteric ganglia of the large intestine from rhesus monkeys, guinea-pigs and man. *Z. Zellforsch,* 106:376–397.
4. Bayliss, W. M., and Starling, E. H. (1902): The mechanism of pancreatic secretion. *J. Physiol.,* 28:325–353.
5. Bishop, A. E., Polak, J. M., and Bloom, S. R. (1979): Vasoactive Intestinal Polypeptide innervation of the genital tract of women. *J. Endocrinol.,* 80:33–34.

6. Bloom, S. R. (1978): Somatostatin and gut. *Gastroenterology,* 75:145–147.
7. Bloom, S. R., Christofides, N. D., Bryant, M. G., Buchan, A. M. J., and Polak, J. M. (1979): One motilin or several? *Gastroenterology,* 76(5):1102.
8. Bloom, S. R., Polak, J. M., and Pearse, A. G. E. (1973): Vasoactive intestinal peptide and the watery diarrhea syndrome. *Lancet,* ii:14–16.
9. Bloom, S. R., Polak, J. M., and Welbourn, R. B. (1979): Pancreatic apudomas. *World J. Surg.,* 3:581–595.
10. Bloom, S. R., Polak, J. M., and West, A. M. (1978): Somatostatin content of pancreatic endocrine tumors. In: *Metabolism, Vol. 27 No. 9 Suppl. 1,* edited by J. E. Gerich, S. Raptis, and J. Rosenthal, pp. 1235–1238, Grune & Stratton, New York.
11. Brazeau, P., Vale, W., Burgus, R., Ling, N., Butcher, M. Rivier, J., and Guillemin, R. (1973): Hypothalamic polypeptide that inhibits the secretion of immunoreactive pituitary growth hormone. *Science,* 179:77–79.
12. Bryant, M. G., Bloom, S. R., Polak, J. M., Albuquerque, R. H., Modlin, I., and Pearse, A. G. E. (1976): Possible dual role for vasoactive intestinal peptide gastrointestinal hormone and neuro-transmitter substance. *Lancet,* i:991–993.
13. Buchan, A. M. J., Polak, J. M., Solcia, E., Capella, C., Hudson, H., and Pearse, A. G. E. (1978): Electroimmunocytochemical evidence for the human intestinal I cell as the source of CCK. *Gut,* 19:403–407.
14. Buchan, A. M. J., Polak, J. M., Solcia, E., and Pearse, A. G. E. (1979): Localization of intestinal gastrin in a distinct endocrine cell type. *Nature,* 277:138–140.
15. Burnstock, G. (1972): Purinergic nerves. *Pharmacol. Rev.,* 24:509–581.
16. Capella, C., Solcia, E., Frigerio, B., and Buffa, R. (1975): Endocrine cells of the human intestine—an ultrastructural study. In: *Endocrine Gut and Pancreas,* edited by T. Fujita, pp. 42–59. Elsevier, Amsterdam.
17. Chayvialle, J. A. P., Descos, F., Bernard, C., Martin, A. Barbe, C., and Partensky, C. (1978): Somatostatin in mucosa of stomach and duodenum in gastroduodenal disease. *Gastroenterology,* 75:13–19.
18. Cook, R. D., and Burnstock, G. (1976): The ultrastructure of Auerbach's plexus in the guinea-pig. 1. Neuronal elements. *J. Neurocytol.,* 5:171–194.
19. Creutzfeldt, W., Arnold, R., Creutzfeldt, C., and Frerichs, H. (1979): Experimental production of endocrine pancreatic tumors in the rat. In: *Proceedings of the II European Symposium on Hypoglycaemia, Rome, Jan. 1979,* edited by D. Andreani, P. Lefevre, and V. Marks. Academic Press, New York, *(in press).*
20. Davis, D. R., Dockerty, M. B., and Tiayo, C. W. (1955): The myenteric plexus in regional enteritis: A study of the number of ganglion cells in the ileum in 24 cases. *Surg. Gynaecol. Obstet.,* 101:208–216.
21. Dogiel, S. A. (1899): Uber den Bau der Ganglien in den Geflechten des Darmes und der Gallenblase des Menschen u. der Saügetiere. *Arch. Anat. Phys. Anat. Abt.,:* 130–158.
22. Erspamer, V., and Melchiorri, P. (1973): Active polypeptides of the amphibian skin and their synthetic analogues. *Pure Appl. Chem.,* 35:463–494.
23. Euler, U. S. von, and Gaddum, J. H. (1931): An unidentified depressor substance in certain tissue extracts. *J. Physiol.,* 192:74–87.
24. Fahrenkrug, J., Galbo, H., Holst, J. J., and Schaffalitzky de Muckadell, O. B. (1978): Influence of the autonomic nervous system on the release of vasoactive intestinal polypeptide from the porcine gastrointestinal tract. *J. Physiol. (Lond.),* 280:405–422.
25. Feyrter, F. (1938): *Uber diffuse endokrine epitheliale Organe.* J. A. Barth, Leipzig. pp. 6–17.
26. Forssmann, W. G., Helmstaedter, V., Metz, J., Mühlmann, G., and Feurle, G. E. (1978): Immunohistochemistry and ultrastructure of somatostatin cells with special reference to the gastroenteropancreatic (GEP) system. In: *Metabolism, Vol., 27, No. 9, Suppl. 1,* edited by J. E. Gerich, S. Raptis, and J. Rosenthal, pp. 1179–1191. Grune & Stratton, New York.
27. Fujita, T., and Kobayashi (1977): Structure and function of gut endocrine cells. *Int. Rev. Cytol.,* (Suppl), 6:187–227.
28. Ganda, Om. P., Weir, G. C., Soeldner, J. S., Legg, M. A., Chick, W. L., Patel, Y. C., Ebeid, A. M., Gabbay, K. H., and Reichlin, S. (1977): Somatostatinoma—A somatostatin-containing tumor of the endocrine pancreas. *N. Engl. J. Med.,* 296:963–967.
29. Grimelius, L., Polak, J. M., Solcia, E., and Pearse, A. G. E. (1978): The enteroglucagon cell. In: *Gut Hormones,* edited by S. R. Bloom, pp. 365–368. Churchill Livingstone, Edinburgh.
30. Heidenhain, R. (1870): Untersuchungen über den Bau der Labdrüsen. *Arch. Mikr. Anat.,* 6:368.

31. Hirsch, H. J., Loo, S., Evans, N., Crigler, J. F., Filler, R. M., and Gabbay, K. H. (1977): Hypoglycemia of infancy and nesidioblastosis—studies with somatostatin. *N. Engl. J. Med.* 296:1323–1326.
32. Holst, J. J., Schaffalitzky de Muckadell, O. B., and Fahrenkrug, J. F. (1979): Nervous control of pancreatic exocrine secretion in pigs. *Acta Physiol. Scand.*, 105:33–51.
33. Jessen, K. R., Polak, J. M., Van Noorden, S., Bryant, M. G., Bloom, S. R., and Burnstock, G. (1979): A new approach to the demonstration of the enteric plexus origin of peptide-containing nerves by immunocytochemistry and radioimmunoassay. *Gastroenterology,* 76(5):1161.
34. Kataoka, K. (1974): An electron microscope study on a neuro-endocrine complex in the proventricular mucosa of the finch. *Arch. Histol. Jpn.*, 36:391–400.
35. Kataoka, K. (1977): The neuro-endocrine complex in the gastroentero-pancreatic endocrine system. In: *Paraneurons: New Concepts on Neuro-Endocrine Relations, Archivum Histologicum Japonicum, Vol. 40, Suppl. 1977,* edited by S. Kobayashi and T. Chiba, pp. 119–127. Japan Society of Histological Documentation, Niigata, Japan.
36. Konturek, S. J. (1978): Endogenous opiates and the digestive system. *Scand. J. Gastroenterol.,* 13:257–261.
37. Konturek, S. J., Tasler, J., Cieszkowski, M., Jaworek, J., Coy, D. H., and Schally, A. V. (1978): Inhibition of pancreatic secretion by enkephalin and morphine in dogs. *Gastroenterology,* 74 *(Part I):* 851–855.
38. Kultschitzky, N. (1897): Zur Frage uber den Bau des Darmkanals. *Arch. Mikrosk. Anat.,* 49:7–35.
39. Langley, J. N. (1898): The sympathetic and other related system of nerves. In: *Textbook of Physiology, Vol. 1,* edited by E. A. Schäfer, pp. 475–530. Pentland, Edinburgh.
40. Larsson, L.-I., Hirsch, M. A., Holst, J. J., Ingemansson, S., Kuhl, C., Jensen, S. L., Lundqvist, G., and Rehfeld, J. F. (1977): Pancreatic somatostatinoma—clinical features and physiological implications. *Lancet,* i:666–669.
41. Lehto, V.-P., and Virtanen, I. (1979): Association of intermediate filaments with other cell organelles in carcinoid tumor of the colon. *Experientia,* 35:35–36.
42. Matsuo, Y., Seki, A., and Fukuda, S. (1976): Neuro-endocrine cells in the lamina propria of rat stomach. In: *Endocrine Gut and Pancreas,* edited by T. Fujita, pp. 159–164. Elsevier, Amsterdam.
43. Melchiorri, P. (1978): Bombesin and bombesin-like peptides of amphibian skin. In: *Gut Hormones,* edited by S. R. Bloom, pp. 534–540. Churchill Livingstone, Edinburgh.
44. Moody, A. J., Jacobsen, H., and Sundby, F. (1978): Gastric glucagon and gut glucagon-like immunoreactants. In: *Gut Hormones,* edited by S. R. Bloom, pp. 369–378. Churchill Livingstone, Edinburgh.
45. Pearse, A. G. E. (1966): Common cytochemical properties of cells producing polypeptide hormones, with particular reference to calcitonin and the thyroid C cells. *Vet. Rec.,* 79:587–590.
46. Pearse, A. G. E. (1969): The cytochemistry and ultrastructure of polypeptide hormone-producing cells of the APUD series and the embryologic, physiologic and pathologic implications of the concept. *J. Histochem. Cytochem.,* 17:303–313.
47. Pearse, A. G. E. (1976): Peptides in brain and intestine. *Nature,* 262:92–94.
48. Pearse, A. G. E., and Polak, J. M. (1975): Immunocytochemical localisation of substance P in mammalian intestine. *Histochemistry,* 41:373–375.
49. Pickel, V. M., Reis, D. J., and Leeman, S. E. (1977): Ultrastructural localisation of substance P in neurons of rat spinal cord. *Brain Res.,* 122:534–540.
50. Polak, J. M., Bishop, A. E., and Bloom, S. R. (1978): The morphology of VIPergic nerves in Crohn's disease. *Scand. J. Gastroenterol. (Suppl. 49),* 13:144.
51. Polak, J. M., Bishop, A. E., Bloom, S. R., Buchan, A. M. J., and Timson, C. M. (1978): The VIPergic innervation of the pancreas. *Scand. J. Gastroenterol. (Suppl. 49,)* 13:145.
52. Polak, J. M., and Bloom, S. R. (1978): Peptidergic innervation of the gastrointestinal tract. In: *Gastrointestinal Hormones and Pathology of the Digestive System,* edited by M. Grossman, V. Speranza, N. Basso, and E. Lezoche, pp. 27–49. Plenum Press, New York.
53. Polak, J. M., and Bloom, S. R. (1978): Peptidergic nerves of the gastrointestinal tract. *Invest. Cell Pathol.,* 1:301–326.
54. Polak, J. M., and Bloom, S. R. (1979): Decreased somatostatin content in persistent neonatal hyperinsulinaemic hypoglycaemia. In: *Proceedings of Second International Symposium on Hypoglycaemia,* edited by D. Andreani. Academic Press, New York, *(in press).*

55. Polak, J. M., and Bloom, S. R. (1979): The Neuroendocrine Design of the Gut. In: *Clinics in Endocrinology and Metabolism, Vol. 8,* No. 2, edited by K. Buchanan. W. B. Saunders, London, *(in press).*
56. Polak, J. M., Bloom, S. R., Bishop, A. E., and McCrossan, M. V. (1978): D cell pathology in duodenal ulcers and achlorhydria. *Metabolism, (Suppl. 1),* 27:1239–1242.
57. Polak, J. M., Bloom, S. R., Coulling, I., and Pearse, A. G. E. (1971): Immunofluorescent localisation of enteroglucagon cells in the gastrointestinal tract of the dog. *Gut,* 12:311–318.
58. Polak, J. M., and Buchan, A. M. J. (1979): Motilin—Immunocytochemical localisation indicates possible molecular heterogeneity or the existence of a motilin family. *Gastroenterology,* 76(5):1065–1066.
59. Polak, J. M., Buchan, A. M. J., and Pearse, A. G. E. (1978): Beta-endorphin-like immunoreactivity in neuroendocrine (APUD) cells of the intestinal sub-mucosa of the salamander (Salamandra salamandra). *Scand. J. Gastroenterol. (Suppl. 49),* 13:146.
60. Polak, J. M., Coulling, I., Bloom, S. R., and Pearse, A. G. E. (1971): Immunofluorescence localisation of secretin and enteroglucagon in human intestinal mucosa. *Scand. J. Gastroenterol.,* 6:739–744.
61. Polak, J. M., Ghatei, M. A., Wharton, J., Bishop, A. E., Bloom, S. R., Solcia, E., Brown, M. R., and Pearse, A. G. E. (1978): Bombesin-like immunoreactivity in the gastrointestinal tract, lung and central nervous system. *Scand. J. Gastroenterol., (Suppl. 49),* 13:148.
62. Polak, J. M., Pearse, A. G. E., Grimelius, L., Bloom, S. R., and Arimura, A. (1975): Growth-hormone releasing inhibiting hormone (GH-RIH) in gastrointestinal and pancreatic D cells. *Lancet,* i:1220–1225.
63. Polak, J. M., Wharton, J., Bryant, M. G., and Bloom, S. R. (1979): Peptidergic (VIP) innervation of salivary glands. *Gastroenterology,* 76(5):1219.
64. Said, S. I. (1978): VIP: Overview. In: *Gut Hormones,* edited by S. R. Bloom, pp. 465–468. Churchill Livingstone, Edinburgh.
65. Schultzberg, M., Hokfelt, T., Lundberg, J. M., Terenius, L., Elfvin, L. G., and Elde, R. (1978): Enkephalin-like immunoreactivity in nerve terminals in sympathetic ganglia and adrenal medulla and in adrenal medullary gland cells. *Acta Physiol. Scand.,* 103:475–478.
66. Skrabaneck, P., and Powell, D. (1977): Substance P. In: *Annual Research Reviews,* Vol. I, edited by P. Skrabaneck and D. Powell, pp. 69–101. Churchill Livingstone, Edinburgh.
67. Solcia, E., Polak, J. M., Pearse, A. G. E., Forssmann, W. G., Larsson, L.-I., Sundler, F., Lechago, J., Grimelius, L., Fujita, T., Creutzfeldt, W., Gepts, W., Falkmer, S., Lafranc, G., Heitz, Ph., Hage, E., Buchan, A. M. J., Bloom, S. R., and Grossman, M. I. (1978): Lausanne 1977 classification of gastroenteropancreatic endocrine cells. In: *Gut Hormones,* edited by S. R. Bloom, pp. 40–48. Churchill Livingstone, Edinburgh.
68. Solcia, E., Vassallo, G., and Sampietro, R. (1967): Endocrine cells in the antro-pyloric mucosa of the stomach. *Z. Zellforsch.,* 81:474–486.
69. Søvik, O., Fevang, F. Ø., and Finne, P. H. (1979): Familial nesidioblastosis. *Pediatric Research, (in press).*
70. Sullivan, S. N., Bloom, S. R., and Polak, J. M. (1978): Enkephalin in peripheral neuroendocrine tumours. *Lancet,* i:1155.
71. Sutherland, E. W., and de Duve, C. (1948): Origin and distribution of the hyperglycaemic-glycogenolytic factor of the pancreas. *J. Biol. Chem.,* 175:665–670.
72. Timson, C. M., Polak, J. M., Wharton, J., Ghatei, M. A., Bloom, S. R., Usellini, L., Capella, C., Solcia, E., Brown, M. R., and Pearse, A. G. E. (1979): Bombesin-like immunoreactivity in the avian gut and its localisation to a distinct cell type. *Histochemistry, (in press).*
73. Van Noorden, S., Polak, J. M., Bloom, S. R., and Bryant, M. G. (1979): Vasoactive Intestinal Polypeptide in the pituitary pars nervosa. *Neuropathol. Appl. Neurobiol.,* 5:149–153.
74. Wharton, J., Polak, J. M., Bloom, S. R., Ghatei, M. A., Solcia, E., Brown, M. R., and Pearse, A. G. E. (1978): Bombesin-like immunoreactivity in the lung. *Nature,* 5665:769.
75. Wharton, J., Polak, J. M., Bloom, S. R., Will, J. A., Brown, M. R., and Pearse, A. G. E. (1979): Substance P-like immunoreactive nerves in mammalian lung. *Invest. Cell Pathol.,* 2:3–10.

Gastrointestinal Hormones, edited by
George B. Jerzy Glass.
Raven Press, New York © 1980.

Chapter 3

Problems and Pitfalls in Immunocytochemistry of Gut Peptides

Lars-Inge Larsson

Institute of Medical Biochemistry, University of Aarhus, DK-8000 Aarhus C, Denmark

INTRODUCTION

Numerous hormonal and neuronal peptides have been isolated from the gastrointestinal tract. Knowledge of the cellular and subcellular localization of these peptides is of paramount importance in interpreting their physiological roles. The only technique capable of providing us with such information is immunocytochemistry (ICC).

In ICC studies of gut peptides two problems have appeared particularly severe. The first problem is that most of the gut peptides show similarities in their amino acid sequences, allowing us to group them together in hormone, or, perhaps more correctly, peptide families. Antisera raised against one member of such a family may react with other members as well. Since not all members of a given family can be expected to have been purified and characterized, such cross-reactivities may lead to great difficulties in interpreting staining results. In this context it is essential to remember that most antibodies are directed against only a small sequence of amino acids (usually comprising 3–8 residues). The specificity of an antiserum for a given peptide will, hence, depend on the uniqueness of the sequence against which it is directed. The antigenic site may be either continuous (i.e., a simple straight sequence of amino acids) or discontinuous (i.e., depending on the conformation of the peptide). Broadly speaking, antisera specific for discontinuous antigenic sites may be expected to be more peptide specific than others, since in this case binding will depend on both the sequence and the conformation of the peptide. Most gut peptide antisera, however, seem to be directed against only a limited portion of the molecule and are subjected to the risk of cross-reactivity with known and unknown peptides. A means of avoiding this dilemma has been offered by the introduction of antibodies specific against several distinct regions of gut peptides. Use of such region-specific antibodies allows the demonstration of several antigenic sites of the peptide under investigation (13,16,17). Consequently, region-specific ICC adds considerably to the credibility of peptide localization studies.

The second major problem is related to the need for optimal preservation of both antigenicity and tissue structure. Thus many peptides have been purported to be "localized" to specific cell types, but the "localization" has been documented by electron micrographs of such a poor quality that cell identification is impossible. The adjacent semithin-ultrathin section technique is the one usually employed for identification of gut and pancreatic endocrine cells. This technique, originally developed by Lange (9,10), relies on the ICC demonstration of peptidic antigens in semithin plastic sections and the identification of the immunoreactive cells in adjacent ultrathin sections (2,9,10). The reliability of the technique depends on the degree of morphological preservation and on the quality of the ICC technique. Unfortunately, some authors have chosen to ignore the importance of ultramorphological preservation and numerous journal pages are littered with electron micrographs of severely injured or violently assassinated cells of indeterminable type. Thus, the status of gut peptide localization is actually much more chaotic than would appear from a casual glance at the present review literature. In fact, very few peptides can be said to be unequivocally localized to a particular cell type.

In this chapter some of the minimum standards for ICC studies are discussed. For technical details as well as for further discussion of standards the reader is referred to several recent books and articles dealing primarily with ICC techniques (2,8,13,27,28,29,33–35,37). It is important to realize that even if all of these criteria are met, ICC in itself can no more than any other immunological technique provide an absolute identification of a particular peptide. Therefore, it is desirable to combine ICC techniques with other available biochemical methods to approach as true localizations as possible.

For convenience the discussion to follow has been divided into three parts:

(a) preservation of antigenicity and structure;
(b) quality of the ICC procedure; expressed in terms of specificity, reproducibility, and sensitivity; and
(c) applications of ICC techniques.

PRESERVATION OF ANTIGENICITY AND STRUCTURE

Since the aim of ICC is to provide an exact localization of antigens, this parameter is no less and no more important than the quality criteria. Several different factors have to be considered:

(a) immobilization of antigens with minimal diffusion and loss of reactive molecules;

(b) minimal denaturation of antigens and optimal penetrability of antibodies; and

(c) preservation of structural integrity, permitting clear identification of reactive tissue and cell components at the light and electron microscopic levels.

Antigens differ with respect to chemical and physical properties, making it naive to suggest single standard procedures that fulfill all of the above criteria. Unfortunately, immobilization of antigens as well as acceptable preservation of morphology often requires fixation conditions that lead to severe denaturation of several antigens. An additional problem, which is encountered particularly often in work with isolated cells, is that many fixation procedures make membranes and cytosol compartments poorly penetrable with antibodies, necessitating the use of agents that disrupt membranes through chemical or physical forces (24).

ICC studies of peptides are often carried out on material fixed in aldehydes. Since aldehyde-based fixatives react with primary amino groups, significant denaturation of peptide antigens is bound to occur. Several alternative fixation procedures have, therefore, been suggested. Such procedures include the use of carbodiimides (CDI) (7,30), diethylpyrocarbonate (DEPC) (25), and parabenzoquinone (PBQ) (25). DEPC, used in vapor form, has been valuable for localizing many antigens that are severely denatured after standard aldehyde-fixation procedures. Problems with DEPC are that the fixation is not very efficient for preserving structure and cannot be employed for ultrastructural studies. In addition, some batches of DEPC produce unsatisfactory immobilization of antigens, resulting in significant diffusion. The mechanisms by which PBQ fixates tissues are only incompletely known and prolonged fixation results in the formation of undefined pigments (20). As is evident from published photomicrographs, ultrastructural preservation with both CDI and PBQ is entirely insufficient for cell identification studies.

Studies on the chemistry and efficiency of aldehyde fixation have, so far, offered more worthwhile results than the introduction of new fixatives. The reaction between, e.g., formaldehyde and primary amino groups is known to be incomplete (1,5). Studies employing the fluorescent amino group probe, fluorescamine, show that the efficiency with which formaldehyde reacts with primary amino groups is dependent on pH, temperature, time, and concentration. With the use of the fluorescamine technique, we have been able to show that fixation of freeze-dried tissues with formaldehyde vapors results in a less complete reaction with primary amino groups than standard liquid phase fixation (5,19). In ultrastructural ICC, where morphological integrity is, or should be, a prime criterion, the use of low concentrations of glutaraldehyde has been proposed (9,33). Alternatively, short-time fixation with more concentrated glutaraldehyde or formaldehyde mixtures may be tested at low temperatures (4°C) (9). Use of short aldehyde fixation times in combination with cryostat sectioning, as introduced by Hökfelt et al. (6), has proven very valuable for light and fluorescence microscopic localization of a large body of neuronal and hormonal peptides. This technique is currently used together with freeze-drying procedures in our laboratory and has, so far, been successful with most peptidic antigens tested.

Formaldehyde fixation alone gives a less satisfactory ultrastructural preservation than glutaraldehyde and, sometimes, short-time glutaraldehyde fixation results in destruction of antigenicity. In these cases, fixation combinations have been tested. A combination of formaldehyde, periodic acid, and lysine (PLP) is thought to immobilize glycoproteins and has been successfully exploited for the localization of several pituitary and brain antigens (38). In addition, PLP produces a much more satisfactory ultrastructural preservation than formaldehyde alone. Recently, in studies on the ultrastructural localization of the vasoactive intestinal polypeptide (VIP), we found that simple aldehyde fixation destroys immunoreactivity toward our VIP antibodies (but not necessarily reactivity toward VIP antibodies specific for other regions of the peptide!). A combination fixative consisting of parabenzoquinone, formaldehyde, and glutaraldehyde was found to preserve both antigenicity and ultrastructural integrity (12). This observation may indicate that PBQ in some undefined way protects VIP against the denaturing actions of aldehyde fixatives.

The consensus of the above discussion is that, due to their preservation of structure and antigenicity, aldehyde fixatives are to be preferred whenever possible. Other fixatives may preserve antigenicity but result in unacceptable morphology and incomplete immobilization of antigens. In doubtful cases combinations of fixatives may be valuable. It is important to note that since antisera may bind to different regions of a peptide, it is impossible to design fixatives that work well with all antibodies against a particular peptide. Thus, claims for "generally applicable" or "peptide-specific" fixation procedures are, almost by definition, false.

QUALITY OF THE IMMUNOCYTOCHEMICAL PROCEDURE

Specificity

Immunocytochemistry versus radioimmunochemistry

It is frequently assumed that, with a given antiserum, the specificity of ICC is similar to that of radioimmunoassay (RIA). Thus, in numerous publications

RIA data are cited as proofs for immunocytochemical specificity. As is evident from both theoretical considerations and from empirical data, these assumptions are entirely unjustified. Thus, in RIAs, a radiolabeled ligand is employed. This ligand competes with components in the sample for binding to antibodies. Antibodies unable to bind the ligand are, hence, never detected in RIA systems. Furthermore, the radiolabeled ligand may, at the dilutions and conditions of a RIA system, bind only to a selected population of specific antibodies. The ICC system usually employs lower dilutions of antibodies than the RIA system. In ICC systems the antibodies are added in surplus and do not compete with another ligand for binding to tissue-bound antigen. Furthermore, all antibodies that bind to the tissue sections are demonstrated by immunofluorescence or immunoperoxidase techniques. These differences emphasize the impossibility of direct comparisons between RIA and ICC systems and demonstrate the need for assessing antibody specificity directly at the ICC level.

These theoretical considerations may be practically illustrated by the behavior of one of our antibodies (Ab 2604) in RIA and ICC systems. This rabbit antibody was raised against synthetic human gastrin–17 (SHG I), which contains the same COOH-terminal pentapeptide sequence as cholecystokinin (CCK). In RIA systems, with the use of ^{125}I-SHG I, Ab 2604 showed negligable reactivity with the CCKs (CCK-8: < 0.001 at ID_{50}). When used in an ICC system, however, the antibody was found to react as readily with CCK cells as with gastrin cells. Staining of both cell types was abolished by addition of CCK-33, CCK-8, or SHG I to the antiserum. Presumably, a population of antibodies directed against the COOH-terminal penta- or tetrapeptide sequence was revealed with the noncompetitive ICC technique. Obviously, if the RIA specificity data had been combined only with absorption studies with SHG I, numerous CCK cells would have been read as gastrin cells.

Recently, we introduced the radioimmunocytochemical (RICH) technique in order to increase the ICC specificity and to make ICC and RIA data more easily comparable (18). In contrast with other generally applicable ICC techniques, the RICH techniques rely on the direct detection of antigen-antibody reactions via the use of a radiolabeled antigen (Figs. 1 and 2). Hence, antisera are first allowed to react with radiolabeled antigen. If this reaction is carried out in antibody surplus, then a preponderance of RICH complexes is formed (18). The RICH complex is a bivalent antibody, which binds radiolabeled antigen with only one of its two combining sites and has the remaining site free for reaction with tissue-bound antigen. Thus, when RICH complexes are applied to tissue sections, the antibody will form a "bridge" between tissue-bound antigen and the radiolabeled antigen. Subsequently, the site of antigen-antibody reaction is detected by autoradiography. Antibodies able to bind radiolabeled antigen are, hence, the only antibodies detected and, empirically, the RICH technique has been shown to possess a sensitivity equal or superior to that of other ICC techniques (18). Controls are employed as in other ICC techniques and serve to confirm the specificity of the antigen-antibody reaction, as well as to exclude that radiolabeled antigen itself binds to tissue components. In recent studies

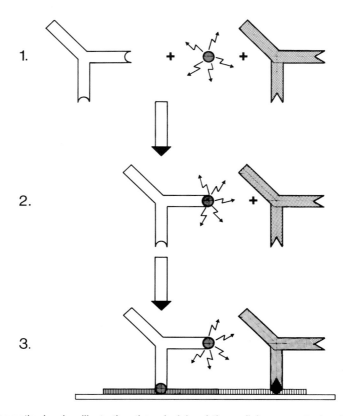

FIG. 1. Schematic drawing illustrating the principle of the radioimmunocytochemical (RICH) technique. (1) An excess of antibodies is allowed to react with radiolabeled antigen, resulting in the formation of RICH complexes (2), consisting of antibodies that bind radiolabeled antigen with one of their antigen-combining sites and have the remaining site free. (3) The remaining site may hence react with tissue bound antigen and the site of reaction is visualized by autoradiography. Note that antibodies *(dotted)* that are unable to bind specific radiolabeled antigen, but may be able to bind to other tissue constituents, are not detected in the RICH technique. Such antibodies are, however, visualized in all other immunocytochemical techniques with the associated risk of unspecific reactions.

employing the above-mentioned Ab 2604 in a RICH-complex with ^{125}I-labeled SHG I, we found that this antibody reacts only with gastrin cells and not with CCK cells (Fig. 2). It is, hence, possible that the use of a specific radiolabeled antigen selects an antibody population specific for that antigen and that RICH and RIA data may be somewhat comparable in terms of specificity.

Controls

A number of different controls have been devised for ICC techniques. The relative importance of these controls may vary with the aim of the investigation.

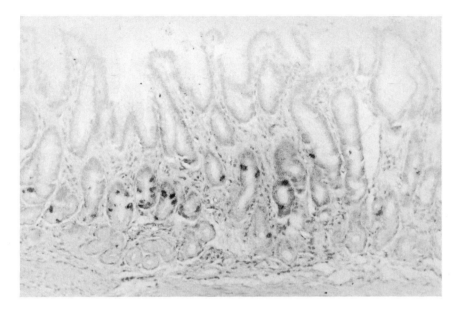

FIG. 2. Gastrin cells of monkey antropyloric mucosa demonstrated with the RICH technique (RICH-complex made of Ab 2604 and ^{125}I-labeled synthetic human gastrin I, courtesy of Prof. J. F. Rehfeld); autoradiography using Kodak NTB-2 emulsion (exposure time, 3 days). For details see ref. 18.

Thus, workers trying to demonstrate autoantibodies or antibodies against ill-defined or uncharacterized antigens tend to put more weight on so-called staining controls and conjugate quality than on specificity controls. This is, however, not acceptable in the field of gastrointestinal peptides since the access to highly purified or synthetic peptides and peptide fragments make specificity controls easily feasible.

Staining Controls

Staining controls form a type of quality control of ICC and serve to exclude autofluorescence, endogenous enzyme activity, and nonspecific binding of the second antibodies. Staining controls are not able to tell whether or not binding of the primary ("peptide") antibody is specific. In indirect immunofluorescence or immunoperoxidase techniques, several staining controls are used.

  (a) deletion of the primary antibody;
  (b) deletion of the secondary antibody;
  (c) deletion of the tertiary antibody;
       (applicable only in the immunoglobulin bridge techniques);
  (d) deletion of all antibodies;

(e) blocking tests; and

(f) substitution of the primary antibody with preimmune or nonimmune serum.

Controls (a) through (d) should result in disappearance of staining. If this very basic criterion is not fulfilled, then ICC staining is impossible. Failure of controls (a) through (d) may be ascribed to, e.g., the use of badly labeled antibodies ("bad conjugates"), defective tissue treatment, or insufficient antibody solutions.

Blocking tests (e) are usually employed only in direct ICC procedures. They serve to demonstrate that the staining observed is due to native antibodies and not to artifactual products obtained through conjugation of antibodies. They are of little significance for peptide localization studies.

In some studies workers are content with controls (a) through (e), but usually a sixth control (f) is added. This control is not a staining control *per se,* but it is not a real specificity control either. Above all, nonimmune or preimmune sera differ from hyperimmune sera in their concentration of IgG molecules. If used, control (f) should preferably be substituted with an immune serum toward an antigen different from the one investigated. Even so, control (f) is of little help and most often only serves to make the list of "controls" more impressive.

Specificity Controls

Specificity controls are the most critical controls in gut peptide ICC. The controls serve to demonstrate the specificity of interaction between the primary antibody and the tissue-bound antigen. They are performed by permitting antisera to react with varying concentrations of pure or synthetic peptides (absorption controls). The absorption of an antiserum against pure antigen, but not against related or unrelated peptides, should result in inactivation of staining. It follows that a successful absorption control also represents the best staining control available. If an absorption control does not abolish staining (provided that suitable quantities of antigen are added), then at least three alternatives exist:

(a) defective staining technique;

(b) presence of antibody populations in the antiserum directed against other antigens; and

(c) binding of the absorbed peptide to tissue components.

Alternative (a) is easily checked by staining controls (a) through (d) or (a) through (f). Alternative (b) may be checked by absorptions against putative contaminants of the antigen. Alternative (c) has been encountered, e.g., in pituitary LH cells, which react with luteinizing hormone-releasing hormone (LH-RH) antisera and where absorption of the antisera with LH-RH actually increases staining intensity (34,35). The phenomenon has been ascribed to the existence of internalized LH-RH receptors in LH cells and may be checked by use of LH-RH-coupled immunosorbents. Judicious use of such immunosorbents results in the removal of LH-RH antibodies from the antisera and in the inactivation of LH cell staining (34,35).

Thus, immunosorbents, consisting of antigens covalently coupled to, e.g., Sepharose 4B, may serve useful purposes in ICC staining and may also be used as models for detecting antibodies and for quantification (3,8,29,36). The rather infrequent use of immunosorbents may be explained by the fact that peptide absorption to tissue constituents, under conditions usually employed, seems to be a comparatively rare phenomenon. Furthermore, rather large quantities of peptides are required for the preparation of immunosorbents. Use of immunosorbents may possibly also cause failure to detect nonspecific reactions due to F_c-binding, since they remove much antibody proteins from the staining medium. Conventional "liquid-state" absorptions are not subject to this risk since the antibody solutions still contain the IgG molecules, binding specific antigens with their F_{ab} segments. Other controls, serving to exclude F_c binding, include enzymatic cleavage of antibodies, releasing the F_c fragments as well as use of control immune sera (type f) containing high IgG concentrations.

If an absorption control results in inactivation of staining, then it is reasonable to assume that the antiserum is able to react with the peptide in question. The control does not, however, in any way exclude the possibility that the antiserum does not also react with other peptides (cf. the example above using gastrin and CCK). Gut peptides are more or less homologous in their amino acid sequences. Hence, gastrin and CCK possess identical COOH-terminal penta-peptide sequences and more or less pronounced structural similarities occur between glucagon, secretin, VIP, gastric inhibitory polypeptide (GIP), glicentin, bombesin, and pancreatic polypeptide (PP). It is therefore imperative that anti-sera against any of these peptides should be checked for cross-reactivity against the others. The occurrence of structural similarities in only one part of the molecule, as in the gastrin-CCK family, makes antibody characterizations (by selective absorptions) easy, whereas the peptides of the "secretin family" show scattered structural similarities along the entire length of their sequences. The mistakes made in the immunolocalization of secretin-like peptides are also numerous. It is impossible to decide whether these mistakes have all been caused by failures to recognize cross-reactivity of antisera against different members of the "secretin family." They serve, however, to emphasize that main difficulties concerning the immunolocalization of these peptides remain and that, as a minimum, careful absorptions against different members of the secretin family should be tried with all antisera.

Region-Specific Antisera

Antisera are usually directed against only a small sequence of amino acids (usually 3–8) of a particular peptide or protein. It is hence improper, but convenient, to refer to antibodies as gastrin antibodies, VIP antibodies, and so forth, as their specificity toward any one peptide relies on the relative uniqueness of the particular (small) peptide sequence they are directed against. Antisera directed against the COOH-terminal tetrapeptide of gastrin react also with CCK and it may be a matter of dispute whether such antisera should be referred to as gastrin or as CCK antisera. By convention, antisera are named after the peptide against which they were raised. This conventional naming of antisera must, however, not be taken to indicate specificity. In order to characterize gastrin- and CCK-immunoreactive structures in gut and brain, we have recently developed a set of antibodies that are specific for different regions (or sequences) of gastrin and CCK (16,17). Use of such antisera is very helpful for directly characterizing peptides, stored in different cell types, and the results obtained are in good agreement with radioimmunochemical and gel chromatographical data.

Judicious use of region-specific antibodies (RSA) offers possibilities for direct immunochemical demonstration of specific amino acid sequences. Combination of data obtained by different RSA allows conclusions about the specificity of the immunolocalization. We believe that the use of these techniques, eventually in conjunction with radioimmunocytochemical detection systems, may wipe out many white spots on the map of gut peptides.

Reproducibility

Although, for obvious reasons, specificity is, and must be, the prime criterion in all ICC techniques, a criterion of reproducibility may be added. Reproducibility in the ICC sense means that results obtained with a given antibody should be reproducible with other antibodies against the same antigen. Nonreproducibility may, for instance, be due to cross-reactivity phenomena, which subsequently have to be checked with absorptions against different peptides or peptide fragments. Quite often, partial nonreproducibility is encountered. Thus, antibodies directed against the COOH-terminal part of gastrin react with numerous antropyloric and duodenal cells. Antibodies directed against the midportion or NH_2-terminal region of gastrin also detect the antropyloric cells but react with only very few duodenal cells. Absorption studies and staining with CCK antisera reveal that the duodenal cells, which react with COOH-terminus-specific gastrin antisera are, in fact, CCK cells. These and similar examples show that antibody characterizations advantageously may be performed as an interaction between tissue staining experiments employing different antisera and by selective absorptions against different peptides and peptide fragments. It is important to realize that RIA data may, at best, give only a very rough estimate of ICC antibody specificity.

Sensitivity

Preferably, antibodies with as high association constants as possible should be used. With such antibodies higher dilutions may be employed and, consequently, nonspecific background staining is suppressed. Use of high avidity antibodies may, however, result in difficulties in ICC double-staining techniques, which require removal of the antibodies prior to a second staining step. In some published techniques, removal of antibodies is incomplete and subsequent reactions may be due to immunoglobulin bridge types of reactions, which do not involve a specific interaction between antibodies and tissue-bound peptides. Fortunately, a recently published technique shows great promise for removal of antibodies of even very high avidity (39).

Sensitivity is a disputed parameter in ICC. Some refer to sensitivity as a function of the dilution of the primary antibody. Thus, sensitivity is expressed in terms of the sensitivity of the detection system. Others feel that sensitivity should be a measure of the minimum amount of detectable antigen (27). In terms of sensitivity of the detection system, the most sensitive techniques are the RICH and immunoglobulin-bridge techniques (18,33). Also, radiolabeled antibodies may be expected to show a quite high degree of sensitivity. Empirically, use of highly sensitive detection systems allows higher dilutions of primary antibodies and largely eliminates unspecific binding. It is uncertain whether high sensitivity of the detection system also means high sensitivity for the demonstration of a particular peptide. Although this is likely to be the case, final proof from quantitation studies is not yet available.

The sensitivity of the detection system is, of course, also dependent on the conditions of microscopy. Fluorochromes, such as fluorescein isothiocyanate (FITC) and tetramethylrhodamine isothiocyanate (TRITC), show a pH-dependent fluorescence yield and well-defined spectral properties which, of course, have to be met for optimal sensitivity (29,33). All too many workers still use suboptimal combinations of filters and lamps and consequently work with lower levels of sensitivity. This line of reasoning may also apply to peroxidase-labeled systems. It has recently been demonstrated that pH optima for the demonstration of horseradish peroxidase are not met in the standard Graham and Karnovsky technique and that choice of buffers and filter systems may also affect the sensitivity of peroxidase detection (21). It has yet to be explored whether modifications introduced in the area of horseradish peroxidase tracing techniques (21) may be applicable to ICC techniques.

APPLICATIONS OF IMMUNOCYTOCHEMICAL TECHNIQUES

The primary importance of ICC rests with its ability to localize biologically important molecules to cellular and subcellular compartments. Thus, starting with McGuigan's original observation on immunolocalization of gastrin to scattered endocrine cells of the antropyloric mucosa (22), numerous endocrine cells producing secretin, GIP, gut-type glucagon, CCK, neurotensin, and so forth, have been demonstrated to be widely distributed in the gastrointestinal tract (Fig. 3). The occurrence of contacts between the lumen and apical portion of these cells suggests that changes in the luminal fluid affect release of hormones.

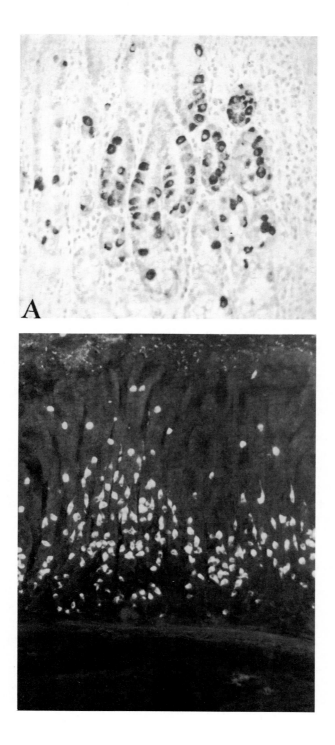

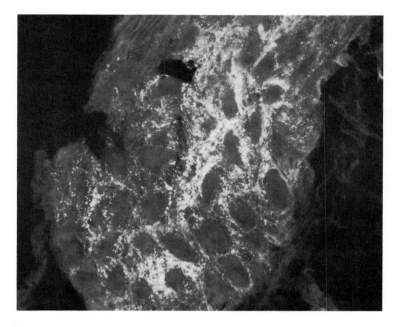

FIG. 4. CCK nerves of guinea pig celiac-superior mesenteric ganglion. Numerous nerve terminals surround nonimmunoreactive ganglionic cell bodies in an innervation-like pattern. The nerves were visualized with Ab 4562, which recognizes the COOH-terminal tetrapeptide of both gastrin and CCK, since radioimmunoassay and chromatographical studies indicate the presence of large amounts of a free tetrapeptide-like component. Radioimmunoassays and immunocytochemistry employing CCK-specific antibodies confirm that these nerves contain true CCK.

The differential distribution of the cells provides us with valuable hints concerning which of the luminal components may affect hormone secretion. The other important contribution of ICC is the identification of a widespread system of neurons that contain peptides such as substance P, somatostatin, VIP, CCK, gastrin, and enkephalin (Fig. 4). Studies at the electron microscopic level have shown that substance P (4) as well as VIP (12) is localized to granulated vesicles in the neuron terminal and, hence, may be released on nerve stimulation. Furthermore, studies on the distribution and topography of peptidergic nerves may indicate their physiological function. Thus, certain nerve terminals (e.g., those of substance P and enkephalin neurons) are primarily associated with neuronal cell bodies and smooth musculature (31), whereas, e.g., VIP nerve terminals in addition show a most intimate relationship with blood vessels (14).

FIG. 3. Gastrin cells of human **(a)** and guinea pig **(b)** antropyloric mucosa visualized with the peroxidase-antiperoxidase (PAP) technique **(a)** or with immunofluorescence **(b)**. For details see ref. 16.

Recent ICC studies have also identified a new type of peptide-synthesizing cell: the paracrine cell, which may be intermediate between an endocrine cell and a neuron. Thus, somatostatin cells of the gastric mucosa of both man and rat were shown to possess long cytoplasmic processes that contacted gastrin cells and parietal cells (15) (Fig. 5). Similar processes have been detected in other endocrine cells of the gut (15) but the demonstration of somatostatin cell processes induced a chain of thought that such cell processes may be the morphological substrate for a local regulatory (paracrine) mechanism.

A new and most exciting possibility, suggested by ICC studies, is that both endocrine cells and nerves may elaborate more than one type of biological messenger. Thus, ICC evidence for the simultaneous occurrence of more than one hormone has been obtained in, e.g., pituitary gonadotrophs and corticotrophs (23), thyroid calcitonin cells (40), antropyloric gastrin cells (11,31), and PP cells (11) (Fig. 6). So far, however, these data must be treated with caution. First, the contributions of cross-reacting unidentified peptides (e.g., prohormones) cannot yet be excluded and secondly, problems with the ICC specificity have already caused the deletion of two cell types from the list of potentially multihormonal cells. Thus, VIP was reported to be stored together with bombesin in a particular intestinal endocrine cell type (26), but subsequent studies indicate that this cell contains neither true VIP nor bombesin! Reports concerning the occurrence of GIP in glucagon cells (32) must likewise be regarded with doubt,

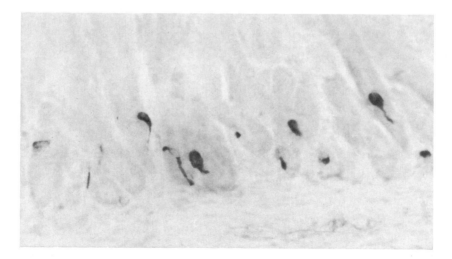

FIG. 5. Somatostatin-containing cells of rat antropyloric mucosa. Note the presence of long cytoplasmic extensions from the cell bodies. Some of these processes have been found to terminate on cells, whose functions are profoundly affected by somatostatin. It is believed that somatostatin may be released locally (paracrine secretion) from these processes to affect the functions of, e.g., gastrin cells, which are located in the neighborhood of, but not adjacent to, somatostatin cells. These paracrine cells may thus represent intermediates between neurons and endocrine cells. For details see ref. 15.

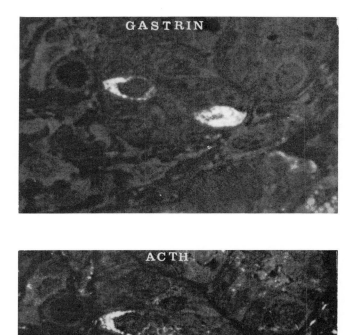

FIG. 6. Adjacent 0.3-μm thick plastic sections, showing the localization of gastrin and ACTH-like immunoreactivity to the same endocrine cell type of the rat antropyloric mucosa. Although data indicating a differential processing of the two types of immunoreactivity are now available, much evidence needs still to be collected before it can be firmly stated that the gastrin cell is a multihormonal cell. For details see ref. 11.

since recent studies show that GIP shares an antigenic site with the postulated glucagon precursor, glicentin (Larsson and Moody, *to be published*). Future developments involving, above all, the use of region-specific antisera may, however, be expected to resolve many of these contradictory data.

On the background of this explosive development, it may not be too surprising that the problems and pitfalls have been numerous. It seems obvious now, however, that a critical methodological approach must be undertaken and that many of the data obtained must be consolidated or revised by the use of refined cytochemical and biochemical tools.

SUMMARY

This chapter deals with the efforts spent in making ICC an exact tool for the identification of peptide messengers in endocrine, paracrine, and neuronal cell populations. Particular emphasis is placed on the treatment of peptide antigens as chemicophysically distinct entities and on the use of antibodies as region-specific detection reagents. Use of ultrasensitive and specific techniques in the elucidation of the cellular and subcellular localization of peptides is reviewed and suggestions for future explorations are given.

CONCLUSIONS

Dealing with immunological techniques is dealing with biological material, subject to all types of natural variations. The goal must be to control and minimize the influences of such variations. ICC has for a long time dwelt in a dark, no man's land between imprecise staining histology and exact biochemistry. Wizards and sorceresses of this dark land have produced brilliant fluorescent images that sometimes reflected the truth and sometimes were false. It is the hope of the author that the present review may remove some of the magic surrounding ICC.

PROJECTIONS FOR THE FUTURE

Recognition of antibodies as region-specific, or sometimes even sequence-specific detection reagents, realization of the diversity of antibody populations present in immune sera, and understanding of peptide antigens as chemical individuals, differing in chemicophysical properties, should assist the investigator in his efforts toward a precise localization of these biologically important molecules. Our technical arsenal for this venture is excellent, featuring immunocytochemical techniques such as the PAP and RICH methods of unsurpassed sensitivity and specificity, availability of synthetic peptides and peptide fragments, and a large variety of fixation techniques, which can be tailor-made to suit the preservation of various peptides.

An important challenge to ICC is now to optimize these techniques, making them exact and scientifically impeccable. Most important will be the development of regionspecific antibodies to more gut and pancreatic peptides, enabling us to arrive at an exact identification of their cellular and subcellular stores. Labeled antigen techniques, such as, e.g., the RICH technique, may be very valuable in this respect since labeled peptide fragments may be used to select antibodies of desired specificity out of the usually mixed antibody soup called immune serum.

A biologically important problem that needs solving is the identification of the peptide-producing cell systems of the gut and pancreas, including endocrine and paracrine cells and neurons. Only when we know the extent, distribution, and, most importantly, the cellular destinations of paracrine and neuronal cell processes in the gut are we in a position to interpret the physiological roles of the many new peptides found in this organ. Recently, ICC has also challenged the old one hormone-one cell concept. These findings, perhaps more than any others, have caused us to look critically at our techniques. Thus, with the exception of the pituitary and cerebral ACTH/MSH/β-LPH/β-endorphin system, unequivocal evidence for the existence of multihormonal cells has yet to be obtained. Such evidence must necessarily be obtained at both the cellular and subcellular levels, employing region-specific ICC, as well as at the molecular biology level, including identification of responsible mRNA species.

REFERENCES

1. Baker, J. R. (1970): *Principles of Biological Microtechniques. A study of Fixation and Dyeing.* Methuen, London.
2. Bussolati, G., and Canese, M. G. (1972): Electron microscopical identification of the immuno-fluorescent gastrin cells in the cat pyloric mucosa. *Histochemie,* 29:198–206.
3. Capel, P. J. A. (1975): The defined antigen substrate spheres (DASS) system and some of its applications. *Ann. N. Y. Acad. Sci.,* 254:108–118.
4. Chan-Palay, V., and Palay, S. I. (1977): Ultrastructural identification of substance P cells and their processes in rat sensory ganglia and their terminals in the spinal cord by immunocytochemistry. *Proc. Natl. Acad. Sci. USA,* 74:4050–5054.
5. Håkanson, R., Larsson, L.-I. and Sundler, F. (1974): Fluorescamine: A novel reagent for the histochemical detection of amino groups. *Histochemistry,* 39:15–23.
6. Hökfelt, T., Fuxe, K., Goldstein, M., and Joh, T. H. (1973): Immunohistochemical localization of three catecholamine synthesizing enzymes: Aspects on methodology. *Histochemie,* 33:231–254.
7. Kendall, P. A., Polak, J. M., and Pearse, A. G. E. (1971): Carbodiimide fixation for immunohisto-chemistry: Observations on the fixation of polypeptide hormones. *Experientia,* 27:1104–1106.
8. Knapp, W., and Ploem, J. S. (1974): Microfluorometry of antigen-antibody interactions in immunofluorescence using the defined antigen substrate spheres (DASS) system. Sensitivity, specificity, and variables of the method. *J. Immunol. Methods,* 5:259–273.
9. Lange, R. H. (1971): A light and electron microscopic study, including immunohistochemistry of non-β-cells in the islets of Langerhans (frog, rat), with special reference to the number of cell types. *Mem. Soc. Endocrinol.,* 19:457–467.
10. Lange, R. H. (1973): Histochemistry of the islets of Langerhans. In: *Handbuch der Histochemie,* Vol. VIII, Suppl., edited by W. Graumann and K. Neumann, Gustav Fischer Verlag, Stuttgart.
11. Larsson, L.-I. (1977): Corticotropin-like peptides in central nerves and in endocrine cells of gut and pancreas. *Lancet,* ii:1321–1323.
12. Larsson, L.-I. (1977): Ultrastructural localization of a new neuronal peptide (VIP). *Histochemistry,* 54:173–176.
13. Larsson, L.-I. (1979): Peptide immunocytochemistry. *Prog. Histochem. Cytochem., (in press).*
14. Larsson, L.-I. Fahrenkrug, J. Schaffalitzky de Muckadell, O., Sundler, F., Håkanson, R., and Rehfeld, J. F. (1976). Localization of vasoactive intestinal polypeptide (VIP) to central and peripheral neurons. *Proc. Natl. Acad. Sci. USA,* 73:3197–3200.
15. Larsson, L.-I., Goltermann, N., de Magistris, L., Rehfeld, J. F., and Schwartz, T. W. (1979): Gastric somatostatin cells: Morphological substrate for local (paracrine) functions. *Science,* 205:1393–1394.
16. Larsson, L.-I., and Rehfeld, J. F. (1977): Characterization of antral gastrin cells with region-specific antisera. *J. Histochem. Cytochem.,* 25:1317–1321.
17. Larsson, L.-I., and Rehfeld, J. F. (1977): Evidence for a common evolutionary origin of gastrin and cholecystokinin. *Nature,* 269:335–338.
18. Larsson, L.-I., and Schwartz, T. W. (1977): Radioimmunocytochemistry—A novel immunocyto-chemical principle. *J. Histochem. Cytochem.,* 25:1140–1148.

19. Larsson, L.-I., Sundler, F., and Håkanson, R. (1975): Fluroescamine as a histochemical reagent: Demonstration of polypeptide hormone-secreting cells. *Histochemistry,* 44:245–251.
20. Lorentz, K. (1976): On the nature of protein benzoquinone complexes. *Experientia,* 32:1502–1503.
21. Malmgren, L., and Olsson, Y. (1978): A sensitive method for histochemical demonstration of horseradish peroxidase in neurons following retrograde axonal transport. *Brain Res.,* 148:279–294.
22. McGuigan, J. E. (1968): Gastric mucosal intracellular localization of gastrin by immunofluorescence. *Gastroenterology,* 55:315–327.
23. Moriarty, G. C., and Garner, L. L. (1977): Immunocytochemical studies of cells in the rat adenohypophysis containing both ACTH and FSH. *Nature,* 265:356–358.
24. Ohtsuki, I., Manzi, R. M., Palade, G. E., and Jamieson, J. D. (1978): Entry of macromolecular tracers into cells fixed with low concentrations of aldehydes. *Biol. Cellulaire,* 31:119–126.
25. Pearse, A. G. E., and Polak, J. M. (1975): Bifunctional reagents as vapour- and liquid-phase fixatives for immunohistochemistry. *Histochem. J.,* 7:179–186.
26. Pearse, A. G. E., Polak, J. M., and Bloom, S. R. (1977): The newer gut hormones. *Gastroenterology,* 72:746–761.
27. Petrusz, P., DiMeo, P., Ordronneau, P., Weaver, C., and Keefer, D. A. (1975): Improved immunoglobulin-enzyme bridge method for light microscopic demonstration of hormone-containing cells of the rat adenohypophysis. *Histochemistry,* 46:9–26.
28. Petrusz, P., Sar, M., Ordronneau, P., and DiMeo, P. (1976): Specificity in immunocytochemical staining. *J. Histochem. Cytochem.,* 24:1110–1112.
29. Ploem, J. S. (1975): General introduction. *Ann. N.Y. Acad. Sci.,* 254:4–20.
30. Polak, J. M., Kendall, P. A., Heath, C. M., and Pearse, A. G. E. (1972): Carbodiimide fixation for electron microscopy and immunoelectron cytochemistry. *Experientia,* 28:368–370.
31. Polak, J. M., Sullivan, S. N., Bloom, S. R., Facer, P., and Pearse, A. G. E. (1977): Enkephalin-like immunoreactivity in the human gastrointestinal tract. *Lancet,* i:972–974.
32. Smith, P. H., Merchant, F. W., Johnson, D. G., Fujimoto, W. Y., and Williams, R. H. (1977): Immunocytochemical localization of a gastric inhibitory polypeptide-like material within A-cells of the endocrine pancreas. *Am. J. Anat.,* 149:585–590.
33. Sternberger, L. A. (1974): *Immunocytochemistry.* Prentice-Hall, Englewood Cliffs, N.J.
34. Sternberger, L. A. (1977): Immunocytochemistry of neuropeptides and their receptors. In: *Peptides in Neurobiology* edited by H. Gainer, pp. 61–97. Plenum Press, New York and London.
35. Sternberger, L. A., and Hoffman, G. E. (1978): Immunocytology of luteinizing hormone-releasing hormone. *Neuroendocrinology,* 25:111–128.
36. Streefkerk, J. G., van der Ploeg, M., and van Duijn, P. (1975): Agarose beads as matrices for proteins in cytophotometric investigations of immunohistoperoxidase procedures. *J. Histochem. Cytochem.,* 23:243–250.
37. Swaab, D. F., Pool, C. W., and Van Leeuwen, F. W. (1977). Can specificity ever be proved in immunocytochemical staining? *J. Histochem. Cytochem.,* 25:388–391.
38. Tabuchi, K., Kirsch, W. M., and Nakane, P. K. (1976): The fine structural localization of S-100 protein in rodent cerebellum. *J. Neurol. Sci.,* 28:65–76.
39. Tramu, G., Pillez, A., and Leonardelli, J. (1978): An efficient method of antibody elution for the successive or simultaneous localization of two antigens by immunocytochemistry. *J. Histochem. Cytochem.,* 26:322–324.
40. Van Noorden, S., Polak, J. M., and Pearse, A. G. E. (1977): Single cellular origin of somatostatin and calcitonin in the rat thyroid gland. *Histochemistry,* 53:243–247.

Gastrointestinal Hormones, edited by
George B. Jerzy Glass.
Raven Press, New York © 1980.

Chapter 4

Cellular Synthesis and Release of Gastro-Entero-Pancreatic Hormones

Norman S. Track, *Cora Creutzfeldt, and *Werner Creutzfeldt

*Departments of Surgery and Clinical Biochemistry, University of Toronto, and Mount Sinai Hospital, Toronto, Ontario, Canada; and *Division of Endocrinology and Metabolism, Department of Medicine, University of Goettingen, Goettingen, German Federal Republic*

INTRODUCTION

The gastro-entero-pancreatic (GEP) endocrine system represents an interesting group of cells for the study of hormone synthesis and release. Each of these endocrine cells is identified by its unique ultrastructural appearance, immunohistochemical staining characteristics, and hormone content. The cells are distributed sparsely in the GEP regions of the gastrointestinal (GI) tract. Hormone synthesis, storage, and release is the major function of these cells. An understanding of these cellular functions can be achieved by the study of these cells' responses to different types of nutrition.

Current knowledge about the synthesis and release of hormones from GEP endocrine cells is outlined and control mechanisms for some of the GEP endocrine cells is discussed.

HORMONE SYNTHESIS

Insulin-Producing Cells

Insulin-producing cells are the best studied of the GEP endocrine system. Incubation of human insulinoma tissue led to the discovery of proinsulin (44); this observation was extended rapidly to pancreatic B cells. The extensive studies of Steiner's group led to a comprehensive scheme of events for the synthesis and storage of insulin (45). The process commences by the translation of specific preproinsulin messenger RNA on membrane-bound ribosomes (28). The first 20 amino acids are a signal region to direct the growing polypeptide chain out of the rough endoplasmic reticulum and into the Golgi zone. Once in the Golgi zone, this portion is lost, leaving the proinsulin to be packaged into secretory granules. Conversion of proinsulin into insulin and C peptide occurs in secretory granules.

Secretory granules play an important role in the management of proinsulin/insulin within insulin-producing cells. Pancreatic B cells with mainly mature, electron-dense secretory granules contain less than 5% proinsulin. Fewer secretory granules and a lower insulin content are observed after glucose stimulation. Treatment with tolbutamide leads to a significant degranulation of pancreatic B cells, a lower insulin content, and to the presence of more insulin in the cytoplasm of the B cell (9). These tolbutamide-induced characteristics are similar to those found naturally with human insulinoma tissue. The major functional abnormality of human insulinomas is their defective storage capacity for insulin (11). This abnormality is manifest in lower insulin contents, lower degrees of cellular granulation, and higher proinsulin percentages. The insulinoma studies emphasize the relationship between degree of granulation and both insulin content and proinsulin percentage. Insulinoma cells with the highest insulin contents have the most granules and the lowest proinsulin percentages, whereas those with the lowest insulin contents are virtually agranular and have elevated proinsulin percentages. Another feature of the human insulinoma cell is its ability to synthesize proinsulin/insulin at a faster rate than pancreatic B cells (9). This faster rate is associated with the decreased storage capacity of these cells.

Studies of (pro)insulin synthesis established the concept of hormones being synthesized as precursors and subsequently cleaved into smaller, biologically active forms. Heterogeneous forms of a number of GEP hormones have been identified [e.g., glucagon (32), gastrin (32), cholecystokinin (CCK) (38,41)]; however, biosynthetic relationships are not as clear as for proinsulin/insulin. A prime example of this is gastrin.

Gastrin-Producing Cells

Four major immunoreactive forms of gastrin have been identified: component I, big gastrin (G-34), little gastrin (G-17), and minigastrin (G-14) (cf. ref. 7). G-17 predominates in antral tissue (95% G-17: 5% G-34) whereas G-34 makes a more significant contribution in duodenal tissue (60% G-17: 40% G-34). These different antral and duodenal gastrin component distributions suggest that there are major differences between antral and duodenal gastrin-producing cells. No consistent gastrin component distribution pattern has been found in human gastrinoma tissue (12).

The size distribution of gastrin components suggests that component I and G-34 are precursors of G-17. The diffuse distribution of antral gastrin-producing G cells is the major problem to be overcome to study gastrin synthesis. Culture of antral (13,17,25) and gastrinoma (23,49) tissues has been one approach to solve this problem. Although gastrin synthesis was demonstrated by both increased contents of immunoreactive gastrin (IRG) and incorporation of radioactive tryptophan into gastrin (G-17), these experiments unfortunately provide no information about the precursor relationship of component I and G-34 to G-17.

Another approach to circumvent the diffuse cell problem has been to perform *in vivo* feeding experiments. In this approach it is possible to introduce a physiological stimulus intragastrically and assess its effect on gastrin synthesis (content) at specific times postprandially. Feeding experiments in both humans (30) and animals (40,48) indicate that after an initial depletion of antral gastrin an immedi-

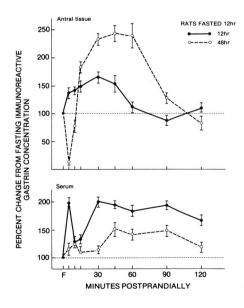

FIG. 1. Antral tissue **(top)** and serum **(bottom)** immunoreactive gastrin postprandial responses. Rats were fasted for 12 (●——————●) or 48 (○— — — —○) hr. Gastrin responses are expressed as percent change from basal concentrations for comparative purposes. Note how the length of fasting affects the gastrin response patterns. For complete details see ref. 48.

ate replenishing of gastrin stores occurs. The effect of fasting (starvation) on postprandial responses is illustrated in Fig. 1. Fasting has a dramatic effect on antral gastrin content (24,26). Extension of the period fasted from 12 to 48 hr causes a significant decrease in gastrin content (ng immunoreactive gastrin (IRG)/mg protein)(12 hr, 71.0 ± 4.6, $n = 14$; 48 hr, 30.2 ± 5.3, $n = 16$)(48). For comparative purposes the postprandial responses are expressed as percent change from basal concentrations. Rats fasted 12 hr have a significantly higher antral gastrin content 5 to 45 min postprandially; from 6 to 120 min it is not different from the basal content. Rats fasted 48 hr have an initial decrease in gastrin content 5 min postprandially; 15 min postprandially the content is almost double the basal. The highest contents are found between 30 and 60 min postprandially. Both experiments demonstrate a postprandial gastrin synthetic response.

HORMONE RELEASE

Release Mechanisms

Classically, endocrine cells were thought to respond to stimulation by releasing their hormones solely into the circulation. Present knowledge reveals that this view is simplistic. GEP endocrine cells are classified as either open or closed endocrine cells (Fig. 2) (16). Open endocrine cells possessing a luminal exposure are affected by circulating, luminal, and intercellular factors; they possess the potential to release their hormones into the circulation (endocrine), into the lumen (exocrine) or intercellularly (paracrine) (Fig. 2, left). For additional information on this subject, see Chapter 38 by L. Hanssen and J. Myren, pp. 855–862, *this volume*. Gastro-entero endocrine cells are open cells. Closed endocrine cells are affected by circulating or intercellular factors; they possess the potential to release their hormones into the circulation (endocrine) or intercellularly (paracrine) (Fig. 2, right). Pancreatic endocrine cells clustered in the islets of Langerhans are closed cells. Hormones operating by paracrine interactions affecting neighboring cells will probably not appear in the circulation. Because of these different release mechanisms available in GEP endocrine cells, reliance on circulating hormone responses is no longer appropriate to assess the status of a CEP hormone. Luminal and paracrine hormone release may be more important mechanisms in certain GEP endocrine cells or in response to specific types of nutrition.

Insulin Release

A wealth of information has been generated about the release of insulin (5, 22,29,34,43). Insulin is released in a biphasic pattern, with neither phase being dependent on insulin synthesis. A number of interrelated factors control insulin release. Cyclic AMP and calcium ions are intimately involved in the release

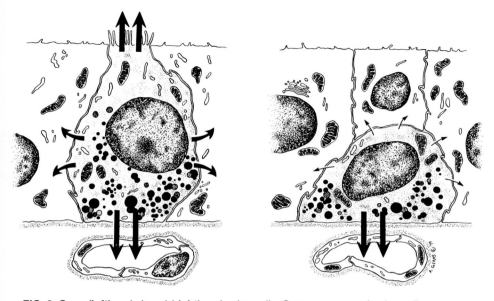

FIG. 2. Open **(left)** and closed **(right)** endocrine cells. Gastro-entero endocrine cells are open cells with luminal exposure, whereas pancreatic endocrine cells are closed cells. Open cells possess the potential to release their hormones into the circulation (endocrine), into the lumen (exocrine), or intercellularly (paracrine). Closed cells do not have the potential for luminal release.

process; glucose metabolites and other hormones [e.g., glucagon, gastric inhibitory polypeptide (GIP)] are major regulatory factors. Correct organization of all these contributing factors results in the orderly process of insulin release.

A close correlation exists between insulin release and the ultrastructural appearance of the B cell secretory granules (39). Insulin is released by emiocytosis. During the release phase there is not a substantial loss of insulin content. Newly synthesized proinsulin/insulin is not released until after 60 min of incubation (cf. ref. 50). The glucose concentration of the incubation medium determines the percentage of newly synthesized proinsulin released—low percentages with normoglycemia and higher percentages with hyperglycemia (50). The enzymatic converting capacity of the B cell secretory granules is not adequate to deal with the extra proinsulin produced under hyperglycemic conditions (27).

The importance of insulin secretory granules in determining the nature of the secreted products is seen clearly in studies of newly synthesized proinsulin/insulin release from human insulinoma tissue (9). Human insulinoma cells synthesize and release proinsulin/insulin within 15 min. Release of newly synthesized products occurs at a faster rate than that observed for pancreatic B cells; also, proinsulin constitutes a much higher proportion of the released products.

Gastrin Release

A number of factors are involved in regulating gastrin release (53). Gastric pH, gastric distention, protein, and the vagus are regulatory factors. Gastrin is released into the circulation in a biphasic pattern (7,48). Nutritional status has a major influence on this release pattern. A clear postprandial biphasic release pattern is observed in rats fasted 12 hr (Fig. 1). The first response peak is absent in rats fasted 48 hr. Postprandial serum responses in both groups are associated with a significant increase in antral gastrin contents.

These increases in gastrin content are excessive to support solely endocrine gastrin release; however, this large increase in gastrin content may be necessary to support luminal gastrin release. Human (14) and animal (51,52) studies provide evidence for luminal gastrin release. Electrical stimulation of the feline vagus causes a minor increase in circulating gastrin, whereas the major gastrin response is detected in the gastric juice. Human studies suggest that luminal gastrin release influences gastric acid secretion. Therefore, under certain physiological conditions the antral G cells may respond to stimulation by releasing gastrin into both the circulation and the lumen. Gastrin synthesis is necessary to satisfy these gastrin release commitments. For additional information on this subject see Chapter 6 by G. Nilsson, pp. 127–167 *(this volume)*.

Studies of immunoreactive gastrin (IRG) components in basal and postprandial conditions reveal some interesting features about gastrin component release. In the basal state, G-34 constitutes approximately 70% of the IRG (7); this is derived from antral and duodenal sources that are 95% and 60% G-17. Even allowing for the longer circulating half-life of G-34, it is not clear why the basal G-34 level is so high. Postprandially, the G-17 contribution increases to approximately 70%. A similar discrepancy between tissue and circulating gastrin component distributions is seen with gastrinoma patients (12). Gastrin component distributions are unique for each gastrinoma. Gastrinoma tissue component distribution patterns are not related to those found in the blood. Despite the large effort invested in the study of gastrin components, the discrepancy between tissue and circulating gastrin component distributions remains to be resolved.

G Cell Cycle

From an ultrastructural study of feline antral G cells in different activity states, a G cell cycle was proposed (15). The initial proposal is based solely on changes in the electron density of the G cell granules. In the fasting state, G cells contain mainly dark, electron-dense granules. Immediately after stimulation, G cells contain electron-lucent granules. G cell granules varying in electron density from electron-dense to electron-lucent are encountered after refeeding. If the granule electron density is associated with antral gastrin content, then antral tissue from fasting animals should have the highest gastrin content, tissue from animals immediately after stimulation the lowest, and animals during re-feeding somewhere in between.

Interpretation of the G cell cycle is somewhat controversial because studies exploring the G cell cycle have not been standardized (1,35–37,42,48). To examine the validity of the G cell cycle it is necessary to challenge animals with a physiological stimulus, measure both circulating and tissue gastrin contents, and perform ultrastructural analyses by routine, reproducible techniques. Failure to fulfill these basic requirements casts doubt on the meaningfulness and applicability of results to the G cell cycle.

Consideration of the G cell cycle raises several important questions. Is the electron density of G cell granules directly related to gastrin content? Examination of antral gastrin contents and antral G cell granule density indices from fasting and postprandial animals is shown in Fig. 3. The high mean G cell

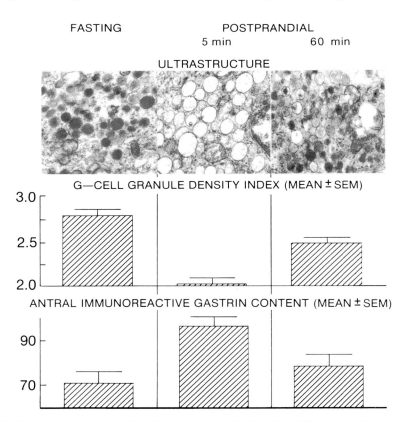

FIG. 3. Ultrastructural and antral gastrin responses to feeding. **Top:** Ultrastructural appearance of granules in G cells from fasting rats and 5 and 60 min postprandially. **Middle:** G cell granule density indices. **Bottom:** Antral gastrin contents (ng immunoreactive gastrin/mg protein). For complete details see ref. 48. Note the lack of a direct relationship between G cell granule electron density and antral gastrin content.

granule density index for rats fasted 12 hr reflects the predominance of electron-dense granules in their antral G cells. A mean antral gastrin content of 71.0 ± 4.6 ng IRG/mg protein is found for fasting rats. Five minutes postprandially, the striking absence of electron-dense granules is reflected by the lower mean granule density index; surprisingly, this index occurs with a mean antral gastrin content of 97.5 ± 7.1 ng IRG/mg protein. The 60-min postprandial mean granule density index and mean antral gastrin content lie between those calculated for fasting and 5-min postprandial rats. If a strict relationship existed between granule electron density and gastrin content then low indices should be associated with low gastrin contents. This is not observed.

By what type of cellular release mechanism(s) does gastrin exit from G cells? The answer to this question is not straightforward. The initial study of the G cell cycle did not discover any evidence of emiocytosis and proposed a process of cytoplasmic dissolution of granules (15). Several subsequent studies claim to have evidence for emiocytosis in antral G cells (21,42). These studies have employed sodium bicarbonate to stimulate G cell activity; sodium bicarbonate is a doubtful gastrin releaser (2). It is argued that evidence for emiocytosis is lacking beause these release phenomena occur so infrequently and thereby escape detection (36). Whatever the reason, gastrin release by emiocytosis has not yet been documented. Seeing that the G cell possesses the capacity for different types of release (endocrine, luminal, and paracrine), it may be that the G cell can release gastrin by different cellular mechanisms.

GEP Hormone Release and Total Parenteral Nutrition

Total Parenteral Nutrition (TPN) Effects on GEP Hormone Release

TPN provides an unique opportunity to study the digestive system and GEP hormone release in the absence of oral nutrient intake. Gastric acid secretion (47) and pancreatic exocrine secretions (20) are reduced after TPN. Increased plasma insulin concentrations are found in human subjects maintained on TPN (18). Animal studies reveal decreased antral gastrin (19) and increased serum secretin (20).

Of particular interest is the way in which GEP endocrine cells adapt to the absence of oral nutrients and respond to continuous intravenous nutrients. Plasma GEP hormone concentrations over a 10-day period of TPN in rats are presented in Fig. 4. The most dramatic response is seen with gastrin; plasma gastrin decreases to undetectable at day 6. By day 10 gastrin is detectable and almost back to the starting concentration. The changes in plasma insulin and glucagon are expected in response to the continuous intravenous infusion of 30% dextrose/12% amino acids. The immediate increase in insulin may cause the initial decrease observed with GIP.

These different hormonal responses to TPN may reflect basic metabolic adjustments to the intravenous nutrients and the anatomical location of the cells.

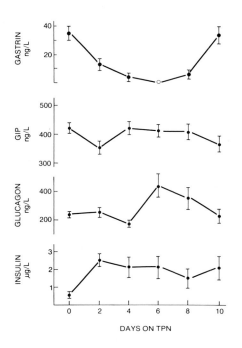

FIG. 4. The effect of total parenteral nutrition (TPN) upon plasma GEP hormone concentrations. Rats were maintained on TPN (30% dextrose plus 12% amino acids) for increasing lengths of time from 2 to 10 days. Plasma gastrin, GIP, glucagon, and insulin were measured by RIA. Note the dramatic decrease of plasma gastrin found at day 6. The insulin and glucagon responses are expected in response to the intravenous diet.

Carbohydrate metabolism is controlled by pancreatic endocrine hormones; its regulation is fundamental to life. Pancreatic endocrine cells do not receive luminal nutrients so that absence of such stimulation will not affect them. Antral G cells are exposed to gastric luminal contents and display a dramatic loss of gastrin activity while they adapt to intravenous nutrients. Jejunal K cells producing GIP do not seem to be affected by the TPN.

Coordination of GEP Hormone Release

The stomach is a major control center for digestion and the ingestion of nutrients is the initial stimulus for GEP hormone release. For a number of hormones active digestion/absorption of nutrients in the stomach and upper small intestine is necessary for hormone release. The stomach and upper small intestine generate signals (hormones) that activate a properly coordinated sequence of digestive events. Introduction of nutrients into the stomach and subsequently the upper small intestine causes rapid release of some GEP hormones. Since carbohydrate releases GIP (4), neurotensin (3), and enteroglucagon (31) within 15 min, it seems that carbohydrate absorption alone cannot stimulate these jejunal/ileal hormones. Fat ingestion releases motilin within 15 min, whereas intraduodenal instillation of fat has no effect on plasma motilin concentrations (8). These findings suggest that gastric hormones may act as control signals for hormone release for jejunal and ileal endocrine cells. The concept of gastric hormones regulating hormone release in the small and large intestines is presented in Fig. 5.

Support for this conjecture comes from a recent report of a gastrin-releasing protein isolated from the fundic portion of the stomach (33). Despite the luminal exposure of the antral gastrin-producing G cells, there is still a gastric hormone involved in the regulation of gastrin release. Hormones located in the small intestine regulate pancreatic function. Chymodenin, a releasing protein isolated from the upper small intestine, releases chymotrypsinogen specifically from pancreatic acinar cells (6). Another small intestinal hormone, GIP, regulates pancreatic endocrine function. GIP enhances glucose-induced insulin release (10)

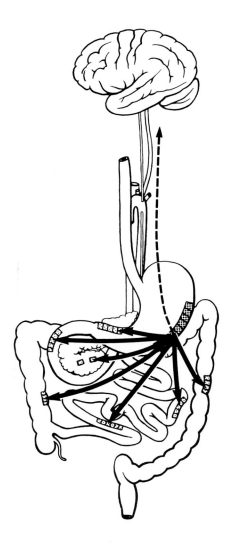

FIG. 5. Diagrammatic representation of how gastric hormones may regulate the release of different GEP hormones. See text for further explanation.

and may influence glucagon release. These isolated releasing hormones could be the first of a series of gastro-entero regulatory hormones that control nutrient-induced hormone release from GEP endocrine cells. It is possible that such regulatory hormones are involved in the capacity of the gastro-entero region to send signals to the brain. GEP hormones or releasing factors could be transported to the brain to regulate satiety. It is of interest that several GEP hormones have been detected in brain tissues. Furthermore, brain concentrations of CCK are lower in obese mice than in their lean littermates, suggesting that CCK and perhaps other GEP hormones may be involved in satiety and body weight control (46).

SUMMARY

Gastro-entero-pancreatic endocrine cells produce a large number of hormones. To date, insulin- and gastrin-producing cells are the best studied. Insulin synthesis proceeds by a tightly coordinated series of events; very little is known about gastrin synthesis. In response to appropriate stimulation both pancreatic B cells and antral G cells release their hormonal products in a biphasic manner. Insulin release is not dependent on insulin synthesis; gastrin release is dependent on gastrin synthesis as evidenced by the doubling of antral gastrin contents postprandially. Thus, although the observed hormone responses are comparable for both cells, different cellular mechanisms are operative to produce them. Insulin is released by emiocytosis; gastrin release by emiocytosis has not been documented and may occur by cytoplasmic dissolution of G cell granules. Changes in G cell granule electron density are not related directly to antral gastrin content. Total parenteral nutrition causes a dramatic change in plasma gastrin concentrations; insulin, glucagon, and GIP responses are appropriate for the intravenous carbohydrate/amino acid nutrients. Gastro-entero releasing hormones seem to be active in coordinating GEP hormone release.

PROJECTIONS FOR THE FUTURE

To delve deeper into the understanding of GEP hormone turnover it is necessary to study representative, or marker, hormones from different areas of the GEP endocrine system. The ability of different nutrients (carbohydrate, fat, protein) delivered orally or intravenously to stimulate their synthesis and release will reveal how comparable the response mechanisms are throughout the GEP system.

For detailed studies of GEP hormone synthesis it will be necessary to develop techniques to isolate and concentrate GEP endocrine cells. Assessment of the GEP hormone releasing potential of gastro-entero proteins will provide further insight into the role gastro-entero hormones play in regulating GEP hormone release.

ACKNOWLEDGMENTS

The studies reported were supported in part by the Atkinson Charitable Foundation, the Hospital for Sick Children Foundation, the Mount Sinai Institute, the Canadian Medical Research Council, and the Deutsche Forschungsgemeinschaft (Bonn-Bad Godesberg, Grant Cr 20/7).

REFERENCES

1. Bastie, M. J., Balas, D., Senegas-Balas, F., Bertrand, C., Pradayrol, L., Frexinos, J., and Ribet, A. (1979): A cyto-physical study of the G-cell secretory cycle in the antrum mucosa of the hamster and of the rat. *Scand. J. Gastroenterol.,* 14:35–48.
2. Becker, H. D., Reeder, D. D., and Thompson, J. C. (1973): The effect of changes in antral pH on the basal release of gastrin. *Proc. Soc. Exp. Bio.. Med.,* 143:238–240.
3. Bloom, S. R., Blackburn, A. M., Besterman, H. S., Sarson, D. L., and Polak, J. M. (1978): Measurement of neurotensin in man: A new circulating peptide hormone affecting insulin release and carbohydrate metabolism. *Diabetologia,* 15:220 (Abstr.).
4. Cataland, S., Crockett, S. E., Brown, J. C., and Mazzaferri, E. L. (1974): Gastric inhibitory polypeptide (GIP) stimulation by oral glucose in man. *J. Clin. Endocrinol. Metab.,* 39:223–228.
5. Charles, M. A., Lawecki, J., Pictet, R., and Grodsky, G. M. (1975): Insulin secretion: Interrelationships of glucose, cyclic adenosine 3':5'-monophosphate, and calcium. *J. Biol. Chem.,* 250:6134–6140.
6. Chang, R., Glaser, C. B., and Adelson, J. (1978): Structural studies of chymodenin, a hormonelike gastrointestinal polypeptide related to GIP and glucagon. *Scand. J. Gastroenterol. (Suppl. 13),* 49:36 (Abstr.).
7. Christiansen, L. A., Lindkaer Jensen, S., Rehfeld, J. F., Stadil, F., and Christensen, K. C. (1978): Antral content and secretion of gastrin in pigs. *Scand. J. Gastroenterol.,* 13:719–725.
8. Collins, S. M., Lewis, T. D., Fox, J. E. T., Track, N. S., and Daniel, E. E. (1979): Motilin release. *Can. J. Physiol. Pharmacol., (in press).*
9. Creutzfeldt, C., Track, N. S., and Creutzfeldt, W. (1973): *In vitro* studies of the rate of proinsulin and insulin turnover in seven human insulinomas. *Eur. J. Clin. Invest.,* 3:371–384.
10. Creutzfeldt, W. (1979): The incretin concept today. *Diabetologia,* 16:75–86.
11. Creutzfeldt, W., Arnold, R., Creutzfeldt, C., Deuticke, U., Frerichs, H., and Track, N. S. (1973): Biochemical and morphological investigations of 30 human insulinomas. *Diabetologia,* 9:217–231.
12. Creutzfeldt, W., Arnold, R., Creutzfeldt, C., and Track, N. S. (1975): Pathomorphologic, biochemical, and diagnostic aspects of gastrinomas (Zollinger-Ellison syndrome). *Hum. Pathol.,* 6:47–76.
13. De Schryver-Kecskemeti, K., Greider, M. H., Saks, M. K., Rieders, E. R., and McGuigan, J. E. (1977): The gastrin-producing cells in tissue cultures of the rat pyloric antrum. *Lab. Invest.,* 37:406–410.
14. Fiddian-Green, R. G., Farrell, J., Havlichek, D., Jr., Kothary, P., and Pittenger, G. (1978): A physiological role for luminal gastrin? *Surgery,* 83:663–668.
15. Forssmann, W. G., and Orci, L. (1969): Ultrastructure and secretory cycle of the gastrinproducing cell. *Z. Zellforschung.,* 101:419–432.
16. Fujita, T. (1974): *Gastro-entero-pancreatic Endocrine System.* Georg Thieme, Stuttgart.
17. Harty, R. F., van der Vijver, J. C., and McGuigan, J. E. (1977): Stimulation of gastrin secretion and synthesis in antral organ culture. *J. Clin. Invest.,* 60:51–60.
18. Jeejeebhoy, K. N., Anderson, G. H., Nakhooda, A. F., Greenberg, G. R., Sanderson, I., and Marliss, E. B. (1976): Metabolic studies in total parenteral nutrition with lipid in man. *J. Clin. Invest.,* 57:125–136.
19. Johnson, L. R., Copeland, E. M., Dudrick, S. J., Lichtenberger, L. M., and Castro, G. A. (1975): Structural and hormonal alterations in the gastro-intestinal tract of parenterally fed rats. *Gastroenterology,* 68:1177–1183.
20. Johnson, L. R., Schanbacher, L. M., Dudrick, S. J., and Copeland, E. M. (1977): Effect of

long-term parenteral feeding on pancreatic secretion and serum secretin. *Am. J. Physiol.,* 233:E524–E529.

21. Kobayashi, S., and Fujita, T. (1974): Emiocytotic granule release in the basal-granulated cells of the dog induced by intraluminal application of adequate stimuli. In: *Gastro-entero-pancreatic Endocrine System,* edited by T. Fujita, pp. 49–53. Georg Thieme, Stuttgart.
22. Lazarus, N. R., and Davis, B. (1975): Model for extrusion of insulin B-granules. *Lancet,* i:143–147.
23. Lichtenberger, L. M., Lechago, J., Dockray, G. J., and Passaro, E., Jr. (1975): Culture of Zollinger-Ellison tumor cells. *Gastroenterology,* 68:1119–1126.
24. Lichtenberger, L. M., Lechago, J., and Johnson, L. R. (1975): Depression of antral and serum gastrin concentration by food deprivation in the rat. *Gastroenterology,* 68:1473–1479.
25. Lichtenberger, L. M., Shorey, J. M., and Trier, J. S. (1978): Organ culture studies of rat antrum: Evidence for an antral inhibitor of gastrin release. *Am. J. Physiol.,* 235:E410–E415.
26. Lichtenberger, L. M., Welsh, J. D., and Johnson, L. R. (1976): Relationship between the changes in gastrin levels and intestinal properties in the starved rat. *Am. J. Dig. Dis.,* 21:33–38.
27. Lin, B. J., Nagy, B. R., and Haist, R. E. (1972) Effect of various concentrations of glucose on insulin biosynthesis. *Endocrinology,* 91:309–311.
28. Lomedico, P. T., Chan, S. J., Steiner, D. F., and Saunders, G. F. (1977): Immunological and chemical characterization of bovine preproinsulin. *J. Biol. Chem.,* 252:7971–7978.
29. Malaisse, W. J. (1973): Insulin secretion: Multifactorial regulation for a single process of release. *Diabetologia,* 9:167–173.
30. Malmström, J., and Stadil, F. (1976): Gastrin content and gastrin release. *Scand. J. Gastroenterol. (Suppl.),* 37:71–76.
31. Matsuyama, T., and Foa, P. P. (1974): Plasma glucose, insulin, pancreatic and enteroglucagon levels in normal and depancreatised dogs. *Proc. Soc. Exp. Biol. Med.,* 147:97–102.
32. Melani, F. (1974): Pro-hormones in tissues and in circulation. *Horm. Metab. Res.,* 6:1–8.
33. McDonald, T. J., Nilsson, G., Vagne, M., Ghatei, M., Bloom, S. R., and Mutt, V. (1978): A gastrin releasing peptide from the porcine non-antral gastric tissue. *Gut,* 19:767–774.
34. Montague, W., Howell, S. L., and Green, I. C. (1975): Insulin release and the microtubular system of the islets of Langerhans. *Biochem. J.,* 148:237–243.
35. Mortensen, N. J. McM., and Morris, J. F. (1977): The effect of fixation conditions on the ultrastructural appearance of gastrin cell granules in the rat gastric pyloric antrum. *Cell Tissue Res.,* 176:251–263.
36. Mortensen, N. J. McM., Morris, J. F., and Owen, C. J. (1978): Gastrin and the ultrastructure of G-cells after stimulation with acetylcholine. *Cell Tissue Res.,* 192:513–525.
37. Mortensen, N. J. McM., Morris, J. F., and Owens, C. J. (1979): Gastrin and the ultrastructure of G-cells in the fasting rat. *Gut,* 20:41–50.
38. Muller, J. E., Straus, E., and Yalow, R. S. (1977): Cholecystokinin and its COOH-terminal octapeptide in the pig brain. *Proc. Natl. Acad. Sci. USA,* 74:3035–3037.
39. Orci, L. (1974): A portrait of the pancreatic B-cell. *Diabetologia,* 10:163–187.
40. Reeder, D. D., Watayou, T., Booth, R. A. D., and Thompson, J. C. (1975): Depletion of antral gastrin after food in rats. *Am. J. Surg.,* 129:67–70.
41. Rehfeld, J. F. (1978): Immunochemical studies of cholecystokinin. *J. Biol. Chem.,* 253:4022–4030.
42. Sato, A. (1978): Quantitative electron microscopic studies of the kinetics of secretory granules in G-cells. *Cell Tissue Res.,* 187:45–59.
43. Sharp, G. W. G., Wollheim. C., Muller, W. A., Gutzeit, A., Trueheart, P. A., Blondel, B., Orci, L., and Renold, A. E. (1975): Studies on the mechanism of insulin release. *Fed. Proc.,* 34:1537–1548.
44. Steiner, D. F. (1977): Insulin today. *Diabetes,* 26:322–340.
45. Steiner, D. F. (1967): Evidence for a precursor in the biosynthesis of insulin. *Trans. N.Y. Acad. Sci. Ser. II,* 30:60–68.
46. Straus, E., and Yalow, R. S. (1979): Cholecystokinin in the brains of obese and nonobese mice. *Science,* 203:68–69.
47. Thor, P. J., Copeland, E. M., Dudrick, S. J., and Johnson, L. R. (1977): Effect of long-term parenteral feeding on gastric secretion in dogs. *Am. J. Physiol.,* 232:E39–E43.
48. Track, N. S., Creutzfeldt, C., Arnold, R., and Creutzfeldt, W. (1978): The antral gastrin-producing G-cell: Biochemical and ultrastructural responses to feeding. *Cell Tissue Res.,* 194:131–139.

49. Track, N. S., Creutzfeldt, C., Junge, U., and Creutzfeldt, W. (1975): Gastrin turnover in gastrinoma tissue: *In vitro* incubation, subcellular fractionation and monolayer culture studies. In: *Gastrointestinal Hormones,* edited by J. C. Thompson, pp 403–424. University of Texas Press, Austin.

50. Track, N. S., Frerichs, H., and Creutzfeldt, W. (1974): Release of newly synthesized proinsulin and insulin from granulated and degranulated isolated rat pancreatic islets. The effect of high glucose concentration. *Horm. Metab. Res. (Suppl.),* 5:97–103.

51. Uvnäs-Wallensten, K. (1976): Gastrin release and HCl secretion induced by electrical vagal stimulation in the cat. *Acta Physiol. Scand. (Suppl.),* 438:1–39.

52. Uvnäs-Wallensten, K. (1977): Occurrence of gastrin in gastric juice, in antral secretion, and in antral perfusates of cats. *Gastroenterology,* 73:487–491.

53. Walsh, J. H., and Grossman, M. I. (1975): Gastrin. *N. Engl. J. Med.,* 292:1324–1334.

Isolation, Characterization, Structure-Activity Relation and Biological Functions of the Gastrointestinal Hormones and Peptides

Gastrointestinal Hormones, edited by
George B. Jerzy Glass.
Raven Press, New York © 1980.

Chapter 5

Secretin: Isolation, Structure, and Functions

Viktor Mutt

Department of Biochemistry II, Karolinska Institute, Stockholm, Sweden

INTRODUCTION

In 1825 Leuret and Lassaigne (233) described their discovery that, in the dog, instillation of dilute acetic acid into the upper intestine resulted in dilatation of the duodenal orifices of the pancreatic and bile ducts and in a flow of pancreatic juice and of bile into the intestine. They also suggested that since the chyme is normally acidic, it could physiologically produce the same effects as the acetic acid under the experimental conditions.

Leuret and Lassaigne do not seem, however, to have quite recognized the great importance of their own observation, and their work was largely overlooked by later workers.

The stimulation of pancreatic secretion by duodenal acidification was rediscovered in Pavlov's laboratory by Becker (23) and extensively investigated there by Dolinsky (97). Attempts to demonstrate a neural mechanism that could explain the action of the acid were unsuccessful (289,391,392) and this led to the discovery by Bayliss and Starling in 1902 that acid extracts of the mucosa of the upper intestine contained a substance that if injected into the bloodstream caused the pancreas to secrete (19,20). Bayliss and Starling named this substance *secretin.* It was evident to them that many other substances, chemically different from, but functionally analogous to, secretin would be found to act as chemical messengers between various organs and therefore they suggested that a new term, *hormone,* be created to describe such messengers. The word itself, derived from the Greek ὁρμάω ("I arouse to activity") was suggested to them by W. B. Hardy (22,344).

ISOLATION OF SECRETIN

Soon after the discovery of secretin, work started in many laboratories with the object of isolating this substance. During the course of this work, many important observations concerning the nature of secretin were made. However, the methods necessary for isolating it from the complex mixtures of polypeptides that are found in extracts of intestinal tissue were not available before the mid-1950s, by which time they had been developed in other areas of biochemistry. The early work has been reviewed by several authors (e.g., refs. 124,129,134,262) and will not be discussed here except when it has had a direct influence on subsequent developments.

The only secretin that has been isolated hitherto is porcine secretin (197). Highly purified preparations of both bovine and chicken secretin have recently been obtained in our laboratory, but some further purification is necessary before meaningful comparisons of these substances with porcine secretin can be carried out. The possibility cannot be excluded that one or more variant forms of porcine secretin may exist in addition to the form isolated by us. Legge et al. (228) found secretin activity in two fractions on countercurrent distribution in the system water-2-butanol-acetic acid-dichloroacetic acid (1,000:860:19:8 v/v), and Newton et al. (275) found three components, two major and one minor, using the system 2-butanol-water-dichloroacetic acid (100:100:1 v/v). We too have consistently found relatively small amounts of secretin-like activity in several side fractions from the isolation of secretin. However, until some of these active materials are isolated, it is only a matter of conjecture as to whether they are isohormones of secretin, large molecular forms incorporating the "ordinary" secretin, or just simply secretins artefactually modified or tenaciously adsorbed to other peptide material. It is, of course, also possible that secretin-like activity may be exerted by substances chemically very different from secretin, as indeed has been shown to be the case for dopamine (157).

The method that we worked out for the isolation of secretin starts with the observation of Bayliss and Starling that its activity is fairly thermostable and that if the upper intestinal mucosa is briefly boiled in water then active secretin may be extracted from the coagulated material with acid, but not with water (20). Our method starts with the collection and heating for 8 to 10 min in boiling water of the uppermost meter of hog intestines as soon as feasible. The heating step serves to inactivate the proteolytic enzymes of the intestines and also to coagulate the bulk of the structural proteins that are thereby rendered insoluble in the extraction step. The material is then frozen, minced, and extracted with cold 0.5 M acetic acid. Carrying out the extraction with cold acid may be expected to be less destructive to acid-labile peptide linkages and other structures than extraction at higher temperatures. After filtration, peptides, including secretin, are adsorbed from the extract to alginic acid, eluted with 0.2 M HCl, and precipitated from the eluate with NaCl at saturation (195). This precipitate, CTIP (*c*oncentrate of *t*hermostable *i*ntestinal *p*eptides), which constitutes by weight about one-thousandth of that of the (boiled) intestinal tissue (both wet weight) has been used as the starting material for the isolation of secretin and subsequently of several other intestinal polypeptides as well. As pointed out previously (264,266), there is no reason to believe that CTIP should contain all types of polypeptide hormones that may occur in intestinal tissue. By definition it would not contain thermolabile hormones.

Salting out of secretin from aqueous solution with NaCl at saturation was originally used by Weaver et al. (389) and by Penau and Simonnet (284) for the separation of secretin from histamine and other toxic substances that remain in solution.

The secretin may, of course, be isolated from CTIP by a variety of techniques. In the one currently in use in our laboratory, the first step is dissolving CTIP in water to a 5% (w/v) solution, addition of 2 volumes of 95% ethanol, and adjustment of the pH of the solution to 7.2 ± 0.1 as measured by a glass electrode (261), at which stage a precipitate forms. This precipitate contains little secretin activity as measured by bioassay, and has hitherto been routinely filtered off and discarded. The solubility properties of this precipitate suggest that it could contain peptides of higher molecular weight than those remaining in solution.

It is now increasingly evident that many, possibly all, peptide hormones are formed by proteolytic cleavage of larger precursor forms, either extracellularly as in the case of angiotensin (325) and bradykinin (306), or intracellularly, as shown first for insulin by Steiner and co-workers (345) and subsequently for numerous other hormones by different workers (167). It is not improbable that the precipitate may contain larger molecular forms of the known (and yet unknown) intestinal hormones, and we have recently started to investigate this possibility.

Peptides, among them secretin, are recovered from the filtrate in aqueous solution and reprecipitated with NaCl. This precipitate, which is by weight about one-fifth that of CTIP, is chromatographed on Sephadex G-25 (fine) in 0.2 M acetic acid (264) and the fraction containing the bulk of the secretin (and cholecystokinin) bioactivity is saturated with NaCl. The precipitate that forms is dissolved in water and reprecipitated at pH 4 with NaCl. This precipitate is by weight one-fifteenth to one-tenth of the original CTIP, but roughly half of the secretin activity of the latter had already been lost into the various side fractions prior to precipitation. The precipitate is extracted with methanol (50 ml/g), with the bulk of the secretin passing into solution and the bulk of the cholecystokinin (CCK) remaining undissolved. The undissolved material is filtered off, washed on the filter with ether, and, after removal of the ether *in vacuo,* used for the purification of CCK (see below) and of gastric inhibitory peptide (GIP).

The pH of the filtrate is brought to 7.5 ± 0.1 (261), as measured by a glass electrode, and the precipitate that forms is collected. This "AMESNI" (*a*cid *me*thanol *s*oluble, *n*eutral *i*nsoluble) fraction has been the starting material for the purification of chymodenin by J. Adelson (2). The filtrate is, after acidification, precipitated with 3 volumes of ether and the precipitate is reprecipitated from water with NaCl.

This precipitate, containing secretin and also motilin (55) and vasoactive intestinal peptide (VIP) (314), is chromatographed on carboxymethyl cellulose in either 0.02 M NH₄HCO₃ (261) or sodium (0.025 M) ortophosphate of pH 8 ± 0.1 (314). The fraction containing the bulk of the secretin activity is acidified to pH 2.5 and the secretin is adsorbed to alginic acid and eluted into 0.2 M HCl. After exchange of chloride for acetate, the material is lyophilized and then subjected to countercurrent distribution over 200 transfers in the system butanol/0.1 M phosphate pH 7 ± 0.1 (197). The secretin activity will be found in tubes 60 to 100. The contents of these tubes are dissolved in water and the secretin is recovered in lyophilized form by the use of alginic acid as in the preceding purification step. The material is essentially pure; we use this term to mean that no ambiguity because of impurities present will arise if it is used for the determination of the amino acid sequence of the polypeptide. One milligram of this material is obtained from approximately 70 kg of boiled intestinal tissue (from 1,000 hogs). A further, slight, purification may be achieved by chromatography in 0.2 M acetic acid on Sephadex G-25, by rechromatography in 0.02 M NH₄HCO₃ on carboxymethyl cellulose, or by high pressure liquid chromatography *(unpublished).*

STRUCTURE OF SECRETIN

The amino acid sequence of secretin was determined by a combination of selective enzymatic degradations and Edman degradations (269,270), as is usual in sequence work on polypeptides. The only real difficulty was that the work had to be carried out on small amounts of material that we had available. Because of this, the synthesis of secretin by Bodanszky et al. (33), which was carried out in parallel with our sequence work, greatly facilitated the latter, since the correctness of proposed sequences could be either confirmed or refuted by comparison of the synthetic with the natural peptides. An unusual feature in the sequence work was the use of thrombin to selectively cleave only one of the four arginyl bonds that are susceptible to tryptic cleavage in secretin. This was useful for the alignment of the five tryptic peptides in the peptide chain, particularly as the bond cleaved by thrombin was cleaved at a slower rate by trypsin than the other three arginyl bonds.

The amino acid sequence of (porcine) secretin is H S D G T F T S E L S R L R D S A R L Q R L L Q G L V ■, using the one-letter notation for amino acid residues recommended by the IUPAC-IUB Commission on Biochemical Nomenclature (181), with ■ indicating that the C-terminal residue is in amide form. The expanded form is seen in Fig. 1.

It is evident that secretin is a heptacosapeptide amide composed of 11 different types of amino acid residues in the proportions Ala_1, Arg_4, Asp_2, Glu_3, Gly_2, His_1, Leu_6, Phe_1, Ser_4, Thr_2, Val_1, the C-terminal valine and the side chain carboxyls of two of the glutamic acid residues being in amide form. Consequently, of the amino acid residues commonly found in proteins those of cysteine/cystine, isoleucine, lysine, methionine, proline, tryptophan, and tyrosine are absent from secretin. Because of the absence of tryptophan and tyrosine, the light absorbance of secretin solutions is low at 280 nm. Concerning the secondary structure of secretin, Bodanszky and co-workers have obtained evidence indicating that secretin exists in a preferred conformation in aqueous solution. Optical rotatory dispersion and circular dichroism spectra indicate that there is a helical region in the chain. Investigation of secretin fragments originally seemed to suggest that this helical region was present within the N-terminal half of the molecule (34) but more recent work suggests that it exists in the C-terminal part instead (32). Porcine secretin shows sequence similarities to several other porcine hormonal peptides. Most marked is its similarity to glucagon (50) (14 identities), and then to VIP (271) and GIP (54) (nine identities in each case):

```
Secretin    H S D G T F T S E L S R L R D S A R L Q R L L Q G L V ■
Glucagon  H S Q G T F T S D Y S K Y L D S R R A Q D F V Q W L M N T
VIP         H S D A V F T D N Y T R L R K Q M A V K K Y L N S I L N ■
GIP          Y A E G T F I S D Y S I A M D K I R Q Q D F V N W L L A Q Q
              K G K K S D W K H N I T Q
```

A certain degree of sequence similarity may be found between secretin and motilin (265) and somatotropin (1) and lipotropin (123), respectively. If one considers not only identical amino acid residues in the same positions in the different hormones but also those acids that, although different, have similar chemical properties (e.g., isoleucine in position 26 of VIP as compared with leucine in the same position in secretin), then the similarities between secretin and the other peptides mentioned above become still more marked.

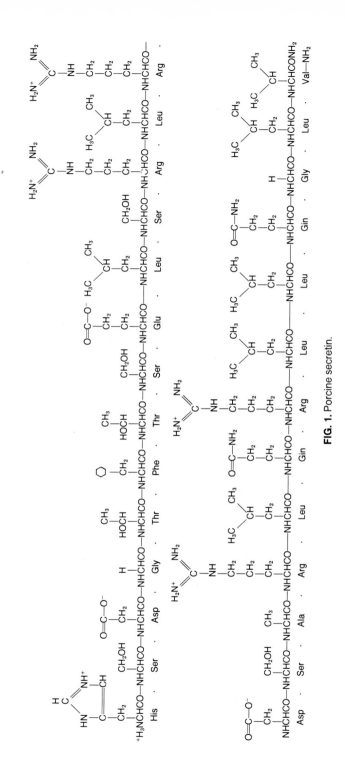

FIG. 1. Porcine secretin.

SYNTHESIS OF SECRETIN

The first organic-chemical synthesis of secretin was accomplished by Bodanszky et al. in 1966 (33) (see Chapter 18 by M. Bodanszky and V. Kwei, pp. 413–432, *this volume*). The synthetic material was hormonally active but distinctly weaker than the natural product. An improved synthesis yielded a preparation (283) that was found to be equipotent with natural secretin in stimulating pancreatic secretion in dogs (379). Following his synthesis of glucagon (402), Wünsch (403) synthesized secretin by a method other than that used by the previous workers. Subsequently still other syntheses have been described (160,206,382,406).

In our laboratory we have had the opportunity to compare the effects of the materials synthesized by Ondetti et al. (283) and by Wünsch (403) on pancreatic bicarbonate secretion in anesthetized cats (272). Both synthetic materials were within experimental error equipotent with the natural product.

Biosynthesis of secretin by the hybrid DNA method (180) has not been described at the time of writing of this chapter (February 1979).

OCCURRENCE OF SECRETIN

Bayliss and Starling injected acid extracts of upper intestinal mucosa from mammals, birds, reptiles, amphibians, and teleostian and elasmobranch fish intravenously into dogs and observed that in each case a secretin-like stimulation on pancreatic secretion took place. They concluded that secretin occurs in all species of vertebrates (21) and nothing in the later work has invalidated this assumption. Partially purified preparations of material showing secretin-like activity have been obtained from the intestines of the Chimaera monstrosa (276), lampreys (17), the pike (94), the cod (95), and the chicken (277). The function of secretin in birds is puzzling. Bayliss and Starling observed that on injecting a secretin-containing extract of dog intestine intravenously into a goose only a slight stimulation of pancreatic secretion occurred and they were inclined to ascribe the absence of any greater effect to the goose's being in the process of fattening for Christmas (21). Angelucci et al. (7) found that porcine secretin did not stimulate pancreatic secretion in the chicken and Dockray (96) found that in the turkey porcine secretin was a weak stimulant of pancreatic secretion, whereas porcine VIP was a strong stimulant and chicken VIP a still stronger one. This would indicate that in birds VIP might have the function that secretin has in mammals. However, this leaves the role of secretin in the bird unexplained. Chicken secretin seems to have an activity at least as high as about one-fourth of that of porcine secretin when assayed in the anesthetized cat in doses causing a moderate stimulation of pancreatic secretion. At higher dose levels porcine secretin, however, appears to be much stronger than chicken secretin (A. Nilsson, *unpublished*). Material with secretin-like activity has been extracted also from the intestine of an invertebrate, *Octopus vulgaris* (227).

Recent work (30) on the distribution of the S cells, which are known to contain material with secretin-like immunoreactivity (336), and investigations on the occurrence of radioimmunoassayable secretin in tissue extracts of the alimentary tract (30,352) confirm earlier findings (253) that secretin occurs in the tissue of the upper intestine, either exclusively or quite predominantly.

PHYSIOLOGY, PHARMACOLOGY, AND PHYSIOLOGICAL RELEASE OF SECRETIN

Bayliss and Starling found that in addition to stimulating pancreatic secretion in dogs secretin also stimulated the flow of hepatic bile (20). Incidentally, secretion of bile into the intestine of a dog following acidification of the upper intestine of the animal had been previously described by Rutherford in 1880 (311). Other workers, using crude preparations, ascribed a variety of actions to secretin, including effects on hemopoiesis and on blood sugar concentrations. These early claims have been reviewed by Mellanby (252) and by Still (347). Using purer preparations, Ågren found no effects of secretin other than the two described by Bayliss and Starling; except for some stimulation of upper intestinal secretion (4), Still had reached the same conclusion (347). In the early 1950s the question was whether pure secretin stimulated pancreatic secretion exclusively, i.e., whether the stimulating actions that secretin preparations exhibited on biliary and intestinal secretion were actions of secretin itself or of some other substance(s) contained in preparations. That the picture would in reality turn out to be much more complicated could be anticipated from the work of Gregory and Tracy on gastrin. It had been expected that when gastrin would be isolated it would stimulate gastric acid secretion and nothing else, and that all the other effects found for partially purified preparations would be due to the effects of contaminants. However, it was soon found that gastrin, as such, exhibited some half a dozen effects in addition to the stimulation of gastric acid secretion. Among these effects was the stimulation, although weak, of the flow of pancreatic juice in dogs (131,133). An analogous picture was true for secretin. In addition to stimulating pancreatic secretion, secretin was found to stimulate, at least in some species, the secretion of hepatic bile, of the Brunner glands, of pepsinogen, and of gastric mucus. It also released insulin, had cardiovascular actions, caused lipolysis in adipose tissue, relaxed the lower esophageal sphincter, delayed gastric emptying, and inhibited gastrin-induced gastric acid secretion (see refs. 132,175,263). In some instances regarding its effects or lack of effects on blood calcium concentration discrepancies were present between the findings of different workers (48,178,324,396). The picture is still more complicated due to species variations in the effects of secretin as well as to interactions of secretin with nerve impulses and other hormones. Grossman has pointed out that a distinction must be made between the physiological effects of peptide hormones and their pharmacological actions, which are manifest only on the administration of large doses of exogenous hormone that cause plasma concentrations in excess of those ever reached under physiological conditions (138). This is an important consideration. In addition, some of the actions that occur physiologically may be of little significance. Of the many actions of secretin, Grossman considers only stimulation of pancreatic secretion of water and bicarbonate and potentiation of the pancreozymic effect of CCK to be of physiological importance. The discovery, in Pavlov's laboratory, that the pancreatic juice differed in composition depending on the mechanism by which the pancreas was stimulated preceded the discovery of secretin. Stimulation of the vagus (215) resulted in a juice rich in enzymes, whereas stimulation by duodenal acidification resulted in a juice high in bicarbonate but low in enzyme concentration (385). This was pointed out by Babkin and Sawitsch already in 1908 (11). Several authors, although working with very crude secretin preparations, soon found that secretin stimulated the secretion of juice with a low protein and consequently low enzyme content (90,258). These observations would become truly significant if they could be reproduced by the use of purer preparations. Mellanby concluded that pancreatic secretion was controlled by two mechanisms: secretin stimulating the secretion of water and bicarbonate, and the vagus that of enzymes (250). This hypothesis was generally accepted until the discovery of pancreozymin (CCK-PZ) by Harper and Raper (154). Lagerlöf concluded that secretin did not stimulate enzyme secretion in man (220). Using one of our partially purified preparations of secretin, we came to the same conclusion in regard to pancreatic secretion both in man (390) and in the cat (194). Anyone observing the very different effects of secretin and CCK-PZ at least in man, cat, and dog, has been inclined to conclude that secretin does not stimulate the secretion of enzymes. However, the theoretical discussion as to whether secretin has an effect, however slight, on enzyme secretion goes on (164,398). In fact recent work on dispersed guinea pig pancreatic acinar cells indicates that it has such an effect (303). This may be true, however, for only a small number of species (305), since the mechanisms of stimulation of pancreatic secretion appear to show quite pronounced species differences. From work done mainly in dogs and cats (230), it has been concluded that vagal stimulation results in the secretion of enzymes, but of only little water. However, Hickson (168) found that in the pig the vagus had an almost secretin-like effect on fluid secretion.

The demonstration of VIP-containing nerves in the pancreas (60,223,356) points to the possibility of VIP exerting local stimulatory effects on pancreatic secretion in mammals (173). In birds, at any rate in the turkey, it has been shown that intravenously administered porcine VIP is by far a more potent stimulant of pancreatic secretion than is porcine secretin, but the reverse was found in mammals (96). A few years ago a rather unexpected possibility became apparent, namely that secretin, although an excellent stimulant of pancreatic secretion, was normally of no importance for this effect.

Actually such a possibility had since long been implicit in the question as to whether the intestinal contents ever become sufficiently acidic in relation to meals for the acid to significantly stimulate pancreatic secretion. Thomas and Crider investigated this problem in dogs and found that the pH had to fall to 5 or below for pancreatic secretion to occur. They concluded that "under some physiological conditions the activity of the intestinal contents during digestion is adequate to stimulate the pancreas" (364). Later, however, Thomas and his co-workers considered acidification of the intestine to be inadequate as a physiological mechanism for the stimulation of pancreatic secretion (287,363). Meyer et al. (255) found that in dogs the threshold pH for the intestinal contents to stimulate pancreatic secretion was 4.5 and Brooks and Grossman (51) found that such a low pH was reached only in the proximal duodenum. This would result in the release of only a small fraction of the secretin present in the mucosa of the small intestine. Considerations of this sort led Wormsley to discuss the possibility, rather unlikely, that secretin might not be an important factor for normal digestion (400). In this discussion Wormsley seemed to assume that the only mechanism for the release of secretin was duodenal acidification, an assumption that may not necessarily be valid.

Grossman and Konturek (141) came to the conclusion that gastric acid nevertheless did drive pancreatic bicarbonate secretion. Although the amounts of secretin released by acid would be small, their action would be greatly potentiated by the CCK that would be released simultaneously with secretin during a meal. Such a potentiation of the secretin effect by CCK had been shown to occur following administration of the exogenous hormones in the cat (53), the dog (165), and in man (399). Meyer et al. (254) further showed in dogs that exogenous secretin was potentiated by endogenous CCK. The action of secretin on the pancreas has been found to be potentiated also by vagal impulses in cats (53), but apparently not in the dog (162).

The assumption that the pancreatic secretion resulting from introduction of acid into the upper intestine was due to the release of secretin, and also to some extent of CCK (386) was well founded but nevertheless not proven. Only recently it has been confirmed beyond any doubt. When radioimmunoassays (RIAs) for secretin became available, it was found in several laboratories that intraduodenal acidification led to increased plasma concentrations of immunoreactive secretin in man (29,35,205,280), dog (37,280), and in the pig (28). It was also found, however, in several laboratories that no rise in plasma secretin concentration could be noted consistently following an ordinary meal so that doubt was cast again on the importance of secretin in normal digestion (79,205). Quite recently, however, several laboratories have reported the finding of an increase in plasma secretin concentration in connection with ordinary meals (77,145,318,319). These increases were small but probably sufficient for the degree of stimulation of pancreatic secretion provided in the secretin activity is potentiated by CCK and/or vagal impulses. Recent discussions of the various interactions of secretin and of other gastrointestinal hormones, with each other and with nervous impulses, have been published by Grossman (138), Makhlouf (245), Konturek (209), and Matsuo and Seki (249). A finding from one laboratory that plasma secretin concentrations do not increase but actually decrease in connection with meals (58) is difficult to interpret.

If the majority view is accepted that plasma secretin levels do increase in connection with meals, then the question arises whether some other agent in addition to acid is involved in its release. In one report intraduodenal glucose was claimed to result in raised plasma secretin levels (82) but this has not been confirmed (58,78). Boden et al. found in anesthetized dogs that intraduodenal administration of glucose solutions of various concentrations (37) or of an 8.5% amino acid mixture, 5% fructose, 40% sucrose, 9% NaCl, 50 mM sodium oleate, or oleic acid in bile (36) did not result in increases in plasma secretin levels. Hanssen et al. (151) found in man that intraduodenally administered cattle bile stimulates pancreatic secretion with concomitant increases in plasma secretin concentration. This drew attention to the old controversy between the findings of Mellanby, who claimed that intraduodenal bile stimulated secretin release (251), and that of other workers who did not find such an effect (365). Another controversial question is whether vagal or other nervous impulses are involved in secretin release. Konturek et al. (210) found that vagotomy in dogs reduced the pancreatic secretory response to intraduodenal acidification but not to exogenous secretin. This suggested that vagal innervation played a permissive role in the release of secretin from the intestinal mucosa but did not interact with it at the level of the pancreatic cells. O'Connor et al. (280) observed that in man premedication with scopolamine prevented rise in plasma immunoreactive secretin in response to duodenal acidification. Ward and Bloom, however, did not find that vagotomy in man significantly affected secretin release in response to duodenal acidification (387). Topical application of local anesthetics to the mucosa of the proximal small intestine in dogs strongly inhibited pancreatic secretion evoked by duodenal acidification (320,335).

EFFECTS OF SECRETIN ON BILE SECRETION

A large number of investigations have been carried out in different species on the effects of secretin on hepatic biliary secretion. This may seem strange since it has been often stated that the bile secretion is regulated mainly by the synthesis and the excretion of bile acids (340), rather than by the intestinal hormones (193,327,330). One reason for the interest in secretin in this connection is that secretin and bile acids apparently stimulate secretion from the anatomically different areas of the biliary system. This results in different composition of the bile secreted. It is mainly through the analysis of these differences that the current concept of the bile production has evolved, namely, that its secretion arises partly from the hepatocytes into the canaliculi and partly from the cells of the ductuli and ducts into the ductular lumen. The canalicular secretion is in part dependent and in part independent of bile acids, whereas ductular secretion is responsive to stimulation with secretin (75,112,393). This simple picture as approximation is correct, but does not account for all the facts. The magnitude of the fraction of total biliary secretion stimulated by secretin varies greatly from species to species, and may in some of them be of definite physiological importance. In some species in which ductular secretion is of little importance, it may normally acquire importance under certain pathological conditions.

In the rabbit no choleretic effect of secretin could be observed by several investigators (3,200,327,331). Esteller et al. (115), however had recently demonstrated its weak stimulating effect. In rats, no effect was observed on intravenous injection of secretin (312,330,331) but a small yet significant effect could be seen on its injection into the hepatic artery (12).

There is no doubt that secretin has a choleretic effect in man (5,140,211, 236,294,384), monkey (114,119,142,236,350), pig (202,278), dog (57,192,236, 291,295,348,395), cat (4,327), guinea pig (118,253), and sheep (70). In most of these species the volume of bile obtainable by maximal stimulation with secretin is about one-fifth to one-tenth of the volume of the pancreatic juice (393) that can be obtained, under similar conditions. The exception is the sheep, where the volume of bile has been found to exceed that of the pancreatic juice (70) during maximal stimulation. Grossman et al. (140) found that in man secretin stimulated the flow of bile with a low concentration of bile acids. In discussing the question of the part of the biliary apparatus stimulated by secretin, the authors referred to the work of Grossman and Ivy on the pancreas in which a suggestive evidence had been obtained that the hormone acted on the ductules rather than on the acinar cells (139).

Working with dogs, Wheeler and Ramos (395) agreed with other investigators on the important role played by bile salts in bile production. They suggested that the flow and composition of bile after secretin were modified by the addition to it of a fluid rich in bicarbonates resembling in certain respects pancreatic juice. Preisig et al. found that the bile secreted in response to stimulation with taurocholate was slightly hypotonic, whereas it was hypertonic in response to secretin (295). Wheeler and Mancusi-Ungaro (394) found that the choleretic action of secretin was stronger when it was infused into the hepatic artery (which supplies the ductules system) than when it was infused into the splenic vein. They further found that the washout volume of sulfobromophtalein administered to the animals on transition from low basal to highly stimulated bile secretion was distinctly smaller with secretin than with taurocholate. This suggested that secretin acted at some site of the biliary tract distal to the canaliculi. O'Maille et al. (281) found that excretion of bromosulphtalein administered to dogs in excess of its basal biliary excretion rate could be increased if bile flow was increased by the administration of taurocholate but not by secretin. They also concluded that taurocholate was acting at the canalicular, and secretin at the ductular level. Nahrwold found that in dogs the epithelium of the large bile ducts secretes in response to secretin (273). Rous and McMaster had previously found that the common duct of the dog could secrete alkaline fluid (308).

That the bicarbonate concentration of bile is increased by secretin has been found not only in dogs (192,395) but also in cats (327), sheep (70), and in man (384), as well as in the isolated perfused livers of the pig (153) and calf (288). Working with the isolated perfused pig liver preparation Hardison and Norman (153) found that the anion composition of the bile secreted in response to secretin remained fairly constant over a wide range of secretin doses. They concluded that secretin stimulated the secretion of a fluid with a fixed electrolyte composition and that ion-exchange and reabsorption processes did not play any role under normal conditions. They might do so under conditions of stasis or with elevation of biliary pressure.

That secretin and bile acids stimulate secretion from different areas of the biliary system is further suggested by their different effects on the biliary clearance of erythritol or mannitol. Forker (118) found that the biliary clearance of erythritol in guinea pig increased when the flow of bile was increased by the administration of exogenous bile acids, but not through stimulation with secretin. Prandi et al. (294) obtained evidence suggesting that in man erythritol clearance was also a measure of canalicular bile acid dependent and independent bile secretion. Strasberg et al. (350) found the same to be true for Rhesus monkeys, and Morris (259), for dogs. From all this it is tempting to state that secretin has no effect at the canalicular level and therefore does not influence either the erythritol clearance or the secretion of bile acids and pigments. As to the validity of using the erythritol clearance as a measure of canalicular bile secretion, Russel et al. (310) found that in dogs there was, a definite increase in this clearance during secretin choleresis. This increase was small compared with that during taurocholate choleresis. This implied, according to these workers, either a canalicular action of secretin on, or a certain degree of ductular permeability for erythritol. Strong evidence for the latter mechanism was also obtained by Barnhart and Combes (16).

There are, however, several observations that do not wholly confirm such a statement and suggest that secretin may, at least in some species, by some mechanism, influence processes at the canalicular level. In man Konturek et al. (211) found that when the flow of bile was increased by secretin the concentration of bile acids fell yet the total output of bile acids increased. In dogs Soloway et al. (339) observed that although exogenous secretin had a choleretic effect after termination of its administration, both bile and bile acid secretion fell below the basal secretory rate established during the preinfusion period. Jablonski et al. (183) found that secretin, given alone, lowered the output of bile acids in the isolated perfused pig liver, that CCK or pentagastrin did not influence this output, and that secretin given together with CCK or with pentagastrin increased the output. Consequently, it appeared that all three substances had an effect on bile secretion at the canalicular level. These workers also found that CCK and pentagastrin potentiated the effect of secretin on bile water and bicarbonate secretion so that the combined effect of secretin and either of the other two substances was greater than that of the sum of the effects of the substances given alone. This finding differed from an earlier observation from the same laboratory where the effects were found to be simply additive (122). The effect of secretin or other intestinal hormones on the secretion of bile acids from isolated hepatocytes (8,323) does not seem to have been investigated.

An interesting observation concerning the effect of secretin, and CCK, on the composition of hepatic bile in monkeys was made by Gardiner et al. (119), who found that the amount of bile salt secreted during secretin choleresis increased in relation to that of cholesterol and phospholipid. CCK increased the proportion of bile salt to phospholipid, but not to cholesterol.

Secretin and VIP were found to inhibit net absorption of water from the guinea pig gallbladder *in vitro,* and to induce its net secretion (260). Similar results were found for the gallbladder in anesthetized cats (185,186).

Little is known about the effects of secretin on biliary secretion in nonmammalian species. In anesthetized chickens Linari et al. (238) found that porcine secretin did not stimulate but actually inhibited the secretion of bile. In the turkey, porcine secretin was found to stimulate the secretion of hepatic bile but with little effect on its bicarbonate concentration (169). For further information see Chapter 24 by W. Y. Chey, pp. 562–612, *this volume.*

EFFECTS OF SECRETIN ON INSULIN RELEASE AND SECRETION

Another action of secretin, for which the extent of investigation seems to be out of proportion to its physiological significance, or rather insignificance, is the stimulation of insulin secretion. Again, this may be explained by the light that these investigations have shed on basic physiological mechanisms.

Four years after the discovery of secretin and 15 before the isolation of insulin Moore et al. (257) discussed the possibility that not only the external but also the internal secretion of the pancreas might be controlled "by a hormone or secretin." This possibility was subsequently investigated by many workers and conflicting findings were reported. Some preparations of secretin were found to influence blood sugar concentrations. This effect was no longer seen when purer preparations became available (4,252,347). La Barre described a factor in porcine small intestinal extracts that lowered blood sugar concentrations in rabbits and in normal dogs but not, or only weakly, in pancreatectomized dogs (217). He named this presumably insulin-releasing substance incretin. Later, he claimed however, that secretin itself could be cleaved into "excretin" and "incretin," and that incretin did have a blood sugar lowering effect also in pancreatectomized dogs (218,219). Laughton and Macallum (224) made observations suggesting the existence of an incretin, in concordance with La Barre's view. Other workers, however, could not, in careful studies, find any evidence for the regulation of blood sugar concentrations by intestinal factors (239) and interest for the possible existence of such factors declined. This remained low until 1954, when Scow and Cornfield (326) showed that in rats the increases in blood sugar concentrations following the administration of glucose were of much lesser magnitude if the sugar was given orally than if it was given intravenously.

In 1963, Arnould et al. (9) observed with a bioassay that in dogs oral glucose administration caused greater increase of plasma insulin-like activity as maintained by the degree of glycemia attained, than predicted by results obtained from work in which glucose was administered parenterally. Further work was greatly facilitated by the development of the radioimmunoassay by Yalow and Berson (405). Elrick et al. (110) found that in man there were no significant differences in plasma glucose concentration changes following oral as compared with intravenous administration of small doses of glucose, but the plasma immunoreactive insulin concentration increased far more following oral than intravenous administration. They suggested that these differences might be due to the oral glucose activating some gastrointestinal or liver factor. McIntyre et al. (242) compared in two normal subjects the effects of intravenously and intrajejunally administered glucose on plasma immunoreactive insulin and glucose concentrations. They found that following intrajejunal administration the glucose concentrations increased less and the insulin concentrations increased more than following intravenous administration. They considered that the most likely explanation for this was induction by glucose of the release of a humoral substance from the jejunal wall which, together with the rise in blood glucose concentration, stimulated insulin release from the pancreatic islets. As to the nature of this humoral substance, Dupré et al. (107) found that in man intravenous administration of a partially purified preparation of secretin, together with glucose, clearly resulted in a swifter return to basal values of the blood sugar concentrations than if glucose was given without the secretin preparation. This indicated that either secretin itself and/or some other substance in the preparation used was responsible for the accelerated glucose assimilation. Later, Dupré et al. (108) showed that in man both portal and peripheral blood concentrations of immunoreactive insulin increased after administration of essentially pure secretin. Unger et al. (377) demonstrated that in dogs injections of secretin into the portal vein resulted in increased concentrations of insulin-like immunoreactivity in pancreaticoduodenal vein blood and Pfeiffer et al. (286) observed that secretin could cause insulin release from rabbit and dog pancreatic slices *in vitro.* Hinz et al. (170) found that secretin did not stimulate release of insulin from isolated rat pancreatic islets but stimulated its release from pieces of pancreatic tissue. This was interpreted to mean that the presence of exocrine pancreatic tissue was necessary for the insulin-releasing effect of secretin. Later, however, Danielsson and Lernmark (85) as well as Best et al. (25) found that secretin did release insulin from isolated mouse islets.

That exogenous secretin released insulin in man has been confirmed by many investigators (43,46,187,285,299). Stahlheber et al. (342) found also in dogs that the administration of synthetic as well as exogenous natural secretin resulted in increased plasma insulin concentrations.

In 1962 Lechin (226) observed that in man and in normal dogs plasma potassium concentrations decreased following the administration of secretin but that no such effect occurred in alloxan diabetic or pancreatectomized dogs. He suggested that this might be explained by insulin release caused either by secretin or some contaminant in the preparation used.

Working with the perfused rat pancreas, Curry et al. (84) showed that the release of insulin in response to glucose infusion occurred in two phases—one early, but rapidly subsiding, and a second, prolonged and lasting over the duration of the glucose infusion. Porte and Pupo (290) obtained evidence suggesting that in man insulin was stored in a two-pool system—one for the acute release and the other for longer term responses. Lerner and Porte (232) found that in man, in contrast with insulin release by glucose, the release by secretin was uniphasic and apparently occurred only from a stored, readily available pool. On the other hand Kraegen et al. (214) and Dudl et al. (106) presented evidence for a two-phase action on insulin release also by secretin. Whenever the administration of exogenous secretin has been found to increase plasma insulin concentrations it has not usually been found to be accompanied by changes in blood glucose concentrations (e.g., 108,299). However, in a few cases in man Jarrett and Cohen (187) observed small and transient depressions in blood glucose concentrations following the administration of essentially pure secretin, and Kaess and Schlierf (198) made similar observations, using a less highly purified secretin. Deckert (86) and also Enk (111) reported that whereas diabetic patients responded to the administration of glucose with lower increases in plasma insulin concentrations than the non-diabetics, there was no difference in their insulin responses to exogenous secretin. Raptis et al. (299) found that only patients with subclinical and with maturity-onset diabetes had an insulin response to secretin indistinguishable from nondiabetic persons, but that this response was depressed, although not abolished, in juvenile diabetics. Deckert and Worning (87) suggested that glucose and secretin act on different release receptors on the β cell.

It is evident from the above findings that secretin, without any doubt, can release insulin from the β cell. However, it seems to be almost as clear from other investigations that this is mainly a pharmacological action, of no, or, at the most, of very limited physiological importance. No effects on plasma insulin concentrations were observed in man on release of endogenous secretin by duodenal acidification (45,198,244).

In the isolated perfused porcine pancreas Lindkaer Jensen et al. (188) found that the threshold doses of secretin for insulin release were more than a hundred times higher than for stimulation of exocrine pancreatic secretion. Yet Chisholm et al. (82) observed that oral administration of glucose resulted in increases in plasma immunoreactive secretin concentrations, which were followed by increases in insulin concentrations. This was indeed suggestive of a physiological role of secretin in insulin release. However, Sum and Preshaw (353) demonstrated that intraduodenal glucose infusion did not stimulate exocrine pancreatic secretion in man just as had been shown for dogs by Wang and Grossman (386). Other workers were unable to obtain any increases in plasma concentrations of immunoreactive secretin following oral glucose (78), and Turner (373) suggested that the antibodies used by Chisholm et al. (82) were reacting with incretin as well as with secretin. Turner reported that neither secretin nor CCK-PZ released insulin from an *in vitro* preparation of rabbit pancreas, whereas glucagon and a glucagon-free extract of porcine duodeno-jejunal mucosa caused such release. This suggested that incretin be used as a name for the uncharacterized active substance in the extract. Incretin has, however, like enterogastrone (130,191), now become a concept rather than a name for a specific peptide. Turner and co-workers have partially purified an incretin that they have referred to as IRP (insulin-releasing peptide) (374) and have discussed the possible identity of IRP with GIP. Whereas secretin is a weak incretin, GIP is a strong one (56) and VIP at any rate is stronger than secretin (189). There are indications for the existence of other, as yet uncharacterized incretins (117,234,256,409).

Apart from its effects on insulin release, a synergistic effect of secretin on the actions of insulin on glycolysis and calcium efflux in human voluntary muscle has been described by Chisholm et al. (81). An observation in which secretin was found to increase insulin bioactivity and immunoreactivity in dog plasma *in vitro* (91) does not seem to have found an explanation. Santeusanio et al. (315) reported that administration of secretin to dogs resulted in a fall of plasma glucagon concentrations. No effect of secretin administration on plasma glucagon could be found, however, in man by Dudl et al. (106) and no effect on glucagon release from the perfused pig pancreas could be observed by Jensen et al. (188). In the latter preparation VIP released glucagon at low but not at high, and insulin at high but not at low concentrations of glucose in the perfusing fluid. Shima et al. (333) found that in man secretin in doses that should produce plasma concentrations in the range occurring physiologically after a meal did not influence plasma concentrations of either glucagon or insulin.

MECHANISM OF ACTION OF SECRETIN

The information available at present does not allow a detailed understanding as to how secretin or any other polypeptide hormone exerts its action(s). However, for secretin, as for other hormones, observations have been made that provide partial answers to certain problems.

A problem, early recognized, was the source of the bicarbonate secreted by the pancreas under the influence of secretin. This was elegantly solved by Ball and co-workers, who injected radioactive (^{11}C) bicarbonate into dogs secreting pancreatic juice under the influence of secretin, and found that the ratio, approximately 5 to 1, of the concentration of radioactive bicarbonate in the pancreatic juice to that in the plasma was the same as for total juice bicarbonate to plasma bicarbonate (14). This indicated that the main part of the bicarbonate secreted was derived from plasma and not from metabolic activities of the pancreatic gland.

The pancreas is a composite organ, and the question soon arose as to which of its different cells were responsive to stimulation by secretin. Grossman and Ivy (139) showed that alloxan-diabetic dogs had a decreased pancreatic response to secretin but an apparently normal response to CCK-PZ. Since alloxan had been shown by Goldner and Gomori (120) to lead to destructive changes in the ductular epithelial but not in the acinar cells Grossman and Ivy suggested that secretin acted on the ductular, and CCK-PZ on the acinar cells. Subsequent work has supported this concept, but because of the augmentation of the effects of CCK by secretin and vice versa it would seem that secretin has also direct actions on acinar cells, and CCK on ductular ones (136). It has indeed been shown that the acinar cells of the guinea pig have receptors for secretin (303).

In contrast with many, although not all, peptide hormones, such as gastrin (370), CCK (268), or parathyrin (292) from which fragments show activities on a molar basis equal to or higher than those of the undegraded hormones, essentially the whole peptide chain of secretin appears to be necessary for a substantial degree of pancreatic stimulatory activity. During the stepwise synthesis by Bodanszky et al. (33) of porcine secretin, which started from its C-terminal valine amide, we found in the anesthetized cat that the sequence 2–27, i.e., deshistidine secretin, seemed not to have more than about 1% of the activity of the 1–27 sequence (267). Recently it has been shown that in the dog deshistidine secretin has the same ability as secretin to stimulate pancreatic secretion, but is only about 1% as potent (337).

Although several analogs and derivatives of secretin have been described, with considerable degree of secretin-like activity, none as yet have shown stronger activity than secretin itself. An analog in which the histidine had been replaced by tyrosine (407) was found to have an activity similar to that of deshistidine secretin. However, another analog in which the secretin chain had been lengthened by a tyrosine residue had an activity as high as one-fourth of that of secretin (407). Replacement of the phenylalanine in position 6 by tyrosine resulted in an analog (143) that in doses that weakly stimulated pancreatic secretion appeared to have about 10% of the secretin activity. However, the dose-response curves for this analog and for secretin were not parallel (76). An analog in which the Gly^4-Thr^5 sequence of secretin had been replaced by the Ala^4-Val^5 sequence of VIP had essentially the same activity as secretin, whereas an analog in which the His^1-Ser^2-Asp^3 sequence of secretin had been replaced by the Tyr^1-Ala^2-Glu^3 sequence of GIP had very low, although clearly demonstrable, activity (404).

Glucagon and secretin have some actions in common, i.e., both hormones stimulate lipolysis in rat adipose tissue (225,309). However, neither exhibits what, presumably, is the main action of the other, i.e., stimulation of pancreatic secretion in the case of secretin and activation of hepatic glycogenolysis in the case of glucagon. VIP, however, exhibits, although rather weakly, the main actions of both secretin and glucagon.

As pointed out in connection with the determination of the amino acid sequence (271) of VIP, an analysis of the structural similarities and differences of VIP, glucagon, and secretin might give some indication about which amino acid residues in these peptides may be of importance for secretin-like and glucagon-like activities. For instance, looking at the N-terminal tripeptide sequences of glucagon (histidylserylglutaminyl-), secretin (histidylserylaspartyl-), and VIP (histidylserylaspartyl-), it is evident that all three have identical structures in positions 1 and 2 but in position 3 the two stimulators of pancreatic secretion, VIP and secretin, have a residue of aspartic acid, whereas the nonstimulating glucagon has a residue of glutamine. Consequently it might be reasonable to investigate whether or not the aspartic acid residue in position 3 might be necessary for a peptide to have secretin-like activity. There is some evidence from synthetic work that this might be so. Before the discovery of VIP, in connection with their synthesis of secretin (33), Bodanszky and co-workers sent us a sample of 3-asparaginyl secretin and this was found to have very weak secretin-like activity (267). The same has subsequently been found to be true of the 3-glutaminyl and 3-glutamyl (404) analogs, the latter observation showing that it is not sufficient to have an acidic group in position 3; this group must be in the correct geometric relation to the other structures. This was indeed already indicated by the finding that an analog with very weak secretin activity results if the Asp^3 to Gly^4 linkage is by the β-carboxyl of the aspartic acid rather than by the α-carboxyl. Such a conversion of α-aspartyl to β-aspartyl is the basis of one of the *in vitro* inactivation mechanisms for secretin (184, 206,282). Whether or not this has any importance *in vivo* is not known.

Following the discovery by Sutherland and co-workers of the role of adenosine-3', 5'-monophosphate (cyclic AMP) as the intracellular second messenger for the actions of catecholamines and certain peptide hormones (297,357), much work has been carried out on individual peptide hormones to define if, and if so to what extent, their actions are mediated by cyclic AMP, or guanosine 3',5' monophosphate (cyclic GMP). Also, secretin has been extensively investigated in this connection, but a clear picture has not been obtained. There is, however, a considerable amount of indirect evidence that some of the actions of secretin may be mediated by cyclic AMP. Case et al. found that in the perfused cat pancreas dibutyryl cyclic AMP stimulated in a secretin-like fashion the secretion of water and bicarbonate, but not of enzymes. It was also found that the action of small doses of secretin was markedly enhanced by theophylline, which is known, among its other actions, to inhibit the enzyme phosphodiesterase that inactivates cyclic AMP (73,74). Case et al. then showed that following administration of secretin to anesthetized cats there was an increase in the concentrations of cyclic AMP in pancreatic tissue (72). These increases occurred, however, in two phases—an initial rise and fall in parallel with the effect of the secretin on pancreatic secretion, and then a second rise without stimulation of secretion, suggesting that there was no simple relationship between pancreatic cyclic AMP concentrations and secretion.

Bhoola and Lemon found that in the cat pancreas adenylate cyclase, the enzyme that catalyzes the formation of cyclic AMP from adenosine triphosphate is activated by secretin, but not by PZ (26), and Bonting et al. (40) found that imidazole, known to stimulate phosphodiesterase activity, inhibits secretin action.

In dogs Tompkins et al. (369) reported that theophylline increased pancreatic responses to secretin, but the opposite was found by Guelrud et al. (142). More recently Domschke et al. (98) found that secretin increased cyclic AMP levels in pancreatic tissue in dogs and that this increase was parallel with pancreatic secretion of cyclic AMP and bicarbonate. In the rabbit pancreas theophylline was found to have a secretin-like action (203) on cyclic AMP.

In homogenates of rat pancreatic tissue secretin was shown by two groups of investigators to stimulate adenylate cyclase activity (247,313). Other investigators found this to be true for fragments of rat pancreatic tissue (89).

In vivo secretin has been found to increase the cyclic AMP concentrations of rat pancreatic tissue (304). In man Domschke et al. (98) reported that secretin administration caused parallel increases in pancreatic secretion of bicarbonate and cyclic AMP. In rat adipose tissue stimulation of lipolysis by secretin was found to be accompanied by an increased adenylate cyclase activity in "ghosts" of fat cells (307) and apparently also in cell-free homogenates of rat adipose tissue (65).

Seemingly contradictory findings have been obtained by various workers concerning the involvement of cyclic AMP in secretin-stimulated choleresis. Levine and Hall (236) have recently reviewed the earlier work and pointed out that there might be important species variations in this respect. They, themselves, obtained evidence for a regulatory role of cyclic AMP in choleresis in man and baboons, but not in dogs. Poupon et al. (293) could find no evidence for cyclic AMP being involved in secretin choleresis in dogs or rats.

One group of investigators found that secretin, in high concentrations, activated guanyl cyclase in homogenates of several, but not all, types of rat tissue. Some of the tissues in which activation was observed (i.e., brain cortex and skeletal muscle) are not known to be target tissues for secretin (367).

Although convincing evidence seems to have been presented in some cases for secretin action to be accompanied by increases in tissue concentrations of cyclic AMP, nothing is yet known about how such concentration changes result in the known physiological actions of secretin, if any. The problem of cyclic nucleotides in relation to secretin and to other gastrointestinal hormones has been the object of several recent reviews (e.g. 199,235). It has also been discussed by several workers at a conference on stimulus-secretion coupling in the gastrointestinal tract (72).

Whether or not dopamine, which by itself exhibits secretin-like actions on both biliary (156) and pancreatic (126,157) secretion, is in any way involved in mediating the activities of secretin is not known (18).

BIOASSAY OF SECRETIN

If secretin is to be used for clinical or physiological work it must be quantitated in terms of its bioactivity. Since preparations that have lost their bioactivity may still be immunoreactive, only bioassay seems to be useful for this purpose. Secretin shows many types of bioactivity and it may be that several of these could be used as the basis for its bioassay. In practice the only activity that has been used is stimulation of pancreatic secretion, with the pancreatic response to graded doses of secretin being registered. Since there is a great variation in the response of the pancreas, even among individuals of the same species, it has long been recognized that the estimation of the strength of an unknown preparation has to be done by comparing the pancreatic responses of graded doses of the unknown with the responses to a standard preparation (125,146). There is still no accepted international reference standard of secretin available but there is reason to believe that such a preparation will be available before long. (Personal communication from Prof. D. R. Bangham, National Institute for Biological Standards and Control, Holly Hill, Hampstead, London NW3 6RB England.)

The biological activity of secretin is usually expressed in clinical units (4). Pure lyophilized secretin acetate is assumed to have 4 clinical units (c.u.) per microgram. Recalculated to the free secretin base this would be 5 c.u./μg. The dose for the clinical secretin test is usually considered to be 1 c.u./kg body weight but there is some ambiguity in this regard. Recently Domschke et al. (98) found that in man maximal flow of pancreatic juice was obtained by the administration of 0.5 c.u./kg body weight/hr. The response may be registered either by measuring the volume of juice secreted (125) or by titration of the alkali content (146). Different species of animals have been used: dogs, anesthetized (125,182,237) or conscious (341) cats, anesthetized (63,146,182,252) or conscious (208), anesthetized rabbits (99) and anesthetized rats (159,237, 241,322,359). The use of the isolated, perfused cat pancreas for the assay of secretin and substances with "secretin-like" activity in tissues and biological fluids has been described by Scratcherd et al. (328) and the effects of secretin on the isolated and perfused dog pancreas have been reported by Nardi et al. (274), Hermon-Taylor (166), Stock et al. (349), and by Kowalewski and Kolodej (212). Heatley (159) has discussed the problems involved in assaying secretin in crude extracts of intestinal tissue that may contain CCK and that would potentiate the action of secretin, thereby giving erroneously high values.

In our own work we have used cats anesthetized with Placidyl® for periods of up to a week for titration of the alkali secreted in response to secretin (196). We have also used minks (unpublished experiments in collaboration with K. Burlin), and although we have found them to be a poor substitute for cats, they can be used at times when the latter are not available.

RADIOIMMUNOASSAY OF SECRETIN

The first RIA of secretin seems to have been described by Young et al. (408), who worked with antisera obtained in rabbits after immunization with porcine secretin conjugated to rabbit serum albumin. Radioiodination of the tracer was carried out by a slight modification of the chloramine T method of Hunter and Greenwood (177). Since secretin contains no residue of tyrosine it was assumed that the histidine residue was iodinated. The absence of tyrosine in secretin has led to various attempts to iodinate derivatives or analogs of secretin that contain such residues. Raptis et al. (298) used 6-tyrosyl secretin (143), Yanaihara et al., N$^\alpha$-tyrosylsecretin and (Tyr^1)-secretin (407), Urbach et al. (378), des-tyrosyl-β-alanylsecretin. Numerous publications have, however, described the radioiodination of secretin as such, as it had been done in the original work of Young et al. (408). Indeed Straus et al. (351), Rayford et al. (301), and Schaffalitzky de Muckadell and Fahrenkrug (316,317) found that there was no advantage in the use of 6-tyrosyl-secretin over secretin itself. In most of the cases some modification of the chloramine T technique (177) has been used for the iodination [Teale et al. (362), Boden and Chey (35), Tai et al. (360), Straus et al. (351), Hanssen and Torjesen (152), Byrnes and Marjason (68), Rayford et al. (301), Fahrenkrug et al. (116), and Burhol et al. (62)]. Others [Holohan et al. (172) and Bloom et al. (28)] have used the lactoperoxidase procedure (368) for oxidizing the iodide. Schaffalitzky de Muckadell and Fahrenkrug (316) prepared their iodinated tracers by either iodinating secretin with the chloramine T, lactoperoxidase, or by the gaseous diffusion (67) methods, or by preparation of the ^{125}I-labeled 3-(4-hydroxyphenyl) propionyl derivative (38) of secretin. They found that the chloramine T method was the easiest and gave the most reproducible results.

Antibodies to secretin have been generated in rabbits by immunization with secretin coupled to bovine serum albumin (28,35,62,116,205,298,321,378), to rabbit serum albumin (408), to ovalbumin (68,362), or to guinea pig serum albumin (351). Antibodies in guinea pigs to secretin coupled to guinea pig serum albumin have been described by Straus et al. (351). Unconjugated secretin adsorbed to microfine carbon particles has been used for antibody production in rabbits by Buchanan et al. (59), and secretin mixed with polyvinylpyrrolidone by Yanaihara et al. (407). Secretin as such has been used by Fahrenkrug et al. (116) and Burhol and Waldum (62). These two groups of workers compared antibody production in rabbits with secretin and with secretin conjugated to bovine serum albumin. They found no evidence for any difference in immunization efficiency between the two types of antigen. For additional information, see Chapter 34 by T. M. Chang and W. Y. Chey, pp. 797–817, *this volume.*

CLINICAL USE OF SECRETIN

The great early interest in the purification of secretin was in no small part due to the obvious potential that the hormone had as a diagnostic aid in the investigation of pancreatic function. The first to use it for this purpose seem to have been Chiray et al. (80), who worked with a preparation produced by Penau and Simonnet (284). Using material of much higher purity and constant activity, prepared by Ågren and Hammarsten (4), Lagerlöf carried out an extensive investigation of human pancreatic activity in health and disease (220,220a). Comprehensive investigations were also carried out by Diamond et al. (92,93). The "secretin test," and later the "secretin pancreozymin test" (64,355) of pancreatic function, in which the response of the pancreas to known amounts of the hormone(s) is determined as to the volume of juice secreted and its concentration in bicarbonate and various enzymes, has played an important role in the diagnosis of pancreatic disease and continues to do so (39,100,147,148,231, 302,354,358,375,380,388,410). Recent discussions of the test with special reference to specific topics were reported for pancreatic cancer by Löffler et al. (240) and Dreiling (101), for cirrhosis of the liver by Van Goidsenhoven et al. (381) and Turnberg and Grahame (372), and for pancreatic hypersecretory states by Dreiling and Bordalo (102) and Dreiling et al. (103). Comprehensive discussions of the test were published by Dreiling and Janowitz (104), Lagerlöf (221), and Zimmerman et al. (411). Since the pancreatic juice is collected by duodenal intubation, the use of a double lumen tube, one bore of which is for removal of the gastric juice and the other for collection of the duodenal aspirate, has been essential (92,220). Later improvements, or modifications, of the original methodology include the infusion of a nonabsorbable marker into the duodenum, permitting correction of the volume of the duodenal juice for incomplete recovery (221a,222) use of larger doses of secretin than in the ordinary procedure (41, 149,155,222,397), the use of stimulation by infusion rather than by bolus injection of the hormone(s) (15,144,329,397), and more recently by the direct cannulation of the papilla of Vater under duodenoscopic visualization, which permits collection of pancreatic juice contaminated by other duodenal fluids (42,128,213). It is, however, not only in the secretin-pancreozymin test that secretin has been found to be useful. In 1949 McNeer and Ewing (243) in collaboration with Papanicolaou identified exfoliated cells from a pancreatic carcinoma in the duodenal aspirate of a jaundiced patient. They suggested that cytological study of duodenal aspirates might prove to be of value in the diagnosis of jaundiced patients. Independently of this observation Lemon and Byrnes (229) pointed out that cytological analysis of duodenal aspirates might be of value in the diagnosis of cancer of the biliary tract and the pancreas. Other workers made similar observations at that time but published them later (44).

Raskin et al. (300) reported on a series of 356 duodenal intubations in which they had encountered carcinoma in 55 cases and in 33 of these malignant cells were recovered. They considered stimulation of pancreatic secretion with secretin to be essential for the success of the method. Dreiling et al. (105) found that the study of exfoliated cells obtained from duodenal drainage was of great value for the diagnosis of cancer of the pancreas and the biliary tract. Goldstein et al. (121), Cabre-Fiol and Vilardell (69), Asnaes and Johansen (10), and Nundy et al. (279) have also found the method useful. Kozu et al. (213) and Hatfield et al. (158) described the selective collection of pancreatic juice for cytodiagnosis by cannulation of the papilla of Vater. A review of pancreatic cytology has been published by Butler (66).

Secretin has also been found to be of value for angiographic visualization of the pancreas (24,201,361,376).

Rather unexpectedly secretin has been found to be of value also in the differential diagnosis of the Zollinger-Ellison syndrome (gastrinoma) (412) in relation to other gastrin hypersecretory states. Usually, secretin depresses the plasma levels of immunoreactive gastrin (150). However, Isenberg et al. (179) observed that in some, but not all, patients with gastrinoma exogenous secretin increases plasma gastrin concentrations. This paradoxical effect of secretin has been repeatedly confirmed (13,47,204,366).

In addition to its accepted diagnostic uses there have been suggestions for the therapeutic use of secretin. Secretin has been shown to strongly inhibit the secretion of gastric acid in dogs (127,401), if this secretion was stimulated by gastrin, but less strongly if stimulated by feeding (334). In rats exogenous secretin has also been shown to be an efficient inhibitor of pentagastrin-stimulated gastric acid secretion (371). In cats, however, secretin is a weak inhibitor of acid secretion (346) and in the chicken it does not inhibit it at all, but stimulates it instead (61). In man secretin has been found to inhibit acid secretion, an effect weaker than in the dog, but stronger than in the cat (52). However, apart from its effects on acid secretion the pancreatic juice secreted in response to secretin will neutralize gastric acid as much as in the duodenal bulb (6). Grossman (135) suggested that the possibility of using exogenous secretin for the treatment of duodenal ulcer disease should be investigated and pointed out that long-term treatment with secretin might act as a "medical gastrectomy" (137). A few such investigations have been carried out. In cats Konturek (207) found that peptic ulcers induced by the administration of large doses of pentagastrin could be prevented by the administration of secretin, and similar results were obtained in rats (190). In man the observations are not conclusive. Some investigators have reported at least suggestive results in favor of such a form of treatment (88,171), whereas others in collaboration with Grossman found no differences between treatment with secretin or placebo (161). Shepherd et al. (332) reported favorable results in the treatment of the gastric hypersecretion in some patients with chronic renal failure. Stanley et al. (343) showed that pentagastrin-induced parietal cell hyperplasia in rats (83) could be prevented by secretin. As pointed out by Demling et al. (88), the stimulatory effect of secretin on pepsin secretion might, however, be a problem in any long-term use of exogenous secretin. It should be mentioned that Henriksen et al. have found that exogenous secretin and CCK given together augmented each other's inhibitory actions on pentagastrin-stimulated gastric acid secretion in man (163). Recently interest in secretin for the treatment of ulcer disease has declined because of the efficiency of the histamine H_2-blockers (27,49) in preventing gastric secretion of acid.

Another possible use for secretin has been suggested by the recent work of Hughes et al. (176), who showed that daily administration of secretin and CCK to dogs prevented the intestinal mucosal hypoplasia due to prolonged parenteral nutrition. It is not clear from this study whether the preventive effect was due to trophic actions of secretin or CCK or both, or whether it was due to the pancreatic secretion entering the intestinal lumen because of hormonal stimulation, which the authors consider more plausible. That secretin may have trophic effects on the pancreas in rats has recently been shown by Solomon et al. (338).

Pathophysiologically, secretin has been implicated as the causative agent in the "pancreatic cholera" (248) or WDHA syndrome (246) [*w*atery *d*iarrhea, *h*ypokalemia (296,383) *a*chlorhydria (113)]. Extracts of tumor tissue from patients with this syndrome were found to exhibit a secretin-like stimulating activity on the exocrine pancreas in dogs (413). However, it has been found later that material with VIP-like immunoreactivity could have been obtained from such tumor extracts (31) and that VIP had secretin-like action on the exocrine pancreas. (The action of VIP on the pancreas, at least in the anesthetized cat, differs from the action of secretin by having a distinctly shorter duration, but this may be difficult to quantify.) Besides VIP, GIP also has been stated to occur in such tumors (109) and in one patient increased plasma concentrations of both VIP and GIP have been described (216).

Another indication for a pathological role of secretin comes from veterinary medicine. It has been suggested that endogenous secretin could be a significant etiologic factor in the development of the ruminal atony, seen in ruminants suffering from acute lactic acid acidosis (174).

SUMMARY AND CONCLUSIONS

The amino acid sequence is, as yet, known only for porcine secretin, and is as follows:

His-Ser-Asp-Gly-Thr-Phe-Thr-Ser-Glu-Leu-Ser-Arg-Leu-Arg-Asp-Ser-Ala-Arg-Leu-Gln-Arg-Leu-Leu-Gln-Gly-Leu-Val-NH_2

All secretin fragments have been found to be either inactive or to have weak activity compared with the intact molecule.

Secretin has demonstrated many pharmacological actions. Physiologically, it is believed to stimulate, in mammals, the pancreatic secretion of water and bicarbonate, and to potentiate the stimulating action of CCK on pancreatic enzyme secretion. There is fairly strong evidence that this physiological action of secretin on the pancreas is in some way mediated by cyclic AMP.

The only known physiological mechanism for the release of secretin is acidification of the upper intestine.

Secretin has been used for the diagnosis of pancreatic disease for over half a century and here its value is unquestionable. Despite such long use the methodology has not stagnated, and new approaches have been suggested. Rather unexpectedly secretin has found use in the differential diagnosis of the Zollinger-Ellison syndrome from other gastrin hypersecretory states.

Secretin has not yet found any accepted place in therapy, but there have been recent suggestions, for its use in the treatment of duodenal ulcer disease.

PROJECTIONS FOR THE FUTURE

Porcine secretin is chemically related to the porcine hormonal peptides glucagon, GIP, VIP, and also PHI (see Chapter 43 [II] by K. Tatemoto, pp. 995–997, *this volume*). There is no reason to believe that all peptides belonging to this group have already been isolated from even the porcine species. A search for additional members may yield results that will be interesting from functional, evolutionary, and perhaps also other aspects. Isolation of secretin and its related peptides from other species may give additional valuable information.

For 77 years it has been an established fact that secretin stimulates pancreatic secretion in mammals, and this has always been held to be its main function. This may well be so. However, the puzzling finding that secretin in birds is a weak stimulant of pancreatic secretion as compared with VIP, which is a strong stimulant, raises suspicion that in this class of vertebrates secretin may have some quite other function than stimulation of pancreatic secretion, and this may be true in mammals as well.

It is known that many, perhaps all, hormones are biosynthesized in larger precursor forms. This has been shown for glucagon, closely related to secretin chemically, but not as yet for secretin itself. The identification of such secretin precursor(s) will certainly satisfy intellectual curiosity and may possibly lead to practical applications.

For many peptide hormones, releasing factors of hormonal nature have been described. No such factor has been described for secretin as yet, but it is unlikely that none of these exists.

REFERENCES

1. Adelson, J. W. (1971): Enterosecretory proteins. *Nature,* 229:321–325.
2. Adelson, J. W. (1975): Chymodenin: An overview. In: *Gastrointestinal Hormones,* edited by J. C. Thompson, pp. 563–574. University of Texas Press, Austin and London.
3. Affolter, H., Piller, M., and Gubler, A. (1964): Tierexperimentelle Untersuchungen über die Wirkung von gereinigtem Sekretin und Cholecystokinin-pankreozymin, sowie von Decholin auf die Gallensekretion. *Gastroenterologia,* 101:247–258.
4. Ågren, G. (1934): Uber die pharmakodynamischen Wirkungen und chemischen Eigenschaften des Secretins. *Skand. Arch. Physiol.,* 70:10–87.
5. Ågren, G., and Lagerlöf, H. (1937): The biliary response in the secretin test. *Acta Med. Scand.,* XCII:359–366.
6. Andersson, S., and Grossman M. I. (1965): Effect of vagal denervation of pouches on gastric secretion in dogs with intact or resected antrums. *Gastroenterology,* 48:449–462.

7. Angelucci, L., Balderi, M., and Linari, G. (1970): The action of caerulein on pancreatic and biliary secretions of the chicken. *Eur. J. Pharmacol.,* 11:217–232.
8. Anwer, M. S., Kroker, R., and Hegner, D. (1975): Bile acids secretion and synthesis by isolated rat hepatocytes. *Biochem. Biophys. Res. Commun.,* 64:603–609.
9. Arnould, Y., Bellens, R., Franckson, J. R. M., and Conard, V. (1963): Insulin response and glucose-C^{14} disappearance rate during the glucose tolerance test in the unanesthetized dog. *Metabolism,* 12:1122–1131.
10. Asnaes, S., and Johansen, A. (1970): Duodenal exfoliative cytology. Duodenal drainage smears after stimulation with secretin. *Acta Pathol. Microbiol. Scand. (Suppl.),* 212:11–14.
11. Babkin, B. P., and Sawitsch, W. W. (1908): Zur Frage über den Gehalt an festen Bestandteilen in dem auf verschiedene Sekretionserreger erhaltenen pankreatischen Saft. *Hoppe-Seyler's Z. Physiol. Chem.,* 56:321–342.
12. Balabaud, C., Noel, M., and Dangoumau, J. (1977): Influence de la sécrétine sur la cholérèse chez le rat. *J. Pharmacol.,* 8:191–196.
13. Bali, J. P., Balmes, J. L., Fournajoux, J., Cayrol, B., and Khazrai, H. (1972): Effects of secretin on immuno-reactive serum gastrin in two cases of Zollinger-Ellison Syndrome. *Digestion,* 7:277–283.
14. Ball, E. G., Tucker, H. F., Solomon, A. K., and Vennesland, B. (1941): The source of pancreatic juice bicarbonate. *J. Biol. Chem.,* 140:119–129.
15. Banwell, J. G., Northam, B. E., and Cooke, W. T. (1967): Secretory response of the human pancreas to continuous intravenous infusion of secretin. *Gut,* 8:50–57.
16. Barnhart, J. L., and Combes, B. (1978): Erythritol and mannitol clearances with taurocholate and secretin-induced cholereses. *Am. J. Physiol.,* 234:E146–E156.
17. Barrington, E. J. W., and Dockray, G. J. (1970): The effect of intestinal extracts of lampreys (*Lampetra fluviatilis* and *Petromyzon marinus*) on pancreatic secretion in the rat. *Gen. Comp. Endocrinol.,* 14:170–177.
18. Bastie, M. J., Vaysse, N., Brenac, B., Pascal, J. P., and Ribet, A. (1977): Effects of catecholamines and their inhibitors on the isolated canine pancreas. *Gastroenterology,* 72:719–723.
19. Bayliss, W. M., and Starling, E. H. (1902): On the causation of the so-called "peripheral reflex secretion" of the pancreas. *Proc. Roy. Soc.,* 69:352–353.
20. Bayliss, W. M., and Starling, E. H. (1902): The mechanism of pancreatic secretion. *J. Physiol.,* 28:325–353.
21. Bayliss, W. M., and Starling, E. H. (1903): On the uniformity of the pancreatic mechanism in vertebrata. *J. Physiol.,* 29:174–180.
22. Bayliss, W. M. (1915): *Principles of General Physiology.* Longmans, Green, London.
23. Becker, N. M. (1893): Contributions á la physiologie et á la pharmacologie de la glande pancréatique. *Arch. Sci. Biol. St. Petersburg,* II: 433–461.
24. Bennet, J., Chérigié, E., Caroli, J., Doyon, D., Economopoulos, P., Plessier, J., and Stoopen, M. (1967): La pancréatographie après stimulation par la sécrétine intra-artérielle. *Ann. Radiol.,* 10:617–625.
25. Best, L., Atkins, T. W., and Matty, A. J. (1976): Effect of gastrointestinal hormones on the phasic release of insulin from isolated islets of normal and obese hyperglycaemic mice. *J. Endocrinol.,* 65:57–58p.
26. Bhoola, K. D., and Lemon, M. J. C. (1973): Studies on the activation of adenylate cyclase from the submaxillary gland and pancreas. *J. Physiol.,* 232:83–84p.
27. Black, J. W., Duncan, W. A. M., Durant, C. J., Ganellin, C. R., and Parsons, E. M. (1972): Definition and antagonism of histamine H_2-receptors. *Nature,* 236:385–390.
28. Bloom, S. R. (1975): The development of a radioimmunoassay for secretin. In: *Gastrointestinal Hormones,* edited by J. C. Thompson, pp. 257–268. University of Texas Press, Austin and London.
29. Bloom, S. R., and Ogawa, O. (1973): Radioimmunoassay of human peripheral plasma secretin. *J. Endocrinol.,* 58:xxiv–xxv.
30. Bloom, S. R., and Polak, J. M. (1978): Gut hormone overview. In *Gut Hormones,* edited by S. R. Bloom, pp. 3–18. Churchill Livingstone, Edinburgh, London, and New York.
31. Bloom, S. R., Polak, J. M., and Pearse, A. G. S. (1973): Vasoactive intestinal peptide and watery-diarrhea syndrome. *Lancet,* ii:14–16.
32. Bodanszky, M., and Fink, M. L. (1976): Studies on the conformation of secretin. The position of the helical stretch. *Bioorg. Chem.,* 5:275–282.
33. Bodanszky, M., Ondetti, M. A., Lewine, S. D., Narayanan, V. L., von Salza, M., Sheehan,

J. T., Williams, N. J., and Sabo, E. F. (1966): Synthesis of a heptacosapeptide amide with the hormonal activity of secretin. *Chem. Industr.,* 42:1757–1758.

34. Bodanszky, A., Ondetti, M. A., Mutt, V., and Bodanszky, M. (1969): Synthesis of secretin. IV. Secondary structure in a miniature protein. *J. Am. Chem. Soc.,* 91:944–949.
35. Boden, G., and Chey, W. Y. (1973): Preparation and specificity of antiserum to synthetic secretin and its use in a radioimmunoassay (RIA). *Endocrinology,* 92:1617–1624.
36. Boden, G., Essa, N., and Owen, O. E. (1975): Effects of intraduodenal amino acids, fatty acids, and sugars on secretin concentrations. *Gastroenterology,* 68:722–727.
37. Boden, G., Essa, N., Owen, O. E., Reichle, F. A., and Saraga, W. (1974): Effects of intraduodenal administration of HCl and glucose on circulating immunoreactive secretin and insulin concentrations. *J. Clin. Invest.,* 53:1185–1193.
38. Bolton, A. E., and Hunter, W. M. (1973): The labelling of proteins to high specific radioactivities by conjugation to a ^{125}I-containing acylating agent. *Biochem. J.,* 133:529–539.
39. Bondar, Z. A., and Tuzhilin, S. A. (1974): The diagnostic significance of excretory pancreatic tests. *Am. J. Gastroenterol.,* 62:488–469.
40. Bonting, S. L., Case, R. M., de Pont, J. J. H. H. M., Kempen, H. J. M., and Scratcherd, T. (1974): Further evidence that secretin stimulates pancreatic secretion through adenosine 3',5'-monophosphate (cyclic AMP). *J. Physiol.,* 240:34–35.
41. Bordalo, O., Noronha, M., Lamy, J., and Dreiling, D. (1976): Standardund verstärkter Sekretintest bei der chronischen Pankreatitis. *Münch. Med. Wochenschr.,* 118:415–420.
42. Bornschein, W. (1978): Endoskopische quantitative Pankreassekretions-analyse als kurztest (Sekretin-caerulein-Kurztest/SCKT/). *Z. Castroenterol.,* 16:582–592.
43. Bottermann, P., Souvatzoglou, A., and Schwarz, K. (1967): Stimulierung der Beta-cytotropenwirkung von Tolbutamid durch Sekretin beim Menschen. *Klin. Wochenschr.,* 45:549–550.
44. Bowden, L., and Papanicolaou, G. N. (1959): Exfoliated pancreatic cancer cells in the duct of Wirsung. *Ann. Surg.,* 150:296–298.
45. Boyns, D. R., Jarrett, R. J., and Keen, H. (1966): Intestinal hormones and plasma-insulin. *Lancet,* 1:409–410.
46. Boyns, D. R., Jarrett, R. J., and Keen, H. (1967): Intestinal hormones and plasma insulin: An insulinotropic action of secretin. *Br. Med. J.,* 2:676–678.
47. Bradley, E. L. III., and Galambos, J. T. (1976): Diagnosis of gastrinoma by the secretin suppression test. *Surg. Gynecol. Obstet.,* 143:784–788.
48. Bradley, E. L. III., Wenger, J., Smith, R. B. III., and Galambos, J. T. (1975): Serum calcium responses to exogenous secretin. *Arch. Surg.,* 110:1221–1223.
49. *Br. Med. J.* (1978): Cimetidine for ever (and ever and ever . . .)? Editorial. 1:1435–1436.
50. Bromer, W. W., Sinn, L. G., and Behrens, O. K. (1957): The amino acid sequence of glucagon. V. Location of amide groups, acid degradation studies and summary of sequential evidence. *J. Am. Chem. Soc.,* 79:2807–2810.
51. Brooks, A. M., and Grossman, M. I. (1970): Postprandial pH and neutralizing capacity of the proximal duodenum in dogs. *Gastroenterology,* 59:85–89.
52. Brooks, A. M., and Grossman, M. I. (1970): Effect of secretin and cholecystokinin on pentagastrin-stimulated gastric secretion in man. *Gastroenterology,* 59:114–119.
53. Brown, J. C., Harper, A. A., and Scratcherd, T. (1967): Potentiation of secretin stimulation of the pancreas. *J. Physiol.,* 190:519–530.
54. Brown, J. C., and Dryburgh, J. R. (1971): A gastric inhibitory polypeptide II: The complete amino acid sequence. *Can. J. Biochem.,* 49:867–872.
55. Brown, J. C., Mutt, V., and Dryburgh, J. R. (1971): The further purification of motilin, a gastric motor activity stimulating polypeptide from the mucosa of the small intestine of hogs. *Can. J. Physiol. Pharmacol.,* 49:399–405.
56. Brown, J. C., and Pederson, R. A. (1976): GI hormones and insulin secretion. In: *Proceedings of the V International Congress of Endocrinology, Hamburg,* edited by V. H. T. James, pp. 568–570. Excerpta Medica, Amsterdam.
57. Brunner, H., Slat, B., Kretschmer, G., Funovics, J., and Grabner, G. (1975): Secretin-induced bile secretion, bile acid output and blood supply to the liver in the dog. *Eur. Surg. Res.,* 7:205–211.
58. Buchanan, K. D., Henry, R. W., McLoughlin, J. C., O'Connor, F. A., Calvert, H., and Doherty, C. C. (1978): Control of circulating secretin levels by oral nutrients or fluid in healthy human subjects. *Scand. J. Gastroenterol. (Suppl. 49),* 13:33.
59. Buchanan, K. D., Teale, J. D., and Harper, G. (1972): Antibodies to unconjugated synthetic and natural secretins. *Horm. Metab. Res.,* 4:507.

60. Buffa, R., Capella, C., Solcia, E., Frigerio, B., and Said, S. I. (1977): Vasoactive intestinal peptide (VIP) cells in the pancreas and gastro-intestinal mucosa. *Histochemistry,* 50:217–227.
61. Burhol, P. G. (1974): Gastric stimulation by intravenous injection of cholecystokinin and secretin in fistula chickens. *Scand. J. Gastroenterol.,* 9:49–53.
62. Burhol, P. G., and Waldum, H. L. (1978): Production and evaluation of secretin antibodies. *Acta Hepato-Gastroenterol.,* 25:139–143.
63. Burn, J. H., and Holton, P. (1948): The standardization of secretin and pancreozymin. *J. Physiol.,* 107:449–455.
64. Burton, P., Evans, D. G., Harper, A. A., Howat, H. T., Oleesky, S., Scott, J. E., and Varley, H. (1960): A test of pancreatic function in man based on the analysis of duodenal contents after administration of secretin and pancreozymin. *Gut,* 1:111–124.
65. Butcher, R. W., and Carlson, L. A. (1970): Effects of secretin on fat mobilizing lipolysis and cyclic AMP levels in rat adipose tissue. *Acta Physiol. Scand.,* 79:559–563.
66. Butler, E. B. (1972): Pancreatic cytology. *Clin. Gastroenterol.,* 1:53–60.
67. Butt, W. R. (1972): The iodination of follicle-stimulating and other hormones for radioimmunoassay. *J. Endocrinol.,* 55:453–454.
68. Byrnes, D. J., and Marjason, J. P. (1976): Radioimmunoassay of secretin in plasma. *Horm. Metab. Res.,* 8:361–365.
69. Cabre-Fiol, V., and Vilardell, F. (1974): Citodiagnóstico del cáncer de páncreas. *Rev. Esp. Enferm. Apar. Dig.,* XLIII:351–364.
70. Caple, I., and Heath, T. (1972): Regulation of output of electrolytes in bile and pancreatic juice in sheep. *Aust. J. Biol. Sci.,* 25:155–165.
71. Case, R. M., and Goebell, H. (1976): *Stimulus-Secretion Coupling in the Gastrointestinal Tract.* MTP Press Ltd, Lancaster, England.
72. Case, R. M., Johnson, M., Scratcherd, T., and Sherratt, H. S. A. (1972): Cyclic adenosine $3',5'$-monophosphate concentration in the pancreas following stimulation by secretin, cholecystokinin-pancreozymin and acetylcholine. *J. Physiol.,* 223:669–684.
73. Case, R. M., Laundy, T. J., and Scratcherd, T. (1969): Adenosine $3',5'$-monophosphate (cyclic AMP) as the intracellular mediator of the action of secretin on the exocrine pancreas. *J. Physiol.,* 204:45–47p.
74. Case, R. M., and Scratcherd, T. (1972): The actions of dibutyryl cyclic adenosine $3',5'$-monophosphate and methyl xanthines on pancreatic exocrine secretion. *J. Physiol.,* 223:649–667.
75. Chenderovitch, J. (1973): Bile secretion. *Clin. Gastroenterol.,* 2:31–47.
76. Chey, W. Y., and Hendricks, J. (1974): Biological actions of a synthetic secretin and 6-tyrosyl-secretin in rats and dogs. In: *Endocrinology of the Gut,* edited by W. Y. Chey and F. P. Brooks, pp. 107–115. C. B. Slack, Inc. New Jersey.
77. Chey, W. Y., Lee, Y. H., Hendricks, J. G., Rhodes, R. A., and Tai, H.-H. (1978): Plasma secretin concentrations in fasting and postprandial state in man. *Am. J. Dig. Dis.,* 23:981–988.
78. Chey, W. Y., Oliai, A., and Boehm, M. (1974): Radioimmunoassay (RIA) of secretin ii. Studies on correlation between RIA secretin levels and biological investigations. In: *Endocrinology of the Gut,* edited by W. Y. Chey and F. P. Brooks, pp. 320–326. C. B. Slack, Thorofare, New Jersey.
79. Chey, W. Y., Tai, H.-H., Rhodes, R., Lee, K. Y., and Hendricks, J. (1975): Radioimmunoassay of secretin: Further studies. In: *Gastrointestinal Hormones,* edited by J. C. Thompson, pp. 269–281. University of Texas Press, Austin and London.
80. Chiray, M. M., Salmon, A.-R., and Mergier, A. (1926): Action de la sécrétine purifiée sur la sécrétion externe du pancréas de l'homme. *Bull. Soc. Med. Hop. Paris,* 50:1417–1426.
81. Chisholm, D. J., Klassen, G. A., Dupre, J., and Pozefsky, T. (1975): Interaction of secretin and insulin on human forearm metabolism. *Eur. J. Clin. Invest.,* 5:487–494.
82. Chisholm, D. J., Young, J. D., and Lazarus, L. (1969): The gastrointestinal stimulus to insulin release. I. Secretin. *J. Clin. Invest.,* 48:1453–1460.
83. Crean, G. P., Marshall, M. W., and Rumsey, R. D. E. (1969): Parietal cell hyperplasia induced by the administration of pentagastrin (ICI 50,123) to rats. *Gastroenterology,* 57:147–155.
84. Curry, D. L., Bennett, L. L., and Grodsky, G. M. (1968): Dynamics of insulin secretion by the perfused rat pancreas. *Endocrinology,* 83:572–584.
85. Danielsson, Å., and Lernmark, Å. (1974): Effects of pancreozymin and secretin on insulin release and the role of the exocrin pancreas. *Diabetologia,* 10:407–409.
86. Deckert, T. (1968): Insulin secretion following administration of secretin in patients with diabetes mellitus. *Acta Endocrinol.,* 59:150–158.

87. Deckert, T., and Worning, H. (1970): Insulin secretion after administration of secretin to normal and diabetic subjects and patients with chronic pancreatitis. *Diabetologia,* 6:42.
88. Demling, L., Domschke, W., Domschke, S., Belohlavek, D., Baenkler, H. W., Frümorgen, P., Lingenberg, G., Wünsch, E., and Jaeger, E. (1975): Treatment of duodenal ulcer with a long-acting synthetic secretin: A pilot trial. *Acta Hepato-Gastroenterol.,* 22:310–313.
89. Deschodt-Lanckman, M., Robberecht, P., De Neef, Ph., Labrie, F., and Christophe, J. (1975): In vitro interactions of gastrointestinal hormones on cyclic adenosine 3',5'-monophosphate levels and amylase output in the rat pancreas. *Gastroenterology,* 68:318–325.
90. De Zilwa, L. A. E. (1904): On the composition of pancreatic juice. *J. Physiol.,* 81:230–233.
91. Diaco, J. F., Miller, L. D., Kuo, P. T., Feng, L. Y., and Sugerman, H. J. (1971): Effects of secretin on serum immunoreactive insulin and insulin-like activity. *Ann. Surg.,* 173:578–582.
92. Diamond, J. S., Siegel, S. A., Gall, M. B., and Karlen, S. (1939): The use of secretin as a clinical test of pancreatic function. *Am. J. Dig. Dis.,* 6:366–372.
93. Diamond, J. S., Siegel, S. A., and Kantor, J. L. (1940): The secretin-test in the diagnosis of pancreatic diseases with a report of one hundred thirty tests. *Am. J. Dig. Dis.,* 7:435–444.
94. Dockray, G. J. (1974): Extraction of a secretinlike factor from the intestines of pike (Esox lucius). *Gen. Comp. Endocrinol.,* 23:340–347.
95. Dockray, G. J. (1975): Comparative studies on secretin. *Gen. Comp. Endocrinol.,* 25:203–210.
96. Dockray, G. J. (1976): Hormonal regulation of the exocrine pancreas in birds. *Gen. Comp. Endocrinol.,* 29:289.
97. Dolinsky, M. J. (1894): Etudes sur l'excitabilité sécrétoire spécifique de la muqueuse du canal digestif. *Arch. Sci. Biol.,* 3:399–427.
98. Domschke, S., Domschke, W., Rösch, W., Konturek, S. J., Wünsch, E., and Demling, L. (1976): Bicarbonate and cyclic AMP content of pure human pancreatic juice in response to graded doses of synthetic secretin. *Gastroenterology,* 70:533–536.
99. Dorchester, J. E. C., and Haist, R. E. (1952): A method of secretin assay. *J. Physiol.,* 118:182–187.
100. Dreiling, D. A. (1955): The technique of the secretin test: Normal ranges. *J. Mount Sinai Hosp.,* 21:363–372.
101. Dreiling, D. A. (1975): Secretion analysis: Secretin testing in pancreatic cancer. *J. Surg. Oncol.,* 7:101–105.
102. Dreiling, D. A., and Bordalo, O. (1973): Secretory patterns in minimal pancreatic inflammatory pathologies. *Med. Chir. Dig.,* 2:269–274.
103. Dreiling, D. A., Greenstein, A., and Bordalo, O. (1973): Newer concepts of pancreatic secretory patterns. Pancreatic secretory mass and pancreatic secretory capacity: pancreatic hypersecretion. *Mount Sinai J. Med.,* 40:666–676.
104. Dreiling, D. A., and Janowitz, H. D. (1962): The measurement of pancreatic secretory function. In: *The Exocrine Pancreas,* Ciba Found. Symposium, edited by A. V. S. de Reuch and M. P. Cameron, pp. 225–258. London.
105. Dreiling, D. A., Nieburgs, H. E., and Janowitz, H. D. (1960): The combined secretin and cytology test in the diagnosis of pancreatic and biliary tract cancer. *Med. Clin. North Am.,* 44:801–815.
106. Dudl, R. J., Lerner, R. L., Ensinck, J. W., and Williams, R. H. (1973): The effect of secretin on pancreatic glucoregulatory hormones in man. *Horm. Metab. Res.,* 5:250–253.
107. Dupré, J. (1964): An intestinal hormone affecting glucose disposal in man. *Lancet,* ii:672–673.
108. Dupré, J., Rojas, L., White, J. J., Unger, R. H., and Beck, J. C. (1966): Effects of secretin on insulin and glucagon in portal and peripheral blood in man. *Lancet,* ii:26–27.
109. Elias, E., Polak, J. M., Bloom, S. R., Pearse, A. G. E., Welbourn, R. B., Booth, C. C., Kuzio, M., and Brown, J. C. (1972): Pancreatic cholera due to production of gastric inhibitory polypeptide. *Lancet,* ii:791–793.
110. Elrick, H., Stikkler, L., Hlad, C. J. Jr., and Arai, Y. (1964): Plasma insulin response to oral and intravenous glucose administration. *J. Clin. Endocrinol. Metab.,* 24:1076–1082.
111. Enk, B. (1976): Secretin-induced insulin response. *Acta Endocrinol.,* 82:312–317.
112. Erlinger, S., and Dhumeaux, D. (1974): Mechanisms and control of secretion of bile water and electrolytes. *Gastroenterology,* 66:281–304.
113. Espiner, E. A., and Beaven, D. W. (1962): Non-specific islet-cell tumour of the pancreas with diarrhoea. *Q. J. Med.,* 31:447–471.

114. Esteller, A., Lisbona, F., Martinez de Victoria, E., and Murillo, A. (1977): Algunos aspectos de la secreción biliar en cuatro especies de primates (P. mandrillus, P. papio, M. mulatta, E. patas). *Rev. Espanol. Fisiol.,* 33:31–35.
115. Esteller, A., Lopez, M. A., and Murillo, A. (1977): The effect of secretin and cholecystokinin-pancreozymin on the secretion of bile in the anaesthetized rabbit. *Q. J. Exp. Physiol.,* 62:353–359.
116. Fahrenkrug, J., Schaffalitzky de Muckadell, O. B., and Rehfeld, J. F. (1976): Production and evaluation of antibodies for radioimmunoassay of secretin. *Scand. J. Clin. Lab. Invest.,* 36:281–287.
117. Felber, J. P., Zermatten, A., and Dick, J. (1974) Modulation, by food, of hormonal system regulating rat pancreatic secretion. *Lancet,* ii:185–188.
118. Forker, E. L. (1967): Two sites of bile formation as determined by mannitol and erythritol clearance in the guinea pig. *J. Clin. Invest.,* 46:1189–1195.
119. Gardiner, B. N., Conaway, C., and Small, D. M. (1975): Effects of secretin and cholecystokinin on relative composition of hepatic bile in Rhesus monkeys. *Surg. Forum,* 26:437–439.
120. Goldner, M. G., and Gomori, G. (1943): Alloxan diabetes in the dog. *Endocrinology,* 33:297–308.
121. Goldstein, H., Ventzke, L. E., and Wernett, C. (1968): Value of exfoliative cytology in pancreatic carcinoma. *Gut,* 9:316–318.
122. Gordon, E. M., Douglas, M. C., Jablonski, P., Owen, J. A., Sali, A., and Watts, J. McK. (1972): Gastroduodenal hormones and bile-secretion studies in the isolated perfused pig liver. *Surgery,* 72:708–721.
123. Gráf, L. (1976): Isolation and evolution of the gastrointestinal hormones. *Acta Physiol. Acad. Sci. Hung.,* 47:285–298.
124. Greengard, H. (1948): Hormones of the gastrointestinal tract. In: *The Hormones, Physiology, Chemistry and Applications,* edited by G. Pincus, K. V. Thimann, pp. 201–254. Academic Press, New York.
125. Greengard, H., and Ivy, A. C. (1938): The isolation of secretin. *Am. J. Physiol.,* 124:427–434.
126. Greengard, H., Roback, R. A., and Ivy, A. C. (1942): The effect of sympathomimetic amines on pancreatic secretion. *J. Pharmacol. Exp. Ther.,* 74:309–318.
127. Greenlee, H. B., Longhi, E. H., Guerrero, J. D., Nelsen, T. S., El-Bedri, A. L., and Dragstedt, L. R. (1957): Inhibitory effect of pancreatic secretin on gastric secretion. *Am. J. Physiol.,* 190:396–402.
128. Gregg, J. A., and Sharma, M. M. (1978): Endoscopic measurement of pancreatic juice secretory flow rates and pancreatic secretory pressures after secretin administration in human controls and in patients with acute relapsing pancreatitis, chronic pancreatitis, and pancreatic cancer. *Am. J. Surg.,* 136:569–574.
129. Gregory, R. A. (1962): *Secretory Mechanisms of the Gastro-Intestinal Tract.* E. Arnold, Ltd, London.
130. Gregory, R. A. (1967): Enterogastrone-a reappraisal of the problem. In: *Gastric Secretion. Mechanisms and Control,* edited by T. K. Shnitka, J. A. L. Gilbert, R. C. Harrison, pp. 469–477. Oxford, Oxford University Press.
131. Gregory, R. A. (1968–69): Gastrin-the natural history of a peptide hormone. *Harvey Lectures Ser.,* 64:121–155.
132. Gregory, R. A. (1974): The Bayliss-Starling Lecture 1973. The gastrointestinal hormones: A review of recent advances. *J. Physiol.,* 241:1–32.
133. Gregory, R. A., and Tracy, H. J. (1964): The constitution and properties of two gastrins extracted from hog antral mucosa. *Gut,* 5:103–117.
134. Grossman, M. I. (1950): Gastrointestinal hormones. *Physiol. Rev.,* 30:33–90.
135. Grossman, M. I. (1966): Treatment of duodenal ulcer with secretin: a speculative proposal. *Gastroenterology,* 50:912–913.
136. Grossman, M. I. (1970): Gastrin, cholecystokinin, and secretin act on one receptor. *Lancet,* i:1088–1089.
137. Grossman, M. I. (1972): Gastrointestinal hormones: Some thoughts about clinical applications. *Scand. J. Gastroenterol.,* 7:97–104.
138. Grossman, M. I. (1973): Specrtrum of biological actions of gastrointestinal hormones. In: *Frontiers in Gastrointestinal Hormone Research,* edited by S. Andersson, pp. 17–28. Almqvist & Wiksell, Stockholm.

139. Grossman, M. I., and Ivy, A. C. (1946): Effect of alloxan upon external secretion of the pancreas. *Proc. Soc. Exp. Biol. Med.,* 63:62–63.
140. Grossman, M. I., Janowitz, H. D., Ralston, H., and Kim, K. S. (1949): The effect of secretin on bile formation in man. *Gastroenterology,* 12:133–138.
141. Grossman, M. I., and Konturek, S. J. (1974): Gastric acid does drive pancreatic bicarbonate secretion. *Scand. J. Gastroenterol.,* 9:299–302.
142. Guelrud, M., Rudick, J., and Janowitz, H. D. (1971) Endogenous cyclic AMP and pancreatic enzyme secretion. *Gastroenterology,* 60:671.
143. Guiducci, M. (1974): Solid phase synthesis of porcine secretin and 6-tyrosyl-secretin. In: *Endocrinology of the Gut,* edited by W. Y. Chey and F. P. Brooks, pp. 103–106. Charles B. Slack, Thorofare, New Jersey.
144. Gullo, L., Costa, P. L., and Labò, G. (1978): A comparison between injection and infusion of pancreatic stimulants in the diagnosis of exocrine pancreatic insufficiency. *Digestion,* 18:64–69.
145. Häcki, W. H., Greenberg, G. R., and Bloom, S. R. (1978): Role of secretin in man. I. In: *Gut Hormones,* edited by S. R. Bloom, pp. 182–192. Churchill Livingstone, Edinburgh/London/New York.
146. Hammarsten, E., Wilander, O., and Ågren, G. (1928): Versuche zur Reinigung von Sekretin. *Acta Med. Scand.,* 68:239–247.
147. Hanscom, D. H., Jacobson, B. J., and Littman, A. (1967): Output of protein after pancreozymin. A test of pancreatic function. *Ann. Intern. Med.,*
148. Hanscom, D. H., Littman, A., and Pinto, J. V. (1963): Dose-response relationship to pancreozymin in normal subjects and in patients with chronic pancreatitis. *Gastroenterology,* 45:209–214.
149. Hansky, J. (1971): Pancreatic function tests: Comparison of standard and augmented secretin. *Aust. N. Z. J. Med.,* 2:109–113.
150. Hansky, J., Soveny, C., and Korman, M. G. (1971): Effect of secretin on serum gastrin as measured by immunoassay. *Gastroenterology,* 61:62–68.
151. Hanssen, L. E., Osnes, M., Flaten, O., and Myren, J. (1978): Response of plasma secretin and pure pancreatic juice to intraduodenal bile infusions in man. *Scand. J. Gastroenterol. (Suppl. 49)* 13:80.
152. Hanssen, L. E., and Torjesen, P. (1977): Radioimmunoassay of secretin in human plasma. *Scand. J. Gastroenterol.,* 12:481–488.
153. Hardison, W. G., and Norman, J. C. (1967): Effect of bile salt and secretin upon bile flow from the isolated perfused pig liver. *Gastroenterology,* 53:412–417.
154. Harper, A. A., and Raper, H. S. (1943): Pancreozymin, a stimulant of the secretion of pancreatic enzymes in extracts of the small intestine. *J. Physiol.,* 102:115–125.
155. Hartley, R. C., Gambill, E. E., and Summerskill, W. H. J. (1965): Pancreatic volume and bicarbonate output with augmented doses of secretin. *Gastroenterology,* 48:312–317.
156. Harty, R. F., Rose, R. C., and Nahrwold, D. L. (1974): Stimulation of hepatic bile secretion by dopamine. *J. Surg. Res.,* 17:359–363.
157. Hashimoto, K., Satoh, S., and Takeuchi, O. (1971): Effect of dopamine on pancreatic secretion in the dog. *Br. J. Pharmacol.,* 43:739–746.
158. Hatfield, A. R. W., Whittaker, R., and Gibbs, D. D. (1974): The collection of pancreatic fluid for cytodiagnosis using a duodenoscope. *Gut,* 15:305–307.
159. Heatley, N. G. (1968): The assay of secretin in the rat. *J. Endocrinol.,* 42:535–547.
160. Hemmasi, B., and Bayer, E., (1977): The solid phase synthesis of porcine secretin with full biological activity. *Int. J. Pept. Protein Res.,* 9:63–70.
161. Henn, R. M., Selcon, S., Sturdevant, R. A. L., Isenberg, J. I., and Grossman, M. I. (1976): Experience with synthetic secretin in the treatment of duodenal ulcer. *Am. J. Dig. Dis.,* 21:921–926.
162. Henriksen, F. W. (1969): Effect of vagotomy or atropine on the canine pancreatic response to secretin and pancreozymin. *Scand. J. Gastroenterol.,* 4:137–144.
163. Henriksen, F. W., Jörgensen, S. P., and Möller, S. (1974): Interaction between secretin and cholecystokinin on inhibition of gastric secrection in man. *Scand. J. Gastroenterol.,* 9:735–740.
164. Henriksen, F. W., and Möller, S. (1971): Effect of secretin on the pancreatic secretion of protein. *Scand. J. Gastroenterol. (Suppl.),* 9:181–187.
165. Henriksen, F. W., and Worning, H. (1967): The interaction of secretin and pancreozymin on the external pancreatic secretion in dogs. *Acta Physiol. Scand.,* 70:241–249.

166. Hermon-Taylor, J. (1968): A technique for perfusion of the isolated canine pancreas. Responses to secretin and gastrin. *Gastroenterology,* 55:488–501.
167. Hew, C.-L., and Yip, C. C. (1976): Biosynthesis of polypeptide hormones. *Can. J. Biochem.,* 54:591–599.
168. Hickson, J. C. D. (1970): The secretion of pancreatic juice in response to stimulation of the vagus nerves in the pig. *J. Physiol.,* 206:275–297.
169. Himes, J. A., Bruss, M. L., Simpson, C. F., and Cornelius, C. E. (1976): Hypercholeresis in turkeys following the ingestion of crotalaria spectabilis seeds. *Cornell Vet.,* 66:521–565.
170. Hinz, M., Katsilambros, N., Schweitzer, B., Raptis, S., and Pfeiffer, E. F. (1971): The role of the exocrine pancreas in the stimulation of insulin secretion by intestinal hormones. *Diabetologia,* 7:1–5.
171. Höj, L., Holst, J. J., and Rune, S. J. (1973): A trial of exogenous secretin in the treatment of duodenal ulcer pain. *Scand. J. Gastroenterol.,* 8:279–281.
172. Holohan, K. N., Murphy, R. F., Flanagan, R. W. J., Buchanan, K. D., and Elmore, D. T. (1973): Enzymic iodination of the histidyl residue of secretin: A radioimmunoassay of the hormone. *Biochim. Biophys. Acta,* 322:178–180.
173. Holst, J. J., Schaffalitzky de Muckadell, O. B., and Fahrenkrug, J. (1979): Nervous control of pancreatic exocrine secretion in pigs. *Acta Physiol. Scand.,* 105:33–51.
174. Horn, G. W., and Huber, T. L. (1975): Duodenal acidification: Stimulus for the release of intestinal hormones in sheep. *J. Anim. Sci.,* 41:1199–1205.
175. Hubel, K. A. (1972): Secretin: A long progress note. *Gastroenterology,* 62:318–341.
176. Hughes, C. A., Bates, T., and Dowling, R. H. (1978): Cholecystokinin and secretin prevent the intestinal mucosal hypoplasia of total parenteral nutrition in the dog. *Gastroenterology,* 75:34–41.
177. Hunter, W. M., and Greenwood, F. C. (1962): Preparation of iodine-131 labelled human growth hormone of high specific activity. *Nature,* 194:495–496.
178. Isenberg, J. I., Brickman, A. S., and Moore, E. W. (1973): The effect of secretin on serum calcium in man. *J. Clin. Endocrinol.,* 37:30–33.
179. Isenberg, J. I., Walsh, J. H., Passaro, E. Jr., Moore, E. W., and Grossman, M. I. (1972): Unusual effect of secretin on serum gastrin, serum calcium, and gastric acid secretion in a patient with suspected Zollinger-Ellison syndrome. *Gastroenterology,* 62:626–631.
180. Itakura, K., Hirose, T., Crea, R., Riggs, A. D., Heyneker, H. L., Bolivar, F., and Boyer, H. W. (1977): Expression in Escherichia coli of a chemically synthesized gene for the hormone somatostatin. *Science,* 198:1056–1063.
181. IUPAC-IUB Commission on biochemical nomenclature (CBN) (1962): A one-letter notation for amino acid sequences. *Eur. J. Biochem.,* 5:151–153.
182. Ivy, A. C., and Janecek, H. M. (1959): Assay of Jorpes-Mutt secretin and cholecystokinin. *Acta Physiol. Scand.,* 45:220–230.
183. Jablonski, P., Sali, A., and Watts, J. McK. (1974): Gastro-intestinal hormones and bile secretion in the perfused pig liver: The effects of secretin, cholecystokinin and pentagastrin. *Aust. N.Z.J. Surg.,* 44:173–178.
184. Jaeger, E., Knof, S., Scharf, R., Lehnert, P., Schulz, I., and Wünsch, E. (1978): Chemical evidence for the mechanism of inactivation of secretin. *Scand. J. Gastroenterol., (Suppl. 49),* 13:93.
185. Jansson, R., Steen, G., and Svanvik, J. (1978): Effects of intravenous vasoactive intestinal peptide (VIP) on gallbladder function in the cat. *Gastroenterology,* 75:47–50.
186. Jansson, R., and Svanvik, J. (1977): Effects of intravenous secretin and cholecystokinin on gallbladder net water absorption and motility in the cat. *Gastroenterology,* 72:639–643.
187. Jarrett, R. J., and Cohen, N. M. (1967): Intestinal hormones and plasma insulin. *Lancet,* ii:861–863.
188. Jensen, S. L., Fahrenkrug, J., Holst, J. J., Kühl, C., Nielsen, O. V., and Schaffalitzky de Muckadell, O. B. (1978): Secretory effects of secretin on isolated perfused porcine pancreas. *Am. J. Physiol.,* 235:E381–E386.
189. Jensen, S. L., Fahrenkrug, J., Holst, J. J., Nielsen, O. V., and Schaffalitzky de Muckadell, O. B. (1978): Secretory effects of VIP on isolated perfused porcine pancreas. *Am. J. Physiol.,* 235:E387–E391.
190. Joffe, S. N. (1976): Effect of GIH secretin on secretagogue-induced duodenal ulcers. *Br. J. Surg.,* 63:152.
191. Johnson, L. R., and Grossman, M. I. (1968): Secretin: the enterogastrone released by acid in the duodenum. *Am. J. Physiol.,* 215:885–888.

192. Jones, R. S., and Grossman, M. I. (1969): Choleretic effects of secretin and histamine in the dog. *Am. J. Physiol.,* 217:532–535.
193. Jonson, G., Sundman, L., and Thulin, L. (1964): The influence of chemically pure secretin on hepatic bile output. *Acta Physiol. Scand.,* 62:287–290.
194. Jorpes, E., and Mutt, V. (1954): On the action of highly purified preparations of secretin and of pancreozymin. *Arkiv Kemi,* 7:553–559.
195. Jorpes, J. E., and Mutt, V. (1961): Process for the production of gastrointestinal hormones and hormone concentrate. U.S.A. Patent no. 3.013.944.
196. Jorpes, J. E., and Mutt, V. (1966): On the biological assay of secretin. The reference standard. *Acta Physiol. Scand.,* 66:316–325.
197. Jorpes, J. E., Mutt, V., Magnusson, S., and Steele, B. B. (1962): Amino acid composition and N-terminal amino acid sequence of porcine secretin. *Biochem. Biophys. Res. Commun.,* 9:275–279.
198. Kaess, H., and Schlierf, G. (1969): Veränderungen des Blutzuckers und der Plasmainsulinkonzentration nach Stimulierung der endogenen Sekretinfreisetzung. *Diabetologia,* 5:228–232.
199. Kimberg, D. V. (1974): Cyclic nucleotides and their role in gastrointestinal secretion. *Gastroenterology,* 67:1023–1064.
200. Kirchmayer, S., Tarnawski, A., Droźdź, H., and Cicheka, K. (1972): Effect of cholecystokininpancreozymin and secretin on the volume, composition, and enzymatic activity of hepatic bile in rabbits. *Gut,* 13:709–712.
201. Kisseler, B., Leistner, G. H., and Barth, E. (1965): The roentgenologic diagnosis of pancreatic disease. *Radiology,* 85:59–63.
202. Klapdor, R., Schliewe, and Valerius, H. (1975): Zur Physiologie der Galleexkretion beim Zwergschwein. *Res. Exp. Med.,* 166:241–251.
203. Knodell, R. G., Toskes, P. P., Reber, H. A., and Brooks, F. P. (1970): Significance of cyclic AMP in the regulation of exocrine pancreas secretion. *Experientia,* 26:515–517.
204. Kolts, B. E., Herbst, C. A., and McGuigan, J. E. (1974): Calcium and secretin-stimulated gastrin release in the Zollinfer-Ellison syndrome. *Ann. Intern. Med.,* 81:758–762.
205. Kolts, B. E., and McGuigan, J. E. (1977): Radioimmunoassay measurement of secretin halflife in man. *Gastroenterology,* 72:55–60.
206. König, W., Geiger, R., Wissmann, H., Bickel, M., Obermeier, R., Teetz, W., and Uhmann, R. (1977): Chemical and biological properties of porcine secretin analogues modified in positions 3 and 4. *Gastroenterology,* 72:797–800.
207. Konturek, S. J. (1968): The effect of secretin on gastric acid secretion and peptic ulcers induced by pentagastrin in cats with intact or resected duodenum. *Am. J. Dig. Dis.,* 13:874–881.
208. Konturek, S. J. (1969): Comparison of pancreatic responses to natural and synthetic secretins in conscious cats. *Am. J. Dig. Dis.,* 14:557–565.
209. Konturek, S. J. (1978): Current concepts of neuro-hormonal control of pancreatic secretion. *Ir. J. Med. Sci.,* 147:1–10.
210. Konturek, S. J., Becker, H. D., and Thompson, J. C. (1974): Effect of vagotomy on hormones stimulating pancreatic secretion. *Arch. Surg.,* 108:704–708.
211. Konturek, S. J., Dabrowski, A., Adamczyk, B., and Kulpa, J. (1969): The effect of secretin, gastrin-pentapeptide, and histamine on gastric acid and hepatic bile secretion in man. *Am. J. Dig. Dis.,* 14:900–907.
212. Kowalewski, K., and Kolodej, A. (1975): Simultaneous study of gastric and pancreatic secretion in a preparation perfused ex vivo. *Surg. Gynecol. Obstet.,* 141:595–601.
213. Kozu, T., and Kondo, T. (1972): The duodenoscopic collection of the intrapancreatic juice. *Arch. Fr. Mal. App. Dig.,* 61:233c.
214. Kraegen, E. W., Chisholm, D. J., Young, J. D., and Lazarus, L. (1970): The gastrointestinal stimulus to insulin release. II. A dual action of secretin. *J. Clin. Invest.,* 49:524–529.
215. Kudrewecki, W. W. (1890): *Materiale zur Physiologie der Bauchspeicheldrüse.* Diss, St. Petersburg.
216. Kunert, H., Kuhn, F. M., Schwemmle, K., and Ottenjann, R. (1976): VIP-und GIP-produzierender pankreatumor. *Dtsch. Med. Wochenschr.,* 101:920–923.
217. La Barre, M. J. (1932): Sur le possibilités d'un traitment du diabète par l'incrétine. *Bull. Acad. Med. Belg.,* 12:620–634.
218. La Barre, J. (1936): *La Sécrétine.* Son role physiologique, ses propriétés thérapeutiques. Masson et Cie, Paris.

219. La Barre, J., and Ledrut, J. (1934): A propos de l'action hypoglycémiante des extraits duodénaux. *Compt. Rend.,* 115:750–752.
220. Lagerlöf, H. O. (1942): Pancreatic function and pancreatic disease studied by means of secretin. *Acta Med. Scand. (Suppl.),* CXXVIII.
221a. Lagerlöf, H. O. and Mutt, V. (1970): Secretin and cholecystokinin-pancreozymin: Chemistry, Physiology, Pharmacology, and Clinical Applications. In: Progress in Gastroenterology, Vol II, edited by G. B. J. Glass, pp. 125–148, Grune & Stratton, 1970.
221. Lagerlöf, H. O. (1967): Pancreatic secretion: pathophysiology. In: *Handbook of Physiology, sect. 6, Alimentary Canal, Vol. 2,* edited by C. F. Code, pp. 1027–1042. Washington DC.
222. Lagerlöf, H. O., Schütz, H. B., and Holmer, S. (1967): A secretin test with high doses of secretin and correction for incomplete recovery of duodenal juice. *Gastroenterology,* 52:67–77.
223. Larsson, L.-I., Fahrenkrug, J., Holst, J. J., and Schaffalitzky de Muckadell, O. B. (1978): Innervation of the pancreas by vasoactive intestinal polypeptide (VIP) immunoreactive nerves. *Life Sci.,* 22:773–780.
224. Laughton, N. B., and Macallum, A. B. (1932): The relation of the duodenal mucosa to the internal secretion of the pancreas. *Proc. Roy. Soc. (Lond.) ser. B.,* CXI:37–46.
225. Lazarus, N. R., Voyles, N. R., Devrim, S., Tanese, T., and Recant, L. (1968): Extra-gastrointestinal effects of secretin, gastrin, and pancreozymin. *Lancet,* ii:248–250.
226. Lechin, F. (1962): An effect of secretin on serum potassium. *Acta Physiol. Latin Am.,* 12:370–374.
227. Ledrut, J., and Ungar, G. (1937): Action de la sécrétine chez l'octopus vulgaris. *Arch. Int. Physiol.,* XLIV:205–211.
228. Legge, J. W., Morieson, A. S., Rogers, G. E., and Marginson, M. A. (1957): The chromatography and countercurrent distribution of secretin. *Aust. J. Exp. Biol.,* 35:569–582.
229. Lemon, H. M., and Byrnes, W. W. (1949): Cancer of the biliary tract and pancreas. *J.A.M.A.,* 141:254–257.
230. Lenninger, S., and Ohlin, P. (1971): The flow of juice from the pancreatic gland of the cat in response to vagal stimulation. *J. Physiol.,* 216:303–318.
231. Lenti, G., and Emanuelli, G. (1976): Klinische Bedeutung verschiedener Tests für die Diagnose chronischer pankreaserkrankungen. *Münch. Med. Wochenschr.,* 118:405–408.
232. Lerner, R. L., and Porte, D. Jr. (1970): Uniphasic insulin responses to secretin stimulation in man. *J. Clin. Invest.,* 49:2276–2280.
233. Leuret, F., and Lassaigne, J.-L. (1825): *Recherches Physiologiques et Chimiques pour Servir a l'Histoire de la Digestion.* Madame Huzard, Paris.
234. Levin, S., Goldberg, N., Pehlevanian, M., and Adachi, R. (1978): Nutrient independent "incretin": secretion from the isolated, perfused rat intestine and from the human intestine. *Scand. J. Gastroenterol. (Suppl. 49),* 13:114.
235. Levine, R. A. (1970): The role of cyclic AMP in hepatic and gastrointestinal function. *Gastroenterology,* 59:280–300.
236. Levine, R. A., and Hall, R. C. (1976): Cyclic AMP in secretin choleresis. Evidence for a regulatory role in man and baboons but not in dogs. *Gastroenterology,* 70:537–544.
237. Lin, T. M., and Alphin, R. S. (1962): Comparative bio-assay of secretin and pancreozymin in rats and dogs. *Am. J. Physiol.,* 203:926–928.
238. Linari, G., and Linari, B. (1975): Effetto di alcuni polipeptidi sulla secrezione pancreatica del pollo. *Boll. Soc. Ital. Biol. Sper.,* 51:1146–1151.
239. Loew, E. R., Gray, J. S., and Ivy, A. C. (1940): The effect of acid stimulation of the duodenum upon experimental hyperglycemia and utilization of glucose. *Am. J. Physiol.,* 128:298–308.
240. Löffler, A., Stadelmann, O., Miederer, S. E., and Sobbe, A. (1974): Diagnostik des pankreaskarzinoms. *Dtsch. Med. Wochenschr.,* 99:1976–1983.
241. Love, J. W. (1957): A method for the assay of secretin using rats. *Q. J. Exp. Physiol.,* 42:279–284.
242. McIntyre, N., Holdsworth, C. D., and Turner, D. S. (1964): New interpretation of oral glucose tolerance. *Lancet,* ii:20–21.
243. McNeer, G., and Ewing, J. H. (1949): Exfoliated pancreatic cancer cells in duodenal drainage. *Cancer,* 2:643–645.
244. Mahler, R. J., and Weisberg, H. (1968): Failure of endogenous stimulation of secretin and pancreozymin release to influence serum-insulin. *Lancet,* i:448–451.

245. Makhlouf, G. M. (1974): The neuroendocrine design of the gut. The play of chemicals in a chemical playground. *Gastroenterology*, 67:159–184.
246. Marks, I. N., Bank, S., Louw, J. H. (1967): Islet cell tumor of the pancreas with reversible watery diarrhea and achlorhydria. *Gastroenterology*, 52:695–708.
247. Marois, C., Morisset, J., and Dunnigan, J. (1972): Presence and stimulation of adenyl cyclase in pancreatic homogenate. *Rev. Can. Biol.*, 31:253–257.
248. Matsumoto, K. K., Peter, J. B., Schultze, R. G., Hakim, A. A., and Franck, P. T. (1966): Watery diarrhea and hypokalemia associated with pancreatic islet cell adenoma. *Gastroenterology*, 50:231–242.
249. Matsuo, Y., and Seki, A. (1978): The coordination of gastrointestinal hormones and the automatic nerves. *Am. J. Gastroenterol.*, 69:21–50.
250. Mellanby, J. (1925): The mechanism of pancreatic digestion—the function of secretin. *J. Physiol.*, 60:85–91.
251. Mellanby, J. (1926): The secretion of pancreatic juice. *J. Physiol.*, 61:419–435.
252. Mellanby, J. (1928): The isolation of secretin—its chemical and physiological properties. *J. Physiol.*, LXVI:1–18.
253. Mellanby, J., and Huggett, A. S. G. (1926): The relation of secretin formation to the entrance of acid chyme into the small intestine—the properties of secretin. *J. Physiol.*, 61:122–130.
254. Meyer, J. H., Spingola, L. J., and Grossman, M. I. (1971): Endogenous cholecystokinin potentiates exogenous secretin on pancreas of dog. *Am. J. Physiol.*, 221:742–747.
255. Meyer, J. H., Way, L. W., and Grossman, M. I. (1970): Pancreatic bicarbonate response to various acids in duodenum of the dog. *Am. J. Physiol.*, 219:964–970.
256. Moody, A. J., Markussen, J., Fries, A. S., Steenstrup, C., and Sundby, F. (1970): The insulin releasing activities of extracts of pork intestine. *Diabetologia*, 6:135–140.
257. Moore, B., Edie, E. S., and Abram, J. H. (1906): On the treatment of diabetes mellitus by acid extract of duodenal mucous membrane. *Biochem. J.*, 1:28–39.
258. Morel, L., and Terroine, E. (1909): Variations de l'alcalinité et du pouvoir lipolytique du suc pancréatique, au cours de sécrétions provoquées par des injections répétées de sécrétine. *Compt. Rend. Soc. Biol.*, 66:36–38.
259. Morris, T. Q. (1973): Hepatic circulatory adjustments during non-taurocholate associated canalicular cho3lereses. *Gastroenterology*, 64:163.
260. Morton, I. K. M., Phillips, S. J., Saverymuttu, S. H., and Wood, J. R. (1976): Secretin and vasoactive intestinal peptide inhibit fluid absorption and induce secretion in the isolated gallbladder of the guinea-pig. *J. Physiol.*, 266:65–66p.
261. Mutt, V. (1959): Preparation of highly purified secretin. *Arkiv Kemi*, 15:69–74.
262. Mutt, V. (1959): On the preparation of secretin. *Arkiv Kemi*, 15:75–95.
263. Mutt, V. (1974): The intestinal hormones in 1973. In: *Proc. 4th Int. Symp. London*, edited by S. Taylor, pp. 100–116. William Heinemann Medical Books Ltd, London.
264. Mutt, V. (1976): Further investigations on intestinal hormonal polypeptides. *Clin. Endocrinol., (Suppl.)*, 5:175–183s.
265. Mutt, V. (1978): Progress in intestinal hormone research. In: *Gastrointestinal Hormones and Pathology of the Digestive System*, edited by M. Grossman, V. Speranza, N. Basso, and E. Lezoche, pp. 133–146. Plenum Publishing Corporation.
266. Mutt, V. (1978): Hormone isolation. In: *Gut Hormones*, edited by S. R. Bloom, pp. 21–27. Churchill Livingstone, Edinburgh, London, and New York.
267. Mutt, V., and Jorpes, J. E. (1967): Contemporary developments in the biochemistry of the gastrointestinal hormones. *Rec. Progr. Horm. Res.*, 23:483–503.
268. Mutt, V., and Jorpes, J. E. (1968): Structure of porcine cholecystokinin-pancreozymin. 1. Cleavage with thrombin and with trypsin. *Eur. J. Biochem.*, 6:156–162.
269. Mutt, V., Jorpes, J. E., and Magnusson, S. (1970): Structure of porcine secretin. The amino acid sequence. *Eur. J. Biochem.*, 15:513–519.
270. Mutt, V., Magnusson, S., Jorpes, J. E., and Dahl, E. (1965): Structure of porcine secretin. I. Degradation with trypsin and thrombin. Sequence of the tryptic peptides. The C-terminal residue. *Biochemistry*, 4:2358–2362.
271. Mutt, V., and Said, S. I. (1974): Structure of the porcine vasoactive intestinal octacosapeptide. The amino-acid sequence. Use of kallikrein in its determination. *Eur. J. Biochem.*, 42:581–589.
272. Mutt, V., and Söderberg, U. (1959): On the assay of secretin. *Arkiv Kemi*, 15:63–68.

273. Nahrwold, D. L. (1971): Secretion by the common duct in response to secretin. *Surg. Forum,* 22:386–387.
274. Nardi, G. L., Greep, J. M., Chambers, D. A., McCrae, C., and Skinner, D. B. (1963): Physiologic peregrinations in pancreatic perfusion. *Ann. Surg.,* 158:830–839.
275. Newton, G. G. F., Love, J. W., Heatley, N. G., and Abraham, E. P. (1959): Purification of secretin. *Biochem. J.,* 71:6p.
276. Nilsson, A. (1970): Gastrointestinal hormones in the holocephalian fish Chimaera monstrosa (L.) *Comp. Biochem. Physiol.,* 32:387–390.
277. Nilsson, A. (1974): Isolation, amino acid composition and terminal amino acid residues of the vasoactive intestinal octacosapeptide from chicken intestine. Partial purification of chicken secretin. *FEBS Lett.,* 47:284–289.
278. Norman, J. C., Franco, F. O., Brown, M. E., Saravis, C. A., Ackroyd, F. W., and McDermott, W. V. Jr. (1966): Techniques of obtaining and preparing the porcine liver for experimental and clinical temporary ex vivo perfusion. *J. Surg. Res.,* 6:117–120.
279. Nundy, S., Shirley, D., Beales, J. S. M., O'Higgins, N., Heaf, R., Pearse, E. E., Lavender, J. P., and Baron, J. H. (1974): Simultaneous combined pancreatic test. *Br. Med. J.,* 1:87–90.
280. O'Connor, F. A., Buchanan, K. D., Connon, J. J., and Shahidullah, M. (1976): Secretin and insulin: Response to intraduodenal acid. *Diabetologia,* 12:145–148.
281. O'Maille, E. R. L., Richards, T. G., and Short, A. H. (1966): Factors determining the maximal rate of organic anion secretion by the liver and further evidence on the hepatic site of action of the hormone secretin. *J. Physiol.,* 186:424–438.
282. Ondetti, M. A., Deer, A., Sheehan, J. T., Pluscec, J., and Kocy, O. (1968): Side reactions in the synthesis of peptides containing the aspartylglycyl sequence. *Biochemistry,* 7:4069–4074.
283. Ondetti, M. A., Narayanan, V. L., von Saltza, M., Sheehan, J. T., Sabo, E. F., and Bodanszky, M. (1968): The synthesis of secretin. III. The fragment condensation approach. *J. Am. Chem. Soc.,* 90:4711–4716.
284. Penau, H., and Simonnet, H. (1925): Secrétine duodénale et insuline. *Bull. Soc. Chim. Biol. (Paris),* VII:17–25.
285. Pfeiffer, E. F., Raptis, S., and Fussgänger, R. (1973): Gastrointestinal hormones and islet function. In: *Secretin, Cholecystokinin, Pancreozymin and Gastrin,* edited by J. E. Jorpes and V. Mutt, pp. 259–310. Springer-Verlag, Berlin, Heidelberg, New York.
286. Pfeiffer, E. F., Telib, M., Ammon, J., Melani, F., and Ditschuneit, H. (1965): Direkte Stimulierung der Insulin-sekretion in vitro durch Sekretin. *Dtsch. Med. Wochenschr.,* 90:1663–1669.
287. Pincus, I. J., Thomas, J. E., Hausman, D., and Lachman, P. O. (1948): Relationship between the pH of the duodenal content and pancreatic secretion. *Proc. Soc. Exp. Biol. Med.,* 67:497–501.
288. Pissidis, A. G., Bombeck, G. T., Merchant, F., and Nyhus, L. M. (1969): Hormonal regulation of bile secretion: A study in the isolated, perfused liver. *Surgery,* 66:1075–1084.
289. Popielski, L. B. (1901): Über das peripherische reflektorische Nervencentrum des Pankreas. *Pflüg. Arch. Ges. Physiol.,* 86:215–246.
290. Porte, D. Jr., and Pupo, A. A. (1969): Insulin responses to glucose: Evidence for a two pool system in man. *J. Clin. Invest.,* 48:2309–3219.
291. Post, J. A., and Hanson, K. M. (1975): Hepatic, vascular and biliary responses to infusion of gastrointestinal hormones and bile salts. *Digestion,* 12:65–77.
292. Potts, J. T. Jr., Tregear, G. W., Keutmann, H. T., Niall, H. D., Sauer, R., Deftos, L. J., Dawson, B. F., Hogan, M. L., and Aurbach, G. D. (1971): Synthesis of a biologically active N-terminal tetratriacontapeptide of parathyroid hormone. *Proc. Natl. Acad. Sci. USA,* 68:63–67.
293. Poupon, R. E., Dol, M.-L., Dumont, M., and Erlinger, S. (1978): Evidence against a physiological role of cAMP in choleresis in dogs and rats. *Biochem. Pharmacol.,* 27:2413–2416.
294. Prandi, D., Erlinger, S., Glasinović, J.-C., and Dumont, M. (1975): Canalicular bile production in man. *Eur. J. Clin. Invest.,* 5:1–6.
295. Preisig, R., Cooper, H. L., and Wheeler, H. O. (1962): The relationship between taurocholate secretion rate and bile production in the unanesthetized dog during cholinergic blockade and during secretin administration. *J. Clin. Invest.,* 41:1152–1162.
296. Priest, W. M., and Alexander, M. K. (1957): Islet-cell tumour of the pancreas with peptic ulceration, diarrhea, and hypokalaemia. *Lancet,* ii:1145–1147.

297. Rall, T. W., Sutherland, E. W., and Berthet, J. (1957): The relationship of epinephrine and glucagon to liver phosphorylase. *J. Biol. Chem.*, 224:463–475.
298. Raptis, S., Leitze, M., Schlegel, W., and Pfeiffer, E. F. (1975): Secretin radioimmunoassay using ¹²⁵J-6-tyrosyl-secretin (6TS). *Horm. Metab. Res.*, 7:447.
299. Raptis, S., Schröder, K. E., Faulhaber, J. D., and Pfeiffer, E. F. (1968): Stimulierung der Insulinsekretion durch Sekretin bei Diabetikern. *Dtsch. Med. Wochenschr.*, 93:2420–2424.
300. Raskin, H. F., Wenger, J., Sklar, M., Pleticka, S., and Yarema, W. (1958): The diagnosis of cancer of the pancreas, biliary tract, and duodenum by combined cytologic and secretory methods. *Gastroenterology*, 34:996–1008.
301. Rayford, P. L., Curtis, P. J., Fender, H. R., and Thompson, J. C. (1976): Plasma levels of secretin in man and dogs: Validation of a secretin radioimmunoassay. *Surgery*, 79:658–665.
302. Rick, W. (1970): Der Sekretin-pankreozymin-test in der Diagnostik der Pankreasinsuffizienz. *Internist*, 11:110–117.
303. Robberecht, P., Conlon, T. P., and Gardner, J. D. (1976): Interaction of porcine vasoactive intestinal peptide with dispersed pancreatic acinar cells from the guinea pig. *J. Biol. Chem.*, 251:4635–4639.
304. Robberecht, P., Deschodt-Lanckman, M., De Neef, Ph., Borgeat, P., and Christophe, J. (1974): In vivo effects of pancreozymin, secretin, vasoactive intestinal polypeptide and pilocarpine on the levels of cyclic AMP and cyclic GMP in the rat pancreas. *FEBS Lett.*, 43:139–143.
305. Robberecht, P., Deschodt-Lanckman, M., Lammens, M., De Neef, Ph., and Christophe, J. (1977): "In vitro" effects of secretin and vasoactive intestinal polypeptide on hydrolase secretion and cyclic AMP levels in the pancreas of five animal species. A comparison with caerulein. *Gastroenterol. Clin Biol.*, 1:519–525.
306. Rocha e Silva, M., Beraldo, W. T., and Rosenfeld, G. (1949): Bradykinin, a hypotensive and smooth muscle stimulating factor released from plasma globulin by snake venoms and by trypsin. *Am. J. Physiol.*, 156:261–273.
307. Rodbell, M., Birnbaumer, L., and Pohl, S. L. (1970): Adenyl cyclase in fat cells. III. Stimulation by secretin and the effects of trypsin on the receptors for lipolytic hormones. *J. Biol. Chem.*, 245:718–722.
308. Rous, P., and McMaster, P. D. (1921): Physiological causes for the varied character of stasis bile. *J. Exp. Med.*, 34:75–96.
309. Rudman, D., and Del Rio, A. E. (1969): Lipolytic activity of synthetic porcine secretin. *Endocrinology*, 85:214–217.
310. Russell, T. R., Searle, G. L., and Jones, R. S. (1975): The choleretic mechanisms of sodium, taurocholate, secretin, and glucagon. *Surgery*, 77:498–504.
311. Rutherford, W. (1878/1880): On the physiological actions of drugs on the secretion of bile. *Trans. Roy. Soc. Edinburgh*, XXIX:133–263.
312. Rutishauser, S. C. B. (1976): An analysis of the reported choleretic effect of secretin in the rat. *J. Physiol.*, 257:59p.
313. Rutten, W. J., de Pont, J. J. H. H. M., and Bonting, S. L. (1972): Adenylate cyclase in the rat pancreas properties and stimulation by hormones. *Biochim. Biophys. Acta*, 274:201–213.
314. Said, S. I., and Mutt, V. (1972): Isolation from porcine-intestinal wall of a vasoactive octacosapeptide related to secretin and to glucagon. *Eur. J. Biochem.*, 28:199–204.
315. Santeusanio, F., Faloona, G. R., and Unger, R. H. (1972): Suppressive effect of secretin upon pancreatic alpha cell function. *J. Clin. Invest.*, 51:1743–1749.
316. Schaffalitzky de Muckadell, O. B., and Fahrenkrug, J. (1976): Preparation of ¹²⁵I-labelled synthetic porcine secretin for radioimmunoassay. *Scand. J. Clin. Lab. Invest.*, 36:661–668.
317. Schaffalitzky de Muckadell, O. B., and Fahrenkrug, J. (1977): Radioimmunoassay of secretin in plasma. *Scand. J. Clin. Lab. Invest.*, 37:155–162.
318. Schaffalitzky de Muckadell, O. B., and Fahrenkrug, J. (1978): Role of secretin in man. III. In: *Gut Hormones*, edited by S. R. Bloom, pp. 197–200. Churchill Livingstone, Edinburgh, London, New York.
319. Schafmayer, A., Teichmann, R. K., Rayford, P. L., and Thompson, J. C. (1978): Physiologic release of secretin measured in peripheral and portal venous blood of dogs. *Digestion*, 17:509–515.
320. Schapiro, H., and Woodward, E. R. (1965): Inhibition of the secretin mechanism by local anesthetics. *Am. Surg.*, 31:139–141.

321. Schlegel, W., and Raptis, S. (1976): A reliable method for generating antibodies against pancreozymin, secretin and gastrin. *Clin. Chim. Acta,* 73:439–444.
322. Schmidt, H. A., Goebell, H., and Johannson, F. (1972): Pancreatic and gastric secretion in rats studied by means of duodenal and gastric perfusion. *Scand. J. Gastroenterol.,* 7:47–53.
323. Schwarz, L. R., Schwenk, M., Pfaff, E., and Greim, H. (1976): Excretion of taurocholate from isolated hepatocytes. *Eur. J. Biochem.,* 71:369–373.
324. Schwille, P. O., Scholz, D., Samberger, N. M., and Kayser, P. E. (1975): Studies on the calcemic effect of intravenous secretin in humans. *Acta Hepato-Gastroenterol.,* 22:192–200.
325. Schwyzer, R. (1960): The chemistry and pharmacology of angiotensin. *Vit. Horm.,* 18:237–288.
326. Scow, R. O., and Cornfield, J. (1954): Quantitative relations between the oral and intravenous glucose tolerance curves. *Am. J. Physiol.,* 179:435–438.
327. Scratcherd, T. (1965): Electrolyte composition and control of biliary secretion in the cat and rabbit. In: *The Biliary System,* edited by W. Taylor, pp. 515–529. Blackwell Scientific Publications, Oxford.
328. Scratcherd, T., Case, R. M., and Smith, P. A. (1975): A sensitive method for the biological assay of secretin and substances with "secretin-like" activity in tissues and biological fluids. *Scand. J. Gastroenterol.,* 10:821–828.
329. Seiffert, U. B., Roth, W. D., and Alt, A. (1974): Eine Pankreasfunktions-prüfung bei kombinierter kontinuierlicher Stimulation mit Sekretin und Pankreozymin. *Z. Gastroenterol.,* 12:87–94.
330. Shaw, H. M., and Heath, T. (1972): The significance of hormones, bile salts and feedings in the regulation of bile and other digestive secretions in the rat. *Aust. J. Biol. Sci.,* 25:147–154.
331. Shaw, H. M., and Heath, T. J. (1974): Regulation of bile formation in rabbits and guinea pigs. *Q. J. Exp. Physiol.,* 59:93–102.
332. Shepherd, A. M. M., Stewart, W. K., Thjodleifsson, B., and Wormsley, K. G. (1974): Further studies of gastric hypersecretion in chronic renal failure. *Br. Med. J.,* 1:96–98.
333. Shima, K., Kurokawa, M., Sawazaki, N., Tanaka, R., and Kumahara, Y. (1978): Effect of secretin on plasma insulin and glucagon in man. *Endocrinol. Jpn.,* 25:461–465.
334. Sjödin, L. (1972): Influence of secretin and cholecystokinin on canine gastric secretion elicited by food and by exogenous gastrin. *Acta Physiol. Scand.,* 85:110–117.
335. Slayback, J. B., Swena, E. M., Thomas, J. E., and Smith, L. L. (1967): The pancreatic secretory response to topical anesthetic block of the small bowel. *Surgery,* 61:591–595.
336. Solcia, E., Capella, C., Buffa, R., Frigerio, B., Usellini, L., and Fontana, P. (1978): Endocrine cells of the gut and related growths. In: *Gut Hormones,* edited by S. R. Bloom, pp. 77–81. Churchill Livingstone, Edinburgh, London, and New York.
337. Solomon, T. E., Beyerman, H. C., and Grossman, M. I. (1977): Potency of des-histidyl[1]-secretin for pancreatic secretion in dogs. *Clin. Res.,* 25A 574.
338. Solomon, T. E., Petersen, H., and Grossman, M. I. (1978): Trophic effects of secretin on stomach and pancreas. *Scand. J. Gastroenterol. (Suppl. 49),* 13:172.
339. Soloway, R. D., Clark, M. L., Powell, K. M., Senior, J. R., and Brooks, F. P. (1972): Effects of secretin and bile salt infusions on canine bile composition and flow. *Am. J. Physiol.,* 222:681–686.
340. Sperber, I. (1959): Secretion of organic anions in the formation of urine and bile. *Pharmacol. Rev.,* 11:109–134.
341. Spingola, L. J., and Grossman, M. I. (1973): Bioassay. In: *Peptide Hormones,* edited by S. A. Berson, and R. S. Yalow, pp. 1066–1068. American Elsevier, New York.
342. Stahlheber, H., Reiser, M., Lehnert, P., Forell, M. M., Bottermann, P., and Jaeger, E. (1975): Die Wirkung von natürlichem und Synthetischem sekretin auf die Insulinsekretion. *Klin. Wochenschr.,* 53:339–341.
343. Stanley, M. D., Coalson, R. E., Grossman, M. I., and Johnson, L. R. (1972): Influence of secretin and pentagastrin on acid secretion and parietal cell number in rats. *Gastroenterology,* 63:264–269.
344. Starling, E. H. (1905): The Croonian Lecture on the chemical correlation of the function of the body. I. *Lancet,* ii:339–341.
345. Steiner, D. F., and Oyer, P. E. (1967): The biosynthesis of insulin and a probable, precursor of insulin by a human islet cell adenoma. *Proc. Natl. Acad. Sci. USA,* 57:473–480.

346. Stening, G. F., Johnson, L. R., and Grossman, M. I. (1969): Effect of secretin on acid and pepsin secretion in cat and dog. *Gastroenterology,* 56:468–475.
347. Still, E. U. (1931): Secretin. *Physiol. Rev.,* 11:328–357.
348. Still, E. U., McBean, J. W., and Ries, F. A. (1931): Studies on the physiology of secretin. *Am. J. Physiol.,* 99:94–100.
349. Stock, C., Stoebner, P., Kachelhoffer, J., and Grenier, J.-F. (1973): Perfusion de pancréas isolé chez le chien. *Ann. Biol. Clin.,* 31:377–385.
350. Strasberg, S. M., Ilson, R. G., Siminovitch, K. A., Brenner, D., and Palaheimo, J. E. (1975): Analysis of the components of bile flow in the Rhesus monkey. *Am. J. Physiol.,* 228:115–121.
351. Straus, E., Urbach, H.-J., and Yalow, R. S. (1975): Comparative reactivities of ^{125}I-secretin and ^{125}I-6-tyrosyl secretin with guinea pig and rabbit anti-secretin sera. *Biochem. Biophys. Res. Commun.,* 64:1036–1040.
352. Straus, E., and Yalow, R. S. (1978): Immunoreactive secretin in gastrointestinal mucosa of several mammalian species. *Gastroenterology,* 75:401–404.
353. Sum, P. T., and Preshaw, R. M. (1967): Intraduodenal glucose infusion and pancreatic secretion in man. *Lancet,* ii:340–341.
354. Sun, D. C. H. (1963): The use of pancreozymin-secretin test in the diagnosis of pancreatitis and tumors of the pancreas. *Gastroenterology,* 45:203–208.
355. Sun, D. C. H., and Shay, H. (1960): Pancreozymin-secretin test. The combined study of serum enzymes and duodenal contents in the diagnosis of pancreatic disease. *Gastroenterology,* 38:570–581.
356. Sundler, F., Alumets, J., Håkanson, R., Fahrenkrug, J., and Schaffalitzky de Muckadell, O. B. (1978): Peptidergic (VIP) nerves in pancreas. *Histochemistry,* 55:173–176.
357. Sutherland, E. W., Øye, I., and Butcher, R. W. (1965): The action of epinephrine and the role of the adenyl cyclase system in hormone action. *Rec. Progr. Horm. Res.,* 21:623–646.
358. Szadkowski, M. (1972): The pancreozymin-secretin test of pancreatic function in different age groups of healthy humans. *Acta Med. Pol.,* XIII:427–438.
359. Tachibana, S. (1971): The bioassay of secretin in the rat. *Jpn. J. Pharmacol.,* 21:325–336.
360. Tai, H. H., Korsch, B., and Chey, W. Y. (1975): Preparation of ^{125}I-labelled secretin of high specific radioactivity. *Anal. Biochem.,* 69:34–42.
361. Taylor, D. A., Macken, K. L., and Fiore, A. S. (1966): Angiographic visualization of the secretin-stimulated pancreas. *Radiology,* 87:525–526.
362. Teale, J. D., Buchanan, K. D., and Harper, G. (1972): A radioimmunoassay for secretin using antibodies raised to pure natural and synthetic secretins. *Gut,* 13:849–850.
363. Thomas, J. E. (1950): *The External Secretion of the Pancreas.* C. C. Thomas, Springfield, Illinois.
364. Thomas, J. E., and Crider, J. O. (1940): A quantitative study of acid in the intestine as a stimulus for the pancreas. *Am. J. Physiol.,* 131:349–356.
365. Thomas, J. E., and Crider, J. O. (1943): The effect of bile in the intestine on the secretion of pancreatic juice. *Am. J. Physiol.,* 138:548–552.
366. Thompson, J. C., Reeder, D. D., Bunchman, H. H., Becker, H. D., and Brandt, E. N. Jr. (1972): Effect of secretin on circulating gastrin. *Ann. Surg.,* 176:384–391.
367. Thompson, W. J., Johnson, D. G., Lavis, V. R., and Williams, R. H. (1974): Effects of secretin on guanyl cyclase of various tissues. *Endocrinology,* 94:276–278.
368. Thorell, J. I., and Johansson, B. G. (1971): Enzymatic iodination of polypeptides with ^{125}I to high specific activity. *Biochim. Biophys. Acta,* 251:363–369.
369. Tompkins, R. K., and Kuchenbecker, S. L. (1973): Relationship of cyclic AMP to secretin stimulation of the pancreas. *J. Surg. Res.,* 14:172–176.
370. Tracy, H. J., and Gregory, R. A. (1964): Physiological properties of a series synthetic peptides structurally related to gastrin I. *Nature,* 204:935–938.
371. Tumpson, D. B., and Johnson, L. R. (1969): Effect of secretin and cholecystokinin on the response of the gastric fistula rat to pentagastrin. *Proc. Soc. Exp. Biol. Med.,* 131:186–188.
372. Turnberg, L. A., and Grahame, G. (1974): Secretion of water and electrolytes into the duodenum in normal subjects and in patients with cirrhosis: The response to secretin and pancreozymin. *Gut,* 15:273–277.
373. Turner, D. S. (1969): Intestinal hormones and insulin release: In vitro studies using rabbit pancreas. *Horm. Metab. Res.,* 1:168–174.

374. Turner, D. S., and Marks, V. (1972): Enhancement of glucose-stimulated insulin release by an intestinal polypeptide in rats. *Lancet,* i:1095–1097.
375. Tympner, F., Domschke, W., Koch, H., and Demling, L. (1974): Sekretin-Pankreozymin-Test. *Dtsch. Med. Wochenschr.,* 99:1611–1615.
376. Udén, R. (1976): Secretin and epinephrine combined in celiac angiography. *Acta Radiol. Diagn.,* 17:17–40.
377. Unger, R. H., Ketterer, H., Eisentraut, A., and Dupré, J. (1966): Effect of secretin on insulin secretion. *Lancet,* ii:24–26.
378. Urbach, H.-J., Domschke, W., Reiss, M., Domschke, S., Rosselin, G., Wünsch, E., Jaeger, E., Moroder, L., and Demling, L. (1976): Superior immunoreactivity of ^{125}I-(des-Tyrβ-Ala)-secretin with rabbit anti-secretin sera compared to ^{125}I-secretin and ^{125}I-6-tyrosyl secretin. *Horm. Metab. Res.,* 8:459–461.
379. Vagne, M., Stening, G. F., Brooks, F. P., and Grossman, M. I. (1968): Synthetic secretin: Comparison with natural secretin for potency and spectrum of physiological actions. *Gastroenterology,* 55:260–267.
380. Vandermeers-Piret, M. C., Vandermeers, A., Rathé, J., Christophe, J., van der Hoeden, R., Wettendorff, P., and Delcourt, A. (1974): A comparison of enzyme activities in duodenal aspirate following injection of secretin, caerulein, and cholecystokinin. *Digestion,* 10:191–204.
381. Van Goidsenhoven, G. E., Henke, W. J., Vacca, J. B., and Knight, W. A. Jr. (1963): Pancreatic function in cirrhosis of the liver. *Am. J. Dig. Dis.,* 8:160–173.
382. van Zon, A., and Beyerman, H. C. (1976): Synthesis of the gastrointestinal peptide hormone secretin by the repetitive excess mixed anhydride (REMA) method. *Helv. Chim. Acta,* 59:1112–1126.
383. Verner, J. V., and Morrison, A. B. (1958): Islet cell tumor and a syndrome of refractory watery dirrhea and hypokalemia. *Am. J. Med.,* 25:374–380.
384. Waitman, A. M., Dyck, W. P., and Janowitz, H. D. (1969): Effect of secretin and acetazolamide on the volume and electrolyte composition of hepatic bile in man. *Gastroenterology,* 56:286–294.
385. Walter, A. A. (1899): Excitabilité sécrétoire spécifique de la muqueuse du canal digestif. *Arch. Sci. Biol.,* VII:1–86.
386. Wang, C. C., and Grossman, M. I. (1951): Physiological determination of release of secretin and pancreozymin from intestine of dogs with transplanted pancreas. *Am. J. Physiol.,* 164:527–545.
387. Ward, A. S., and Bloom, S. R. (1975): Effect of vagotomy on secretin release in man. *Gut,* 16:951–956.
388. Watanabe, S. (1973): Pancreozymin-secretin test. *J. Jpn. Soc. Intern. Med.,* 62:32–45.
389. Weaver, M. M., Luckhardt, A. B., and Koch, F. C. (1926): Preparation of potent vasodilatin free pancreatic secretin. *J.A.M.A.,* 87:640–645.
390. Werner, B., and Mutt, V. (1954): The pancreatic response in man to the injection of highly purified secretin and of pancreozymin. *Scand. J. Clin. Lab. Invest.,* 6:228–236.
391. Wertheimer, E., and Lepage, L. (1901): Sur le fonctions réflexes des ganglions abdominaux du sympathique dans l'innervation sécrétoire du pancréas. *J. Physiol. Pathol. Gén.,* 3:335–348.
392. Wertheimer, E., and Lepage, L. (1901): Sur les fonctions réflexes des ganglions abdominaux du sympathique dans l'innervation sécrétoire du pancréas. *J. Physiol. Pathol. Gén.,* 3:363–374.
393. Wheeler, H. O. (1968): Water and electrolytes in bile. In: *Handbook of Physiology,* sect. 6, Alimentary Canal vol. 5, edited by C. F. Code pp. 2409–2431. Washington DC.
394. Wheeler, H. O., and Mancusio-Ungaro, P. L. (1966): Role of bile ducts during secretin choleresis in dogs. *Am. J. Physiol.,* 210:1153–1159.
395. Wheeler, H. O., and Ramos, O. L. (1960): Determinants of the flow and composition of bile in the unanaesthetized dog during constant infusions of sodium taurocholate. *J. Clin. Invest.,* 39:161–170.
396. Windeck, R., Brown, E. M., Gardner, D. G., and Aurbach, G. D. (1978): Effect of gastrointestinal hormones on isolated bovine parathyroid cells. *Endocrinology,* 103:2020–2026.
397. Wormsley, K. G. (1968): Response to secretin in man. *Gastroenterology,* 54:197–209.
398. Wormsley, K. G. (1968): The action of secretin on the secretion of enzymes by the human pancreas. *Scand. J. Gastroenterol.,* 3:183–188.

399. Wormsley, K. G. (1969): A comparison of the response to secretin, pancreozymin and a combination of these hormones, in man. *Scand. J. Gastroenterol.,* 4:413–417.
400. Wormsley, K. G. (1973): Is secretin secreted? *Gut,* 14:743–751.
401. Wormsley, K. G., and Grossman, M. I. (1964): Inhibition of gastric acid secretion by secretin and by endogenous acid in the duodenum. *Gastroenterology,* 47:72–81.
402. Wünsch, E. (1967): Die Totalsynthese des Pankreas-hormons Glukagon. *Z. Naturforsch.,* 225:1269–1275.
403. Wünsch, E. (1972): Zur Synthese von biologisch voll-aktivem Sekretin. *Naturwissenschaften,* 59:239–246.
404. Wünsch, E., Jaeger, E., Moroder, L., and Schulz, I. (1977): Progress in the problem of structure activity relations of gastrointestinal hormones. In: *Hormonal Receptors in Digestive Tract Physiology,* edited by S. Bonfils, P. Fromageot, G. Rosselin, pp. 19–27. North-Holland, Amsterdam, New York, Oxford.
405. Yalow, R. S., and Berson, S. A. (1960): Immunoassay of endogenous plasma insulin in man. *J. Clin. Invest.,* 39:1157–1175.
406. Yanaihara, N., Kubota, M., Sakagami, M., Sato, H., Mochizuki, T., Sakura, N., Hashimoto, T., Yanaihara, C., Yamaguchi, K., Zeze, F., and Abe, K. (1977): Synthesis of phenolic group containing analogues of porcine secretin and their immunological properties. *J. Med. Chem.,* 20:648–655.
407. Yanaihara, N., Sato, H., Kubota, M., Sakagami, M., Hashimoto, T., Yanaihara, C., Yamaguchi, K., Zeze, F., Abe, K., and Kaneko, T. (1976): Radioimmunoassay for secretin using N^α-tyrosylsecretin and (Tyr[1])-secretin. *Endocrinol. Jpn.,* 23:87–90.
408. Young, J. D., Lazarus, L., Chisholm, D. J., and Atkinson, F. F. V. (1968): Radioimmunoassay of secretin in human serum. *J. Nucl. Med.,* 9:641–642.
409. Zermatten, A., and Felber, J.-P. (1974): Sensitivity to glucose of an intestinal factor stimulating insulin release. *Horm. Metab. Res.,* 6:272–274.
410. Zieve, L., Silvis, S. E., Mulford, B., Blackwood, W. D., McHale, A., and Doizaki, W. (1966): Secretion of pancreatic enzymes. I. Response to secretin and pancreozymin. *Am. J. Dig. Dis.,* 11:671–684.
411. Zimmerman, M. J., Dreiling, D. A., and Janowitz, H. D. (1973): The secretin test. In: *Secretin, Cholecystokinin, Pancreozymin and Gastrin,* edited by J. E. Jorpes and V. Mutt, pp. 219–246. Springer-Verlag, Berlin, Heidelberg, New York.
412. Zollinger, R. M., and Ellison, E. H. (1955): Primary peptic ulcerations of the jejunum associated with islet cell tumors of the pancreas. *Ann. Surg.,* 142:709–728.
413. Zollinger, R. M., Tompkins, R. K., Amerson, J. R., Endahl, G. L., Kraft, A. R., and Moore, F. T. (1968): Identification of the diarrheogenic hormone associated with non-beta islet cell tumors of the pancreas. *Ann. Surg.,* 168:502–521.

Gastrointestinal Hormones, edited by
George B. Jerzy Glass.
Raven Press, New York © 1980.

Chapter 6

Gastrin: Isolation, Characterization, and Functions

Göran Nilsson

*Department of Physiology, Faculty of Veterinarian Medicine, Swedish University of
Agricultural Sciences, Uppsala; and Department of Experimental Surgery,
Serafimerlasarettet, Stockholm, Sweden*

DISCOVERY AND PURIFICATION OF GASTRIN

In his appearance at the Royal Society in May 1905 (60), Edkins presented the following preliminary communication: "On the analogy of what has been held to be the mechanism at work in the secretion of pancreatic juice by Bayliss and Starling, it is probable that, in the process of absorption of digested food in the stomach, a substance may be separated from the cells of the mucous membrane which, passing into the blood or lymph, later stimulates the secretory cells of the stomach to functional activity." Between the discoveries of secretin (10) and gastrin the name *hormone* was proposed for intrinsic substances that exert action at a site other than that of their formation and release (see 81).

Edkins' theory soon met opposition. Zeljony and Savich (285), working in Pavlov's laboratory, demonstrated that the introduction of Liebig's extract into the isolated pyloric antrum produced a gastric secretion that could be prevented by the previous administration of atropine or by the painting of the pyloric mucosa with cocaine, indicating a nervous mode of stimulation. Other workers demonstrated that extracts from tissues of different origin induced acid secretion when given to dogs with gastric pouches. Popielski (188) attributed this action to a substance widely distributed in the body called *vasodilatin*. Later Dale and Laidlaw (45) identified histamine having such a distribution in the body. Others demonstrated that histamine is also present in the pyloric antrum (207) and that it is a powerful stimulator of gastric secretion (189). As a consequence, the gastrin hypothesis was no longer attractive and disappeared from the scene and did not reappear until the end of the 1930s.

Komarov (138) then assumed that gastrin like secretin might be a polypeptide and therefore separable from histamine in extracts. Other laboratories soon established that a stimulant of protein nature could be extracted from the antral mucosa, although the preparations obtained were relatively crude and not always successful in stimulating acid secretion. In 1961, Gregory and Tracy (96) described a method of extraction that regularly yielded gastrin preparations active in stimulating acid secretion. The procedure was not, however, suitable as a

G 34   PYR-LEU-GLY-PRO-GLN-GLY-PRO-PRO-HIS-LEU-VAL-ALA-ASP-PRO-SER-LYS-LYS

         -GLN-GLY-PRO-TRP-LEU-GLU-GLU-GLU-GLU-ALA-TYR-GLY-TRP-MET-ASP-PHE-NH$_2$
                                                               I
                                                                R

G 17   PYR-GLY-PRO-TRP-LEU-GLU-GLU-GLU-GLU-GLU-ALA-TYR-GLY-TRP-MET-ASP-PHE-NH$_2$
                                                                 I
                                                                 R

G 14   TRP-LEU-GLU-GLU-GLU-GLU-GLU-ALA-TYR-GLY-TRP-MET-ASP-PHE-NH$_2$
                                                                 I
                                                                 R

NT-G 17   PYR-GLY-PRO-TRP-LEU-GLU-GLU-GLU-GLU-GLU-ALA-TYR-GLY
                                                            I
                                                             R

FIG. 1. Amino acid sequences of chemically identified forms of human gastrin. The radical (R) at tyrosine in gastrin type I corresponds to H and in gastrin II to SO$_3$H. Note that amino acids 26–28 are SER-PRO-HIS instead of HIS-PRO-PRO as previously reported. (By kind permission of Drs. R. A. Gregory and J. Dockray).

basis for the final isolation of the hormone. Such a method was evolved during the next few years and resulted in 1964 (97) in the final identification of two heptadecapeptides named gastrins I and II and differing only in the presence of sulfate on the tyrosine of gastrin II (Fig. 1). Determination of the structure (94) as well as synthesis (1) of the gastrins followed.

Gregory and Tracy (97) isolated their gastrins from the mucosa of hogs. In subsequent studies, gastrin heptadecapeptides have been isolated also from dog, cat, sheep, cow (136), and man (15) and found to differ by only one or two amino acid substitutions in the middle of the linear peptide chain, requiring the change of only one base of the codon triplet per substitution (Fig. 2). Following the introduction of radioimmunological methods for gastrin determinations in tissue extracts and in body fluids, gastrin was demonstrated to exist also in a larger and less acidic form than the heptadecapeptide. This gastrin, originally presented as "big gastrin" (282), has been isolated from human gastrinoma extracts and from hog antral mucosa and the amino acid sequence determined (98).

The "big gastrin," which has 34 amino acids, consists of the heptadecapeptide amide (G-17) covalently linked at its N-terminus by two lysyl residues to a further heptadecapeptide, the N-terminus of which is, as in free G-17, pyroglutamyl (Fig. 1).

As for G-17, two forms of G-34 exist with and without the sulfated tyrosine. Gregory and Tracy (99) also isolated small amounts of a sulfated and unsulfated minigastrin peptide, which later was shown to be a C-terminal tetradecapeptide fragment of G-17 (Fig. 1).

In addition to the above-mentioned forms of gastrin, Yalow and Berson (284) have reported a gastrin-like component emerging in the void volume of Sephadex G-50 columns and named it "big big gastrin" (BBG). The existence of this component has been the subject of some discussion (162) and it has been suggested (197) that BBG may be formed as a result of interference in the radioimmunoassay (RIA) by large proteins eluted in the void volume.

Another component having gastrin-like immunoreactivity and emerging on Sephadex columns in the region of proinsulin has been indicated by Rehfeld and Stadil (199) and named component I. Gregory (94) has also reported a pair of inactive gastrin fragments present in hog antral mucosa that was demonstrated to have the N-tridecapeptide sequence of G-17 (Fig. 1). This fragment seems to have been identified in the serum in later work by Dockray and Walsh

| Human | PYR - GLY - PRO - TRP - LEU - GLU - GLU - GLU - GLU - GLU - ALA - TYR - GLY - TRP - MET - ASP - PHE - NH$_2$ |
| | 1   2   3   4   5   6   7   8   9   10 11 12 13 14 15 16 17 |

Cat	ALA
Pig	MET
Dog	MET ALA
Cow / Sheep	VAL ALA

FIG. 2. Heptadecapeptide gastrin isolated from various species.

(55). Other findings (200) indicate that gastrin may be even more heterogenous. Repeated filtrations of serum on large Sephadex columns suggest the existence of no less than 20 different gastrins, i.e., six component I:s, six G-34s, four G-17s, and four G-14s. For additional information on this subject see Chapter 19 by J. F. Rehfeld, pp. 433–450, *this volume.* The elution pattern on Sephadex of the most common gastrin forms is illustrated in Fig. 3.

The related gastrin forms have been demonstrated to exist in serum as well as in tissue extracts. In pyloric mucosa, G-17 is the predominant gastrin form (> 90%), whereas G-34 is the most abundant circulating gastrin form. The reason for this discrepancy is not fully understood, although it has been suggested that differences in clearance rates from the circulation as well as selective release of G-34 from tissues may be contributing factors.

The physiological significance of the different gastrin peptides isolated and suggested cannot at present be fully evaluated. Although G-34 may be the predominating form in serum, it will, due to its less pronounced biological activity, probably be less important than G-17 in activating the parietal cells to cause acid secretion (261). In cats, minigastrin seems to play the indicated role of G-17 (258). The carboxyl-terminal portion of the gastrin molecule has all the biological actions of the G-17 molecule (246). However, fragments as small as the C-terminal dipeptide amide have a certain activity (19).

For a more detailed description of structure-activity relationships for gastrin-like molecules, see references 168 and 247. When activity is expressed as the exogenous dose needed to induce a certain level of a maximal response, the molar potency will increase with the chain length from G-13 to G-34 (48,

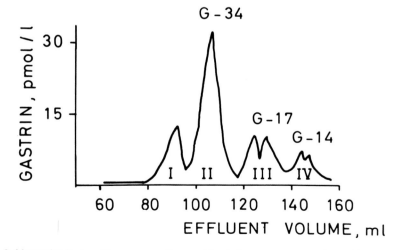

FIG. 3. Molecular forms of immunoreactive gastrins in human serum evaluated by gel filtration on Sephadex G-50 superfine columns (10 × 2000 mm). The elution was monitored by radioimmunoassay, using gastrin antiserum 2604 that measures components I–III with equimolar potency. (With permission of J. F. Rehfeld.)

265). Expressed as blood level needed to obtain a fraction of the maximal response, G-17 is the most potent on a molar basis (48,265).

The gastrin-like peptide most often used clinically and in research is pentagastrin. This commercially available synthetic pentapeptide consists of the C-terminal tetrapeptide amide of gastrin and beta-alanine and an N-terminal blocking group, tertiary butyl oxycarbonyl. The biological effect in stimulating acid secretion is comparable with that of the C-terminal pentapeptide amide of gastrin.

The C-terminal pentapeptide amide sequence of gastrin is identical with that of cholecystokinin-pancreozymin (CCK-PZ) and this fragment has all the biological actions of the two hormones. Among the gastrin-like peptides identified, the ratio of potency for gallbladder and pancreas stimulation to potency for acid secretory effect does not vary with chain length but is essentially constant for G-4 through G-34.

TISSUE DISTRIBUTION OF GASTRIN

The antral mucosa is no doubt the richest source of gastrin in all species investigated. However, several reports exist that extra-antral tissues also contain gastrin-like activity.

Through use of biological methods for gastrin determination, gastrin-like activities were found in the duodenal mucosa of man, dog, cat, and hog in several studies (69,108,138,139,149,255), whereas some authors failed to demonstrate gastrin in this location in dogs and hogs (61,96,253,254) and only occasionally in cats (253). The gastrin distribution was more extensively studied by Nilsson et al., using radioimmunological technique. Gastrin-like immunoreactivity was found in the duodenum of man, dog, cat, and hog (177) and in monkey, rat, rabbit, and guinea pig (172).

The studies (Table 1 and Fig. 4) showed that within the mucosa of duodenum, a concentration gradient of gastrin was apparent with decreasing concentrations in distal direction. This gradient continued farther down in the jejunum. Within the remaining portion of the mucosa of the small intestine, minute amounts of gastrin-like immunoreactivity were detected, whereas no such activity was noted in the mucosa of the large intestine. Low concentrations of gastrin-like immunoreactivity were also found in the buccal mucosa, tongue, and esophagus in man, dog, cat, and hog, as well as in the pancreas of man. In the latter case, the immunoreactivity was further characterized and revealed to consist of heptadecapeptide gastrin and a minor portion of G-34. Radioimmunological determinations have revealed gastrin-like immunoreactivity in pancreatic extracts from man in other studies also (103,198) and in hog (186), whereas others have not been able to detect gastrin in the pancreas of the hog, dog, and cat (177). The total amounts of extra-antral gastrin in the species investigated were low or 0.1 to 7%, except for the duodenal gastrin content in man, which in the small autopsy material available showed considerable individual variations. Great amounts of duodenal gastrin in man has also been indicated by Lai (149),

TABLE 1. *Average concentration and range of gastrin-like immunoreactivity in mμg/g wet tissue in various species*

Extracted tissue	Human (4)	Dog (3)	Cat (5)	Hog (4)
Tongue	—	0	2 (0–9.6)	4.6 (2.3–7.0)
Proximal esophagus (PO)	0.2 (0–0.3)	0.3 (0–0.5)	0.9 (0–3.9)	1.4 (0.1–3.5)
Middle esophagus (MO)	0.3 (0–0.8)	0.6 (0.5–0.9)	0.5 (0–1.4)	2.1 (0.7–3.1)
Distal esophagus (DO)	0.8 (0–2.3)	0.6 (0.4–0.7)	0.4 (0–1.5)	1.8 (0.8–3.6)
Corpus I (C I)	0.3 (0–0.8)	0.5 (0–1.4)	0.6 (0–1.2)	2.0 (0.7–3.4)
Corpus II (C II)	3 (0–7)	87.3 (2–215)	224 (0–769)	23 (7.1–40.0)
Corpus III (C III)	0.1 (0–0.3)	0.2 (0.1–0.2)	0	1.2 (1.0–1.4)
Corpus IV (C IV)	0.6 (0.5–0.7)	0.2 (0–0.5)	0.2 (0–1.1)	0.6 (0.3–0.8)
Corpus V (C V)	2.3 (1.1–4.2)	19.4 (8–27)	39 (0–26)	48 (24–87)
Antrum (A)	1486 (66–3016)	648 (239–913)	2052 (171–4806)	22085 (8764–39374)
Proximal duodenum (PD)	752 (92–1888)	7.1 (3.3–10.9)	24.4 (6.5–72.1)	49.2 (30.7–60.4)
Middle duodenum (MD)	507 (43–1446)	4.1 (3.2–5.4)	4.7 (0.8–11.0)	27.4 (21.9–37.1)
Distal duodenum (DD)	267 (1–1053)	2.1 (1.9–2.2)	4.4 (1.1–11.6)	20.1 (13.1–28.1)
Intestine I (In I)	6 (4.0–10.0)	2.0 (1.3–2.7)	3.3 (0.6–11.2)	10.4 (6–15.1)
Intestine II (In II)	3.8 (2.0–7.0)	0.6 (0.5–0.8)	1.4 (0.8–2.5)	4.7 (3.5–6.2)
Intestine III (In III)	3.8 (2.0–4.3)	1.4 (1.1–1.8)	0.7 (0.3–1.6)	4.2 (2.9–5.9)
Intestine IV (In IV)	2.1 (1.2–3.1)	0.5 (0.4–0.6)	0.2 (0–0.6)	5.1 (2.8–7.2)
Intestine V (In V)	1.7 (1.2–2.4)	0.3 (0.1–0.4)	—	4.8 (2.6–6.4)
Intestine VI (In VI)	1.8 (1.2–2.7)	0.2 (0.1–0.3)	—	4.0 (2.0–7.1)
Intestine VII (In VII)	0.7 (0.4–0.9)	0.2 (0.1–0.4)	—	3.0 (1.4–4.8)
Intestine VIII (In VIII)	0.6 (0.2–0.9)	0.2 (0.1–0.5)	—	2.9 (1.3–4.6)
Intestine IX (In IX)	0.5 (0.3–0.7)	0.2 (0.1–0.3)	—	1.9 (0.7–3.9)
Intestine X (In X)	0.5 (0.3–0.8)	0.1 (0–0.3)	—	1.8 (0.6–3.7)
Colon	0	0		
Pancreas	0.4 (0.3–0.5)	0	0	0
Kidney	0	0	0	0
Liver	0	0	0	0
Lung	0	0	0	0

Adapted from ref. 177. The data are to be related to Fig. 4. Figures under the species indicate number of specimens.

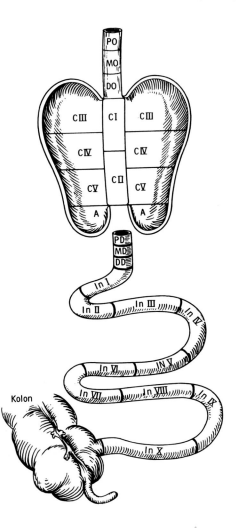

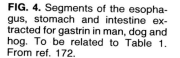

FIG. 4. Segments of the esophagus, stomach and intestine extracted for gastrin in man, dog and hog. To be related to Table 1. From ref. 172.

using biological technique and by Bloom and Polak (22), who determined duodenal gastrin by RIA.

According to the observations related above, gastrin-like activities of significant order have been demonstrated in several species in the mucosa of both the antrum and the duodenum with biological as well as immunological techniques. In these tissues and in pancreatic islet tissue of man, morphological data exist that correlate them to the gastrin content.

In the antral and duodenal mucosa, gastrin is supposed to be produced, stored, and released from the so-called G cells identified by different groups by immunohistological technique and using antisera specific against synthetic gastrin (28,

43,164,206). In the antral mucosa, the G cells are essentially located in the junctional area between the mucous cells of the glandular neck and the mucoid cells, i.e., in the intermediate third of the glands. This distribution compares favorably with observations by Broomé et al. (24). They determined the gastrin-like activity in extracts from longitudinal sections of the antral mucosa and submucosa of cats and dogs.

Ultrastructural investigations of the G cell in the antrum and duodenum reveal characteristics that are essentially common among species (29,77,206,221). The cells generally have a pyramidal form and are surrounded by mucoid cells. The apical pole of the cells is in contact with the lumen of the mucosal gland and projects microvilli into the lumen. A few electron-dense granules are located in this part of the cell as organelles such as lamellar endoplasmic reticulum with ribosomes and the Golgi apparatus. At the basal portion of the cell adjacent to a capillary vessel, granules are stored. Accordingly, the gastrin-containing cells seem to be in close connection with both the blood circulation and the lumen of the gastrointestinal tract. (See Fig. 5.)

The cellular origin of the gastrin present in pancreatic extracts is subject to

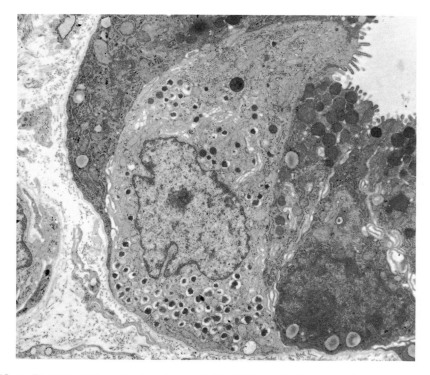

FIG. 5. Electron micrograph of a single cat G cell demonstrating microvillous structures of the luminal end. (Courtesy of Dr. Enrico Solcia.)

discussion. The islet D_1 cells (271) or IV type islet cell (51) or endocrine cells in the ductular system (42) may be the candidates. For additional information see Chapter 1 by E. Solcia et al., pp. 1–18 and Chapter 2 by J. Polak and S. R. Bloom, pp. 19–52, *this volume.*

METABOLISM OF GASTRIN

Information on the metabolism of gastrin essentially originates from experiments in dogs. Registering the decline in plasma gastrin concentration following pulse injections of extracts from a gastrin tumor, Straus and Yalow (232) found the half-life of G-17, G-34, and BBG to be 3, 9, and 90 min, respectively. Similar results for G-17 (196,211) have been obtained by other workers, whereas the half-life for G-34 in an infusion study was estimated to be 15 min (265). The half-life for G-13 seems to be similar to that of G-17 (48). In man, the half-life of endogenous gastrin was found to be less than 10 min in experiments where the stomach of pernicious anemia patients was acidified (281). In studies where synthetic human G-17 was infused in man, a biexponential disappearance was found with half-lives of 7.5 and 12.6 min (212). Half-lives of natural G-17 and G-34 were found to be 5 and 42 min, respectively (270).

In another study, the clearance rate of G-17-I was assessed in normal man and in patients having duodenal ulcer disease. In both groups, the disappearance half-life for G-17 averaged 6.2 min, indicating that clearance of exogenous gastrin is not altered in patients with duodenal ulcer disease (268).

Studies in which G-34 and G-17 were infused into man and plasma samples chromatographed following different periods of time revealed no evidence of conversion of G-34 to G-17. Nor were there any increases in G-34 following the infusion of G-17 (268).

Several studies indicate that the kidney is very efficient in removing gastrin from the circulation. For example, nephrectomy in dogs (32) and rat (113) or renal artery ligation in rats (113) produces an increased disappearance rate. Also, studies in patients suffering from uremia or in human subjects who are nephrectomized suggest a role for the kidney in eliminating gastrin (141). Minute amounts of gastrin have been found in urine, indicating that metabolism takes place in the kidney. The enzymatic activities involved in the kidney metabolism of gastrin are not well understood. The C-terminal dipeptide amide Asp-Phe-NH_2 has been demonstrated to be removed from the gastrin tetrapeptide when incubated with kidney homogenates of rat (269). Possibly also several other enzymatic activities take part in the kidney destruction of gastrin. In addition to the kidney, several other organs have the ability to convert and remove gastrin from the circulation. Several studies in intact animals or in man have measured gastrin concentrations in blood before and after the passage through the liver. The main conclusion from such experiments is that small synthetic analogs such as tetra- and pentagastrin are rapidly removed, whereas the disappearance of G-17 and larger forms of gastrin proceeds at a slower rate.

Minor gastrin forms such as pentagastrin and the tetrapeptide of gastrin will appear in bile; both are unchanged and are present in the deaminated form (280). The deamidation seems to be achieved by a specific amidase that removes the C-terminal amide group and can be demonstrated in homogenates of liver (213,269). Some evidence exists that the gastric fundus eliminates gastrin and that the extraction rate will increase when acid is secreted by the stomach (71).

A considerably more efficient mechanism eliminating gastrin into the lumen is present in the pyloric antrum, which seems to deliver more gastrin to the lumen when the gastric content is acid than when neutral (3). The significance of fragments of endogenous peptides in the lumen of the gastrointestinal tract is so far not fully understood. One possibility may be that elimination into the lumen simply represents a mode of removing active peptides from the circulation or releasing tissues, resulting in a degradation of the peptide fragment to amino acids that will be absorbed and take part in the synthesis of new peptides. According to another possibility, which has gained some experimental support, gastrin in the gastric lumen may bind specifically to parietal cell receptors located luminally (110) and may hypothetically exert an effect. Other studies (130) suggest that gastrin present in the intestinal lumen may exert trophic effects on the intestinal mucosa that cannot be ascribed to gastrin transported to the site of action by the blood circulation. For other information on this subject see Chapter 38B by Miller and Go, pp. 863–876, *this volume.*

In a very recent study (236), it has been shown that not only kidney, liver, and the gastrointestinal tract remove considerable amounts of gastrin. A great arteriovenous difference for gastrin across the head and the rear leg was also noted.

RELEASE OF GASTRIN

Nervous Mechanisms

On the basis of experiments where secretion of acid from the stomach was taken as evidence for gastrin release, Uvnäs in 1942 (252) suggested that vagal excitation causes the release of gastrin in cats. Uvnäs' experiments initially met criticism (7,124,185), since vagal activation by sham-feeding or insulin hypoglycemia in dogs failed to induce acid secretion in vagally denervated gastric pouches (124).

A number of other studies, in time have supported Uvnäs' theories. In 1950 Glass and Wolf (91a) studied gastric secretion in human subjects in response to insulin hypoglycemia before and after antrectomy. Their results gave reason for the conclusion that a gastrin mechanism might be involved in the stimulation of acid secretion in man. Burstall and Schofield (27) showed that acid gastric juice indeed was secreted from vagally denervated pouches at vagal activation when a sensitive method for detection of acid was used. Another explanation of previous discrepancies was offered by Woodward et al. (278), who demonstrated that low pH in the antrum might reduce the secretion of acid from the stomach. Later, Maung Pe Thein and Schofield (159) presented results showing that denervation of the antrum as well as acidification diminished the acid secretion from Heidenhain pouches in dogs in response to sham-feeding. In other studies (180), Olbe showed that vagal stimulation by sham-feeding or low doses of insulin were inefficient in stimulating acid secretion following surgical removal of the pyloric antrum and the duodenal bulb and that subthreshold amounts of exogenous gastrin would potentiate the acid response to sham-feeding in such dogs (179).

Evidence for a vagal release of gastrin was also provided by Fyrö (84), who found that electrical vagal stimulation in cats reduced the gastrin-like activity content of the antral and duodenal mucosae. In 1972, final proof for vagal release of gastrin was given by Nilsson et al. (176), who demonstrated in dogs that sham-feeding significantly elevates the plasma concentration of gastrin (Fig. 6). Similar results were later reported for vagal excitation induced by insulin hypoglycemia (242) or electrical vagal stimulation (151). Attempts have been made to estimate the amounts of gastrin released following electrical stimulation of vagal nerves. Fyrö, using a bioassay technique for determination of the antral gastrin content, found that approximately 50% of the gastrin-like activity was released at electrical excitation (84). In experiments performed in a similar manner using RIA for gastrin determination, less than 1% of the gastrin content seemed to be released (256).

The related contradictory results (84,256) may be explained by recent discoveries of a peptide in the stomach acting as a potent releaser of gastrin (161). In Fyrö's (84) experiments, vagal stimulation may have released both antral gastrin and the gastrin-releasing peptide. This would result in a greater loss of gastrin-like activity, i.e., ability to induce acid secretion, than in the study by Uvnäs et al. (256), where the gastrin content in antral extracts was determined by a specific gastrin RIA.

Traditionally, vagal impulses causing release of gastrin are supposed to be mediated by cholinergic mechanisms. Nilsson et al. (176) and Csendes et al. (44) found that atropinization more or less abolished the gastrin response induced by sham-feeding (176) and insulin hypoglycemia (44). Atropine in high doses may pass the blood-brain barrier in amounts sufficient to influence cholinergic functions in the central nervous system (CNS). Whether the inhibition observed in these experiments was due to central or peripheral inhibition therefore could not be determined. However, other experiments support the concept that atropine may block cholinergic mechanisms centrally during sham-feeding and insulin stimulation. Electrical excitation of peripheral portions of divided vagal nerves in cats induces a release of gastrin that is not prevented by prior administration

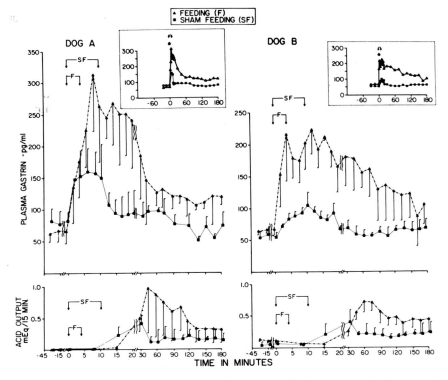

FIG. 6. Plasma gastrin concentration and acid output from Pavlov pouches before and after stimulation by sham-feeding for 10 min or test meal. From ref. 176.

of high doses (0.2–2 mg/kg) of atropine (257). These results in addition provide strong evidence that cholinergic mechanisms are not involved in the peripheral stimulation of vagal gastrin release. Also, other studies favor this concept. In man, small doses of atropine that would not have significant central effects will enhance the release of gastrin induced by sham-feeding (74). Such results in fact establish the possibility that there exist cholinergic mechanisms with the ability to exert an inhibiting influence on the release of gastrin.

Evidence in favor of such a hypothesis had been obtained far earlier in other experiments. Walsh et al. (273) found that test meal stimulation in man produced a considerably greater gastrin response in atropinization experiments than in controls. In the intact dog atropinization with low doses of atropine also enhances the release of gastrin on test meal stimulation (117), whereas large doses to some extent reduce the initial and increase the late gastrin response (176). Until explained, these results seem to be in opposition to other data presented by the Grossman group (46) indicating that local release of gastrin from the antrum induced by both distention and chemicals is prevented by atropinization. In contrast, in cats atropinization with large doses unequivocally inhibits the test meal-induced gastrin response (239). Following vagotomy, gastrin response to test meal stimulation is considerably increased (50,123,140). Atropine reduced the postvagotomy enhancement of gastrin release, suggesting a cholinergic involvement in this phenomenon (50). Another suggested evidence for a cholinergic mechanism inhibiting gastrin release is the observation that bethanechol inhibits release of gastrin induced by bombesin (240,241).

In summary, the observations related above give experimental support for the existence of intracerebral cholinergic mechanisms involved in the release of gastrin and peripheral cholinergic mechanisms mediating inhibitory influences on gastrin release. They also indicate species differences in the influence of atropine on the meal-induced gastrin response. Assuming that peripheral cholinergic mechanisms do not mediate the stimulation of the antral G cells, other nervous mechanisms have to be postulated. Recent studies demonstrate that catecholamine-containing fibers exist in the vagal nerves (155,170). In man the administration of adrenalin causes release of gastrin that can be blocked by β-adrenergic blocking agents (223). Similarly, in the rat the β-receptor agonist isoprenaline induces release of gastrin that may be counteracted by β-blocking substances (157). In addition, dopamine also seems to influence plasma gastrin concentration by evoking a considerable release (109). At present, it is not possible to conclude whether or not adrenergic mechanisms will contribute to the physiological regulation of vagal release of gastrin.

Recent studies with immunohistochemical techniques have indicated that a great number of peptides are present within the vagal as well as other peripheral nerves (156). In the vagal nerve the gastrin-like immunoreactivity has been identified as G-17 (259). Possibly such peptide neurons may mediate the peripheral vagal excitation that is induced by the sight, smell, and taste of food.

Local Release from the Antrum

In dogs gastrin release following a meal is considerably greater than that obtained by vagal stimulation induced by sham-feeding (176). (See Fig. 6). A similar relationship seems to exist also in man. According to the traditional view, essentially developed from studies in dogs, when reaching the stomach the food will release gastrin by distention and chemical excitation. Using acid secretion from fundic pouches as evidence for gastrin release, Olbe (179) showed that distention of transplanted antral pouches induced secretion of acid gastric juice. In more recent studies, determinations of plasma gastrin concentration following antral pouch distention have indicated release of gastrin to the blood (46). Recent studies have provided results that question the role of gastric distention in causing gastrin release. Thus, no significant increase in plasma gastrin levels has been seen at such a stimulation in man (76). These results appear to be in contrast with previous observations on dogs with isolated pouches of the pyloric antrum.

Results of studies on the chemical release of gastrin from the antrum were most commonly based on those in which the rates of acid secretion were supposed to reflect the release of antral gastrin. In extensive studies on dogs, Elwin (66) found that certain amino acids were more potent than others in inducing acid secretion when instilled into pyloric pouches. The position and availability of the amino groups seem to be critical for the ability of the amino acids to act in a stimulatory way. For example, glycine, which is a potent stimulant, was considerably less active when the amino group was methylated yielding the amino acid sarcosine. Also, the stimulatory action of alanine was reduced when the amino group was present in the α instead of the β position.

In more recent studies, Grossman et al. (237) tested the ability of a large number of amino acids to release gastrin. These results provide direct evidence that amino acids indeed cause gastrin release. However, discrepancies were found between the ability of individual amino acids to stimulate acid secretion and to elevate serum gastrin concentration, which suggested direct stimulatory effect of some of the amino acids on parietal cells. Other studies show that the ability to release gastrin is not exclusively a property of amino acids but can be accomplished also by larger peptide fragments (47,66). Also, ingested fats have been demonstrated to release gastrin, whereas carbohydrates seem to lack gastrin-releasing properties (202). According to studies by Elwin (65), solutions of various alcohols induce acid secretion when instilled into pyloric pouches in dogs. For different alcohols, a relationship between chemical structure and excitatory action on the oxyntic glands was demonstrated and taken as evidence for gastrin release. In man ethanol is a poor releaser of gastrin (13) and a weak stimulant of acid secretion (35).

Other studies have been performed in order to further clarify the mechanism by which local stimulation induces release of gastrin from the pyloric mucosa. One concept was based on the observations by Zeljony and Savich (285) that treatment of antral mucosa with a solution of cocaine inhibited acid secretion induced by a secretagogue. It has been assumed that there may exist mucosal surface receptors activated by the chemical stimulants and transmitting the impulses via a short neuron to the submucosal plexus. From there a common nervous pathway would conduct nervous impulses of mucosal as well as vagal origin to the gastrin-releasing cell. The morphological basis for neurons connecting the mucosal surface and submucosal plexa has never been demonstrated. On the other hand, it has been shown that atropine may reduce the release of gastrin induced with both chemical and mechanical stimulation of the antral mucosa (46).

According to another concept, there are no such interneurons but certain chemicals will diffuse into the mucosa to reach the gastrin cell and cause gastrin release. Organic bases and acids will be differently dissociated at different pHs. They will diffuse optimally when the local pH of the antrum will equal the pH at which the organic substances are charged and uncharged to a similar extent. At further dissociation, the ability to diffuse will become reduced (2). In the light of the finding that gastrin cells seem to have contact with the gastric lumen, one may perhaps modify the speculation by Andersson and Elwin (2) by suggesting that amino acids when less charged will more easily enter the gastrin cell and intracellularly contribute to gastrin release. From these observations it seems evident that food in the stomach considerably contributes to the release of gastrin. The role played by mechanical antral stimulation in causing gastrin release is, however, unclear and it would seem as if chemical stimulation of the gastrin-releasing mechanism plays a significant role. One may, however, wonder to which extent free amino acids and digested peptide fragments having gastrin-releasing properties will be present in the stomach during the first 15 min after a meal. At this time, the plasma gastrin peak concentration is reached and the secretion of acid gastric juice is about to start.

At present it is, therefore, more likely that other mechanisms may be more efficient in causing gastrin release during a meal. It has been shown recently that a factor may be extracted from the fundic portion of the stomach that when given to dogs acts as an extremely potent releaser of gastrin (161). Similar properties have been described for the amphibian peptide bombesin (20,116). Bombesin-like immunoreactivity has been found in extracts of the fundic mucosa and other portions of the gastrointestinal tract (271) (see also Chapter 29 by P. Melchiorri, pp. 717–728, *this volume*). Whether the principle under isolation (161) is indeed a mammalian form of bombesin or a peptide of other chemical structure remains to be established. The existence of a peptide in the gastric mucosa having gastrin-releasing properties may perhaps explain the release of gastrin observed by Debas et al. (49) on stimulation of the fundic mucosa and interpreted as an oxynto-pyloric reflex.

Extragastric Release

In most species except possibly man (22,149,177), the extragastric tissue amounts of gastrin are low. Older studies, however, indicate that extragastric gastrin may be released. For example, vagal excitation in cats decreases the duodenal content of gastrin (84). Also, acid response to sham-feeding in dogs may still be considerable following the resection of the pyloric antrum but is abolished following subsequent resection of the duodenal bulb (180,217). In recent studies, the effect of a test meal has been studied on gastrin release before and after the resection of the pyloric antrum with gastroduodenostomy. Interestingly, postantrectomy levels of basal plasma gastrin were essentially unchanged and test meal stimulation released amounts of gastrin that were surprisingly high considering the amounts of gastrin normally present in the duodenum. Subsequent resection of the duodenal bulb resulted in a decrease in basal levels of gastrin and test meal stimulation no longer caused release of gastrin (218).

These studies indicate that gastrin release may take place from extraantral sources of gastrin in the dog and cat and that such release essentially occurs from the upper portion of the duodenum corresponding to the duodenal bulb. Release of gastrin from extraantral sources has been demonstrated in man (230). It is not known to which extent the extraantral gastrin sources participate in the release of gastrin under normal conditions. In dogs, significant release of extraantral gastrin most likely does not occur in the intact animal. Following antrectomy, the gastrin release following test meal stimulation will originate primarily from a duodenum that had increased its gastrin content to compensate for antrum loss. This concept is supported by results from other studies in which the duodenal content of gastrin was determined in normal and in antrectomized dogs. Following removal of the antrum, gastrin content in proximal duodenum was increased severalfold as compared with controls (173). It is not known whether such a compensatory increase of gastrin also exists in man. Since gastrin is released after antrectomy, surgery in man should include removal of the duodenal bulb in order to remove gastrin-releasing tissues.

MECHANISMS INHIBITING RELEASE OF GASTRIN

Effects of Antral Acidity on Gastrin Release

Woodward et al. (278) were the first to provide experimental evidence that reduction of the antral pH inhibits gastric secretion. During the subsequent years, many studies were presented offering evidence for either inhibition of gastrin release from the antrum for the release of a humoral factor, an antral chalone, reducing the secretion of gastric juice (243) (see Chapter 42 by Glass). In 1972 Nilsson et al. (176), using radioimmunological technique, showed that gastrin responses to sham-feeding were considerably greater when the acid secretion was prevented from reaching the antral mucosa by drainage through a gastric fistula (Fig. 7). Other experiments have indicated that elevation of the intraantral pH does not influence the release of gastrin under basal conditions (46,111). Although gastrin release to the blood under stimulated conditions may be prevented by low acidity in the antrum, it is not known how the gastrin release is reduced. In this context, it may be relevant to consider the observations made by Jordan et al. (133,134) in 1972 that indicated that gastrin-like immunoreactivity was present in gastric juice. In a subsequent study, Andersson and Nilsson (3) showed in dogs with isolated pouches of the pyloric antrum that antral perfusates contain high concentrations of gastrin-like immunoreactivity. A puzzling observation was that acid perfusates contained considerably higher concentrations of gastrin-like immunoreactivity than did the neutral ones. Also, the biological gastrin-like activity in stimulating acid secretion was considerably

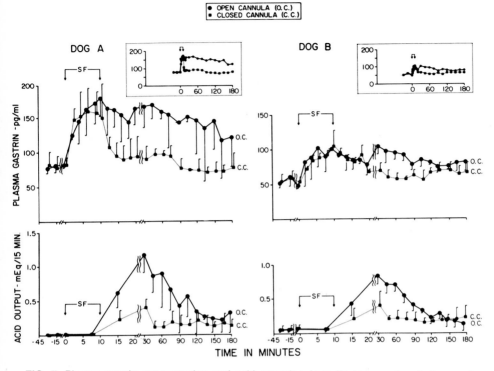

FIG. 7. Plasma gastrin concentration and acid secretion from Pavlov pouches before and after sham-feeding for 10 min with or without gastric cannula open. From ref. 176.

greater in acid than in neutral perfusates. The interpretation of these observations is difficult. They may indicate that at a low pH within the pyloric antrum gastrin is delivered into the gastric cavity rather than into the blood. The connection of the apical portion of the antral G cell to the gastric lumen that has been demonstrated offers a morphological basis for such an elimination mechanism (Fig. 5).

A brief elevation of the intraantral pH in dogs induced by perfusion of antral pouches with more alkaline solutions or the administration of antacids in man does not elevate basal plasma gastrin levels. The long-term hypochlorhydria or achlorhydria will result, however, in elevations of basal plasma gastrin concentration. Also, plasma gastrin levels will reach concentrations that are greater than the average gastrin response following stimulation by a meal under such conditions (283). The mechanism responsible for this gastrin increase as yet has not been identified. However, hyperplasia of G cells has been demonstrated in such patients (41). Although reduction of the intraantral pH in normal man does not influence the plasma gastrin concentrations, the administration of acid to hypochlorhydric hypersecretors of gastrin will efficiently reduce the gastrin concentration in blood (281).

Other Factors

In addition, nervous and humoral factors exist that can reduce the secretion of gastrin from the antrum. Nervous factors possibly influencing gastrin release have been discussed on page 136, *this volume*. A number of peptides such as secretin (245), glucagon (12), vasoactive intestinal peptide (VIP) (193), gastric inhibitory peptide (GIP) (193), calcitonin (11), and somatostatin (21) have been shown to suppress gastrin release following parenteral administration. The question of whether these humoral factors inhibit release of gastrin under physiological conditions is not settled.

GASTRIN INTERACTIONS

Straaten (231) was the first to suggest that a pyloric mechanism participates in the activation of the parietal cells under vagal stimulation. Later, Uvnäs in experiments on cats expanded this concept and suggested that vagal excitation releases gastrin and that gastrin and vagal excitation act synergistically on the HCl-secreting glands (252).

Subsequent studies by Olbe in dogs demonstrated that following surgical removal of the antrum and duodenal bulb vagal stimulation by sham-feeding no longer induced acid secretion (180). However, this was fully restored when amounts of exogenous gastrin that *per se* did not evoke gastric secretion were administered during the sham-feeding stimulation (179). In other studies (4) acid secretion in response to gastrin was studied in fully innervated gastric pouches that later were converted to vagally denervated (Heidenhain type) pouches by transection of the gastric wall. Following the vagal denervation, acid responses to gastrin were considerably reduced. The above results indicate that gastrin plays a contributory role in the activation of gastric secretion following vagal stimulation in the dog and the cat.

It appears from the later studies by Olbe on the interrelationship between vagal excitation and gastrin that gastrin is less important in man in causing gastric secretion during vagal stimulation. The surgical removal of the antrum and the duodenal bulb did not substantially reduce the acid secretory response to sham-feeding or to the exogenous gastrin administration in man (137). In contrast to gastrin, histamine induces a maximal acid response from vagally denervated gastric pouches in dogs (4). In man, on the other hand, vagotomy will reduce the maximal acid response to both pentagastrin and histamine. When histamine and gastrin are given to dogs with vagally denervated gastric pouches, these two substances will potentiate each other's effects (184). The physiological role of gastrin for the activation of acid secretion is beyond doubt. However, the mechanism of the stimulation of acid by gastrin in oxyntic cells is not yet resolved.

Gastrin, in the rat, activates the histidine decarboxylase activity in the gastric mucosa, which will result in the formation of histamine from histidine. Also, cholinergic excitation will induce the formation of histamine, although this does not seem to occur to the same extent in animals that have undergone resection of gastrin-releasing tissues (131,238). Although there is a general agreement that gastrin may induce the formation of histamine, there are still certain controversies whether the formed histamine is indeed involved in the physiological stimulation of the parietal cells. If so, the knowledge of the final mechanism for activation of the HCl glands is still incomplete. The presence of parietal cell receptors for both cholinergic factors and histamine has been shown. Since no specific inhibitor of gastrin is available, receptors for gastrin have been only postulated.

EFFECTS OF GASTRIN

The effects of exogenous gastrin on a great number of physiological gastrointestinal functions have been examined. A considerable number of these functions has been shown to be modified and influenced by gastrin. It is not possible at present to classify these effects as either physiological or purely pharmacological. In relatively few cases, only plasma levels of gastrin observed following gastrin administration have been correlated with the effects observed and compared with the levels present during physiological stimulation. Nor had it been possible to decide whether different gastrin forms demonstrated in blood had selective actions on different target organs. A number of gastrin effects described are discussed here.

The secretion of water and electrolytes from the stomach appears to be the main physiological effect of gastrin. However, stimulatory effects have also been reported on such secretions from the pancreas (228), liver (132), Brunner's glands (229), and small intestine (88).

In the small intestine, gastrin may, in addition, inhibit the absorption of water and electrolytes (91). Stimulation of enzyme output by gastrin has been shown in secretions from the stomach (70) and pancreas (228). It is not settled as yet whether the output of pepsin from the stomach represents a true secretion of pepsin or whether it is secondary to the activation of acid secretion. Johnson (126) instilled solutions of hydrochloric acid into vagally denervated fundic pouches in dogs and obtained a secretion of pepsin that could not be further stimulated by the administration of gastrin. These results indicate a minor role for gastrin in activating pepsin secretion. Data suggesting a minor role of gastrin in pepsin secretion have also been presented by Olbe et al. (182). In addition to activation of the oxyntic cells of the stomach to secrete acid, gastrin exerts a well-established trophic effect on the mucosa of the stomach. In rats surgical removal of the antrum causes an atrophy of the gastric mucosa (40), as well as a decrease in the mucosal content of DNA and RNA that may be prevented by pentagastrin (127). Other evidence for a trophic effect of gastrin on gastrointestinal tissues has been obtained by starvation experiments in rats during which gastrin content and plasma gastrin concentration will become lowered. The atrophy of the tissues in the stomach, small intestine, and pancreas that develops in such experiments may be prevented also if pentagastrin gastrin is administered to the gastrointestinal tract intraluminally (130). In man surgical removal of gastrin-releasing tissues causes an approximately 50% reduction of the maximal secretory capacity of the stomach. Continuous administration of pentagastrin during the postoperative period will partially prevent this reduction in the acid secretory capacity (181). In patients having gastrinomas a hyperplasia of the gastric mucosa and an increase in mucosal volume, number of parietal cells, and rate of acid secretion is present (171).

In this context, it may be pertinent to mention the existence of a mechanism controlling the production of gastrin in the duodenum and possibly also in the antrum. As stated earlier, after antrectomy there is an increase of gastrin content in the upper duodenum (173). When the entire stomach is surgically removed this increase is less pronounced (171). The above results suggest that mechanisms may exist that exert controlling effects on the production of tissue gastrin, and that such mechanisms are located at least partially in the acid-producing portion of the stomach.

In addition to effects on different exocrine secretory organs, gastrin has been claimed to exert stimulatory and inhibitory effects on smooth muscles and to influence the blood flow in the gastrointestinal tract and the metabolism of histamine. These effects have been noted in certain species but not in others. Some effects of gastrin are listed in Table 2 together with pertinent references.

GASTRIN IN PATHOLOGICAL CONDITIONS IN MAN

By the use of RIA, the gastrin concentration in blood has been studied in a great number of pathological conditions associated or not associated with the hypersecretion of acid gastric juice.

Zollinger-Ellison Syndrome, or Gastrinoma

In 1955 Zollinger and Ellison (286) reported on two patients having recurrent aggressive peptic ulcer disease, hypersecretion of acid gastric juice despite repeated gastric surgery, and tumors of the pancreatic islet cells of non-beta cell origin. Although cases of peptic ulcer disease with acid hypersecretion and islet cell tumors (25,78,93,191,208,235) had been reported previously, Zollinger and Ellison were the first to suggest that a humoral factor from the pancreatic

TABLE 2. *Investigations demonstrating stimulatory or inhibitory effects of gastrin*

Target effect	Tissue	References Stimulatory effects	Inhibitory effects
Water and electrolyte secretion	Stomach	60	
	Brunner's glands	229	
	Small intestine	88	91
	Large intestine	64	64
	Pancreas	228	
	Liver	132	
Enzyme secretion	Stomach	70	
	Pancreas	228	
Smooth muscle activity	Lower esophageal sphincter	30	
	Stomach	118	
	Small intestine	14	
	Ileo-cecal sphincter		59
	Gallbladder	260	
	Sphincter of Oddi		153
Trophic actions Growth	Gastric mucosa	40	
	Mucosa of small intestine	130	
	Mucosa of large intestine	130	
	Pancreas	129	
Amino acid uptake	Gastric mucosa	128	
Histamine metabolism Release of histamine	Gastric mucosa	135	
Histidine decarboxylase activity		6	

tumor might be the cause of the ulcer disease. They originally suggested glucagon to be the humoral factor responsible. Later, materials having gastrin-like biological properties were isolated from islet cell tumors (102,105) and in 1969 (101) and 1972 (98) Gregory et al. reported the amino acid composition of G-17 (101) and G-34 (98) gastrins isolated from Zollinger-Ellison tumor tissue.

Before the era of RIA, the Zollinger-Ellison disease was considered rare and relatively few cases were reported in the literature. After gastrin determinations in plasma had become possible, the disease had been detected in a large number of patients. It is now evident that the disease may often have a moderate course. Without the demonstration of hypergastrinemia it may therefore sometimes be difficult to distinguish it from duodenal ulcer disease. The discussion of the gastrinoma from the surgical point of view will be found in Chapter 30 by F. Stadil, pp. 729–740.

Gastrinoma Tumors

The tumors associated with the Zollinger-Ellison syndrome are generally called gastrinomas. They are usually small and with morphological features in common with carcinoid tumors (190). Due to their size both primary and metastatic tumors may be difficult to find during operation or at autopsies. On the basis of microscopical findings, it may be difficult to distinguish between benign and malignant forms. This is why the differentiation may be based on the presence of metastatic spread. On evaluating a greater number of registered cases, Ellison and Wilson (62) in 1964 reported that 61% of the tumors were malignant. Another 10% had diffuse islet cell hyperplasia or microadenomatosis. A diffuse hyperplasia was sometimes observed together with discrete adenomas or carcinomas. Considering that cases exist having a much milder course than the classic form described, it is not unreasonable to assume that the frequency of malignancy of gastrinomas may be lower than the 61% reported. Even if metastatic spread has occurred, the immediate prognosis for the patient is relatively good, since tumors in patients with total gastrectomy seem to grow slowly.

The most common localization of the gastrinomas is in the pancreas, although tumors have been reported to exist in the duodenum (90,92,178,244,273) in 10% of the cases and sometimes in the stomach (152,205). According to present concepts, pancreatic tumor gastrin is produced by the rare islet D_1 cells of the pancreas (261), by IV type islet cells (51), or by endocrine cells in the ductular system (42). Whether these cell types or others of the antral G type that have been found in pancreatic tumor (42,43) constitute the origin of pancreatic gastrinomas remains an open question. Although morphological identification of tumors may fail, a certain way to identify a gastrinoma is by demonstrating the presence of gastrin in tissue extracts of the tumor by RIA. Hyperplastic islet of the pancreas (41) is a morphological finding occurring in most gastrinoma patients.

Plasma Gastrin Levels in Gastrinoma

The levels of gastrin in plasma of normal man varied markedly during the first years of plasma gastrin determinations in various laboratories. As more experience has been gained in the use of the method, most laboratories today seem to report normal plasma levels to be below 100 pg/ml, the average concentration being about 50 pg/ml. In gastrinoma the basal levels will exceed 200 pg/ml and often become greater than 1,000 pg/ml. However, lower levels have also been reported in patients who had undergone a complete surgical removal of the stomach (83,224) or the excision of a parathyroid adenoma (251). In the low range of hypergastrinemia there will be an overlapping in gastrin values between those duodenal ulcer patients whose gastrin elevation is due to a tumor and those having it for other reasons. Different gastrin forms present in plasma of these patients have been determined. The principal circulating form has, however, been shown to be the G-34 peptide in both groups (199,201,283). In contrast, the extractions of tumors have provided a greater yield of the G-17 peptide (283). Separation of gastrin forms present in plasma of patients with hypergastrinemia therefore does not provide a way of differentiating the gastrinoma patients from those having hypergastrinemia of other causes. Instead, other tests have appeared to be more valuable. The intravenous infusion of calcium produces in gastrinoma patients an acid secretory response from the stomach that is exaggerated (9) and a release of gastrin from the tumor (43, 194,248). However, an increase in plasma gastrin concentration will occur also in patients with duodenal ulcer disease of other origins, so that overlapping results may be seen in the gastrin response to calcium infusion. Therefore, a secretin test in combination with test meal stimulation is at present the most preferable diagnostic procedure for detecting gastrinoma patients. In the absence of gastrinoma, the intravenous administration of secretin suppresses basal levels of gastrin in plasma or produces no effect at all (107). However, the gastrinoma patients in most cases will respond with an increase in plasma gastrin concentration that is optimal 5 to 10 min following the i.v. administration of secretin (41,121,201,210). Whereas the plasma gastrin level in gastrinoma patients may rise considerably following the injection or infusion of secretin, the test meal stimulation in general is less efficient in increasing the gastrin concentration (18,233). This is in contrast with the more pronounced gastrin responses in patients with hypergastrinemia due to hypersecretion of gastrin from the antral mucosa. Thus, the increase of gastrin plasma level following the administration of secretin and lack of or moderate gastrin response to a test meal strongly indicate the presence of a gastrinoma.

Acid Secretion in Gastrinoma

Basal acid hypersecretion is generally present in patients with gastrinoma, whereas stimulated acid responses may be relatively less elevated. The basal hypersecretion of acid is a consequence of the parietal cell hyperplasia induced by gastrin and by the continuous gastrin stimulation of the acid-secreting glands. When determination of basal and maximal acid secretions is performed, the high ratio of basal to peak stimulated secretion may be significant. Different methods of performing and interpreting calculations of acid responses have been reviewed elsewhere (120). Determination of acid secretion alone is, however, not sufficient to establish the diagnosis of gastrinoma since certain patients lack hypersecretion of acid and in others gastric hypersecretion may be difficult to establish because of prior surgery.

Ulcerations in Gastrinoma

A few gastrinoma patients do not have peptic ulcerations, although a massive hypersecretion of acid may be present. Approximately 75% of the patients have bulbar or postbulbar ulceration. In certain cases in which the hypersecretion is massive, ulcerations may be seen even in distal duodenum and jejunum. In addition to ulcerations, radiological examinations may reveal large gastric folds, dilution of barium contrast due to the excessive acid secretion, and blunting and irregularity of the mucosal folds of the duodenum and jejunum as well as dilatation of the lumen.

Diarrhea and Steatorrhea in Gastrinoma

Approximately one-third to three-quarters of the gastrinoma patients have diarrhea (63,120), which may be the only symptom in approximately 10% of patients. Steatorrhea has also been reported (120). The mechanism underlying the diarrhea and steatorrhea is not completely understood. The daily infusion of large amounts of acid into the stomach of dogs over a 5-week period has been demonstrated to produce both symptoms (183). The diarrhea observed is therefore not exclusively a direct effect of the hypersecretion of gastrin, although gastrin has been demonstrated to stimulate intestinal motility and decrease the small bowel absorption. In patients having acid hypersecretion delivery of excessive amounts of acid to the intestine with damage of the bowel mucosa, decreased absorption of water from the intestine and increased intestinal motility may together be responsible for the diarrhea. In addition, delivery of a large volume of acid to the intestine may stimulate the intestinal motility mechanically and chemically. Decreased small bowel absorption may develop from damage of intestinal mucosa as well as a direct effect of gastrin. Most likely as a result of inactivation of lipase, precipitation of bile salts, and mucosal damage evoked by a low pH in the bowel lumen, steatorrhea will develop in some cases of gastrinoma (112,215). That gastric acid secretion is a factor in producing diarrhea is also indicated by the findings that diarrhea will disappear following total gastrectomy and may be relieved by continuous nasogastric aspiration (35,52, 58,169,214,220). The diarrhea in Zollinger-Ellison disease should be distinguished from the massive watery diarrhea without acid hypersecretion that is present in pancreatic cholera (267), another syndrome caused by an islet cell endocrine tumor originally called Verner-Morrison syndrome (263) or WDHA syndrome (158).

Association of Gastrinoma with Other Endocrine Tumors

Endocrine disorders of nonpancreatic origin have been reported (62,274) to be associated with gastrinoma, with an incidence of 10 to 40%. Different terms such as multiple endocrine adenoma syndrome, pluriglandular syndrome, or multiple endocrine neoplasia type I have been suggested (39). The most common endocrine disease associated with Zollinger-Ellison syndrome appears to be hyperparathyroidism, which is found in approximately 20% of gastrinoma patients (120). In this condition, the coexisting hypercalcemia may exert a stimulatory action on the gastrin-releasing tumor. Following removal of the parathyroid adenoma, the calcium level in blood will become normal, which leads to a reduction of plasma gastrin level to the normal range and a reduced gastric acid secretion (54,163,251). Despite the normalized gastrin and gastric acid secretion, such patients may still respond with an abnormal elevation of plasma gastrin level following administration of secretin or calcium (248). Except for cases of gastrinoma, hyperparathyroidism does not seem to be associated frequently with duodenal ulcer disease (31).

In addition to hyperparathyroidism, simultaneous endocrine disorders of the adrenals, ovaries, pituitary, and thyroid have been reported (39). The pathological lesions found in these conditions have been carcinomas, single or multiple adenomas, or diffuse hyperplasia. In some cases the multiple endocrine disorders have been reported as a familiar disease (276).

Treatment of the Zollinger-Ellison Syndrome

Tumors causing this syndrome are frequently too small in diameter to permit detection when conventional tumor diagnostic procedures or palpation during operation are used. The chances that a single resectable tumor will be found at operation have been estimated to be less than one in five (120). Recently, intraportal catheterization in combination with gastrin RIA is being used in an attempt to localize the tumor or tumors and to obtain a better basis for a radical surgical resection. Successful results with this technique have been reported (225). However, the localization of the tumor or tumors still constitutes a great problem so that total gastrectomy has often remained the operation of choice, and gave good immediate results. The overall 5 and 10 year survival rate have been reported to be 55 and 42%, respectively, whereas partial resections of the stomach have been less successful (79).

It has been claimed that removal of the whole stomach will induce a regression of metastatic tumors that may even disappear (82). The mechanism of this effect is not understood. Secretin has been demonstrated to cause release of gastrin from the gastrinoma. Possibly, the acid gastric juice secreted in response to the tumor gastrin may release secretin, which not only causes release of gastrin but also exerts a trophic effect on the gastrinoma (267). Another possibility may be that the previously mentioned fundic factor that influences tissue concentration and release of gastrin in dogs (161) may also be present in man and stimulate the gastrin tumor. Removal of this factor that may be secreted in great amounts could lead to decrease of the tumor size. Medical treatment of the Zollinger-Ellison syndrome has been tried but, as a general rule, patients respond to it less well. Recent use of the H_2-receptor antagonist, cimetidine, is promising and may be tried when surgery is contradicted (225).

Antral G Cell Hyperplasia

There are indications that certain patients may have a hypersecretion of gastrin that is not due to a gastrin-producing tumor. Berson and Yalow (281) were the first to describe patients with such a hypersecretion. Polak et al. (187) found evidence for antral G cell hyperplasia in certain patients having hypergastrinemia without gastrinoma. From these observations they inferred that there may exist two different types or stages of the Zollinger-Ellison syndrome, one of which was due to a hyperplasia of the antral G cells. In another study (37) reporting a case with hypergastrinemia and hyperplastic changes of the antrum, this was called type I Zollinger-Ellison syndrome, in contradistinction to type II Zollinger-Ellison syndrome, which would include cases of gastrinoma. Still other workers reported similar cases and preferred for them the descriptive terms of antral gastrin cell hyperplasia and gastrinoma (86).

The present knowledge of the frequency of antral G cell hyperplasia is incomplete. However, most laboratories dealing with gastrin determinations in duodenal ulcer patients will occasionally face the problem of distinguishing a possible antral G cell hyperplasia from a gastrinoma. One way seems to be the determination of the gastrin responses to the administration of secretin and a test meal. The failure of secretin to raise the plasma gastrin concentration with a good gastrin response to feeding would indicate antral G cell hyperplasia rather than gastrinoma. (See page 149.) Hypergastrinemia associated with hypersecretion of acid has also been reported in patients with a retained antrum, i.e., remaining antral mucosa in the duodenal stump that is not exposed to the acid content of the stomach (142), in gastric-outlet obstruction (75), and in alterations of the gastrin metabolism secondary to renal failure or nephrectomy (53,141,160). Also following intestinal resection (80,277), increased gastrin levels have been observed under basal conditions and following meal stimulation.

Peptic Esophagitis

In peptic esophagitis there is a reflux of acid gastric juice into the esophagus and a decreased pressure of the lower esophageal sphincter (33). According to one concept, gastrin exerts a physiological control of the cardiac region by maintaining the lower esophageal sphincter pressure (30,154). Insufficiency of the sphincter might then be due to a defect of the gastrin-controlling mechanism (11). No correlations between fasting gastrin plasma concentrations and basal lower esophageal pressure have been established, however (56). Nor do patients suffering from this disease have low gastrin levels (73,148). Other studies (104) indicate that amounts of gastrin greater than those required for maximal acid secretion have to be given in order to induce an increase in the sphincter pressure. This suggests that factors other than gastrin may be responsible for this pathological condition. For a more detailed discussion of this problem, see Chapter 26 by R. S. Fischer and S. Cohen, pp. 613–638, *this volume.*

Gastrin in Ulcer Disease

Relatively few systematic attempts have been made to quantitatively correlate immunohistochemical findings in gastrin-releasing tissues with numbers of parietal cells as well as functional data on the gastrin release under basal and stimulated conditions with estimations of the acid secretory rates of the parietal cells.

According to a recent Norwegian study (226,227) that included patients with duodenal or gastric ulcer disease or gastric cancer, large individual variations were found in the overall antral G cell density in the antral area corresponding with the distribution of G cells and in the total G cell mass and these variables were not significantly related to diagnosis, age, or sex. Nor were there any significant differences in the number of duodenal G cells among the groups examined.

In most of the groups investigated an increase in density of G cells was found from the proximal through the distal portions of the antrum. In the gastric ulcer patients the density of the distal portion of the antrum did not differ from that of the middle and proximal antral portions. These results compare favorably with observations made by Emås et al. (67), who determined gastrin activity in mucosal specimens from the distal portion of the pyloric antrum and found less gastrin-like activity in the gastric than in the duodenal ulcer patients. Data comparing gastrin contents in the antral mucosae of normals with those in patients with ulcer disease are sparse. Emås et al. (67) did not find any difference between normals and duodenal ulcer patients on measuring gastrin in the extracts of the distal pyloric antrum. Nor was such a difference noted in a study based on radioimmunological determinations of gastrin (115), whereas gastric ulcer patients had lower mucosal contents of gastrin in the distal antrum. Some controversies exist as to the duodenal contents of gastrin in health and disease. When a biological technique for gastrin determination was used, no difference was found between normals and patients having duodenal ulcer (67), whereas gastric ulcer patients had reduced duodenal gastrin amounts. Similar results were reported by Arnold et al. (5) and by Stave et al. (226), whereas Connon (34) found slightly increased concentrations of duodenal gastrin in gastric ulcer patients and highly increased concentrations in patients with duodenal ulcer. Also, Polak et al. (187) reported increased duodenal G cell density in the latter group of patients. The overall impression from these studies is that the estimation of the number of G cells or of the gastrin concentration in a single or in a few antral biopsies has to be interpreted cautiously. Great variations also exist in the extent of the endocrine area of the stomach. There are no well documented findings as to the relationship between the G cell mass and the release of gastrin following physiological stimulation. Preliminary reports (226) do not indicate that the meal-induced gastrin response correlates with the immunoreactive G cell mass.

Duodenal Ulcer

Other studies in which plasma gastrin concentrations were determined in normals and in patients with duodenal ulcer revealed no differences under basal conditions (143,249,266). Following stimulation with a protein meal, however, several studies indicated a greater gastrin response in duodenal ulcer patients than in a healthy man (143,249,263). An explanation may be that the pH-dependent antral mechanism inhibiting gastrin release may be less efficient in duodenal ulcer patients than in normals (272).

Patients with duodenal ulcers have an increased parietal cell mass (38) and respond more than normals to pentagastrin stimulation (119). Since gastrin appears to be the only agent known to induce parietal cell hyperplasia (127), gastrin must be considered until disproved as a possible cause of the parietal cell hyperplasia. This, in combination with the greater release of gastrin following test meal stimulation in duodenal ulcer due probably to a deficient inhibition of gastrin release, is the most convincing evidence indicating a relationship between gastrin and duodenal ulcer.

Gastric Ulcer

Patients with gastric ulcer differ from duodenal ulcer patients in certain respects. Gastric secretion is normal or below the normal rate (279). Although the gastrin content, at least in the distal part of the antrum, is lower than in normals and duodenal ulcer patients, the plasma gastrin concentration is often elevated to various extents (89,250). The levels of basal gastrin in plasma of these patients seem to be inversely related to the basal rate of gastric acid secretion. In general, patients having combined and distal antral or duodenal ulcers appear to have higher rates of acid secretion and normal range of fasting gastrin levels.

Effects of Ulcer Treatment on Tissue and Plasma Gastrin Concentrations

Medical Treatment

The effects of the pharmacological treatment of ulcer disease on gastrin levels in the tissue and blood have not been adequately studied. In man, acute administration of anticholinergics such as atropine does not essentially reduce basal levels of gastrin in normals and in ulcer patients, whereas the gastrin response to test meal stimulation becomes enhanced under these conditions (270).

A number of studies exist on the effect of antacids on basal plasma gastrin concentration in man. Results obtained with the administration of calcium-containing antacids are conflicting. Some authors found increases of plasma gastrin concentrations following acute administration of large doses of calcium carbonate (195,209). Antacids containing calcium carbonate (0.25 g) as one of several components and administered in adequate amounts do not significantly influence plasma gastrin concentrations (175). As a whole, acute administration of antacids, except for sodium bicarbonate, does not significantly influence plasma gastrin concentration. No systematic studies have been performed on the long-term antacid effect. Creutzfeldt et al. (42) found that treatment of normals with antacids for 4 weeks elevated the antral gastrin concentration when determined by RIA.

The effect of the H_2 antagonist, cimetidine, on gastrin concentration in plasma has been studied by several groups prior, during, and after treatments of various length. Richardson et al. (203) found some elevation of the gastrin response to a meal following acute administration of cimetidine. This was most likely due to the reduced secretion of acid gastric juice. Long-term treatment studies (76,222) with cimetidine indicate elevations of basal as well as meal-stimulated plasma gastrin levels that decrease when therapy is discontinued.

Surgical Treatment

Vagotomy. Truncal, selective gastric, or highly selective parietal cell vagotomies relatively uniformly lead to an increase in plasma gastrin concentration (123,147,166). As mentioned earlier in this chapter, removal of a vagal mechanism inhibiting gastrin release may contribute to this increase.

Gastric resection. Following antrectomy, basal plasma concentrations of gastrin are somewhat reduced (166), the reduction being greater with Billroth II than with Billroth I anastomosis (230). According to one study, basal and postprandial plasma gastrin levels are higher after antrectomy if removal of the gastric antrum is combined with vagotomy. This indicates that extraantral gastrin release may also be under a vagal inhibitory control.

SUMMARY AND CONCLUSIONS

Gastrin, originally isolated as a factor stimulating the secretion of gastric acid juice, has been demonstrated to exist in different molecular shapes in tissue extracts as well as in body fluids. In addition to stimulating acid secretion, several other effects have been attributed to gastrin. The physiological significance of effects other than stimulating the secretion and growth of parietal cells remains to be proven. In stimulating the acid secretion gastrin acts synergistically with vagal impulses on the HCl glands.

The possible role of gastrin in causing duodenal ulcer disease is not fully established except for cases where a gastrin-producing tumor, gastrinoma, is present. The existence of cases having hyperplastic changes of the pyloric gland area that may induce hypersecretion of gastric secretion has also been described.

PROJECTIONS FOR THE FUTURE

Future studies in gastrin research face a number of stimulating but complicated problems. The true role of gastrin in stimulating acid secretion has to be resolved. What sequence of events is involved when gastrin and vagal impulses excite the HCl glands? Does the contribution of gastrin to this stimulation consist mainly in causing an ignition of the stimulation process or is gastrin, in addition, required to maintain secretion once initiated? The role of the different gastrins already isolated or indicated from separation studies has to be established. Do they simply represent metabolic forms of gastrin or do they indeed have separate effects on different physiological parameters?

Great interest has been directed toward paracrine effects of gastrointestinal hormones. The paracrine role of gastrin, if any, has to be revealed. The effects of different sorts of long-term treatment of ulcer disease in influencing gastrin production and release are not known and should be the subject of future investigation.

ACKNOWLEDGMENTS

The author's studies in this review have been supported by grants (04X3521) from the Swedish Medical Research Council.

The secretarial assistance of Mrs. Ewa Kallerman is gratefully acknowledged.

REFERENCES

1. Anderson, J. C., Harton, M. A., Gregory, R. A., Hardy, P. M., Kenner, G. W., MacLeod, J. K., Preston, J., Sheppard, R. C., and Morley, J. S. (1964): The antral hormone gastrin. Synthesis of gastrin. *Nature,* 204:933–934.
2. Andersson, S., and Elwin, C. E. (1971): Relationship between antral acidity and gastrin releasing potency of chemical stimulants. *Acta Physiol. Scand.,* 83:437–445.
3. Andersson, S., and Nilsson, G. (1974): Appearance of gastrin in perfusates from the isolated gastric antrum of dogs. *Scand. J. Gastroenterol.,* 9:619–621.
4. Andersson, S., and Olbe, L. (1964): Gastric acid secretory responses to gastrin and histamine in dogs before and after vagal denervation of the gastric pouch. *Acta Physiol. Scand.,* 60:51–56.
5. Arnold, R. Creutzfeldt, C., Track, N. S., and Creutzfeldt, W. (1974): Gastrin and duodenalulcus. *Verh. Dtsch. Ges. Im. Med.,* 80:368–377.
6. Aures, D., Johnson, L. R., and Way, L. W. (1970): Gastrin: Obligatory intermediate for activation of gastric histidine decarboxylase. *Am. J. Physiol.,* 219:214–216.
7. Babkin, B. P., and Schachter, M. (1944): The chemical phase of gastric secretion and the surgery of the stomach. *McGill Med. J.,* 13:127–138.
8. Ballard, H. S., Frame, B., Hartsock, R. J. (1964): Familial multiple endocrine adenoma peptic ulcer complex. *Medicine (Balt.),* 43:481–516.
9. Basso, N., Passaro, E Jr. (1970): Calcium-stimulated gastric secretion in the Zollinger-Ellison syndrome. *Arch. Surg.,* 101:399–402.
10. Bayliss, W. M., and Starling, E. H. (1902): The mechanism of pancreatic secretion. *J. Physiol.,* 28:325–353.
11. Becker, H. D., Reeder, D. D., Scurry, M. T., and Thompson, J. C. (1974): Inhibition of gastrin release and gastric secretion by calcitonin in patients with peptic ulcer. *Am. J. Surg.,* 127:71–75.
12. Becker, H. D., Reeder, D. D., Thompson, J. C. (1973): Effect of glucagon on circulating gastrin. *Gastroenterology,* 65:28–35.
13. Becker, H. D., Reeder, D. D., Thompson, J. C. (1974): Gastrin release by ethanol in man and in dogs. *Ann. Surg.,* 179:906–909.
14. Bennet, A. (1965): Effect of gastrin on isolated smooth muscle preparations. *Nature,* 208:170–173.
15. Bentley, P. H., Kenner, G. W., and Sheppard, R. C. (1966): Structures of human gastrins I and II. *Nature,* 209:583–585.
16. Bergegårdh, S., Nilsson, G., and Olbe, L. (1976): The effect of antral distension on acid secretion and plasma gastrin in duodenal ulcer patients. *Scand. J. Gastroenterol.,* 11:475–479.
17. Berson, S. A., Walsh, J. H., and Yalow, R. S. (1973): Radioimmunoassay of gastrin in human

plasma and regulation of gastrin secretion. In: *Frontiers in Gastrointestinal Hormone Research,* edited by S. Andersson, pp. 57–68. Almqvist & Wiksell, Stockholm.

18. Berson, S. A., and Yalow, R. S. (1972): Radioimmunoassay in gastroenterology. *Gastroenterology,* 62:1061–1084.

19. Bertaccini, G. (1973): Pharmacological actions of kinins occurring in amphibian skin. In: *Pharmacology and the Future of Man: Proceedings of the 5th International Congress of Pharmacology, San Francisco 1972. Vol. 5,* pp. 336–346. S. Karger, Basel.

20. Bertaccini, G., Melchiorri, P., Erspamer V., and Sopranzi, N. (1974): Gastrin release by bombesin in the dog. *Br. J. Pharmacol.,* 52:219–225.

21. Bloom, S. R., Mortimer, C. H., Thorner, M. O., Besser, G. M., Hall, R., Gomez-Pan, A., Roy, V. M., Russel, R. C. G., Coy, D. H., Kastin, A. J., and Schally, A. V. (1974): Inhibition of gastrin and gastric acid secretion by growth-hormone release-inhibiting hormone. *Lancet,* ii:1106–1109.

22. Bloom, S. R., and Polak, J. M. (1978): *Gut Hormone Overview,* pp. 3–18. Churchill & Livingstone, Edinburgh.

23. Bonfils, S., and Bader, J. P. (1970): The diagnosis of Zollinger-Ellison syndrome with special reference to the multiple endocrine adenomas. In: *Progress in Gastroenterology, Vol. II.,* edited by G. B. J. Glass, pp. 332–355. Grune & Stratton, New York.

24. Broomé, A., Fyrö, B., and Olbe, L. (1968): Localization of gastrin activity in the gastric antrum. *Acta Physiol. Scand.,* 74:331–339.

25. Brown, C. H., Neville, W. E., and Hazard, J. B. (1950): Islet-cell adenoma without hypoglycemia, causing duodenal obstruction. *Surgery,* 27:616–620.

26. Burns, G. P., and Schenk, W. G. (1969): Effect of digestion and exercise on intestinal blood flow and cardiac output. *Arch. Surg.,* 98:790–794.

27. Burstall, P. A., and Schofield, B. (1954): The effects of pyloric antrectomy on the secretory response of Heidenhain pouches in dogs to central vagal stimulation. *J. Physiol. (Lond.),* 123:168–186.

28. Bussolati, G., and Pearse, A. G. E. (1970): Immunofluorescent localization of the gastrin-secreting G-cells in the pyloric antrum of the pig. *Histochemie,* 21:1–4.

29. Capella, C., and Solcia, E. (1972): The endocrine cells of the pig gastrointestinal mucosa and pancreas. *Arch. Histol. Jpn.,* 35:1–29.

30. Castell, D. O., and Harris, L. D. (1970): Hormonal control of gastroesophageal sphincter strength. *N. Engl. J. Med.,* 282:886–889.

31. Christiansen, J. (1974): Primary hyperparathyroidism and peptic ulcer disease. *Scand. J. Gastroenterol.,* 9:111–114.

32. Clendinnen, B. G., Reeder, D. D., Brandt, E. N. Jr., and Thompson, J. C. (1973): Effect of nephrectomy on the rate and pattern of the disappearance of exogenous gastrin in dogs. *Gut,* 14:462–467.

33. Cohen, S., Harris, L. D. (1971): Does hiatal hernia affect competence of the gastroesophageal sphincter? *N. Engl. J. Med.,* 284:1053–1056.

34. Connon, J. J., Ardill, J., and McFarland, R. J. (1975): Tissue gastrin in peptic ulceration. *Gut,* 16:407.

35. Cook, H. B., and French, A. B. (1968): Physiologic responses to gastric acid in Zollinger-Ellison syndrome. *Am. J. Dig. Dis.,* 13:191–203.

36. Cooke, A. R. (1972): Ethanol and gastric function. *Gastroenterology,* 62:501–502.

37. Cowley, D. J., Dymock, I. W., Boyes, B. E., Wilson, R. Y., Stagg, B. H., Lewin, M. R., Polak, J. M., and Pearse, A. G. E. (1973): Zollinger-Ellison syndrome type 1: clinical and pathological correlations in a case. *Gut,* 14:25–29.

38. Cox, A. J. (1952): Stomach size and its relation to chronic peptic ulcer. *Arch. Pathol.,* 54:407–422.

39. Craven, D. E., Goodman, A. D., and Carter, J. H. (1972): Familial multiple endocrine adenomatosis: multiple endocrine neoplasia type I. *Arch. Intern. Med.,* 129:567–569.

40. Crean, G. P., Marshall, M. W., and Rumsey, R. D. E. (1969): Parietal cell hyperplasia induced by the administration of pentagastrin (ICI 50,123) to rats. *Gastroenterology,* 57:147–155.

41. Creutzfeldt, W., Arnold, R., Creutzfeldt, C., and Track, N. S. (1975): Pathomorphological, biochemical and diagnostic aspects of gastrinomas (Zollinger-Ellison syndrome). *Hum. Pathol.,* 6:47–76.

42. Creutzfeldt, W., Arnold, R., and Creutzfeldt, C. (1974): Gastrin producing cells. In: *Endocrinology of the Gut,* edited by W. Y. Chey, and S. P. Brooks, pp. 35–62. C. B. Slack, Thorofare, New Jersey.

43. Creutzfeldt, W., Arnold, R., Creutzfeldt, C., Feurle, G., and Ketterer, H. (1971): Gastrin and G-cells in the antral mucosa of patients with pernicious anemia, acromegaly and hyperparathyroidism and in a Zollinger-Ellison tumour of the pancreas. *Eur. J. Clin. Invest.,* 1:461–479.

44. Csendes, A., Walsh, J. H., and Grossman, M. I. (1972): Effects of atropine and of antral acidification on gastrin release and acid secretion in response to insulin and feeding in dogs. *Gastroenterology,* 63:257–263.

45. Dale, H. H., and Laidlaw, P. P. (1910): The physiological action of β-imidazolylethylamine. *J. Physiol.,* 41:318–344.

46. Debas, H. T., Csendes, A., Walsh, J. H., and Grossman, M. I. (1974): Release of antral gastrin. In: *Endocrinology of the Gut,* edited by W. Y. Chey and S. P. Brooks, pp. 222–232. C. B. Slack, Thorofare, New Jersey.

47. Debas, H. T., Walsh, J. H., and Grossman, M. I. (1974): Release of antral gastrin by large polypeptides. *Clin. Res.,* 22 171-A (Abstr.).

48. Debas, H. T., Walsh, J. H., and Grossman, M. I. (1974): Pure human minigastrin: secretory potency and disappearance rate. *Gut,* 15:686–689.

49. Debas, H. T., Walsh, J. H., and Grossman, M. I. (1975): Evidence for oxynto-pyloric reflex for release of antral gastrin. *Gastroenterology,* 68:687–690.

50. Debas, H. T., Walsh, J. H., and Grossman, M. I. (1976): After vagotomy atropine suppresses gastrin release by food. *Gastroenterology,* 70:1082–1084.

51. Deconinick, J. F., Potvliege, P. R., and Gepts, W. (1971): The ultra-structure of the human pancreatic islets. I. The islets of adults. *Diabetologia,* 7:266–282.

52. Deleu, J., Tytgat, H., and Van Goidsenhover, G. E. (1964): Diarrhea associated with pancreatic islet-cell tumours. *Am. J. Dig. Dis.,* 9:97–108.

53. Dent, R. I., Hirsch, H., James, J. H., and Fischer, J. E. (1972): Hypergastrinemia in patients with acute renal failure. *Surg. Forum,* 23:312–313.

54. Dent, R. I., James, J. H., Wang, C., Deftos, L. J., Talamo, R., and Fischer, J. E. (1972): Hyperparathyroidism: gastric acid secretion and gastrin. *Am. Surg.,* 176:360–369.

55. Dockray, G. J., and Walsh, J. H. (1974): Amino terminal gastrin fragment in serum of Zollinger-Ellison syndrome patient. *Gastroenterology,* 68:222–230.

56. Dodds, W. J., Hogan, W. J., Miller, W. N., Arndorfer, R. C., and Barreras, R. F. (1974): Relationship between serum gastrin levels and lower esophageal sphincter pressure in fasting subjects. *Gastroenterology,* 66:686.

57. Donaldson, R. M., von Eigen, P. R., and Dwight, R. W. (1957): Gastric hypersecretion peptic ulceration and islet cell tumour of the pancreas (The Zollinger-Ellison syndrome). *N. Engl. J. Med.,* 257:965–970.

58. Edemads, J. G., Mathews, R. E., McPhedran, N. T., and Ezrin, C. (1962): Diarrhea caused by pancreatic islet cell tumours. *Can. Med. Assoc. J.,* 86:847–851.

59. Editorial. (1970): Treating like with like. *N. Engl. J. Med.,* 282:565–566.

60. Edkins, J. S. (1905): On the chemical mechanism of gastric secretion. *Proc. R. Soc. (Lond.),* 76:376.

61. Elliot, D. W., Endahl, G. L., Knoernshild, H. E., Grant, G. N., Goswitz, J. T., and Zollinger, R. M. (1963): Relation of antrum to pancreatic-induced gastric hypersecretion. *Surgery,* 54:9–18.

62. Ellison, E. H., and Wilson, S. D. (1964): The Zollinger-Ellison syndrome: Reappraisal and evaluation of 260 registered cases. *Ann. Surg.,* 160:512–528.

63. Ellison, E. H., and Wilson, S. D. (1967): Ulcerogenic tumour of the pancreas. *Proc. Clin. Cancer,* 3:225–244.

64. El Masri, S. H., Lewin, M. R., and Clark, C. G. (1977): In vitro effects of gastrin on the movement of electrolytes across the human colon. *Scand. J. Gastroenterol.,* 12:999–1002.

65. Elwin, C. E. (1969): Stimulation of gastric acid secretion by irrigation of the antrum with some aliphatic alcohols. *Acta Physiol. Scand.,* 75:1–11.

66. Elwin, C. E. (1974): Gastric acid responses to antral application of some amino acids, peptides, and isolated fractions of a protein hydrolysate. *Scand. J. Gastroenterol.,* 9:239–247.

67. Emås, S., Borg, I., and Fyrö, B. (1971): Antral and duodenal gastrin activity in non ulcer and ulcer patients. *Scand. J. Gastroenterol.,* 6:39–43.

68. Emås, S., and Fyrö, B. (1965): Vagal release of gastrin in cats following reserpine. *Acta Physiol. Scand.,* 63:358–369.

69. Emås, S., and Fyrö, B. (1968): Gastrin-like activity in different parts of the gastro-intestinal tract of the cat. *Acta Physiol. Scand.,* 74:359–367.

70. Emås, S., and Grossman, M. I. (1967): Effect of truncal vagotomy on acid and pepsin responses to histamine and gastrin in dogs. *Am. J. Physiol.,* 34:133–144.
71. Evans, J. C. W., Reeder, D. D., Becker, H. D., and Thompson, J. C. (1974): Extraction of circulating endogenous gastrin by the gastric fundus. *Gut,* 15:112–115.
72. Farooq, O., Walsh, J. H. (1975): Atropine enhances serum gastrin response to insulin in man. *Gastroenterology,* 68:662–666.
73. Farrell, R. L., Castell, D. O., McGuigan, J. E. (1974): Measurements and comparisons of lower esophageal sphincter pressures and serum gastrin levels in patients with gastroesophageal reflux. *Gastroenterology,* 67:415–422.
74. Feldman, M., Richardson, C. T., Taylor, I. A., and Walsh, J. H. (1978): Neural regulation of gastrin and pancreatic polypeptide release in man. *Clin. Res.,* 26:497 A (abstr.).
75. Feurle, G., Ketterer, H., Becker, H. D., and Creutzfeldt, W. (1972): Circadian serum gastrin concentrations in control persons and in patients with ulcer disease. *Scand. J. Gastroenterol.,* 7:177–183.
76. Forrest, J. A. H., Fettes, M., McLoughlin, G., and Heading, R. C. (1978): The effect of long-term cimetidine on gastric acid secretion, serum gastrin and gastric emptying. In: *Cimetidine,* edited by C. Wastell and P. Lance, pp. 57–65. Churchill Livingstone, Edinburgh.
77. Forssman, W. G., Pictet, R., Renold, A. E., and Rouiller, C. (1969): The endocrine cells in the epithelium of the gastrointestinal mucosa of the rat. *J. Cell Biol.,* 40:692–715.
78. Forty, F., and Barrett, G. M. (1952): Peptic ulceration of the third part of the duodenum associated with islet-cell tumours of the pancreas. *Br. J. Surg.,* 40:60–63.
79. Fox, P. S., Hofmann, J. W., Decosse, J. J., and Wilson, S. D. (1974): The influence of total gastrectomy on survival in malignant Zollinger-Ellison tumour. *Ann. Surg.* 180:558–566.
80. Frederick, P. L., Sizer, J. S., and Osborne, M. P. (1965): Relation of massive bowel resection to gastric secretion. *N. Engl. J. Med.,* 272:509–514.
81. Friedman, M. H. F. (1954): The significance of the discovery of secretin. *Gastroenterology,* 26:795–801.
82. Friesen, S. R. (1967): Effect of total gastrectomy on the Zollinger-Ellison tumour: observations by second-look procedures. *Surgery,* 62:609–613.
83. Friesen, S. R., Bolinger, R. E., Pearse, A. G. E. and McGuigan, J. E. (1970): Serum gastrin levels in malignant Zollinger-Ellison syndrome after total gastrectomy and hypophysectomy. *Ann. Surg.,* 172:504–519.
84. Fyrö, B. (1967): Reduction of antral and duodenal gastrin activity by electrical vagal stimulation. *Acta Physiol. Scand.,* 71:334–340.
85. Ganguli, P. C., Cullen, D. R., and Irvine, W. J. (1971): Radioimmunoassay of plasmagastrin in pernicious anaemia, achlorhydria without pernicious anaemia, hypochlorhydria and in controls. *Lancet,* i:155–158.
86. Ganguli, P. C., Elder, J. B., Polak, J. M., and Pearse, A. G. E. (1974): Antral-gastrin-cell hyperplasia in peptic-ulcer disease. *Lancet,* i:1288–1289.
87. Ganguli, P. C., Polak, J. M., Pearse, A. G. E., Elder, J. B., and Hegarty, M. (1974): Antral-gastrin-cell hyperplasia in peptic-ulcer disease. *Lancet,* i:583–586.
88. Gardner, J. D., Peskin, G. W., Cerda, J. J., and Brooks, F. P. (1967): Alterations of In Vitro fluid and electrolyte absorption by gastrointestinal hormones. *Am. J. Surg.,* 113:57–64.
89. Gedde-Dahl, D. (1974): Radioimmunoassay of gastrin: fasting serum levels in human with normal and high gastric secretion. *Scand. J. Gastroenterol.,* 9:41–47.
90. Gerber, B. C., and Shields, T. W. (1960): Simultaneous duodenal carcinoma and non-beta cell tumours of the pancreas. Two tumours of high ulcerogenic potential. *Arch. Surg.,* 81:379–388.
91. Gingell, J. C., Davies, M. W., and Shields, R. (1968): Effect of synthetic gastrin-like pentapeptide upon the intestinal transport of sodium, potassium and water. *Gut,* 9:111–116.
91a. Glass, G. B. J., and Wolf, S. (1950): Hormonal mechanisms in nervous mechanism of gastric acid secretion in humans. *Proc. Soc. Exp. Biol. Med.,* 73:535–537.
92. Goodman, J. M. (1964): Duodenal submucosal islet-cell adenoma and chronic gastroduodenitis. *Am. J. Surg.,* 10:726–729.
93. Gordon, B. S., and Olivetti, R. G. (1947): Carcinoma of the islets of Langerhans: Review of the literature and report of two cases. *Gastroenterology,* 9:409–424.
94. Gregory, H., Hardy, P. M., Jones, D. S., Kenner, G. W., and Sheppard, R. C. (1964): The antral hormone gastrin. Structure of gastrin. *Nature,* 204:931–933.
95. Gregory, R. A. (1974): The gastrointestinal hormones: A review of recent advances. *J. Physiol. (Lond.),* 241:1–32.

96. Gregory, R. A., and Tracy, H. J. (1961): The preparation and properties of gastrin. *J. Physiol. (Lond.),* 156:523–543.
97. Gregory, R. A., and Tracy, H. J. (1964): The constitution and properties of two gastrins extracted from hog antral mucosa. *Gut,* 5:103–117.
98. Gregory, R. A., and Tracy, H. J. (1972): Isolation of two "big gastrins" from Zollinger-Ellison tumour tissue. *Lancet,* ii:797–799.
99. Gregory, R. A., and Tracy, H. J. (1974): Isolation of two minigastrins from Zollinger-Ellison tumour tissue. *Gut,* 15:683–685.
100. Gregory, R. A., and Tracy, H. J. (1974): The chemistry of the gastrins: some recent advances. In: *International Symposium on Gastrointestinal Hormones,* edited by J. C. Thompson, pp. 13–24. Austin, University of Texas Press.
101. Gregory, R. A., Tracy, H. J., Agarwal, K. L., and Grossman, M. I. (1969): Aminoacid constitution of two gastrins isolated from Zollinger-Ellison tumour tissue. *Gut,* 10:603–608.
102. Gregory, R. A., Tracy, H. J., French, J. M., and Sircus, W. (1960): Extraction of a gastrin-like substance from a pancreatic tumour in a case of Zollinger-Ellison syndrome. *Lancet,* i:1045–1048.
103. Greider, M. H., and McGuigan, J. E. (1971): Cellular localization of gastrin in the human pancreas. *Diabetes,* 20:389–396.
104. Grossman, M. I. (1973): What is physiological? *Gastroenterology,* 65:994.
105. Grossman, M. I., Tracy, H. J., and Gregory, R. A. (1961): Zollinger-Ellison syndrome in a Bantu-woman with isolation of gastrin-like substance from primary and secondary tumours. II. Extraction of gastrin-like activity from tumours. *Gastroenterology,* 41:87–91.
106. Hansky, J. (1977): Hypergastrinemia, hyperacidity and peptic ulceration. *Rendic. Gastroenterol.,* 9:11. (Abstr.).
107. Hansky, J., Soveny, C., and Korman, M. G. (1971): Effect of secretin on serum gastrin as measured by immunoassay. *Gastroenterology,* 61:62–68.
108. Harper, A. A. (1946): The effect of extracts of gastric and intestinal mucosa on the secretion of HCl by the cat's stomach. *J. Physiol. (Lond.),* 105:31P.
109. Hayes, J. R. (1978): Stimulation of gastrin release by dopamine and serotonin. In: *Second International Symposium on Gastrointestinal Hormones,* edited by J. Myren, E. Schrumpf, L. E. Hanssen, and M. Vatn, p. 84. 13.Suppl. 49.
110. Hedenbro, J. L., Fink, A. S., and Fiddian-Grean, R. (1978): Directions of access to gastrin receptor sites in canine parietal mucosa. In: *Second International Symposium on Gastrointestinal Hormones,* edited by J. Myren, E. Schrumpf, L. E. Hanssen, and M. Vatn, *Scand. J. Gastroenterol.* (Suppl. 49) 13:84 (Abstr.).
111. Higgs, R. H., Smyth, R. D., and Castell, D. O. (1974): Gastric alkalinization: effect on lower-esophageal-sphincter pressure and serum gastrin. *N. Engl. J. Med.,* 291:486–490.
112. Hoffman, A. F. (1966): A physicochemical approach to the intraluminal phase of fat absorption. *Gastroenterology,* 50:56–64.
113. Hohnke, L. A., and Wilder, D. E. (1978): Evidence for renal modulation of serum gastrin concentration in the rat. In: *Second International Symposium on Gastrointestinal Hormones,* edited by J. Myren, E. Schrumpf, L. E. Hanssen, and M. Vatn, p. 89. 13.Suppl. 49. (abstr.).
114. Howitz, J., and Rehfeld, J. F. (1974): Serum-gastrin in vitiligo. *Lancet,* i:831–833.
115. Hughes, W. S., Snyder, N., and Hernandez, A. (1977): Antral gastrin concentration in upper-gastrointestinal disease. *Am. J. Dig. Dis.,* 3:201–208.
116. Impicciatore, M., Debas, H., Walsh, J. H., Grossman, M. I., and Bertaccini, G. (1974): Release of gastrin and stimulation of acid secretion by bombesine in dogs. *Rendiconti,* 6:99–101.
117. Impicciatore, M., Walsh, J. H., and Grossman, M. I. (1977): Low doses of atropine enhance serum gastrin response to food in dogs. *Gastroenterology,* 72:995–996.
118. Isenberg, J. I., and Grossman, M. I. (1969): Effect of gastrin and SC 15396 on gastric motility in dogs. *Gastroenterology,* 56:450–455.
119. Isenberg, J. I., Grossman, M. I., Maxwell, V., and Walsh, J. H. (1975): Increased sensitivity to stimulation of acid secretion by pentagastrin in duodenal ulcer. *J. Clin. Invest.,* 55:330–337.
120. Isenberg, J. I., Walsh, J. H., and Grossman, M. I. (1973): Zollinger-Ellison syndrome. *Gastroenterology,* 65:140–165.
121. Isenberg, J. I., Walsh, J. H., Passaro, E. Jr., Moore, E. W., and Grossman, M. I. (1972): Unusual effect of secretin on serum gastrin, serum calcium and gastric acid secretion in a patient with suspected Zollinger-Ellison syndrome. *Gastroenterology,* 62:626–631.

122. Jacobson, E. D., Swan, K. G., and Grossman, M. I. (1967): Blood flow and secretion in the stomach. *Gastroenterology,* 52:414–420.
123. Jaffe, B. M., Clendinnen, B. G., Clarke, R. J., and Williams, J. A. (1974): The effect of selective and proximal gastric vagotomy on serum gastrin. *Gastroenterology,* 66:944–953.
124. Janowitz, H. D., and Hollander, F. (1951): Critical evidence that vagal stimulation does not release gastrin. *Proc. Soc. Exp. Biol. Med.,* 76:49–52.
125. Johnson, G. J., Summerskill, W. H. J., Anderson, V. E., and Keating, F. R. (1967): Clinical and genetic investigation of a large kindred with multiple endocrine adenomatosis. *N. Engl. J. Med.,* 277:1379–1386.
126. Johnson, L. R. (1973): Effect of gastric mucosal acidification on the action of pepsigogues. *Am. J. Physiol.,* 225:1411–1415.
127. Johnson, L. R. (1974): Gut hormones on growth of gastrointestinal mucosa. In: *Endocrinology of the Gut,* edited by W. H. Chey, and F. P. Brooks, pp. 163–177. Charles B. Slack, Thorofare, New Jersey.
128. Johnson, L. R., Aures, D., and Yuen, L. (1969): Pentagastrin-induced stimulation of protein synthesis in the gastrointestinal tract. *Am. J. Physiol.,* 217:251–254.
129. Johnson, L. R., Castro, G. A., Lichtenberger, L. M., Copeland, E. M., and Dudrick, S. J. (1974): The significance of the trophic action of gastrin. *Gastroenterology,* 66:718.
130. Johnson, L. R., Copeland, E. M., and Dudrick, S. J. (1978): Luminal gastrin stimulates growth of distal rat intestine. In: *Second International Symposium on Gastrointestinal Hormones,* edited by J. Myren, E. Schrumpf, L. E. Hanssen, and M. Vatn, *Scand. J. Gastroenterol. (Suppl 49.)* 13:95. (abstr.).
131. Johnson, L. R., Jones, R. S., Aures, D., and Håkansson, R. (1969): Effect of antrectomy on gastric histidine decarboxylase activity in the rat. *Am. J. Physiol.,* 216:1051–1053.
132. Jones, R. S., and Grossman, M. I. (1970): Choleretic effects of cholecystokinin, gastrin II and caerulein in dog. *Am. J. Physiol.,* 219:1014–1018.
133. Jordan, P. H. Jr., and Yip, B. S. S. C. (1972): The presence of gastrin in fasting and stimulated gastric juice of man. *Surgery,* 72:352–356.
134. Jordan, P. H. Jr., and Yip, B. S. S. C. (1972): The canine secretory response to gastrin extracted from gastric juice of man. *Surgery,* 72:624–629.
135. Kahlson, G., Rosengren, E., Svahn, D., and Thunberg, R. (1964): Mobilization and formation of histamine in the gastric mucosa as related to acid secretion. *J. Physiol.,* 174:400–416.
136. Kenner, G. W., and Sheppard, R. C. (1973): Gastrins of various species. In: *Frontiers in Gastrointestinal Hormone Research,* edited by S. Andersson, pp. 137–142. Almquist and Wiksell, Stockholm.
137. Knutsson, U., and Olbe, L. (1974): The effect of exogenous gastrin on the acid sham feeding response in antrum-bulb-resected duodenal ulcer patients. *Scand. J. Gastroenterol.,* 9:231–238.
138. Komarov, S. A. (1938): Gastrin. *Proc. Soc. Exp. Biol. Med.,* 38:514–516.
139. Komarov, S. A. (1942): Studies on gastrin-II. Physiological properties of the specific gastric secretagogue of the pyloric mucous membrane. *Rev. Can. Biol.,* 1:377–401.
140. Korman, M. G., Brough, B. J., and Hansky, J. (1972): Gastrin and acid studies in the pouch dog. II. Effect of truncal vagotomy on response to food and insulin hypoglycemia. *Scand. J. Gastroenterol.,* 7:525–529.
141. Korman, M. G., Layer, M. C., and Hansky, J. (1972): Hypergastrinaemia in chronic renal failure. *Br. Med. J.,* 1:209–210.
142. Korman, M. G., Scott, D. H., Hansky, J., and Wilson, H. (1972): Hypergastrinaemia due to an excluded gastric antrum: a proposed method for differentiation from the Zollinger-Ellison syndrome. *Aust. NZ. J. Med.,* 3:266–271.
143. Korman, M. G., Soveny, C., and Hansky, J. (1971): Serum gastrin in duodenal ulcer. *Gut,* 12:899–902.
144. Korman, M. G., Soveny, C., and Hansky, J. (1972): Extragastric gastrin. *Gut,* 13:346–348.
145. Korman, M. G., Strickland, R. G., and Hansky, J. (1971): Serum gastrin in chronic gastritis. *Br. Med. J.,* 2:16–18.
146. Kraft, A. R., Tompkins, R. K., Endahl, G. L., and Zollinger, R. M. (1969): Alterations in membrane transport produced by diarrheogenic nonbeta islet cell tumours of the pancreas. *Surg. Forum,* 20:338–340.
147. Kronborg, O., Stadil, F., Rehfeld, J. F., and Christiansen, P. M. (1973): Relationship between serum gastrin concentrations and gastric acid secretion in duodenal ulcer patients before and after selective and highly selective vagotomy. *Scand. J. Gastroenterol.,* 8:491–496.

148. Kun, T. L., and Sturdevant, R. A. L. (1973): Gastrin and gastroesophageal spincter incompetence. In: *Proceedings of the Fourth International Symposium on Gastrointestinal Motility, Banff, Alberta, Canada, Sept. 6–8, 1973,* edited by E. Daniel, pp. 125–130. Mitchell Press, Vancouver, Canada.

149. Lai, K. S. (1964): Studies on gastrin-II. Quantitative study of the distribution of gastrin-like activity along the gut. *Gut,* 5:334–336.

150. Lamers, C. B. H. (1976): The Zollinger-Ellison syndrome. Observations on 18 patients. In: *Some Aspects of the Zollinger-Ellison Syndrome and Serum Gastrin,* edited by G. B. H. Lamers, pp. 17–48. Krips Repro Meppel, Amsterdam.

151. Lanciault, H. G., Bonoma, C., and Brooks, F. (1973): Vagal stimulation gastrin release and acid secretion in anaesthetized dogs. *Am. J. Physiol.,* 226:546–552.

152. Larsson, L. I., Ljungberg, O., Sundler, F., Håkansson, R., Borg, I., Rehfeld, J. F., and Holst, J. (1973): Antro pyloric gastrinoma associated with pancreatic nesidioblastosis and proliferation of islets. *Virchows Arch. Pathol. Anat.,* 360:305–314.

153. Lin, T. M., and Spray, G. F. (1969): Effect of pentagastrin cholecystokinin, caerulein and glucagon on the choledochal resistence and bile flow of conscious dog. *Gastroenterology,* 56:1178.

154. Lipshutz, W. H., Gaskins, R. D., Lukash, W. M., and Sode, J. (1973): Pathogenesis of lower-esophageal sphincter incompetence. *N. Engl. J. Med.,* 289:182–184.

155. Lundberg, J. M., Ahlman, H., Dahlström, A., and Kewenter, J. (1976): Catecholamine containing nerve fibres in the human abdominal vagus. *Gastroenterology,* 70:472–474.

156. Lundberg, J. M., Hökfelt, T., Nilsson, G., Terenius, L., Rehfeld. J., Elde, R., and Said, S. (1978). Peptide neurons in the vagus, splanchnic and sciatic nerves. *Acta Physiol. Scand.,* 104:499–501.

157. Lundell, L., Svensson, S. E., and Nilsson, G. (1976): Further studies on the mode of action of isoprenaline on gastric secretion in conscious rat. *Br. J. Pharmacol.,* 58:17–25.

158. Marks, I. N., Bank, S., and Louw, J. H. (1967): Islet cell tumour of the pancreas with reversible watery diarrhea and achlorhydria. *Gastroenterology,* 52:695–707.

159. Maung Pe Thein and Schofield, B. (1959): Release of gastrin from the pyloric antrum following vagal stimulation by sham-feeding in dogs. *J. Physiol. (Lond.),* 148:291–305.

160. Maxwell, J. G., Moore, J. G., Dixon, J., and Stevens, L. E. (1971): Gastrin levels in anephric patients. *Surg. Forum,* 22:305–306.

161. McDonald, T. J., Nilsson, G., Vagne, M., Ghatei, M., Bloom, S. R., and Mutt, V. (1978): A gastrin releasing peptide from the porcine nonantral gastric tissue. *Gut,* 19:767–774.

162. McGuigan, J. E. (1976): The absence of big, big gastrin in human serum as determined by immune absorption techniques. In: *First International Symposium on Gastrointestinal Hormones.* Asilomar. Ao 96.

163. McGuigan, J. E., Colwell. J. A., and Franklin, J. (1974): Effect of parathyroidectomy on hypercalcemic hypersecretory peptic ulcer disease. *Gastroenterology,* 66:269–272.

164. McGuigan, J. E., and Greider, M. H. (1971): Correlative immunochemical and light microscopic studies of the gastrin cell of the antral mucosa. *Gastroenterology,* 60:223–236.

165. McGuigan, J. E., and Trudeau, W. L. (1970): Serum gastrin concentration in pernicious anemia. *N. Engl. J. Med.,* 282:358–361.

166. McGuigan, J. E., and Trudeau, W. L. (1972): Serum gastrin levels before and after vagotomy and pyloroplasty or vagotomy and antrectomy. *N. Engl. J. Med.,* 286:184–188.

167. McGuigan, J. E., and Trudeau, W. L. (1973): Serum and tissue gastrin concentrations in patients with carcinoma of the stomach. *Gastroenterology,* 64:22–25.

168. Morley, J. S. (1968): Structure-function relationships in gastrin-like peptides. *Proc. R. Soc. (Lond.) Biol.,* 170:97–111.

169. Moshal, M. G., Broitman, S. A., and Zamcheck, N. (1970): Gastrin and absorption. A review. *Am. J. Clin. Nutr.,* 23:336–342.

170. Muryobayashi, T., Mori, J., Fujiwara, M., and Shimamoto, K. (1968): Fluorescence histochemical demonstration of adrenergic nerve fibers in the vagus nerve of cats and dogs. *Jpn. J. Pharmacol.,* 18:285–293.

171. Neuburger, P. H., Lewin, M., and Bonfils, S. (1972): Parietal and chief cell populations in four cases of the Zollinger-Ellison syndrome. *Gastroenterology,* 63:937–942.

172. Nilsson, G. (1976): Regulationsmechanismen der Magensäuresekretion. In: *Vagotomie,* edited by H. Burge, et al., pp. 14–25. George Thieme Verlag, Stuttgart.

173. Nilsson, G., and Brodin, K. (1977): Increase of gastrin concentration in duodenal mucosa of dogs following resection of the gastric antrum. *Acta Physiol. Scand.,* 99:510–512.

174. Nilsson, G., and Brodin, K. (1978): Evidences for a mechanism influencing tissue gastrin concentration in dogs. In: *Second International Symposium on Gastrointestinal Hormones,* edited by J. Myren, E. Schrumpf, L. E. Hansen, and M. Vatn, *Scand. J. Gastroenterol. (Suppl. 49.)* 13:134 (Abstr.).

175. Nilsson, G., Hjelmquist, U., and Brodin, E. (1978): Effect of oral administration of calcium carbonate, camalox and novalucol on plasma gastrin concentration in duodenal ulcer patients. *Acta Pharm. Toxicol.,* 44:81–84.

176. Nilsson, G., Simon, J., Yalow, R. S., and Berson, S. A. (1972): Plasma gastrin and gastric acid responses to sham-feeding and feeding in dogs. *Gastroenterology,* 63:51–59.

177. Nilsson, G., Yalow, R. S., and Berson, S. A. (1973): Distribution of gastrin in the gastrointestinal tract on human, dog, cat and hog. In: *Frontiers in Gastrointestinal Hormone Research,* pp. 95–101. Almqvist and Wiksell, Stockholm.

178. Oberhelman, H. A., and Nelson, T. S. (1964): Surgical consideration of the management of ulcerogenic tumours of the pancreas and duodenum. *Am. J. Surg.,* 108:132–140.

179. Olbe, L. (1964): Potentiation of sham-feeding response in Pavlov pouch dogs by subthreshold amounts of gastrin with and without acidification of denervated antrum. *Acta Physiol. Scand.,* 61:244–254.

180. Olbe, L. (1964): Effect of resection of gastrin releasing regions on acid response to sham-feeding and insulin hypoglycemia in Pavlov pouch dogs. *Acta Physiol. Scand.,* 62:169–175.

181. Olbe, L. (1974): Differences between human and animal gastric acid secretion. Syllabus for American Gastroenterological Association Postgraduate Course on Peptic Ulcer Disease, San Francisco. *American Gastroenterological Association,* pp. 6–10.

182. Olbe, L., Ridley, P. T., and Uvnäs, B. (1967): Effects of gastrin and histamine on vagally induced acid and pepsin secretion in antrectomized dogs. *Acta Physiol. Scand.,* 72:492–497.

183. Parker, P. E., Soergel, K., and Ellison, E. H. (1963): Effects of excessive hydrochloric acid on canine intestinal tract. *Surg. Forum,* 14:333–334.

184. Passaro, E. P. Jr., Gillespie, I. E., and Grossman, M. I. (1963): Potentiation between gastrin and histamine in stimulation of gastric secretion. *Proc. Soc. Exp. Biol.,* 114:50–52.

185. Pevsner, L., and Grossman, M. I. (1955): The mechanism of vagal stimulation of gastric acid secretion. *Gastroenterology,* 28:493–499.

186. Pointer, J. P., Accary, J., Vatier, M., Dubrasquet, M., and Bonfils, S. (1973): Detection of gastrin in normal pancreas by radioimmunoassay. *Horm. Metab. Res.,* 5:303–304.

187. Polak, J. M., Stagge, B., and Pearse, A. G. E. (1972): Two types of Zollinger-Ellison syndrome: immunofluorescent, cytochemical and ultrastructural studies of the antral and pancreatic gastrin cells in different clinical states. *Gut,* 13:501–512.

188. Popielski, L. (1912): Die Wirkung der Organextrakte und die Theorie der Hormone. *Münich Med. Wochenschr.,* 59:534–535.

189. Popielski, L. (1920): β-imidazolyläthylamin und die organextrakte; β-imidazolyläthylamin als mächtiger Erreger der Magendrüsen. *Pflüg. Arch. Physiol.,* 178:214–236.

190. Ptak, T., and Kirsner, J. B. (1970): The Zollinger-Ellison syndrome, polyendocrine adenomatosis and other endocrine associated associations with peptic ulcer. *Adv. Int. Med.,* 16:213–242.

191. Rabinovitch, J., and Achs, S. (1945): Tumours of the islands of Langerhans. *Arch. Pathol.,* 40:74–77.

192. Rawson, A. B., England, M. T., Gillam, G. G., French, J. M., and Stammers, F. A. R. (1960): Zollinger-Ellison syndrome with diarrhea and malabsorption. *Lancet,* ii:131–134.

193. Rayford, P. L., Villar, H. V., Reeder, D. D., and Thompson, J. C. (1974): Effect of GIP and VIP on gastrin release and gastric secretion. *Physiologist,* 17:319.

194. Reeder, D. D., Becker, I. D., and Thompson, J. C. (1974): Effect of intravenously administered calcium on serum gastrin and gastric secretion in man. *Surg. Gynecol. Obstet.,* 138:847–851.

195. Reeder, D., Conlee, J. L., and Thompson, J. C. (1972): Changes in gastric secretion and serum gastrin concentration in duodenal ulcer patients after oral calcium antacid. In: *Gastrointestinal Hormones. International Symposium at Erlangen 1971,* edited by L. Demling, pp. 19–22. George Thieme Verlag, Stuttgart.

196. Reeder, D. D., Jackson, B. M., Brandt, L. N. Jr., and Thompson, J. C. (1972): Rate and pattern of disappearance of exogenous gastrin in dogs. *Am. J. Physiol.,* 222:1571–1574.

197. Rehfeld, J. F. (1976): Circulating forms of gastrin in normals and DU. In: *First International Symposium on Gastrointestinal Hormones.* Asilomar A 126.

198. Rehfeld, J. F., and Iversen, J. (1973): Secretion of immunoreactive gastrin from the isolated, perfused canine pancreas. *VIII Congress of the International Diabetes Federation, Brussels.* Excerpta Medica, Amsterdam International Congress Series No. 280, p. 119 (Abstr.).
199. Rehfeld J. F., and Stadil, F. (1973): Gel filtration studies on immunoreactive gastrin in serum from Zollinger-Ellison patients. *Gut,* 14:369–373.
200. Rehfeld, J. F., Stadil, F., Malmström, J., and Miyata, M. (1975): Gastrin heterogeneity in serum and tissue. A progress report. In: *Gastrointestinal Hormones,* edited by J. C. Thompson, pp. 43–58. Univ. of Texas Press, Austin, Texas.
201. Rehfeld, J. F., Stadil, F., and Vikelsoe, J. (1974): Immunoreactive gastrin components in human serum. *Gut,* 15:102–111.
202. Richardson, C. T., Walsh, J. H., Hicks, M. I., and Fordtran, J. S. (1976): Studies on the mechanisms of food-stimulated gastric acid secretion in normal human subjects. *J. Clin. Invest.,* 58:623–631.
203. Richardson, C. T., Walsh, J. H., and Hicks, M. I. (1976): The effect of cimetidine, a new histamine H_2-receptor antagonist, on meal-stimulated acid secretion, serum gastrin and gastric emptying in patients with duodenal ulcer. *Gastroenterology,* 71:19–23.
204. Rooney, P. J., Kennedy, A. C., Hayes, J. R., Buchanan, K. D., Webb, J., Lee, P., and Dick, W. C. (1973): Hypergastrinaemia in rheumatoid arthritis. *Scott Med. J.,* 18:32.
205. Royston, C. M. S., Brew, D. S. J., Garnham, J. R., Stagg, B. H., and Polak, J. M. (1972): The Zollinger-Ellison syndrome due to an infiltrating tumour of the stomach. *Gut,* 13:638–642.
206. Rubin, W. (1972): Endocrine cells in the normal human stomach. *Gastroenterology,* 62:784–800.
207. Sacks, J., Ivy, A. C., Burgess, J. P., and Vandolah, J. E. (1932): Histamine as the hormone for gastric secretion. *Am. J. Physiol.,* 101:331–338.
208. Sailer, S., and Zinninger, M. (1946): Massive islet cell tumour of the pancreas without hypoglycemia. *Surg. Gynecol. Obstet.,* 82:301–305.
209. Scholten, Th., Rehlinghaus, U., Fritsch, W.-P., and Hansamen, T. U. (1976): Zur gastrinfreisetzung durch kalziumhaltige Antazida. *Med. Welt,* 27:1332–1333.
210. Schrumpf, E., Petersen, H., Berstad, A., Myren, J., and Rosenlund, B. (1973): The effect of secretin on plasma gastrin in the Zollinger-Ellison syndrome. *Scand. J. Gastroenterol.,* 8:145–150.
211. Schrumpf, E., and Semb, I. S. (1973): The metabolic clearance rate and half-life of synthetic human gastrin in dogs. *Scand. J. Gastroenterol.,* 8:203–207.
212. Schrumpf, E., Semb, I. S., and Vold, H. (1973): Metabolic clearance and disappearance rates of synthetic human gastrin in man. *Scand. J. Gastroenterol.,* 8:731–734.
213. Seelig, H. P. (1972): Gastrin Inaktivierung und Abbau. Stuttgart, *Gastroenterologie und Stoffwechsel.*
214. Shafer, W. (1964): Nonbeta islet-cell carcinoma of the pancreas presenting as diarrhea, report of a case. *Ann. Intern. Med.,* 61:539–543.
215. Shimoda, S. S., Saunders, D. R., and Rubin, C. E. (1968): The Zollinger-Ellison syndrome with steatorrhea. II. The mechanisms of fat and vitamin B_{12} malabsorption. *Gastroenterology,* 55:705–723.
216. Singleton, J. W., Kern, F., and Wadell, W. R. (1965): Diarrhea and pancreatic islet cell tumour: Report of a case with severe jejunal mucosal lesion. *Gastroenterology,* 49:197–208.
217. Sjödin, L. (1972): Potentiation of the gastric secretory response to sham-feeding in dogs by infusions of gastrin and pentagastrin. *Acta Physiol. Scand.,* 85:24–32.
218. Sjödin, L., and Nilsson, G. (1976): Role of antrum and duodenum in the control of postprandial gastric acid secretion and plasma gastrin concentration in dogs. *Gastroenterology,* 69:928–934.
219. Snyder, N., Scurry, M., and Hughes, W. (1974): Hypergastrinemia in familial multiple endocrine adenomatosis. *Ann. Intern. Med.,* 80:321–325.
220. Soergel, K. H. (1969): Mechanism of diarrhea in the Zollinger-Ellison syndrome. In: *Noninsulin Producing Tumours of the Pancreas. Modern Aspects on Zollinger-Ellison Syndrome and Gastrin,* edited by L. Demling and R. Oltenjann, pp. 152–161. Georg Thieme Verlag, Stuttgart.
221. Solcia, E., Vassalo, G., and Capella, C. (1969): Studies on the G-cells of the pyloric mucosa, the probable site of gastrin secretion. *Gut,* 10:379–388.
222. Spence, R. W., McCormick, D. A., Oliver, J. M., and Celestin, L. R. (1978): Cimetidine.

In: *The Westminister Symposium 1978,* edited by C. Wastell and P. Lance, pp. 153–169. Churchill Livingstone, Edinburgh.

223. Stadil, F., and Rehfeld, J. F. (1973): Release of gastrin by epinephrine in man. *Gastroenterology,* 65:210–215.

224. Stadil, F., Rehfeld, J. F., and Thaysen, E. H. (1971): Variations in the concentrations of serum gastrin in the Zollinger-Ellison syndrome. In: *Gastrointestinal Hormones and Other Subjects,* edited by E. H. Thaysen, pp. 125–129. Munksgaard, Copenhagen.

225. Stadil, F., and Stage, J. G. (1978): Treatment of the Zollinger-Ellison syndrome. In: *Second International Symposium on Gastrointestinal Hormones,* edited by J. Myren, E. Schrumpf, L. E. Hanssen, and M. Vatn, *Scand. J. Gastroenterol., (Suppl. 49),* 13:174. (Abstr.).

226. Stave, R., and Brandtzaeg, P. (1978): Immunohistochemical investigation of gastrin-producing cells, (G-cells). Estimation of antral density mucosal distribution, and total mass of G-cells in resected stomachs from patients with peptic ulcer disease. *Scand. J. Gastroenterol.,* 13:199–203.

227. Stave, R., Myren, J., Brandtzaeg, P., and Gjone, E. (1978): Quantitative studies of gastrin cells (G-cells) and parietal cells in relation to gastric acid secretion in patients with peptic ulcer disease. *Scand. J. Gastroenterol.,* 13:293–298.

228. Stening, G. F., and Grossman, M. I. (1969): Gastrin-related peptides as stimulants of pancreatic and gastric secretion. *Am. J. Physiol.,* 217:262–266.

229. Stening, G. F., and Grossman, M. I. (1969): The hormonal control of Brunner's glands. *Gastroenterology,* 56:1047–1052.

230. Stern, D. H., and Walsh, J. H. (1973): Gastrin release in postoperative ulcer patients: evidence for release of duodenal gastrin. *Gastroenterology,* 64:363–369.

231. Straaten, T. (1933): Die Bedeutung der Pülorusdrüsenzone für die Magensaftsekretion. Ein experimenteller Beitrag zur Resektionsbehandlung des Geschwurleidens. *Arch. Klin. Chir.,* 176:236–251.

232. Straus, E., and Yalow, R. S. (1974): Studies on the distribution and degradation of heptadeca-peptides, big, and big big gastrin. *Gastroenterology,* 66:936–943.

233. Straus, E., and Yalow, R. S. (1975): Differential diagnosis of hypergastrinemia. In: *Gastrointestinal Hormones,* edited by J. C. Thompson, pp. 99–113. University of Texas Press, Austin, Texas.

234. Strickland, R. G., Bhathal, P. S., Korman, M. G., and Hansky, J. (1971): Serum gastrin and the antral mucosa in atrophic gastritis. *Br. Med. J.,* 4:451–453.

235. Ström, R. (1953): A case of peptic ulcer and insulinoma. *Acta Chir. Scand.,* 104:252–260.

236. Strunz, U. T., Walsh, J. H., and Grossman, M. I. (1978): Removal of gastrin by various organs in dogs. *Gastroenterology,* 74:32–33.

237. Strunz, U. T., Walsh, J. H., and Grossman, M. I. (1978): Stimulation of gastric acid secretion and gastrin release in dogs by individual amino acids. *Proc. Soc. Exp. Biol. Med.,* 157:440–441.

238. Svensson, S. E. (1970): Secretory behaviour and histamine formation in the rat Heidenhain pouch following antrectomy. *J. Physiol.,* 207:699–708.

239. Svensson, S. O., Emås, S., Dörner, M., and Kaess, H. (1976): Cholinergic release of gastrin by feeding in cats. *Gastroenterology,* 70:742–746.

240. Taylor, I. L., Walsh, J. H., Carter, D. C., Chew, P., and Grossman, M. I. (1977): Bethanecol and atropine both inhibit the gastrin response to bombesin. *Clin. Res.,* 25:574. (Abstr.).

241. Taylor, I. L., Walsh, J. H., Carter, D. C., Wood, J., and Grossman, M. I. (1978): Effect of atropine and bethanechol on release of pancreatic polypeptide (PP) and gastrin by bombesin in dog. In: *Second International Symposium on Gastrointestinal Hormones,* edited by J. Myren, E. Schrumpf, L. E. Hanssen, and M. Vatn. *Scand. J. Gastroenterol.* (Suppl. 49) 13:183 (Abstr.).

242. Tepperman, B. L., Walsh, J. H., and Preshaw, R. M. (1972): Effect of antral denervation on gastrin release by sham-feeding and insulin hypoglycemia in dogs. *Gastroenterology,* 63:973–980.

243. Thompson, J. C. (1962): The inhibition of gastric secretion by the duodenum and by the gastric antrum. *J. Surg. Res.,* 2:181–196.

244. Thompson, J. C., Hirose, F. M., Lemnu, C. A. E., and Davidson, W. D. (1968): Zollinger-Ellison syndrome in a patient with multiple carcinoid-islet cell tumours of the duodenum. *Am. J. Surg.,* 115:177–184.

245. Thompson, J. C., Reeder, D. D., Bunchman, H. H., Becker, H. D., and Brandt, E. N. (1972): Effect of secretin on circulating gastrin. *Ann. Surg.,* 176:384–393.

246. Tracy, H. J., and Gregory, R. A. (1964): Physiological properties of a series of synthetic peptides structurally related to gastrin I. *Nature,* 204:935–938.
247. Trout, H. H. III, and Grossman, M. I. (1971): Penultimate aspartyl unnecessary for stimulation of acid secretion by gastrin-related peptide. *Nature New Biol.,* 234:256.
248. Trudeau, W. L., and McGuigan, J. E. (1969): Effects of calcium on serum gastrin levels in the Zollinger-Ellison syndrome. *N. Engl. J. Med.,* 281:862–866.
249. Trudeau, W. L., and McGuigan, J. E. (1970): Serum gastrin levels in patients with peptic ulcer disease. *Gastroenterology,* 59:6–12.
250. Trudeau, W. L., and McGuigan, J. E. (1971): Relations between serum gastrin levels and rates of gastric hydrochloric acid secretion. *N. Engl. J. Med.,* 282:408–412.
251. Turbey, W. J., and Passaro, E. Jr. (1972): Hyperparathyroidism in the Zollinger-Ellison syndrome. *Arch. Surg.,* 105:62–66.
252. Uvnäs, B. (1942): The part played by the pyloric region in the cephalic phase of gastric secretion. *Acta Physiol. Scand. (Suppl.),* 13:1–86.
253. Uvnäs, B. (1943): The secretory excitant from the pyloric mucosa. *Acta Physiol. Scand.,* 6:97–107.
254. Uvnäs, B. (1945): Further attempts to isolate a gastric secretory excitant from the pyloric mucosa of pigs. *Acta Physiol. Scand.,* 9:296–305.
255. Uvnäs, B. (1945): The presence of a gastric secretory excitant in the human gastric and duodenal mucosa. *Acta Physiol. Scand.,* 10:97–101.
256. Uvnäs, B., Uvnäs-Wallensten, K., and Nilsson, G. (1975): Release of gastrin on vagal stimulation in the cat. *Acta Physiol. Scand.,* 94:167–176.
257. Uvnäs-Wallensten, K., and Andersson, H. (1977): Effect of atropine and methiamide on vagally induced gastric acid secretion and gastrin release in anaesthetized cats. *Acta Physiol. Scand.,* 99:496–502.
258. Uvnäs-Wallensten, K., and Rehfeld, J. F. (1977): Type of gastrin released by vagal stimulation in anaesthetized cats. *Gastroenterology,* 72:825. (Abstr.).
259. Uvnäs-Wallensten, K., Rehfeld, J. F., Larsson, L. I., and Uvnäs, B. (1977): Heptadecapeptide gastrin in the vagal nerve. *Proc. Natl. Acad. Sci. USA,* 74:5707–5710.
260. Vagne, M., and Grossman, M. I. (1968): Cholecystokinetic potency of gastrointestinal hormones and related peptides. *Am. J. Physiol.,* 215:881–884.
261. Vassallo, G., Solcia, F., Bussolati, G., Polak, J. M., and Pearse, A. G. E. (1972): Non-G-cell gastrin-producing tumours of the pancreas. *Virchows Arch. Abt. B. Zellpath.,* 11:66–79.
262. Verner, J. V. (1968): Clinical syndromes associated with non-insulin producing tumours of the pancreatic islets. In: *Non-Insulin-Producing Tumours of the Pancreas. International Symposium at Erlangen,* edited by L. Demling and R. Ottenjann, pp. 165–183. Georg Thieme Verlag, Stuttgart.
263. Verner, J. V., and Morrison, A. B. (1958): Islet cell tumour and a syndrome of refractory watery diarrhea and hypokalemia. *Am. J. Med.,* 25:374–380.
264. Walsh, J. H. (1978): Biological activity and clearance of gastrin peptides in dog and man: Effects of varying chain length of peptide fragments. In: *Gastrointestinal Hormones and Pathology of the Digestive System,* edited by M. I. Grossman, V. Speranza, N. Basso, and E. Lezoche, pp. 85–89. Plenum Press, New York.
265. Walsh, J. H., Debas, H. T., and Grossman, M. I. (1974): Pure human big gastrin: immunochemical properties, disappearance half time, and acid-stimulating action in dogs. *J. Clin. Invest.,* 54:477–485.
266. Walsh, J. H., and Grossman, M. I. (1973): Circulating gastrin in peptic ulcer disease. *Mt. Sinai Med. J. NY,* 50:374–381.
267. Walsh, J. H., and Grossman, M. I. (1975): Gastrin. *N. Engl. J. Med.,* 292:1324–1332.
268. Walsh, J. H., Isenberg, J. I., Ansfield, J., and Maxwell, V. (1976): Clearance and acid-stimulating action of human big and little gastrins in duodenal ulcer subjects. *J. Clin. Invest.,* 57:1125–1131.
269. Walsh, J. H., and Laster, L. (1973): Enzymatic deamidation of the C-terminal tetrapeptide amide of gastrin by mammalian tissues. *Biochem. Med.,* 8:432–449.
270. Walsh, J. H., Maxwell, V., and Isenberg, J. I. (1975): Biological activity and clearance of human big gastrin in man. *Clin. Res.,* 23:259A.
271. Walsh, J. H., Reeve, J. R., Vigna, S. R., Chew, P., Wong, H. C., and Dockray, G. J. (1978): Identification of different forms of bombesin-like immunoreactivity in mammalian gut. In:

Second International Symposium on Gastrointestinal Hormones, edited by J. Myren, E. Schrumpf, L. E. Hanssen, and M. Vatn, *Scand. J. Gastroenterol., (Suppl. 49),* 13:191 (Abstr.).

272. Walsh, J. H., Richardson, C. T., and Fordtran, S. (1975): pH dependence of acid secretion and gastrin release in normal and ulcer subjects. *J. Clin. Invest.,* 55:462–468.

273. Walsh, J. H., Yalow, R. S., and Berson, S. A. (1971): The effect of atropine on plasma gastrin response to feeding. *Gastroenterology,* 60:16–21.

274. Way, L., Goldman, L., and Dunphy, J. E. (1968): Zollinger-Ellison syndrome. An analysis of twenty-five cases. *Am. J. Surg.,* 116:293–304.

275. Weichert, R., Reed, R., and Creech, O., Jr. (1967): Carcinoid-islet cell tumours of the duodenum. *Ann. Surg.,* 165:660–669.

276. Wermer, P. (1967): The diagnosis of polyadenomatosis of endocrine glands. *Symposium on Radiology and the Endocrine System,* 5:349–354.

277. Winawer, S. J., Broitman, S. A., Wolochow, D. A., Osborne, M. P., and Zamcheck, N. (1966): Successful management of massive small-bowel resection based on assessment of absorption defects and nutritional needs. *N. Engl. J. Med.,* 272:72–78.

278. Woodward, E. R., Lyon, E. S., Landor, J., and Dragstedt, L. R. (1954): The physiology of the gastric antrum; experimental studies on isolated antrum pouches in dogs. *Gastroenterology,* 27:766–785.

279. Wormsley, K. G., and Grossman, M. I. (1965): Maximal histalog test in control subjects and patients with peptic ulcer. *Gut,* 6:427–435.

280. Wyllie, J. H., Stagg, B. H., and Termperley, J. M. (1974): Inactivation of pentagastrin by the liver. *Br. J. Surg.,* 61:22–26.

281. Yalow, R. S., and Berson, S. A. (1970): Radioimmunoassay of gastrin. *Gastroenterology,* 58:1–14.

282. Yalow, R. S., and Berson, S. A. (1970): Size and charge distinctions between endogenous human plasma gastrin in peripheral blood and heptadecapeptide gastrins. *Gastroenterology,* 58:609–615.

283. Yalow, R. S., and Berson, S. A. (1971): Further studies on the nature of immunoreactive gastrin in human plasma. *Gastroenterology,* 60:203–214.

284. Yalow, R. S., and Berson, S. A. (1972): And now, big big gastrin. *Biochem. Biophys. Res. Commun.,* 48:391–395.

285. Zeljony, G. P., and Savich, V. (1911): Concerning the mechanisms of gastric secretion. In: *Proc. Soc. Rus. Physc. St. Petersburg.* Quoted by Babkin, Secretory mechanisms of the digestive glands, New York, Hoeber, 1950.

286. Zollinger, R. M., and Ellison, E. M. (1955): Primary peptic ulceration of the jejunum associated with islet cell tumours of the pancreas. *Ann. Surg.,* 142:709–728.

Gastrointestinal Hormones, edited by
George B. Jerzy Glass.
Raven Press, New York © 1980.

Chapter 7

Cholecystokinin: Isolation, Structure, and Functions

Viktor Mutt

Department of Biochemistry II, Karolinska Institute, Stockholm, Sweden

Working in Starlings' laboratory, Okada noted that in dogs not only the secretion of hepatic bile but also the expulsion of gallbladder bile into the intestine was stimulated by intestinal acidification (302). In 1928 Ivy and Oldberg described experiments with dogs and cats suggesting that the tissue of the upper intestine contained a substance that on release into the bloodstream would cause gallbladder contraction. They named this hormone cholecystokinin (200), and the following year Ivy et al. (199) described attempts to chemically separate cholecystokinin and secretin that had been extracted together from the upper intestinal tissues of dogs and pigs.

Since it must have been immediately obvious that applications in clinical medicine could be expected for cholecystokinin, it is puzzling that for many years only little interest was directed toward its chemical identification. During the 15-year period following its discovery, apart from the laboratory in which it was discovered, only Ågren seems to have shown interest in this problem (3).

In 1943 an important contribution toward the characterization of cholecystokinin was made, although this was not recognized at that time. Following on the observation by Harper and Vass (166) that in cats in which the extrinsic nerves to the intestine had been sectioned, introduction of food into the intestine still led to a stimulation of pancreatic enzyme secretion, Harper and Raper demonstrated that extracts of porcine intestinal tissue contained a substance, distinct from secretin, that was able, on intravenous administration, to stimulate the secretion of pancreatic enzymes. They named this hormone pancreozymin (165). Later work led to the isolation from hog intestinal tissue (217) of a substance that exhibited the properties ascribed to cholecystokinin (200) as well as to pancreozymin (165), and no evidence has been obtained for the existence of any substance showing only one of these activities. This does not prove that no such substance(s) may occur in the intestinal tissue, but such a possibility does not seem to be likely. Since cholecystokinin was discovered earlier than pancreozymin, it has been suggested that cholecystokinin-pancreozymin (CCK-PZ) be named cholecystokinin (CCK) for short, it being understood that CCK has both cholecystokinetic and pancreozyminic activities (157).[1] Later work in various laboratories *(vide infra)* was to show that, in analogy with what had been found concerning other polypeptide hormones (364), CCK occurred in tissue extracts in forms of different sizes, the smaller ones being presumably derived by fragmentation of the larger forms. It was further found that CCK could be extracted not only from intestinal but also from cerebral tissue.

ISOLATION AND PRIMARY STRUCTURE OF CCK

The first CCK to be isolated was the porcine. In our work on secretin it was found that its crude preparations also contained pancreozymin activity, and that on following our procedure for the isolation of secretin to the step where extraction of it into methanol takes place the bulk of the pancreozymin activity remains unextracted. This methanol-insoluble fraction was the starting material for our work on the isolation of pancreozymin. The first step entailed adsorption of the active material to carboxymethyl cellulose from a pH 6.5 phosphate buffer, 0.02 M in sodium. Elution was carried out by making the buffer 0.2 M in NaCl and the activity was precipitated from the eluate by saturating the latter with NaCl. In animal experiments we had found that this material was still quite toxic but that these toxic reactions could be essentially eliminated by dissolving it in 75% ethanol and precipitating with 2 volumes of butanol. Butanol is known to be an excellent solvent for lipids (279) and this makes us believe that the toxic impurities were of lipid nature. The butanol-precipitated material was next chromatographed in a sodium pyrophosphate-orthophosphate buffer (0.005 M in pyrophosphate) at pH 9.1 on diethylaminoethyl (DEAE) cellulose (216). [Originally we used triethylaminoethyl (TEAE) cellulose but further work showed this to have no distinct advantages over the use of DEAE cellulose.] From the eluate the active material was adsorbed to alginic acid (at pH 2.5), eluted with 0.2 M HCl, and after exchange of chloride for acetate on DEAE-Sephadex, lyophilized. This material has been extensively used clinically under the name "10% pure CCK." The percentage is of course approximate and is determined on the basis of activity. Following on the finding that this type of preparation contained substantial quantities of gastric inhibitory peptide (GIP) (52), an additional purification step, chromatography on Sephadex G50 in 0.25 M phosphate buffer at pH 8 (218) has been added. The eluate from this Sephadex column was desalted by passage, in 0.2 M acetic acid, through Sephadex G-25 (coarse) and the eluate was lyophilized. The yield of the lyophilized material was about 1 mg from 30 kg of boiled intestinal tissue, and the yield in activity, based on the activity of CTIP, is about 5%. Because of the possibility, or rather probability (158), of various interactions, inhibitory as well as augmentatory, of other peptides present in crude preparations with CCK

---

[1] This terminology is used throughout this chapter. Consequently, in referring to published work, "CCK" is used even when the authors in question may have used cholecystokinin-pancreozymin (CCK-PZ) or even just pancreozymin.

(50), the activity measurements may give an approximation only of the actual content of CCK in the materials.

To further purify CCK, the material was chromatographed on Amberlite CG 50 II (BDH) in phosphate buffer of pH 7.5 and 0.05 M in sodium (218). The peptide material was adsorbed from the eluate to alginic acid, eluted with 0.2 M HCl, and, after exchange of chloride for acetate, lyophilized. Approximately 15 mg was obtained from 100 mg chromatographed. The lyophilized material was predominantly a mixture of two forms of CCK that may be separated by chromatography on carboxymethyl cellulose in dilute ammonium bicarbonate solution, one form eluting in 0.02 M, and the other at a higher concentration of the bicarbonate (285). The peptides were recovered from the eluates by lyophilization and relyophilized from 0.2 M acetic acid. In this chromatography, as in others, unaccounted for losses occurred, and from 10 mg of the mixture only about 3 mg of the CCK eluting in 0.02 M bicarbonate, and slightly less of the other form, were obtained. Acid hydrolyzates of the material eluted with 0.02 M ammonium bicarbonate contained 16 different types of amino acid residues in the proportions: Ala_1, Arg_3, Asp_5, Glu_1, Gly_2, His_1, Ile_2, Leu_2, Lys_2, Met_3, Phe_1, Pro_2, Trp_1, Tyr_1, Ser_5, Val_1.

It was found that one of the aspartic acids was derived from a residue of asparagine in the peptide chain; the glutamic acid, from a residue of glutamine; and the phenylalanine, from C-terminal phenylalanine amide. It was further found that the phenolic group of the tyrosine residue was esterified with sulfuric acid in the peptide. The sequence was found to be (286)

K A P S G R V S M I K N L Q S L D P S H R I S D R D Y² M G W M D F ■

This form of CCK is conveniently referred to as CCK-33. The variant eluting at a higher concentration of ammonium bicarbonate was found to have the sequence of CCK-33 with an N-terminal extension by the hexapeptide Y I Q Q A R (284). Figure 1 shows the amino acid sequence of CCK-39 in expanded form.

We found (218) that the C-terminal tryptic peptide of CCK (CCK-8), and all other fragments incorporating it, exhibited, as did CCK itself, both cholecystokinetic and pancreozyminic activities. Work with synthetic CCK-8 showed it to be, also on a molar basis, several times stronger in terms of its activity than the whole molecule (304). Recently, it has been found by several workers, using various types of chromatographies of small intestinal tissue extracts in combination with radioimmunoassays (RIAs), that CCK-8 and other, larger, fragments of CCK occur in free form in intestinal tissue of various species (91,169,330,368).

Following on the demonstration by Vanderhaeghen et al. (383) of gastrin-like immunoreactivity in cerebral tissue of man and several other species, Dockray, using different antibodies directed preferentially toward either gastrin or

---

² The amino acid residues are referred to by one-letter symbols (*Eur. J. Biochem.*, 5:151–153), the symbol ■ indicates that the carboxyl group of the C-terminal acid residue is in amide form and * that the phenolic group of the tyrosine residue is esterified with sulfuric acid.

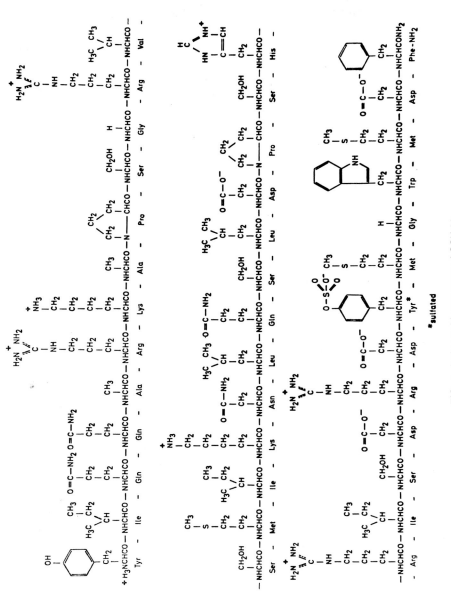

FIG. 1. Amino acid sequence of CCK-39.

*sulfated

CCK-8, showed that the gastrin-like immunoreactivity in extracts of cerebral tissue from rats, pigs, and dogs was due to peptides resembling CCK more than gastrin (90). Also with the aid of RIA, Muller et al. provided evidence for the existence of both intact CCK and CCK-8 in pig cerebral cortical tissue (281). Later, Straus and Yalow found both of these peptides in cerebral tissue of the monkey and the dog, in addition to that of the pig (368). Using sequence-specific antibodies, Rehfeld (329,330) found that in man and in the pig the quantitatively predominant part of the CCK-like immunoreactivity seemed to be due to CCK-8, CCK-33, and a gastrin-like group of substances occurring in much smaller quantities. Robberecht et al. (337) using, i.e., a radioreceptor assay in which the concentrations of CCK-like peptides were measured by their ability to inhibit binding of [^{3}H]cerulein to rat pancreatic plasma membranes, found that the $10^5 \times$ g pellet of human cerebral cortical gray matter contained a peptide closely resembling CCK-8. Del Mazo (265) also found immunoreactive CCK, in greatly varying concentrations, in the central nervous system (CNS) of rats and cats and, recently, Dockray isolated two peptides with CCK-like immunoreactivities and bioactivities from ovine cerebral tissue. One of them was found to be identical in every respect to porcine CCK-8, but the other, although apparently having the same sequence, nevertheless differed from it in several of its chromatographic properties (92). The biosynthetic relationships between the larger and the smaller forms of CCK are not yet clear. Recently, Straus et al. described the partial purification, from canine and porcine cerebral cortical extracts, of an enzyme distinct from trypsin but apparently belonging to the group of trypsin-like enzymes, i.e., enzymes that show strong preference for the cleavage of arginyl and lysyl peptide bonds (367). This enzyme was found to form from porcine CCK-33 what, as evidenced by their chromatographic and immunological properties, appeared to be CCK-12 and CCK-8. Unlike trypsin, it did not attack human gastrin-34 (G-34). It is not unusual for trypsin-like enzymes to show greatly restricted specificity as compared with trypsin itself. Thus, in CCK-33 only one of the four bonds that are cleaved by trypsin is also cleaved by thrombin (285); in secretin, similarly, only one of four (287); and in porcine vasoactive intestinal peptide (VIP) only one of the five bonds is cleaved by pancreatic kallikrein (288).

It may be mentioned that *in vitro* conversion of CCK-39 to CCK-33 may be achieved by degrading the former with dipeptidylaminopeptidase I, since this enzyme removes dipeptides from the N-terminus of a polypeptide until a N-terminal residue of arginine or lysine is reached (252).

Organic chemical syntheses have been described for CCK-8 and its nonsulfated analog (304), CCK-12 (303), the N-terminal hexapaptide of CCK (41), and the unsulfated analog of CCK-33 (404).

OCCURRENCE OF CCK

Although the larger forms of CCK, CCK-39, and CCK-33 have to date been isolated from one species only—the pig, and the C-terminal octapeptide,

CCK-8, from one other—the sheep, there is no reason to believe that CCK does not occur in all mammalian species and beyond.

Nilsson (299) found that intestinal extracts of the holocephalian fish *Chimaera monstrosa* exhibit CCK-like activity on the guinea pig gallbladder *in situ.* This activity, like that of porcine CCK, is destroyed by trypsin but not by chymotrypsin. Barrington and Dockray (23) showed that intestinal extracts of lamprey (*Lampetra fluviatilis* and *Petromyzon marinus*) stimulate pancreatic enzyme secretion in a CCK-like fashion in rats, that extracts of eel intestine (24) stimulate contraction of the rabbit gallbladder *in vitro,* and rat pancreatic secretion *in vivo.* Likewise, it has been shown that the salmon gallbladder responds to CCK, although it cannot distinguish it from gastrin (384).

The cells that synthesize or store CCK in the intestinal mucosa have been found (53,317) to resemble the I cells of the modified Wiesbaden classification (361). It has also been found, in several mammalian species, that these cells are most numerous in the duodenum and proximal jejunum, but absent from the distal ileum (53). This is in accordance with what has been shown for the pancreozyminic activity in small intestinal extracts (164).

However, CCK, or at any rate material with CCK-like immunoreactivity, is not confined to these intestinal cells. Cerebral CCK (92,330,368) has been found in high concentration in the synaptosomal pellet obtained on differential centrifugation of homogenates of rat cerebral cortical tissue (315). Grube et al. (160) found material showing CCK-like immunoreactivity in extracts of human and rat pancreatic tissue, and in the glucagon-containing A cells of the islets. Larsson and Rehfeld (239,240), using region-specific antisera against gastrin and CCK, found that the intestinal mucosa contained three distinct types of cells that reacted with an antiserum against the C-terminal tetrapeptide of gastrin and of CCK. The material in one of these cell types reacted in addition with a specific anti-CCK serum, directed toward the non-C-terminal part of the CCK sequence, but did not react with the corresponding antigastrin serum. This cell type was considered to be the CCK cell. Of the remaining two cell types, one reacted with the specific serum against gastrin but not with that against CCK. This cell was considered to be a gastrin cell. The third type, finally, did not react with either of the specific antisera. It was therefore considered to contain either the C-terminal tetrapeptide as such or this peptide, lengthened N-terminally by a sequence different from both that of gastrin and of CCK. This would mean that this cell contained a yet unknown member of the gastrin-CCK group of peptides.

PHYSIOLOGICAL AND PHARMACOLOGICAL ACTIONS OF CCK

Originally discovered because of its ability to cause gallbladder contraction (200), CCK was soon found to have several other actions also. First it was found to induce contractions of the guinea pig ileum (219); then an indication was obtained that it might inhibit the spincter of Oddi, while increasing the tone and motility of the duodenum (345).

It was observed that partially purified preparations of pancreozymin stimulated gallbladder contraction (98,394). This could have been due to contamination of the pancreozymin preparations by CCK and it was rather unexpected when it was found that the pancreozyminic activity was an inherent property of CCK (217).

Since then a long and growing number of activities have been described for CCK but there is reason to believe that many of these are pharmacological rather than physiological. Grossman considers that only *stimulation of gallbladder contraction, stimulation of pancreatic enzyme secretion, augmentation of the effect of secretin on pancreatic bicarbonate secretion,* and *inhibition of gastric emptying* have definitely been shown to be physiological actions of CCK, but that there is reasonably good evidence that its *trophic effect on the pancreas* might also be physiological (159). Pharmacological effects may of course be of practical usefulness, and, like physiological effects, may reveal various biological mechanisms.

Effects on the Sphincter of Oddi

There is some uncertainty concerning the effect of CCK on the sphincter of Oddi. Toouli et al. (375) pointed out that in experiments in which the tonicity of the sphincter is measured by the resistance it offers to the flow of water through the common duct into the duodenum, an increased flow rate may be obtained not only by relaxation of the sphincter but also by rhythmic contraction and relaxation of its musculature. They reported on experiments *in vitro* in which both the canine and human common bile duct muscles contracted in response to CCK. Sarles et al. (346) made similar observations in rabbits. Other workers have described experiments suggesting a direct relaxing effect of CCK on the sphincter in cats (309), and also in rabbits and dogs (293). From a recent review (363) it may be seen that the inverse functional relationship between the motility changes of the gallbladder and that of the sphincter of Oddi is a long standing and complicated problem.

Effects on the Discharge and Synthesis of Pancreatic Enzymes

Another unsolved question is whether CCK stimulates only the discharge of enzymes and zymogens from the pancreas or whether it also stimulates their *de novo* synthesis. Investigating the synthesis of amylase in slices of pigeon pancreas, Hokin and Hokin (185) concluded that only discharge was stimulated by CCK and similar results have quite recently been obtained using mouse pancreatic slices (56). Dickman et al. found (84) that stimulation of enzyme discharge with pilocarpine did not influence the rate of incorporation into proteins of radioactive amino acids by bovine pancreatic slices. Others have, however, obtained evidence that enzyme synthesis is also stimulated by CCK. Rothman and Wells found that in rats the synthesis of amylase, chymotrypsinogen, and trypsinogen was stimulated by CCK in a nonparallel fashion (341). Reggio et al. reported that the synthesis of protein by the rat pancreas was increased by treating the animals with CCK (327) and Leroy et al. (242) found that in rats the synthesis of pancreatic amylase increased in response to intraperitoneally administered CCK in a dose-related manner in the dose range 1 to 4 IDU (Ivy dog units) per kg body weight.

These divergent findings are suggestive of a difference in the effect of CCK *in vitro* and *in vivo* (278). However, Rosenfeld et al. (338) described stimulation by CCK of amylase synthesis in porcine pancreatic minces, although, as they pointed out, the degree of purity of the CCK preparation they used was not very high. It cannot therefore be excluded that the observed effect could have been due to some factor other than CCK. Mongeau et al. showed that administration of CCK to rats causes a transient decrease in protein synthesis but that this is soon followed by an increase over basal values (272). Rothman and Wells found in rats that not only did the pancreatic content of amylase, chymotrypsinogen, and trypsinogen increase following treatment with CCK, but also that the total weight of the pancreatic glands increased. They attributed this to hypertrophy of the pancreatic cells (341).

Trophic Effects on the Exocrine Pancreas

Intense work on the trophic effects of gastrointestinal hormones has followed on the findings by Crean et al. that treatment of rats with pentagastrin results in hyperplasia of the gastric fundic cells (71) and of Johnson et al. that pentagastrin in rats stimulates protein synthesis in gastric and duodenal (but not in liver or muscle) tissue (209). Mainz et al. found that in rats treatment with CCK resulted in both hypertrophy and hyperplasia of pancreatic cells (258).

Barrowman and Mayston (25) observed in rats an increase in the pancreatic content of both DNA and RNA during treatment with CCK, and that the content of amylase and proteolytic enzymes also increased, but not the content of lipase. Johnson and Guthrie (212) found that in rats DNA synthesis was stimulated by CCK-8 in fundic mucosa, duodenal mucosa, and pancreatic tissue. Only the effect on the pancreas was elicited with hormone concentrations within the probable physiological range. A recent review discusses the trophic actions of CCK and other gastrointestinal hormones (208). More recently Fölsch et al. (118) investigated the effects of repeated administration of secretin and CCK to rats. In accordance with the earlier findings of Barrowman and Mayston (25), they found that the pancreatic contents of amylase and trypsinogen increased during the period of treatment with the hormone, whereas the content of lipase did not change. This pattern was also seen in the pancreatic juice. Secretin in the doses used was not found to result in changes in pancreatic weight. Ihse et al., on the other hand, found that long-term treatment with either CCK or CCK-8 resulted in a parallel increase of the pancreatic content of amylase, lipase, and trypsinogen (195). Petersen et al. (310) investigated the effects of chronic administration of CCK, secretin, and pentagastrin on not only the weight, but also the functional properties of the rat pancreas. It was found that all three substances increased pancreatic weight, but that this increase was small after secretin and pentagastrin and quite substantial after CCK. The increase in weight was accompanied by parallel increases in the maximal pancreatic output of protein and bicarbonate in response to CCK. The output of bicarbonate in response to secretin did not change after CCK treatment but there was some increase in fluid output. Pentagastrin did not cause noticeable changes in secretory responses to either secretin or CCK. Secretin treatment influenced neither the pancreatic secretory responses to CCK nor the maximal responses to secretin itself. However, the secretin-treated animals had become less sensitive to secretin, larger doses of it being necessary to obtain a given secretory response. The conclusion of the authors was that in the rat changes produced by CCK were consistent with it having a selective trophic effect on the acinar cells. Treatment of rats with a combination of secretin and CCK (the CCK analog cerulein was used) had a strikingly different effect than treatment with either CCK or secretin alone. In addition to the trophic effect of CCK on the acinar cells, a trophic effect on the ductular cells was now clearly distinguishable, the maximal bicarbonate output in response to secretin being almost doubled (311). CCK does not seem to be a trophic hormone for the endocrine pancreas (118,195).

Stimulatory Effects on Bicarbonate and Water Secretion and Insulin Secretion by the Pancreas

It had long been assumed that CCK stimulated pancreatic enzyme secretion exclusively and that all stimulation of secretion of water and bicarbonate was due to secretin. Heatley, however, observed that in rats a highly purified preparation of CCK stimulated the secretion not only of enzymes but also of fluid. Since then it has been found that CCK, as such, in several species has a certain stimulatory effect on the secretion of bicarbonate and water. This was most clearly demonstrated for dogs by Debas and Grossman, using CCK-33, CCK-39, and cerulein.

The finding that CCK stimulated insulin secretion in dogs (266,379) man (314), and from isolated rat pancreatic islets (182), as well as the secretion of glucagon from the latter preparation, and in dogs (379) caused great interest. The observations were important although later work showed that the effects were due mainly to the presence of GIP in the CCK preparations used. Nevertheless it has been shown that CCK itself does raise, although weakly, the plasma concentrations of both insulin and glucagon in dogs (122). Indeed it has also been found that the C-terminal tetrapeptide amide common to CCK, gastrin, and cerulein stimulates insulin secretion in dogs (221) and in man (328). A recent report claims that in the perfused rat pancreas pretreatment with cerulein increases the insulin response to a subsequent dose of glucose (305). Insulin and glucagon (or more strictly substances showing insulin- and glucagon-like immunoreactivities) are not the only hormones released by CCK; release of calcitonin in pigs (55,69) and of somatostatin in dogs (196) have been described. It may be mentioned that one group of workers have described a hypocalcemic action of CCK in rats (369).

The secretion of all the enzymes present in pancreatic juice is not stimulated by CCK. Nakajima et al. found that secretion of γ-glutamyl transpeptidase present in pancreatic juice is not stimulated (292). On the other hand, the secretion of several enzymes of intestinal origin seems to be stimulated by CCK (294). Intestinal alkaline phosphatase secretion was found to be stimulated both in man (102,390,391) and dogs (101), as was secretion of intestinal disacchari-dases (100). Götze et al. described the release in rats of enterokinase in response to administration of CCK and pointed out the probable physiological importance of this release in parallel with the release of trypsinogen from the pancreas (151). Release of enterokinase in man after the administration of either CCK or secretin has also been described (280). Eddeland and Wehlin have observed a parallel stimulation by CCK in man of the secretion of trypsinogen and pan-creatic trypsin inhibitor (103). Wahlin et al. (387) found that CCK stimulated glycoprotein secretion from the mouse gallbladder epithelium.

Inhibition of Gastric Emptying and Effects on the Sphincters

Debas et al. (79) found that in dogs administration of CCK in doses resulting in plasma CCK concentrations within the physiological range inhibited the emp-tying of 0.15 M solutions of NaCl instilled into the stomach. This is consistent with the earlier findings of Chey et al. (63) that in man secretin and CCK inhibited gastric emptying. Yamagishi and Debas (405) found that this inhibition was due to both relaxation of the proximal part of the stomach (207,382) and stimulation of the pyloric sphincter (47,116,197). In this area of investigation, species differences and differences due to experimental designs seem to be pro-nounced. Behar et al. (32) found that in the cat CCK usually causes relaxation of the pyloric sphincter, whereas the opossum sphincter *in vitro* usually contracts in response to CCK (18,115). The lower esophageal sphincter was found to be inhibited by CCK *in vitro* in 46 cats of 50 tested (31). Stimulation of gastric antral muscle in the dog by CCK was described by Morgan et al. (275). In the isolated guinea pig, stomach motor activity was stimulated both in the antrum and in the fundus, although differently. In the antrum the amplitude and frequency of rhythmic contractions were stimulated, whereas in the fundus the basal tension was elevated (136,138).

Increase of Intestinal Blood Flow

An intestinal lymphagogue action of CCK in the rat has been described by Turner and Barrowman (377), who consider it to be due to the increased intestinal blood flow, which had been demonstrated by several authors on stimulation with CCK. A wider discussion of the effects of CCK on blood flow in the splanchnic area may be found in a recent article by Thulin and Samnegård (374).

Stimulation of Hepatic Bile Secretion

CCK has been shown to stimulate the secretion of hepatic bile in several species: dogs (104,127,215,323,358), rabbits (229,283), guinea pigs (117), monkeys (131), and rats (74). The type of response, in the dog, i.e., stimulation of bicarbonate secretion (215), and no effect on erythritol clearance (358) that occurs indicates that, at any rate, the choleretic action of CCK, like that of secretin, is exerted, at least predominantly, on the ductule cells.

Since both CCK and secretin stimulate hepatic biliary secretion, and gastrin also has some such effect (215), the questions arise as to which other peptides may do so, whether or not there exists an unidentified hepatocrinin (125) with such stimulation as its main function, and whether there are intestinal peptides acting on hepatocytes in addition to, or instead of, on the ductular cells. Fritz and Brooks (127) and Jones (214) demonstrated stimulation of canalicular bile secretion in dogs by insulin but this effect seemed to be mediated by the vagi (214). In the monkey a difference in the effects of secretin and CCK on the composition of the bile secreted has been described (131): the CCK increased the secretion of cholesterol but secretin left it unaffected.

Effects on the Intestinal Transit Time

In clinical investigations it was found that the intestinal transit time of a barium sulfate contrast meal was greatly shortened by the administration of CCK (20,273,276,307). Dahlgren found in dogs that duodenal motor activity was stimulated by CCK (73) and Hedner et al. (174) found the same for the upper small intestine of guinea pigs and cats. Using an intraluminal pressure recording technique, Gutiérrez et al. (162) found that the basal motor activity of both the duodenum and the jejunum was stimulated by CCK, and that this could be counteracted by secretin. Dinoso et al. (88) observed that in man the motor activity of the sigmoid colon was also stimulated by CCK, but the activity of the rectum was not influenced, whereas Waller et al. (388) found that the motor activity of the pelvic colon was not influenced by CCK.

Effects on Gastric Secretion

Many investigators have dealt with the actions of CCK on gastric secretion, but because of the limited availability of the (essentially) pure CCK much of this work had been carried out with preparations containing various amounts of other peptides, including GIP (51). Surprisingly, this does not seem to have led to any serious mistakes, since the observations, as a rule, have been confirmed by the later use of synthetic CCK-8 or the CCK analogue cerulein. An exception to this statement is the finding by Magee and Dutt (256) that (essentially) pure CCK-33 augmented metacholine stimulated pepsin secretion from innervated dog gastric mucosa whereas "10 per cent pure" CCK did not do so. Nakajima and Magee (291) had earlier found that in Heidenhain pouch dogs the partially purified CCK-preparation strongly inhibited pepsin(ogen) secretion, whether stimulated by mecholyl or by secretin. They further found (256) that whereas both the essentially pure and the "10% pure" CCK inhibited pentagastrin stimulated acid secretion both from innervated and denervated dog gastric mucosa, metacholyl stimulated acid secretion from both types of mucosa was not inhibited but rather augmented under these conditions.

The picture appears complex but most of it can be explained by the similarity in structure of CCK and gastrin. Preshaw and Grossman (318) noted that in dogs with chronic gastric and pancreatic fistulas the administration of small doses of CCK preparation sometimes stimulated the secretion of gastric acid, whereas Murat and White (282) and Magee and Nakamura (257) found in dogs with Heidenhain pouches that these doses inhibited gastric acid secretion. In man, low doses of CCK were also found to stimulate acid secretion (61,402), whereas in the rat (64) and the cat (392) stimulation was noted over a wide range of CCK doses. Stimulation by CCK was also seen in the isolated mucosa of the bullfrog (77) and the mud puppy *Necturus maculosus* by one (35), but not by another group of investigators (290). In dogs with Heidenhain pouches, Jordan and Peterson noted the secretion of gastric acid in response to feeding was inhibited by CCK. The same was noted by Gillespie and Grossman (143) in response to hog gastrin and to small doses of histamine and by Bedi et al. (30) in response to pentagastrin and gastrin, whereas the secretion from the gastric remnant was stimulated rather than inhibited. Pentagastrin-stimulated acid secretion was also inhibited by CCK in man (48,63), whereas in the rat this inhibition was not very impressive (376), and in the cat it did not occur at all (392). Johnson and Grossman (211) found, however, that inhibition of pentagastrin stimulated secretion of gastric acid in dogs with Heidenhain pouches occurred with pure CCK (CCK-33) and that the kinetics of the inhibition were of the competitive type. This fits with the structures of CCK and gastrin, as does the finding that secretin inhibits gastrin-stimulated secretion and noncompetitively (210). This is in conflict with a puzzling finding of Berstad and Petersen (37), that in man secretin also inhibits pentagastrin-stimulated acid secretion in an apparently competitive fashion.

Effects on Food Intake

The finding by Gibbs et al. (142) that on intraperitoneal administration to rats a partially purified preparation of CCK, as well as CCK-8, suppressed, in a dose-related fashion, the food intake of the animals has been followed by a large number of investigations on the effects of CCK on food intake. Investigations both supporting (17,234,255,297) and refuting (83,144) the possibility that CCK acts as a satiety signal in rats have been published. Two groups of investigators did not find any effect of CCK on satiety in man (145,153).

Malagelada et al. (260) have made the interesting observation that the pancreas in man, under physiological condition, may be more sensitive to CCK than is the gallbladder.

MECHANISM OF ACTION OF CCK

Structural Aspects

It is not yet known how CCK exerts any of its many actions. However, although there is mostly unanimous information as to which parts of its structure are essential for activity, there is a very large amount of often contradictory information on the manner in which various cellular mechanisms are activated by CCK.

The investigations concerning the structural requirements for CCK activity were greatly simplified by the finding that, in a manner analogous to gastrin (155), a C-terminal fragment of the hormone exhibited the cholecystokinetic and pancreozyminic activities of the whole molecule. There is no evidence at present that the N-terminal part of CCK has any activity of its own, except possibly by modifying the actions of the C-terminal part (380). Of course the absence of information does not exclude the possibility that some as yet undiscovered activity may be related to it.

The C-terminal part of the CCK molecule shows a striking degree of sequence homology with the corresponding part of gastrin (155) and with cerulein (10):[3]

C-terminal octapeptide of porcine CCK	D Ẏ M G W M D F ■
C-terminal octapeptide of porcine gastrin II (sulfated)	E A Ẏ G W M D F ■
Cerulein	E Q D Ẏ T G W M D F ■

STRUCTURAL REQUIREMENTS FOR CHOLECYSTOKINETIC ACTIVITY

Comparisons of the biological activities of these three peptides and their various analogs, fragments, and derivatives have yielded important information on the structures necessary for CCK activity. For cholecystokinetic activity it has been shown that sulfation of the phenolic group of the tyrosine residue is important, although not absolutely essential. There are some differences among the

---

[3] Symbols as on p. 172. The N-terminal amino acid residue of cerulein shown as glutamyl is actually pyroglutamyl.

findings from different laboratories concerning the activity ratios of the sulfated peptides to their nonsulfated analogs. In part this may be due to species variations in gallbladder responsiveness. Ondetti et al. (304) found that CCK-8 was some 150 times more potent than its unsulfated analog, if assayed on the guinea pig gallbladder *in vivo* or *in vitro,* and Johnson et al. (213) found the same effects of these peptides on the gallbladder of conscious cats. Using isolated cat gallbladder, however, Chowdhury et al. (65) found the sulfated peptide to be almost a thousand times more active than the unsulfated. This led Fara and Erde (112) to compare the effects of cerulein and nonsulfated cerulein on the guinea pig gallbladder. They found that the differences in activity between these peptides were more pronounced *in vitro* than *in vivo,* indicating the possibility that the sulfation of the nonsulfated and/or desulfation of the sulfated peptide might be taking place *in vivo.* Apart from sulfation, the position in the peptide chain of the tyrosine-*O*-sulfated residue is also important. Whereas CCK, cerulein, and gastrin II all have identical C-terminal pentapeptide sequences and all contain a residue of tyrosine-*O*-sulfate, in the two strongly cholecystokinetic peptides, CCK and cerulein, this sulfated residue is displaced from the pentapeptide by an intervening amino acid residue—methionine in CCK and threonine in cerulein—but in the weakly cholecystokinetic gastrin it is linked directly to the pentapeptide. The importance of this configuration for cholecystokinetic activity has been substantiated by synthetic work. When the tyrosine-*O*-sulfate residue in CCK-8 was translocated with either of its neighboring amino acid residues, a drastic loss in cholecystokinetic activity resulted (304). In a teleost fish, the salmon, however, the gallbladder does not seem to distinguish between the CCK-cerulein types and the gastrin types of peptides (384), both being equally potent stimulators of gallbladder contraction. Yet the sulfated peptides are here also more potent than the unsulfated ones. The sulfation seems to be less important, however, for activity in peptides with the gastrin type of structural relationship between the C-terminal pentapeptide and the tyrosine residue. Vagne and Grossman (380) found that in conscious dogs the sulfated and nonsulfated porcine heptadecapeptide gastrins had the same potency for stimulation of gallbladder contraction. However, when tested on the guinea pig gallbladder *in vivo* and *in vitro* (4), the sulfated gastrin was at least ten times stronger than the nonsulfated, and the same was true for the cat gallbladder *in vitro* (65).

Comparison of Sulfated and Nonsulfated CCKs with Regard to Gastric Acid Secretion

Kaminski et al. (220) showed that both CCK-7 and CCK-8 stimulated the secretion of hepatic bile in dogs, but that their nonsulfated analogs were inactive. Yet, both sulfated and nonsulfated CCKs were approximately equipotent with respect to stimulation of gastric acid secretion. Johnson et al. (213), on the other hand, found that sulfated cerulein was about six times stronger than nonsulfated in this respect. Gregory and Tracy (156) did not note any differences, among the gastrin type of peptides, between the sulfated and nonsulfated gastrin heptadecapeptides in their potency for stimulation of gastric acid secretion in dogs. Also, Stening and Grossman (366) found them to be equipotent in this respect. However, the sulfated gastrin was found to be ten times as potent as the nonsulfated in stimulating acid secretion of the isolated bullfrog mucosa (393). And Brooks et al. (49) found that desulfated cerulein, in contrast with cerulein, did not inhibit pentagastrin-stimulated acid secretion in either denervated or innervated gastric pouches in conscious dogs.

Effects on Muscular Contraction

Vizi et al. (386) found that both gastrin- and CCK-like peptides elicited reciprocal responses of the two muscle layers of the guinea pig ileum *in vitro*. The contraction of the longitudinal muscle was always accompanied by relaxation of the circular muscle, and *vice versa*. The sulfated forms of both types of peptides were more potent in these effects than the nonsulfated ones.

STRUCTURAL REQUIREMENTS FOR THE PANCREOZYMINIC ACTIVITY OF CCK

The structural requirements for the pancreozymic activity of CCK appear to be essentially the same as for the cholecystokinetic one. In dogs the difference in potency of sulfated and nonsulfated peptides appears, however, to be considerably less marked for the sulfated one (213,366). In the rat Dockray (89) carried out a careful comparative study of the effects on pancreatic secretion of fluid and protein of pentagastrin, porcine sulfated and nonsulfated heptadecapeptide gastrins, their C-terminal hexapeptides, the C-terminal dodeca and octapeptides of CCK (CCK-12 and CCK-8), and the unsulfated analog of CCK-8. The peptides showed the same calculated maximal responses in stimulating both fluid and protein secretion. They varied greatly in potency, however. In all cases the sulfated peptides were stronger stimulants than the corresponding nonsulfated ones. Also, those peptides in which the sulfated tyrosine residue was displaced from the C-terminal pentapeptide by an intervening methionine residue were stronger than those in which the sulfated tyrosine was attached directly to the pentapeptide. Interestingly, there were differences in the relative potencies of the peptides in respect to the two actions studied. Thus, CCK-8 was about 4,000 times stronger than pentagastrin as a stimulant of fluid secretion from the pancreas, but "only" 2,500 times stronger as a stimulant of protein secretion.

In view of the importance of the tyrosine-O-sulfated residue for CCK activity, Bodanszky and co-workers investigated whether it is essential that the sulfate residue be attached explicitly to tyrosine. They found that replacing tyrosine-O-sulfate by serine-O-sulfate (43) almost, but not quite, abolished activity, indicative of the importance of tyrosine. Later work, however, showed that if the tyrosine-O-sulfate was replaced by ε-hydroxynorleucine-O-sulfate, then the heptapeptide had quite substantial CCK activity. This suggests that the correct distance between the sulfuric acid group and the peptide chain might be the essential requirement for CCK activity (42).

Next to nothing is known about the tertiary structure of CCK. Investigations, with the aid of fluorescence spectroscopy, of the tyrosine-tryptophan distance in the desulfated analog of CCK-7 have indicated the existence of some kind of folded conformation in this heptapeptide (351).

Effects on Opiate Receptors

In view of some similarity of the amino acid sequence of the N-terminal pentapeptide, Y̊ M G W M, of CCK-7 with that of methionine enkephalin, Y G G F M (191), Schiller et al. (350) investigated the effect of CCK-7 on the opiate receptors in rat brain and guinea pig ileum. CCK-7 itself was found to have no measurable activity in this regard, but its unsulfated analog was clearly active, although its potency was only about 0.5% of that of (Met[5]) enkephalin.

MEDIATORS OF CCK EFFECTS

Motor Effects

In 1933 Jung and Greengard (219) found that the action of CCK on the isolated guinea pig gallbladder was not inhibited by atropine, and this has been confirmed by later work. They also mentioned, however, that the ileum behaved like the gallbladder, but this has not been confirmed. Naito et al. (289) found that atropinization prevented the stimulating effect of a CCK preparation on the motor activity of the upper intestine of rabbits, dogs, and guinea pigs. Hedner et al. (174), using essentially pure CCK, confirmed this for the guinea pig ileum *in vitro,* and found it to be true also of the peristaltic movements of the cat duodenum *in vivo.* Bennet (33) described experiments suggesting that in stimulating contractions of the guinea pig ileum gastrin acted via the release of acetylcholine from postganglionic parasympathetic nerves, and Vizi et al. (385) and Del Tacca et al. (371) found the same for the action of the CCK-like peptides. The latter authors, however, suggested that some other mediator(s) in addition to acetylcholine might also be involved. Hedner and Rorsman (175) concluded that the stimulating effect of CCK on both muscle layers of the guinea pig ileum is mediated via a cholinergic neural pathway without cholinergic synapses. Vizi et al. (386), however, found that the effect of CCK on the circular layer involved transmission over at least one ganglion. Yau et al. (406), although conceding that release of acetylcholine was involved in the action of CCK on intestinal muscle, found that much lower concentrations of atropine were necessary to block the actions of exogenous acetylcholine than of exogenous CCK, and pointed to the possibility that CCK also might have a direct action on the muscle potentiated by the simultaneously released acetylcholine. Frigo et al. (126) found that administration of both CCK and cerulein stimulated the peristaltic reflex of the guinea pig small and large intestines *in vitro* but at concentrations lower than those that caused contraction of the intestinal muscles. Inhibition of the reflex by acetylcholine was partially counteracted by CCK in the ileum, but not in the colon. Gerner and Haffner (137) found that in the isolated guinea pig stomach CCK stimulated rhythmic antral activity and raised fundal basal pressure. The antral motor effects were significantly blocked by atropine but the fundal were unaffected, suggesting that the former were mediated through local cholinergic pathways and the latter were independent of such. More recently, Gerner et al. (138) found that the stimulating effects of both histamine and CCK on the fundic muscle were not inhibited by the histamine H_2 receptor inhibitor cimetidine, but were inhibited by the H_1 receptor inhibitor mepyramine, suggesting the possibility that CCK in this area acted via H_1 receptors. Fara et al. (113) have, however, found that the effect of CCK on the dog antral muscle is only weakly and partially inhibited by atropine and suggested that CCK in that area acted on a noncholinergic receptor. Morgan et al. (275) have come to a similar conclusion. Amer (5) found that the action of CCK on rabbit gallbladder strips was not prevented by either cholinergic or α- or β-adrenergic blockade, indicating that CCK was acting independently of the autonomic nervous system. The gallbladder strips were relaxed by exogenous 3',5'-cyclic adenosine monophosphate (cyclic AMP). Gallbladder contraction stimulated by either acetylcholine or α-adrenergic receptor agonists was followed by a fall in tissue cyclic AMP concentrations, whereas the action of CCK did not result in statistically significant decreases in cyclic AMP concentrations, although insignificant decreases could be observed. Amer suggested that CCK either acted independently of cyclic AMP or lowered a small tissue pool of it, presumably by locally activating the cyclic AMP-hydrolyzing phosphodiesterase. A paradoxical result was obtained with imidazole, the administration of which led to gallbladder contraction but, contrary to what might have been expected, tissue cyclic AMP concentrations rose. Subsequently, Amer and McKinney described experiments in which CCK did in fact activate phosphodiesterase in several rabbit tissues, including gallbladder (8). These tissues also contained a phosphodiesterase that hydrolyzed 3',5'-cyclic guanosine monophosphate (cyclic GMP), and this phosphodiesterase was inhibited by CCK. By direct measurement of tissue cyclic AMP concentrations and phosphodiesterase activity, Andersson et al. (11) confirmed that in the isolated guinea pig gallbladder CCK led to decreased tissue cyclic AMP concentrations. In the isolated cat sphincter of Oddi, on the other hand, CCK increased tissue cyclic AMP concentrations. This was not due to inhibition of phosphodiesterase, the activity of which was increased on the contrary as in the gallbladder, but presumably to an activation also of adenylate cyclase, the action of which then prevailed over that of the diesterase (12). The authors considered this increase in cyclic AMP concentration to be involved in the mechanism of sphincter relaxation. In strips of guinea pig gallbladder *in vitro,* Andersson et al. (16)

found that lanthanum, possibly by displacing a fraction of membrane-bound Ca^{2+} or by preventing the flow of Ca^{2+} ions across the plasma membrane, inhibited the contractile effects of both CCK and acetylcholine. Later, Amer found (6) that CCK and acetylcholine increased the guanyl cyclase activity of rabbit gallbladder muscle *in vitro* and raised the tissue concentrations of cyclic GMP. This increase preceded gallbladder contraction, which was consistent with a possible "second messenger" role for cyclic GMP in gallbladder contraction. Andersson et al. (14) confirmed that CCK induced both a fall in the guinea pig gallbladder tissue concentration of cyclic AMP and an increase in cyclic GMP. However, although neither the contraction of the gallbladder nor the fall in its cyclic AMP concentration was influenced by indomethacin, the rise in cyclic GMP was completely abolished by it. These findings seem to make it highly improbable that the CCK-induced rise in cyclic GMP is in any way involved in the mechanism by which the gallbladder contracts, with the "phospholipid effect." Hokin and Hokin (185) discovered that addition of either cholinergic agents or CCK to slices of pigeon gallbladder *in vitro* stimulated not only the secretion of amylase by the slices but also the incorporation of inorganic phosphate into certain phospholipids of the tissue. At first it seemed highly probable that a causal relationship existed between phospholipid synthesis and enzyme secretion, but the later work by Hokin (184) and others (26) has made this improbable, at least at low rates of enzyme secretion. It has been suggested that the phospholipid effect is instead due to increased hormone-stimulated synthesis of phospholipids during the formation of new intracellular membranes (184). Andersson et al. (13) observed that certain prostaglandins, particularly E_2, exhibited several CCK-like actions. Further investigations, however, have made it unlikely that prostaglandins mediate the effects of CCK (15).

Pancreozyminic Effects

Regarding the pancreozyminic action of CCK, Harper and Raper showed that in cats this was not inhibited by atropine or by section of the vagus or the splanchnic nerves (165). Davies et al. (76) found that the respiration of cat pancreatic fragments *in vitro* was stimulated by CCK, and Dickman and Morril (85) showed the same to be true for the mouse pancreas. Danielsson and Sehlin (75) found that in fragments of exocrine mouse pancreas *in vitro*, CCK increased the oxidation of D-glucose, L-alanine, and L-leucine. Insulin increased the oxidation of D-glucose but not that of the amino acids.

For more than a decade numerous investigations have been concerned with the problem of whether, how, and to what extent cyclic nucleotides and/or calcium are involved in the pancreozyminic actions of CCK. Much information has been obtained, but the picture is still far from clear. In 1968 Kulka and Sternlicht (235) found that cyclic AMP, its mono- and dibutyryl derivatives, and theophylline (an inhibitor of the phosphodiesterase hydrolyzing cyclic AMP to 5'-adenosine monophosphate) stimulated the secretion of amylase from mouse pancreas *in vitro,* whereas 3'-adenosine monophosphate inhibited amylase secretion, whether stimulated by cyclic AMP or by CCK. Ridderstap and Bonting (333) demonstrated that protein secretion of the isolated rabbit pancreas was stimulated by theophylline and by exogenous cyclic AMP.

Theophylline also potentiated pancreozymin-induced secretion. Stimulation of pancreatic enzyme secretion by theophylline from the rabbit pancreas *in vitro* was described by Knodell et al. (230). This seemed to suggest that cyclic AMP might be acting as a "second messenger" in mediating the pancreozyminic effect of CCK (370). Very soon, however, other findings were described that made such a role for cyclic AMP seem doubtful. Case and Scratcherd (60), working with the isolated perfused cat pancreas found that dibutyryl cyclic AMP stimulated the secretion of water and bicarbonate, but not of enzymes. Theophylline in low doses had an effect similar to that of cyclic AMP, although in high doses it would slightly stimulate enzyme secretion. These findings suggested that the effect on the pancreas of secretin but hardly that of CCK, might be mediated by cyclicAMP (60). It may be mentioned that already in 1966 Vaille et al. (381) had found caffeine to have a secretin-like effect on rat pancreatic secretion. Subsequently, Case et al. (59) found that in anesthetized cats and in the perfused isolated cat pancreas administration of secretin or CCK would result in a short, transient rise in pancreatic tissue cyclic AMP concentration, which, after returning to control values, would be followed by a second, slow and prolonged cyclic AMP rise, apparently unrelated in time to enzyme secretion. These findings were interpreted as suggesting that although cyclic AMP might be involved in the response of the pancreas to CCK, secretin, and acetylcholine, no simple relationship existed between cyclic AMP concentration and pancreatic secretion. Benz et al. (34) found that cyclic AMP or its dibutyryl derivative did not stimulate amylase release from pieces of guinea pig pancreas *in vitro,* and that CCK did not increase pancreatic cyclic AMP concentration. Bauduin et al. (27) observed that exogenous cyclic AMP did stimulate, very weakly, the secretion of enzymes from pieces of rat pancreas *in vitro,* and that there were several metabolic differences in the pancreatic tissue stimulation by cyclic AMP, CCK, or cholinergic agents. The authors considered it doubtful whether cyclic AMP functioned as an important mediator of the physiological stimulants on the enzyme secretion.

During the following years an equal number of papers were published suggesting that cyclic AMP had a "second messenger" role in pancreatic enzyme secretion as those suggesting that it did not. Pederson et al. (308) showed that in cats theophylline enhanced the stimulating effect of CCK on pancreatic protein secretion, and Guelrud et al. (161) demonstrated that in dogs theophylline had a pancreozyminic effect, presumably by increasing endogenous cyclic AMP concentration. Bhoola and Lemon (38), however, found that in the cat pancreas secretin stimulated adenylate cyclase activity but that CCK did not. Marois et al. (261) showed that both secretin and CCK stimulated adenylate cyclase in homogenates of rat pancreatic tissue. Rutten et al. (344) made the same observation but found that a hundred times higher concentration of CCK than that of secretin was necessary to obtain a similar degree of activation and Kempen et al. (228) described experiments suggesting that this might in part be artifactual because of a greater lability of CCK than of secretin receptors. Morisset and Webster (278) found that dibutyryl cyclic AMP stimulated the secretion of protein by the rat pancreas in vivo, but the stimulation was weak compared with that by pancreozymin and was not followed by a new protein synthesis as is seen on stimulation by hormones. Haig (163) found that exogenous cyclic AMP did not stimulate amylase release from rat pancreas slices and Heisler et al. (179) found that CCK had a biphasic effect on the cyclic AMP concentrations of rat pancreas fragments in vitro, an increase being followed by decrease. Deschodt-Lanckman et al. (81) demonstrated that secretin and VIP increased the cyclic AMP content of rat pancreatic fragments in vitro, and that these increases could be prevented by CCK.

Following the demonstration of the presence of different protein kinases in the rat pancreas dependent on cyclic AMP and cyclic GMP, respectively (241), and of phosphodiesterases capable of hydrolyzing cyclic AMP and cyclic GMP (335), Robberecht et al. (336) on further investigation found that in rats administration of CCK resulted in rapid rises in pancreatic cyclic GMP concentrations, whereas cyclic AMP concentrations were not affected. The latter did, however, rise following administration of secretin or of VIP. The increased cyclic GMP concentrations following CCK returned to basal values before the stimulated secretion of amylase did so. Since then many investigators have confirmed that CCK is capable of raising cyclic GMP levels in pancreatic tissue. Haymovits and Scheele (172) found that in guinea pig and rabbit pancreatic lobules in vitro, CCK led to increases in cyclic GMP concentrations, whereas cyclic AMP concentrations were not changed. The increases in cyclic GMP concentrations were swift, whereupon the high levels initially reached fell but remained distinctly elevated throughout the period of hormonal stimulation. The authors considered it probable that cyclic GMP was an intracellular mediator of the action of CCK on the pancreatic acinar cell. It has been repeatedly confirmed that cyclic GMP concentrations increase on stimulation of the pancreas with CCK. However, the work on cyclic nucleotides has often included investigations of the effects of CCK on intracellular calcium.

Role of Calcium

Interest in the importance of calcium for pancreatic secretion has been at least as great as the interest in the cyclic nucleotides. Birmingham et al. (39) showed that ACTH-stimulated steroid secretion from rat adrenal glands incubated in vitro was dependent on the presence of Ca^{2+} in the medium. Douglas and Rubin, working with isolated perfused cat adrenal glands, found that the acetylcholine-stimulated release of catecholamines from the medullae was in some way dependent on Ca^{2+}, i.e., that calcium was involved in "stimulus secretion coupling" (93). Hokin (183) found that omission of Ca^{2+} from the incubation medium prevented acetylcholine from stimulating amylase release from pigeon pancreas slices. It was shown in dogs (409) and in man (148) that CCK-stimulated enzyme secretion resulted in increased secretion of Ca^{2+} by the pancreas.

Robberecht and Christophe (334) found that the basal secretion of lipase and amylase from perfused rat pancreatic fragments was slowly but reversibly depressed by omitting calcium from the perfusing fluid. The secretory response to CCK was also depressed but not completely inhibited, by using a calcium-free medium. However, Kanno (222), also working with the perfused rat pancreas *in vitro,* found essentially complete inhibition of CCK- or acetylcholine-induced enzyme secretion when a calcium-free perfusion fluid was used. This suggested that influx of calcium into the acinar cells might be a prerequisite for amylase release. Benz et al. (34), working with pieces of guinea pig pancreas *in vitro,* found that if a calcium-free medium was used then the basal secretion of amylase was not affected. However, the normal increase in response to betanechol did not occur. Matthews and Petersen (263) found that when segments of mouse pancreas *in vitro* were exposed to CCK or to acetylcholine an influx of Na^+ and also a small influx of Ca^{2+} occurred. Using the same type of pancreatic tissue that had been preincubated with $^{45}Ca^{2+}$, Matthews et al. (264) found that there was a marked efflux of calcium from the cells on treatment with pancreozymin or acetycholine. Similar findings had been reported by Case and Clausen (58). Argent et al. (19), working with a saline-perfused preparation of the cat pancreas, found amylase secretion to consist partly of a small continuous basal secretion and partly of secretion that could be stimulated by CCK. Calcium secretion in the juice varied with the secretion of amylase. Perfusion with calcium-free solutions reduced the basal secretion of amylase and progressively decreased the stimulated secretion until it was completely abolished. Electrolyte secretion was also reduced during the calcium-free perfusion, but could be completely restored to the normal values by adding calcium to the perfusate; the effects on enzyme secretion were only partly reversible. Case and Clausen (58) preincubated *in vitro* uncinate pancreatic processes of young rats with $^{45}Ca^{2+}$. They found that CCK then released both amylase and $^{45}Ca^{2+}$ in a dose-related fashion, but did not influence the rate of calcium uptake. In a calcium-free medium, efflux of cellular $^{45}Ca^{2+}$ still took place in response to CCK, but amylase release was abolished. The CCK-induced amylase release in a calcium-containing medium was inhibited if Na^+ in the medium was replaced by Li^+. This suggested that a Na^+ concentration gradient across the plasma membrane was of importance for enzyme secretion. The authors suggested that the primary action of CCK might be to increase the influx of Na^+ into the cell by changing membrane permeability. This would result in Ca^{2+} release from intracellular stores, leading to localized intracellular rises in Ca^{2+} concentration that initiate enzyme secretion. Beaudoin (29), working with pieces of rat pancreas *in vitro,* proposed a model however, in which both sodium and calcium were taken up by the cell prior to enzyme secretion. These authors and also Heisler et al. (178) discussed the possibility that cyclic AMP might in some way be involved in the mobilization or conservation of intracellular calcium. Such a possibility had indeed been suggested earlier by Rasmussen and Tenenhouse (324). In 1974 it was shown that the divalent cation ionophore A23187 (225) caused enzyme secretion from rat (325), mouse (399), and rabbit (355) pancreas *in vitro* provided the incubation medium contained calcium. This effect was not inhibited by atropine. Eimerl et al. (106) suggested that only the secretion of digestive enzymes was stimulated, since the basal secretion of lactic dehydrogenase was not affected. These authors suggested that calcium was acting as the second messenger and cyclic GMP as the third messenger in transporting information from the hormone-activated receptor to the enzyme secretory apparatus of the cell. The ionophore has since then found extensive use in the investigations of CCK action. Heisler (177) reported that it did not influence cyclic AMP concentrations in rat pancreas *in vitro* but that it stimulated a rapid Ca^{2+}-dependent increase in cyclic GMP, which preceded the onset of protein secretion. They suggested that the CCK receptor might be functioning as a calcium ionophore and that influx of extracellular Ca^{2+} in some way stimulated the synthesis of cyclic GMP. At present there is a fair degree of agreement among different workers that stimulation of enzyme secretion by CCK is associated with changes in cellular calcium concentrations, but there is disagreement concerning the nature of these changes. Some workers, like Kanno (222) and Beaudoin (29), working with perfused rat pancreas *in vitro,* and Kondo and Schulz (231), working with dispersed rat pancreatic acinar cells, consider that influx of extracellular calcium is increased, others claim that calcium influx is not noticeably affected and only efflux is increased, reflecting release of calcium from intracellular stores. This has been stated to be the case for the perfused cat pancreas *in vitro* (58), the isolated rabbit pancreas and pancreatic fragments *in vitro* (356), the mouse pancreas *in vitro* (397), isolated acinar cells of the rabbit pancreas (332), isolated guinea pig acinar cells (132,251), and isolated rat acinar cells (133). Gardner et al. (132) found that the relative potency with which CCK and several peptides related to it stimulate calcium efflux from guinea pig isolated pancreatic acinar cells is the same as that of their pancreozyminic activity. As to where the intracellular calcium stores are located, evidence points to the mitochondriae (68,251), microsomes (251), and various cellular membranes (359).

Calcium and Secretion of Enzymes

Kanno and Yamamoto (226), as well as Petersen and Ueda (313,378), working with the isolated perfused rat pancreas found that lowering the Ca^{2+} concentration of the perfusing fluid strikingly inhibited the CCK-induced secretion of enzymes. This only slightly inhibited the secretin-induced secretion of fluid. On the other hand, lowering the $NaHCO_3$ concentration abolished the secretin-stimulated secretion of fluid but inhibited only weakly the CCK-induced secretion of enzymes and of fluid. Petersen and Ueda (312), working with segments of mouse and rat pancreas *in vitro,* came to the conclusion that release of calcium from the cell membrane was involved in CCK-stimulated enzyme secretion, whereas the influx of Na^+, observed earlier by Case and Clausen (58), was of importance for acinar fluid secretion and thereby only indirectly for enzyme secretion. Kanno and Saito (225) found CCK-stimulated enzyme secretion from the perfused rat pancreas to be dependent on the K^+ concentration in the perfusing fluid. They postulated that entry of calcium and sodium into the cell takes place simultaneously by way of a carrier complex containing one Ca^{2+} to four Na^+.

Effects on the Transmembrane Electrical Potentials

Another area where discrepancies exist in the observations of different workers pertains to the effect of CCK on the transmembrane electrical potentials of the pancreatic acinar cells. Kanno (222) found that CCK and acetylcholine hyperpolarized the acinar cells of rats, whereas Dean and Matthews (78) found that CCK, but not secretin, depolarized the acinar cells of mice. Nishiyama and Petersen (300) showed that the acinar cells of cat, mouse, rabbit, and rat pancreas were always depolarized *in vitro* by CCK, but that in some case this was followed by hyperpolarization. The depolarization is assumed to have increased the permeability of the plasma membrane. Kanno (223), however, later found hyperpolarization to occur, although this was sometimes after the transient depolarization of the membranes. Iwatsuki and Petersen (202) found that the cells within a pancreatic acinus of the mouse are electrically coupled when at rest. They are uncoupled by secretagogues like cerulein, this being associated with cell membrane depolarization. Greenwell (154) found that CCK in the mouse pancreas caused depolarization of the acinar cell membranes. It had no effect on ductule cell membranes, whereas secretin caused hyperpolarization of ductule cell membranes without affecting acinar cell membranes.

Effects on Isolated Pancreatic Cells

Earlier, Benz et al. (34) had found that elevation of the K^+ concentration increased amylase release from pieces of guinea pig pancreas *in vitro,* but Williams et al. (396) found that this did not apply to dissociated pancreatic acinar cells. Other functional differences between dissociated cells and pieces of pancreatic tissue have been described. For instance, Williams et al. (396) found that isolated mouse pancreatic cells, unlike pancreatic guinea pig cells, did not respond to cerulein by secreting amylase, whereas a preparation of mouse pancreatic acini did respond (398). Haig (163), referring to the discovery by Wharton (395) that the acinar cells obtain their blood supply through a portal system from the islets, has discussed the possibility that islet cell hormones participate in the regulation of acinar function, a regulation that would be absent from isolated acinar cells. Despite such shortcomings, isolated acinar cells have been found to be most useful in investigations of CCK action. Christophe et al. (66) found that CCK-8 as well as carbamylcholine-stimulated calcium efflux, increase of cyclic GMP concentrations, and amylase secretion in guinea pig dispersed acinar cells. Neither calcium efflux nor changes in cyclic GMP concentrations were caused by secretin. This suggested that in pancreatic acinar cells the initial steps of CCK action were mobilization of intracellular calcium, followed by increase in cyclic GMP concentrations and then enzyme release. Gardner and Jackson (134), investigating the secretion of amylase from such cells, concluded that there were two mechanisms for stimulated amylase release: one by CCK or cholinergic agents mediated by GMP, and one by either secretin or VIP, mediated by cyclic AMP. The maximally effective concentrations for VIP were a hundred, and for secretin a thousand times higher than those for CCK-8. This seemed to leave no room for changes in cyclic AMP concentrations due to CCK. Recently Long and Gardner (247) described experiments showing that although CCK does not increase cyclic AMP concentrations in isolated acinar cells, it does so in cell homogenates. In intact cells it inhibits the increase in response to VIP and secretin. Results of recent experiments by Bauduin et al. suggest that dibutyryl cyclic AMP stimulated enzyme secretion is qualitatively similar to physiological hormone stimulated secretion and not due to some toxic effect on the pancreatic cells (28). Heisler (176) found that the α, β-methylene analog of ATP [Ap(CH$_2$) pp] prevented CCK- or acetylcholine-stimulated enzyme secretion, but not secretion stimulated by cyclic AMP.

Messenger Role of Cyclic AMP and Cyclic GMP

Although there is no doubt that CCK can lead to increased concentrations of cyclic GMP in pancreatic acinar cells, little is understood of how this initiates enzyme secretion, or indeed if it does so. Of possible relevance in this connection are the findings of Lambert et al. (237) that CCK increases orthophosphate incorporation into rat pancreatic proteins, especially into the membrane proteins of the zymogen granules. Also, the findings of MacDonald and Ronzio (253) that rat pancreatic zymogen granule membrane polypeptides were phosphorylated by a pancreatic protein kinase that was stimulated, although weakly, by cyclic GMP, but not at all by cyclic AMP are relevant to the role of cyclic AMP in the mechanism of cellular secretion. Lambert et al. have recently found that guanosine triphosphatase activity in rat pancreatic plasma membranes was stimulated by CCK. (238). Not all experiments, however, support a direct messenger role for either cyclic AMP or cyclic GMP. Jamieson had, for instance, found that certain substances increase pancreatic cyclic GMP concentrations without stimulation of enzyme secretion, whereas other substances stimulate enzyme secretion without affecting cyclic GMP concentrations (203).

Recent discussions of the intracellular messengers for CCK are to be found, i.e., in the articles by Chandler (62) and Case (57). A complicating factor in the structure-function relationships for CCK is the finding, by different groups of workers, that bombesin, a tetradecapeptide with a structure very different from that of CCK (9), nevertheless exerts CCK-like pancreozyminic activities on pancreatic fragments from rats and mice (82,201) and on isolated guinea pig acinar cells (204).

An interesting line of investigation should be the irreversible activation of pancreatic secretory cell receptors by photolabeling with hormone analogs, as described by Galardy and Jamieson (130).

INHIBITION OF CCK ACTIVITY

Beaudoin et al. (29) found that CCK-stimulated amylase secretion from pieces of rat pancreas *in vitro* could be inhibited approximately 75% by tetracaine, whereas secretion stimulated by dibutyryl cyclic AMP was not influenced. Rudick et al. (343) and Kelly et al. (227) found in dogs that isoproterenol strongly inhibited CCK-induced pancreatic enzyme secretion.

The partial purification from porcine ileal extracts of an anticholecystokinetic peptide (ACP) has been described by Sarles et al. (347) and the effects on pancreatic secretion of somatostatin and of an intestinal peptide with C-terminal somatostatin, is discussed in this volume by Pradayrol, pp. 984–988.

PHYSIOLOGICAL RELEASE OF CCK

Ivy and Oldberg (200) found that introduction of dilute HCl into the upper intestine of dogs resulted in gallbladder contraction. Introduction of olive oil, egg yolk, or cream did not result in contraction, but if these materials had been predigested with "pancreatin," contraction ensued.

Two years before the discovery by Harper and Raper of pancreozymin, Thomas and Crider (372) had observed in dogs that infusion of various proteolytic digests of proteins resulted in the secretion of a pancreatic juice rich in enzymes. They assumed that the effect was transmitted from the intestine to the pancreas via nervous pathways.

A decade later Wang and Grossman, working with dogs in which the pancreas had been subcutaneously autotransplanted (389), investigated the effects on secretion from the transplants of the introduction of various substances into the intestine. It was assumed that the secretion of fluid and bicarbonate was due to the stimulation by the released secretin, and the secretion of enzymes by the released CCK. The main conclusions from this work were that acid mainly stimulated the release of secretin, but to a considerable extent also that of CCK. Peptones and amino acid mixtures, on the other hand, stimulated predominantly the release of CCK, and less that of secretin. Of the individual amino acids, leucine, phenylalanine, and tryptophan were strong stimulants of CCK release, whereas all the others were either inactive or weak stimulants. It was further found that corn oil and sodium oleate were moderately efficient stimulants, whereas the carbohydrates starch, dextrose, and maltose were essentially inactive.

The authors mentioned that the same substances that stimulated the release of secretin and pancreozymin also seemed to stimulate the release of CCK. Later work has mainly confirmed, but also modified and extended, these early observations. Meyer and Grossman (267) showed in dogs that whereas L-phenylalanine stimulated pancreatic secretion, D-phenylalanine was almost or completely inactive. Meyer et al. (271) then found that, in dogs, intraduodenal L-phenylalanine mimicked the effects of intravenous CCK. The authors pointed out that since it had been shown that CCK by itself stimulated the pancreatic secretion of bicarbonate and fluid, it was probable that the phenylalanine was specifically releasing CCK, and not, as had been assumed in the work of Wang and Grossman (389), that of both CCK and secretin.

By introducing dilute HCl into the intestine of dogs secreting pancreatic juice under maximal stimulation with exogenous secretin, Barbezat and Grossman (22) confirmed that the acidification of the intestinal contents resulted in an increased secretion of protein into the pancreatic juice, presumably because of the release of endogenous CCK. It could be estimated that the acid released five times as much secretin, however, as CCK.

Meyer and Jones (268) investigated, in dogs, the effect on pancreatic secretion of intraduodenal perfusion of fats and products of fat digestion. They found that triglycerides as such did not stimulate pancreatic secretion, unless preceded by lipolysis. Fatty acids with less than nine carbon atoms did not stimulate, whereas those with longer chains stimulated in a dose-related fashion within the concentration range of 5 to 160 mM. The composition of the secreted pancreatic juice suggested that fatty acids released not only CCK but also some secretin. In contrast, α-monooleate seemed to stimulate the release of CCK only.

An investigation in dogs of the effects on pancreatic secretion of various synthetic peptides was performed by Meyer et al. (269), who concluded that some but by no means all peptides stimulate secretion. Of the peptides tested, glycylphenylalanine, glycyltryptophan, and phenylalanylglycine stimulated secretion, whereas di- and tri-glycine had no effect.

In man di Magno et al. found that perfusion of the duodenum and proximal distal jejunum with an amino acid solution resulted in pancreatic enzyme secretion, whereas no such effect could be elicited from the ileum (87). Simultaneous intraintestinal and intravenous infusions of the amino acid solution resulted in a lower pancreatic response than perfusion of the intestine only. This effect was ascribed to the release of glucagon by the intravenously administered amino acids. Given by intravenous infusion only, a solution of amino acids and sorbitol was found to increase the secretion of pancreatic enzymes (128).

Malagelada et al. (259) showed that in man intraduodenal glycerol did not have any effect on pancreatic secretion, whereas intraduodenal fatty acids stimulated both pancreatic enzyme secretion and gallbladder contraction. The release efficiency was dependent on the chain length of the fatty acids. The authors found further that low loads of fatty acids stimulated enzyme secretion without gallbladder contraction, which is of interest in view of the earlier findings of a greater sensitivity to CCK of the pancreas as compared with the gallbladder (260). When bile acids were administered simultaneously with the fatty acids their concentration exhibited a complicated relation to pancreatic secretion, partly because of concentration-dependent effects on micelli formation.

Go et al. (146) found in man that the output of pancreatic enzymes was significantly higher in response to the intraduodenal administration of a mixture of amino acids than to micellar fatty acids. They also found that phenylalanine, methionine, and valine, tested individually, were the strongest CCK releasers, whereas the effect of tryptophan was less marked. In dogs Meyer et al. (270), however, confirmed that intraduodenal tryptophan and phenylalanine were potent stimulators of pancreatic enzyme secretion. Valine and leucine were comparatively weak stimulants.

Ertan et al. (111) showed that in man jejunal perfusion of an amino acid solution stimulated pancreatic enzyme secretion and discharged gallbladder bile into the intestine, as it was done by intravenous CCK. Later Ertan et al. (110) found that the effect of the amino acid solution was inhibited by intraduodenal application of atropine or a topical anesthetic, suggesting that a local cholinergic mechanism might have been involved in CCK release. Earlier, Hong et al. (188) had found that duodenal application of procaine inhibited gallbladder contraction in response to instillation of dilute HCl into the duodenum. They did not find, however, that atropine had any inhibitory effect. Konturek et al. (232) demonstrated that in dogs truncal vagotomy depressed the stimulant effect on pancreatic enzyme secretion of intraduodenal amino acids or fatty acids without influencing the effect of exogenous CCK. This suggested that vagal innervation played a permissive role for the release of CCK from the duodenal mucosa. Quite recently, Solomon and Grossman (362) have found, however, that in dogs neither atropinization of the intestine nor truncal vagotomy influences the stimulatory effect on protein secretion of perfusion of the upper intestine with sodium oleate from a subcutaneously autotransplanted pancreas. This suggested that the release of CCK was not mediated by cholinergic pathways and that in those experiments where vagotomy or atropinization had diminished the pancreatic responses to intestinal perfusion with presumptive CCK releasers, this must have been due to mechanisms other than decreased CCK release. There is every reason to believe that gallbladder contraction and secretion of pancreatic enzymes are related to plasma CCK concentrations. Yet it is obvious that other factors may influence these functions (363) and that direct measurement of plasma CCK concentrations would be valuable in following the CCK release. As yet little has been done in this field. Nevertheless, Reeder et al. (326) have shown that intraduodenal instillation of phenylalanine or fat in dogs resulted in increased plasma concentrations of CCK-like immunoreactivity.

CCK-LIKE IMMUNOREACTIVITY

Forell and Stahlheber found that the secretion of pancreatic enzymes, especially of lipase and trypsinogen, in subjects secreting pancreatic juice following secretin stimulation was greatly increased if bile was introduced into the duodenum (120). Wormsley (403) confirmed this observation and demonstrated that the effect could be obtained by the bile acid component of the bile. The stimulation of pancreatic enzyme secretion by the bile acids was not associated, however with gallbladder contraction. Wormsley suggested that this might be due either to the role of bile acids, which in some way inhibit the cholecystokinetic action of CCK, or else that the amount of CCK released was adequate to stimulate the pancreas but not the gallbladder. The latter possibility finds support in the observation of Malagelada et al. (260) that the pancreas is more sensitive to CCK than is the gallbladder. Intraduodenal infusion of salts of calcium (186) or magnesium (187) has been found to stimulate pancreatic secretion in man, similarly to intravenously administered CCK. Kanno and Imai (224), working with the isolated and perfused rat duodenum, found that intraluminal instillation of a soybean extract released CCK, identified by bioassay, into a vascular perfusing solution provided that the latter contained calcium. If calcium was removed from the perfusion solution, the secretion of CCK stopped, and started again on readdition of calcium.

Release of CCK has been described in dogs in response to jejunal distention (67) and intraduodenal sorbitol (96). In rats it has been shown that intraduodenal administration of trypsin or chymotrypsin inhibitors or removal of the bile and pancreatic juice from the intestine resulted in a striking increase in pancreatic enzyme secretion (159,194). The possibility has been discussed that active proteolytic enzymes in the duodenum may in some way inhibit CCK release.

A new aspect of the physiological CCK release is the possible involvement of a bombesin-related peptide in this process. Bombesin has been found in dogs to increase plasma concentrations of immunoreactive CCK (114), and bombesin-like immunoreactive material was present in the tissues of the mammalian gastrointestinal tract (108). Recently, a peptide exhibiting bombesin-like bioactivity, but chemically not identical to bombesin, has been isolated in our laboratory from porcine gastric and intestinal tissue. (See Chapter 43II by T. McDonald, pp. 975–977, *this volume.*)

Inhibition, in man, of meal-induced CCK-release by somatostatin has been described by Schlegel et al. (353).

ASSAY OF CCK

Bioassay

Two different properties of CCK, the cholecystokinetic and the pancreozyminic, have been the basis of the various techniques described for its bioassay. Ivy and Oldberg originally worked with dogs and cats in which the cystic duct was clamped and the dome of the gallbladder was cannulated. The cannula was connected to a glass tube of a narrow inner diameter. On injection of CCK the pressure in the gallbladder and thereby the length of the column of bile in the glass tube increased in a dose-related fashion (200). The "Ivy dog unit" was defined as that amount of cholecystokinin activity that would under specified conditions increase the intragallbladder pressure by one cm of bile. Ivy and Janecek have described the methodology of their assay in detail (198). In practice the assay of CCK by this and all other methods has always been carried out by comparing the activity of the preparation to be tested with that of a standard preparation (140). We used the assay technique of Ivy and coworkers at first, and although we now use another technique for practical reasons, we have continued to express the activity of our various CCK preparations in Ivy dog units. Pure CCK-33 is, perhaps somewhat arbitrarily, assumed to have an activity of 3 IDU per microgram (80) and may be used as a reference substance for local standard preparations. In the standardization of CCK it is necessary to remember that its activity is easily lost on oxidation and that it is therefore necessary to use water that is as far as possible free of molecular chlorine. As an additional precaution, in our laboratory we make up the CCK solutions to be bioassayed in "physiological saline" in which 100 μg per ml of cysteine HCl have been dissolved. In the case of the C-terminal acidic fragments of CCK cysteine, is used instead of cysteine HCl.

The guinea pig gallbladder has often been used *in vitro* for the assay of CCK (139,192,219). Ljungberg (246) worked out a method in which the contractions in response to CCK of the guinea pig gallbladder *in situ* were recorded via a strain gauge transducer. We have used this method extensively in our laboratory and found it to be quite convenient and reliable. Many other methods have, however, also been described. Amer and Becvar used strips of rabbit gallbladder *in vitro* (7). Berry and Flower (36) also used rabbit gallbladder strips but found that their sensitivity could be increased by using a superfusion technique. Improved versions of the latter have been described (205,262). Vizi et al. (386) recommended the use of the longitudinal muscle of the guinea pig ileum for CCK assay. They found the sensitivity of it to be in the range of 10^{-9} M CCK. The segments of the guinea pig ileum had already earlier been used by Gershbein et al. (139).

The pancreozyminic action of CCK has been determined in several bioassays, as in the methods of Burn and Holton (54) and Crick et al. (72), using anesthetized cats, and those of Lin and Grossman (244), who used anesthetized, and Singer et al. (360) conscious dogs. Instead of determining some enzymatic activity in the pancreatic juice it is simpler to determine total protein (173,217), although determination of enzymes may of course be of interest for other reasons, such as investigations of parallel or nonparallel secretion (340).

Lin and Alphin (243) compared the pancreatic response to CCK of anesthetized dogs and rats and conscious rats, and concluded that dogs, because of their greater sensitivity, and because they give more reproducible results, remain the animals of choice for CCK and secretin bioassay. Many laboratories, however, lack facilities for work with dogs, and methods using rats have been worked out. Heatley (173) used anesthetized rats and continuous flushing of the cannulated common duct.

Collection of the rat pancreatic juice, although contaminated with duodenal secretions, by continuous perfusion of the duodenum has been described (119,189,342,354), and the technique may well be found useful for bioassays of CCK, as a similar technique using gastric perfusion has been of value for the bioassay of gastrin (141,236).

Quite other methods may find application for the assay of CCK. For instance, it has been suggested (167) that $^{45}Ca^{2+}$ efflux from isolated pancreatic acinar cells could form the basis of a bioassay procedure.

Radioimmunoassay

Several groups of workers have described radioimmunoassay (RIA) procedures for CCK. A factor to take into account is that gastrin and CCK have identical C-terminal sequences and that some antibodies to CCK will react with the common C-terminal sequence of the two hormones (254). Agarwal et al. (1) solved the problem for gastrin by raising antibodies toward a fragment of the gastrin molecule that lacks sequence homology with CCK.

The first RIA for CCK was described 10 years ago by Young et al. (407). They immunized rabbits with a partially purified preparation of CCK that was conjugated to rabbit serum albumin. Their method suffered from the disadvantage that essentially pure CCK seems not to have been available for use as a tracer and that they therefore had used for this purpose the same material that they had used for immunization after iodinating it with ^{131}I by the chloramine T procedure of Hunter and Greenwood (193). Reeder et al. (326) described a somewhat similar RIA procedure, but this group of workers soon modified their procedure, and now use essentially pure CCK-33 as the tracer (373). Go et al. (147) immunized guinea pigs with a partially purified CCK preparation and used essentially pure CCK-33 as a tracer. They found that their antibodies reacted with porcine but not with human CCK and suggested that there were species differences among the CCKs. Harvey et al. (168) immunized rabbits, guinea pigs, and sheep with partially purified CCK and used CCK-33 as a tracer. One series of antibodies obtained in rabbits proved to be particularly useful since it reacted with CCK-33 as well as with its C-terminal fragments CCK-12 and CCK-8 but not with gastrin. This indicated that its specificity was not directed toward the C-terminal pentapeptide common to both CCK and gastrin. Schlegel and co-workers generated antibodies in rabbits against essentially pure porcine CCK-33 conjugated to bovine serum albumin (354) and used ^{125}I CCK-39 as a tracer (352).

Rehfeld (329), using a partially purified preparation of CCK for immunization, raised antibodies to CCK in guinea pigs and rabbits. The peptide preparation was used as such for the guinea pigs, but conjugated to bovine serum albumin for the rabbits. The antibodies from different animals were characterized as to their specificity and it was found that some reacted with both CCK and gastrin whereas others reacted with CCK only. Further work showed that the antibodies reacting with both gastrin and CCK recognized the 30–33 sequence of CCK-33 whereas those reacting with CCK only were of two types, one recognizing the 20–25 sequence and the other the 20–30 sequence.

As a tracer Rehfeld used CCK-33 acylated with ^{125}I-hydroxyphenyl propionic acid according to Bolton and Hunter (44). Different antibodies, with specificities for different regions of the gastrin sequence, one region being the C-terminal pentapeptide, common to gastrin and CCK, were put to excellent use by Dockray (90). He showed that the gastrin-like immunoreactive material discovered in cerebral tissue by Vanderhaeghen et al. (383) was in fact CCK-like.

Muller et al. (281) immunized a goat with a partially purified preparation of porcine CCK, and found that the antibodies that were formed were directed preferentially toward the N-terminal part of the CCK-33 sequence, since they reacted strongly with CCK-33 but very poorly with CCK-8. These antibodies reacted with material in extracts of porcine upper intestinal tissue but not in corresponding extracts from several other species. In contrast with this, antibodies raised in rabbits to the C-terminal tetrapeptide of gastrin (and of CCK) reacted with CCK-33, CCK-8, and material in intestinal tissue extracts from all species investigated. These findings were interpreted as indicating that the CCKs from various species were identical in their C-terminal parts but varied N-terminally. This is in accordance with the earlier findings of Go et al. (147) and also with the later findings of Straus and Yalow (368) concerning cerebral CCK. RIAs for CCK have also been described by Englert (107) and del Mazo (265).

CLINICAL USES OF CCK

The use of CCK in the secretin-pancreozymin test of pancreatic function has been referred to in the Chapter 5 on secretin (pp. 85–126, *this volume*). Its use for roentgenological examination of the gallbladder and for collection of bile by duodenal drainage was suggested by Duncan et al. (97).

Diagnostic Uses of CCK

The first clinical work with CCK from our laboratory was carried out with preparations that had an activity of only 20 to 25 IDU per milligram. Nevertheless, provided that the material was injected slowly intravenously no toxic side reactions were observed. This material had been obtained by following approximately, not in detail, the procedure outlined on p. 171 to the stage of precipitation from 75% ethanol with butanol. Although we never investigated the problem in detail we have the impression that this precipitation was essential for the removal of highly toxic material of lipid character, which remained in the supernatant, since the CCK preparations prior to this step could at times show serious toxi effects. It was found by several workers that injection of CCK in a dose of one IDU per kg b.w. in most cases resulted in contraction of the gallbladder.

This could be followed roentgenologically, provided that the gallbladder had been filled with bile containing some opaque medium [references to this early work may be found in the articles by Jorpes and Mutt (216), and Backlund (20)]. When it became apparent that CCK could be purified much further we continued the purification first one step further (chromatography on TEAE, and later on DEAE cellulose, p. 171). This material found extensive use in many countries under the name "10% pure" CCK. During the last 2 years one further purification step has been taken, namely, chromatography on Sephadex G50 (p. 171), and the product was then about 30% pure when based on [HS]bioactivity. The losses in the next step, which would give a mixture of essentially pure CCK-33, and CCK-39, have been until now prohibitive, but recent developments in methodology suggest that this may not always remain so.

Blau et al. (40) demonstrated that it was possible to visualize the pancreas by scanning techniques following pancreatic uptake of γ-emitting amino acid analogs. This uptake was enhanced by the administration of CCK, an hour before that of the radioactive amino acid, ^{75}Se-selenomethionine. This technique of pancreatic scanning has found fairly wide application (45,94,129,150,319, 322,401). One of the major difficulties associated with its use was the high background uptake of radioactivity by the liver, and various substractive procedures that had to be devised to compensate for this (322 and 129).

Functional tests based on intraduodenal of the radioactive selenium, taken up by the pancreas on stimulation with CCK secretion, have been described (94,408). Pointer (316) demonstrated in rats that secretion of the radioactive selenium took place not only into the pancreatic juice but also into the bile. Others (86,109) have found that stimulation of pancreatic enzyme secretion by the intrajejunal or intraduodenal perfusions of amino acid solutions, presumably acting via release of endogenous CCK, might be useful for the diagnosis of pancreatic disease in man.

Several investigators have found CCK to be valuable for the differential diagnosis of various types of acalculous biliary disease. This is a large and specialized clinical field, and here essentially only references to some of the more important articles can be given. The references to additional work may be found in the articles quoted. Nathan et al. (296), Nora et al. (301), Goldstein et al. (149), and Neschis et al. (298) have all found CCK to be of diagnostic usefulness in this field. Dunn et al. (99), however, claimed that "cholecystokinin cholecystography, as currently employed, is not helpful in the diagnosis and management of patients with possible acalculous gallbladder disease." Recently Nathan et al. (295) have described the normal findings in oral and CCK cholecystography in 200 control subjects.

Cozzolino et al. (70) described the "cystic duct syndrome." Here the injections of CCK were followed by a typical attack of gallbladder pains in patients without gallstones but with some obstruction of the cystic duct. Reid et al. (331), however, maintained that while a positive pain reaction after CCK was of some diagnostic significance, a negative reaction did not exclude the obstruction of the outflow, even by small concrements. A test for patency of the cystic duct has been developed by Eikman et al. (105). The gallbladder is stimulated to empty by the injection of CCK, and a radiolabeled biliary marker is injected intravenously. The uptake of the label into the liver and the gallbladder regions is then followed. If the cystic duct is obstructed, the uptake of the marker into the gallbladder is absent or greatly reduced. A similar technique has been described by Paré et al. (306).

Several workers consider microscopy and chemical analysis of the bile recovered by duodenal drainage during stimulation of gallbladder contraction with CCK to be of diagnostic value. Steinitz and Talis (365) found this to be indispensable for detection of amebas in the biliary tract. Freeman et al. (123) found that both duodenal drainage during CCK administration and CCK cholangiography were of diagnostic value in patients without gallstones but with pain in the right upper quadrant of the abdomen. Foss and Laing (121) have recently described a technique in which the drainage tube is introduced into the duodenum with the aid of fiber-endoscopy. They found duodenal drainage to give important information in cases of gallbladder disease with normal oral cholecystograms. Frenkel et al. (124) found CCK useful for the diagnosis of cystadenoma.

CCK has also been used for accelerating the passage of contrast medium through the small intestine (274,277,307).

Therapeutic Uses of CCK

The use of CCK in therapy has been limited. It has been used in surgery to flush out concrements from the common duct without operation (21,339). Possibly the swift and repetitive, at short intervals, gallbladder emptying achieved by CCK could in some cases be used for removal of small concrements also from the gallbladder. Cerulein, acting like CCK, has been used for the treatment of paralytic ileus (2).

In dog experiments Herzog and Nelson (181) showed that the rate of elimination of an orally given cholecystographic agent from the liver was increased by the administration of CCK. Apparently, CCK did not act directly on the liver, but by emptying the gallbladder and thereby accelerating the enterohepatic bile acid circulation.

Whether or not CCK could have any preventive action on the cholestasis that may occur in immature newborn infants given parenteral alimentation does not seem to have been investigated (321). Hughes et al. (190) have shown in dogs that the administration of exogenous secretin and CCK can prevent the intestinal mucosal hypoplasia that develops on long-term total parenteral nutrition, and that there is some reason to believe that the pancreatic insufficiency that develops in man may likewise be prevented (233).

Harvey and Read (171) have suggested that saline purgatives act by releasing CCK.

Geller et al. (135) have found that in patients with chronic relapsing pancreatitis the capacity of the hepatocytes to take up bromosulftalein is decreased and that it can be improved by the administration of CCK.

Plasma CCK Levels in Disease

There is no conclusive evidence that pathological concentrations, increased or decreased, of plasma CCK play a causative role in any disease, although there are indications that such changes in CCK concentrations may be involved in certain cases. Wilson et al. (400) described a patient with severe gastric hypersecretion and diarrhea in whom the plasma gastrin concentrations were normal but the CCK concentrations were three to four times higher than normal. Long and Weiss (248) found that patients with pancreatic insufficiency had much more rapid gastric emptying after fatty meals than control subjects, whereas there was no such difference if the fats had been enzymatically hydrolyzed. It is known that CCK is released by fatty acids, but not by unhydrolyzed fats.

It is not improbable that plasma CCK concentrations may, in a secondary fashion, play a role in the development of biliary disease. Hepner (180) found in man that a predominantly carbohydrate diet, known to release CCK inefficiently or not at all, resulted in greatly decreased gallbladder emptying, which was associated with increased pools of the primary bile acids. Recently Duane and Hanson (95) have shown that among control subjects on a standard diet there are considerable individual variations in gallbladder emptying and in the small intestinal transit times. Both these processes are important for the regulation of bile acid pool sizes in man. On the other hand, the question as to whether or not regular gallbladder emptying prevents gallstone formation does not yet seem to have a simple answer (245,357).

Controversial reports have appeared concerning the behavior of CCK in celiac disease. Low-Beer et al. (250) found that patients with this disease showed normal gallbladder contractions in response to exogenous CCK, but sluggish contractions in response to fatty meals. This suggests that the release or synthesis of endogenous CCK was here impaired. Di Magno et al. (86) found that both gallbladder contraction and secretion of pancreatic enzymes in response to intraduodenal infusions of amino acid solutions were impaired, and that responses to exogenous CCK were normal. Braganza and Howat (46), on the other hand, found that in a substantial percentage of these patients, gallbladder contractions in response to exogenous CCK were impaired. Low-Beer et al. (249) subsequently came to the same conclusion, and found, in addition, that the patients had very high plasma concentrations of CCK as compared with controls. The additional increases in these concentrations during meals were sluggish, however, as compared with the swift increases in controls. They concluded that the gallbladder was less sensitive to CCK in these patients, possibly because of the constantly high plasma concentrations to which it was being subjected.

Moderately increased plasma concentrations of CCK have been described in cholecystectomized patients (206).

A clinical picture showing gallbladder atony, chronic cholecystitis, and pancreatitis has been attributed by Rafes to CCK deficiency (320). Harvey and Read (170) found that in patients with the irritable colon syndrome administration of CCK resulted in increased colonic motor activity, which in a minority of the patients was associated with typical attacks of their pain. Waller et al. (388), however, found that CCK did not affect colonic motility in man.

Sarles and Sahel (348) have suggested that selective release of CCK resulting in the secretion of viscous enzyme-rich pancreatic juice may be involved in the etiology of the calcifying pancreatitis of chronic alcoholics. Savion and Zelinger (349) have shown in rat pancreatic slices that supramaximal stimulation of enzyme secretion results in increased lysosomal activity and the production of a myocardial depressant factor.

SUMMARY AND CONCLUSIONS

Cholecystokinin (CCK), originally isolated from porcine intestinal tissue in the form of a 33-residue peptide (CCK-33), has been found to occur in this tissue also in a larger form, CCK-39, in which CCK-33 is lengthened from its N-terminus by a hexapeptide. The amino acid sequence of CCK-39 is Tyr-Ile-Gln-Gln-Ala-Arg-Lys-Ala-Pro-Ser-Gly-Arg-Val-Ser-Met-Ile-Lys-Asn-Leu-Gln-Ser-Leu-Asp-Pro-Ser-His-Arg-Ile-Ser-Asp-Arg-Asp-Tyr (SO_3)-Met-Gly-Trp-Met-Asp-Phe-NH_2.

All the known biological activities of CCK are exerted in full force by its C-terminal fragments, starting with the heptapeptide. Shorter fragments show only weak activity. The heptapeptide has been reported to be on a molar basis several times stronger than either CCK-33 or CCK-39. Structural requirements for activity are, i.e., esterification of the phenolic group of the tyrosine residue with sulfuric acid, and the proper position of the tyrosine-O-sulfate residue in relation to C-terminal pentapeptide amide.

The C-terminal dodecapeptide, CCK-12, is swiftly formed *in vitro* by tryptic degradation of either CCK-33 or CCK-39, and is slowly degraded further to CCK-8.

Convincing evidence has been presented for the occurrence of free CCK-8 in intestinal tissue, and it has been isolated from sheep cerebral tissue. Cerebral tissue, especially that of the neocortex, is rich in CCK.

Little is yet known about the enzymes that *in vivo* convert the larger forms of CCK to the smaller ones.

CCK has been found to exhibit a large number of pharmacological actions. There is strong evidence that it plays a major physiological role in stimulating pancreatic enzyme secretion and gallbladder emptying. Other of its physiologically important actions seem to be potentiation of the effect of secretin on the pancreas, inhibition of emptying of the stomach, and a trophic effect on the pancreas.

CCK seems to act directly on the acinar cells of the pancreas and on the muscle of the gallbladder but via release of acetylcholine on the muscles of the small intestine. In actions on the pancreas and the gallbladder it effects changes in intracellular concentrations of cyclic nucleotides and in transmembrane fluxes of Na^+ and Ca^{2+} ions. How this is related to gallbladder contraction and pancreatic enzyme secretion is, as yet, far from clear.

It has been shown that acidification of the upper intestine releases not only secretin but also CCK. Other CCK releasers are fatty acids but not unhydrolyzed fats, and certain peptides and amino acids. The latter differ greatly in their releasing efficiency. Tryptophan and phenylalanine are strong releasers; valine, leucine and methionine are moderate ones, and the other amino acids are weak or ineffective.

CCK has found considerable clinical use in the diagnosis of pancreatic and gallbladder disease, and because of its accelerating effect on intestinal transit, in roentgenological investigations of the intestine. There are a few suggestions also for its therapeutic use, but more work is necessary to evaluate these possibilities and to enlarge the scope of its diagnostic and therapeutic applications.

PROJECTIONS FOR THE FUTURE

The history of CCK has been dramatic. First described as a hormone involved in the physiological control of gallbladder function, it was soon found to have other actions, among which, quite unexpectedly, was the important control of pancreatic enzyme secretion, an activity that had been believed to be exerted by a specific hormone, pancreozymin.

Also unexpectedly, CCK was found to be chemically related to another hormone, gastrin, and to occur not only in intestinal but also in cerebral tissue.

Future work will elucidate its function in the CNS, and there is little point in speculation at this stage. Possibly, it acts as a neurotransmitter. However, its enzyme-releasing and trophic activities elsewhere, as well as its actions on blood flow, depolarizing or hyperpolarizing effects on the membranes of certain cells, and effects on cellular sodium and calcium fluxes do not make it improbable that it can have actions other than, or in addition to, neurotransmitter function.

Concerning its cholecystokinetic and pancreozyminic activities, it will be of interest to find out whether these can be separated by synthetic modifications of the CCK structure. It will also be of interest if peptides will be discovered that have only one or the other of these activities, or if these activities are in fact being exerted by so similar cellular mechanisms as to make such separation impossible.

Another interesting question is which other peptides of the gastrin-cholecystokinin group still remain to be isolated—from mammalian tissues and from species further away.

REFERENCES

1. Agarwal, K. L., Grudzinski, S., Kenner, G. W., Rogers, N. H., Sheppard, R. C., and McGuigan, J. E. (1971): Immunochemical differentiation between gastrin and related peptide hormones through a novel conjugation of peptides to proteins. *Experientia,* 27:514–515.
2. Agosti, A., Bertaccini, G., Paulucci, R., and Zanella, E. (1971): Caerulein treatment for paralytic ileus. *Lancet,* i:395.
3. Ågren, G. (1939): On preparation of cholecystokinin. *Scand. Arch. Physiol.,* 81:234–243.
4. Amer, M. S. (1969): Studies with cholecystokinin. II. Cholecystokinetic potency of porcine gastrins I and II and related peptides in three systems. *Endocrinology,* 84:1277–1281.
5. Amer, M. S. (1972): Studies with cholecystokinin *in vitro.* III. Mechanism of the effect on the isolated rabbit gall bladder strips. *J. Pharmacol. Exp. Ther.,* 183:527–534.
6. Amer, M. S. (1974): Cyclic guanosine 3',5'-monophosphate and gallbladder contraction. *Gastroenterology,* 67:333–337.
7. Amer, M. S., and Becvar, W. E. (1969): A sensitive *in vitro* method for the assay of cholecystokinin. *J. Endocrinol.,* 43:637–642.
8. Amer, M. S., and McKinney, G. R. (1972): Studies with cholecystokinin *in vitro.* IV. Effects of cholecystokinin and related peptides on phosphodiesterase. *J. Pharmacol. Exp. Ther.,* 183:535–548.
9. Anastasi, A., Erspamer, V., and Bucci, M. (1971): Isolation and structure of bombesin and alytesin, two analogous active peptides from the skin of the European amphibians *Bombina* and *Alytes. Experientia,* 27:166–167.
10. Anastasi, A., Erspamer, V., and Endean, R. (1968): Isolation and amino acid sequence of caerulein, the active decapeptide of the skin of *Hyla caerulea. Arch. Biochem. Biophys.,* 125:57–68.
11. Andersson, K. E., Andersson, R., and Hedner, P. (1972): Cholecystokinetic effect and concentration of cyclic AMP in gallbladder muscle *in vitro. Acta Physiol. Scand.,* 85:511–516.
12. Andersson, K. E., Andersson, R., Hedner, P., and Persson, C. G. A. (1972): Effect of cholecystokinin on the level of cyclic AMP and of mechanical activity in the isolated sphincter of Oddi. *Life Sci.,* 11:723–732.
13. Andersson, K.-E., Andersson, R., Hedner, P., and Persson, C. G. A. (1973): Parallelism between mechanical and metabolic responses to cholecystokinin and prostaglandin E₂ in extrahepatic biliary tract. *Acta Physiol. Scand.,* 89:571–579.
14. Andersson, K. E., Andersson, R. G. G., Hedner, P., and Persson, C. G. A. (1977): Interrelations between cyclic AMP, cyclic GMP and contraction in guinea pig gallbladder stimulated by cholecystokinin. *Life Sci.,* 20:73–78.
15. Andersson, K.-E., Hedner, P., and Persson, C. G. A. (1974): Differentiation of the contractile effects of prostaglandin E₂ and the C-terminal octapeptide of cholecystokinin in isolated guinea pig gallbladder. *Acta Physiol. Scand.,* 90:657–663.
16. Andersson, K. E., Hedner, P., and Persson, C. G. A. (1974): Effects of lanthanum and calcium antagonists on contractile responses of isolated guinea pig gallbladder. *Acta Physiol. Scand.,* 91:16A–17A.
17. Anika, S. M., Houpt, T. R., and Houpt, K. A. (1977): Satiety elicited by cholecystokinin in intact and vagotomized rats. *Physiol. Behav.,* 19:761–766.
18. Anuras, S., Cooke, A. R., and Christensen, J. (1974): An inhibitory innervation at the gastroduodenal junction. *J. Clin. Invest.,* 54:529–535.
19. Argent, B. E., Case, R. M., and Scratcherd, T. (1973): Amylase secretion by the perfused cat pancreas in relation to the secretion of calcium and other electrolytes and as influenced by the external ionic environment. *J. Physiol.,* 230:575–593.
20. Backlund, V. (1970): Die Verwendung des Cholecystokinins in der Röntgendiagnostik. *Der Radiologe,* 10:36–39.
21. Backlund, V., and Peterson, H.-I. (1965): Die Verwendung des Cholecystokinins in der Chirurgie der Gallengänge. *Der Radiologe,* 5:100–104.
22. Barbezat, G. O., and Grossman, M. I. (1975): Release of cholecystokinin by acid. *Proc. Soc. Exp. Biol. Med.,* 148:463–467.
23. Barrington, E. J. W., and Dockray, G. J. (1970): The effect of intestinal extracts of lampreys *(Lampetra fluviatilis* and *Petromyzon marinus)* on pancreatic secretion in the rat. *Gen. Comp. Endocrinol.,* 14:170–177.

24. Barrington, E. J. W., and Dockray, G. J. (1972): Cholecystokinin-pancreozyminlike activity in the eel *(Anguilla anguilla L.). Gen. Comp. Endocrinol.,* 19:80–87.
25. Barrowman, J. A., and Mayston, P. D. (1974): The trophic influence of cholecystokinin on the rat pancreas. *J. Physiol.,* 238:73p–75p.
26. Bauduin, H., and Cantraine, F. (1972): "Phospholipid effect" and secretion in the rat pancreas. *Biochim. Biophys. Acta,* 270:248–253.
27. Bauduin, H., Rochus, L., Vincent, D., and Dumont, J. E. (1971): Role of cyclic 3',5'-AMP in the action of physiological secretagogues on the metabolism of rat pancreas in vitro *Biochim. Biophys. Acta,* 252:171–183.
28. Bauduin, H., Stock, C., Launay, J. F., Vincent, D., Potvliege, P., and Grenier, J. F. (1977): On the secretagogue effect of dibutyryl cyclic AMP in the rat exocrine pancreas. *Pflügers Arch.,* 372:69–76.
29. Beaudoin, A. R., Marois, C., Dunnigan, J., and Morisset, J. (1974): Biochemical reactions involved in pancreatic enzyme secretion. I. Activation of the adenylate cyclase complex. *Can. J. Physiol. Pharmacol.,* 52:174–182.
30. Bedi, B. S., Govaerts, J.-P., Master, S. P., and Gillespie, I. E. (1967): Inhibition of gastric acid secretion by intravenous cholecystokinin extract. *Scand. J. Gastroenterol.,* 2:68–76.
31. Behar, J., and Biancani, P. (1977): Effect of cholecystokinin-octapeptide on lower esophageal sphincter. *Gastroenterology,* 73:57–61.
32. Behar, J., Biancani, P., and Zabinski, M. P. (1979): Characterization of feline gastroduodenal junction by neural and hormonal stimulation. *Am. J. Physiol.,* 236:E45–E51.
33. Bennett, A. (1965): Effect of gastrin on isolated smooth muscle preparations. *Nature,* 208:170–173.
34. Benz, L., Eckstein, B., Matthews, E. K., and Williams, J. A. (1972): Control of pancreatic amylase release *in vitro:* Effects of ions, cyclic AMP, and colchicine. *Br. J. Pharmacol.,* 46:66–77.
35. Berkowitz, J. M., Praissman, M., and LeFevre, M. E. (1976): Effects of peptide hormone structure on H^+ secretion by *Necturus* gastric mucosa. *Am. J. Physiol.,* 231:573–578.
36. Berry, H., and Flower, R. J. (1971): The assay of endogenous cholecystokinin and factors influencing its release in the dog and cat. *Gastroenterology,* 60:409–420.
37. Berstad, A., and Petersen, H. (1970): Dose-response relationship of the effect of secretin on acid and pepsin secretion in man. *Scand. J. Gastroenterol.,* 5:647–654.
38. Bhoola, K. D., and Lemon, M. J. C. (1973): Studies on the activation of adenylate cyclase from the submaxillary gland and pancreas. *J. Physiol.,* 232:83p–84p.
39. Birmingham, M. K., Elliott, F. H., and Valère, P. H.-L. (1953): The need for the presence of calcium for the stimulation in vitro of rat adrenal glands by adrenocorticotrophic hormone. *Endocrinology,* 53:687–689.
40. Blau, M., Manske, R. F., and Bender, M. A. (1962): Clinical experience with Se^{75}-selenomethionine for pancreas visualization. *J. Nucl. Med.,* 3:202.
41. Bodanszky, M., Chaturvedi, N., Hudson, D., and Itoh, M. (1972): Cholecystokinin-pancreozymin. I. The synthesis of peptides corresponding to the N-terminal sequence. *J. Org. Chem.,* 37:2303–2307.
42. Bodanszky, M., Martinez, J., Priestley, G. P., Gardner, J. D., and Mutt, V. (1978): Cholecystokinin (pancreozymin). 4.[1] Synthesis and properties of a biologically active analogue of the C-terminal heptapeptide with ε-hydroxynorleucine sulfate replacing tyrosine sulfate. *J. Med. Chem.,* 21:1030–1035.
43. Bodanszky, M., Natarajan, S., Hahne, W., and Gardner, J. D. (1977): Cholecystokinin (pancreozymin). 3.[1] Synthesis and properties of an analogue of the C-terminal heptapeptide with serine sulfate replacing tyrosine sulfate. *J. Med. Chem.,* 20:1047–1050.
44. Bolton, A. E., and Hunter, W. M. (1973): The labelling of proteins to high specific radioactivities by conjugation to a ^{125}I-containing acylating agent. *Biochem. J.,* 133:529–539.
45. Braganza, J., Critchley, M., Howat, H. T., Testa, H. J., and Torrance, H. B. (1972): An appraisal of ^{75}Se-selenomethionine scanning as a test of pancreatic function: A comparison with the secretin-pancreozymin test. *Gut,* 13:844.
46. Braganza, J., and Howat, H. T. (1971): Gallbladder inertia in coeliac disease. *Lancet* i:1133.
47. Brink, B. M., Schlegel, J. F., and Code, C. F. (1965): The pressure profile of the gastroduodenal junction zone in dogs. *Gut,* 6:163–171.
48. Brooks, A. M., and Grossman, M. I. (1970): Effect of secretin and cholecystokinin on pentagastrin stimulated gastric secretion in man. *Gastroenterology,* 59:114–119.

49. Brooks, A. M., Johnson, L. R., Spencer, J., and Grossman, M. I. (1970): Failure of desulfated caerulein to inhibit pentagastrin-stimulated acid secretion. *Am. J. Physiol.,* 219:794–797.
50. Brown, J. C., Harper, A. A., and Scratcherd, T. (1967): Potentiation of secretin stimulation of the pancreas. *J. Physiol.,* 190:519–530.
51. Brown, J. C., Mutt, V., and Pederson, R. A. (1970): Further purification of a polypeptide demonstrating enterogastrone activity. *J. Physiol.,* 209:57–64.
52. Brown, J. C., Pederson, R. A., Jorpes, E., and Mutt, V. (1969): Preparation of highly active enterogastrone. *Can. J. Physiol. Pharmacol.,* 47:113–114.
53. Buffa, R., Solcia, E., and Go, V. L. W. (1976): Immunohistochemical identification of the cholecystokinin cell in the intestinal mucosa. *Gastroenterology,* 70:528–532.
54. Burn, J. H., and Holton, P. (1948): The standardization of secretin and pancreozymin. *J. Physiol.,* 107:449–455.
55. Care, A. D., Bruce, J. B., Boelkins, J., Kenny, A. D., Conaway, H., and Anast, C. S. (1971): Role of pancreozymin-cholecystokinin and structurally related compounds as calcitonin secretogogues. *Endocrinology,* 89:262–271.
56. Carlsöö, B., and Danielsson, Å. (1979): Effects of cholecystokinin-pancreozymin on amylase synthesis and secretion in the mouse pancreas. *Acta Hepato Gastroenterol. (Stuttg.),* 26:37–42.
57. Case, R. M. (1978): Synthesis, intracellular transport and discharge of exportable proteins in the pancreatic acinar cell and other cells. *Biol. Rev.,* 53:211–354.
58. Case, R. M., and Clausen, T. (1973): The relationship between calcium exchange and enzyme secretion in the isolated rat pancreas. *J. Physiol.,* 235:75–102.
59. Case, R. M., Johnson, M., Scratcherd, T., and Sherratt, H. S. A. (1972): Cyclic adenosine 3',5'-monophosphate concentration in the pancreas following stimulation by secretin, cholecystokinin-pancreozymin and acetylcholine. *J. Physiol.,* 223:669–684.
60. Case, R. M., and Scratcherd, T. (1972): The actions of dibutyryl cyclic adenosine 3',5'-monophosphate and methyl xanthines on pancreatic exocrine secretion. *J. Physiol.,* 223:649–667.
61. Celestin, L. R. (1967): Gastrin-like effects of cholecystokinin-pancreozymin. *Nature,* 215:763–764.
62. Chandler, D. E. (1978): Control of pancreatic enzyme secretion: A critique on the role of calcium. *Life Sci.,* 23:323–334.
63. Chey, W. Y., Hitanant, S., Hendricks, J., and Lorber, S. H. (1970): Effect of secretin and cholecystokinin on gastric emptying and gastric secretion in man. *Gastroenterology,* 58:820–827.
64. Chey, W. Y., Sivasomboon, B., Hendricks, J., and Lorber, S. H. (1970): Effects of secretin and cholecystokinin on gastric secretion in rats. *Gastroenterology,* 58:1037.
65. Chowdhury, J. R., Berkowitz, J. M., Praissman, M., and Fara, J. W. (1976): Effect of sulfated and non-sulfated gastrin and octapeptide-cholecystokinin on cat gall bladder *in vitro. Experientia,* 32:1173–1175.
66. Christophe, J. P., Frandsen, E. K., Conlon, T. P., Krishna, G., and Gardner, J. D. (1976): Action of cholecystokinin, cholinergic agents, and A-23187 on accumulation of guanosine 3':5'-monophosphate in dispersed guinea pig pancreatic acinar cells. *J. Biol. Chem.,* 251:4640–4645.
67. Chung, R. S. K., Fromm, D., Trencis, L., and Silen, W. (1970): Gastric and pancreatic responses to jejunal distention. *Gastroenterology,* 59:387–395.
68. Clemente, F., and Meldolesi, J. (1975): Calcium and pancreatic secretion-dynamics of subcellular calcium pools in resting and stimulated acinar cells. *Br. J. Pharmacol.,* 55:369–379.
69. Cooper, C. W., Schwesinger, W. H., Ontjes, D. A., Mahgoub, A. M., and Munson, P. L. (1972): Stimulation of secretion of pig thyrocalcitonin by gastrin and related hormonal peptides. *Endocrinology,* 91:1079–1089.
70. Cozzolino, H. J., Goldstein, F., Greening, R. R., and Wirts, C. W. (1963): The cystic duct syndrome. *JAMA,* 185:920–924.
71. Crean, G. P., Marshall, M. W., and Rumsey, R. D. E. (1969): Parietal cell hyperplasia induced by the administration of pentagastrin (ICI 50,123) to rats. *Gastroenterology,* 57:147–155.
72. Crick, J., Harper, A. A., and Raper, H. S. (1950): On the preparation of secretin and pancreozymin. *J. Physiol.,* 110:367–376.
73. Dahlgren, S. (1966): Cholecystokinin: Pharmacology and clinical use. *Acta Chir. Scand. (Suppl.),* 357:256–260.
74. Dangoumau, J., Balabaud, C., Bussiere-Leboeuf, C., Dallet-Duverge, F., and Noel, M. (1977):

Influence de la pentagastrine, de la cholecystokinine et de la caeruléine sur la cholérèse chez le rat. *J. Pharmacol. (Paris),* 8:197–204.

75. Danielsson, Å., and Sehlin, J. (1974): Transport and oxidation of amino acids and glucose in the isolated exocrine mouse pancreas: Effects of insulin and pancreozymin. *Acta Physiol. Scand.,* 91:557–565.

76. Davidson, W. D., Urushibara, O., and Thompson, J. C. (1969): Action of pancreozymin-cholecystokinin on the isolated gastric mucosa of the bullfrog. *Proc. Soc. Exp. Biol. Med.,* 129:711–713.

77. Davies, R. E., Harper, A. A., and Mackay, I. F. S. (1949): A comparison of the respiratory activity and histological changes in isolated pancreatic tissue. *Am. J. Physiol.,* 157:278–282.

78. Dean, P. M., and Matthews, E. K. (1972): Pancreatic acinar cells: Measurement of membrane potential and miniature depolarization potentials. *J. Physiol.,* 225:1–13.

79. Debas, H. T., Farooq, O., and Grossman, M. I. (1975): Inhibition of gastric emptying is a physiological action of cholecystokinin. *Gastroenterology,* 68:1211–1217.

80. Debas, H. T., and Grossman, M. I. (1973): Pure cholecystokinin: Pancreatic protein and bicarbonate response. *Digestion,* 9:469–481.

81. Deschodt-Lanckman, M., Robberecht, P., De Neef, P., Labrie, F., and Christophe, J. (1975): *In vitro* interactions of gastrointestinal hormones on cyclic adenosine 3′,5′-monophosphate levels and amylase output in the rat pancreas. *Gastroenterology,* 68:318–325.

82. Deschodt-Lanckman, M., Robberecht, P., De Neef, P., Lammens, M., and Christophe, J. (1976): *In vitro* action of bombesin and bombesin-like peptides on amylase secretion, calcium efflux, and adenylate cyclase activity in the rat pancreas. *J. Clin. Invest.,* 58:891–898.

83. Deutsch, J. A., and Hardy, W. T. (1977): Cholecystokinin produces bait shyness in rats. *Nature,* 266:196.

84. Dickman, S. R., Holtzer, R. L., and Gazzinelli, G. (1962): Protein synthesis by beef pancreas slices. *Biochemistry,* 1:574–580.

85. Dickman, S. R., and Morrill, G. A. (1957): Stimulation of respiration and secretion of mouse pancreas *in vitro. Am. J. Physiol.,* 190:403–407.

86. DiMagno, E. P., Go, V. L. W., and Summerskill, W. H. J. (1972): Impaired cholecystokinin-pancreozymin secretion, intraluminal dilution, and maldigestion of fat in sprue. *Gastroenterology,* 63:25–32.

87. DiMagno, E. P., Go, V. L. W., and Summerskill, W. H. J. (1973): Intraluminal and postabsorptive effects of amino acids on pancreatic enzyme secretion. *J. Lab. Clin. Med.,* 82:241–248.

88. Dinoso, Jr., V. P., Meshkinpour, H., Lorber, S. H., Gutiérrez, J. G., and Chey, W. Y. (1973): Motor responses of the sigmoid colon and rectum to exogenous cholecystokinin and secretin. *Gastroenterology,* 65:438–444.

89. Dockray, G. J. (1973): The action of gastrin and cholecystokinin-related peptides on pancreatic secretion in the rat. *Q. J. Exp. Physiol.,* 58:163–169.

90. Dockray, G. J. (1976): Immunochemical evidence of cholecystokinin-like peptides in brain. *Nature,* 264:568–570.

91. Dockray, G. J. (1977): Immunoreactive component resembling cholecystokinin octapeptide in intestine. *Nature,* 270:359–361.

92. Dockray, G. J., Gregory, R. A., Hutchison, J. B., Harris, J. I., and Runswick, M. J. (1978): Isolation, structure and biological activity of two cholecystokinin octapeptides from sheep brain. *Nature,* 274:711–713.

93. Douglas, W. W., and Rubin, R. P. (1961): The role of calcium in the secretory response of the adrenal medulla to acetylcholine. *J. Physiol.,* 159:40–57.

94. Dressler, J., Hör, G., Buttermann, G., and Pabst, H. W. (1975): PankreasFunktionsdiagnostik mit dem [75]Selen-Methionin-Test. *Münch. Med. Wochenschr.,* 117:237–240.

95. Duane, W. C., and Hanson, K. C. (1978): Role of gallbladder emptying and small bowel transit in regulation of bile acid pool size in man. *J. Lab. Clin. Med.,* 92:858–872.

96. Dubich, S. Y., and Kreknin, A. F. (1969): The effect produced by sorbitol on biliation, gastric, duodenal and pancreatic juice secretion under normal conditions and in experimental pancreatitis. *Farmakol. Toksikol.,* 32:75–78.

97. Duncan, P. R., Evans, D. G., Harper, A. A., Howat, H. T., Oleesky, S., Scott, J. E., and Varley, H. (1953): The use of the cholecystokinetic agent in preparations of pancreozymin to study gallbladder function in man. *J. Physiol.,* 121:19p–20p.

98. Duncan, P. R., Harper, A. A., Howat, H. T., Oleesky, S., and Varley, H. (1952): Tests of

gallbladder function in man. The use of preparations containing cholecystokinin. *Gastroenterologia,* 78:349–353.

99. Dunn, F. H., Christensen, E. C., Reynolds, J., Jones, V., and Fordtran, J. S. (1974): Cholecystokinin cholecystography. *JAMA,* 228:997–1003.

100. Dyck, W. P., Bonnet, D., Lasater, J., Stinson, C., and Hall, F. F. (1974): Hormonal stimulation of intestinal disaccharidase release in the dog. *Gastroenterology,* 66:533–538.

101. Dyck, W. P., Hall, F. F., and Ratliff, C. R. (1973): Hormonal control of intestinal alkaline phosphatase secretion in the dog. *Gastroenterology,* 65:445–450.

102. Dyck, W. P., Martin, G. A., and Ratliff, C. R. (1973): Influence of secretin and cholecystokinin on intestinal alkaline phosphatase secretion. *Gastroenterology,* 64:599–602.

103. Eddeland, A., and Wehlin, L. (1978): Secretin/cholecystokinin-stimulated secretion of trypsinogen and trypsin inhibitor in pure human pancreatic juice collected by endoscopic retrograde catheterization. *Hoppe Seylers Z. Physiol. Chem.,* 359:1653–1658.

104. Edholm, P., Jonson, G., and Thulin, L. (1962): Le débit biliaire du foie: Stimulation par la cholécystokinine, la sécrétine et l'alimentation per-orale. *Pathol. Biol.,* 10:447–450.

105. Eikman, E. A., Cameron, J. L., Colman, M., Natarajan, T. K., Dugal, P., and Wagner, H. N., Jr. (1975): A test for patency of the cystic duct in acute cholecystitis. *Ann. Intern. Med.,* 82:318–322.

106. Eimerl, S., Savion, N., Heichal, O., and Selinger, Z. (1974): Induction of enzyme secretion in rat pancreatic slices using the ionophore A-23187 and calcium. *J. Biol. Chem.,* 249:3991–3993.

107. Englert, E., Jr. (1973): Radioimmunoassay (RIA) of cholecystokinin (CCK). *Clin. Res.,* 21:207.

108. Erspamer, V., and Melchiorri, P. (1975): Actions of bombesin on secretions and motility of the gastrointestinal tract. In: *Gastrointestinal Peptides,* edited by J. C. Thompson, pp. 575–589. University of Texas Press, Austin and London.

109. Ertan, A. (1975): Nouvelle méthode d'exploration de la fonction exocrine du pancréas. *Arch. Fr. Mal. App. Dig.,* 64:107–114.

110. Ertan, A., Brooks, F. P., Arvan, D., and Williams, C. N. (1975): Mechanism of release of endogenous cholecystokinin by jejunal amino acid perfusion in man. *Am. J. Dig. Dis.,* 20:813–823.

111. Ertan, A., Brooks, F. P., Ostrow, J. D., Arvan, D. A., Williams, C. N., and Cerda, J. J. (1971): Effect of jejunal amino acid perfusion and exogenous cholecystokinin on the exocrine pancreatic and biliary secretions in man. *Gastroenterology,* 61:686–692.

112. Fara, J. W., and Erde, S. M. (1978): Comparison of *in vivo* and *in vitro* responses to sulfated and non-sulfated ceruletide. *Eur. J. Pharmacol.,* 47:359–363.

113. Fara, J. W., Praissman, M., and Berkowitz, J. M. (1979): Interaction between gastrin, CCK, and secretin on canine antral smooth muscle *in vitro. Am. J. Physiol.,* 236:E39–E44.

114. Fender, H. R., Curtis, P. J., Rayford, P. L., and Thompson, J. C. (1976): Effect of bombesin on serum gastrin and cholecystokinin in dogs. *Surg. Forum,* 26:414–416.

115. Fisher, R., and Cohen, S. (1973): Physiological characteristics of the human pyloric sphincter. *Gastroenterology,* 64:67–75.

116. Fisher, R. S., Lipshulz, W., and Cohen, S. (1973): The hormonal regulation of pyloric sphincter function. *J. Clin. Invest.,* 52:1289–1296.

117. Fischer, W. S., Smith, B. M., and Jones, R. S. (1973): Analysis of bile formation in guinea pigs. *Surg. Forum,* 24:407–408.

118. Fölsch, U. R., Winckler, K., and Wormsley, K. G. (1978): Influence of repeated administration of cholecystokinin and secretin on the pancreas of the rat. *Scand. J. Gastroenterol.,* 13:663–671.

119. Fölsch, U. R., and Wormsley, K. G. (1973): Pancreatic enzyme response to secretin and cholecystokinin-pancreozymin in the rat. *J. Physiol.,* 234:79–94.

120. Forell, M. M., and Stahlheber, H. (1966): Gallefluβ und Pankreassekretion. *Klin. Wochenschr.,* 44:1184–1189.

121. Foss, D. C., and Laing, R. R. (1977): Detection of gallbladder disease in patients with normal oral cholecystograms. *Am. J. Dig. Dis.,* 22:685–689.

122. Frame, C. M., Davidson, M. B., and Sturdevant, R. A. L. (1975): Effects of the octapeptide of cholecystokinin on insulin and glucagon secretion in the dog. *Endocrinology,* 97:549–553.

123. Freeman, J. B., Cohen, W. N., and DenBesten, L. (1975): Cholecystokinin cholangiography and analysis of duodenal bile in the investigation of pain in the right upper quadrant of the abdomen without gallstones. *Surg. Gynecol. Obstet.,* 140:371–376.

124. Frenkel, L. D., Javitt, N. B., and McSherry, C. K. (1971): Cholecystadenoma and the use of cholecystokinin. *J. Pediatr.,* 79:468–470.
125. Friedman, M. H. F., and Snape, W. J. (1945): Comparative effectiveness of extracts of intestinal mucosa in stimulating the external secretions of the pancreas and the liver. *Fed. Proc.,* 4:21–22.
126. Frigo, G. M., Lecchini, S., Falaschi, C., DelTacca, M., and Crema, A. (1971): On the ability of caerulein to increase propulsive activity in the isolated small and large intestine. *Naunyn Schmiedeberg's Arch. Pharmakol.,* 268:44–58.
127. Fritz, M. E., and Brooks, F. P. (1963): Control of bile flow in the cholecystectomized dog. *Am. J. Physiol.,* 204:825–828.
128. Frölich, Ch., Locher, M., and von Oldershausen, H. F. (1973): Die Beeinflussung des exokrinen Pankreas durch die intravenöse Infusion einer Nährlösung. *Klin. Wochenschr.,* 51:1207–1209.
129. Frühling, J., Vincent, J.-L., van der Hoeden, R., and Delcourt, A. (1975): Correlation between isotopic scanning and pancreatic function tests in the diagnosis of pancreatic diseases: Image and digital computer techniques. *Int. J. Nucl. Med. Biol.,* 2:145–152.
130. Galardy, R. E., and Jamieson, J. D. (1975): Photoaffinity labeling of secretagogue receptors in the pancreatic exocrine cell. In: *Gastrointestinal Hormones,* edited by J. C. Thompson, 345–365. University of Texas Press, Austin and London.
131. Gardiner, B. N., Conaway, C., and Small, D. M. (1975): Effects of secretin and cholecystokinin on relative composition of hepatic bile in rhesus monkeys. *Surg. Forum,* 26:437–439.
132. Gardner, J. D., Conlon, T. P., Klaeveman, H. L., Adams, T. D., and Ondetti, M. A. (1975): Action of cholecystokinin and cholinergic agents on calcium transport in isolated pancreatic acinar cells. *J. Clin. Invest.,* 56:366–375.
133. Gardner, J. D., and Hahne, W. F. (1977): Calcium transport in dispersed acinar cells from rat pancreas. *Biochim. Biophys. Acta,* 471:466–476.
134. Gardner, J. D., and Jackson, M. J. (1977): Regulation of amylase release from dispersed pancreatic acinar cells. *J. Physiol.,* 270:439–454.
135. Geller, L. I., Bulgakova, O. S., and Petrenko, V. F. (1978): Effect of pancreozymin on the absorptive function of hepatocytes and the rate of the blood flow in the liver in chronic relapsing pancreatitis. *Klin. Med. (USSR),* 56:72–76.
136. Gerner, T. (1979): Pressure responses to OP-CCK compared to CCK-PZ in the antrum and fundus of isolated guinea-pig stomachs. *Scand. J. Gastroenterol.,* 14:73–77.
137. Gerner, T., and Haffner, J. F. W. (1977): The role of local cholinergic pathways in the motor response to cholecystokinin and gastrin in isolated guinea pig fundus and antrum. *Scand. J. Gastroenterol.,* 12:751–757.
138. Gerner, T., Haffner, J. F. W., and Norstein, J. (1979): The effects of mepyramine and cimetidine on the motor responses to histamine, cholecystokinin, and gastrin in the fundus and antrum of isolated guinea pig stomachs. *Scand. J. Gastroenterol.,* 14:65–72.
139. Gershbein, L. L., Denton, R. W., and Hubbard, B. W. (1953): *In vitro* assay of cholecystokinin concentrates. *J. Appl. Physiol.,* 5:712–716.
140. Gershbein, L. L., Wang, C. C., and Ivy, A. C. (1949): Assay of secretin and cholecystokinin concentrates. *Proc. Soc. Exp. Biol. Med.,* 70:516–521.
141. Ghosh, M. N., and Schild, H. O. (1958): Continuous recording of acid gastric secretion in the rat. *Br. J. Pharmacol.,* 13:54–61.
142. Gibbs, J., Young, R. C., and Smith, G. P. (1973): Cholecystokinin decreases food intake in rats. *J. Comp. Physiol. Psychol.,* 84:488–495.
143. Gillespie, I. E., and Grossman, M. I. (1964): Inhibitory effect of secretin and cholecystokinin on Heidenhain pouch responses to gastrin extract and histamine. *Gut,* 5:342–345.
144. Glick, Z., and Modan, M. (1977): Behavioral compensatory responses to continuous duodenal and upper ileal glucose infusion in rats. *Physiol. Behav.,* 19:703–705.
145. Glick, Z., Thomas, D. W., and Mayer, J. (1971): Absence of effect of injections of the intestinal hormones secretin and cholecystokinin-pancreozymin upon feeding behavior. *Physiol. Behav.,* 6:5–8.
146. Go, V. L. W., Hofmann, A. F., and Summerskill, W. H. J. (1970): Pancreozymin bioassay in man based on pancreatic enzyme secretion: Potency of specific amino acids and other digestive products. *J. Clin. Invest.,* 49:1558–1564.
147. Go, V. L. W., Ryan, R. J., and Summerskill, W. H. J. (1971): Radioimmunoassay of porcine cholecystokinin-pancreozymin. *J. Lab. Clin. Med.,* 77:684–689.
148. Goebell, H., Bode, C., and Horn, H. D. (1970): Einfluβ von Sekretin und Pankreozymin

auf die Calciumsekretion im menschlichen Duodenalsaft bei normaler und gestörter Pankreas-funktion. *Klin. Wochenschr.*, 48:1330–1339.

149. Goldstein, F., Grunt, R., and Margulies, M. (1974): Cholecystokinin cholecystography in the differential diagnosis of acalculous gallbladder disease. *Am. J. Dig. Dis.*, 19:835–849.

150. Goriya, Y., Hoshi, M., Etani, N., Kimura, K., Shichiri, M., and Shigeta, Y. (1975): Dynamic study of exocrine function of the pancreas in diabetes mellitus with scintigraphy using ^{75}Se-selenomethionine. *J. Nucl. Med.*, 16:270–274.

151. Götze, H., Götze, J., and Adelson, J. W. (1978): Studies on intestinal enzyme secretion: The action of cholecystokinin-pancreozymin, pentagastrin and bile. *Res. Exp. Med. (Berl.)*, 173:17–25.

152. Green, G. M., and Lyman, R. L. (1972): Feedback regulation of pancreatic enzyme secretion as a mechanism for trypsin inhibitor-induced hypersecretion in rats. *Proc. Soc. Exp. Biol. Med.*, 140:6–12.

153. Greenway, F. L., and Bray, G. A. (1977): Cholecystokinin and satiety. *Life Sci.*, 21:769–772.

154. Greenwell, J. R. (1975): The effects of cholecystokinin-pancreozymin acetylcholine and secretin on the membrane potentials of mouse pancreatic cells *in vitro*. *Pflügers Arch.*, 353:159–170.

155. Gregory, H., Hardy, P. M., Jones, D. S., Kenner, G. W., and Sheppard, R. C. (1964): The antral hormone gastrin. *Nature*, 204:931–933.

156. Gregory, R. A., and Tracy, H. J. (1964): The constitution and properties of two gastrins extracted from hog antral mucosa. *Gut*, 5:103–117.

157. Grossman, M. I. (1970): Proposal: Use the term cholecystokinin in place of cholecystokinin-pancreozymin. *Gastroenterology*, 58:128.

158. Grossman, M. I. (1973): Spectrum of biological actions of gastrointestinal hormones. In: *Frontiers in Gastrointestinal Hormone Research*, edited by S. Andersson, pp. 17–28. Almqvist & Wiksell, Stockholm.

159. Grossman, M. I. (1977): Physiological effects of gastrointestinal hormones. *Fed. Proc.*, 36:1930–1932.

160. Grube, D., Maier, V., Raptis, S., and Schlegel, W. (1978): Immunoreactivity of the endocrine pancreas. Evidence for the presence of cholecystokinin-pancreozymin within the A-cell. *Histochemistry*, 56:13–35.

161. Guelrud, M., Rudick, J., and Janowitz, H. D. (1971): Endogenous cyclic AMP and pancreatic enzyme secretion. *Gastroenterology*, 60:671.

162. Gutiérrez, J. G., Chey, W. Y., and Dinoso, V. P. (1974): Actions of cholecystokinin and secretin on the motor activity of the small intestine in man. *Gastroenterology*, 67:35–41.

163. Haig, T. H. B. (1974): Regulation of pancreatic acinar function: Effects of cyclic AMP, dibutyryl cyclic AMP, and theophylline in vitro. *Can. J. Physiol. Pharmacol.*, 52:780–785.

164. Harper, A. A., Blair, E. L., and Scratcherd, T. (1962): The distribution and physiological properties of pancreozymin. In: *CIBA Foundation Symposium on The Exocrine Pancreas.*, edited by A. V. S. de Reuck, and M. P. Cameron, 168–185. J. and A. Churchill, London.

165. Harper, A. A., and Raper, H. S. (1943): Pancreozymin, a stimulant of the secretion of pancreatic enzymes in extracts of the small intestine. *J. Physiol.*, 102:115–125.

166. Harper, A. A., and Vass, C. C. N. (1941): The control of the external secretion of the pancreas in cats. *J. Physiol.*, 99:415–435.

167. Harvey, R. F. (1976): Physiology and pathophysiology of cholecystokinin-pancreozymin. *J. Endocrinol.*, 70:5P–6P.

168. Harvey, R. F., Dowsett, L., Hartog, M., and Read, A. E. (1974): Radioimmunoassay of cholecystokinin-pancreozymin. *Gut*, 15:690–699.

169. Harvey, R. F., Dowsett, L., and Read, A. E. (1974): Studies on the nature of cholecystokinin-pancreozymin in small-intestinal mucosal extracts. *Gut*, 15:838–839.

170. Harvey, R. F., and Read, A. E. (1973): Effect of cholecystokinin on colonic motility and symptoms in patients with the irritable-bowel syndrome. *Lancet*, i:7793–7795.

171. Harvey, R. F., and Read, A. E. (1973): Saline purgatives act by releasing cholecystokinin. *Lancet*, i:185–187.

172. Haymovits, A., and Scheele, G. A. (1976): Cellular cyclic nucleotides and enzyme secretion in the pancreatic acinar cell. *Proc. Natl. Acad. Sci. USA*, 73:156–160.

173. Heatley, N. G. (1968): The assay of pancreozymin, and of secretin and pancreozymin simultaneously, in the rat. *J. Endocrinol.*, 42:549–557.

174. Hedner, P., Persson, H., and Rorsman, G. (1967): Effect of cholecystokinin on small intestine. *Acta Physiol. Scand.,* 70:250–254.
175. Hedner, P., and Rorsman, G. (1968): Structures essential for the effect of cholecystokinin on the guinea pig small intestine *in vitro. Acta Physiol. Scand.,* 74:58–68.
176. Heisler, S. (1976): Effects of an ATP analogue (α,β-methylene-adenosine-5'-triphosphate) on cyclic AMP and cyclic GMP levels, ^{45}Ca efflux, and protein secretion from rat pancreas. *Can. J. Physiol. Pharmacol.,* 54:692–697.
177. Heisler, S. (1976): Calcium and cyclic nucleotide involvement in exocrine pancreatic enzyme secretion studied with the ionophore A-23187. *Life Sci.,* 19:233–242.
178. Heisler, S., Fast, D., and Tenenhouse, A. (1972): Role of Ca^{2+} and cyclic AMP in protein secretion from rat exocrine pancreas. *Biochim. Biophys. Acta,* 279:561–572.
179. Heisler, S., Grondin, G., and Forget, G. (1974): The effect of various secretagogues on accumulation of cyclic AMP and secretion of α-amylase from rat exocrine pancreas. *Life Sci.,* 14:631–639.
180. Hepner, G. W. (1975): Effect of decreased gallbladder stimulation on enterohepatic cycling and kinetics of bile acids. *Gastroenterology,* 68:1574–1581.
181. Herzog, R. J., and Nelson, J. A. (1976): The role of cholecystokinin in radiographic opacification of the gallbladder. *Invest. Radiol.,* 11:440–447.
182. Hinz, M., Katsilambros, N., Schweitzer, B., Raptis, S., and Pfeiffer, E. F. (1971): The role of the exocrine pancreas in the stimulation of insulin secretion by intestinal hormones. *Diabetologia,* 7:1–5.
183. Hokin, L. E. (1966): Effects of calcium omission on acetylcholine-stimulated amylase secretion and phospholipid synthesis in pigeon pancreas slices. *Biochim. Biophys. Acta,* 115:219–221.
184. Hokin, L. E. (1967): Metabolic aspects and energetics of pancreatic secretion. *Hdbk. Physiol. Aliment. Canal Sect.,* 6:935–953.
185. Hokin, L. E., and Hokin, M. R. (1956): The actions of pancreozymin in pancreas slices and the role of phospholipids in enzyme secretion. *J. Physiol.,* 132:442–453.
186. Holtermüller, K. H., Malagelada, J.-R., McCall, J. T., and Go, V. L. W. (1976): Pancreatic, gallbladder, and gastric responses to intraduodenal calcium perfusion in man. *Gastroenterology,* 70:693–696.
187. Holtermüller, K. H., Sinterhauf, K., Konicek, S., and Müller, V. (1976): Intraduodenales Magnesium stimuliert die Pankreasenzymsekretion und Gallenblasenentleerung beim Menschen. *Verh. Dtsch. Ges. Inn. Med.,* 82:978–980.
188. Hong, S. S., Magee, D. F., and Crewdson, F. (1956): The physiologic regulation of gall bladder evacuation. *Gastroenterology,* 30:625–630.
189. Hotz, J., Swicker, M., Minne, H., and Ziegler, R. (1975): Pancreatic enzyme secretion in the conscious rat. *Pflügers Arch.,* 353:171–189.
190. Hughes, C. A., Bates, T., and Dowling, R. H. (1978): Cholecystokinin and secretin prevent the intestinal mucosal hypoplasia of total parenteral nutrition in the dog. *Gastroenterology,* 75:34–41.
191. Hughes, J., Smith, T. W., Kosterlitz, H. W., Fothergill, L. A., Morgan, B. A., and Morris, H. R. (1975): Identification of two related pentapeptides from the brain with potent opiate agonist activity. *Nature,* 258:577–579.
192. Hultman, E. H. (1955): A method for the standardization of cholecystokinin in vitro. *Acta Physiol. Scand.,* 33:291–295.
193. Hunter, W. M., and Greenwood, F. C. (1962): Preparation of iodine-131 labelled human growth hormone of high specific activity. *Nature,* 194:495–496.
194. Ihse, I., Arnesjö, B., and Lundquist, I. (1975): Studies on the reversibility of oral trypsin inhibitor induced changes of rat pancreatic exocrine enzyme activity and insulin secretory capacity. *Scand. J. Gastroenterol.,* 10:321–326.
195. Ihse, I., Arnesjö, B., and Lundquist, I. (1976): Effects of exocrine and endocrine rat pancreas of long-term administration of CCK-PZ (cholecystokinin-pancreozymin) or synthetic octapeptide-CCK-PZ. *Scand. J. Gastroenterol.,* 11:529–535.
196. Ipp, E., Dobbs, R. E., Harris, V., Arimura, A., Vale, W., and Unger, R. H. (1977): The effects of gastrin, gastric inhibitory polypeptide, secretin, and the octapeptide of cholecystokinin upon immunoreactive somatostatin release by the perfused canine pancreas. *J. Clin. Invest.,* 60:1216–1219.
197. Isenberg, J. I., and Csendes, A. (1972): Effect of octapeptide of cholecystokinin on canine pyloric pressure. *Am. J. Physiol.,* 222:428–431.

198. Ivy, A. C., and Janecek, H. M. (1959): Assay of Jorpes-Mutt secretin and cholecystokinin. *Acta Physiol. Scand.,* 45:220–230.
199. Ivy, A. C., Kloster, G., Lueth, H. C., and Drewyer, G. E. (1929): On the preparation of "cholecystokinin." *Am. J. Physiol.,* 91:336–344.
200. Ivy, A. C., and Oldberg, E. (1928): A hormone mechanism for gallbladder contraction and evacuation. *Am. J. Physiol.,* 86:599–613.
201. Iwatsuki, N., and Petersen, O. H. (1978): *In vitro* action of bombesin on amylase secretion, membrane potential, and membrane resistance in rat and mouse pancreatic acinar cells. *J. Clin. Invest.,* 61:41–46.
202. Iwatsuki, N., and Petersen, O. H. (1978): Electrical coupling and uncoupling of exocrine acinar cells. *J. Cell Biol.,* 79:533–545.
203. Jamieson, J. D. (1978): Properties of the plasmalemma of pancreatic acinar cells: Secretagogue receptors, cell surface saccharides and their interrelationships for exocytosis. *J. Physiol.,* 285:26P–27P.
204. Jensen, R. T., Moody, T., Pert, C., Rivier, J. E., and Gardner, J. D. (1978): Interaction of bombesin and litorin with specific membrane receptors on pancreatic acinar cells. *Proc. Natl. Acad. Sci. USA,* 75:6139–6143.
205. Johnson, A. G., and McDermott, S. J. (1973): Sensitive bioassay of cholecystokinin in human serum. *Lancet,* ii:589–591.
206. Johnson, A. G., and Marshall, C. E. (1976): The effect of cholecystectomy on serum cholecystokinin bioactivity. *Br. J. Surg.,* 63:153–154.
207. Johnson, L. P., and Magee, D. F. (1965): Cholecystokinin-pancreozymin extracts and gastric motor inhibition. *Surg. Gynecol. Obstet.,* 121:557–562.
208. Johnson, L. R. (1976): The trophic action of gastrointestinal hormones. *Gastroenterology,* 70:278–288.
209. Johnson, L. R., Aures, D., and Yuen, L. (1969): Pentagastrin-induced stimulation of protein synthesis in the gastrointestinal tract. *Am. J. Physiol.,* 217:251–254.
210. Johnson, L. R., and Grossman, M. I. (1969): Characteristics of inhibition of gastric secretion by secretin. *Am. J. Physiol.,* 217:1401–1404.
211. Johnson, L. R., and Grossman, M. I. (1970): Analysis of inhibition of acid secretion by cholecystokinin in dogs. *Am. J. Physiol.,* 218:550–554.
212. Johnson, L. R., and Guthrie, P. (1976): Effect of cholecystokinin and 16,16-dimethyl prostaglandin E_2 on RNA and DNA of gastric and duodenal mucosa. *Gastroenterology,* 70:59–65.
213. Johnson, L. R., Stening, G. F., and Grossman, M. I. (1970): Effect of sulfation on the gastrointestinal actions of caerulein. *Gastroenterology,* 58:208–216.
214. Jones, R. S. (1976): Effect of insulin on canalicular bile formation. *Am. J. Physiol.,* 231: 40–43.
215. Jones, R. S., and Grossman, M. I. (1970): Choleretic effects of cholecystokinin, gastrin II, and caerulein in the dog. *Am. J. Physiol.,* 219:1014–1018.
216. Jorpes, J. E., and Mutt, V. (1961): The gastrointestinal hormones, secretin and cholecystokinin-pancreozymin. *Ann. Intern. Med.,* 55:395–405.
217. Jorpes, E., and Mutt, V. (1966): Cholecystokinin and pancreozymin one single hormone? *Acta Physiol. Scand.,* 66:196–202.
218. Jorpes, E., Mutt, V., and Toczko, K. (1964): Further purification of cholecystokinin and pancreozymin. *Acta Chem. Scand.,* 18:2408–2410.
219. Jung, F. T., and Greengard, H. (1933): Response of the isolated gallbladder to cholecystokinin. *Am. J. Physiol.,* 103:275–278.
220. Kaminski, D. L., Ruwart, M. J., and Jellinek, M. (1977): Structure-function relationships of peptide fragments of gastrin and cholecystokinin. *Am. J. Physiol.,* 233:E286–292.
221. Kaneto, A., Tasaka Y., Kosaka, K., and Nakao, K. (1969): Stimulation of insulin secretion by the C-terminal tetrapeptide amide of gastrin. *Endocrinology,* 84:1098–1106.
222. Kanno, T. (1972): Calcium-dependent amylase release and electrophysiological measurements in cells of the pancreas. *J. Physiol.,* 226:353–371.
223. Kanno, T. (1975): The electrogenic sodium pump in the hyperpolarizing and secretory effects of pancreozymin in the pancreatic acinar cell. *J. Physiol.,* 245:599–616.
224. Kanno, T., and Imai, S. (1976): Stimulus-secretion coupling in the cell secreting cholecystokinin-pancreozymin. In: *Endocrine Gut and Pancreas,* edited by T. Fujita, 245–254. Elsevier, Amsterdam.
225. Kanno, T., and Saito, A. (1978): Influence of external potassium concentration on secretory

responses to cholecystokinin-pancreozymin and ionophore A23187 in the pancreatic acinar cell. *J. Physiol.,* 278:251–263.

226. Kanno, T., and Yamamoto, M. (1977): Differentiation between the calcium-dependent effects of cholecystokinin-pancreozymin and the bicarbonate-dependent effects of secretin in exocrine secretion of the rat pancreas. *J. Physiol.,* 264:787–799.

227. Kelly, G. A., Rose, R. C., and Nahrwold, D. L. (1977): Characteristics of inhibition of pancreatic secretion by isoproterenol. *Surgery,* 82:680–684.

228. Kempen, H. J. M., De Pont, J. J. H. H. M., and Bonting, S. L. (1974): Rat pancreas adenylate cyclase. II. Inactivation and protection of its hormone receptor sites. *Biochim. Biophys. Acta,* 370:573–584.

229. Kirchmayer, S., Tarnawski, A., Droźdź, H., and Cichecka, K. (1972): Effect of cholecystokinin-pancreozymin and secretin on the volume, composition, and enzymatic activity of hepatic bile in rabbits. *Gut,* 13:709–712.

230. Knodell, R. G., Toskes, P. P., Reber, H. A., and Brooks, F. P. (1970): Significance of cyclic AMP in the regulation of exocrine pancreas secretion. *Experientia,* 26:515–517.

231. Kondo, S., and Schulz, I. (1976): Calcium ion uptake in isolated pancreas cells induced by secretagogues. *Biochim. Biophys. Acta,* 419:76–92.

232. Konturek, S. J., Becker, H. D., and Thompson, J. C. (1974): Effect of vagotomy on hormones stimulating pancreatic secretion. *Arch. Surg.,* 108:704–708.

233. Kotler, D. P., and Levine, G. M. (1978): Reversible gastric and pancreatic hyposecretion after long-term total parenteral nutrition. *N. Engl. J. Med.,* 300:241–242.

234. Kraly, F. S., Carty, W. J., Resnick, S., and Smith, G. P. (1978): Effect of cholecystokinin on meal size and intermeal interval in the shamfeeding rat. *J. Comp. Physiol. Psychol.,* 92:697–707.

235. Kulka, R. G., and Sternlicht, E. (1968): Enzyme secretion in mouse pancreas mediated by adenosine-3'5'-cyclic phosphate and inhibited by adenosine-3'-phosphate. *Proc. Natl. Acad. Sci. USA,* 61:1123–1128.

236. Lai, K. S. (1964): Studies on Gastrin. *Gut,* 5:327–341.

237. Lambert, M., Camus, J., and Christophe, J. (1973): Pancreozymin and caerulein stimulate in vitro protein phosphorylation in the rat pancreas. *Biochem. Biophys. Res. Commun.,* 52:935–942.

238. Lambert, M., Svoboda, M., and Christophe, J. (1979): Hormone-stimulated GTPase activity in rat pancreatic plasma membranes. *FEBS Lett.,* 99:303–307.

239. Larsson, L. I., and Rehfeld, J. F. (1978): Distribution of gastrin and CCK cells in the rat gastrointestinal tract. *Histochemistry,* 58:23–31.

240. Larsson, L. I., and Rehfeld, J. F. (1979): A peptide resembling COOH-terminal tetrapeptide amide of gastrin from a new gastrointestinal endocrine cell type. *Nature,* 277:575–578.

241. Van Leemput-Coutrez, M., Camus, J., and Christophe, J. (1973): Cyclic nucleotide-dependent protein kinases of the rat pancreas. *Biochem. Biophys. Res. Commun.,* 54:182–190.

242. Leroy, J., Morisset, J. A., and Webster, P. D. (1971): Dose-related response of pancreatic synthesis and secretion to cholecystokinin-pancreozymin. *J. Lab. Clin. Med.,* 78:149–157.

243. Lin, T. M., and Alphin, R. S. (1962): Comparative bio-assay of secretin and pancreozymin in rats and dogs. *Am. J. Physiol.,* 203:926–928.

244. Lin, T. M., and Grossman, M. I. (1956): Dose response relationship of pancreatic enzyme stimulants: Pancreozymin and metacholine. *Am. J. Physiol.,* 186:52–56.

245. Lindelöf, G., and van der Linden, W. (1965): The role of stasis in experimental gallstone formation. *Acta Chir. Scand.,* 130:494–498.

246. Ljungberg, S. (1969): Biological assay of cholecystokinin in guinea pig gallbladder *in situ. Acta Pharm. Suecica,* 6:599–606.

247. Long, B. W., and Gardner, J. D. (1977): Effects of cholecystokinin on adenylate cyclase activity in dispersed pancreatic acinar cells. *Gastroenterology,* 73:1008–1014.

248. Long, W. B., and Weiss, J. B. (1973): Rapid gastric emptying of fatty meals in pancreatic insufficiency. *Gastroenterology,* 64:763.

249. Low-Beer, T. S., Harvey R. T., Nolan, Y. D., Davies, E. R., and Read, A. E. (1974): Abnormalities of cholecystokinin secretion and gallbladder emptying in coeliac disease. *Gut,* 15:338.

250. Low-Beer, T. S., Heaton, K. W., and Read, A. E. (1970): Gallbladder inertia in adult coeliac disease. *Gut,* 11:1057–1058.

251. Lucas, M., Schmid, G., Kromas, R., and Löffler, G. (1978): Calcium metabolism and enzyme secretion in guinea pig pancreas. *Eur. J. Biochem.,* 85:609–619.

252. McDonald, J. K., Callahan, P. X., and Ellis, S. (1972): Preparation and specificity of dipeptidyl aminopeptidase I. *Methods Enzymol.,* 25:272–281.
253. MacDonald, R. J., and Ronzio, R. A. (1974): Phosphorylation of a zymogen granule membrane polypeptide from rat pancreas. *FEBS Lett.,* 40:203–206.
254. McGuigan, J. E. (1968): Antibodies to the C-terminal tetrapeptide amide of gastrin. *Gastroenterology,* 54:1012–1017.
255. Maddison, S. (1977): Intraperitoneal and intracranial cholecystokinin depress operant responding for food. *Physiol. Behav.,* 19:819–824.
256. Magee, D. F., and Dutt, Br. (1972): Effect of pure and commercial cholecystokinin and an inhibitory polypeptide on gastric secretion. *Am. J. Physiol.,* 222:73–76.
257. Magee, D. F., and Nakamura, M. (1966): Action of pancreozymin preparations on gastric secretion. *Nature,* 212:1487–1488.
258. Mainz, D. L., Black, O., and Webster, P. D. (1973): Hormonal control of pancreatic growth. *J. Clin. Invest.,* 52:2300–2304.
259. Malagelada, J.-R., DiMagno, E. P., Summerskill, W. H. J., and Go, V. L. W. (1976): Regulation of pancreatic and gallbladder functions by intraluminal fatty acids and bile acids in man. *J. Clin. Invest.,* 58:493–499.
260. Malagelada, J. R., Go, V. L. W., and Summerskill, W. H. J. (1973): Differing sensitivities of gallbladder and pancreas to cholecystokinin-pancreozymin (CCK-PZ) in man. *Gastroenterology,* 64:950–954.
261. Marois, C., Morisset, J., and Dunnigan, J. (1972): Presence and stimulation of adenyl cyclase in pancreas homogenate. *Rev. Can. Biol.,* 31:253–257.
262. Marshall, C. E., Egberts, E. H., and Johnson, A. G. (1978): An improved method for estimating cholecystokinin in human serum. *J. Endocrinol.,* 79:17–27.
263. Matthews, E. K., and Petersen, O. H. (1973): Pancreatic acinar cells: Ionic dependence of the membrane potential and acetylcholine-induced depolarization. *J. Physiol.,* 231:283–295.
264. Matthews, E. K., Petersen, O. H., and Williams, J. A. (1973): Pancreatic acinar cells: Acetylcholine-induced membrane depolarization, calcium efflux and amylase release. *J. Physiol.,* 234:689–701.
265. del Mazo, J. (1977): Measurement of immunoreactive CCK-PZ in the GI tract and in the central nervous system of several animal species. *Gastroenterology,* 72:1047.
266. Meade, R. C., Kneubuhler, H. A., Schulte, W. J., and Barboriak, J. J. (1967): Stimulation of insulin secretion by pancreozymin. *Diabetes,* 16:141–144.
267. Meyer, J. H., and Grossman, M. I. (1972): Comparison of d- and l-phenylalanine as pancreatic stimulants. *Am. J. Physiol.,* 222:1058–1063.
268. Meyer, J. H., and Jones, R. S. (1974): Canine pancreatic responses to intestinally perfused fat and products of fat digestion. *Am. J. Physiol.,* 226:1178–1187.
269. Meyer, J. H., Kelly, G. A., and Jones, R. S. (1976): Canine pancreatic response to intestinally perfused oligopeptides. *Am. J. Physiol.,* 231:678–681.
270. Meyer, J. H. Kelly, G. A., Spingola, L. J., and Jones, R. S. (1976): Canine gut receptors mediating pancreatic responses to luminal l-amino acids. *Am. J. Physiol.,* 231:669–677.
271. Meyer, J. H., Spingola, L. J., and Grossman, M. I. (1971): Endogenous cholecystokinin potentiates exogenous secretin on pancreas of dog. *Am. J. Physiol.,* 221:742–747.
272. Mongeau, R., Couture, Y., Dunnigan, J., and Morisset, J. (1974): Early dissociation of protein synthesis and amylase secretion following hormonal stimulation of the pancreas. *Can. J. Physiol. Pharmacol.,* 52:198–205.
273. Monod, M. E. (1964): Action entérokinétique de la cécékine. *Arch. Mal. App. Dig.,* 53:607–608.
274. Monod, M. E. (1971): Modification de la technique d'accélération du transit grêle par la cécékine. *Arch. Fr. App. Dig.,* 60:141–142.
275. Morgan, K. G., Schmalz, P. F., Go, V. L. W., and Szurszewski, J. H. (1978): Electrical and mechanical effects of molecular variants of CCK on antral smooth muscle. *Am. J. Physiol.,* 235:E324–E329.
276. Morin, G., Besancon, Fr., Grall, A., Debray, Ch., and Garat, J.-P. (1966): La cholécystokinine appliquée au radiodiagnostic usuel de l íntestin grêle: nouvelle technique de radiocinématographie complète en quelques minutes, avec 62 observations. *Radiologie,* 9:247–250.
277. Morin, G., Grall, A., Jouve, R., Bellin, A., and Debray, C. (1968): La technique du grêle accéléré par la cécékine. Bilan de 250 examens. *Arch. Mal. App. Dig.,* 57:956–962.
278. Morisset, J. A., and Webster, P. D. (1971): *In vitro* and *in vivo* effects of pancreozymin, urecholine, and cyclic AMP on rat pancreas. *Am. J. Physiol.,* 230:202–208.

279. Morton, R. K. (1950): Separation and purification of enzymes associated with insoluble particles. *Nature,* 166:1092–1095.
280. Moss, S., Lobley, R. W., and Holmes, R. (1972): Enterokinase in human duodenal juice following secretin and pancreozymin. *Arch. Fr. Mal. App. Dig.,* 61:214c.
281. Muller, J. E., Straus, E., and Yalow, R. S. (1977): Cholecystokinin and its COOH-terminal octapeptide in the pig brain. *Proc. Natl. Acad. Sci. USA,* 74:3035–3037.
282. Murat, J. E., and White, T. T. (1966): Stimulation of gastric secretion by commercial cholecystokinin extracts. *Proc. Soc. Exp. Biol. Med.,* 123:593–594.
283. Murillo, A., and Lopez M. A. (1971): Contribución al estudio de la regulación hormonal de la secreción pancreática en el conejo. *Rev. Esp. Fisiol.,* 27:131–138.
284. Mutt, V. (1976): Further investigations on intestinal hormonal polypeptides. *Clin. Endocrinol. (Suppl.),* 5:175s–183s.
285. Mutt, V., and Jorpes, J. E. (1968): Structure of porcine cholecystokinin-pancreozymin. 1. Cleavage with thrombin and with trypsin. *Eur. J. Biochem.,* 6:156–162.
286. Mutt, V., and Jorpes, E. (1971): Hormonal polypeptides of the upper intestine. *Biochem. J.,* 125:57p–58p.
287. Mutt, V., Magnusson, S., Jorpes, J. E., and Dahl, E. (1965): Structure of porcine secretin. I. Degradation with trypsin and thrombin. Sequence of the tryptic peptides. The C-terminal residue. *Biochemistry,* 4:2358–2362.
288. Mutt, V., and Said, S. I. (1974): Structure of the porcine vasoactive intestinal octacosapeptide. The amino-acid sequence. Use of kallikrein in its determination. *Eur. J. Biochem.,* 42:581–589.
289. Naito, S., Iwata, R., and Saito, T. (1963): Etudes sur la cholécystokinine, son mode d'action sur la contraction de la vésicule biliaire. *Presse Med.,* 55:2688–2689.
290. Nakajima, S., Hirschowitz, B. I., Shoemaker, R. L., and Sachs, G. (1971): Inhibition of gastric acid secretion *in vitro* by C-terminal octapeptide of cholecystokinin. *Am. J. Physiol.,* 221:1009–1013.
291. Nakajima, S., and Magee, D. F. (1970): Inhibitory action of cholecystokinin-pancreozymin on gastric pepsin secretion. *Experientia,* 26:159.
292. Nakajima, S., Toda, Y., Hayakawa, T., Suzuki, T., and Noda, A. (1973): Secretory characteristics of pancreatic γ-glutamyl transpeptidase. *Pflügers Arch.,* 345:271–279.
293. Nakayama, S. (1974): The effects of secretin and cholecystokinin on the sphincter muscles. In: *Gastro-Entero-Pancreatic-Endocrine System,* edited by I. Fujika, pp. 145–154. Ikagu Shoiu, Okayama, Japan.
294. Nasset, E. S. (1972): Succus entericus secretion stimulated by cholecystokinin and its C-terminal octapeptide. *Fed. Proc.,* 31:354.
295. Nathan, M. H., Newman, A., and Murray, D. J. (1978): Normal findings in oral cholecystokinin cholecystography. *JAMA,* 240:2271–2272.
296. Nathan, M. H., Newman, A., Murray, D. J., and Camponovo, R. (1970): Cholecystokinin cholecystography. A four year evaluation. *Am. J. Roentg. Radium Ther. Nucl. Med.,* 110:240–251.
297. Nemeroff, C. B., Osbahr, A. J. III., Bissette, G., Jahnke, G., Lipton, M. A., and Prange, A. J., Jr. (1978): Cholecystokinin inhibits tail pinch-induced eating in rats. *Science,* 200:793–794.
298. Neschis, M., King, M. C., and Murphy, R. A. (1978): Cholecystokinin cholecystography in the diagnosis of acalculous extrahepatic biliary tract disorders. *Am. J. Gastroenterol.,* 70:593–599.
299. Nilsson, A. (1970): Gastrointestinal hormones in the holocephalian fish *Chimaera monstrosa* (L.) *Comp. Biochem. Physiol.,* 32:387–390.
300. Nishiyama, A., and Petersen, O. H. (1974): Pancreatic acinar cells: Membrane potential and resistance change evoked by acetylcholine. *J. Physiol.,* 238:145–158.
301. Nora, P. F., McCarthy, W., and Sanez, N. (1974): Cholecystokinin cholecystography in acalculous gallbladder disease. *Arch. Surg.,* 108:507–511.
302. Okada, S. (1914/15): On the secretion of bile. *J. Physiol.,* 49:457–482.
303. Ondetti, M. A., Pluščec, J., Sabo, E. F., Sheehan, J. T., and Williams, N. (1970): Synthesis of cholecystokinin-pancreozymin. I. The C-terminal dodecapeptide. *J. Am. Chem. Soc.,* 92:195–199.
304. Ondetti, M. A., Rubin, B., Engel, S. L., Pluščec, J., and Sheehan, J. T. (1970): Cholecystokinin-pancreozymin. Recent developments. *Am. J. Dig. Dis.,* 15:149–156.
305. Otsuki, M., Sakamoto, Ch., Yuu, H., Maeda, M., Morita, S., Ohki, A., Kobayashi, N., Terashi,

K., Okano, K., and Baba, Sh. (1979): Discrepancies between the doses of cholecystokinin or caerulein-stimulating exocrine and endocrine responses in perfused isolated rat pancreas. *J. Clin. Invest.,* 63:478–484.

306. Paré, P. Shaffer, E. A., and Rosenthall, L. (1978): Nonvisualization of the gallbladder by ^{99m}Tc-HIDA cholescintigraphy as evidence of cholecystitis. *CMAJ.,* 18:384–386.

307. Parker, J. G., and Beneventano, Th. C. (1970): Acceleration of small bowel contrast study by cholecystokinin. *Gastroenterology,* 58:679–684.

308. Pederson, R. A., Pearson, J. A., and Brown, J. C. (1970): The effect of theophylline on the actions of pancreozymin and secretin. *Experientia,* 26:961.

309. Persson, C. G. A., and Ekman, M. (1972): Effect of morphine, cholecystokinin and sympathomimetics on the sphincter of Oddi and intramural pressure in cat duodenum. *Scand. J. Gastroenterol.,* 7:345–351.

310. Petersen, H., Solomon, T., and Grossman, M. I. (1978): Effect of chronic pentagastrin, cholecystokinin, and secretin on pancreas of rats. *Am. J. Physiol.,* 234:E286–E293.

311. Petersen, H., Solomon, T. E., and Grossman, M. I. (1979): Pancreatic secretion in rats after chronic treatment with secretin plus caerulein. *Gastroenterology,* 76:790–794.

312. Petersen, O. H., and Ueda, N. (1976): Pancreatic acinar cells: The role of calcium in stimulus-secretion coupling. *J. Physiol.,* 254:583–606.

313. Petersen, O. H., and Ueda, N. (1977): Secretion of fluid and amylase in the perfused rat pancreas. *J. Physiol.,* 264:819–835.

314. Pfeiffer, E. F. (1969): Intestinal factors controlling insulin secretion. *Excerpta Med. Found.,* 172:419–424.

315. Pinget, M., Straus, E., and Yalow, R. S. (1978): Localization of cholecystokinin-like immunoreactivity in isolated nerve terminals. *Proc. Natl. Acad. Sci. USA,* 75:6324–6326.

316. Pointner, H. (1974): The biliary secretion of radioactive selenium after intravenous injection of ^{75}Se-L-seleno-methionine. *Acta Hepato Gastroenterol.,* 21:380–382.

317. Polak, J. M., Pearse, A. G. E., Bloom, S. R., Buchan, A. M. J., Rayford, P. L., and Thompson, J. C. (1975): Identification of cholecystokinin-secretin cells. *Lancet* ii:1016–1017.

318. Preshaw, R. M., and Grossman, M. I. (1965): Stimulation of pancreatic secretion by extracts of the pyloric gland area of the stomach. *Gastroenterology,* 48:36–44.

319. Quinton, A., Tamarelle, C., Dubarry, J. J., and Blanquet, P. (1974): Tubage et scintigraphie pancréatiques. *Nouv. Presse Med.,* 3:737–739.

320. Rafes, Y. I. (1973): Cholecystokininopancreozymin insuffiency. *Vrach. Delo,* 8:26–31.

321. Rager, R., and Finegold, M. J. (1975): Cholestasis in immature newborn infants: Is parenteral alimentation responsible? *J. Pediatr.,* 86:264–269.

322. Răiciulescu, N., Niculescu-Zinca, D., Belgun, M., and Cocu, F. (1974): Our experience on the technique for pancreatic scanning. *Rev. Roum. Med. Int.,* 11:51–57.

323. Ramorino, M. L., Luzietti, L., and Campioni, N. (1961): Effetti della colecistocinina su l'attivita-'biligenetica del fegato. *Folia Endocrinologica,* 14:266–271.

324. Rasmussen, H., and Tenenhouse, A. (1968): Cyclic adenosine monophosphate, Ca^{++}, and membranes. *Proc. Natl. Acad. Sci. USA,* 59:1364–1370.

325. Reed, P. W., and Lardy, H. A. (1972): A23187: A divalent cation ionophore. *J. Biol. Chem.,* 247:6970–6977.

326. Reeder, D. D., Becker, H. D., Smith, N. J., Rayford, P. L., and Thompson, J. C. (1972): Radioimmunoassay of cholecystokinin. *Surg. Forum,* 23:361–362.

327. Reggio, H., Cailla-Deckmyn, H., and Marchis-Mouren, G. (1971): Effect of pancreozymin on rat pancreatic enzyme biosynthesis. *J. Cell. Biol.,* 50:333–343.

328. Rehfeld, J. F. (1971): Effect of gastrin and its C-terminal tetrapeptide on insulin secretion in man. *Acta Endocrinol.,* 66:169–176.

329. Rehfeld, J. F. (1978): Immunochemical studies on cholecystokinin. *J. Biol. Chem.,* 253:4016–4021.

330. Rehfeld, J. F. (1978): Immunochemical studies on cholecystokinin. *J. Biol. Chem.,* 253:4022–4030.

331. Reid, D. R. K., Rogers, I. M., and Calder, J. F. (1975): The cholecystokinin test: An assessment. *Br. J. Surg.,* 62:317–319.

332. Renckens, B. A. M., Schrijen, J. J., Swarts, H. G. P., De Pont, J. J. H. H. M., and Bonting, S. L. (1978): Role of calcium in exocrine pancreatic secretion. IV Calcium movements in isolated acinar cells of rabbit pancreas. *Biochim. Biophys. Acta,* 544:338–350.

333. Ridderstap, A. S., and Bonting, S. L. (1969): Cyclic AMP and enzyme secretion by the isolated rabbit pancreas. *Pflügers Arch.,* 313:62–70.

334. Robberecht, P., and Christophe, J. (1971): Secretion of hydrolases by perfused fragments of rat pancreas: Effect of calcium. *Am. J. Physiol.,* 220:911–917.
335. Robberecht, P., Deschodt-Lanckman, M., De Neef, Ph., and Christophe, J. (1974): Hydrolysis of the cyclic 3':5'-monophosphates of adenosine and guanosine by rat pancreas. *Eur. J. Biochem.,* 41:585–591.
336. Robberecht, P., Deschodt-Lanckman, M., De Neef, Ph., Borgeat, P., and Christophe, J. (1974): In vivo effects of pancreozymin, secretin, vasoactive intestinal polypeptide and pilocarpine on the levels of cyclic AMP and cyclic GMP in the rat pancreas. *FEBS Lett.,* 43:139–143.
337. Robberecht, P., Deschodt-Lanckman, M., and Vanderhaeghen, J. J. (1978): Demonstration of biological activity of brain gastrin-like peptidic material in the human: Its relationship with the COOH-terminal octapeptide of cholecystokinin. *Proc. Natl. Acad. Sci. USA,* 75:524–528.
338. Rosenfeld, M. G., Abrass, I. B., and Chang, B. (1976): Hormonal stimulation of α-amylase synthesis in porcine pancreatic minces. *Endocrinology,* 99:611–618.
339. Rosenqvist, H. (1964): Cholecystokinin as an adjuvant in biliary surgery. *Opusc. Med.,* 9:108–112.
340. Rothman, S. S. (1977): The digestive enzymes of the pancreas: A mixture of inconstant proportions. *Annu. Rev. Physiol.,* 39:373–389.
341. Rothman, S. S., and Wells, H. (1967): Enhancement of pancreatic enzyme synthesis by pancreozymin. *Am. J. Physiol.,* 213:215–218.
342. Rozé, C., De La Tour, J., Chariot, J., Souchard, M., and Debray, C. (1975): Technique d'étude de la sécrétion pancréatique externe chez le rat. *Biol. Gastroenterol. (Paris),* 8:291–295.
343. Rudick, J., Gonda, M., Rosenberg, I. R., Chapman, M. L., Dreiling, D. A., and Janowitz, H. D. (1973): Effects of beta-adrenergic receptor stimulant (isoproterenol) on pancreatic exocrine secretion. *Surgery,* 74:338–343.
344. Rutten, W. J., De Pont, J. J. H. H. M., and Bonting, S. L. (1972): Adenylate cyclase in the rat pancreas properties and stimulation by hormones. *Biochim. Biophys. Acta,* 274:201–213.
345. Sandblom, P., Voegtlin, W. L., and Ivy, A. C. (1935): The effect of cholecystokinin on the choledochoduodenal mechanism (sphincter of Oddi). *Am. J. Physiol.,* 113:175–180.
346. Sarles, J. C., Bidart, J. M., Devaux, M. A., Echinard, C., and Castagnini, A. (1976): Action of cholecystokinin and caerulein on the rabbit sphincter of Oddi. *Digestion,* 14:415–423.
347. Sarles, H., Demol, P., Bataille, D., Guy, O., and Rosselin, G. (1978): Mise en évidence d'une hormone iléale inhibitrice de la sécrétion pancréatique (ACP: anticholécystokininepeptide). *C.R. Acad. Sc. Ser. D.,* 286:367–369.
348. Sarles, H., and Sahel, J. (1974): Pancréatite chronique calcifiante, alcool et pancréas. *Nouv. Presse Med.,* 3:817–820.
349. Savion, N., and Selinger, Z. (1978): Secretagogue-induced production of myocardial depressant factor in rat pancreatic slices. *J. Physiol.,* 285:27p–28p.
350. Schiller, P. W., Lipton, A., Horrobin, D. F., and Bodanszky, M. (1978): Unsulfated C-terminal 7-peptide of cholecystokinin: A new ligand of the opiate receptor. *Biochem. Biophys. Res. Comm.,* 85:1332–1338.
351. Schiller, P. W., Natarajan, S., and Bodanszky, M. (1978): Determination of the intramolecular tyrosine-tryptophan distance in a 7-peptide related to the C-terminal sequence of cholecystokinin. *Int. J. Peptide Protein Res.,* 12:139–142.
352. Schlegel, W., and Grube, D. (1978): Radioimmunologische Bestimmung (RIA) von Cholecystokinin-Pankreozymin (33-CCK). *Z. Gastroenterol.,* 16:304–310.
353. Schlegel, W., Raptis, S., Dollinger, H. C., and Pfeiffer, E. F. (1977): Inhibition of secretin-, pancreozymin and gastrin release and their biological activities by somatostatin. In: *First International Symposium on Hormonal Receptors in Digestive Tract Physiology,* edited by S. Bonfils et al., pp. 361–377. Elsevier/North-Holland Biomedical Press, Amsterdam.
354. Schmidt, H. A., Goebell, H., and Johannson, F. (1972): Pancreatic and gastric secretion in rats studied by means of duodenal and gastric perfusion. *Scand. J. Gastroenterol.,* 7:47–53.
355. Schreurs, V. V. A. M., de Pont, J.-J. H. H. M., and Bonting, S. L. (1974): Role of calcium in pancreatic enzyme secretion. *J. Cell Biol.,* 63:304a.
356. Schreurs, V. V. A. M., Swartz, H. G. P., De Pont, J. J. H. H. M., and Bonting, S. L. (1976): Role of calcium in exocrine pancreatic secretion. II. Comparison of the effects of carbachol and the ionophore A-23187 on enzyme secretion and calcium movements in rabbit pancreas. *Biochim. Biophys. Acta,* 419:320–330.
357. Scott, V. F., Roth, H. P., Bellon, E. M., and Neiderhiser, D. H. (1972): Effect of regular

emptying of the gallbladder on gallstone formation in the rabbit. *Gastroenterology,* 63:851–855.

358. Shaw, R. A., and Jones, R. S. (1978): The choleretic action of cholecystokinin and cholecystokinin octapeptide in dogs. *Surgery,* 84:622–625.

359. Shelby, H. T., Gross, L. P., Lichty, P., and Gardner, J. D. (1976): Action of cholecystokinin and cholinergic agents on membrane-bound calcium in dispersed pancreatic acinar cells. *J. Clin. Invest.,* 58:1482–1493.

360. Singer, M. V., Dermol, P., Mendes de Oliveira, J. P., and Sarles, H. (1978): Vergleich zweier Methoden zur Bestimmung der Dosis-Wirkungsbeziehung zwischen Cholecystokinin und exokriner Pankreassekretion beim Hund. *Z. Gastroenterol.,* 16:95–100.

361. Solcia, E., Pearse, A. G. E., Grube, D., Kobayashi, S., Bussolati, G., Creutzfeldt, W., and Gepts, W. (1973): Revised Wiesbaden classification of gut endocrine cells. *Rendic. Gastroenterol.,* 5:13–16.

362. Solomon, T. E., and Grossman, M. I. (1979): Effect of atropine and vagotomy on response of transplanted pancreas. *Am. J. Physiol.,* 236:E186–E190.

363. Stasiewicz, J., and Wormsley, K. G. (1974): Functional control of the biliary tract. *Acta Hepatogastroenterol.,* 21:450–468.

364. Steiner, D. F., Kemmler, W., Tager, H. S., and Peterson, J. D. (1974): Proteolytic processing in the biosynthesis of insulin and other proteins. *Fed. Proc.,* 33:2105–2115.

365. Steinitz, H., and Tallis, B. (1971): Amebae in the human biliary tract. *Harefuah,* LXXX: 77–80.

366. Stening, G. F., and Grossman, M. I. (1969): Gastrin-related peptides as stimulants of pancreatic and gastric secretion. *Am. J. Physiol.,* 217:262–266.

367. Straus, E., Malesci, A., and Yalow, R. S. (1978): Characterization of a nontrypsin cholecystokinin converting enzyme in mammalian brain. *Proc. Natl. Acad. Sci. USA,* 75:5711–5714.

368. Straus, E., and Yalow, R. S. (1978): Species specificity of cholecystokinin in gut and brain of several mammalian species. *Proc. Natl. Acad. Sci USA,* 75:486–489.

369. Stulberg, B., Norberg, H. P., and Kaplan, E. L. (1976): Cholecystokinin, a new hypocalcemic agent. *Surg. Forum,* 26:430–431.

370. Sutherland, E. W., Øye, I., and Butcher, R. W. (1965): The action of epinephrine and the role of the adenyl cyclase system in hormone action. *Rec. Progr. Horm. Res.,* 21:623–646.

371. Del Tacca, M., Soldani, G., and Crema, A. (1970): Experiments on the mechanism of action of caerulein at the level of the guinea pig ileum and colon. *Agents Actions,* 14:176–182.

372. Thomas, J. E., and Crider, J. O. (1941): The pancreatic secretagogue action of products of protein digestion. *Am. J. Physiol.,* 134:656–663.

373. Thompson, J. C., Fender, H. R., Ramus, N. I., Villar, H. V., and Rayford, P. L. (1975): Cholecystokinin metabolism in man and dogs. *Ann. Surg.,* 182:496–504.

374. Thulin, L., and Samnegård, H. (1978): Circulatory effects of gastrointestinal hormones and related peptides. *Acta Chir. Scand. (Suppl.),* 482:73–74.

375. Toouli, J., and Watts, J. McK. (1972): Actions of cholecystokinin/pancreozymin, secretin and gastrin on extra-hepatic biliary tract motility *in vitro. Ann. Surg.,* 175:439–447.

376. Tumpson, D. B., and Johnson, L. R. (1969): Effect of secretin and cholecystokinin on the response of the gastric fistula rat to pentagastrin. *Proc. Soc. Exp. Biol. Med.,* 131:186–188.

377. Turner, S. G., and Barrowman, J. A. (1977): The effects of cholecystokinin and cholecystokininoctapeptide on intestinal lymph flow in the rat. *Can. J. Physiol. Pharmacol.,* 55:1393–1396.

378. Ueda, N., and Petersen, O. H. (1977): The dependence of caerulein-evoked pancreatic fluid secretion on the extracellular calcium concentration. *Pflügers Arch.,* 370:179–183.

379. Unger, R. H., Ketterer, H., Dupré, J., and Eisentraut, A. M. (1967): The effects of secretin, pancreozymin, and gastrin on insulin and glucagon secretion in anesthetized dogs. *J. Clin. Invest.,* 46:630–645.

380. Vagne, M., and Grossman, M. I. (1968): Cholecystokinetic potency of gastrointestinal hormones and related peptides. *Am. J. Physiol.,* 215:881–884.

381. Vaille, Ch., Debray, Ch. de la Tour, J. Rozé, Cl., and Souchard, M. (1966): Action de la caféine sur la sécrétion de la bile et du suc pancréatique. *Ann. Pharm. Fr.,* 24:515–522.

382. Valenzuela, J. E. (1976): Effect of intestinal hormones and peptides on intragastric pressure in dogs. *Gastroenterology,* 71:766–769.

383. Vanderhaeghen, J. J., Signeau, J. C., and Gepts, W. (1975): New peptide in the vertebrate CNS reacting with antigastrin antibodies. *Nature,* 257:604–605.

384. Vigna, S. R., and Gorbman, A. (1977): Effects of cholecystokinin, gastrin, and related peptides on coho salmon gallbladder contraction *in vitro. Am. J. Physiol.,* 232:E485–E491.

385. Vizi, S. E., Bertaccini, G., Impicciatore, M., and Knoll, J. (1973): Evidence that acetylcholine released by gastrin and related polypeptides contributes to their effect on gastrointestinal motility. *Gastroenterology,* 64:268–277.

386. Vizi, S. E., Bertaccini, G., Impicciatore, M., Mantovani, P., Zséli, J., and Knoll, J. (1974): Structure-activity relationship of some analogues of gastrin and cholecystokinin on intestinal smooth muscle of the guinea pig. *Naunyn Schmiedebergs Arch. Pharmacol.,* 284:233–243.

387. Wahlin, T. Bloom, G. D., and Danielsson, Å. (1976): Effect of cholecystokinin-pancreozymin (CCK-PZ) on glycoprotein secretion from mouse gallbladder epithelium. *Cell. Tissue Res.,* 171:425–435.

388. Waller, S. L., Carvalhinhos, A., Misiewicz, J. J., and Russell, R. I. (1973): Effect of cholecystokinin on colonic motility. *Lancet,* i:264.

389. Wang, C. C., and Grossman, M. I. (1951): Physiological determination of release of secretin and pancreozymin from intestine of dogs with transplanted pancreas. *Am. J. Physiol.,* 164:527–545.

390. Warnes, T. W., Hine, P., and Kay, G. (1969): Alkaline phosphatase in duodenal juice following secretin and pancreozymin. *Gut,* 10:1049.

391. Warnes, T. W., Hine, P., and Kay, G. (1974): The action of secretin and pancreozymin on small-intestinal alkaline phosphatase. *Gut,* 15:39–47.

392. Way, L. W. (1971): Effect of cholecystokinin and caerulein on gastric secretion in cats. *Gastroenterology,* 60:560–565.

393. Way, L. W., and Durbin, R. P. (1969): Response of the bullfrog mucosa to gastrin I and gastrin II. *Gastroenterology,* 56:1266.

394. Werner, B., and Mutt, V. (1954): The pancreatic response in man to the injection of highly purified secretin and of pancreozymin. *Scand. J. Clin. Lab. Invest.,* 6:228–236.

395. Wharton, G. K. (1932): The blood supply of the pancreas, with special reference to that of the islands of Langerhans. *Anat. Rec.,* 53–54:55–81.

396. Williams, J. A., Cary, P., and Moffat, B. (1976): Effects of ions on amylase release by dissociated pancreatic acinar cells. *Am. J. Physiol.,* 231:1562–1567.

397. Williams, J. A., and Chandler, D. (1975): Ca^{++} and pancreatic amylase release. *Am. J. Physiol.,* 228:1729–1732.

398. Williams, J. A., Korc, M., and Dormer, R. L. (1978): Action of secretagogues on a new preparation of functionally intact, isolated pancreatic acini. *Am. J. Physiol.,* 235:E517–E524.

399. Williams, J. A., and Lee, M. (1974): Pancreatic acinar cells: Use of a Ca^{++} ionophore to separate enzyme release from the earlier steps in stimulus-secretion coupling. *Biochem. Biophys. Res. Commun.,* 60:542–548.

400. Wilson, S. D., Soergel, K., and Go, V. L. W. (1973): Diarrhoea, gastric hypersecretion, and "cholecystokinin-like" hormone. *Lancet* i:1515–1516.

401. Winston, M. A., Guth, P., Endow, J. S., and Blahd, W. H. (1974): Enhancement of pancreatic concentration of ^{75}Se-selenomethionine. *J. Nucl. Med.,* 15:662–666.

402. Wormsley, K. G. (1968): Gastric response to secretin and pancreozymin in man. *Scand. J. Gastroenterol.,* 3:632–636.

403. Wormsley, K. G. (1970): Stimulation of pancreatic secretion by intraduodenal infusion of bile salts. *Lancet,* ii:586–588.

404. Yajima, H., Mori, Y., Kiso, Y., Koyama, K., Tobe, T., Setoyama, M., Adachi, H. Kanno, T., and Saito, A. (1976): Synthesis of (27-Tyr)-cholecystokinin-pancreozymin (CCK-PZ). *Chem. Pharm. Bull.,* 24:1110–1113.

405. Yamagishi, T., and Debas, H. T. (1978): Cholecystokinin inhibits gastric emptying by acting on both proximal stomach and pylorus. *Am. J. Physiol.,* 234:E375–E378.

406. Yau, W. M., Makhlouf, G. M., Edwards, L. E., and Farrar, J. T. (1974): The action of cholecystokinin and related peptides on guinea pig small intestine. *Can. J. Physiol. Pharmacol.,* 52:298–303.

407. Young, J. D., Lazarus, L., and Chisholm, D. J. (1969): Radioimmunoassay of pancreozymin cholecystokinin in human serum. *J. Nucl. Med.,* 10:743–745.

408. Youngs, G. R., Agnew, J. E., Levin, G. E., and Bouchier, I. A. D. (1971): Radioselenium in duodenal aspirate as an assessment of pancreatic exocrine function. *Br. Med. J.,* 2:252–255.

409. Zimmerman, M. J., Dreiling, D. A., Rosenberg, I. R., and Janowitz, H. D. (1967): Secretion of calcium by the canine pancreas. *Gastroenterology,* 52:865–870.

Gastrointestinal Hormones, edited by
George B. Jerzy Glass.
Raven Press, New York © 1980.

Chapter 8

Gastric Inhibitory Polypeptide (GIP): Isolation, Structure, and Basic Functions

J. C. Brown, J. L. Frost, S. Kwauk, S. C. Otte, and
C. H. S. McIntosh

*Department of Physiology, University of British Columbia, Vancouver,
British Columbia, Canada V6T 1W5*

INTRODUCTION

Isolation of a polypeptide with inhibitory activity for H^+ secretion, pepsin secretion, and motor activity in extrinsically denervated pouches of the body of the stomach of dogs has been described (10,14). The polypeptide was isolated from a partially purified preparation of the gastrointestinal hormone cholecystokinin-pancreozymin (CCK-PZ) (GIH Research Laboratory, Karolinska Institute, Stockholm, Sweden) by separation techniques, as outlined briefly in Fig. 1.

Brown and Pederson (13) had earlier presented physiological evidence indicating that these CCK-PZ preparations contained an inhibitory substance for acid secretion in dogs other than the CCK-PZ. Impure CCK-PZ preparations had been described as possessing inhibitory activity for acid secretion stimulated by both exogenous (26) and endogenous (9) gastrin. Similar preparations had also been described as inhibitory for basal and stimulated motor activity of the body of the stomach (8,29) and stimulatory for acid secretion (31,33). The multiparameter studies of Brown and Pederson (13) indirectly demonstrated

```
HEAT COAGULATED HOG DUODENO-JEJUNAL EXTRACT
                        ↓

ACETIC ACID EXTRACT
                    ↓   adjust pH to 2.5
                        adsorption to alginic acid
                        desorption with HCl

        NaCl PRECIPITATE
                    ↓   Methanol extraction

METHANOL INSOLUBLE FRACTION
                    ↓   CM cellulose pH 6.5

        CRUDE CCK-P2
                    ↓   TEAE cellulose pH 9.1

        10% PURE CCK
                    ↓   Sephadex G 50

┌─────────────────────────┐
│ GIP STARTING MATERIAL    │
└─────────────────────────┘
                        adjust pH to 2.5
                    ↓   adsorption to alginic acid
                        desorption with HCl
                        DEAE-Sephadex, acetic acid

        EG STATE I
                    ↓   CM cellulose pH 7.8

        EG STAGE II
                    ↓   Sephadex G 25

        EG STAGE III
                    ↓   Sephadex G 50

        EG STAGE IV
```

FIG. 1. Stages in the purification of GIP.

that in the purification of CCK-PZ, an inhibitory material for gastric acid secretion had been removed.

Purification and amino acid sequencing have been accomplished (3,5) and the acronym GIP (gastric inhibitory polypeptide) was assigned to the 43 amino acid polypeptide (3). The amino acid sequence of GIP:

Tyr–Ala–Glu–Gly–Thr–Phe–Ile–Ser–Asp–Tyr–Ser–Ile–Ala–Met–
Asp–Lys–Ile–Arg–Gln–Gln–Asp–Phe–Val–Asn–Trp–Leu–Leu–Ala–
Gln–Gln–Lys–Gly–Lys–Lys–Ser–Asp–Trp–Lys–His–Asn–Ile–Thr–Gln

was determined by using the dansyl-Edman technique on the tryptic peptides separated by ion exchange chromatography and countercurrent distribution.

Confirmation of sequences and alignment of the tryptic peptides was accomplished by dansyl-Edman procedures on the cyanogen bromide (CNBr) cleaved fragments of the GIP molecule and selected chymotrypsin and thermolysin peptides (6). The tryptic peptides subjected to sequential dansyl-Edman analyses were obtained from digestion of either the complete GIP molecule or the C-terminal CNBr fragment purified by chromatography on Sephadex G25 fine and carboxymethyl cellulose 11 (12). The amino acid composition revealed the presence of six basic amino acid residues, five lysines, and one arginine. If none of the basic amino acids were in the N- or C-terminal position, or in juxtaposition, digestion of the whole molecule with trypsin could be expected to produce seven tryptic peptides. Five major tryptic peptides were obtained and in addition four minor splits occurred. The minor peptides Tr-6 and Tr-7 aided in the alignment of the major tryptic peptides. The presence of an acidic peptide Tr-1 (a weakly staining peptide) is intriguing. Amino acid analyses reveal this to be a dipeptide with alanine and glutamic acid residues. Tr-1 has also been found as a minor peptide after tryptic digestion of the C-terminal cyanogen bromide fragment, suggesting its presence within the sequence 15 to 43, either as a weak enzymatic cleavage site or within the sequence of a structurally related contaminant. Sufficient evidence to support either of these hypotheses is not yet available. The probability that this tryptic peptide was cleaved from a biochemically dissimilar molecule had no support from studies currently in progress.

EGIII (10) has been subjected to a further purification procedure on CM-Sephadex C25 using 0.01 M NH_4HCO_3, pH 7.8 as eluting buffer (Fig. 2). The peak obtained was divided into four fractions and subjected to polyacrylamide

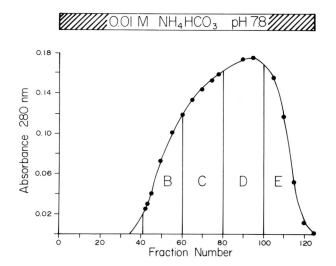

FIG. 2. Chromatography of 10 mg of GIP (EGIII) on carboxymethyl Sephadex C-25. Eluting buffer was 0.01 M NH_4HCO_3, pH 7.8. Fraction size was 1.5 ml.

gel electrophoresis, amino acid analyses, and tryptic digestion followed by high voltage electrophoresis for peptide separation. Polyacrylamide gel electrophoresis revealed no differences among the four fractions and no difference of any significance could be observed after hydrolyses and amino acid analyses. Tryptic digestion followed by high voltage electrophoresis for separation of the peptides revealed that peptide Tr-1 was clearly present in fraction D and to a lesser extent in fractions E, B, and C. Bioassays for gastric acid inhibitory activity and insulinotropic activity lack the sensitivity required to detect minor (<5%) contamination. Accurate interpretation of bioassays can be achieved only when separation and purification of the minor component have been achieved.

EFFECTS OF EXOGENOUS GIP

On the Endocrine Pancreas

It has been shown that GIP is insulinotropic in man (21), dog (41,42), and rat (37,38,40) when administered in doses producing levels in plasma or perfusate of an isolated perfused pancreas, similar to those found postprandially. Isolated pancreatic islets from adult rats are responsive to pharmacological (1–10 μg/ml) concentration of GIP (45,46) but cultured islets from 2 to 5-day-old rats respond to GIP levels as low as 1 ng/ml (25). Single, large injections of GIP in dogs with basal serum glucose levels produced a monophasic peak of insulin release (41). The prevailing glucose concentration was first shown to be important for the insulinotropic action of GIP by Dupré et al. (21). Elevation of serum IR-GIP levels to approximately 1 ng/ml during intravenous glucose infusion increased insulin levels significantly above those obtained with glucose alone. *In vitro* studies demonstrated that a threshold glucose concentration was necessary for GIP to stimulate insulin release from isolated islets (6–8 nM) (45,46) or from the perfused pancreas (5.5 mM) (37).

In order to study the insulinotropic effect of GIP under finely controlled steady-state glucose concentrations, Elahi et al. (23) applied a glucose clamp (48) to normal human volunteers receiving a GIP infusion (6.7 ng/kg 1 min). During basal state glycemia, GIP had no insulinotropic effect. In mild hyperglycemia (54 mg/dl above basal), IRI levels were modestly augmented and in moderate hyperglycemia (143 mg/dl above basal), IRI levels were highly elevated during the GIP infusion. In this study, as in the perfused rat pancreas, the action of GIP has been shown to be on both the initial phase and the prolonged second phase of insulin release. Exogenous GIP is therefore a potent insulinotropic polypeptide and, as discussed elsewhere (11), is at present the major candidate for the gastrointestinal insulinotropic hormone.

High levels of GIP (100 ng/ml) have been shown to stimulate glucagon release from diced rat pancreas and, with these high GIP concentrations, glucose had no suppressive effect on the secretion (7). In streptozotocin-treated rats, the elevated GLI levels were further increased by treatment with GIP. In the isolated perfused pancreas, GIP produced biphasic glucagon release in the presence of 4 mM glucose and also augmented the response to arginine (38,39). A glucagono-tropic action for GIP is therefore evident in the rat, although no such action has been described in man.

Ipp et al, (28) reported that GIP (58 ng/ml) stimulated somatostatin release from the perfused canine pancreas with attached duodenum. However, since somatostatin is also present in the duodenum, the exact site of origin is uncertain.

On the Gastrointestinal Tract

In dogs GIP infusion produced a dose-dependent inhibition of acid secretion from denervated pouches of the body of the stomach (36). Maximum inhibition ($\sim 70\%$) of pentagastrin-stimulated secretion occurred at an infusion rate of 1.0 μg/kg-hr, which produced circulating IR-GIP levels in the range observed after feeding. Acid secretion stimulated by histamine or insulin hypoglycemia were inhibited but to a lesser degree. Pepsin secretion and acetylcholine-stimulated motor activity in pouches of the antrum and body of the stomach are all inhibited by GIP (35). Both gastrin release and meal-stimulated acid secretion from Heidenhain pouches are also reduced by infusion of GIP (55). In man, it has been shown (17) that a single injection of GIP (2 μg/kg) potently inhibited acid secretion, although levels of plasma IR-GIP were supraphysiological. An enterogastrone function for GIP is suggested by available data but the relative insensitivity of innervated stomach preparations to exogenous GIP needs further investigation.

An enterocrinin-like effect of GIP was first reported by Barbezat and Grossman (2) in Thiry-Vella loops of dog upper jejunum or lower ileum. With the use of a triple-lumen gut perfusion technique in man, more physiological doses of GIP also produced a stimulation of intestinal secretion (27). Since GIP does not seem to stimulate adenylate cyclase in either the small intestine (47) or in the colon (56), its effect is unlikely to be mediated by cyclic AMP.

RADIOIMMUNOASSAY FOR GIP

Kuzio et al. (30) developed a radioimmunoassay (RIA) for IR-GIP by using a guinea pig antibody raised against GIP conjugated to albumin by the carbodi-imide technique. An antibody to glutaraldehyde coupled GIP gives similar values for plasma levels of IR-GIP in man (32). At the present time, all available antisera appear to be directed toward the C-terminal portion of the GIP molecule.

Gel filtration of human serum samples and duodenal extracts (7) has shown the existence of at least two molecular forms of IR-GIP. The larger species, approximately 8,000 daltons MW, is a potential precursor of the 5,000 dalton MW form. Attempts are being made to confirm this suggestion.

RELEASE OF GIP

In man, fasting serum levels of IR-GIP range from nondetectable to approximately 500 pg/ml. After either a solid or a liquid mixed meal, circulating levels increase at least fivefold (11,17,19,30). Triglycerides administered orally in man (4,17,19,24) and dog (39) or intraduodenally in dog (35) produced a sustained rise in IR-GIP. There was no accompanying rise in immunoreactive insulin (IRI).

Cataland et al. (16) demonstrated that ingestion of glucose elevated IR-GIP levels to approximately 750 pg/ml within 45 to 60 min, whereas i.v. glucose was without effect. Subsequent studies have confirmed the rapid rise in IR-GIP in response to oral glucose and attempts were made to correlate this with the increase in insulin secretion. Andersen et al. (1) studied the insulinotropic action of endogenous GIP, using the glucose clamp technique to maintain glucose at 125 mg/dl above basal. After administration of i.v. glucose alone, there was no change in IR-GIP from mean basal levels of 305 pg/ml. After oral glucose ingestion, IR-GIP levels began to rise within 10 min and peaked at 40 min (752 pg/ml). The insulin response to i.v. glucose was typically biphasic, and after oral glucose IRI levels rose dramatically above the levels achieved by hyperglycemia induced by i.v. glucose alone. The time courses of GIP and IRI were almost identical. When euglycemia was maintained after oral glucose by simultaneously infusing insulin, no increase in IRI was seen despite stimulated levels of IR-GIP. Andersen et al. concluded that "GIP is, at a minimum, a major component among the physiological stimuli to insulin secretion" (1).

Duodenal perfusion of an amino acid mixture in man (52) and dog (34) has also been shown to stimulate IR-GIP release and to be accompanied by augmented insulin secretion. Peak IR-GIP levels (15 min) preceded the insulin peak (30 min). Intravenous amino acids had no effect on IR-GIP levels and stimulated IRI to a lesser degree than when administered intraduodenally. An amino acid mixture that stimulated CCK release had little effect on either IR-GIP or insulin (54).

A possible interaction between GIP and other gastrointestinal hormones is indicated by the observation that gastrin and CCK potentiate intraduodenal glucose-stimulated IR-GIP release (49). Although an indirect effect via stimulated acid secretion cannot be excluded, available evidence has indicated that GIP release was not stimulated by intraduodenal acid (7). Both somatostatin and glucagon inhibit IR-GIP release and a possible role as local (paracrine) and feedback modulators, respectively, should be considered (22,39). A feedback regulation of GIP secretion by insulin has also been suggested to occur (7,17, 19,20). IR-GIP levels achieved after oral triglyceride were reduced by simultaneous i.v. glucose infusion (17,20) and by i.v. insulin (7) but no effect of endogenously released insulin on glucose stimulated IR-GIP secretion was observed (1).

CELLULAR LOCALIZATION OF GIP

Immunocytochemical studies with antibodies raised against natural porcine GIP have been used to identify GIP-containing cells in the gastrointestinal tract of man, pig, and dog (15,18,43,44,51). GIP cells were predominantly localized in the lower and middle zone of the mucosal crypts of the duodenum and the jejunum. At the electron microscopic level, the cell of origin has been identified as the K cell, characterized by round or slightly ovoid granules having an osmiophilic core and less dense matrix, and with an average diameter of 300 nm (15). Hyperplasia of GIP cells has been reported in genetically obese (ob/ob) mice (47) and in patients with celiac disease (18). GIP-like immunoreactive material has also been identified in pancreatic A cells (50).

Release of IR-GIP by selective small bowel perfusion of human subjects has confirmed the histological localization of the GIP cells (53). The integrated IR-GIP levels (ng.min^{-1}.ml^{-1}) were: duodenum, 111 ± 21; proximal jejunum, 69 ± 5; mid-jejunum, 47 ± 7; and ileum, 25 ± 6.

SUMMARY AND CONCLUSIONS

The biological assay used in the purification of GIP was the inhibition of pentagastrin-stimulated acid secretion in the extrinsically denervated pouch of the body of the stomach of dogs. The role of GIP as a physiological inhibitor of acid secretion in the innervated stomach now appears doubtful. The role of cholinergic innervation in the action of GIP as an enterogastrone must be established. It is possible that GIP contributes to the overall regulation of gastric secretion, which is not apparent when the hormone is tested in isolation from other factors with which it may interact.

The primary action of GIP is in the control of insulin secretion. It has been proven that the polypeptide fulfills all the requirements as an insulinotropic hormone. The pathophysiology of GIP is an active area of research and attention to date has focused on the hypersecretion observed in obesity, maturity-onset diabetes, and pancreatitis. Whether or not GIP hypersecretion is causative or passive in these situations remains to be clarified.

PROJECTIONS FOR THE FUTURE

The nature of the large molecular weight (approximately 8,000 daltons) IR-GIP remains to be clarified. Is this a hormone precursor or a separate unrelated entity? Several groups have now produced their own antisera to GIP, necessitating careful characterization of each, especially when the respective RIA is applied to studies of the pathophysiology of GIP. A successful synthesis is awaited both to confirm the published amino acid sequence and to increase the availability of the hormone. Can GIP completely account for the gastrointestinal contribution to the regulation of insulin secretion or are other factors involved? The glucose-dependent nature of the insulinotropic action of GIP may be indicative of the necessity for other potentiating factors for the various effects of GIP to be manifested, suggesting that the specific physiological effect of the hormone depends on the prevailing conditions. Interaction of GIP and certain amino acids at the β-cell also requires further investigation. A glucagonotropic action for GIP in the rat has also been described, but these observations need to be extended to other species.

Inhibition of acid secretion by the hormone in the innervated stomach is weak, but in the denervated preparation potent inhibition is seen. This must be reconciled.

REFERENCES

1. Andersen, D. K., Elahi, D., Brown, J. C., Tobin, J. D., and Andres, R. (1978): Oral glucose augmentation of insulin secretion: interactions of gastric inhibitory polypeptide with ambient glucose and insulin levels. *J. Clin. Invest.,* 63:153–161.
2. Barbezat, G. O., and Grossman, M. I. (1971): Intestinal secretion: stimulation by peptides. *Science,* 174:422–424.
3. Brown, J. C. (1971): A gastric inhibitory polypeptide I. The amino acid composition and tryptic peptides. *Can. J. Biochem.,* 49:255–261.
4. Brown, J. C. (1974): In: *Endocrinology 1973,* edited by S. Taylor, pp. 276–284. Heinemann, London.
5. Brown, J. C., and Dryburgh, J. R. (1971): A gastric inhibitory polypeptide. II. The complete amino acid sequence. *Can. J. Biochem.,* 49:867–872.
6. Brown, J. C., and Dryburgh, J. R. (1974): *Chemistry of Gastric Inhibitory Polypeptide (GIP) and Motilin: Endocrinology of the Gut.* edited by W. Y. Chey and F. P. Brooks, pp. 14–21. Charles B. Slack,
7. Brown, J. C., Dryburgh, J. R., Ross, S. A., and Dupre, J. (1975): Identification and actions of gastric inhibitory polypeptide. *Recent Prog. Horm. Res.,* 31:487–532.
8. Brown, J. C., Johnson, L. P., and Magee, D. F. (1967): The inhibition of induced motor activity in transplanted fundic pouches. *J. Physiol.,* 188:45–52.
9. Brown, J. C., and Magee, D. F. (1967): Inhibitory action of cholecystokinin on acid secretion from Heidenhain pouches, induced by endogenous gastrin. *Gut,* 8:29–31.
10. Brown, J. C., Mutt, V., and Pederson, R. A. (1970): Further purification of a polypeptide demonstrating enterogastrone activity. *J. Physiol.,* 209:57–64.
11. Brown, J. C., and Otte, S. C. (1978): Gastrointestinal hormones and the control of insulin secretion. *Diabetes,* 27:782–789.
12. Brown, J. C., and Pederson, R. A. (1970): Cleavage of a gastric inhibitory polypeptide with cyanogen bromide and the physiological action of the C-terminal fragment. *J. Physiol.,* 210:52–53P.
13. Brown, J. C., and Pederson, R. A. (1970): A multiparameter study on the action of preparations containing cholecystokinin-pancreozymin. *Scand. J. Gastroenterol.,* 5:537–541.
14. Brown, J. C., Pederson, R. A., Jorpes, J. E., and Mutt, V. (1969): Preparation of highly active enterogastrone. *Can. J. Physiol. Pharmacol.,* 47:113–114.
15. Buffa, R., Polak, J. M., Pearse, A. G. E., Solcia, E., Grimelius, L., and Capella, C. (1975): Identification of the intestinal cell storing gastric inhibitory peptide. *Histochemistry,* 43:249–255.
16. Cataland, S., Crockett, S. E., Brown, J. C., and Mazaferri, E. L. (1974): Gastric inhibitory polypeptide (GIP) stimulation by oral glucose in man. *J. Clin. Endocrinol. Metab.,* 39:223–228.
17. Cleator, I. G. M., and Gourlay, R. M. (1975): Release of immunoreactive gastric inhibitory polypeptide (IR-GIP) by oral ingestion of food substances. *Am. J. Surg.,* 130:128–135.
18. Creutzfeldt, W., Ebert, R., Arnold, R., Frerichs, H., and Brown, J. C. (1976): Gastric inhibitory

polypeptide (GIP), gastrin and insulin: response to test meal in coeliac disease and after duodeno-pancreatectomy. *Diabetologia,* 12:279–286.

19. Creutzfeldt, W., Ebert, R., Willms, B., Frerichs, H., and Brown, J. C. (1978): Gastric inhibitory polypeptide (GIP) and insulin in obesity: Increased response to stimulation and defective feedback control of serum levels. *Diabetologia,* 14:15–24.

20. Crockett, S. E., Mazzafferri, E. L., and Cataland, S. (1976): Gastric inhibitory polypeptide (GIP) in maturity onset diabetes mellitus. *Diabetes,* 25:931–935.

21. Dupré, J., Ross, S. A., Watson, D., and Brown, J. C. (1973): Stimulation of insulin secretion by gastric inhibitory polypeptide in man. *J. Clin. Endocrinol. Metab.,* 37:826–828.

22. Ebert, R., Arnold, R., and Creutzfeldt, W. (1977): Lowering of fasting and food stimulated serum immunoreactive gastric inhibitory polypeptide (GIP) by glucagon. *Gut,* 18:121–127.

23. Elahi, D., Andersen, D. K., Brown, J. C., Debas, H. T., Herschcopf, R. J., Raizes, G. S., Tobin, J. D., and Andres, R. (1979): Pancreatic alpha and beta cell responses to GIP infusion in normal man. *Am. J. Physiol.,* 237(2):E185–191.

24. Falko, J. M., Crockett, S. E., Cataland, S., and Mazzaferri, E. L. (1975): Gastric inhibitory polypeptide (GIP) stimulated by fat ingestion in man. *J. Clin. Endocrinol. Metab.,* 41:260–265.

25. Fujimoto, W. Y., Ensinck, J. W., Merchant, F. W., Williams, R. H., Smith, P. H., and Johnson, D. G. (1978): Stimulation by gastric inhibitory polypeptide of insulin and glucagon secretion by rat islet cultures. *Proc. Soc. Exp. Biol. Med.,* 157:89–93.

26. Gillespie, I. E., and Grossman, M. I. (1964): Inhibitory effect of secretin and cholecystokinin on Heidenhain pouch responses to gastrin extract and histamine. *Gut,* 5:342–345.

27. Helman, C. A., and Barbezat, G. O. (1977): The effect of gastric inhibitory polypeptide on human jejunal water and electrolyte secretion. *Gastroenterology,* 72:376–379.

28. Ipp, E., Dobbs, R. E., Harris, V., Arimura, A., Vale, W., and Unger, R. H. (1977): The effects of gastrin, gastric inhibitory polypeptide, secretin, and the octapeptide of cholecystokinin upon immunoreactive somatostatin release by the perfused pancreas. *J. Clin. Invest.,* 60:1216–1219.

29. Johnson, L. P., and Magee, D. F. (1965): Cholecystokinin-pancreozymin extracts and gastric motor inhibition. *Surg. Gynecol. Obstet.,* 121:557–562.

30. Kuzio, M., Dryburgh, J. R., Malloy, K. M., and Brown, J. C. (1974): Radioimmunoassay for gastric inhibitory polypeptide. *Gastroenterology,* 66:357–364.

31. Magee, D. F., and Nakamura, M. (1966): Action of pancreozymin preparations on gastric secretion. *Nature,* 212:1487–1488.

32. Morgan, L. M., Morris, B. A., and Marks, V. (1978): Radioimmunoassay of gastric inhibitory polypeptide. *Ann. Clin. Biochem.,* 15:172–177.

33. Murat, J. E., and White, T. T. (1966): Stimulation of gastric secretion by commercial cholecystokinin extracts. *Proc. Soc. Exp. Biol. Med.,* 123:593–594.

34. O'Dorisio, T. M., Cataland, S., Stevenson, M., and Mazzaferri, E. L. (1976): Gastric Inhibitory Polypeptide (GIP). Intestinal distribution and stimulation by amino acids and medium-chain triglycerides. *Am. J. Dig. Dis.,* 21:761–765.

35. Pederson, R. A. (1972): Thesis: The isolation and action of gastric inhibitory polypeptide. University of British Columbia.

36. Pederson, R. A., and Brown, J. C. (1972): Inhibition of pentagastrin-, histamine- and insulin-stimulated canine gastric secretion by pure gastric inhibitory polypeptide. Gastroenterology, 62:393–400.

37. Pederson, R. A., and Brown, J. C. (1976): The insulinotropic action of gastric inhibitory polypeptide in the isolated perfused rat pancreas. *Endocrinology,* 99:780–785.

38. Pederson, R. A., and Brown, J. C. (1978): Interaction of gastric inhibitory polypeptide, glucose, and arginine on insulin and glucagon secretion from the perfused rat pancreas. *Endocrinology,* 103:610–615.

39. Pederson, R. A., Dryburgh, J. R., and Brown, J. C. (1975): The effect of somatostatin on release and insulinotropic action of gastric inhibitory polypeptide. *Can. J. Physiol. Pharmacol.,* 53:1200–1205.

40. Pederson, R. A., Dryburgh, J. R., Brown, J. C., and Dupree, A. H. (1978): GIP effects on the isolated pancreas. In: *Gut Hormones,* pp. 283–287. Churchill Livingstone, Edinburgh.

41. Pederson, R. A., Schubert, H. E., and Brown, J. C. (1975): The insulinotropic action of gastric inhibitory polpyeptide. *Can. J. Physiol. Pharmacol.,* 53:217–223.

42. Pederson, R. A., Schubert, H. E., and Brown, J. C. (1975): Gastric Inhibitory Polypeptide. Its physiologic release and insulinotropic action in the dog. *Diabetes,* 24:1050–1056.
43. Polak, J. M., Bloom, S. R., Kuzio, M., Brown, J. C., and Pearse, A. G. E. (1973): Cellular localization of gastric inhibitory polypeptide in the duodenum and jejunum. *Gut,* 14:284–288.
44. Polak, J. M., Pearse, A. G. E., Grimelius, L., and Marks, V. (1975): Gastrointestinal apudosis in obese hyperglycaemic mice. *Virchows. Archiv. (Cell Pathol.),* 19:135–140.
45. Schauder, P., Brown, J. C., Frerichs, H., and Creutzfeldt, W. (1975): Gastric inhibitory polypeptide: effect on glucose-induced insulin release from isolated rat pancreatic islets in vitro. *Diabetologia,* 11:483–484.
46. Schauder, P., Schindler, B., Panten, U., Brown, J. C., Frerichs, H., and Creutzfeldt, W. (1977): Insulin release from isolated rat pancreatic islets induced by α-ketoisocaproic acid, L-leucine, D-glucose or D-glyceraldehyde: effect of gastric inhibitory polypeptide or glucagon. *Mol. Cell. Endocrinol.,* 7:115–123.
47. Schwartz, C. J., Kimberg, D. V., Sheerin, H. E., Field, M., and Said, S. I. (1974): Vasoactive intestinal peptide stimulation of adenylate cyclase and active electrolyte secretion in intestinal mucosa. *J. Clin. Invest.,* 54:536–544.
48. Sherwin, R. S., Kramer, K. J., Tobin, J. D., Insel, P. A., Liljenquist, J. E., Berman, M., and Andres, R. (1974): A model of the kinetics of insulin in man. *J. Clin. Invest.,* 53:1481–1492.
49. Sirinek, K. R., Cataland, S., O'Dorisio, T. M., Mazzaferri, E. L., Crockett, S. E., and Pace, W. G. (1977): Augmented gastric inhibitory polypeptide response to intraduodenal glucose by exogenous gastrin and cholecystokinin. *Surgery,* 82:438–442.
50. Smith, P. H., Merchant, F. W., Johnson, D. G., Fujimoto, W. Y., and Williams, R. H. (1977): Immunocytochemical localization of a gastric inhibitory polypeptide-like material within A-cells of the endocrine pancreas. *Am. J. Anat.,* 149:585–590.
51. Solcia, E., Polak, J. J., Buffa, R., Capella, C. and Pearse, A. G. E. (1975): Endocrine cells of the intestinal mucosa. In: *Symposium Gastrointestinal Hormones,* edited by J. C. Thompson, pp. 155–168. University of Texas Press, Austin and London,
52. Thomas, F. B., Mazzaferri, E. L., Crockett, S. E., Mekhjian, H. S., Gruemer, H. D., and Cataland, S. (1976): Stimulation of secretion of gastric inhibitory polypeptide and insulin by intraduodenal amino acid perfusion. Gastroenterology, 70:523–527.
53. Thomas, F. B., Shook, D. F., O'Dorisio, T. M., Cataland, S., Mekhjian, H. S., Caldwell, A. H., and Mazzaferri, E. L. (1977): Localization of gastric inhibitory polypeptide release by intestinal glucose perfusion in man. Gastroenterology, 72:49–54.
54. Thomas, F. B., Sinar, D., Mazzaferri, E. L., Cataland, S., Mekhjian, H. S., Caldwell, J. H., and Fromkes, J. J. (1978): Selective release of gastric inhibitory polypeptide by intraduodenal amino acid perfusion in man. Gastroenterology, 74:1261–1265.
55. Villar, H. V., Fender, H. R., Rayford, P. L., Bloom, S. R., Ramus, N. I., and Thompson, J. C. (1976): Suppression of gastrin release and gastric secretion by gastric inhibitory polypeptide (GIP) and vasoactive intestinal polypeptide (VIP). *Ann. Surg.,* 184:97–102.
56. Waldman, D. B., Gardner, J. D., Zfass, A. M., and Makhlouf, G. M. (1977): Effects of vasoactive intestinal peptide, secretin and related peptides on rat colonic transport and adenylate cyclase activity. *Gastroenterology,* 73:518–523.

Gastrointestinal Hormones, edited by
George B. Jerzy Glass.
Raven Press, New York © 1980.

Chapter 9

Motilin: Isolation, Structure, and Basic Functions

Christopher H. S. McIntosh and John C. Brown

Faculty of Medicine, Department of Physiology, The University of British Columbia, Vancouver, British Columbia, Canada

ENTERAL pH AND THE CONTROL OF GASTRIC MOTILITY

The control of gastric motility and emptying is primarily mediated by a myogenic mechanism and modulated by hormonal and neuronal elements (18). One segment of this control involves a pH-dependent enteral reflex of poorly understood nature.

Instillation of acid into the duodenum causes inhibition of gastric motor activity (6,14) and delayed gastric emptying (62). Vagotomy (53,68) or ganglionectomy (58) abolished this effect, indicating the involvement of a neural mechanism. The rapid onset of inhibition (17) is support for this hypothesis, although a humoral mechanism probably involving secretin cannot be excluded (15).

Stimulation of gastric emptying by duodenal perfusion with sodium bicarbonate (63) and increased gastric motor activity on diversion of the acid gastric contents away from the duodenum (68) suggest that alkaline conditions in the duodenum may initiate a stimulatory reflex for motor activity. Evidence for the involvement of a hormonal factor in such a reflex resulted from dog experiments, in which increased motor activity of denervated and transplanted pouches of stomach corpus occurred when the duodenal pH was raised by 1.0 pH unit (11). In the denervated pouch preparation, intraduodenal administration of pig pancreatic juice produced a similar response (11). The explanation for the mechanism of this reflex was proposed to be that "either such solutions prevent the release of an inhibitory humoral agent, or they release a stimulatory humoral agent for motor activity."

ISOLATION AND AMINO ACID SEQUENCE OF MOTILIN

The search for a possible stimulatory factor for gastric motor activity began with a screening of various crude preparations of secretin and cholecystokinin (CCK) (7). One of these extracts, Pancreozymin (CCK-PZ) (Boots), stimulated motor activity and a partial purification by gel filtration produced a fraction with gastric motor stimulatory activity distinct from CCK-PZ activity (13). A polypeptide was finally purified from a side fraction produced during the isolation of secretin by Mutt and Jorpes as starting material and by sequential gel filtration and ion-exchange chromatographic separations, and the name *motilin* was chosen for the polypeptide because of its ability to stimulate motor activity in fundic pouches (7,12).

Amino acid analysis of motilin demonstrated the absence of histidine, tryptophan, and cystine and the presence of a high content of glutamate or glutamine (12). The complete amino acid sequence (Fig. 1) was determined by the subtractive dansyl-Edman technique on peptides produced by cleavage of the molecule with cyanogen bromide, trypsin, chymotrypsin, and thermolysin (8,9).

A successful synthesis of a 13-norleucine (nleu) analog of motilin has been achieved (71,72). A comparison of tryptic peptides of the synthetic and natural material showed that the natural peptide TR3 was less acidic than previously reported, suggesting the presence of an amidated glutamic acid. Kinetic studies with leucine aminopeptidase gave Met-Gln-Glu-Lys as the sequence (60). More recent work utilizing a radioimmunoassay (RIA) for motilin to follow the purification of motilin has revealed that two peaks of immunoreactivity may be eluted from cellulose CM22, with characteristics indicative of both the amidated and the deamidated glutamic acid forms (10). Whether motilin is synthesized *in vivo* with all glutamic acid residues amidated and whether deamidation occurs solely during isolation remains to be clarified. However, synthetic 14-Gln-15-Glu and 14-Gln-15-Gln do not differ significantly from porcine motilin in either biological or immunological activity (73).

```
PHE-VAL-PRO-ILE-PHE-THR-TYR-GLY-GLU-LEU-GLN
 1   2   3   4   5   6   7   8   9   10  11


-ARG-MET-GLU-GLU-LYS-GLU-ARG-ASN-LYS-GLY-GLN
 12  13  14  15  16  17  18  19  20  21  22
```

```
-ARG-MET-|GLN|-GLU-LYS-GLU-ARG-ASN-LYS-GLY-GLN
 12  13  | 14|  15  16  17  18  19  20  21  22
```

FIG. 1. Amino acid sequences of porcine motilin. (Data from refs. 8 and 60.)

CELLULAR LOCALIZATION OF MOTILIN

Motilin was initially localized to 5-hydroxytryptophan (5-HT) containing enterochromaffin (EC) cells in a number of species (49,52). These studies utilized antibodies raised against natural porcine motilin for immunofluorescent staining. Most cells were detected in the duodenum and upper jejunum, although motilin cells were also detected in the upper ileum (49) and rabbit gallbladder (32).

Subsequently, substance P has also been found in gastrointestinal EC cells and it was concluded that motilin was localized in duodenal type EC cells (EC$_2$) and substance P in EC$_1$ cells (31,48,51). Further confusion arose when studies using antisera raised against synthetic motilin did not detect any motilin in 5-HT staining EC cells but a further cell group, possibly a subpopulation of D$_1$ cells, stained for motilin (28,50,67).

Clearly, further investigations are needed to resolve these contradictions, especially since there appear to be differences between antisera raised against natural or synthetic motilin in the RIA (5,26,74).

RIA FOR MOTILIN

RIAs for motilin have been developed with antibodies raised against natural porcine motilin (5,26) and synthetic (14-Met) motilin (74). Species differences in relative gastrointestinal distribution may occur, since the jejunal:duodenal:ileal ratios have been reported as 100:7:0.04 (pig), 100:442:1.3 (man), and 100:156:28 (dog) (5,26,74). Yanaihara's group also found a much broader distribution of motilin, with relatively high amounts in the stomach, adrenals, salivary gland, gallbladder, pineal body, and pituitary (74).

Motilin-like immunoreactivity has been detected in plasma from dogs and humans (5,10,35). Fasting human levels show a broad and skew distribution (5) and an age dependence, with infants (1–60 weeks old) having levels three to four times those of adults (44). Part of the wide variation may be explained by spontaneous fluctuations that occur in the fasted state (35).

Only one molecular form of motilin has been detected in plasma and duodenal extracts (5). However, it is possible that antibodies with different specificities may detect other forms of motilin.

EFFECTS OF EXOGENOUS MOTILIN

Gastroi..testinal Motility and Gastric Emptying

Studies on strips of rabbit duodenal and colonic circular muscle and fundic muscle from human stomach have shown that porcine motilin potently increased the contractile response (61,65). Synthetic 13-leucine or 13-norleucine analogs were equipotent to natural motilin (24,64,65), and 13-nleu-motilin potentiated acetylcholine-induced contractions (66). Guinea pig and rat preparations were refractory, raising the possibility that, if these species possess a motilin-like peptide, the structure and organ receptor specificities may be different from those in responsive animals.

Pharmacological blockade of ganglia by hexamethonium or axonal conduction by tetrodotoxin and atropinization had no effect on motilin-induced contraction (64). The authors concluded that motilin acted directly on the muscle cell. The contractile response to motilin is blocked by the calcium transport antagonist verapamil (64), but since motilin has no effect on calcium uptake it may cause a redistribution of intracellular calcium (57). Motilin-induced contractions are associated with a concomitant increase in intracellular cyclic GMP concentration (23), whereas increasing endogenous cyclic AMP content by isobutyl-theophylline is accompanied by a reduction in tone and negation of the tone-enhancing effect of motilin (59). The adenyl cyclase/guanyl cyclase system may therefore also be involved.

Motilin-induced changes in electrical events have been demonstrated. In isolated strips of duodenal muscle, 13-norleucine motilin causes membrane depolarization. Slow fluctuations of membrane potential, characteristic of minute-rhythm type, appeared and trains of spikes occurring at the crests of these rhythms were associated with muscular contraction (54).

In the isolated perfused dog stomach and duodenum, motilin has been found to produce no effect on duodenal slow wave (pacemaker) frequency and a 10% reduction in that of the stomach antrum (29,70). An increase in spike activity occurred that could be blocked by atropine.

In vivo studies with motilin showed it to be a powerful stimulator of motor activity in fundic and antral pouches of the stomach of conscious dogs at doses as low as 50 ng/kg. Experiments performed with an interrupted infusion of motilin showed that both antral and fundic pouches exhibited tachyphylaxis

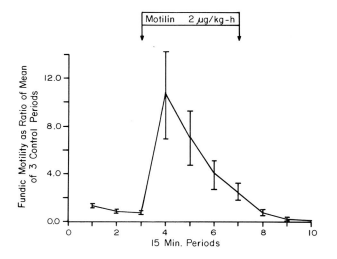

FIG. 2. Effect of a 1-hr infusion of motilin (2 μg/kg-h) on fundic pouch motor activity. Mean ± SE. (From ref. 19, with permission.)

(Figs. 2 and 3). Cholinergic blockade with atropine caused a strong reduction in fundic motor activity in response to motilin (Fig. 4). It was therefore suggested that motilin might act via release of an intermediate, possibly acetylcholine, and the tachyphylaxis was due to depleted stores of this intermediate (19).

Itoh et al. (34,35) performed elegant studies on the possible involvement of motilin in the control of interdigestive migrating myoelectric complexes. Strain

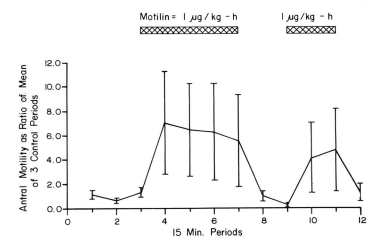

FIG. 3. Effect of an infusion of motilin (1 μg/kg-h) on antral pouch motor activity. Mean ± SE. (From ref. 19, with permission.)

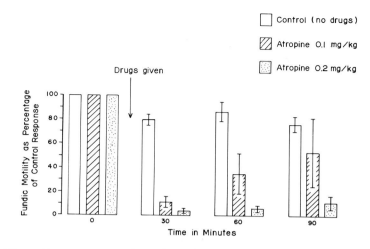

FIG. 4. Effect of intravenous injections of atropine 0.1 and 0.2 mg/kg on fundic pouch motor activity responses to intravenous injections of motilin (2 mg). Responses at time 0 defined as 100%. Mean ± SE. (From ref. 19, with permission.)

gage force transducers were chronically implanted throughout the gastrointestinal tract, enabling continuous multiple site recording of motor activity. In the digestive state, motilin had no effect on motor activity, whereas in the interdigestive state a pattern of activity resembling naturally occurring interdigestive contractions occurred. These were inhibited by ingestion of food or intravenous pentagastrin. Duodenal acidification also inhibited the regular occurrence of contractions and motilin restored the motor pattern. Motilin measurements showed parallel changes in plasma immunoreactive motilin and gastric motor activity. Other workers also showed that intravenous motilin produces premature migrating complexes in the spontaneous interdigestive sequence (70). They have also suggested that motilin does not act directly on motor activity but rather interacts with a hypothetical center controlling this activity.

Gastric emptying of liquid, but not solid, meals was stimulated by motilin infusion in dogs (20). Conversely, in man, 13-norleucine motilin inhibited gastric emptying of a liquid meal (56), whereas porcine motilin stimulated solid emptying (4). The reason for these different results is not clear but may purely reflect species differences. Debas et al. (20) also provided evidence that, at least in the dog, the effect of motilin is on the body of the stomach and is modulated by vagal tone.

The effects of motilin on smooth muscle have prompted a number of studies on its possible involvement in control of the lower esophageal sphincter pressure (LES). In both conscious and anesthetized dogs, motilin induced strong phasic pressure changes in the LES (34,35,36,37,41). At doses over 50 ng/kg, repetitive high amplitude contractions occurred (41). The motilin response was sensitive to atropine and hexamethonium, suggesting action on preganglionic cholinergic neurons. Similar observations have been made in man (40,55) and in the opossum (30).

Evidence that endogenous motilin release coincides with LES pressure changes is not so convincing. Both good (22) and poor (27,33) correlations between the two parameters have been reported.

Gastric and Pancreatic Secretion

During investigations on the effect of motilin on gastric motility, it was observed that pepsin secretion was also stimulated (12). 13-Norleucine motilin also stimulated pepsin secretion in dogs (38,39) and in humans (56,61). An increased gastric mucosal blood flow, measured by augmented aminopyrine clearance, correlated with the pepsin secretion and it was speculated that the motilin effect may be mediated by this increase (38). A direct effect on peptic cells is equally possible.

Infusion of motilin (1 μg/kg/hr) in dogs had little effect on basal acid secretion but potentiated secretion stimulated by synthetic human gastrin (19). Konturek et al. (39) found that 13-norleucine motilin (50 ng/kg/hr) also had little effect on basal secretion but strongly inhibited pentagastrin, histamine, or peptone meal-stimulated acid secretion. The reasons for the discrepancy may be related to differences in biological actions of 13-methionine and 13-norleucine motilin or to the dose used.

A stimulatory effect on basal volume, bicarbonate, and protein output from the pancreas and inhibition of secretin-stimulated bicarbonate output in conscious dogs have also been reported (39) but no effect of 13-norleucine motilin was found on human pancreatic secretion (21).

SECRETION OF MOTILIN

Response to Changes in Gastrointestinal pH

In dogs with extrinsically denervated pouches of stomach fundus and antrum, the infusion of 50 ml of Tris into the duodenum resulted in a rapid increase in motilin levels from 294 ± 44 pg/ml to 498 ± 100 pg/ml at a time when duodenal pH increased by 0.7 pH units. This was accompanied by increased motor activity of the body of the stomach. Maximum motilin levels (916 ± 96 pg/ml) were reached at 5 min, when motor activity was also maximal but duodenal pH had returned to the pre-infusion level (10,26). The motilin response to alkalinization of the gastrointestinal tract in man has been contradictory. Hellemans et al. (33) found increased circulating motilin in response to antral perfusion with sodium bicarbonate and delayed increases in response to intraduodenal sodium hydroxide. Conversely, duodenal alkalinization with Tris decreased motilin levels in man (43,69). Although species differences may account for the conflicting results, failure to obtain sufficient pH change, the site of buffer application, or assay differences may also be responsible.

Increases in circulating IR-motilin occurred in response to intraduodenal acid in dog (10) and in man (16,33,42,43). This response depended on the rate of perfusion (16). Since the motilin response is not accompanied by changes in stomach motility (10), it has been suggested that an antagonistic humoral agent could be released simultaneously.

Response to Feeding

In man a small but significant decrease in motilin occurred 30 to 45 min after feeding glucose or a mixed meal (25,45). Increases in motilin have been reported after oral (3,43) or intravenous administration of fat (3).

Miscellaneous

Infusions of secretin (45) and somatostatin inhibit motilin release.

MOTILIN PATHOLOGY

The original localization of motilin to the EC-cell suggested it may be involved in the carcinoid syndrome. Normal serum levels have been found in patients with lung, gastric, and ileal argentaffin carcinoid tumors (47). It has been suggested that since "motilin cells are distinct from enterochromaffin cells" it is unlikely that motilin is increased in any form of carcinoids (67). Polak et al. (50) suggested, however, that motilin might play a role in duodenal-jejunal carcinoids.

Elevated basal motilin levels have been reported in patients with postinfective tropical malabsorption (387 ± 76 pg/ml) and pancreatic disease (211 ± 32 pg/ml) (1,2).

SUMMARY AND CONCLUSIONS

Motilin research is in a very active phase but, although a great deal of information on its actions is available, little is known of the physiological mode of secretion.

The potent actions on gastrointestinal muscle contraction, both *in vivo* and *in vitro,* suggest that motilin is important in the control of gastrointestinal motility and gastric emptying. It is not clear whether this is a direct effect or whether it occurs via an intermediate. The correlation between motilin levels and interdigestive migrating myoelectric complexes implicate it in the control of "debris" removal from the small bowel, a function that may be of considerable importance.

One of the major controversies of the present time concerns the differences observed between man and dog, in particular the effect of duodenal pH on circulating motilin levels. It is possible that this reflects a species response difference or that current antisera are not really suited to human studies. The variable and small changes observed in response to feeding indicate this is a strong possibility. Alternatively, motilin may act in a paracrine fashion and measurement of peripheral plasma levels would not reflect the true, local concentration of the peptide.

PROJECTIONS FOR THE FUTURE

A number of intriguing observations require more detailed study.

The differences obtained in cellular localization by immunohistochemical techniques using two different antisera raises the possibility of the existence of two motilin-like molecules. Chromatographic profiles of gut extracts measured with the two antisera may indicate whether or not this is so.

The finding of high concentrations of motilin-like-immunoreactivity in the pineal and the pituitary should be confirmed, since it may be one more example of a dual neural/gut location for a peptide. The significance may be more difficult to elucidate.

Studies on the release of motilin into the circulation should be correlated with the known actions of this peptide. Selective catheterization of small bowel veins with concurrent motility measurements may indicate whether local concentrations more closely reflect the motilin response to feeding and whether these correlate with motility changes.

REFERENCES

1. Bloom, S. R., Besterman, H. S., Adrian, T. E., Christofides, N. D., Sarson, D. L., Mallinson, C. N., Pera, A., South, M., Madigliani, R., and Guerin, S. (1978): Gut hormone profile in pancreatic disease. *Gastroenterology,* 74:10 (Abstr.).
2. Bloom, S. R., Besterman, H. S., Cook, G. C., Sarson, D. L., and Christofides, N. D. (1978): Gut hormone profile in post-infective tropical malabsorption (acute tropical sprue). *Gastroenterology,* 74:1010 (Abstr.).
3. Bloom, S. R., Christofides, N. D., Besterman, H. S., Adrian, T. E., and Ghatei, M. A. (1978): Release of motilin in man by oral and intravenous nutriments. *Gastroenterology,* 74:1010 (Abstr.).
4. Bloom, S. R., Christofides, N. D., Modlin, I., and Fitzpatrick, M. L. (1978): Effect of motilin on gastric emptying of solid meals in man. *Gastroenterology,* 74:1010 (Abstr.).
5. Bloom, S. R., Mitznegg, P., and Bryant, M. G. (1976): Measurement of human plasma motilin. *Scand. J. Gastroenterol. (Suppl. 39),* II:47–52.
6. Boldyreff, W. N. (1904): Thesis, St. Petersburg. Quoted by Babkin (1904). *Die Aussere Sekretion der Verdannugsdrüsen,* Ed. 2. J. Springer, Berlin.
7. Brown, J. C. (1967): Presence of a gastric motor-stimulating property in duodenal extracts. *Gastroenterology,* 52:225–229.
8. Brown, J. C., Cook, M. A., and Dryburgh, J. R. (1972): Motilin, a gastric motor activity-stimulating polypeptide: final purification, amino acid composition, and C-terminal residues. *Gastroenterology,* 62:401–404.
9. Brown, J. C., Cook, M. A., and Dryburgh, J. R. (1973): Motilin, a gastric motor activity stimulating polypeptide: the complete amino acid sequence. *Can. J. Biochem.,* 51:533–537.
10. Brown, J. C., and Dryburgh, J. R. (1978): Isolation of motilin. In: *Gut Hormones,* edited by S. R. Bloom, Churchill Livingstone Press.

11. Brown, J. C., Johnson, L. P., and Magee, D. F. (1966): Effect of duodenal alkalinization on gastric motility. *Gastroenterology,* 50:333–339.
12. Brown, J. C., Mutt, V., and Dryburgh, J. R. (1971): The further purification of motilin, a gastric motor activity-stimulating polypeptide from the mucosa of the small intestine of hogs. *Can. J. Physiol. Pharmacol.,* 49:399–405.
13. Brown, J. C., and Parkes, C. O. (1967): Effect on fundic pouch motor activity of stimulatory and inhibitory fractions separated from pancreozymin. *Gastroenterology,* 53:731–736.
14. Brunemeier, E. H., and Carlson, A. J. (1915): Reflexes from the intestinal mucosa to the stomach. *Am. J. Physiol.,* 36:191–195.
15. Chey, W. Y., Hitanant, S., and Hendricks, J. (1970): Effect of secretin and cholecystokinin on gastric emptying and gastric secretion in man. *Gastroenterology,* 58:820–827.
16. Collins, S. M., Lewis, T. P., Track, N., Fox, J., and Daniel, E. E. (1978): Release of Motilin. *Gastroenterology,* 74:1020 (Abstr.).
17. Cooke, A. R. (1974): Duodenal acidification: role of the first part of the duodenum in gastric emptying and secretion in dogs. *Gastroenterology,* 67:85–92.
18. Cooke, A. R. (1975): Control of gastric emptying and motility. *Gastroenterology,* 68:804–816.
19. Cook, M. A. (1972): Ph.D. Thesis: The isolation, structure and physiological actions of motilin. University of British Columbia.
20. Debas, H. T., Yamagishi, T., and Dryburgh, J. R. (1977): Motilin enhances gastric emptying of liquids in dogs. *Gastroenterology,* 73:777–780.
21. Domschke, S., Domschke, W., Schmack, B., Tympner, F., Junge, O., Wunsch, E., Jaeger, E., and Demling, L. (1976): Effects of 13-nle-motilin on salivary, gastric, and pancreatic secretions in man. *Am. J. Dig. Dis.,* 21:789–792.
22. Domschke, W., Lux, G., Mitznegg, P., Rosch, W., Domschke, S., Bloom, S. R., Wunsch, E., and Demling, L. (1976): Relationship of plasma motilin response to lower esophageal sphincter pressure in man. *Scand. J. Gastroenterol. (Suppl. 39),* II:81–84.
23. Domschke, W., Strunz, U., Mitznegg, P., Domschke, S., Springel, W., Ruppin, H., Wunsch, E., and Demling L. (1978): Pharmacology of motilin. In: *Gut Hormones,* edited by S. R. Bloom, Churchill Livingstone Press.
24. Domschke, W., Strunz, U., Mitznegg, P., Ruppin, H., Domschke, S., Schubert, E., Wunsch, E., Jaeger, E., and Demling, L. (1974): 13-Norleucin-motilin-Analyse der Wirkungen auf den gastrointestinal trakt. *Naturwissenschaflen,* 61:370.
25. Dryburgh, J. R. (1977): Ph.D. Thesis: Immunological techniques in the investigation of the physiological functions of gastric inhibitory polypeptide and motilin. University of British Columbia.
26. Dryburgh, J. R., and Brown, J. C. (1975): Radioimmunoassay for motilin. *Gastroenterology,* 68:1169–1176.
27. Eckardt, V., and Grace, N. D. (1976): Lower esophageal sphincter pressure and serum motilin levels. *Am. J. Dig. Dis.,* 21:1008–1011.
28. Forssman, W. G., Yanaihara, N., Helmstaedter, V., and Grube, D. (1976): Differential demonstration of the motilin-cell and the enterochromaffin-cell. *Scand. J. Gastroenterol. (Suppl. 39),* II:43–45.
29. Green, W. E. R., Ruppin, H., Wingate, D. L., Domschke, W., Wunsch, E., Demling, L., and Ritchie, H. D. (1976): Effects of 13-nle motilin on the electrical and mechanical activity of the isolated perfused canine stomach and duodenum. *Gut,* 17:362–370.
30. Gutierrez, J. G., Thanik, K. D., Chey, W. Y., and Yajima, H. (1976): The effect of motilin on the lower esophageal sphincter of the opossum. *Gastroenterology,* 70:958 (Abstr.).
31. Heitz, P. U., Kasper, M., Kreg, G., Polak, J. M., and Pearse, A. G. E. (1978): Immunoelectron cytochemical localization of motilin in human duodenal enterochromaffin cells. *Gastroenterology,* 74:713–717.
32. Heitz, Ph., Polak, J. M., Kasper, M., Timson, C. N., and Pearse, A. G. E. (1977): Immunoelectron cytochemical localization of motilin and substance P in rabbit bile duct enterochromaffin (EC) cells. *Histochemistry,* 50:319–325.
33. Hellemans, J., Vantrappen, G., and Bloom, S. R. (1976): Endogenous motilin and the LES pressure. *Scand. J. Gastroenterol. (Suppl. 39),* II:67–73.
34. Itoh, Z., Honda, R., Hiwatashi, K., Takeuchi, S., Aizawa, I., Takayanagi, R., and Couch, E. F. (1976): Motilin-induced mechanical activity in the canine alimentary tract. *Scand. J. Gastroenterol. (Suppl. 39),* II:93–110.

35. Itoh, Z., Takeuchi, S., Aizawa, I., Takayanagi, R., Mori, H., Taminato, T., Seino, Y., Imura, H., and Yanaihara, N. (1978): Recent advances in motilin research: its physiological and clinical significance. In: *Gastrointestinal Hormones and Pathology of the Digestive System,* edited by M. Grossman, V. Speranza, N. Basso, and E. Lezoche. Plenum Press, New York.
36. Jennewein, H. M., Bauer, R., Hummelt, H., Lepsin, G., Siewert, R., and Waldeck, F. (1976): Motilin effects on gastrointestinal motility and lower esophageal sphincter (LES) pressure in dogs. *Scand. J. Gastroenterol. (Suppl. 39),* II:63–65.
37. Jennewein, H. M., Hummelt, H., Siewert R., and Waldeck, F. (1975): The motor-stimulating effect of natural motilin on the lower esophageal sphincter, fundus, antrum, and duodenum in dogs. *Digestion,* 13:246–250.
38. Koch, H., Domschke, S., Belohlavek, D., Domschke, W., Wunsch, E., Jaeger, E., and Demling, L. (1976): Gastric mucosal blood flow and pepsin secretion in dogs-stimulation by 13-Nle-motilin. *Scand. J. Gastroenterol., (Suppl. 39),* II:93–96.
39. Konturek, S. J., Dembinski, A., Krol, R., and Wunsch, E. (1976): Effects of motilin on gastric and pancreatic secretion in dogs. *Scand. J. Gastroenterol. (Suppl. 39),* II:57–61.
40. Lux, G., Rosch, W., Domchke, S., Domschke, W., Wunsch, E., Jaeger, E., and Demling, L. (1976): Intravenous 13-Nle-motilin increases the human lower esophageal sphincter pressure. *Scand. J. Gastroenterol. (Suppl. 39),* II:75–79.
41. Meissner, A. J., Bowes, K. L., Zwick, R., and Daniel, E. E. (1976): Effect of motilin on the lower oesophageal sphincter. *Gut,* 17:923–932.
42. Mitznegg, P., Domschke, W., Wunsch, E., Bloom, S. R., Domschke, S., and Demling, L. (1976): Release of motilin after duodenal acidification. *Lancet,* i:888–889.
43. Mitznegg, P., Bloom, S. R., Christofides, N., Besterman, H., Domschke, W., Domschke, S., Wunsch, E., and Demling, L. (1976): Release of motilin in man. *Scand. J. Gastroenterol. (Suppl. 39),* II:53–56.
44. Mitznegg, P., Domschke, W., Schubert, E., Domschke, W., Sprugel, W., Wunsch, E., and Demling L. (1977): Age dependence in fasting plasma motilin: elevation in infants. *Gastroenterology,* 72:1103 (Abstr.).
45. Mitznegg, P., Bloom, S. R., Domschke, W., Haeki, W. I., Domschke, S., Belohlavek, D., Wunsch, E., and Demling, L. (1977): Effect of secretin on plasma motilin in man. *Gut,* 18:468–471.
46. Mitznegg, P., Bloom, S. R., Domschke, W., Domschke, S., Wunsch, E., and Demling, L. (1977): Pharmacokinetics of motilin in man. *Gastroenterology,* 72:413–416.
47. Modlin, I. M., Bloom, S. R., and Christofides, N. (1977): Plasma motilin in carcinoid tumors. *Lancet,* ii:979.
48. Pearse, A. G. E. (1976): The cellular origin of motilin in the gastrointestinal tract. *Scand. J. Gastroenterol. (Suppl. 39),* II:35–38.
49. Pearse, A. G. E., Polak, J. M., Bloom, S. R., Adams, C., Dryburgh, J. R., and Brown, J. C. (1974): Enterochromaffin cells of the mammalian small intestine as the source of motilin. *Virchows Archiv. (Cell Pathol.),* 16:111–120.
50. Polak, J. M., Buchan, A. M. J., Dryburgh, J. R., Christofides, N., Bloom, S. R., and Yanaihara, N. (1978): Immunoreactive motilins? *Lancet,* i:1364–1365.
51. Polak, J. M., Heitz, P., and Pearse, A. G. E. (1976): Differential localization of substance P and motilin. *Scand. J. Gastroenterol. (Suppl. 39),* II:39–42.
52. Polak, J. M., Pearse, A. G. E., and Heath, C. M. (1975): Complete identification of endocrine cells in the gastrointestinal tract using semithin-thin sections to identify motilin cells in human and animal intestine. *Gut,* 16:225–229.
53. Quigley, J. P., and Meschan, I. (1938): The role of the vagus in the regulation of the pyloric sphincter and adjacent portions of the gut, with special reference to the process of gastric evacuation. *Am. J. Physiol.,* 123:166.
54. Riemer, J., Kolling, K., and Mayer, C. J. (1977): The effect of motilin on the electrical activity of rabbit circular duodenal muscle. *Pfluegers Arch.* 372:243–250.
55. Rosch, W., Lux, G., Domschke, S., Domschke, W., Wunsch, E., Jaeger, E., and Demling L. (1976): Effect of 13-nle-motilin on lower esophageal sphincter pressure (LES) in man. *Gastroenterology,* 70:931 (Abstr.).
56. Ruppin, H., Domschke, S., Domschke, W., Wunsch, E., Jaeger, E., and Demling, L. (1975): Effects of 13-nle-motilin in man—inhibition of gastric evacuation and stimulation of pepsin secretion. *Scand. J. Gastroenterol.,* 10:199–202.

57. Ruppin, H., Mayer, C. J., Domschke, W., Wunsch, E., and Demling, L. (1977): Lack of effect of 13-norleucine motilin on net calcium uptake of isolated rabbit duodenal muscle. *Gastroenterology*, 72:1123 (Abstr.).
58. Schapiro, H., and Woodward, E. R. (1959): Pathways of enterogastric reflex. *Proc. Soc. Exp. Biol. Med.*, 101:407–409.
59. Schubert, E., Mitznegg, P., Strunz, U., Domschke, W., Domschke, S., Wunsch, E., Jaeger, E., Demling, L., and Hein, F. (1975): Influence of the hormone analogue 13-nle-motilin and of 1-methyl-3-isobutylxanthine on tone and cyclic 3',5'-AMP content of antral and duodenal muscles in the rabbit. *Life Sci.*, 16:263–272.
60. Schubert, H., and Brown, J. C. (1974): Correction to the amino acid sequence of porcine motilin. *Can. J. Biochem.*, 52:7–8.
61. Seyawa, T., Nakano, M., Kai, Y., Kawatani, H., and Yajima, H. (1976): Effect of synthetic motilin and related polypeptides on contraction of gastrointestinal smooth muscle.
62. Serdinokov, A. (1899): One of the conditions available for the passage of food into the intestine. Dissertation St. Petersburg. Reported by Pavlov, I. P. In: *The Work of the Digestive Glands*, translated by W. H. Thompson. Lippincott, Philadelphia.
63. Shay, H., and Gershon-Cohen, J. (1934): Experimental studies in gastric physiology in man. II. A study of pyloric control. Role of acid and alkali. *Surg. Gynecol. Obstet.*, 58:935–955.
64. Strunz, U., Domschke, W., Mitznegg, P., Domschke, P., Schubert, E., Wunsch, E., Jaeger, E., and Demling, L. (1975): Analysis of the motor effects of 13-norleucine motilin on the rabbit, guinea pig, rat, and human alimentary tract *in vitro. Gastroenterology*, 68:1485–1491.
65. Strunz, U., Domschke, W., Domschke, S., Mitznegg, P., Wunsch, E., Jaeger, E., and Demling, L. (1976): Gastroduodenal motor response to natural motilin and synthetic position 13-substituted motilin analogues: a comparative in vitro study. *Scand. J. Gastroenterol., (Suppl. 39)*, II:199–203.
66. Strunz, U., Domschke, W., Domschke, S., Mitznegg, P., Wunch, E., Jaeger, E., and Demling, L. (1976): Potentiation between 13-Nle-motilin and acetylcholine on rabbit pyloric muscle in vitro. *Scand. J. Gastroenterol. (Suppl. 39)*, II:29–33.
67. Sundler, F., Alumets, J., Hakanson, R., Sjolund, K., and Yanaihara, N. (1978): Motilin and carcinoid tumors. *Lancet*, i:1101.
68. Thomas, J. E., Crider, J. O., and Morgan, C. J. (1934): A study of reflexes involving the pyloric sphincter and antrum and their role in gastric evacuation. *Am. J. Physiol.*, 108:683–700.
69. Track, N. S., Collins, S., Lewis, T., and Daniell, E. E. (1978): Motilin release and upper gastrointestinal motility in man. In: *Gut Hormones*, edited by S. R. Bloom. Churchill Livingstone Press, London, Edinburgh, and New York.
70. Wingate, D. L., Ruppin, H., Green, W. E. R., Thompson, H. H., Domschke, W., Wunsch, E., Demling, L., and Ritchie, H. D. (1976): Motilin-induced electrical activity in the canine gastrointestinal tract. *Scand. J. Gastroenterol. (Suppl. 39)*, II:111–118.
71. Wunsch, E. (1976): Syntheses of motilin analogues. *Scand. J. Gastroenterol. (Suppl. 39)*, II:19–24.
72. Wunsch, E., Brown, J. C., Deimer, K-H., Drees, F., Jaeger, E., Musiol, J., Scharf, R., Stocker, H., Thamm, P., and Wendlberger, G. (1973): The total synthesis of norleucine-13-motilin. *Z. Naturtauschung*, 28:235–240.
73. Yajima, H., Kai, Y., Ogawa, H., Kubota, M., Mori, Y., and Koyama, K. (1977): Structure-activity relationships of gastrointestinal hormones: motilin, GIP, and [27-TYR]CCK-PZ. *Gastroenterology*, 72:793–796.
74. Yanaihara, C., Sato, H., Yanaihara, N., Naruse, S., Forssmann, W. E., Helmstaedter, V., Fujita, T., Yamaguichi, W., and Abe, K. (1978): Motilin,-Substance P-and somatostatin-like immuno-reactivities in extracts from dog, tupaia and monkey brain and GI tract. In: *Gastrointestinal Hormones and Pathology of the Digestive System*, edited by M. Grossman, V. Speranza, N. Basso, and E. Lezoche. Plenum Press, New York.

Gastrointestinal Hormones, edited by
George B. Jerzy Glass.
Raven Press, New York © 1980.

Chapter 10

Vasoactive Intestinal Peptide (VIP): Isolation, Distribution, Biological Actions, Structure-Function Relationships, and Possible Functions

Sami I. Said

Veterans' Administration Medical Center, Dallas, Texas 75216; and University of Texas Health Science Center, Dallas, Texas 75235

DISCOVERY

In 1967, Said and co-workers reported that supernates of aqueous extracts of mammalian lungs were highly vasoactive (122). This vasoactivity (systemic vasodilation, hypotension) could not be explained on the basis of the histamine and prostaglandin content of lung tissue, and was thought largely attributable to one or more peptides. In order to isolate these vasoactive peptides, Said went to V. Mutt's laboratory in Stockholm. Together, they extracted and partially purified a vasodilator peptide from porcine lung (129,130). On the premise that the same peptide might occur in other organs, they then turned their search to intestinal extracts, which were more readily available to them.

Using the same bioassay that guided their extraction of the lung peptide (measurement of femoral blood flow and arterial blood pressure), they discovered that peptide fractions from porcine duodenum contained a vasodilator principle (131), which they soon purified to homogeneity and named vasoactive intestinal peptide (VIP) (132,133). Said and Mutt recognized (131) that the presence of a vasodepressor component in intestinal extracts had actually been noted first by Bayliss and Starling, almost 70 years earlier, during their experiments leading to the discovery of secretin (4a).

ISOLATION

The relative speed with which VIP was isolated after its discovery was probably related to the close association of this peptide with secretin. The same techniques that enabled Mutt and Jorpes to extract and purify secretin yielded a VIP-rich peptide fraction (Fig. 1) (107,133). Three additional separation procedures (chromatography on Sephadex G-25, a second chromatography on carboxy-methyl cellulose, and countercurrent distribution) produced a highly purified preparation of VIP, from which traces of impurities could be virtually eliminated by a final chromatography on Sephadex G-25 (Figs. 2–4).

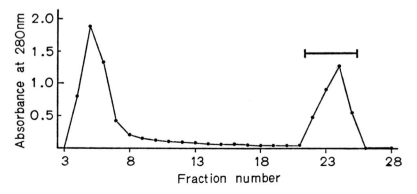

FIG. 1. Chromatography on CM-cellulose of 12 g of methanol-soluble intestinal peptide fraction as used for the isolation of secretin. For details, see ref. 133. Fractions 9 to 18 contain the bulk of the secretin activity, whereas vasoactivity (VIP) was concentrated in fractions 22 to 25, indicated by the *bar*. (From ref. 133, with permission.)

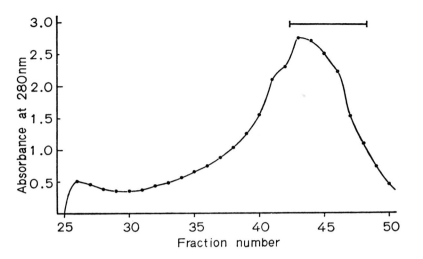

FIG. 2. Chromatography on Sephadex G-25 (fine) of 4.6 g of material of the type recovered from fractions 22 to 25 of Fig. 1. For details, see ref. 133. Fractions 43 to 48, indicated by the *bar,* were combined for further processing. (From ref. 133, with permission.)

DISTRIBUTION IN THE GASTROINTESTINAL TRACT

Although isolated and chemically characterized only from the upper small intestine, VIP now is believed to occur throughout the gastrointestinal tract. This belief is based on the demonstration of VIP-immunoreactivity by radioim-

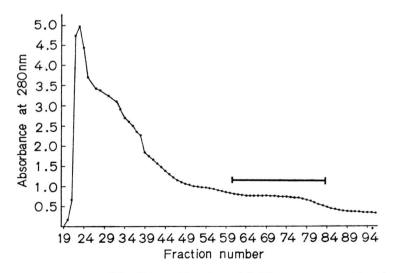

FIG. 3. Chromatography on CM-cellulose of 2 g of material of the type recovered from fractions 43 to 48 of Fig. 2. For details, see ref. 133. Fractions 61 to 83, indicated by the *bar,* were combined for further processing. (From ref. 133, with permission.)

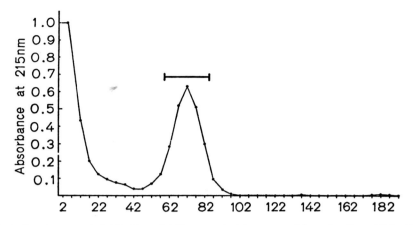

FIG. 4. Countercurrent distribution of 140 mg material recovered from fractions 61 to 83 of Fig. 3. For details, see ref. 133. Fractions 60 to 85, indicated by the *bar,* contained VIP in highly purified form and were combined for further processing. (From ref. 133, with permission.)

munoassay (RIA) of tissue extracts (124) and by immunofluorescence (114). Higher concentrations of the peptide are present in the colon, ileum, and jejunum than in the upper portions of the gut, and relatively high levels are also found in the pancreas (124). VIP in both gut and pancreas is contained mainly within nerve elements (see below), but is also present in specific endocrine cells called D_1 cells (Figs. 5 and 6) (22,23,32). In the intestinal wall, the peptide is located predominantly in the nerve-rich muscular layer, whereas the mucosa contains a relatively small proportion, and epithelium itself has less than 1% of the total peptide content (5,59,60).

OCCURRENCE OUTSIDE THE GASTROINTESTINAL TRACT

VIP in the Nervous System

Several years after its discovery and isolation, VIP was also discovered in high concentrations in neural cell lines (132) and in normal nervous tissues (21,96,136).

FIG. 5. A. VIP cells of a guinea pig islet stained (deep blue in the original preparation) with the immunoperoxidase technique using 1-Cl-4-naphthol. Note unstained B cells and slight nonspecific staining of acinar cells and groups of islet A cells. Unlike VIP cells, the latter cells retained their staining when the anti-VIP serum was absorbed with VIP. PAF fixative; ×320. **B.** VIP cells in a small islet of the dog uncinate process. Immunoperoxidase with 1-Cl-4-napthol, PAF; ×350. **C.** Two blackened cells (likely corresponding to VIP cells of **A**) and a group of A cells (brown; **top right**) stained with Grimelius' silver in a guinea pig islet. Bouin's fixative; ×750. **D.** Immunofluorescent VIP cell in a crypt of the human duodenum, PAF; ×550. **E.** Two immunofluorescent VIP cells in fundic glands of the dog stomach, PAF; ×550. (Courtesy of Professor E. Solcia, Pavia, Italy; from ref. 22, reproduced with permission.)

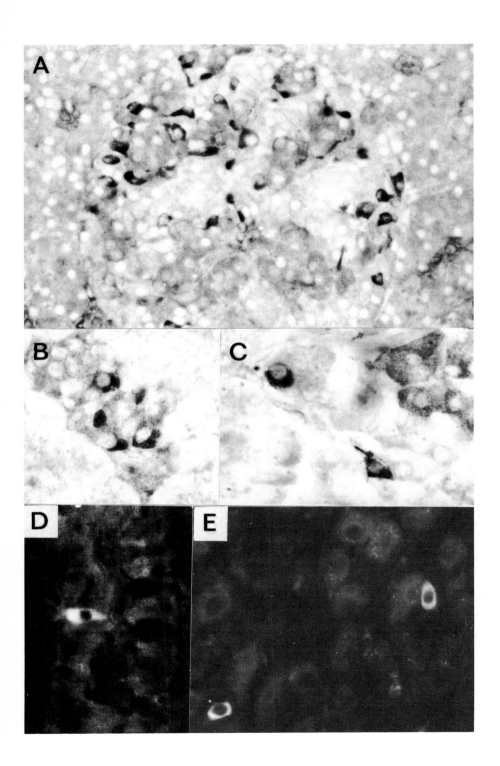

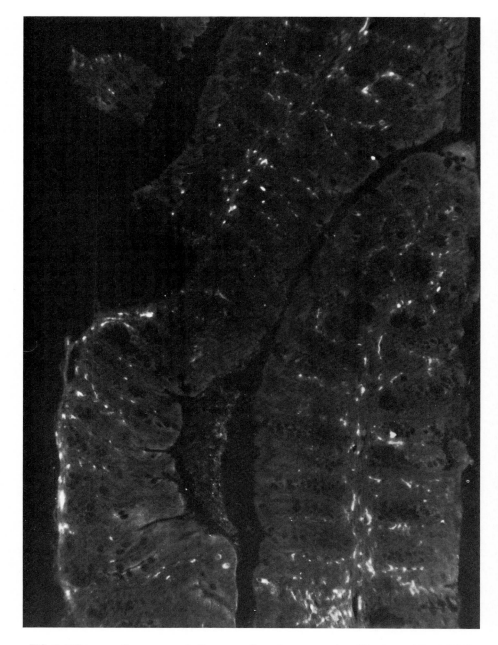

FIG. 6. VIP-immunofluorescence in fine nerve fibers in mouse colon. (Courtesy of Dr. J. Polak, London, England.)

In the brain, the peptide has a discrete regional distribution: highest levels of VIP-immunoreactivity (in rat and dog brain) are found in the cerebral cortex, hypothalamus (suprachiasmatic nucleus, anterior hypothalamic area), amygdala, hippocampus, and corpus striatum (5,136,141). [The cerebral cortex is rich in another gastrointestinal hormone, cholecystokinin-pancreozymin (CCK-PZ)]. Immunohistochemical techniques have confirmed and extended these findings: VIP-positive fibers are present in all these areas, and VIP-positive cell bodies are demonstrable in the cerebral cortex and amygdaloid cortex (58,69). In human brain, the distribution of immunoreactive VIP is similar, except that the highest content (per milligram extracted protein) is in the physiologically important median eminence (140). In all mammalian species examined, little VIP was found in the cerebellum or in the brainstem. Human cerebrospinal fluid (CSF) contains measurable levels of VIP; in one report, these levels were 10 times higher than in plasma (52).

Radioreceptor assay of tissue extracts shows that the VIP in the gastrointestinal tract and in brain is biologically active; in both locations (5), the peptide content is similar when measured by radioreceptor assay or by RIA (5).

VIP occurs widely in the peripheral nervous system and in nerves supplying multiple organs, where it is a major component of the "peptidergic" system of nerves. Such sites where immunoreactive VIP has been demonstrated include:

(a) The submucous (Meissner's) and myenteric (Auerbach's) plexuses in the intestinal wall (58,96,113) and nerves supplying the smooth muscle of the esophagus (161). At least some of the VIP nervous elements in small intestine are intrinsic to this organ, as they are seen in organotypic tissue cultures of fetal intestine, which are devoid of extrinsic innervation (147). The peptide is also demonstrable in nerve cell bodies in the fetal esophagus at an early stage of development (161)

(b) Nerve fibers in the pancreas (93,155) that, in some species (e.g., dog), go directly to acinar cells, islet, and blood vessels

(c) Nerves to the gallbladder (156)

(d) Cell bodies and nerve fibers in sympathetic ganglia, especially in mesenteric ganglia of guinea pig (71)

(e) Nerves in the urogenital organs (1,72,94,95), especially in the vagina and endometrium in the female; in the epididymis and vas deferens in the male; and in the trigonum of the urinary bladder, around the ureteral opening and in the ureteric submucosa and smooth muscle layers, in both sexes. VIP-positive nerve fibers are also present in the kidney, mainly in the cortex, around blood vessels (72)

(f) Nerve terminals in the walls of the cerebral vessels (92)

(g) Nerves in the tracheobronchial tree and upper airways, especially around seromucous glands, blood vessels, and smooth muscle (160)

(h) Peripheral nerves, e.g., the sciatic (65) and the vagus nerves (98,136)

VIP in Other Organs and Tissues

Human placenta has been found to contain immunoreactive VIP in concentrations that were at least two orders of magnitude higher than in peripheral venous blood (2,44). In the same study, VIP levels in cord blood were about three times those in normal plasma.

The adrenal medulla (and possibly also the adrenal cortex), lung (134), and upper airways (160) are among other organs in which VIP or a VIP-like peptide has been shown to exist. Organs with little or no detectable VIP include liver and skeletal muscle (136).

VIP is concentrated within mast cells (of rat peritoneum and lung) (33), where it appears to be associated with histamine, and in platelets (64).

SUBCELLULAR LOCALIZATION

Subcellular fractionation of homogenates of VIP-rich parts of the brain (cerebral cortex, hypothalamus, striatum) showed VIP to be concentrated in the synaptosomal fraction (isolated presynaptic nerve terminals) (66,128). Also concentrated in this fraction were two of the established neurotransmitters, dopamine and norepinephrine (66). This subcellular localization of VIP has been confirmed in other cell fractionation studies (6), and a vesicular localization has been reported in rat hypothalamus (49). The same conclusion was reached from ultrastructural immunoperoxidase studies on intestinal nerves (91). The localization of VIP in synaptosomal and vesicular fractions, from which it can be released (49,66), is in keeping with a role for the peptide in synaptic function.

VIP IN THE ANIMAL KINGDOM

In all mammalian species examined, including pig, dog, rabbit, rat, guinea pig, and man, RIA and immunofluorescence techniques have established the presence of VIP or a closely related peptide. In the chicken, the only nonmammalian species from which the peptide has been isolated, its structure is remarkably similar to the porcine peptide; each has 28 amino acid residues and they differ only in four positions. The wide occurrence of VIP in the animal kingdom, even in more primitive species, is further evidenced by its presence in nervous structures of the earthworm *(Lumbricus terrestris)* (157).

BIOLOGICAL ACTIONS

Although the wide distribution of VIP was not appreciated for several years after its discovery, the multiplicity of its biological actions was already recognized in the title of the first report on its isolation (132).

The full range of actions of VIP probably remains only partially known; actions that have been described (123,125,126) are summarized in Table 1 and further described below.

TABLE 1. *Biological actions of VIP*

Cardiovascular system:	Vasodilation (including peripheral, splanchnic, coronary, extracranial, and cerebral vessels), hypotension, moderate inotropic effect
Respiratory system:	Bronchodilation, augmented ventilation, stimulation of adenylate cyclase activity
Digestive system:	
Esophagus	Relaxation of lower sphincter
Stomach	Relaxation of fundic smooth muscle, suppression of acid, and pepsin secretion
Pancreas, liver	Stimulation of water and bicarbonate secretion (secretin-like action), increased bile flow
Gallbladder	Relaxation of isolated smooth muscle, inhibition of contractile effect of CCK-PZ
Small and large intestine	Inhibition of absorption, stimulation of water and ion secretion, stimulation of adenylate cyclase activity, relaxation of smooth muscle of colon
Metabolism:	Stimulation of glycogenolysis, lipolysis, and adenylate cyclase activity (in liver, pancreatic acini and adipocytes), hyperglycemia
Endocrine function:	
Pancreas	Release of insulin, glucagon, and somatostatin
Pituitary-hypothalamus	Stimulation of release of prolactin, GH, and LH
Adrenal	ACTH-like action (stimulation of steroidogenesis and adenylate cyclase activity)
Central nervous system:	Arousal, excitation of cerebral cortical and spinal cord neurons, hyperthermia, regional stimulation of adenylate cyclase activity

Cardiovascular System

The vasodilator-hypotensive effect of VIP is one of its more remarkable actions and was the basis for its bioassay during isolation from both hog and chicken intestine (Fig. 7).

Vasodilation is induced by VIP in numerous vascular beds, including the peripheral systemic, e.g., femoral; the splanchnic, e.g., mesenteric, pancreatico-

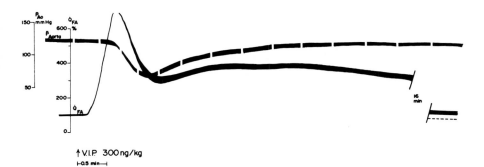

FIG. 7. Vasodilator effect of VIP in anesthetized dog. Infusion of peptide (300 ng/kg) into a superficial branch of a femoral artery caused a greater than fivefold increase in femoral arterial blood flow *(continuous tracing),* measured by an electromagnetic flow probe, and a 60 mm Hg fall in mean aortic blood pressure *(interrupted tracing).* Infusion lasted 30 sec *(bar)* but flow and pressure had barely returned to control values 16 min later.

duodenal, and hepatic (131,132,159) [although intestinal blood flow may be decreased with the hypotension (99)]; the coronary (166); and the carotid (external and internal) vessels. In rabbits, blood flow to cerebral gray matter is moderately increased (68). In dogs, blood flow in the coronary and carotid vessels increase markedly and at dose levels (0.5 μg or less per kilogram) that are too low to increase flow elsewhere or to reduce arterial blood pressure. VIP does not increase total renal blood flow, and its effect on the pulmonary circulation remains ill defined. In doses sufficient to cause generalized vasodilation, infusions of VIP result in a fall in arterial blood pressure, especially diastolic pressure.

VIP has a moderate inotropic effect on heart muscle, determined by an increase in left ventricular dP/dt in anesthetized dogs in which the heart action was kept constant by pacing and left ventricular preload and afterload did not change, and by an increase in tension of isometrically contracting isolated strips of cat papillary muscle (127). The inotropic activity of VIP is comparable with that of glucagon, but larger doses are required to elicit this than the coronary vasodilator effect.

Respiratory System

VIP induces augmentation of ventilation (132). The respiratory stimulation is independent of any reflexes provoked by hypotension since it follows intracarotid infusions of the peptide in doses that are too small to lower blood pressure. Direct evidence for chemoreceptor stimulation was reported in anesthetized dogs (132).

VIP also relaxes isolated tracheobronchial smooth muscle, an effect that may be related to its ability to promote cyclic AMP accumulation in these preparations (55). Administration of the peptide by aerosol to anesthetized dogs prevents or markedly attenuates the bronchoconstrictor action of prostaglandin $F_{2\alpha}$ and of histamine, given over the subsequent 2 hr (67). Given as an aerosol, VIP had either a negligible or no effect on heart rate or blood pressure (67).

Gastrointestinal System

Motility

VIP relaxes smooth muscle of the lower esophageal sphincter in anesthetized opossums (117), awake baboons (149), and man (43). It also relaxes isolated smooth muscle preparations of gastric fundus, gallbladder, colon, and rectum, and opposes *in vitro* and *in vivo* the contractile action of CCK-PZ on the gallbladder (76,77,106,112,120,121). The VIP-induced relaxation of gastrointestinal (and tracheobronchial) smooth muscle is unaffected by blockade of adrenergic or cholinergic receptors (112).

Secretion

Two of the most potent actions of VIP influence gastrointestinal secretion: it inhibits histamine- and pentagastrin-stimulated secretion of gastric acid and pepsin (100,102,163), but stimulates water and electrolyte secretion by small and large intestine (3,31,87,103,116,164). The peptide stimulates adenylate cyclase activity in intestinal mucosa (148,150–152), isolated enterocytes (61,89) and their membrane preparations (80,165), and colonic tumor cell lines (90). The latter effect is of special interest in relation to the postulated role of VIP in the watery-diarrhea syndrome (8,10).

VIP is a secretin-like partial agonist in dog and man with an efficacy of 20 to 30% that of secretin (42,101); in the cat, VIP may be a full agonist (84). In all species, it has low potency (about 10%), compared with secretin, as a stimulant of pancreatic flow and bicarbonate secretion (133), but augments submaximal responses to secretin (99–102). VIP also enhances pancreatic flow response to the octapeptide of CCK-PZ and, in large doses, promotes the flow of bile, but less effectively than secretin (101).

Metabolism

Metabolic effects of VIP include stimulation of glycogenolysis (with approximately 20% the potency of glucagon) (81), hyperglycemia (81), stimulation of lipolysis in rat adipocytes (36,56,138), and stimulation of adenylate cyclase activity in plasma membrane preparations from liver, fat cells (88), enterocytes, exocrine pancreas (78,88), pituitary (63), and brain (20,35) (see also pp. 259–261, *this chapter*).

Endocrine Function

Pancreas

In the perfused cat and porcine pancreas, and in the presence of critical concentrations of glucose, VIP stimulates the secretion of insulin and of glucagon (97,146). These results have been confirmed in anesthetized dogs, where the stimulation of insulin and of glucagon occurred with doses of peptide that were too low to cause hyperglycemia (79,110).

The effects of VIP on islet cell function may be more complex, as it has been shown also to stimulate the release of somatostatin in the isolated canine pancreas (75). In addition, the peptide stimulates adenylate cyclase activity in crude islet membranes (57).

Adrenal

VIP exerts an ACTH-like action on adrenal cortical tumor cells in culture. The steroidogenic effectiveness of the two peptides was comparable, but the potency of VIP was $1:100$ that of ACTH. The peak increase in cyclic AMP production associated with maximal steroidogenesis was several times smaller with VIP than with ACTH (85,86).

Pituitary-Hypothalamic Hormones

The presence of high levels of VIP in hypothalamic nuclei (58,141), in the median eminence of human hypothalamus (140), and in hypophyseal portal plasma (almost 20 times the level in peripheral plasma) (135) has stimulated investigations of the possible influence of this peptide on hypothalamic-pituitary function. These investigations have revealed that intraventricular injections of VIP (in doses of 4 ng or higher) in conscious, female ovariectomized rats, raised plasma levels of prolactin, growth hormone (GH), and luteinizing hormone (LH), without affecting blood pressure (162). The same authors could not detect release of any of these hormones when hemipituitaries were incubated with the peptide *in vitro* for 2½ hr, and concluded that the site of action of VIP was at the level of the hypothalamus. Two other groups of workers, however, reported VIP-induced prolactin release *in vitro* (80,119).

VIP also activates rat pituitary adenylate cyclase, in a dose-related manner, the enzyme activity reaching four times its control value at peptide concentrations of 10^{-6} M (63).

Central Nervous System

VIP causes arousal in anesthetized animals. This observation was first noted during the bioassay of intestinal peptide fractions even before VIP was fully isolated: injections of VIP-rich fractions lightened the depth of anesthesia in dogs and necessitated booster doses of anesthetic. Electroencephalographic confirmation of this effect was obtained in subsequent experiments in which VIP was infused into the carotid circulation.

More recently, it has been found that VIP, applied iontophoretically, excited deep, spontaneously active cortical neurons in rat cerebral cortex and caused depolarization of motoneurons and dorsal root terminals in the isolated amphibian spinal cord. The threshold dose was 10^{-6} M and the effects were comparable with those of another gastrointestinal-neural peptide, substance P (111).

Given by intraventricular injection (10^{-4} μg) in the cat, VIP elicits shivering and a hyperthermic response (30). In this respect, its action is similar to that of methionine-enkephalin, and opposite to those of neurotensin and bombesin (the latter three peptides, like VIP, occur naturally in the brain and in the gut).

VIP also stimulates adenylate cyclase activity in certain parts of the brain (20,37,115). This effect was demonstrated in homogenates of rat cerebral cortex, hypothalamus, and hippocampus, all VIP-rich, as well as in homogenates of cerebellar cortex, where VIP content is low (20,37). The enzyme stimulation was dose-dependent and was inhibited by Ca^{2+}, but was unaffected by guanine nucleotides.

Other Effects

Infusions of VIP in dogs and man produced a slight hypercalcemia (41); the mechanism of this effect has not been clarified. Flushing of the face was observed during infusion in human subjects and in pigs (41,104).

INHIBITION OF ACTIONS

Somatostatin inhibits VIP-stimulated intestinal secretion and cyclic AMP accumulation in rats (25). Somatostatin may also inhibit the release of VIP, especially from VIP-secreting tumors.

Partial VIP sequences so far tested have been relatively weak agonists of the peptide, and hence also weak inhibitors of its actions (20,158). No analogs have been synthesized that are effective inhibitors. Whenever such compounds become available, they would be useful in elucidating the physiological and pathophysiological significance of VIP and in alleviating the effects of its hypersecretion.

INACTIVATION

Porcine VIP is rapidly removed or inactivated in the circulation. From experiments in pigs and man the half-life was estimated to be approximately 1.2 min (41,104).

Some inactivation probably takes place during passage through the liver. This conclusion is based on: (a) attenuation of the hypotensive, respiratory-stimulant, and secretin-like potency of the peptide when it is given by portal vein infusion, as compared with systemic infusion (82); (b) the existence of large portal-systemic concentration gradients of the peptide in the normal state (27), and even larger gradients during experimental conditions causing VIP release from the gut (7, 50,83,104,139,142); and (c) elevations of circulating levels of the peptide in patients with hepatic failure (46,74). No significant hepatic inactivation of VIP was found, however, when its ability to inhibit pentagastrin-stimulated gastric acid secretion was measured during portal and systemic infusions of the peptide (154).

STRUCTURE AND STRUCTURE-FUNCTION RELATIONSHIPS

An examination of the chemical characteristics and structure of gastrointestinal hormones can yield insights into their actions and possible functional interrelationships. On the basis of their amino acid composition and sequence, as well as the methods leading to their isolation from crude tissue extracts, two distinct groups (or "families") of gastrointestinal hormones have been identified (11,107,108)! Each of these groups consists of hormones that are not only structurally related but that also exhibit similar biological actions. One group includes secretin, VIP, glucagon and, to some extent, gastric inhibitory polypeptide (GIP) (Fig. 8). The other group includes gastrin, CCK-PZ, cerulein, and others. There are less pronounced sequence similarities between VIP and a number of other peptides, including CCK-PZ, motilin, substance P, and ACTH (86,108).

Peptides showing the most extensive structural similarities to VIP are secretin and glucagon (11,108). VIP and secretin are purified together from intestinal extracts, beginning with the same crude extract, almost to the final steps (107). These three peptides also share important activities (137). Thus, secretin and VIP relax gastrointestinal and other smooth muscle and stimulate bicarbonate secretion; glucagon and VIP stimulate glycogenolysis and myocardial contractility; GIP and VIP inhibit gastric acid secretion and stimulate insulin secretion; and VIP, glucagon, and GIP stimulate intestinal juice secretion.

It is tempting to explain the similarities between members of hormonal "families" on the basis of evolutionary changes from common ancestors (40). Bodanszky, however, emphasizes that major (nonconservative) differences exist between members of the secretin-VIP family, and that these differences, together with corresponding evolutionary changes in hormone receptors that also must be postulated, cannot be explained by simple evolutionary schemes (11).

The importance of certain structural differences between VIP and secretin in determining their respective biological properties can be seen from consideration of the residue in position 15 in both peptides (19). This position is occupied by an acidic aspartyl residue in secretin and by a basic residue, lysine, in VIP. The peptide S_5–27 has secretin-like activity in large doses. Compared with this peptide, synthetic analogs in which lysine (or the neutral asparagine) replaces

	1	2	3	4	5	6	7	8	9	10	11	12	13	14
VIP	His	Ser	Asp	Ala	Val	Phe	Thr	Asp	Asn	Tyr	Thr	Arg	Leu	Arg
SECRETIN	His	Ser	Asp	Gly	Thr	Phe	Thr	Ser	Glu	Leu	Ser	Arg	Leu	Arg
GLUCAGON	His	Ser	Gln	Gly	Thr	Phe	Thr	Ser	Asp	Tyr	Ser	Lys	Tyr	Leu
GIP	Tyr	Ala	Glu	Gly	Thr	Phe	Ile	Ser	Asp	Tyr	Ser	Ile	Ala	Met

	15	16	17	18	19	20	21	22	23	24	25	26	27	28	29
VIP	Lys	Gln	Met	Ala	Val	Lys	Lys	Tyr	Leu	Asn	Ser	Ile	Leu	AsnNH$_2$	
SECRETIN	Asp	Ser	Ala	Arg	Leu	Gln	Arg	Leu	Leu	Gln	Gly	Leu	ValNH$_2$		
GLUCAGON	Asp	Ser	Arg	Arg	Ala	Gln	Asp	Phe	Val	Gln	Trp	Leu	Met	Asn	Thr
GIP	Asp	Lys	Ile	Arg	Gln	Gln	Asp	Phe	Val	Asn	Trp	Leu	Leu	Ala	Gln

FIG. 8. Amino acid sequence of porcine VIP, secretin, glucagon, and GIP. Identities between two or more of the peptides are framed. NH$_2$, amide group at C-terminal end of VIP and secretin.

```
              1                      7                       14
Porcine VIP:  His-Ser-Asp-Ala-Val-Phe-Thr-Asp-Asn-Tyr-Thr-Arg-Leu-Arg
Chicken VIP:  His-Ser-Asp-Ala-Val-Phe-Thr-Asp-Asn-Tyr-Ser-Arg-Phe-Arg
             15                     21                      28
Porcine VIP:  Lys-Gln-Met-Ala-Val-Lys-Lys-Tyr-Leu-Asn-Ser-Ile-Leu-Asn-NH₂
Chicken VIP:  Lys-Gln-Met-Ala-Val-Lys-Lys-Tyr-Leu-Asn-Ser-Val-Leu-Thr-NH₂
```

FIG. 9. Amino acid sequence of porcine and chicken VIP. Different amino acids in positions 11, 13, 26, and 28 are marked by *asterisks*.

aspartic acid have more VIP-like biological activity on smooth muscle and show greater affinity for VIP receptors in pancreatic acinar cells. In other words, such analogs are more VIP-like and less secretin-like than their parent sequence, S_5–27. The nature of the residue in position 15 is, therefore, an important determinant of the biological activities of VIP (19).

Like the porcine peptide, chicken VIP has 28 residues; the sequences of these two variants are identical in all but four positions (11,13,26, and 28) (109), and these differences are rather conservative (Fig. 9) (15). The stepwise synthesis of both peptides, accomplished by Bodanszky et al., has confirmed their amino acid sequences and provided additional information on structure-activity relationships (15–19).

The entire sequence of VIP is not required for significant hormonal activity. Thus, VIP-like biological activity is present in the C-terminal 11-peptide, VIP_{18-28}, and this activity increases with increasing chain length. The 15-peptide, VIP_{14-28}, is substantially more potent as a vasodilator than the 14-peptide, VIP_{15-28}, and the 22-peptide, VIP_{7-28}, is closer still to the parent 28-peptide in biological activity. The synthetic N-terminal peptides VIP_{1-6} and VIP_{1-10} also show distinct, although weak, activity. The presence of VIP-like activity in nonoverlapping N-terminal and C-terminal parts of the sequence implies the existence in VIP of two "message or command sequences" carrying similar instructions (12).

The 17-norleucine analog of the sequence VIP_{14-28} is as active as the methionine-containing "natural sequence," suggesting that the sulfur-containing amino acid in VIP can be replaced without loss of biological activity (18).

Examination of optic rotatory dispersion spectra of VIP in aqueous solutions shows a preferred conformation with no distinct helical character (14). Addition of even small amounts of organic solvent, e.g., trifluoroethanol, however, results in pronounced helix formation. Synthetic VIP fragments also show this tendency, and the readiness of shorter chains to assume helical conformation parallels their biological activity. From these and related observations, Bodanszky concludes that an "active architecture" may be required for the binding of VIP and other hormones to receptors (14).

VIP RECEPTORS

Specific binding of labeled ^{125}I-VIP to surface receptors has been demonstrated in several different sites in gastrointestinal nervous and endocrine tissues. These sites include rat hepatocytes (35), adipocytes (26,56), and dispersed intestinal epithelial cells (enterocytes) (89), cat pancreatic plasma membranes and guinea pig pancreatic (28,29,62,78) acinar cells, and rat and guinea pig brain membranes (118,158). The relationships between receptor binding of VIP to gastrointestinal organs, its ability to stimulate cyclic AMP accumulation in these organs, and its influence on some of their major functional activities are shown in Table 2, together with a comparison of the same data for secretin and glucagon.

VIP binding to these receptor sites is saturable, reversible, temperature-dependent (maximal at 37°C, slower at cooler temperatures), rapid (peaking within 10 min at 37°C), and is preserved by bacitracin. In general, the binding also correlates with the ability of VIP to stimulate cyclic AMP accumulation and functional activity in these tissues (88). One exception to this generalization are liver-cell membranes where VIP binds with high affinity but is a weak stimulant of cyclic AMP production and of glycogenolysis. Pancreatic acinar cells may possess two classes of binding sites, each of which interacts with VIP or secretin but not with glucagon; one class has a high affinity for VIP and low affinity for secretin, and the other has opposite affinities (28,62).

VIP also binds specifically and with high affinity to brain membranes from areas known to be rich in the peptide, including cerebral cortex, hypothalamus, hippocampus, striatum, and thalamus (158). Partial sequences of VIP compete for this binding with an order of potency matching that which they show for binding to pancreatic acinar cells (158).

As in binding to gastrointestinal receptors, VIP binding to brain membranes is saturable, reversible, rapid, and temperature-dependent. It is consistent with

TABLE 2. *VIP, Secretin and glucagon: receptor sites and effects on cyclic AMP accumulation and function in digestive organs*

	VIP	Secretin	Glucagon
Receptors			
Liver	Yes (binding affinity 100 times that of glucagon)	No (acts through VIP receptors)	Yes
Exocrine pancreas	Yes	Yes	No
Intestine	No	No	No
Cyclic AMP accumulation			
Liver	Poorly effective	Ineffective	Highly effective
Exocrine pancreas	Less potent ($\frac{1}{15}$) than secretin	Most potent (> on ducts than on acinar cells)	Ineffective
Intestine	Most potent and effective	0.1% as potent as VIP	Ineffective
Functional effect			
Liver (glycogenolysis)	20% of glucagon	Ineffective	Maximal
Exocrine pancreas (HCO_3^- secretion)	Less potent than secretin	Most potent and effective	Ineffective
Intestine (secretion)	Most potent and effective	Ineffective	Ineffective

the presence of a single class of noninteracting sites (158). In another report, binding data were considered compatible with the existence of two classes of binding sites (118).

As mentioned earlier in this chapter, radioreceptor assay of VIP has confirmed its distribution as measured by RIA and immunofluorescence, and has shown it to be biologically active (5).

MOLECULAR FORMS OF VIP

Although VIP or a VIP-like peptide occurs widely in many body systems, it has been isolated and chemically identified only from the gut. Chromatographic analysis of tissue extracts suggests that all or almost all of the immunoreactive VIP in the brain, peripheral nerves, and other extraintestinal organs is present in one form, which is similar in molecular size to porcine VIP (21,50,94,96). The probable identity or close similarity of the VIP in these organs to the VIP isolated from intestine is further supported by the demonstration of VIP-like biological activity in extracts of these tissues (136), and by the finding that VIP in brain extracts inhibits the binding of "authentic" VIP to liver membranes (5). VIP in the human intestinal muscle layer also appears to be indistinguishable from porcine VIP, not only in molecular size (gel-permeation chromatography), but also in charge (ion-exchange chromatography) (38,39). Intestinal mucosa (with its VIP-containing endocrine cells but no nerves), on the other hand, contains four peptide components with VIP-like immunoreactivity—one with the full chromatographic properties of VIP, and the other three distinguishable mainly by their less basic character (38,39). These results are consistent with the presence of a single molecular form of VIP in neural elements (e.g., in brain, nerve plexuses in intestinal wall, peripheral nerves) that is identical, or closely similar, to the VIP isolated from gut and of one or more other forms that occur in endocrine cells (e.g., intestinal mucosa) (38,39).

Porcine duodenum contains a peptide, isolated on the basis of having a C-terminal isoleucine amide, that resembles VIP in its binding to liver membrane receptors and its ability to stimulate cyclic AMP accumulation in rat adipocytes, but has little VIP-like immunoreactivity (4).

The existence of larger molecular forms ("precursor peptide," "prohormone") of VIP, as has been shown for other peptide hormones, remains a possibility. Similarly, it is also possible that VIP itself, at least under certain conditions or in certain systems, may function as a prohormone (13). The latter possibility implies that biologically active shorter sequences may be formed through enzymatic degradation at key sites, as in the case of the conversion of proinsulin to insulin (13).

RELEASE

Release of immunoreactive VIP has been demonstrated *in vitro* under a variety of experimental conditions, in perfused organs, in animals, and in man.

(a) Intraduodenal infusion of HCl (40–50 ml of 0.1 M solution, made isotonic with NaCl), fat (40 ml of 20% isotonic fat emulsion), or ethanol (60 ml of "86 proof" vodka) caused an increase in peripheral plasma VIP levels in normal human subjects and in postvagotomy patients (9,143). The same stimuli provoked VIP release, evident in portal and peripheral plasma, in anesthetized pigs. In these experiments, infusions of amino acids, isotonic glucose, hypertonic glucose, isotonic saline, or hypertonic saline did not elicit significant VIP release, nor did the ingestion of a mixed meal by the human subject.

(b) Electric stimulation of the vagus nerve in anesthetized female pigs (50, 53,142) caused a release that had an abrupt onset (within 0.5 min), was reproducible, was maximal at a stimulation frequency of 8 Hz, and was blocked by the ganglionic blocker, hexamethonium, but not by atropine. During the release, VIP levels in portal blood almost doubled, and peripheral VIP concentrations increased significantly. Similar release in blood and lymph was reported in calves (48).

(c) Release of circulating VIP was provoked by intravenous infusions of oxytocin (15 mU/kg/min) in dogs (7). VIP levels in portal blood were increased threefold above control levels, and this increase was reduced by hexamethonium and almost totally prevented by the specific neurotoxin, tetrodotoxin (7). This VIP release, therefore, is probably of neural origin and its pathways include a cholinergic mechanism. Reinforcing this conclusion is the observation that neostigmine (20 ng/kg), an inhibitor of cholinesterase, provoked an even greater release of VIP, causing an 11-fold increase in its levels in portal blood. Simultaneously, neostigmine released VIP also from brain, as reflected in elevations in the peptide concentrations in cerebral venous outflow in the same experiments (7), and in CSF in other experiments (45).

(d) Electric field stimulation (5–10 Hz for 600 μsec), parallel to rabbit ileum mounted in Ussing-type chambers, induced VIP release into the mucosal solution; this release was blocked by tetrodotoxin (60). Similar release occurred from the lower esophageal sphincter of opossum with field stimulation of 40 V, 10 Hz, and 5 and 50 msec (E. E. Daniel, *personal communication*).

(e) Distension of gastric fundus in dogs (26) and mechanical stimulation of intestinal mucosa in cats (51) elicited moderate release of VIP in the portal circulation.

(f) Isolated nerve terminals from cerebral cortex, hypothalamus, or striatum of rat brain (all of which are enriched in VIP) release VIP on addition of 55 mM potassium (chemical depolarization) in the presence of Ca^{2+} (66). Similar K^+-induced, Ca^{2+} dependent, release of VIP occurred on perfusion of rat hypothalamus with 47 mM KCl (49).

(g) Intravenous infusions of calcium gluceptate (4.5 mEq) in dogs resulted in a moderate increment in plasma VIP levels (47). Calcium is known to provoke the release of other gastrointestinal hormones, e.g., gastrin, in suspected cases of the Zollinger-Ellison syndrome.

The potential for VIP release by neural elements, especially at nerve terminals, together with its wide distribution in nerve fibers in many organs, implies that VIP release may occur without being reflected in blood or other biological fluids. Whenever increased concentrations of the peptide are demonstrated in blood or organ perfusate, therefore, such findings may represent "overflow" or "spillover" of the peptide from larger "pools" released in the vicinity of nerve endings.

POSSIBLE FUNCTIONS

The wide distribution of VIP, its predominant presence in neurons and nerve terminals, and its ability to influence numerous body functions make it unlikely that the peptide functions as a circulating hormone. Rather, it seems probable that it may serve a number of different functions in different parts of the body as a product of paracrine secretion, i.e., as a local hormone (54). First proposed in relation to a system of cells in the lung, the gastrointestinal tract, and other organs (54), the notion of paracrine secretion can also be extended to the nervous system. In the nervous system, the concept of neurosecretion, i.e., the secretion of peptide hormones and other active products by specialized neurons, was introduced by B. and E. Scharrer (144,145).

Although located in both neurons and endocrine cells, its overwhelming predominance in the former and the evidence for a neuronal origin of its experimental release (see above) suggest that any physiologically meaningful release of VIP is likely to be in relation to its neuronal presence. From the data summarized above, possible functions of VIP could include the following:

(a) VIP may act as a neurotransmitter or, more likely, a neuromodulator in the central nervous system. Consistent with such a role are its selective distribution in brain, its localization in synaptosomal fractions and synaptic vesicles, its release from these fractions with depolarizing stimuli in the presence of Ca^{2+}, the presence of unique VIP receptors in membranes from selected areas of the brain, and the ability of VIP to stimulate adenylate cyclase activity in these areas.

There is at present insufficient information to indicate what particular aspects of cerebral function, if any, may normally be modulated or regulated by VIP. Its high content in the neocortex, however, suggests a role in relation to cortical association neurons (58).

(b) The localization of VIP in certain hypothalamic nuclei, including, in the human brain, the median eminence, its apparent secretion into portal hypophyseal blood, and its ability to stimulate pituitary adenylate cyclase and to promote the secretion of prolactin, LH, and GH point to a possible role for VIP in modulating hypothalamic-pituitary function.

(c) Recent evidence that VIP in peripheral nerves, e.g., the sciatic nerve, travels by axonal transport from the cell body toward the terminals suggests a possible modulator role in the peripheral nervous system as well (65).

(d) The vasodilator activity of VIP in many vascular beds, supplying organs that contain high levels of the peptide, often in nerve terminals innervating these blood vessels, raises the possibility that it may mediate increases in blood flow to these organs, including the gastrointestinal tract.

(e) As a major component of the system of innervation to gastrointestinal organs, VIP may mediate certain responses that have been attributed to "nonadrenergic inhibitory" nerves (34). The latter have been thought to be "purinergic," with the thought that a purine, such as ATP, was their major mediator (24). It seems attractive to postulate that peptides, rather than purines, are the mediators of this system of nerves (73,113,161). Such peptides would include, in addition to VIP, somatostatin, substance P, enkephalins, bombesin, gastrin, and possibly others (70,113,147).

One nonadrenergic inhibitory response that may be mediated by VIP is the relaxation of the lower esophageal sphincter. Other possible regulatory influences of the peptide might include inhibition of gastric acid secretion and motility, inhibition of gallbladder contraction, and stimulation of water and electrolyte secretion from intestine (103), pancreas (101), and other mucosal surfaces (153).

ROLE IN DISEASE

The principal pathological conditions causing VIP hypersecretion are a group of tumors (VIPomas), which are often associated with the watery-diarrhea (pancreatic cholera, Verner-Morrison, WDHH, or WDHA) syndrome. The relationship of this syndrome to VIP hypersecretion has been discussed in recent reports (8,105,137,139a), and is the subject of another chapter in this volume (Chapter 31, by Owyang and Go, pp. 741–748).

VIP release, largely from the gut, has been reported as a result of intestinal ischemia (103) and during hemorrhagic shock (139).

Elevation of plasma (and CSF) VIP levels also occurs in some patients with hepatic cirrhosis and hepatic failure (45,47,74). Whether this elevation is partly the result of increased VIP secretion or due solely to its impaired inactivation has not been determined.

It is too early to know the full effects of gastrointestinal and neurological disorders on the VIP content in blood, CSF, and tissues. Similarly, except for the watery diarrhea syndrome, the possible pathogenetic or mediator role of the peptide remains to be determined.

ACKNOWLEDGMENT

Some of the research cited here was supported by the Veterans' Administration Research Service and by NIH Grants HL 14187 and CA 21570. I am grateful to Mrs. Vicky Roe for her help with the preparation of this manuscript.

SUMMARY AND CONCLUSIONS

VIP was discovered almost 10 years ago in extracts of porcine duodenum, on the basis of its vasodilator action. This peptide is now known to occur widely in the gastrointestinal and nervous systems of mammals and lower animals, and to have a wide spectrum of biological activity. Its actions include suppression of gastric acid secretion, stimulation of intestinal water and ion secretion, promotion of blood flow to splanchnic and other organs, and stimulation of cyclic AMP accumulation in many systems. Specific VIP receptors are found in the gastrointestinal tract and in selected areas of the brain. The peptide may be released by cholinergic agonists, by vagal stimulation, by depolarizing concentrations of K^+, and by other stimuli, and it appears to function mainly as a neural peptide. It is secreted by tumors associated with the "pancreatic cholera" syndrome, arising from pancreatic islet cells, neural tissue or, less commonly, bronchus. Its normal regulatory functions remain to be defined.

PROJECTIONS FOR THE FUTURE

Questions to be answered by future research relate to the physiologic roles of VIP and include these:

1. What are the physiologic stimuli provoking its release?
2. What gastrointestinal (and other) functions (e.g., secretion, blood flow) does it normally control or modulate?
3. What is the relationship between VIP-containing neurons and cholinergic mechanisms?
4. What are the physiologic implications of interactions between VIP and other gastrointestinal hormones (including secretin, glucagon, insulin, somatostatin)?
5. What physiologic links exist between VIP (and other peptides) in the brain and nerves, and local gastrointestinal mechanisms?

REFERENCES

1. Alm, P., Alumets, J., Håkanson, R., and Sundler, F. (1977): Peptidergic (vasoactive intestinal peptide) nerves in the genito-urinary tract. *Neuroscience,* 2:751–754.
2. Attia, R. R., Ebeid, A. M., Murray, P., and Fischer, J. E. (1976): The placenta as a possible source of gut peptide hormones. *Surg. Forum,* 27:432–434.
3. Barbezat, G. O., and Grossman, M. I. (1971): Intestinal secretion: Stimulation by peptides. *Science,* 174:422–424.
4. Bataille, D., Laburthe, M., Dupont, C., Tatemoto, K., Vauclin, N., Rosselin, G., and Mutt, V. (1978): VIP-like effects of a newly isolated intestinal peptide (PIHIA). *Scand. J. Gastroenterol. (Suppl. 49),* 13:13.
4a. Bayliss, W. M., and Starling, E. H. (1902): The mechanism of pancreatic secretion. *J. Physiol. (Lond.),* 28:325–353.
5. Besson, J., Laburthe, M., Bataille, D., Dupont, C., and Rosselin, G. (1978): Vasoactive intestinal peptide (VIP): Tissue distribution in the rat as measured by radioimmunoassay and by radioreceptorassay. *Acta Endocrinologia,* 87:799–810.
6. Besson, J., Rotsztejn, W., Laburthe, M., Epelbaum, J., Beaudet, A., Kordon, C., and Rosselin,

G. (1979): Vasoactive intestinal peptide (VIP): Brain distribution, subcellular localization and effect of deafferentation of the hypothalamus, in male rats. *Brain Res.*, 165:79–86.

7. Bitar, K. N., Zfass, A. M., Saffouri, B., Said, S. I., and Makhlouf, G. M. (1979): Release of VIP from nerves in the gut. *Gastroenterology*, 76, 1101.

8. Bloom, S. R. (1978): VIP and watery diarrhea. In: *Gut Hormones*, edited by S. R. Bloom, pp. 583–588. Churchill Livingstone, New York.

9. Bloom, S. R., Mitchell, S. J., Greenberg, G. R., Christofides, N., Domschke, W., Domschke, S., Mitznegg, P., and Demling, L. (1978): Release of VIP, secretin and motilin after duodenal acidification in man. *Acta Hepatogastroenterol.*, 25:365–368.

10. Bloom, S. R., and Polak, J. M. (1979): Vipomas, Gluganonomas, PPomas. In: *Gastrointestinal Hormones*, edited by G. B. Jerzy Glass, pp. 19–53. Raven Press, New York.

11. Bodanszky, M. (1975): New hormones: The secretin family and evolution. In: *Gastrointestinal Hormones*, edited by J. C. Thompson, pp. 507–518. University of Texas Press, Austin.

12. Bodanszky, M. (1977): The information content of the sequences of secretin and VIP. In: *First International Symposium on Hormonal Receptors in Digestive Tract Physiology, INSERM Symposium No. 3.*, edited by Bonfils et al., pp. 13–18. Elsevier/North-Holland Biomedical Press, New York.

13. Bodanszky, M., Bodanszky, A., Deshmane, S. S., Martinez, J., and Said, S. I. (1979): Is the vasoactive intestinal peptide (VIP) a prohormone? *Bioorg. Chem., in press.*

14. Bodanszky, M., Bodanszky, A., Klausner, Y. S., and Said, S. I. (1974): A preferred conformation in the vasoactive intestinal peptide (VIP). Molecular architecture of gastrointestinal hormones. *Bioorg. Chem.*, 3:133–140.

15. Bodanszky, M., Henes, J. B., Yiotakis, A. E., and Said, S. I. (1977): Synthesis and pharmacological properties of the N-terminal decapeptide of the vasoactive intestinal peptide (VIP). *J. Med. Chem.*, 20:1461–1464.

16. Bodanszky, M., Klausner, Y. S., Lin, C. Y., Mutt, V., and Said, S. I. (1974): Synthesis of the vasoactive intestinal peptide (VIP). *J. Am. Chem. Soc.*, 96:4973–4978.

17. Bodanszky, M., Klausner, Y. S., and Said, S. I. (1973): Biological activities of synthetic peptides corresponding to fragments of and to the entire sequence of the vasoactive intestinal peptide. *Proc. Natl. Acad. Sci. USA*, 70:382–384.

18. Bodanszky, M., Lin, C. Y., and Said, S. I. (1974): The vasoactive intestinal peptide (VIP). The 17-norleucine analog of the sequence 14–28. *Bioorg. Chem.*, 3:320–323.

19. Bodanszky, M., Natarajan, S., Gardner, J. D., Makhlouf, G. M., and Said, S. I. (1978): Synthesis and some pharmacological properties of the 23-peptide 15-lysine-secretin- (5–27). Special role of the residue in position 15 in biological activity of the vasoactive intestinal polypeptide. *J. Med. Chem.*, 21:1171–1173.

20. Borghi, C., Nicosia, S., Giachetti, A., and Said, S. I. (1978): Vasoactive intestinal polypeptide (VIP) stimulates adenylate cyclase in selected areas of rat brain. *Life Sci.*, 24:65–70.

21. Bryant, M. G., Polak, J. M., Modlin, F., Bloom, S. R., Albuquerque, R. H., and Pearse, A. G. E. (1976): Possible dual role for vasoactive intestinal peptide as gastrointestinal hormone and neurotransmitter substance. *Lancet*, i:991–993.

22. Buffa, R., Capella, C., Solcia, E., Frigerio, B., and Said, S. I. (1977): Vasoactive intestinal peptide (VIP) cells in the pancreas and gastrointestinal mucosa. *Histochemistry*, 50:217–227.

23. Buffa, R., Solcia, E., Capella, C., Fontana, P., Trinci, E., and Said, S. I. (1976): Immunohistochemical detection of vasoactive intestinal peptide (VIP) in a specific endocrine cell of the pancreatic islets. *Rendic. Gastroenterol.*, 8:73–75.

24. Burnstock, G. (1972): Purinergic nerves. *Pharmacol. Rev.*, 24:509–581.

25. Carter, R. F., Bitar, K. N., Zfass, A. M., and Makhlouf, G. M. (1978): Inhibition of VIP-stimulated intestinal secretion and cyclic AMP production by somatostatin in the rat. *Gastroenterology*, 74:726–730.

26. Chayvialle, J.-A., Miyata, M., Rayford, P. L., and Thompson, J. C. (1978): Effect of fundic distension on vasoactive intestinal peptide in dogs. *Scand. J. Gastroenterol. (Suppl. 49)*, 13:38.

27. Chayvialle, J.-A., Miyata, M., Rayford, P. L., and Thompson, J. C. (1978): Vasoactive intestinal peptide in portal, right heart, and aortic plasma in dogs. *Scand. J. Gastroenterol. (Suppl. 49)*, 13:39.

28. Christophe, J. P., Conlon, T. P., and Gardner, J. D. (1976): Interaction of porcine vasoactive intestinal peptide with dispersed pancreatic acinar cells from the guinea pig: Binding of radioiodinated peptide. *J. Biol. Chem.*, 251:4629–4634.

29. Christophe, J. P., Robberecht, P., and Deschodt-Lanckman, M. (1977): Hormone-receptor

interactions in the gastrointestinal tract; the pancreatic acinar cell as a model target in gut endocrinology. In: *Progress in Gastroenterology, Vol. 3,* edited by G. B. Jerzy Glass, pp. 241–284. Grune & Stratton, New York.

30. Clark, W. G., Lipton, J. M., and Said, S. I. (1978): Hyperthermic responses to vasoactive intestinal polypeptide (VIP) injected into the third cerebral ventricle of cats. *Neuropharmacology,* 17:883–885.

31. Coupar, I. M. (1976): Stimulation of sodium and water secretion without inhibition of glucose absorption in the rat jejunum by vasoactive intestinal peptide (VIP). *Clin. Exp. Pharmacol. Physiol.,* 3:615–618.

32. Cristina, M. L., Lehy, T., Zeitoun, P., and Dufougeray, F. (1978): Fine structural classification and comparative distribution of endocrine cells in normal human large intestine. *Gastroenterology,* 75:20–28.

33. Cutz, E., Chan, W., Track, N. S., Goth, A., and Said, S. I. (1978): Release of vasoactive intestinal polypeptide in mast cells by histamine liberators. *Nature,* 275:661–662.

34. Daniel, E. E. (1978): Peptidergic nerves in the gut. *Gastroenterology,* 75:142–145.

35. Desbuquois, B. (1974): The interaction of vasoactive intestinal polypeptide and secretin with liver-cell membranes. *Eur. J. Biochem.,* 46:439–450.

36. Desbuquois, B., Laudat, M. H., and Laudat, P. (1973): Vasoactive intestinal polypeptide and glucagon: Stimulation of adenylate cyclase activity via distinct receptors in liver and fat cell membranes. *Biochem. Biophys. Res. Commun.,* 53:1187–1194.

37. Deschodt-Lanckman, M., Robberecht, P., and Christophe, J. (1977): Characterization of VIP-sensitive adenylate cyclase in guinea pig brain. *FEBS Lett.,* 83:76–80.

38. Dimaline, R., and Dockray, G. J. (1978): Multiple immunoreactive forms of vasoactive intestinal peptide in human colonic mucosa. *Gastroenterology,* 75:387–392.

39. Dimaline, R., and Dockray, G. J. (1978): Distribution of molecular forms of vasoactive intestinal peptide in hog gastrointestinal tract. *J. Physiol.,* 285:39P.

40. Dockray, G. J. (1977): Molecular evolution of gut hormones: Application of comparative studies on the regulation of digestion. *Gastroenterology,* 72:344–358.

41. Domschke, S., Domschke, W., Bloom, S. R., Mitznegg, P., Mitchell, S., Lux, G., Strunz, U., and Demling, L. (1978): Pharmacokinetics and pharmacodynamics. In: *Gut Hormones,* edited by S. R. Bloom, pp. 475–478. Churchill Livingstone, New York.

42. Domschke, S., Domschke, W., Rösch, W., Konturek, S. J., Sprügel, W., Mitznegg, P., Wünsch, E., and Demling, L. (1977): Vasoactive intestinal peptide: A secretin-like partial agonist for pancreatic secretion in man. *Gastroenterology,* 73:478–480.

43. Domschke, W., Lux, G., Domschke, S., Strunz, U., Bloom, S. R., and Wünsch, E. (1978): Effects of vasoactive intestinal peptide on resting and pentagastrin-stimulated lower esophageal sphincter pressure. *Gastroenterology,* 75:9–12.

44. Ebeid, A. M., Attia, R., Murray, P., and Fischer, J. E. (1976): The placenta as a possible source of gut peptide hormones. *Gastroenterology,* 70:A–99.

45. Ebeid, A. M., Attia, R. R., Sundaram, P., and Fischer, J. E. (1979): Release of vasoactive intestinal peptide in the central nervous system in man. *Am. J. Surg.,* 137:123–127.

46. Ebeid, A. M., Escourrou, J., Murray, P., and Fischer, J. E. (1978): Pathophysiology of VIP. In: *Gut Hormones,* edited by S. R. Bloom, pp. 479–483. Churchill Livingstone, New York.

47. Ebeid, A. M., Murray, P., Soeters, P. B., Fischer, J. E. (1977): Release of vasoactive intestinal peptide (VIP) by calcium stimulation. *Am. J. Surg.,* 133:140–144.

48. Edwards, A. V., Birchman, P. M., Mitchell, S. J., and Bloom, S. R. (1978): Changes in the concentration of vasoactive intestinal peptide in intestinal lymph in response to vagal stimulation in the calf. *Experientia,* 34:1186–1187.

49. Emson, P. C., Fahrenkrug, J., Schaffalitzky de Muckadell, O. B., Jessell, T. M., and Iversen, L. L. (1978): Vasoactive intestinal polypeptide (VIP): Vesicular localization and potassium evoked release from rat hypothalamus. *Brain Res.,* 143:174–178.

50. Fahrenkrug, J., Galbo, H., Holst, J. J., and Schaffalitzky de Muckadell, O. B. (1978): Influence of the autonomic nervous system on the release of vasoactive intestinal polypeptide from the porcine gastrointestinal tract. *J. Physiol.,* 280:405–422.

51. Fahrenkrug, J., Haglund, U., Jodal, M., Lundgren, O., Olbe, L., and Schaffalitzky de Muckadell, O. B. (1978): Is vasoactive intestinal polypeptide (VIP) a neurotransmitter in the gastrointestinal tract? *Acta Physiol. Scand.,* 102:22A–23A.

52. Fahrenkrug, J., Schaffalitzky de Muckadell, O. B., and Fahrenkrug, A. (1977): Vasoactive intestinal polypeptide (VIP) in human cerebrospinal fluid. *Brain Res.,* 124:581–584.

53. Fahrenkrug, J., Schaffalitzky de Muckadell, O. B., and Holst, J. J. (1978): Nervous release of VIP. In: *Gut Hormones,* edited by S. R. Bloom, pp. 448–491. Churchill Livingstone, New York.

54. Feyrter, F. (1953): *Über die Peripheren Endokrinen (Parakrinen). Drüsen des Menschen,* Verlag für Medizinische Wissenschaften Wilhelm Maudrich, Vienna/Düsseldorf.

55. Frandsen, E. K., Krishna, G. A., and Said, S. I. (1978): Vasoactive intestinal polypeptide promotes cyclic adenosine 3′,5′-mono-phosphate accumulation in guinea pig trachea. *Br. J. Pharmacol.,* 62:367–369.

56. Frandsen, E. K., and Moody, A. J. (1973): Lipolytic action of a newly isolated vasoactive intestinal polypeptide. *Horm. Metab. Res.,* 5:196–199.

57. Frandsen, E. K., and Moody, A. J. (1977): Hormonal activation of adenylate cyclase in broken cell preparations of isolated mouse islets of langerhans. In: *First International Symposium on Hormonal Receptors in Digestive Tract Physiology, INSERM Symposium No. 3,* edited by Bonfils et al., pp. 332. Elsevier/North-Holland Biomedical Press, New York.

58. Fuxe, K., Hökfelt, T., Said, S. I., and Mutt, V. (1977): Vasoactive polypeptide and the nervous system: Immunohistochemical evidence for localization in central and peripheral neurons, particularly intracortical neurons of the cerebral cortex. *Neurosci. Lett.,* 5:241–246.

59. Gaginella, T. S., Mekhjian, H. S., and O'Dorisio, T. M. (1978): Vasoactive intestinal peptide: Quantification by radioimmunoassay in isolated cells, mucosa, and muscle of the hamster intestine. *Gastroenterology,* 74:718–721.

60. Gaginella, T. S., and O'Dorisio, T. M. (1979): Vasoactive intestinal polypeptide: Neuromodulator of intestinal secretion? In: *Mechanisms of Intestinal Secretion,* KROC Foundation Series, Vol. 12, edited by H. J. Binder, pp. 231–247. Alan R. Liss, New York.

61. Gaginella, T. S., Phillips, S. F., Dozois, R. R., and Go, V. L. W. (1978): Stimulation of adenylate cyclase in homogenates of isolated intestinal epithelial cells from hamsters. *Gastroenterology,* 74:11–15.

62. Gardner, J. D. (1979): Receptors for gastrointestinal hormones. *Gastroenterology,* 76:202–214.

63. Giachetti, A., Borghi, C., Nicosia, S., and Said, S. I. (1979): Vasoactive intestinal polypeptide (VIP) activates rat pituitary adenylate cyclase. *Fed. Proc.,* 38:1129.

64. Giachetti, A., Goth, A., and Said, S. I. (1978): Vasoactive intestinal polypeptide (VIP) in rabbit platelets and rat mast cells. *Fed. Proc.,* 37:657.

65. Giachetti, A., and Said, S. I. (1979): Axonal transport of vasoactive intestinal peptide in sciatic nerve. *Nature,* 281:574–575.

66. Giachetti, A., Said, S. I., Reynolds, R. C., and Koniges, F. C. (1977): Vasoactive intestinal polypeptide in brain: Localization in and release from isolated nerve terminals. *Proc. Natl. Acad. Sci. USA,* 74:3424–3428.

67. Hara, N., Geumei, A., Chijimatsu, Y., and Said, S. I. (1975): Vasoactive intestinal peptide aerosol protects against histamine- and prostaglandin $F_{2\alpha}$-induced bronchoconstriction. *Clin. Res.,* 23:347A.

68. Heistad, D. D., Marcus, M. L., Said, S. I., and Gross, P. M. (1979): Effect of acetylcholine and vasoactive intestinal peptide on cerebral blood flow. *Fed. Proc.,* 38:954.

69. Hökfelt, T., Elde, R., Fuxe, K., Johansson, O., Ljungdahl, Å., Goldstein, M., Luft, R., Efendic, S., Nilsson, G., Terenius, L., Ganten, D., Jeffcoate, S. L., Rehfeld, J., Said, S. I., Perez de la Mora, M., Possani, L., Tapia, R., Teran, L., and Palacios, R. (1978): Aminergic and peptidergic pathways in the nervous system with special reference to the hypothalamus. In: *The Hypothalamus,* edited by S. Reichlin, R. J. Baldessarini, and J. B. Martin, pp. 69–135. Raven Press, New York.

70. Hökfelt, T., Elde, R., Johansson, O., Ljungdahl, Å., Schultzberg, M., Fuxe, K., Goldstein, M., Nilsson, G., Pernow, B., Terenius, L., Ganten, D., Jeffcoate, S. L., Rehfeld, J., and Said, S. I. (1978): Distribution of peptide-containing neurons. In: *Psychopharmacology: A Generation of Progress,* edited by M. A. Lipton, A. DiMascio, and K. F. Killam, pp. 39–66. Raven Press, New York.

71. Hökfelt, T., Elfvin, L.-G., Schultzberg, M., Fuxe, K., Said, S. I., Mutt, V., and Goldstein, M. (1977): Immunohistochemical evidence of vasoactive intestinal polypeptide-containing neurons and nerve fibers in sympathetic ganglia. *Neuroscience,* 2:885–896.

72. Hökfelt, T., Schultzberg, M., Elde, R., Nilsson, G., Terenius, L., Said, S. I., and Goldstein, M. (1978): Peptide neurons in peripheral tissues including the urinary tract: Immunohistochemical studies. *Acta Pharmacol. Toxicol.,* 43:79–89.

73. Humphrey, C. S., and Fischer, J. E. (1978): Peptidergic versus purinergic nerves. *Lancet,* i:390.
74. Hunt, S., Vaamonde, C. A., Rattassi, T., Berian, M. G., Said, S. I., and Papper, S. (1979): Circulating levels of vasoactive intestinal polypeptide (VIP) in liver disease. *Arch. Intern. Med.,* 139:994–996.
75. Ipp, E., Dobbs, R. E., and Unger, R. H. (1978): Vasoactive intestinal peptide stimulates pancreatic somatostatin release. *FEBS Lett.,* 90:76–78.
76. Jansson, R. (1978): Effects of gastrointestinal hormones on concentrating function and motility in the gallbladder. An experimental study in the cat. *Acta Physiol. Scand. (Suppl.),* 456:1–38.
77. Jansson, R., Steen, G., and Svanvik, J. (1978): Effects of intravenous vasoactive intestinal peptide (VIP) on gallbladder function in the cat. *Gastroenterology,* 75:47–50.
78. Jensen, R. T., and Gardner, J. D. (1978): Cyclic nucleotide-dependent protein kinase activity in acinar cells from guinea pig pancreas. *Gastroenterology,* 75:806–816.
79. Kaneto, A., Kaneko, T., Kajinuma, H., and Kosaka, K. (1977): Effect of vasoactive intestinal polypeptide infused intrapancreatically on glucagon and insulin secretion. *Metabolism,* 26:781–786.
80. Kato, Y., Iwasaki, Y., Iwasaki, J., Abe, H., Yanaihara, N., and Imura, H. (1978): Prolactin release by vasoactive intestinal polypeptide in rats. *Endocrinology,* 103:554–558.
81. Kerins, C., and Said, S. I. (1973): Heyperglycemic and glycogenolytic effects of vasoactive intestinal polypeptide. *Proc. Soc. Exp. Biol. Med.,* 143:1014–1017.
82. Kitamura, S., Yoshida, T., and Said, S. I. (1975): Vasoactive intestinal polypeptide: Inactivation in liver and potentiation in lung of anesthetized dogs. *Proc. Soc. Exp. Biol. Med.,* 148:25–29.
83. Konturek, S. J., Domschke, S., Domschke, W., Wünsch, E., and Demling, L. (1977): Comparison of pancreatic responses to portal and systemic secretin and VIP in cats. *Am. J. Physiol.,* 232:E156–E158.
84. Konturek, S. J., Radecki, T., and Pucher, A. (1976): Comparison of endogenous and exogenous VIP and secretin in stimulation of pancreatic secretion. *J. Physiol. (Lond.),* 255:497–509.
85. Kowal, J., Horst, I., Pensky, J., and Alfonzo, M. (1977): Vasoactive intestinal peptide (VIP): An ACTH-like activator of adrenal steroidogenesis. *Clin. Res.,* 25:464A.
86. Kowal, J., Horst, I., Pensky, J., and Alfonzo, M. (1977): A comparison of the effects of ACTH, vasoactive intestinal peptide, and cholera toxin on adrenal cAMP and steroid synthesis. *Ann. NY Acad. Sci.,* 297:314–328.
87. Krejs, G. J., Barkley, R. M., Read, N. W., and Fordtran, J. S. (1977): Intestinal secretion induced by vasoactive intestinal polypeptide. *J. Clin. Invest.,* 78:1337–1345.
88. Laburthe, M., Bataille, D., Rousset, M., Besson, J., Broer, Y., Zweibaum, A., and Rosselin, G. (1978): The expression of cell surface receptors for VIP, secretin and glucagon in normal and transformed cells of the digestive tract. In: *(FEBS) Federation of European Biochemical Societies, 11th Meeting, Copenhagen, 1977,* edited by P. Nicholls, pp. 271–290. Pergamon Press, Oxford New York.
89. Laburthe, M., Besson, J., Hui Bon Hoa, D., and Rosselin, G. (1977): Récepteurs du peptide intestinal vasoactif (VIP) dans les enterocytes: Liaison specifique et stimulation de 1" AMP cyclique. *C.R. Acad. Sci. Paris,* 284:2139–2142.
90. Laburthe, M., Rousset, M., Boissard, C., Chevalier, G., Zweibaum, A., and Rosselin, G. (1978): Vasoactive intestinal peptide: A potent stimulator of adenosine 3′5′-cyclic monophosphate accumulation in gut carcinoma cell lines in culture. *Proc. Natl. Acad. Sci. USA,* 75:2772–2775.
91. Larsson, L.-I. (1977): Ultrastructural localization of a new neuronal peptide (VIP). *Histochemistry,* 54:173–176.
92. Larsson, L.-I., Edvinsson, L., Fahrenkrug, J., Håkanson, R., Owman, Ch., Schaffalitzky de Muckadell, O. B., and Sundler, F. (1976): Immunohistochemical localization of a vasodilatory polypeptide (VIP) in cerebrovascular nerves. *Brain Res.,* 113:400–404.
93. Larsson, L.-I., Fahrenkrug, J., Holst, J. J., and Schaffalitzky de Muckadell, O. B. (1978): Innervation of the pancreas by vasoactive intestinal polypeptide (VIP) immunoreactive nerves. *Life Sci.,* 22:773–780.
94. Larsson, L.-I., Fahrenkrug, J., and Schaffalitzky de Muckadell, O. B. (1977): Vasoactive intestinal polypeptide occurs in nerves of the female genito-urinary tract. *Science,* 197:1374–1375.

95. Larsson, L.-I., Fahrenkrug, J., and Schaffalitzky de Muckadell, O. B. (1977): Occurrence of nerves containing vasoactive intestinal polypeptide immunoreactivity in the male genital tract. *Life Sci.,* 21:503–508.
96. Larsson, L.-I., Fahrenkrug, J., Schaffalitzky de Muckadell, O. B., Sundler, F., Håkanson, R., and Rehfeld, J. F. (1976): Localization of vasoactive intestinal polypeptide (VIP) to central and peripheral neurons. *Proc. Natl. Acad. Sci. USA,* 73:3197–3200.
97. Lindkaer-Jensen, S., Fahrenkrug, J., Holst, J. J., Nielsen, O. V., and Schaffalitzky de Muckadell, O. B. (1978): Secretory effects of VIP on isolated perfused porcine pancreas. *Am. J. Physiol.,* 235:E387–E391.
98. Lundberg, J. M., Hökfelt, T., Nilsson, G., Pettersson, G., Kewenter, J., Ahlman, H., Edin, R., Dahlström, A., Terenius, L., and Said, S. I. (1979): Substance, P-, VIP- and enkephalin-like immunoreactivity in the human vagus nerve. *Gastroenterology,* 77:468–471.
99. Mailman, D. (1978): Effects of vasoactive intestinal polypeptide on intestinal absorption and blood flow. *J. Physiol.,* 279:121–132.
100. Makhlouf, G. M., and Said, S. I. (1975): The effect of vasoactive intestinal peptide (VIP) on digestive and hormonal function. In: *Gastrointestinal Hormones,* edited by J. C. Thompson, pp. 599–610. University of Texas Press, Austin.
101. Makhlouf, G. M., Yau, W. M., Zfass, A. M., Said, S. I., and Bodanszky, M. (1978): Comparative effects of synthetic and natural vasoactive intestinal peptide on pancreatic and biliary secretion and on glucose and insulin blood levels in the dog. *Scand. J. Gastroenterol.,* 13:759–765.
102. Makhlouf, G. M., Zfass, A. M., Said, S. I., and Schebalin, M. (1978): Effects of synthetic vasoactive intestinal peptide (VIP), secretin and their partial sequences on gastric secretion. *Proc. Soc. Exp. Biol. Med.,* 157:565–568.
103. Modigliani, R., Bernier, J. J., Matuchansky, C., and Rambaud, J.-C. (1977): Intestinal water and electrolyte transport in man under the effect of exogenous hormones of the gut and the prostaglandins, and in patients with endocrine tumors of the pancreas. In: *Progress in Gastroenterology,* edited by G. B. Jerzy-Glass, pp. 285–319. Grune & Stratton, New York.
104. Modlin, I. M., Bloom, S. R., and Mitchell, S. J. (1978): Plasma vasoactive intestinal polypeptide (VIP) levels and intestinal ischemia. *Experientia,* 34:535–536.
105. Modlin, I. M., Bloom, S. R., and Mitchell, S. J. (1978): Experimental evidence for VIP as the cause of the watery diarrhea syndrome. *Gastroenterology,* 75:1051–1054.
106. Morgan, K. G., Schmalz, P. F., and Szurszewski, J. H. (1978): The inhibitory effects of vasoactive intestinal polypeptide on the mechanical and electrical activity of canine antral smooth muscle. *J. Physiol.,* 282:437–450.
107. Mutt, V. (1978): Hormone isolation. In: *Gut Hormones,* edited by S. R. Bloom, pp. 21–27. Churchill Livingstone, New York.
108. Mutt, V., and Said, S. I. (1974): Structure of the porcine vasoactive intestinal octacosapeptide: The amino-acid sequence. Use of kallikrein in its determination. *Eur. J. Biochem.,* 42:581–589.
109. Nilsson, A. (1975): Structure of the vasoactive intestinal octacosapeptide from chicken intestine. The amino acid sequence. *FEBS Lett.,* 60:322–325.
110. Ohneda, A., Ishii, S., Horigome, K., Chiba, M., Sakai, T., Kai, Y., Watanabe, K., and Yamagata, S. (1977): Effect of intrapancreatic administration of vasoactive intestinal peptide upon the release of insulin and glucagon in dogs. *Horm. Metab. Res.,* 9:447–452.
111. Phillis, J. W., Kirkpatrick, J. R., and Said, S. I. (1977): Vasoactive intestinal polypeptide excitation of central neurons. *Can. J. Physiol. Pharmacol.,* 56:337–340.
112. Piper, P. J., Said, S. I., and Vane, J. R. (1970): Effects on smooth muscle preparations of unidentified vasoactive peptides from intestine and lung. *Nature,* 225:1144–1146.
113. Polak, J. M., and Bloom, S. R. (1978): Peptidergic innervation of the gastrointestinal tract. *Adv. Exp. Med. Biol.,* 106:27–49.
114. Polak, J. M., Pearse, A. G. E., Garaud, J.-C., and Bloom, S. R. (1974): Cellular localization of a vasoactive intestinal peptide in the mammalian and avian gastrointestinal tract. *Gut,* 15:720–724.
115. Quik, M., Iversen, L. L., and Bloom, S. R. (1978): Effect of vasoactive intestinal peptide (VIP) and other peptides on cAMP accumulation in rat brain. *Biochem. Pharmacol.,* 27:2209–2213.
116. Racusen, L. C., and Binder, H. J. (1977): Alteration of large intestinal electrolyte transport by vasoactive intestinal polypeptide in the rat. *Gastroenterology,* 73:790–796.

117. Rattan, S., Said, S. I., and Goyal, R. K. (1977): Effect of vasoactive intestinal polypeptide (VIP) on the lower esophageal sphincter pressure (LESP). *Proc. Soc. Exp. Biol. Med.,* 155:40–43.

118. Robberecht, P., De Neef, P., Lammens, M., Deschodt-Lachkman, M., and Christophe, J.-P. (1978): Specific binding of vasoactive intestinal peptide to brain membranes from the guinea pig. *Eur. J. Biochem.,* 90:147–154.

119. Ruberg, M., Rotsztejn, W. H., Arancibia, S., Besson, J., and Enjalbert, A. (1978): Stimulation of prolactin release by vasoactive intestinal peptide (VIP). *Eur. J. Pharmacol.,* 51:319–320.

120. Ryan, J., and Cohen, S. (1977): Effect of vasoactive intestinal polypeptide on basal and cholecystokinin-induced gallbladder pressure. *Gastroenterology,* 73:870–872.

121. Ryan, J. P., and Ryave, S. (1978): Effect of vasoactive intestinal polypeptide on gallbladder smooth muscle *in vitro. Am. J. Physiol.,* 234:E44–E46.

122. Said, S. I. (1967): Vasoactive substances in the lung. In: *Proceedings of the Tenth Aspen Emphysema Conference, Aspen, Colorado, June 7–10, 1967, U.S. Public Health Serv. Publication 1787,* pp. 223–228.

123. Said, S. I. (1974): Smooth-muscle relaxant activity of vasoactive intestinal polypeptide. In: *Proceedings of the International Endocrinol. Symposium,* pp. 297–301. William Heinemann, London.

124. Said, S. I. (1975): Vasoactive intestinal polypeptide: Widespread distribution in normal gastrointestinal organs. In: *57th Annual Meeting the Endocrine Society,* June 18–20, New York.

125. Said, S. I. (1975): Vasoactive intestinal polypeptide (VIP): Current status. In: *Gastrointestinal Hormones,* edited by J. C. Thompson, pp. 591–597. University of Texas Press, Austin.

126. Said, S. I. (1978): VIP: Overview. In: *Gut Hormones,* edited by S. R. Bloom, pp. 465–469. Churchill Livingstone, New York.

127. Said, S. I., Bosher, L. P., Spath, J. A., and Kontos, H. A. (1972): Positive inotropic action of newly isolated vasoactive intestinal polypeptide (VIP). *Clin. Res.,* 20:39.

128. Said, S. I., and Giachetti, A. (1977): Vasoactive intestinal polypeptide: Distribution in normal tissues and preliminary report on its subcellular localization in brain. In: *First International Symposium on Hormonal Receptors in Digestive Tract Physiology,* edited by Bonfils, pp. 417–423. Elsevier/North-Holland Biomedical Press, New York.

129. Said, S. I., and Mutt, V. (1969): A peptide fraction from lung tissue with prolonged peripheral vasodilator activity. *Scand. J. Clin. Invest. (Suppl. 107),* 24:51–56.

130. Said, S. I., and Mutt, V. (1969): Long acting vasodilator peptide from lung tissue. *Nature,* 224:699–700.

131. Said, S. I., and Mutt, V. (1970): Potent peripheral and splanchnic vasodilator peptide from normal gut. *Nature,* 225:863–864.

132. Said, S. I., and Mutt, V. (1970): Polypeptide with broad biological activity: Isolation from small intestine. *Science,* 169:1217–1218.

133. Said, S. I., and Mutt, V. (1972): Isolation from porcine-intestinal wall of a vasoactive octacosapeptide related to secretin and to glucagon. *Eur. J. Biochem.,* 28:199–204.

134. Said, S. I., and Mutt, V. (1977): Relationship of spasmogenic and smooth muscle relaxant peptides from normal lung to other vasoactive compounds. *Nature,* 265:84–86.

135. Said, S. I., and Porter, J. C. (1979): Vasoactive intestinal polypeptide: Release into hypophyseal portal blood. *Life Sci.,* 24:227–230.

136. Said, S. I., and Rosenberg, R. N. (1976): Vasoactive intestinal polypeptide: Abundant immunoreactivity in neural cell lines and normal nervous tissue. *Science,* 192:907–908.

137. Said, S. I., and Zfass, A. M. (1978): Gastrointestinal hormones. *D.M.,* 24:1–40.

138. Saito, Y., Matsuoka, N., Shirai, K., Yamamoto, M., Kumagai, A., and Yanaihara, N. (1978): Effects of adrenergic blocking agents on lipolysis and adenylate cyclase activity induced by vasoactive intestinal polypeptide (VIP). *Endocrinol. Jpn.,* 25:403–405.

139. Sakio, H., Matsuzaki, Y., and Said, S. I. (1979): Release of vasoactive intestinal polypeptide during hemorrhagic shock. *Fed. Proc.,* 38:1114.

139a. Said, S. I. (1979): Vasoactive intestinal polypeptide (VIP) as a mediator of the watery diarrhea syndrome. *World J. Surg.,* 3:559–563.

140. Samson, W. K., Said, S. I., Graham, J. W., and McCann, S. M. (1978): Vasoactive intestinal polypeptide concentrations in median eminence of hypothalamus. *Lancet,* ii:901–902.

141. Samson, W. K., Said, S. I., and McCann, S. M. (1979): Radioimmunologic localization of

vasoactive intestinal polypeptide (VIP) in hypothalamic and extra-hypothalamic sites in the rat brain. *Neurosci. Lett.,* 12:265–270.

142. Schaffalitzky de Muckadell, O. B., Fahrenkrug, J., and Holst, J. J. (1977): Release of vasoactive intestinal polypeptide (VIP) by electric stimulation of the vagal nerves. *Gastroenterology,* 72:373–375.

143. Schaffalitzky de Muckadell, O. B., Fahrenkrug, J., Holst, J. J., and Lauritsen, K. B. (1977): Release of vasoactive intestinal polypeptide (VIP) by intraduodenal stimuli. *Scand. J. Gastroenterol.,* 12:793–799.

144. Scharrer, B. (1978): Peptidergic neurons: facts and trends. *Gen. Comp. Endocrinol.,* 34:50–62.

145. Scharrer, E., and Scharrer, B. (1954): Hormones produced by neurosecretory cells. *Recent Prog. Horm. Res.,* 10:183–232.

146. Schebalin, M., Said, S. I., and Makhlouf, G. M. (1977): Stimulation of insulin and glucagon secretion by vasoactive intestinal peptide. *Am. J. Physiol.,* 232:E197–E200.

147. Schultzberg, M., Dreyfus, C. F., Gershon, M. D., Hökfelt, T., Elde, R. P., Nilsson, G., Said, S. I., and Goldstein, M. (1978): VIP-, enkephalin-, substance P- and somatostatin-like immunoreactivity in neurons intrinsic to the intestine: Immunohistochemical evidence from organotypic tissue cultures. *Brain Res.,* 155:239–248.

148. Schwartz, C. J., Kimberg, D. V., Sheerin, H. E., Field, M., and Said, S. I. (1974): Vasoactive intestinal peptide stimulation of adenylate cyclase and active electrolyte secretion in intestinal mucosa. *J. Clin. Invest.,* 54:536–544.

149. Siegel, S. R., Brown, F. C., Castell, D. O., Johnson, L. F., and Said, S. I. (1978): Effects of vasoactive intestinal polypeptide (VIP) on the lower esophageal sphincter in awake baboons: Comparison with glucagon and secretin. *Clin. Res.,* 26:326A.

150. Simon, B., Czygan, P., Spaan, G., Dittrich, J., and Kather, H. (1978): Hormone-sensitive adenylate cyclase in human colonic mucosa. *Digestion,* 17:229–233.

151. Simon, B., and Kather, H. (1978): Activation of human adenylate cyclase in the upper gastrointestinal tract by vasoactive intestinal polypeptide. *Gastroenterology,* 74:722–725.

152. Simon, B., and Kather, H. (1978): Stimulation of human colonic adenylate cyclase. *Digest. Dis.,* 23:93–94.

153. Stoff, J. S., Silva, P., Rosa, R., Fischer, J., and Epstein, F. H. (1977): Active chloride transport in shark rectal gland mediated by cyclic AMP: Role of vasoactive intestinal peptide (VIP). *Clin. Res.,* 25:509A.

154. Strunz, U. T., Walsh, J. H., Bloom, S. R., Thompson, M. R., and Grossman, M. I. (1977): Lack of hepatic inactivation of canine vasoactive intestinal peptide. *Gastroenterology,* 73:768–771.

155. Sundler, F., Alumets, J., Håkanson, R., Fahrenkrug, J., and Schaffalitzky de Muckadell, O. B. (1978): Peptidergic (VIP) nerves in pancreas. *Histochemistry,* 55:173–176.

156. Sundler, F., Alumets, J., Håkanson, R., Ingemansson, S., Fahrenkrug, J., and Schaffalitzky de Muckadell, O. (1977): VIP innervation of the gallbladder. *Gastroenterology,* 72:1375–1377.

157. Sundler, F., Håkanson, R., Alumets, J., and Walles, B. (1977): Neuronal localization of pancreatic polypeptide (PP) and vasoactive intestinal peptide (VIP) immunoreactivity in the earthworm (Lumbricus Terrestris). *Brain Res. Bull.,* 2:61–65.

158. Taylor, D. P., and Pert, C. B. (1979): Vasoactive intestinal polypeptide: Specific binding to rat brain membranes. *Proc. Natl. Acad. Sci., USA,* 76:660–664.

159. Thulin, L., and Samnegård, H. (1978): Circulatory effects of gastrointestinal hormone and related peptides. *Acta Chir. Scand.,* 482:73–74.

160. Uddman, R., Alumets, J., Densert, O., Håkanson, R., and Sundler, F. (1978): Occurrence and distribution of VIP nerves in the nasal mucosa and tracheobronchial wall. *Acta Otolaryngol.,* 367:1–6.

161. Uddman, R., Alumets, J., Edvinsson, L., Håkanson, R., and Sundler, F. (1978): Peptidergic (VIP) innervation of the esophagus. *Gastroenterology,* 75:5–8.

162. Vijayan, E., Samson, W. K., Said, S. I., and McCann, S. M. (1979): Vasoactive intestinal peptide: Evidence for a hypothalamic site of action to release growth hormone, leuteinizing hormone, and prolactin in conscious ovarectomized rats. *Endocrinology,* 104:53–57.

163. Villar, H. V., Fender, H. R., Rayford, P. L., Bloom, S. R., Ramus, N. I., and Thompson, J. C. (1976): Suppression of gastrin release and gastric secretion by gastric inhibitory polypeptide (GIP) and vasoactive intestinal polypeptide (VIP). *Ann. Surg.,* 184:97–102.

164. Waldman, D. B., Gardner, J. D., Zfass, A. M., and Makhlouf, G. M. (1977): Effects of vasoactive intestinal peptide, secretin, and related peptides on rat colonic transport and adenylate cyclase activity. *Gastroenterology,* 73:518–523.
165. Walling, M. W., Mircheff, A. K., Vanos, C. H., and Wright, E. M. (1978): Subcellular distribution of nucleotide cyclases in rat intestinal epithelium. *Am. J. Physiol.,* 235:E539–E545.
166. Yoshida, T., Geumei, A. M., Schmitt, R. J., and Said, S. I. (1974): Vasoactive intestinal peptide: A potent coronary vasodilator. *Fed. Proc.,* 33:378.

Gastrointestinal Hormones, edited by
George B. Jerzy Glass.
Raven Press, New York © 1980.

Chapter 11

Pancreatic Polypeptide: Isolation, Chemistry, and Biological Function

Tsung-Min Lin

The Lilly Research Laboratories, Indianapolis, Indiana 46206

HISTORICAL NOTE

The fortuitous discovery of pancreatic polypeptide (PP) did not follow the traditional pattern by which other classic gastrointestinal hormones were found. The peptide was isolated before any knowledge of its action or function was known. In the late 1960s, Kimmel et al. (46) of The University of Kansas were engaged in the isolation and characterization of chicken insulin and Chance et al. (17) of the Lilly Research Laboratories were carrying out the purification of bovine and porcine glucagon and insulin. After gel filtration of the acid alcohol extract of the chicken or bovine pancreas and appropriate displacement chromatography, a pure polypeptide fraction distinct from and having a molecular mass between that of glucagon and insulin was discovered by both groups of investigators.

Since the function of these peptides was unknown, they were tentatively referred to as avian (APP) and bovine (BPP) pancreatic polypeptide, respectively. In 1971 the partial amino acid sequence of APP was reported by Kimmel et al. (47) while Chance (17) accomplished, in addition to BPP, the isolation and amino acid sequence analysis of porcine (PPP), ovine (OPP), and human (HPP) pancreatic polypeptides.

No sooner had PPs been discovered than studies of their biological actions began. The glycogenolytic and gastric actions of APP were first reported by Kimmel et al. (47) in 1971 and the broad spectrum of gastrointestinal actions of BPP was reported by Lin and Chance (57) in 1972. Antisera to APP, BPP, PPP, and HPP soon became available for investigational use, thus giving accelerated impetus to our rapidly expanding knowledge about the physiology, morphology, and clinical implications of PP.

CHEMISTRY

Isolation and Purification

The initial steps in the preparation of BPP and APP were about the same. The finely ground pancreas was extracted with acid-ethanol. For APP (44) the supernatant solution containing the peptide was carried through such steps as binding to Sephadex G-25, elution with ammonium acetate, filtration over Sephadex G-50 in equilibrium with 1 M acetic acid, and chromatography on DEAE cellulose. Final purification of APP was accomplished by countercurrent distribution and chromatography on CM-cellulose with urea-containing buffers. After the fats from the acid-ethanol extract of beef pancreas were removed, BPP was precipitated by ethanol ether and chromatographed over Sephadex G-50, DEAE, and finally Sephadex G-25.

The homogeneity of PPs was verified by polyacrylamide disc-gel electrophoresis. After proper staining, this resulted in a single band of significant intensity representing PP as a pure protein moiety.

Amino Acid Sequence

When pure PPs were subjected to amino acid sequence analysis, it became obvious that APP and BPP were homologs, each containing 36 amino acid residues in a straight chain and having identities at 15 of the 36 positions (16, 17,44,47,58) (Table 1).

The pancreatic polypeptide isolated from the pancreas of hog, sheep, or human are very similar to BPP and structures of these peptides differ from that of BPP in only one or two residues at positions 2, 6, 11, or 23 (16) (Table 2). Recently Chance et al. *(unpublished data)* found that porcine and canine pancreatic polypeptides were identical. To date, the structures of PPs in five mammalian and one avian species are known.

TABLE 1. *Amino acid sequence of BPP and APP[a]*

BPP	Ala	Pro	Leu	Glu	Pro	Glu	Tyr	Pro	Gly	Asp	Asn	Ala
APP	Gly	Pro	Ser	Gln	Pro	Thr	Tyr	Pro	Gly	Asp	Asp	Ala
	Thr	Pro	Glu	Gln	Met	Ala	Gln	Tyr	Ala	Ala	Glu	Leu
	Pro	Val	Glu	Asp	Leu	Ile	Arg	Phe	Tyr	Asp	Asn	Leu
	Arg	Arg	Tyr	Ile	Asn	Met	Leu	Thr	Arg	Pro	Arg	Tyr-NH₂
	Gln	Gln	Tyr	Leu	Asn	Val	Val	Thr	Arg	His	Arg	Tyr-NH₂

[a]Identical amino acid residues at identical positions of BPP and APP are underlined (16, 44,58).

TABLE 2. *Pancreatic polypeptide: Species variation in mammals*

1	2	3	4	5	6	7	8	9	10	11	12
Ala–	Pro–	Leu–	Glu–	Pro–	Glu–	Tyr–	Pro–	Gly–	Asp–	Asn–	Ala–

13	14	15	16	17	18	19	20	21	22	23	24
Thr–	Pro–	Glu–	Gln–	Met–	Ala–	Gln–	Tyr–	Ala–	Ala–	Glu–	Leu–

25	26	27	28	29	30	31	32	33	34	35	36
Arg–	Arg–	Tyr–	Ile–	Asn–	Met–	Leu–	Thr–	Arg–	Pro–	Arg–	Tyr–NH₂

	2	6	11	23
Bovine (BPP):	Pro	Glu	Asn	Glu
Ovine (OPP):	Ser	Glu	Asn	Glu
Human (HPP):	Pro	Val	Asn	Asp
Canine (CPP): + Porcine (PPP):	Pro	Val	Asp	Glu

From refs. 15–18.

When the sequences of APP and chicken glucagon are aligned (Table 3), eight identities can be found. But in mammalian species the amino acid sequences of PPs and of beef or porcine glucagon have only two identities at positions 10 and 29. Moreover, the structures of the mammalian PPs isolated, so far, are unrelated to any of the gastrointestinal hormones known.

TABLE 3. *Amino acid sequences of APP and chicken glucagon*[a]

APP	Gly	Pro	Ser	Gln	Pro	Thr	Tyr	Pro	Gly	Asp	Asp	Ala
G		His	Ser	Gln	Gly	Thr	Phe	Thr	Ser	Asp	Tyr	Ser
	1					6						12
APP	Pro	Val	Glu	Asp	Leu	Ile	Arg	Phe	Tyr	Asp	Asn	Leu
G	Lys	Tyr	Leu	Asp	Ser	Arg	Arg	Ala	Gln	Asp	Phe	Val
	13											24
APP	Gln	Gln	Tyr	Leu	Asn	Val	Val	Thr	Arg	His	Arg	TyrNH$_2$
G	Gln	Trp	Leu	Met	Ser	Thr						
	25					30						36

G, Chicken glucagon
[a] Identical amino acid residues are underlined.

Physicochemical Properties

The NH$_2$-terminal segment of all the pancreatic polypeptides (residues 1 to 16) contains three or four proline residues with side chain carboxyl groups fairly regularly spaced, and has essentially no amino acids with hydrophobic side chains. The center segment (residues 17 to 31) consists of alternating hydrophobic polar pairs of singlets, whereas the COOH-terminus is polar and highly basic. X-ray studies (76,100) indicated that the APP molecules were partially helical and were arranged as a compact dimer about the crystalographic twofold axis. According to Frank, physicochemical properties of BPP were similar to those of APP (B. H. Frank, Lilly Research Laboratories, *unpublished study*).

BIOLOGICAL ACTIVITY

Metabolic Effects

Since APP and BPP were originally isolated as contaminants of insulin or glucagon, a logical approach to determining the biological action of PP was to examine its effect on carbohydrate and lipid metabolism. Studies on APP were carried out in unanesthetized, nonfasted chicken wherein simultaneous liver glycogen, blood glucose, and plasma glycerol levels were estimated at varying periods after intravenous injection of APP. Like glucagon, APP was an effective glycogenolytic agent. But unlike glucagon, which was hyperglycemic and hyperglycerolemic, APP caused hypoglycerolemia and had no effect on plasma glucose level (39).

In the absence of glycemic alterations, glucose-6-phosphate must be shunted into metabolic pathways other than that of hydrolysis. The observed hepatic glycogenolysis concomitant with decrease in blood glycerol levels in response to APP suggests that hepatic lipogenesis may be stimulated by APP.

BPP was given intravenously to dogs (57,63) and rats (85). In contrast to the actions of glucagon and insulin that produced hyper- and hypoglycemia, respectively, in these animals, BPP had no effect on blood sugar at doses that caused marked gastrointestinal actions. BPP failed to release insulin from isolated pancreas *in vitro* and no effect of BPP on lipid metabolism has been reported (85). In the New Zealand obese mice the hyperinsulinemia, hyperglycemia, and weight gain were returned to normal by intraperitoneal injection of small (1 μg, t.i.d) doses of APP or BPP in 30 days. It was suggested that PPs may have an effect on metabolism and appetite (31).

In addition to hyperglycemic and hyperglycerolemic actions, glucagon caused transient hyperkalemia, diuresis, and increased excretion of electrolytes from the kidney (63,64) and the small intestine (7). BPP differed from glucagon in having no diuretic action, no effect on Na, K, Mg, and Ca excretion in the urine of the conscious dog (Fig. 1), and no effect on the concentrations of Na, K, Ca, and Mg in the jejunum and ileum of the barbitalized dog (Lin and Bloomquist, *unpublished study*).

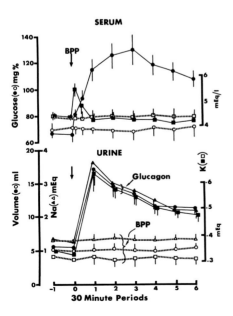

FIG. 1. Effect of BPP and glucagon on glucose and K in serum and excretion of Na and K in urine of dogs. Note the lack of hyperglycemic, hyperkalemic, and diuretic effects of BPP. *Solid lines and symbols* denote changes caused by glucagon, and *dotted lines and symbols* denote changes caused by BPP. Values represent means ± SE of four experiments in four dogs. (From ref. 63, with permission.)

Gastrointestinal Actions

Action on Gastric Secretion

Since insulin stimulates (43,70) and glucagon inhibits (56,79) gastric secretion, it was pertinent to study the gastric action of PP.

The effect of BPP was studied in the conscious dog with vagally innervated gastric fistula and vagally denervated Heidenhain pouch. BPP had both stimulatory and inhibitory effects, depending on the conditions of the animals (57,61,63). When the dogs were fasted, BPP slowly stimulated gastric volume and acid secretion, reaching the peak at the end of a 2-hr intravenous infusion (Fig. 2). When gastric acid secretion was induced by continuous infusion of the C-terminal pentapeptide of gastrin (PG), the steady secretion of HCl was significantly inhibited in a dose-related manner. Both the inhibitory and stimulatory effects of BPP occurred only when the doses were very large (20–100 μg/kg/hr).

In both cases, the vagally innervated portion of the stomach was more sensitive to the actions of BPP than the Heidenhain pouch, suggesting a possible interaction between PP and the vagal mechanism. The action of PP on pepsin secretion has not been reported.

The C-terminal tyrosyl amide residue appeared to be important for the action of BPP on the stomach. The Des-C-Tyr-NH$_2$ BPP (BPP 1–35), the fragment of BPP devoid of the Tyr-amide at the 36th position, had no inhibitory effect on acid secretion (Fig. 3) induced by PG (57,63).

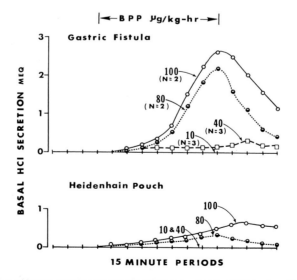

FIG. 2. Stimulation of basal gastric HCl (mean mEq) secretion by BPP in dog. Note the sluggishness of the gastric responses and the difference in the sensitivity of gastric fistula and the Heidenhain pouch to BPP. (From ref. 63, with permission.)

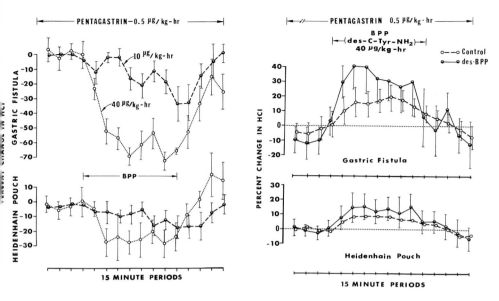

FIG. 3. Effect of BPP **(A)** and des-tyrosyl-NH₂ **(B)** on gastric HCl secretion induced by the C-terminal pentapeptide of gastrin. Note the lack of significant effect of des-tyrosyl-NH₂ BPP. Values are means ± SE of four tests in four dogs. (From ref. 63, with permission.)

Results from structure-function studies further indicated that the C-terminal hexapeptide, fragment 31–36, also significantly inhibited gastric acid secretion in four dogs at a dose of 20 and 40 μg/kg/hr (ref. 58 and Lin, Evans, and Chance, *unpublished study*). However, the molar dose required for the hexapeptide was greater than that for BPP. The minimal effective fragment that mimics the action of BPP is unknown.

Gastric actions of APP were studied in anesthetized chickens and rats. Given in single intravenous doses, APP caused sharp increases in proventricular flow that persisted for at least 90 min (39,47). The increase in volume was accompanied by increased concentration of HCl and pepsin (39). This suggests that APP may be a true gastric secretagogue in the chicken. However, the doses of APP (12–50 μg/kg i.v.) that evoked the secretion in the stomach were probably pharmacological. A final assessment of the physiological role of APP in the regulation of gastric secretion in the chicken must await further elucidation under physiological conditions at low doses.

The action of APP on the proventriculus does not require vagal innervation. Like BPP, which stimulated secretion from the vagally denervated Heidenhain pouch, APP also increased acid secretion from the proventriculus after bilateral vagotomy (39). No inhibitory effect of APP on avian gastric secretion has been reported. APP also stimulated gastric secretion of anesthetized rats. But the sensitivity of rats was much less than that of the chicken to its isologous peptide,

APP. When equal doses of pentagastrin and APP were compared in the rat for gastric secretory activity, the pentapeptide was more potent than PP.

The mechanism by which BPP and APP affect gastric secretion is unknown. It is unlikely that BPP has a direct effect on the oxyntic cells. BPP at concentrations of 2.5 to 5.0 $\times$ 10^{-7} M failed to inhibit or stimulate the spontaneous or histamine-induced acid secretion from the isolated gastric mucosa of the bullfrog, *Rana catesbeiana* (Warrick and Lin, *unpublished study*).

Action on Pancreatic Secretion

APP consistently had no effect on pancreatic secretion in the anesthetized chicken (39). But BPP and PPP both showed profound effects on pancreatic secretion in the acute and chronic pancreatic fistula dogs.

Again, BPP showed both stimulatory and inhibitory actions on the dog pancreas, depending on the experimental condition (63). In fasted dogs pancreatic volume, bicarbonate, and enzyme outputs were all decreased by BPP (57,59,63). Over a wide dose range of BPP, the water and bicarbonate responses induced by secretin were initially augmented during the early part of PP infusion and then returned to control levels as infusion of PP continued (Fig. 4). The nature of the biphasic or "reversal" effects of BPP on secretin-induced volume and bicarbonate responses is not understood. The stimulatory effect of PP at very low doses or in the early phase of intravenous infusion suggests that PP may act as a weak agonist on the water and electrolyte-secreting mechanism of the pancreas and then becomes an antagonist as the dose is increased.

While a biphasic response of water and bicarbonate to BPP was taking place,

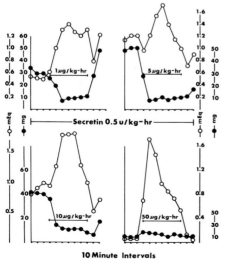

FIG. 4. Examples of biphasic action of BPP on water-bicarbonate (mEq) secretion when dogs were stimulated by continuous infusion of secretin alone. Note consistent suppression of protein output at all doses in the dogs. (From ref. 63, with permission.)

the total protein or enzyme output was consistently inhibited over a wide range of doses. This inhibition of enzyme output occurred even when pancreatic volume output was increased by two to eightfold in the initial phase of PP infusion. This could happen only when the decrease in enzyme concentration was much greater than the increase in pancreatic volume. In this sense the inhibition of protein secretion represents a true suppression of enzyme release by PP (Fig. 5).

Pancreatic volume, bicarbonate, and protein secretions induced by cholecystokinin (CCK) and secretin were all inhibited by BPP in the conscious dog (63,91). The minimal dose required for significant inhibition was approximately 0.25 µg/kg/hr, suggesting that the inhibition of enzyme release by CCK may be a selective or specific effect of PP. This is further supported by the observation that pancreatic volume, bicarbonate, and protein secretion induced by intraduodenal infusion of amino acids for the release of endogenous CCK was inhibited by PP in a dose-related manner (60).

The C-terminal tyrosyl amide that was important for the action of PP on the stomach was also crucial for inhibition of pancreatic secretion. The Des-C-Tyr-NH$_2$ BPP had no inhibitory effect on volume, electrolyte, or enzyme secretion.

PPP differs from BPP by having valine and aspartic acid instead of glutamic acid and asparagine, respectively, in the 6th and 11th positions. PPs isolated from dog and hog pancreata are chemically identical. PPP or CPP inhibited all the parameters of pancreatic secretion in the dog (91). Surprisingly, when

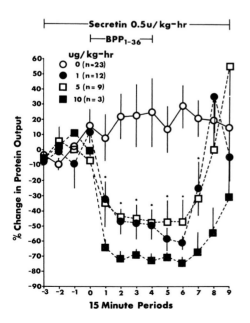

FIG. 5. Inhibition of protein secretion from the pancreas of the dog stimulated by steady infusion of secretin. Values represent the means ± SE in three dogs. N, number of tests at each dose. (From ref. 63, with permission.)

the dose-response inhibitory effects of BPP and PPP on pancreatic secretion in the same dogs were compared, BPP was more active than PPP. This suggests that a natural homolog of CPP was even more potent than the dog's own PP for inhibition of its pancreatic secretion (Lin and Evans, *unpublished study*).

The mechanism by which BPP inhibits pancreatic secretion is unknown. BPP was tested *in vitro* on the pancreatic slices of the guinea pig for its effect on Ca^{2+} efflux and amylase release induced by CCK or carbacholine. The results, so far, have been negative, suggesting that the inhibitory effect of PP on enzyme secretion induced by CCK may be unrelated to the efflux of intracellular calcium (J. D. Gardner, *personal communication*). It was alleged that BPP exerts a trophic effect causing significant increase in DNA synthesis in the rat pancreas (32). Physiologically it is not conceivable that an inhibitor that opposes the action of CCK on enzyme release will at the same time have a trophic effect, like that of CCK, on pancreatic DNA synthesis. Further confirmation of the observation is needed.

Action on Gastrointestinal Motility

The first indication of the biological activity of BPP came from the observation that intravenous administration of large (50–100 μg/kg) doses of BPP caused immediate nausea, retching followed by vomiting, and defecation in dogs with chronic gastric, pancreatic, or bile fistulae (58,59). However, the feces were well formed and not accompanied by an excessive amount of water. It is not known whether the vomiting and defecation were caused by a central mechanism or by a peripheral action.

BPP has both excitatory and inhibitory actions on the gut. Large doses caused increased gut motility in the antrum, duodenum, and colon of the dog (57). However, at either low intravenous doses or by slow intravenous infusion, BPP relaxed the intraluminal pressure in the dog antrum, pylorus, duodenum, ileocecal sphincter, and descending colon (58). Amplitude of contraction recorded with microstrain gauges and action potentials recorded with unipolar electrodes were both suppressed by small doses of BPP (Fig. 6). APP was found to inhibit the amplitude and frequency of contraction of the turkey gizzard (19).

Action on Gallbladder, Choledocho-Duodenal Sphincter, and Bile Flow

In conscious dogs with fistulae in the common bile duct, gallbladder, choledochal sphincter, and stomach, the intraluminal pressure in the gallbladder was reduced and the choledochal resistance was increased by slow infusion of BPP under basal conditions (57–60). The gastric fistula, which was kept open during the experiment, was stimulated to secrete acid. However, the bile flow was not affected by BPP at doses of 20 to 40 μg/kg/hr. APP was found to have no effect on bile flow and gallbladder pressure in anesthetized chickens (39).

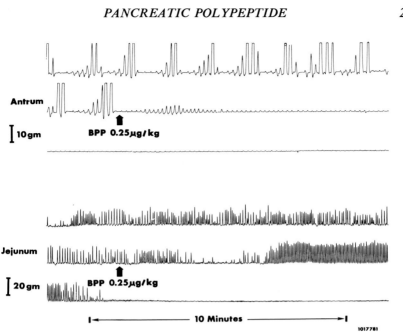

FIG. 6. Inhibition of gastrointestinal motility of the conscious dog by a low dose of BPP. Motility was recorded with pressure transducer strain gages anchored to the serosal surface of the gut. (From Lin and Bloomquist, *unpublished data*.)

Effect on Gastric Emptying, Food Intake, and Bowel Movement in the Small Intestine

In the rat, gastric emptying of a pectin meal containing phenol red was enhanced by BPP. The maximal effect was seen 45 min after BPP was given intraperitoneally. The average emptying of a 2-ml meal was enhanced by 13% over a 15-min period at the dose range of BPP of 1 to 100 μg/kg.

Conflicting results were reported concerning the effect of BPP on bowel movement in the small intestine of the rat. One study showed that the movement of the charcoal meal was enhanced by intraperitoneal injection of 10 μg/kg of BPP (60,62). In another study, PP was found to have no effect on the transit time of a test substance containing $^{51}CrO_4$ (34). A role for BPP in the regulation of food intake in the mouse was proposed (31,65). The dose used in one of the studies (65) ranged from 10 to 100 μg/kg/day for 12 days. In view of the size of the dose and the pharmacological actions of BPP on enhancement of gastric emptying and bowel propulsion in the small intestine of the rat, an assessment of the role of PP in the physiological regulation of food intake must await a definite answer to the following questions: (a) Is the PP in a physiological dose range that causes a rise of plasma PP level no greater than that which can be induced by a meal? (b) Is the reduction of body weight in the obese mice truly due to an effect of PP on the appetite center and not to an indirect effect on gut motility that reduces the availability of food for absorption or assimilation?

Miscellaneous Actions

In the anesthetized chicken, APP had no effect on blood pressure, electrocardiogram, and respiratory movement (39). The actions of BPP on these parameters have not been studied.

MORPHOLOGY OF PP CELLS: IMMUNOHISTOCHEMICAL IDENTIFICATION

Soon after antisera to APP (47), BPP, and HPP (15,59) were successfully developed, immunohistochemical identification of the cells producing PP began.

Avian PP Cells

Larsson et al. (53), using the immunofluorescence technique to reveal APP-producing cells, found that they were disseminated in the exocrine parenchyma of the chicken pancreas. The APP cells were polygonal or spindle-shaped and often had prolonged processes in between the exocrine cells (53).

The staining property of APP cells was different from those of the A (glucagon), B (insulin), D (somatostatin), and EC (enterochromaffin) cells (53). APP cells had the capacity to take up and decarboxylate L-DOPA. Ultrastructurally, they had the typical appearance of polypeptide hormone-producing cells in that they contained numerous cytoplasmic granules.

APP-like immunoreactivity was found in the acid alcohol extracts of the pancreas of eight avian species, the turtle, and the alligator (49). No APP immuno-cross-reactivity was found in the pancreas of mammals and amphibians or in the extracts of the liver, proventriculus, gizzard, heart, spleen, and intestine of the chicken and duck (49).

There was an indication of structural differences between the PP of various avian species since their cross-reactivity with anti-chicken PP serum was incomplete (49).

Mammalian PP Cells

PP-producing cells in mammalian tissues were identified by immunohistochemical procedures using antiserum to HPP, BPP, or PPP.

In the human pancreas the PP cells showed strong immunofluorescence after reacting with anti-HPP serum (51). The HPP cells were located mainly at the

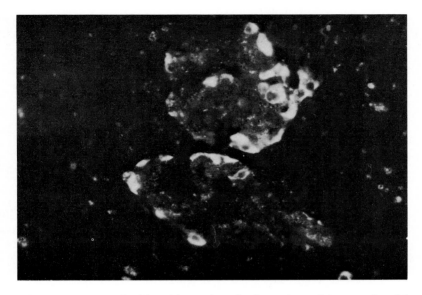

FIG. 7. Human pancreas. An islet of Langerhans is shown to contain several peripherally located PP cells (immunofluorescence technique employing an antiserum to human PP). (Courtesy of Dr. L. I. Larsson, Aarhus, Denmark.)

periphery of the islets (Fig. 7); some were also found scattered in the exocrine parenchyma and even in the epithelium of the ducts (28,51).

In addition to the human pancreas (27,51,68,74,75), PP-producing cells were identified in the pancreata of the dog (26,28,52), rat (52,71,80,84,88), opposum (52), chinchilla (52), rabbit (26), guinea pig (52,71,84,88), mouse (52), shrew (25), and a few lower forms such as the lizard (78) and teleost fishes (97) (Fig. 8).

In addition to the pancreas, PP cells were found in the mucosa of the stomach (9,52,88) (Fig. 9), duodenum (25,73), ileum (9), colon, and rectum (14). PP immunoreactivity was demonstrated in the neural ganglia of the earthworm (87).

In most species, the distribution of PP cells in the pancreas was similar to that in man. The cells were located mainly along the periphery of the islets (9,10,27,40,52,68,73), although in the sheep pancreas (Fig. 8C), PP cells formed a large proportion of the cell population and clustered as one pool at one end of the islets. The rest of the PP cells were scattered throughout the exocrine parenchyma of the pancreas.

Generally, PP cells were numerous in the uncinate process adjacent to the duodenum and were scarce in the body and caudal part of the pancreas (26,40, 51,52,68,73). For this reason the uncinate process contained four to five times as much PP as that in the tail by immunoassay.

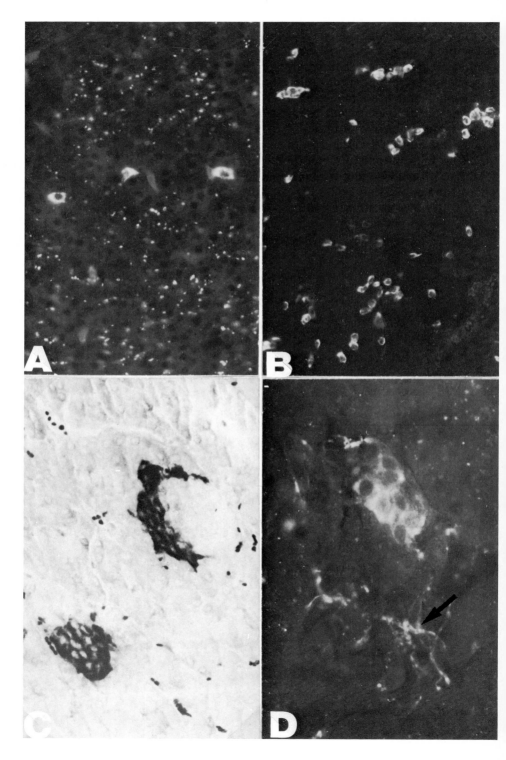

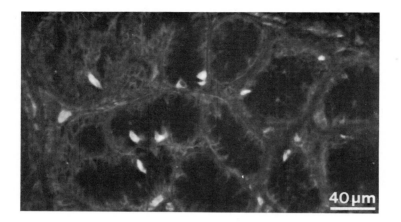

FIG. 9. Paraffin section of the dog antral mucosa, treated with the indirect immunofluorescent technique using anti-BPP serum. Several fluorescent cells are seen in the epithelium of the glands. (Courtesy of Dr. L. Orci, Geneva, Switzerland.)

Histochemically the mammalian PP cells were faintly argyrophilic with the Grimelius silver technique, which stained the A, B, and D cells black (8,28,51). The immunoflourescence of the PP cells was often elongated or irregularly shaped, giving off processes that passed closely between the nonfluorescent islets or exocrine parenchyma cells or epithelial cells of the ducts in the pancreas (51).

The cross-reactivity of anti-HPP or anti-BPP serum with PP was quite specific. The anti-HPP serum raised in rabbits did not cross-react with APP, insulin, proinsulin, glucagon, somatostatin, secretin, gastrin, CCK, GIP, VIP, or GLI (18,41). No immunofluorescent cells were observed when anti-PP serum was adsorbed with BPP or PPP prior to incubation (41).

Ultrastructurally the cytoplasm of the PP cells contained electron-dense granules with tight limiting membrane (8,40,52,53) that had the ability to take up and decarboxylate amine precursors (52,53), features that were characteristic

FIG. 8. Sections from the pancreas of several vertebrates. **A.** Duck pancreas. Immunofluorescence with a specific antiserum to avian PP reveals endocrine cells that occur scattered in the exocrine parenchyma. ×500. **B.** Cat pancreas. In the duodenal lobe (uncinate process) PP cells occur singly or in small groups that are disseminated among the exocrine cells. HPP immunofluorescence; ×236. **C.** Sheep pancreas. In this species, PP cells occur predominantly in islets where they constitute a large proportion of the cells. Ovine PP cells usually tend to be clustered at one pool of the islet. HPP immunoperoxidase staining; note the pseudoperoxidase reaction of red cells; ×400. **D.** Opposum pancreas. PP cells occur in both insular and extrainsular locations. Opposum PP cells store large amounts of dopamine which may be visualized by the Falck-Hillarp fluorescence cytochemical technique. This technique also demonstrates norepinephrine in adrenergic nerve endings (arrow) ×570. (Courtesy of L. I. Larsson, Aarhus, Denmark.)

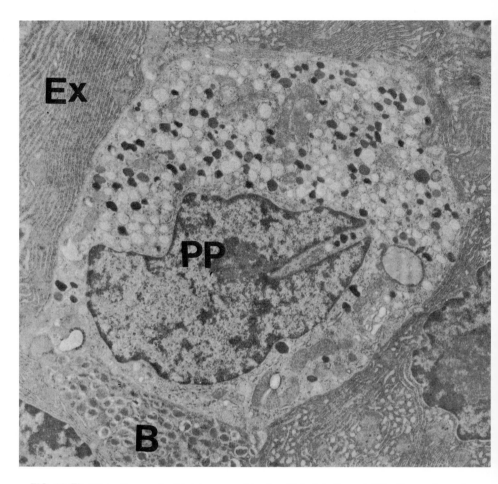

FIG. 10. Electron micrograph of cat pancreas (duodenal lobe). In the cat, PP cells are characterized by the presence of a lobated nucleus and by numerous cytoplasmic granules of highly variable electron density. Cat PP cells are identical with the previously described F (or X) cells. Ultrastructural cytochemistry has proven that the PP cell granules constitute the chief source of PP. Note the close association between the PP cells and the exocrine zymogen (Ex) cells. At the bottom of this electron micrograph a portion of an insulin-producing **(B)** cell is seen. ×11,500. (Courtesy of Dr. L. I. Larsson, Aarhus, Denmark.)

of polypeptide hormone-producing cells. In many species, the nucleus of the PP cells was located as shown in Fig. 10 (25,51). The staining and immunochemical properties and the ultrastructure of the PP cells set them apart from the A, B, D, and EC cells. There has been confusion over the nomenclatural classification of the cells producing PP. These had been called variously D, D_1, F, or L-like cells. But at this juncture no designation serves the purpose better than the simple terms "PP-producing" or "PP-cells."

Embryological Development of PP Cells

In the human fetus, PP cells were observed as early as at 10 weeks of gestation (20,73), whereas in the rat, PP cells were observed before birth. Rat PP cells appeared at parturition and then abruptly increased in number on the 5th to 7th days postnatally. In the rat pancreas, PP cells appeared much later than insulin (B)- and glucagon (A)-producing cells, whereas in man they developed later than somatostatin-, secretin, and glucagon-producing cells.

PP immunoreactivity was found in the pancreas or alimentary tract of the highly developed cartilagenous and bony fishes but not in those of the lower forms (92). Thus, in the phylogeny of the endocrine pancreas, development of PP cells is preceded by that of insulin, somatostatin, and probably glucagon.

REGULATION OF RELEASE OF PANCREATIC POLYPEPTIDE

Basal Plasma Levels of PP

Under fasting conditions, the plasma levels of PP in dogs and man were mostly in the range of 10 to 50 pmoles/liter (23,24,83,89); in exceptional cases basal levels were as low as 8 and as high as 313 pmoles/liter in man (94). Floyd et al. (11,24) found that in healthy persons plasma concentration of PP increased significantly ($p < 0.05$–0.005) with age. A highly significant correlation ($p < 0.01$) between age and basal serum HPP concentration in normal subjects was also reported by Taylor et al. (94). In both sexes PP concentrations in males were significantly higher than those in females (96). Normal concentrations of APP ranging from 476 to 1428 pmoles/liter under fasting conditions (45,49) were many times higher than those of HPP and CPP.

Effect of Food

Food is the natural and one of the most effective stimulants of PP release. Kimmel et al. reported that plasma APP concentration rose to 950 to 2857 pmoles/liter after feeding (45,49). Lin (59) and Chance et al. (18) found that plasma PP levels in the dog increased severalfold after a meal; a large meal (900 g) caused an increase from 50 pmoles/liter to 3,200 pg/ml (720 pmoles/liter). With 400 g of meat Taylor et al. (92) and Lin et al. (18) saw an increase of 100 to 200 pmoles/liter after feeding. In man, Floyd et al. (21) found that ingestion of 500 g of cooked beef caused an increase of approximately 150 pmoles/liter of HPP (21,23,24). Schwartz (83), Adrian (2,5), and Taylor et al. (89,92) reported increments of 100 to 400 pmoles/liter of PP after a meal. These observations have been confirmed and expanded by subsequent studies (36,48,99).

Both the quantity and quality of the food had an important effect on the release of PP. Of the food constituents, protein appeared to be more effective than fats and carbohydrates for the release of PP in the chicken (45) and man (2,24,89). Fat had a modest stimulatory effect on PP release (2,24,48) and appeared to be more effective than ingestion of glucose (2,24). Only ingested protein, fat, and glucose had the ability to release PP; protein, fat, and glucose given intravenously were ineffective (2,24).

Although a modest increase in plasma PP levels was seen when a mixture of 10 amino acids was infused intravenously (24), the possibility of releasing insulin or glucagon by some of the amino acids, and the subsequent effects of insulin or glucagon on plasma PP concentration, could not be ruled out.

Ingested carbohydrate or glucose caused a modest but significant rise of plasma PP levels in the chicken (45) and man (2,24,86,89,99). Given as a 600-g glucose test meal the peak concentration of PP was seen within 15 to 30 min in human plasma (24,86,89). Floyd et al. (24) found that 3 hr after ingestion of glucose, there was a drastic rise in PP concentration that coincided with a sharp fall in blood glucose. On the other hand, hyperglycemia induced by intravenous infusion of glucose definitely decreased plasma levels of PP (24,67,86,99).

Intraduodenal infusion of dilute HCl was reported to have no significant effect on PP release (24,99), but others found that HCl increased secretion of PP in dog (36) and man (37,67).

Evidence for the effect of individual amino acids on release of PP *in vivo* or *in vitro* is still unclear. Intravenous infusion of L-arginine in man caused a slight decrease of PP level that was accompanied by a sharp rise in blood sugar and glucagon (24). An amino acid mixture stimulated the isolated slices of the uncinate process of dog pancreas to secrete PP but individual amino acids such as arginine, leucine, lysine, phenylalanine, tyrosine, and tryptophan were ineffective (29).

There is an indication that the adenylate cyclase system may play a role in the release of PP. Although arginine (30) or glucose (30,42) alone failed to release PP from isolated pancreas, they released PP with the aid of cyclic AMP (30).

Effect of Gastrointestinal Hormones or Peptides

Established gastrointestinal hormones such as gastrin, CCK, and secretin and a number of candidate gastrointestinal hormones have been studied for their action on release of PP.

Most studies showed that gastrin had little effect on PP release (42,81,89), although PP concentration was increased by bolus injection of pentagastrin (24). Taylor et al. (89) reported that in man there was no significant increase in serum PP concentration during infusion of gastrin G-17 or highly purified CCK alone or of the two in combination. This was despite the fact that the highest doses of CCK and G-17 achieved maximal rates of pancreatic and gastric secretion, respectively. Endogenous release of gastrin by alkalinization of the stomach also did not significantly alter the PP levels in plasma (81). Secretion of PP was stimulated by impure secretin (1,86) but not by the highly purified secretin. Endogenous secretin induced by intraduodenal infusion of dilute HCl also did not significantly alter HPP concentration (89). The same is true for CCK; impure CCK caused a significant rise of HPP, whereas synthetic C-octapeptide of CCK had no such effect (77). Since exogenous gastrin did not stimulate PP release, the increase of plasma PP concentration following distention of the stomach with glucose or saline (89) or of the antrum with balloon (81) cannot be explained on the basis of endogenous release of gastrin.

Other candidate hormones of the gut such as GIP and VIP were reported to cause secretion of PP from the isolated pancreas (42), whereas somatostatin (2,24,35,42,66,86,99), which was known to suppress the release of gastrin, secretin, glucagon, and CCK, definitely decreased secretion of PP *in vitro* and in pig, dog, and man. Motilin was found to have no significant effect on the basal and prandial levels of HPP (69).

Bombesin-like immunoreactivity has recently been identified in the gut. In addition to being the most potent stimulus of gastrin release in man and dog (95), bombesin was a potent releaser of PP (93). Cerulein, the tetradecapeptide isolated from the skin of *Hyla caerulea,* was reported to stimulate the release of PP in man (1,2) and *in vitro* (42).

The finding by Floyd et al. (24) that PP was released by insulin has been confirmed (1,67,86). The stimulatory effect of insulin and other hypoglycemic agents and the inhibitory effect of hyperglycemia are probably mediated mainly by a vagal mechanism.

Action of the Autonomic Nervous System

The effect of tease-feeding on plasma levels of PP in the dog was first observed by Lin (59) and Chance et al. (18). Tease-feeding for 10 min increased the mean PP concentration from a basal value of 25.8 pmoles/liter to 55.5 pmoles/liter in 15 min; in 30 min PP peaked at 65 pmoles/liter and the effect of a 10-min tease-feeding lasted for 45 to 60 min. Taylor et al. (89) conducted modified sham-feeding in man and found net increase of HPP concentration of about 15 pmoles/liter in 15 min. Schwartz et al. (81) sham-fed patients with gastrostomy and found that the mean HPP level was raised by about 47 pmoles/liter in 30 min. Thus in comparison with the effect of intragastric food, the effect of sham- or tease-feeding is relatively modest but significant.

The cephalic phase of PP release in man was abolished in vagotomized patients (81,89) and by anticholinergics. Of the anticholinergics, propantheline (89), atropine (36,81,82,90,93), or benzilonium (81) all effectively blocked the release of PP by food. The effect of bombesin on secretion of PP was blocked by atropine (93). Some studies showed that truncal vagotomy abolished the early or cephalic phase of PP response and diminished the delayed PP response to food (38,83). Other studies showed that only the cephalic phase of PP release was decreased;

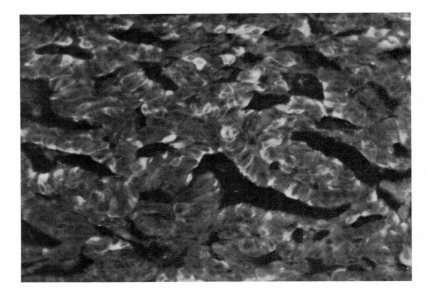

FIG. 11. Human pancreas. A pancreatic endocrine tumor consisting almost exclusively of PP cells and associated with the Verner-Morrison syndrome. HPP immunofluorescence; ×256. (Courtesy of Dr. L. I. Larsson, Aarhus, Denmark.)

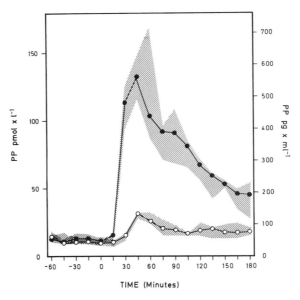

FIG. 12. Plasma PP concentrations, median concentration and interquartile range *(hatched area)* in eight normal subjects during insulin hypoglycemia (0.2 μ/kg) without (●) or with (○) atropine (0.03 mg/kg i.m.) injected 25 min before insulin. (From ref. 82, with permission.)

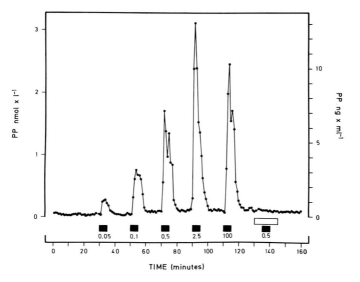

FIG. 13. The effect of increasing doses of acetylcholine on PP concentrations in the perfusate from an isolated porcine pancreas. Note the inhibitory action of atropine on PP release *(open bar)*. (From ref. 82, with permission.)

the food-stimulated PP response was unaffected by a previous vagotomy (89). Vagotomy did not significantly alter basal concentration of PP (90).

Indeed, the action of vagal mediation for PP release can be mimicked by administration of insulin (82), cholinergics (42,82,93), or electrical stimulation of the vagus (92). In man PP release effected by insulin was blocked by atropine (Fig. 12), whereas in pigs PP release induced by acetylcholine or electrical stimulation (Fig. 13) was diminished by atropine or hexamethonium (82). The secretion of PP from the isolated pancreas was also enhanced by acetylcholine (29,42).

In patients suffering from autonomic neuropathy the PP response to insulin was significantly diminished (55). The release of HPP by distention of the antrum or fundus with a balloon (81) or by water load (1,69,89) was mainly if not entirely due to a gastro-vagal reflex. The stimulatory effect of food on PP release in the chicken was completely abolished by anesthesia (45).

Whereas the cholinergic mechanism definitely increased the secretion of PP, the adrenergic agents did not seem to have any significant effect on PP release (42).

PANCREATIC POLYPEPTIDE UNDER PATHOLOGICAL CONDITIONS

Since PP is produced by specific cells, abnormal concentrations of this hormone in plasma can occur when there is a change in the PP cell population, altered sensitivity of the cells to stimuli, or altered capacity of the cells to secrete PP.

In patients with both mature-onset and juvenile-onset diabetes the high levels of PP were not significantly changed by treatment with insulin or sulfonyl ureas (22,23). In fact, hyperplasia of PP cells in the pancreas of juvenile diabetics was reported (72).

Tissue concentrations of PP were grossly elevated in insulinomas (72) and glucagonoma tumors (50) of man. Basal plasma levels of PP were also higher than normal in patients with insulinoma (24). In other forms of multiple endocrine adenomas or apudomas (4), grossly elevated concentrations of PP were found in vipomas (4,72), gastrinomas (50,54,72), and carcinoid tumors (4,50,54).

Basal levels of PP in patients with duodenal ulcer (DU) or Zollinger-Ellison syndromes (ZES) were all significantly higher than those in normal subjects and in patients with gastric ulcer (1,3,38,89), but the PP responses to food (3,89) or insulin (1) in DU patients and normals were the same.

The pancreas was probably the major source of circulating PP. Partial pancreatectomy reduced fasting levels of APP and markedly decreased PP response to feeding in the chicken (45), whereas total pancreatectomy led to undetectable levels of PP in DU patients (3).

In patients with tumors causing the watery diarrhea syndrome, Larsson et al. (50) found that the serum VIP levels were within the normal range, whereas the HPP levels were elevated a thousand times. Large amounts of HPP were measured in the tumor tissue (11–16 nmoles/g wet wt. vs. 200–250 pmoles/g in normal pancreas, Fig. 11), whereas VIP content was low. This led to a number of speculations that HPP might be the agent causing the watery diarrhea syndrome. Lin and Bloomoquist *(unpublished study)* measured the pharmacological effect of BPP at doses 100 to 400 times of that required for inhibition of pancreatic secretion on electrolyte effluxes in the jejunum and ileum of the nembutalized dog, and found that volume of secretion and concentrations of Na, K, Ca, and Mg in the intestinal juice were unaffected by BPP. This suggests that BPP is unlikely to be the causative factor in the watery diarrhea syndrome. In one case of watery diarrhea syndrome that was controlled by prednisolone, plasma VIP levels were halved but HPP levels remained high and unchanged (54).

Based on observations of high content of HPP in pancreatic tumors and high plasma levels of HPP in patients with ZES, insulinomas, or glucagonomas, Polak et al. (72) suggested that measurements of plasma PP levels should be a new aid in the diagnosis of pancreatic tumors. This holds true only if hyperplasia of PP cells is invariably associated with other types of tumors in the pancreas. In fact, the cell types in most endocrine pancreatic tumors are mixed and each cell type produces, stores, and secretes its own peptide. Hyper- or hypofunction of one cell type in a mixed pancreatic tumor associated with a clinical symptom does not necessarily imply that other cell types in the tumor also undergo the same changes in functional state. Thus Floyd et al. (24) reported that high HPP levels in a patient with insulinoma remained elevated despite surgical removal of the tumor. Moreover, Floyd (24) and Larsson et al. (50) were unable to find increased concentrations of HPP in most of the pancreatic tumors.

By the same token the usefulness of a fasting serum HPP concentration of >240 pmoles/liter as a marker of pancreatic gastrinoma (72) is doubtful. Taylor et al. (94) reported that in 22 unoperated ZES patients the basal serum HPP concentrations were not over 240 pmoles/liter. There also was no significant correlation between the basal serum gastrin and HPP concentrations in the ZES patients.

METABOLISM AND FATE OF PANCREATIC POLYPEPTIDE

There is the suggestion that three HPP immunoreactive fractions are present in the plasma of normal subjects, each representing about one-third of the total immunoreactivity and differing in molecular weights between 1,500 to 100,000 (6). The nature of these fractions remains to be studied.

Under basal conditions, the half-time ($t_{1/2}$) for disappearance of a single intravenous bolus of BBP in four dogs averaged 5.2 min (Lin, Chance, and Evans, *unpublished data*). The $t_{1/2}$ disappearance of a steady-state BPP established by slow infusion of BPP into the dog was found by Taylor et al. (21) to be 5.5 ± 1.0 min; the metabolic clearance rate was 25.6 ± 1.0 min kg^{-1}, and the volume of distribution was 209 ± 42 ml kg^{-1}. In man, Adrian et al. (6) found half disappearance time, metabolic clearance rate, and apparent distribution space to be 6.4 to 7.0 min, 5.0 to 5.2 ml kg^{-1}min^{-1}, and 50 to 53 ml, respectively.

Regional concentration of PP was determined in anesthetized pig. In the venous circulation PP levels decreased as follows: hepatic portal > hepatic venous > heart/lung > renal. The hepatic and renal extractions of PP were respectively 36 and 54% (13,100). In man there was no significant difference of basal PP concentration in the splanchnic and hepatic extractions. But in one passage through the kidney, $18.3 \pm 5.5\%$ of PP was extracted; in cirrhotic patients the renal clearance of PP was 158 ± 54 ml/min (13).

QUESTION OF PHARMACOLOGICAL OR PHYSIOLOGICAL ACTION

In considering the pharmacological effects of PPs as possible physiological actions, rigorous scrutiny is needed. Unfortunately, for neither APP nor BPP and PPP, the primary biological function with which all the pharmacological gastrointestinal effects are to be compared is still unknown.

Fortunately, it was learned in the early part of the studies that PP was released by food in the chicken (45,49) and by feeding and tease-feeding in the dog (59,60). The presence of the tyrosine-NH$_2$ in the C-terminal 36th position has rendered PP easy to label with ^{125}I and to assay immunologically in the plasma. It is thus possible for us to compare the plasma levels of PP caused by infusion of exogenous PP with those induced by a physiological stimulus, the meal, and find out at what plasma levels the biological actions of exogenous PP are observed.

Despite the structural homology of APP and BPP or PPP, they share very little in common in their spectra of biological actions, except perhaps a stimulatory effect on gastric secretion. According to Kimmel and Hazelwood et al. (39,47), the dose of APP (6.25–12.5 μg/kg i.v.) required to stimulate proventricular H^+, and pepsin secretion far exceeded that required for metabolic actions. APP was even more effective than pentagastrin for stimulating gastric secretion in the chicken. Hazelwood and Kimmel (39) speculated that action of APP on the proventriculus could be specific.

The plasma level of APP under fasting conditions was hardly detectable; it rose to 950 to 2,857 pmoles/liter after feeding (45,49). However, plasma concentration of APP caused by intravenous injection of the peptide at doses that stimulated proventricular H^+ or pepsin was not determined. Therefore, it cannot be said with certainty whether the action is pharmacological or physiological.

In this type of study it is always better to administer a peptide or a hormone by slow intravenous infusion to stimulate the release of the peptide under normal conditions. Metabolically, BPP differs from APP by having no glycogenolytic and hypoglycerolemic actions (85). Pharmacologically, APP does not have the effects of BPP or PPP on the pancreas, gallbladder, and choledochal sphincter (39,58,59,60). Of the pharmacological actions of BPP on the gut, the effects on the pancreas, gallbladder, choledochal sphincter, antrum, and duodenum in the dog (0.5 μg/kg-hr), and the enhancement of gastric emptying and bowel transit in the small intestine of the rat (1 μg/kg, i.p.) had the lowest dosage requirements. According to Chance et al., an antiserum to rat PP has not been developed to perfection. No attempt will be made to interpret the physiological implication of the results obtained from rats at this juncture.

However, BPP, PPP, and HPP cross-react remarkably well with the antiserum of each other. Lin and Chance (18, *unpublished observations*) found that in the dog peak plasma levels of PP induced by 17.5 and 35 g/kg of a meat meal were respectively 200 and 700 pmoles/liter, and those by 0.25, 0.5, 1.0, and 2.0 μg/kg-hr of BPP were respectively 70, 125, 175, and 275 pmoles/liter. At doses of 0.5, 1.0, and 2.0 μg/kg-hr, respective inhibitions of CCK-secretin-induced pancreatic enzyme secretion by BPP were 32, 46, and 72%. The intraluminal pressure in the gallbladder was significantly decreased and the resistance of the choledochal sphincter was significantly increased by 0.25 to 2.0 μg/kg-hr of BPP. Taylor et al. (91) administered PPP at doses of 100 to 400 pmoles/kg-hr (0.42–1.68 μg/kg-hr) and found respective inhibitions of pancreatic protein secretion of 11.1, 29.2, and 46% in the dog. The mean peak increment in PP concentration in response to a meal of meat was 215 pmoles/liter. In both of these studies, the increments of PP concentrations caused by infusion of PP was smaller than those induced by a physiological stimulus, the meal. This suggests that the PP released at physiological blood concentrations can inhibit pancreatic secretion, reduce gallbladder pressure, and augment the resistance of the choledochal sphincter.

BPP at high doses caused diarrhea and vomiting in the dog, but at low (0.5 μg/kg-hr) doses it inhibited the motility of the upper gastrointestinal tract. This could also be one of the actions of PP under physiological conditions.

The stimulatory and inhibitory effects of BPP on gastric secretion were seen only at doses of 20 to 100 μg/kg-hr. Even at 5 μg/kg-hr, plasma concentration of PP already exceeded the physiological levels of PP induced by a meal. In this sense, the action of PP on gastric secretion in the dog is definitely pharmacological.

Of particular interest is the spectrum of actions of PP (60). It differs from CCK, gastrin, and secretin in its actions on pancreatic secretion, gallbladder tonus, choledochal sphincter resistance, and gut motility. Whatever may be the primary physiological function of PP, it is not unreasonable to assume that PP plays a role in the modulation of the effects of other gastrointestinal hormones at physiological concentrations in the blood.

SUMMARY AND CONCLUSIONS

Chemistry and Occurrence

A polypeptide containing 36 amino acid residues in a straight chain was isolated from the pancreata of several species: the chicken (APP), bovine (BPP), canine (CPP), porcine (PPP), ovine (OPP), and human (HPP). Using immunohistochemical or immunofluorescence techniques, PPs were identified in many species of mammals, birds, reptiles, amphibians, and fishes.

Chemically, APP and the mammalian PPs were homologues having identities in 15 of the 36 positions. The mammalian PPs differed from each other by only one or two residues in the 2, 6, and 23 or 6 and 11 positions.

In the chicken, PP and glucagon had eight amino acid residues in identical positions, but in the mammalians only two identities between PPs and glucagon could be found. The structures of mammalian PPs are unrelated to any of the gastrointestinal hormones known.

Specific immunoreactive PP cells have been identified mainly in the periphery of the pancreatic islets; scattered PP cells were also found in the exocrine parenchyma of the pancreas, the mucosa of the gut, and the neural tissue of earthworm. Immunologically and histochemically, PP cells are different from glucagon (A)-, insulin (B)-, somatostatin (D)-, and enterochromaffin (EC)-producing cells. The main source of PP is the pancreas, extirpation of which leads to drastic lowering of plasma PP levels.

Metabolic Actions

Like glucagon, APP showed glycogenolytic action. But unlike glucagon, APP caused hypoglycerolemia and lacked hyperglycemic effect.

Unlike insulin, glucagon or APP, BPP had no glycemic, lipolytic, glycogeno-lytic, or glycerolemic action in the dog or rat. BPP also differed from glucagon by having no effect on water and electrolyte effluxes in the kidney and the small intestine and hyperkalemic action.

Gastrointestinal Actions

Stomach

APP was a potent stimulator of proventricular secretion of acid and pepsin. BPP stimulated basal acid secretion but inhibited gastrin-induced acid secretion in the dog at high doses. Vagal innervation was not necessary for the action of APP or BPP on the stomach but appeared to enhance the excitatory and inhibitory effects of BPP on gastric secretion.

Pancreas

Water, bicarbonate, and especially protein secretion induced by exogenous or endogenous CCK were all significantly inhibited by BPP or PPP in the dog at very low doses when plasma levels of immunoreactive PP was in the physiological range. On secretin-induced water and bicarbonate responses, BPP had biphasic effects, an initial stimulation followed by inhibition. APP had no effect on the secretion of the chicken pancreas.

For both gastric and pancreatic actions, the C-terminal Tyr-NH_2 residue is important for activity; the des-Tyr-NH_2 BPP was devoid of both gastric and pancreatic actions.

The minimal effective fragment of PP is unknown. The C-terminal hexapeptide of PP was found to mimic the actions of PP on gastric and pancreatic secretion.

Bile Flow and Extrahepatic System

BPP had actions opposite to those of CCK, gastrin, and secretin on the extrahepatic system. It relaxed the gallbladder and augmented the resistance of the choledochal sphincter of the dog under basal conditions. BPP resembled glucagon in action on the gallbladder but differed from glucagon in actions on the sphincter and bile flow in the dog.

Gastrointestinal Motility

BPP had both excitatory and inhibitory effects on gut motility of the dog. The inhibitory effect of PP at low doses appeared to simulate a physiological action. Both the amplitude and frequency of contractions of the turkey gizzard were inhibited by APP. However, gastric emptying and bowel transit in the small intestine of the rat were enhanced by BPP.

Plasma Levels and Release of PP

PP was released by food. Of the foodstuffs, protein was the most effective; fats and carbohydrates had moderate effects in releasing PP. Pure gastrin, CCK, secretin, and motilin had no significant effect on PP release in man and dog. But PP was released by bombesin and cerulein.

Insulin hypoglycemia, sham- and tease-feeding, gastric distention, cholinergics, and electrical stimulation of the peripheral vagal fibers all caused PP release which could be blocked or diminished by anticholinergics or vagotomy.

Abnormally high levels of PP were found in patients with insulinomas, glucagonomas, and other forms of multiple endocrine adenomas or apudomas and in juvenile diabetes. The clinical significance of high plasma PP levels in relation to the diseases mentioned remains to be elucidated.

The $t_{1/2}$ disappearance of plasma PP was approximately 5 to 6 min.

PROJECTIONS FOR THE FUTURE

The immediate task should be the determination of the physiological functions of PP. Only after knowing the physiological effects of PP can meaningful studies on PP be designed.

Of all the pharmacological actions of APP, the stimulation of proventricular secretion and the inhibition of gut motility in the birds appeared to have the lowest dosage requirement. Future experiments should be directed toward the evaluation of these actions of PP under physiological conditions.

Of all the pharmacological actions of BPP and PPP, the inhibition of pancreatic secretion, gut motility, and intraluminal pressure of the gallbladder and the increase in choledochal sphincter resistance had the lowest dosage requirements. Proof that these actions of PP occur when the plasma levels of PP are in the physiological range should be finalized.

Preliminary results showed that in rodents PP enhanced gastric and intestinal transit and reduced body weight. Careful follow-up to clarify this point is necessary. Of particular interest is the mechanism that brings about the reduction of body weight in rodents. Is this a central or peripheral action?

Although established gastrointestinal hormones have, so far, failed to influence the plasma level of PP, and clinical studies, so far, have also failed to establish a firm relationship between plasma levels of PP and any clinical syndrome, efforts to study the interaction of established and candidate hormones with PP and the relationship of PP to clinical conditions should continue.

The involvement of the vagi in cephalic and gastric phases of PP release is an established observation. The physiological and pathophysiological significance of this finding deserves further clarification. Could PP be a marker for "vagality"?

Finally, the mechanism by which PP brought about the observed biological activities is completely obscure. Most intriguing of all is PP's action to suppress pancreatic enzyme secretion in conscious dogs stimulated by CCK. Yet, on pancreatic slices *in vitro,* PP failed to affect the Ca^{2+} extrusion or the activity of the guanylate cyclase system stimulated by CCK.

REFERENCES

1. Adrian, T. E., Besterman, H. S., Christofides, N. D., and Bloom, S. R. (1978): Interaction of gastrointestinal hormones and cholinergic innervation on the release of pancreatic polypeptide. *Scand. J. Gastroenterol. (Suppl. 49):* 13: (Abstr. 1).
2. Adrian, T. E., Besterman, H. S., Mallinson, C. N., Czahkowska, W. M., and Bloom, S. R. (1977): Studies on the release of pancreatic polypeptide and its relationship to pancreatic exocrine function. *J. Endocrinol.,* 75:35P–36P (Abstr.).
3. Adrian, T. E., Bloom, S. R., Bestermann, H. S., Barnes, H. J., Cooke, T. J. C., Russel, R. C. C., and Farber, R. G. (1977): Mechanism of pancreatic polypeptide release in man. *Lancet,* i:161–163.
4. Adrian, T. E., Bloom, S. R., Bestermann, H. S., Polak, J. M., et al. (1978): Pancreatic polypeptide in adrenocarcinomas and apudomas including the carcinoid syndrome. *Scand. J. Gastroenterol. (Suppl. 49),* 13:2 (Abstr. 2).
5. Adrian, T. E., Bloom, S. R., Bryant, M. G., Polak, J. M., Heitz, P. H., and Barnes, A. J. (1976): Distribution and release of human pancreatic polypeptide. *Gut,* 17:940–944.
6. Adrian, T. E., Greenberg, G. R., Bestermann, H. S., Christofides, N. D., and Bloom, S. R. (1978): PP infusion in man: Pharmacokinetics at three dose levels and effects on gastrointestinal and pancreatic hormones. *Scand. J. Gastroenterol. (Suppl. 49),* 13: Abstr. 3.
7. Baetens, D., De Mey, J., and Gepts, W. (1977): Immunohistochemical and ultrastructural identification of the pancreatic polypeptide-producing cell (PP-cell) in the human pancreas. *Cell Tissue Res.,* 185(2):239–246.
8. Baetens, D., Rufener, C., and Orci, L. (1976): Bovine pancreatic polypeptide (BPP) in the pancreas and in the gastrointestinal tract of the dog. *Experientia,* 32(6):785 (Abstr.).
9. Barbezat, G., and Grossman, M. I. (1971): Intestinal secretion: Stimulation by peptides. *Science,* 174:422–424.
10. Berger, D., Crowther, R., Floyd, J. C., Jr., Pek, S., and Fajans, S. S. (1977): Effects of age on fasting levels of pancreatic hormones in healthy subjects. *Diabetes (Suppl. 1),* 26:381.
11. Bergstrom, B. H., Loo, S., Hirsch, H. J., et al. (1977): Ultrastructural localization of pancreatic polypeptide in human pancreas. *J. Clin. Endocrinol. Metab.,* 44(4):795–798.
12. Bloom, S. R., Val, W., Barnes, A. J., Long, R. G., Hanley, J., et al. (1978): New specific long-acting somatostatin analogues in the treatment of pancreatic endocrine tumors. *Scand. J. Gastroenterol. (Suppl. 49),* 13: Abstr. 22.
13. Boden, G., Master, R. W. P., and Owen, O. E. (1978): Hepatic and renal extraction of endogenous human pancreatic polypeptide (HPP). *Scand. J. Gastroenterol. (Suppl. 49),* 13: Abstr. 28.
14. Buffa, R., Capella, C., Fotana, L., Useline, L., and Solcia, E. (1978): Types of endocrine cells in human colon and rectum. *Cell Tissue Res.,* 192:227–240.
15. Chance, R. E. (1971): Proceedings of the fifth anniversary insulin symposium. *Diabetes (Suppl. 2),* 21:536.
16. Chance, R. E., Johnson, M. L., Koppenberger, J. I., et al.: Isolation and characterization of a new pancreatic polypeptide *(unpublished study).*
17. Chance, R. E., and Jones, W. E. (1974): Polypeptide from bovine, ovine, human and porcine pancrease. U.S. Patent No. 3,842,063.
18. Chance, R. E., Lin, T. M., Johnson, M. L., Moon, N. E., and Evans, D. C. (1975): Studies on a new recognized pancreatic hormone with gastrointestinal activities. *Endocrinology (Suppl.),* 96:183 (Abstr. 265).
19. Duke, G. E., and Kimmel, J. R. (1978): Inhibition of gastric motility in turkey by avian pancreatic peptide. *Fed. Proc.,* 37:373 (Abstr. 849).
20. Falkmer, S., and Stefan, Y. (1978): Pancreatic polypeptide (PP): Phylogenetic aspects in gastrointestinal mucosa and endocrine pancreas. *Scand. J. Gastroenterol. (Suppl. 49),* 13: Abstr. 59.
21. Floyd, J. C., Jr., Chance, R. E., Hayasi, M., and Moon, N. E. (1975): Concentration of a

newly recognized pancreatic polypeptide in plasma of healthy subjects and in plasma and tumors of patients with insulin-secreting islet cell tumors. *Clin. Res.*, 23: Abstr. 535.

22. Floyd, J. C., Jr., and Fajans, S. S. (1976): A newly recognized human pancreatic islet polypeptide: Concentrations in healthy subjects and in patients with diabetes mellitus. *Diabetes (Suppl. 1)*, 25:330, (Abstr.).

23. Floyd, J. C., Jr., Fajans, S. S., and Pek, S. (1976): Regulation in healthy subjects of the secretion of a newly recognized pancreatic islet polypeptide. *Clin. Res.*, 24: Abstr. 485.

24. Floyd, J. C., Jr., Fajans, S. S., Pek, S., and Chance, R. E. (1977): A newly recognized pancreatic polypeptide: Plasma levels in health and disease. *Recent Progr. Horm. Res.*, 23:519–570.

25. Forssmann, W. G., Helmstaedter, V., and Chance, R. E. (1977): Ultrastructural and immuno histochemical demonstration of pancreatic polypeptide-containing F-cells in the stomach and pancreas of *Tupaia belangeri. Cell Tissue Res.*, 177:461–492.

26. Forssmann, W. G., Helmstaedter, V., Metz, J., Greenberg, J., and Chance, R. E. (1977): The identification of the F-cell in the dog pancreas as the pancreatic polypeptide producing cell. *Histochemistry*, 50:281–290.

27. Gepts, W. (1977): Histological and histopathological study of the cells which produce pancreatic polypeptide. *J. Ann. Diabetol. Hotel Dieu,* :148–156.

28. Gersell, D. J., Greeder, M. H., and Gingerich, R. L. (1976): Cellular localization of PP in the human and canine pancreas. *Diabetes (Suppl. 1)*, 25: 364, (Abstr.).

29. Gingerich, R. L. (1977): Survey of potential pancreatic polypeptide secretogogues. *Diabetes (Suppl. 1)*, 26: Abstr. 375.

30. Gingerich, R. L., Greeder, M. H., Chance, R. E., and Johnson, M. L. (1976): Secretion of canine pancreatic polypeptide (CPP) *in vitro. Diabetes (Suppl. 1)*, 25: Abstr. 329.

31. Gates, R. J., and Lazarus, N. R. (1977): The ability of pancreatic polypeptide (APP and BPP) to return to normal the hyperglycemia, hyperinsulinaemia and weight gain of New Zealand obese mice. *Horm. Res.*, 8:189–202.

32. Greenberg, G. R., Mitnegg, P., and Bloom, S. R. (1977): Effect of pancreatic polypeptide on DNA synthesis in the pancreas. *Experientia*, 33:1332–1333.

33. Grossman, M. I., et al. (1974): Candidate hormones of the gut. *Gastroenterology*, 67:730–755.

34. Gustavson, S., Johansson, H., Lundquist, G., and Nilsson, F. (1977): Effects of vasoactive intestinal peptide and pancreatic polypeptide on small bowel propulsion in the rat. *Scand. J. Gastroenterol.*, 12:993–997.

35. Gyr, K., Haeckt, W., Kayasseh, L., Girard, J., Rittmann, W. W., and Stadler, G. A. (1977): The effect of somatostatin on endogenous release of secretin and pancreatic polypeptide in dog. *Acta Endocrinol. (Suppl.)*, 212:107.

36. Gyr, K., Kayasseh, L., Hacki, W., Girard, J., et al. (1978): The response of pancreatic polypeptide (PP) by test meal and HCl and its response to somatostatin and atropine in dog. *Scand. J. Gastroenterol. (Suppl. 49)*, 13: Abstr. 71.

37. Hacki, W. H., Halter, F., Gyr, K., and Kayasseh, L. (1978): Release of pancreatic polypeptide by acid in man. *Scand. J. Gastroenterol. (Suppl. 49)*, 13: Abstr. 73.

38. Hansky, J., Ho, P., Korman, M. G., and Stern, A. I. (1978): Pancreatic polypeptide release in man. *Scand. J. Gastroenterol. (Suppl. 49)*, 13: Abstr. 78.

39. Hazelwood, R. L., Turner, S. D., Kimmel, J. R., and Pollock, H. G. (1973): Spectrum effects of a new polypeptide (third hormone?) isolated from the chicken pancreas. *Gen. Comp. Endocrinol.*, 21:485–497.

40. Heitz, P., Polak, J. M., Bloom, S. R., and Pearse, A. G. E. (1976): Identification of the D_1-cell as the source of human pancreatic polypeptide (HPP). *Gut*, 17:755–758.

41. Helmstaedter, V., Muhlman, G., Fuerle, G. E., and Forssmann, W. G. (1978): Ontogenesis of the endocrine cells of the human GEP system. *Scand. J. Gastroenterol. (Suppl. 49)*, 13: Abstr. 87.

42. Iverson, J., Bloom, S. R., Adrian, T. E., and Hermansen, K. (1978): Control of glucagon insulin and pancreatic polypeptide secretion in the isolated pancreas. *Acta Endocrinol. (Suppl.)*, 212:8.

43. Jemerin, E. F., Hollander, F., and Weinstein, V. A. (1943): A comparison of insulin and food as stimuli for the differentiation of vagal and non-vagal gastric pouches. *Gastroenterology*, 1:500–512.

44. Kimmel, J. R., Hayden, J., and Pollock, H. G. (1975): Isolation and characterization of a new pancreatic polypeptide hormone. *J. Biol. Chem.,* 250:9369–9376.
45. Kimmel, J. R., and Pollock, H. G. (1975): Factors affecting blood levels of avian pancreatic polypeptide (APP), a new pancreatic hormone. *Fed. Proc.,* 34: Abstr. 454.
46. Kimmel, J. R., Pollock, H. G., and Hazelwood, R. L. (1968): Isolation and characterization of chicken insulin. *Endocrinology,* 83:1323–1330.
47. Kimmel, J. R., Pollock, H. G., and Hazelwood, R. L. (1971): A new pancreatic polypeptide hormone. *Fed. Proc.,* 30:1550 (Abstr.).
48. Lamers, C., Diemel, J., and Roeffen, W. (1978): Basal and postprandial serum levels of pancreatic polypeptide in Zollinger-Ellison Syndrome, in MEA1- hyperthyroidism and in normal controls. *Scand. J. Gastroenterol. (Suppl. 49),* 13: Abstr. 108.
49. Langslow, D. R., Kimmel, J. R., and Pollock, H. G. (1973): Studies of the distribution of a new avian pancreatic polypeptide and insulin among birds, reptiles, amphibians and mammals. *Endocrinology,* 93:558–565.
50. Larsson, L.-I., Schwartz, T. W., Lundquist, G., Chance, R. E., Sundler, F., Rehfeld, J. F., et al. (1976): Occurrence of human pancreatic polypeptide in pancreatic endocrine tumors. *Am. J. Pathol.,* 85:675–684.
51. Larsson, L. I., Sundler, F., and Hakanson, R. (1975): Immunochemical localization of human pancreatic polypeptide (HPP) to a population of islet cells. *Cell Tissue Res.,* 156:167–171.
52. Larsson, L. I., Sundler, F., and Hakanson, R. (1976): Pancreatic polypeptide-A postulated new hormone: Identification of its cellular storage site by light and electron microscopic immunocytochemistry. *Diabetologia,* 12:211–226.
53. Larsson, L. I., Sundler, F., Hakanson, R., Pollock, H. G., and Kimmel, J. R. (1974): Localization of APP, a postulated new hormone, to a pancreatic endocrine cell type. *Histochemistry,* 42:377–382.
54. Lennon, J., Bloom, S. R., and Sircus, W.: Studies on blood levels of vasoactive inhibitory peptide (VIP) and pancreatic polypeptide (PP) and their relation to clinical behavior in a case of Werner-Morrison syndrome. *Ital. J. Gastroenterol. (in press).*
55. Levitt, N. S., Vinik, A. I., Sive, A. A., and Klaff, L. J. (1978): Gastrointestinal hormones and autonomic neuropathy. *Scand. J. Gastroenterol. (Suppl. 49),* 13: Abstr. 115.
56. Lin, T. M., and Alphin, R. S. (1958): Inhibition of gastric secretion by glucagon and glucose in the dog. *Fed. Proc.,* 17:384 (Abstr.).
57. Lin, T. M., and Chance, R. E. (1972): Spectrum of gastrointestinal actions of a new bovine pancreatic polypeptide (BPP) *Gastroenterology,* 62:852 (Abstr.).
58. Lin, T. M., and Chance, R. E. (1978): Spectrum of gastrointestinal actions of a bovine pancreatic polypeptide (BPP). In: *International Symposium on Gut Hormones,* edited by S. R. Bloom, pp. 242–246. Churchill and Livingstone, Edinburgh.
59. Lin, T. M., and Chance, R. E. (1974): Bovine pancreatic polypeptide (BPP) and avian-pancreatic peptide (APP): Candidate Hormones of the Gut. *Gastroenterology,* 67:737–738.
60. Lin, T. M., and Chance, R. E. (1974): Gastrointestinal actions of a new bovine pancreatic peptide (BPP). In: *Endocrinology of the Gut,* edited by W. Y. Chey and F. P. Brooks, pp. 143–145. Charles B. Slack, Thorofare, New Jersey.
61. Lin, T. M., Chance, R. E., and Evans, D. C. (1973): Stimulatory and inhibitory actions of a bovine pancreatic peptide (BPP) on gastric and pancreatic secretions in dogs. *Gastroenterology,* 64:865 (Abstr.).
62. Lin, T. M., Chance, R. E., Evans, D. C., Spray, G. F., Bloomquist, W. E., and Warrick, M. W. (1977): Gastrointestinal actions of a bovine pancreatic peptide (BPP). First international symposium on gastrointestinal hormones. *Gastroenterology,* 72:A9/819. (Abstr.).
63. Lin, T. M., Evans, D. C., Chance, R. E., and Spray, G. F. (1977): Bovine pancreatic polypeptide action on gastric and pancreatic secretion in dogs. *Am. J. Physiol.,* 1(3): E311–E315.
64. Lin, T. M., Evans, D. C., and Spray, G. F. (1973): Action of glucagon on electrolyte changes in the stomach, kidney and blood of dogs stimulated by pentagastrin or histamine. *Arch. Int. Pharmacodyn. Ther.,* 202:304–313.
65. Malaisse-Lagee, F., Carpentier, J. L., Patel, Y. C., Malaisse, W. J., and Orci, L. (1977): Pancreatic polypeptide: Possible role in the regulation of food intake in the mouse. Hypothesis. *Experientia,* 33:915–917.
66. Marco, J., Hedo, J. A., and Villanueva, M. L. (1977): Inhibitory effect of somatostatin on human pancreatic polypeptide secretion. *Life Sci.,* 21:789–792.

67. Marco, J., Hedo, J. A., and Villanueva, M. L. (1978): Control of pancreatic polypeptide secretion by glucose in man. *J. Clin. Endocrinol. Metab.*, 46:140–145.
68. McCrossan, V. M., Buchan, A. M. J., Timson, C. M., Bloom, S. R., and Pearse, A. G. E. (1977): Two new cells in the human pancreatic islets. *Acta Endocrinol. (Suppl.)*, 212:196.
69. Modlin, I. M., Christofides, N. D., Fitzpatrick, M. L., and Bloom, S. R. (1978): Effect of motilin on gastric emptying of solids in man. *Scand. J. Gastroenterol. (Supp. 49)*, 13: Abstr. 125.
70. Okada, S., Kuramuchi, K., Tsukahara, T., and Ooinoue, T. (1929): Pancreatic secretion: The humoroneural regulation of gastric, pancreatic and biliary secretions. *Arch. Intern. Med.*, 43:446–471.
71. Orci, L., Baetens, D., Ravazzola, M., Stefan, Y., and Malaisse-Lagae, F. (1976): Pancreatic polypeptide and glucagon: non-random distribution in pancreatic islets. *Life Sci.*, 19:1811–1815.
72. Polak, J. M., Bloom, S. R., Adrian, T. E., Heitz, P. L., Bryant, M. G., and Pearse, A. G. E. (1976): Pancreatic polypeptide in insulinomas, gastrinomas, vipomas and glucagonomas. *Lancet,* i:328–330.
73. Paulin, C., and Dubois, P. M. (1978): Immunohistochemical identification and localization of pancreatic polypeptide cells in the pancreas and gastrointestinal tract of the human fetus and adult man. *Cell Tissue Res.,* 188:251–257.
74. Pelletier, G. (1977): Identification of 4 cell types in the human endocrine pancreas by immune-electron-microscopy. *Diabetes,* 26:749–756.
75. Pelletier, G., and Leclerc, R. (1977): Immunohistochemical localization of human pancreatic polypeptide (HPP) in the human endocrine pancreas. *Gastroenterology,* 72:569–571.
76. Pitts, J. E., Jenkins, J. A., Tickle, I. J., Blundell, T. L., and Wood, S. P. (1977): Structural studies on avian pancreatic polypeptide. *Biochem. Soc. Trans.,* 5:1119–1120 (Proceedings).
77. Regan, P. T., Go, V. L. W., and Dimagno, E. P. (1978): Human exocrine pancreatic secretion and pancreatic polypeptide response to CCK and octapeptide of CCK. American Pancreatic Association, Annual Meeting, Nov. 2–3, Chicago, Illinois, Abstr. 46.
78. Rhoten, W. B., and Smith, P. H. (1978): Localization of four polypeptide hormones in the saurian pancreas. *Am. J. Anat.,* 15:595–602.
79. Robinson, R. M., Harris, K., Hlad, C. J., and Eisenman, B. (1957): Effect of glucagon on gastric secretion. *Proc. Soc. Exp. Biol.,* 96:518–520.
80. Rufener, C., Baetens, D., and Orci, L. (1976): Localization of bovine pancreatic polypeptide (BPP)-like immunoreactivity in rat pancreatic monolayer culture. *Experientia,* 32:919–920.
81. Schwartz, T. W., Grotzinger, U., Scoon, I.-M., et al. (1978): Cephalic-vagal and vago-vagal stimulation of pancreatic polypeptide (PP) secretion in man. *Scand. J. Gastroenterol. (Suppl. 49),* 13: Abstr. 161.
82. Schwartz, T. W., Holst, J. J., Fahrenkrug, J., Lindkaer, S., Jessen, O. V., Rehfeld, J. F., Shaffalitzky de Mukadell, O. B., and Stadil, F. (1978): Vagal cholinergic regulation of pancreatic polypeptide secretion. *J. Clin. Invest.,* 61:781–789.
83. Schwartz, T. W., Rehfeld, J. F., Stadil, F., Larsson, L. I., Chance, R. E., and Moon, N. E. (1976): Pancreatic polypeptide response to food in duodenal ulcer patients before and after vagotomy. *Lancet,* i:1102–1105.
84. Schweisthal, M. R., Schweisthal, J. V., and Frost, C. O. (1978): Localization of human pancreatic polypeptide in an argyrophilic fourth cell type in islets of the rat pancreas. *Am. J. Anat.,* 152:257–262.
85. Shaw, W. N. (Lilly Research Laboratories) (1979): *personal communication.*
86. Sive, A. A., Vinik, A. I., Hickman-Van Hoorn, R., and Van Tonder, S. (1978): Secretory response of pancreatic polypeptide in man and pigs. *Scand. J. Gastroenterol. (Suppl. 49),* 13: Abstr. 167.
87. Sundler, F., Hakanson, R., Alumets, J., and Walles, B. (1977): Neuronal localization of pancreatic polypeptide (PP) and vasoactive intestinal peptide (VIP) immunoreactivity in the earthworm *(Lumbrious terrestris).* *Brain Res. Bull.,* 2:61–65.
88. Sundler, F., Hakanson, R., and Larsson, L. I. (1977): Ontogeny of rat pancreatic polypeptide (PP) cells. *Cell Tissue Res.,* 178:303–306.
89. Taylor, I. L., Feldman, M., Richardson, C. T., and Walsh, J. H. (1978): Gastric and cephalic stimulation of human pancreatic polypeptide release. *Gastroenterology,* 75:432–437.

90. Taylor, I. L., Impicciatori, M., and Walsh, J. H. (1977): Effect of atropine and vagotomy on pancreatic polypeptide response to a meal. *Gastroenterology, 72:* Abstr. A116/1139.
91. Taylor, I. L., Solomon, T. E., Walsh, J. H., and Grossman, M. I. (1978): Studies on the metabolism and biologic activity of pancreatic polypeptide (PP). Second international symposium on gastrointestinal hormones. *Scand. J. Gastroenterol.,* 13(49):182.
92. Taylor, I. L., Solomon, T. E., Walsh, J. H., and Grossman, M. I. (1979): Pancreatic polypeptide: Metabolism and effect on pancreatic secretion in dogs. *Gastroenterology,* 76:524–528.
93. Taylor, I. L., Walsh, J. H., Carter, D. C., Wood, J., and Grossman, M. I. (1978): Effect of atropine and bethanechol on release of pancreatic polypeptide (PP) and gastrin by bombesin in dog. *Scand. J. Gastroenterol. (Suppl. 49),* 131: Abstr. 183.
94. Taylor, I. L., Walsh, J. H., Rotter, J., and Passaro, E., Jr. (1978): Is pancreatic polypeptide a marker for Zollinger-Ellison syndrome? *Lancet,* i:845–848.
95. Taylor, I. L., Walsh, J. H., Wood, J., Chew, P., and Grossman, M. I. (1977): Bombesin is a potent stimulant of pancreatic polypeptide (PP) release. *Clin. Res.,* 25: Abstr. 574A.
96. Track, N. S., Watters, L. M., and Gauldie, J. (1978): Motilin and human pancreatic and polypeptide (HPP) plasma concentrations. *Scand. J. Gastroenterol. (Suppl. 49),* 13: Abstr. 187.
97. Van Noorden, S., and Patent, G. J. (1978): Localization of pancreatic polypeptide (PP)-like immunoreactivity in the pancreatic islets of some teleost fishes. *Cell Tissue Res.,* 188:521–525.
98. Villanueva, M. L., Hedo, J. A., and Marco, J. (1977): Heterogeneity of pancreatic polypeptide immunoreactivity in human plasma. *Fed. Eur. Biochem. Soc. Lett.,* 80:99–102.
99. Wilson, R. M., Boden, G., and Owen, O. E. (1978): Pancreatic polypeptide responses to a meal and to intraduodenal amino acids and sodium oleate. *Endocrinology,* 102:859–863.
100. Wood, S. P., Pitts, J. E., Blundell, T. L., Tickle, I. J., and Jenkins, J. A. (1977): Purification, crystallization and preliminary x-ray studies on avian pancreatic polypeptide. *Eur. J. Biochem.,* 78:119–126.

Gastrointestinal Hormones, edited by
George B. Jerzy Glass.
Raven Press, New York © 1980.

Chapter 12

Gut Glucagon-like Immunoreactants (GUT GLIs): Isolation, Structure, and Possible Role

Finn Sundby† and Alister J. Moody

Novo Research Institute, Novo Allé, Bagsvaerd, Denmark

INTRODUCTION

In 1959 Unger et al. (29) developed a radioimmunoassay (RIA) for glucagon based on the method of Berson et al. (2). It soon became evident that the method was not specific for glucagon. Extracts of a number of organs from many animal species, including man, were shown to contain substances that reacted with most, but not all, of the antiglucagon sera available.

These substances extracted from or detected in the intestine are most commonly named gut glucagon cross-reacting material or gut glucagon-like immunoreactants (gut GLIs), a nomenclature specifying the organ of their origin and the immunological property by which they are detected. For review, see Moody (12), Assan (1), Unger (28), Samols and Tyler (20), and Marks and Turner (10).

In the context of this chapter and the chapter on the RIA of gut GLIs in this volume, it is considered appropriate to define a few fundamental terms. These should help anyone reading the chapters and form the basis for a rational and unique nomenclature within this field, the complexity of which increases as more data become available. (See Chapter 36, by Moody and Sundby, pp. 831–839, *this volume.*

¹ ² ³ ⁴ ⁵ ⁶ ⁷ ⁸ ⁹ ¹⁰ ¹¹ ¹² ¹³ ¹⁴ ¹⁵ ¹⁶

His-Ser-Gln-Gly-Thr-Phe-Thr-Ser-Asp-Tyr-Ser-Lys-Tyr-Leu-Asp-Ser-

¹⁷ ¹⁸ ¹⁹ ²⁰ ²¹ ²² ²³ ²⁴ ²⁵ ²⁶ ²⁷ ²⁸ ²⁹

Arg-Arg-Ala-Gln-Asp-Phe-Val-Gln-Trp-Leu-Met-Asn-Thr

FIG. 1. Primary structure of porcine pancreatic glucagon.

DEFINITIONS

Glucagon. When used alone the name glucagon designates the single-chain peptide of 29 amino acid residues, first isolated in a pure, crystalline state from porcine pancreas by Staub et al. (24,25). The primary structure of this glucagon is shown in Fig. 1 according to Bromer et al. (5).

Regardless of its origin, a protein isolated in a pure form and shown to be identical to porcine glucagon is by definition glucagon, but the species and organ of origin should be stated.

If the primary structure of a protein from a species other than pig shows some limited variations from that of glucagon, the protein is considered to be equivalent in that species to glucagon in the pig. In this case the species and the organ/fluid of origin are stated, and the nonidentity to porcine glucagon should be emphasized.

Antiglucagon sera. Throughout this chapter the term antiglucagon sera means antisera raised in rabbits against porcine glucagon, the identical bovine pancreatic glucagon, or mixtures of the two.

The majority of these antisera—the so-called N-terminal, cross-reacting, or unspecific types—react with glucagon and peptides/proteins that definitely are not glucagon, but presumably have a tertiary structure identical to that of the 12–15 amino acid sequence of porcine glucagon.

Another type—the so-called C-terminal or specific antisera—react with glucagon, glucagon fragments, and presumably other proteins containing the structure constituted by the 24–29 sequence of glucagon [for a review, see Moody et al. (14)].

Gut Glucagon-like immunoreactants (gut GLIs). The designation gut glucagon-like immunoreactant (gut GLI) is used for any gut peptide/protein moiety, irrespective of species, that is not glucagon but is able to react with an antiglucagon rabbit serum and compete with radioiodinated porcine glucagon in binding to the serum.

The term "glucagon-like immunoreactants" replaces the previously used "glucagon-like immunoreactivities" to emphasize that the abbreviation "gut GLIs" refers to peptides/proteins containing a definite structure and not to ill-defined substances just cross-reacting with one antiglucagon serum or another (14).

ISOLATION AND STRUCTURE

The demonstration of gut GLIs in intestinal extracts was first reported by Unger et al. in 1961 (30), and their distribution and relative concentration in the gastrointestinal tissues of rat, dog, and man were published by Unger et al. in 1966 (31). Gut GLIs are located in the L cell of the intestinal mucosa (23). The greatest concentration of L cells is found in the lower small intestine and colon, and this distribution of L cells agrees with the amount of gut GLIs extractable from the various sections of the intestine (3).

The first attempt to characterize a gut GLI was reported in 1968 by Unger et al. (32), who showed a jejunal canine extract to contain one peak of gut GLI having a M.W. of approximately 7,000 on gel filtration on Sephadex G-25. Further gel filtration experiments using Biogel P10 revealed, however, the existence of two well-separated peaks of gut GLI, designated peak I and peak II, with M.W.s of 7,000 and 3,000, respectively (33). No attempts were made to further purify and chemically characterize these two substances. A chromatographic pattern of human gut GLI extract similar to that of the dog was reported in 1973 (35).

By combining protein fractionation according to molecular size with the technique of isoelectric focusing, Markussen and Sundby (11) succeeded in demonstrating very pronounced heterogeneity of gut GLI in acid ethanol extracts of pig, rabbit, and rat intestines. Although no pure gut GLI preparation was obtained, this method provided a further parameter—the isoelectric pH of the gut GLIs—for the characterization of these proteins. The still unsolved question was raised: did these many gut GLIs represent native intestinal proteins or were some or most of them produced during the isolation procedure?

Using immunoabsorption to antiglucagon sera of the unspecific type coupled to Sepharose, Murphy et al. (16) succeeded in isolating two gut GLI fractions from an extract of pig ileum. When they were applied to a gel filtration column, a few percent of the total gut GLIs eluted at a position corresponding to a protein of a M.W. of 3,500 (small gut GLI), whereas the main fraction had a M.W. of 12,000 (large gut GLI).

Because of the small amount of the small gut GLI, further investigations were confined to the large gut GLI, which was shown to contain at least three N-terminal amino acids, and was separated into three immunoreactive components by electrophoresis in polyacrylamide gel.

Sasaki et al. (22) have shown a porcine duodenal extract to contain a major gut GLI component in the 2,900 M.W. zone and a minor gut GLI in the 3,500 M.W. zone. The two components are not reported isolated in pure form, but from indirect evidence—biologic, physicochemical, and immunometric— the 3,500 M.W. GLI could not be distinguished from porcine glucagon, whereas the 2,900 M.W. component was readily differentiated from glucagon, e.g., by having an extremely high isoelectric point of >10 as compared with the pI 6.2 of glucagon. Similar results were obtained by Moody et al. (13), who separated an extract of total porcine small intestine by isoelectric focusing. In 1976 Sundby et al. (26) reported the isolation in a highly purified form of one of the several gut GLIs shown to be present in a crude extract of porcine jejunum and ileum. This gut GLI was chosen because it formed the bulk of the extracted GLIs. The number of amino acids was 100, with a M.W. of 11,625.

The isoelectric point was 6.8 to 6.9, and the partial sequence elucidated showed that the N- and the C-terminal sequences of the gut GLI differed from those of porcine glucagon. The amino acid composition was such that the sequence of glucagon could constitute part of the GLI molecule. On a molar basis the gut GLI had the same immunoreactivity as porcine glucagon with the unspecific antiglucagon sera, but less than 0.2% activity using the specific type of antisera. The purified gut GLI, designated porcine gut GLI-1, was further characterized by partial sequence analysis (9). The data support the theory (15) that the gut GLI-1 contains not only the full glucagon sequence, but most likely also the sequence of the possible proglucagon fragment isolated by Tager and Steiner (27), which may explain the nonreactivity with the specific type of antiglucagon sera due to some structural masking in the 24–29 sequence. A comprehensive work on different techniques for extraction and initial purification of porcine gastrointestinal GLIs has been published by Holst (7). No gut GLI was isolated in a pure state, but on indirect evidence, one of the gut GLIs was considered to be identical to the gut GLI-1 of Sundby et al. (26).

POSSIBLE ROLE OF GUT GLIs

The concept of a possible physiological effect of gut GLIs is supported by the fact that these are released into the blood in response to glucose (21) and fat (4) ingestion. Most of the reported biological effects of gut GLIs are identical to those reported for glucagon, which explains the commonly used but misleading designation "enteroglucagon" for the gut GLIs. Some of these effects, *in vitro* as well as *in vivo,* are as follows: (a) glycogenolytic (34), (b) insulin releasing (17), (c) binding to glucagon receptors (18,19,22), and (d) lipolytic (8). For a comprehensive review regarding gut GLIs and their possible physiological role, see the reference by Marks and Turner (10).

So far, however, no biological activity for any gut GLI has been clearly established, and their biological role must at present remain speculative. This failure to establish a role of gut GLIs is largely because only impure preparations have been available, a fact that has been emphasized in the majority of the relevant publications. Some evidence of a clear-cut insulin-releasing effect of a gut GLI is reported by Gutman et al. (6). A crude gut GLI-rich extract of intestinal rat mucosa stimulated insulin release from pancreas pieces *in vitro,* but this effect was abolished by adding antiglucagon sera to the incubation medium, thus indicating a gut GLI component to be the causative agent in the release of insulin.

No biological effect of the highly purified porcine gut GLI-1 of Sundby et al. (26) has been reported. This gut GLI, which has been given the trivial name glicentin by Sundby (*gli* for glucagon-like immunoreactant and *cent* for 100 amino acids) (14,26), has been coupled to human albumin with glutaraldehyde and antisera raised against the complex in rabbits. One of these (R 64) proved useful (15) and this serum was used to detect the presence of glicentin in the A cells of the rat pancreas.

ORIGIN OF GLICENTIN

The presence of the full sequence of glucagon in glicentin (see the preceding paragraph) and of glicentin-like material in A cells of the pancreas supports the concept that glicentin or a closely related molcule is a precursor of glucagon in the pancreatic A cell and of gut GLIs in the intestinal L cells. The two cell types then differ in the degree to which they shorten the common primary gene product before storage and/or secretion of the final peptide (15). The plethora of gut GLIs demonstrated in the past decades could then be the result of a progressive, teleologically determined shortening of such a gut GLI precursor. This would result in the formation of biologically active peptides and inert fragments. An alternative is that the extracted materials are a random mixture of gut GLIs and related peptides formed during extraction and purification.

SUMMARY AND CONCLUSIONS

Gut glucagon-like immunoreactant designates any gut peptide/protein that is not glucagon but is able to react with an antiglucagon rabbit serum and compete with radioiodinated glucagon for binding to the serum.

Extracted gut GLIs are heterogeneous, and so far only one of the several GLIs present in an extract of porcine small intestine has been isolated in a form sufficiently pure to make correct studies of structure and biological effects possible.

This GLI—designated porcine gut GLI-1 or glicentin—has been characterized by partial sequence analysis. The data support the concept that it contains the full glucagon sequence with extension at both the N- and C-terminal ends.

No biological effect of glicentin has been demonstrated, but evidence is presented that glicentin is involved in the biosynthesis of glucagon in the pancreatic A cells and of GLIs in the intestinal L cells.

PROJECTIONS FOR THE FUTURE

It is expected that more gut GLIs will be isolated and characterized, and the native forms of tissue and circulating gut GLIs established. It is hoped that it will be possible to establish specific RIAs for gut GLIs in tissue and in the circulation. The combination of these advances will provide the basis for the establishment of the biological role of gut GLIs, and their therapeutic and diagnostic utility. Establishment of the function of the gut GLIs will add one more piece to a complicated jigsaw puzzle—the mutual relationships between the endocrine secretions of the largest endocrine organ in man, the intestine.

REFERENCES

1. Assan, R. (1973): Gut glucagon. In: *Methods in Investigative and Diagnostic Endocrinology, Vol. 2B,* edited by S. A. Berson and R. S. Yalow, pp. 888–901. North-Holland Publishing Company, Amsterdam.

2. Berson, S. A., Yalow, R. S., Baumann, A., Rothschild, M. A., and Newerly, K. (1956): Insulin-131-I metabolism in human subjects: Demonstration of insulin-binding globulin in the circulation of insulin treated subjects. *J. Clin. Invest.,* 35:170–190.
3. Bloom, S. R., and Polak, J. M. (1978): Gut hormone overview. In: *Gut Hormones,* edited by S. R. Bloom, pp. 3–18. Churchill Livingstone, Edingburgh.
4. Böttger, I., Dobbs, R., Faloona, G. R., and Unger, R. H. (1973): The effects of triglyceride absorption upon glucose, insulin, and gut glucagon-like immunoreactivity. *J. Clin. Invest.,* 52:2532–2541.
5. Bromer, W. W., Sinn, L. G., Staub, A., and Behrens, O. K. (1956): The amino acid sequence of glucagon. *J. Am. Chem. Soc.,* 78:3858–3860.
6. Gutman, R. A., Fink, G., Voyles, N., Selawry, H., Penhos, J. C., Lepp, A., and Recant, L. (1973): Specific biologic effects of intestinal glucagon-like materials. *J. Clin. Invest.,* 52:1165–1175.
7. Holst, J. J. (1977): Extraction, gel filtration pattern, and receptor binding of porcine gastrointestinal glucagon-like immunoreactivity. *Diabetologia,* 13:159–169.
8. Horigome, K., Ohneda, A., Maruhama, Y., Abe, R., and Kai, Y. (1977): Heterogeneity of extractable gut glucagon-like immunoreactivity (GLI) and its lipolytic activity. *Horm. Metab. Res.,* 9:370–374.
9. Jacobsen, H., Demandt, A., Moody, A. J., and Sundby, F. (1977): Sequence analysis of porcine gut GLI-1. *Biochim, Biophys. Acta,* 493:452–459.
10. Marks, V., and Turner, D. S. (1977): The gastrointestinal hormones with particular reference to their role in the regulation of insulin secretion. *Essays Med. Biochem.,* 3:109–152.
11. Markussen, J., and Sundby, F. (1970): Separation and characterization of glucagon-like immunoactive components from gut extracts by electrofocusing. In: *Protides of the Biological Fluids,* edited by H. Peeters, pp. 471–474. Pergamon Press, Oxford.
12. Moody, A. J. (1972): Gastrointestinal glucagon-like immunoreactivity. In: *Glucagon, Molecular Physiology, Clinical and Therapeutic Implications,* edited by P. J. Lefebvre and R. H. Unger, pp. 319–341. Pergamon Press, Oxford.
13. Moody, A. J., Frandsen, E. K., and Sundby, F. (1975): Fractionation of gut glucagon-like activities by isoelectric focusing in polyacrylamide gel. In: *Progress in Isoelectric Focusing and Isotachophoresis,* edited by P. G. Righetti, pp. 179–191. North-Holland Publishing Company, Amsterdam.
14. Moody, A. J., Jacobsen, H., and Sundby, F. (1978): Gastric glucagon and gut glucagon-like immunoreactants. In: *Gut Hormones,* edited by S. R. Bloom, pp. 369–378. Churchill Livingstone, Edinburgh.
15. Moody, A. J., Jacobsen, H., Sundby, F., Frandsen, E. K., Baetens, D., and Orci, L. (1977): Heterogeneity of gut glucagon-like immunoreactants (GLIs). In: *Glucagon: Its Role in Physiology and Clinical Medicine,* edited by P. P. Foa, J. S. Bajaj, and N. L. Foa, pp. 129–135. Springer-Verlag, New York.
16. Murphy, R. F., Buchanan, K. D., and Elmore, D. T. (1973): Isolation of glucagon-like immunoreactivity of gut by affinity chromatography on anti-glucagon antibodies coupled to Sepharose 4B. *Biochim. Biophys. Acta,* 303:118–127.
17. Ohneda, A., Horigome, K., Kai, Y., Itabashi, H., Ishii, S., and Yamagata, S. (1976): Purification of canine gut glucagon-like immunoreactivity (GLI) and its insulin releasing activity. *Horm. Metab. Res.,* 8:170–174.
18. Rehfeld, J. F., Heding, L. C., and Holst, J. J. (1973): Increased gut glucagon release as a pathogenic factor in reactive hypoglycemia. *Lancet,* i:116–118.
19. Rosselin, G., Freychet, P., Bataille, D., and Kitabgi, P. (1974): Polypeptide hormone-receptor interactions. A new approach to the study of pancreatic and gut glucagons. *Isr. J. Med. Sci.,* 10:1314–1323.
20. Samols, E., and Tyler, J. M. (1973): Gut glucagon. In: *Methods in Investigative and Diagnostic Endocrinology, Vol. 2B,* edited by S. A. Berson and R. S. Yalow, pp. 932–937. North-Holland Publishing Company, Amsterdam.
21. Samols, E., Tyler, J., Marri, G., and Marks, V. (1965): Stimulation of glucagon secretion by oral glucose. *Lancet,* ii:1257–1259.
22. Sasaki, H., Rubalcava, B., Baetens, D., Blazquez, E., Srikant, C. B., Orci, L., and Unger, R. H. (1975): Identification of glucagon in the gastrointestinal tract. *J. Clin. Invest.,* 56:135–145.
23. Solcia, E., Polak, J. M., Pearse, A. G. E., Forssmann, W. G., Larsson, L.-I., Sundler, F.,

Lechago, J., Grimelius, L., Fujita, T., Creutzfeldt, W., Gepts, W., Falkmer, S., Lefranc, G., Heitz, Ph., Hage, E., Buchan, A. M. J., Bloom, S. R., and Grossman, M. I. (1978): Lausanne 1977 classification of gastroenteropancreatic endocrine cells. In: *Gut Hormones,* edited by S. R. Bloom, pp. 40–48. Churchill Livingstone, Edinburgh.

24. Staub, A., Sinn, L., and Behrens, O. K. (1953): Purification and crystallization of hyperglycemic glycogenolytic factor (HGF). *Science,* 117:628–629.
25. Staub, A., Sinn, L., and Behrens, O. K. (1955): Purification and crystallization of glucagon. *J. Biol. Chem.,* 214:619–632.
26. Sundby, F., Jacobsen, H., and Moody, A. J. (1976): Purification and characterization of a protein from porcine gut with glucagon-like immunoreactivity. *Horm. Metab. Res.,* 8:366–371.
27. Tager, H. S., and Steiner, D. F. (1973): Isolation of a glucagon-containing peptide: Primary structure of a possible fragment of proglucagon. *Proc. Natl. Acad. Sci. U.S.A.,* 70:2321–2325.
28. Unger, R. H. (1973): Gut glucagon-like immunoreactivity. In: *Methods in Investigative and Diagnostic Endocrinology, Vol. 2B,* edited by S. A. Berson and R. S. Yalow, pp. 906–913. North-Holland Publishing Company, Amsterdam.
29. Unger, R. H., Eisentraut, A. M., McCall, M. S., Keller, S., Lanz, H. C., and Madison, L. L. (1959): Glucagon antibodies and their use for immunoassay of glucagon. *Proc. Soc. Exp. Biol. Med.,* 102:621–623.
30. Unger, R. H., Eisentraut, A. M., Sims, K., McCall, M. S., and Madison, L. L. (1961): Site of origin of glucagon in dogs and humans. *Clin. Res.,* 9:53–60.
31. Unger, R. H., Ketterer, H., and Eisentraut, A. M. (1966): Distribution of immunoassayable glucagon in gastrointestinal tissues. *Metabolism,* 15:865–867.
32. Unger, R. H., Ohneda, A., Eisentraut, A. M., and Exton, J. (1968): Characterization of the responses of circulating glucagon-like immunoreactivity to intraduodenal and intravenous administration of glucose. *J. Clin. Invest.,* 47:48–65.
33. Valverde, I., Rigopoulou, D., Exton, J., Ohneda, A., Eisentraut, A., and Unger, R. H. (1968): Demonstration and characterization of a second fraction of glucagon-like immunoreactivity in jejunal extracts. *Am. J. Med. Sci.,* 225:415–420.
34. Valverde, I., Rigopoulou, D., Marco, J., Faloona, G. R., and Unger, R. H. (1970): Characterization of glucagon-like immunoreactivity (GLI). *Diabetes,* 19:614–623.
35. Valverde, I., Villanueva, M. L., Lozano, I., Román, D., Diaz-Fierros, M., and Marco, J. (1973): Chromatographic pattern of human intestinal glucagon-like immunoreactivity (GLI). *J. Clin. Endocrinol. Metab.,* 36:185–187.

Gastrointestinal Hormones, edited by
George B. Jerzy Glass.
Raven Press, New York © 1980.

Chapter 13

Peptides of the Amphibian Skin Active on the Gut. I. Tachykinins (Substance P-Like Peptides) and Ceruleins. Isolation, Structure, and Basic Functions

Giulio Bertaccini

Institute of Pharmacology, University of Parma, Parma, Italy

Amphibian skin represents a real factory and storehouse of active peptides: many, probably most, of them can be grouped in different families showing well established, peculiar features from both a chemical and a pharmacological point of view. Others, already identified as peptides, still await isolation and a thorough pharmacological study. It is highly probable that still others are present in amphibians and so far have escaped attention of the investigators because of occurrence in insufficient amounts or because of a peculiar pharmacological spectrum of activities that lies beyond the routine screening procedures. In this chapter, two groups of peptides will be described, the so-called tachykinins, which owe their name to the promptness (from the Greek *takus,* fast) of their stimulant action on smooth muscle, and the ceruleins, whose name derives from the first member of the family, cerulein. The large amount of data that appeared in the literature on this topic was reported in recent review articles (10,23,25). In this chapter, only some fundamental works and the most recent papers are quoted.

TACHYKININS

Occurrence and Distribution

The group of tachykinins represents the first distinct family of peptides traced in the amphibian skin and includes the following:

Physalaemin

Physalaemin, the prototype of the group that is the first peptide isolated from amphibian skin, was isolated from methanol extract of the skin of the South American frog *Physalaemus bigilonigerus (fuscumaculatus)*. It is also present in other *Physalaemus* species (*Physalaemus centralis* and *Physalaemus bresslaui*). The concentration of the peptide ranges between 370 and 700 μg per g of dry skin.

A very similar peptide (at least from a chemical point of view, since no detailed pharmacological studies are yet available), is Lys^5, Thr^6-physalaemin, which was found by Nakajima and Erspamer *(unpublished)* in extracts of the Australian frog *Uperoleia rugosa*.

Uperolein

Uperolein is another peptide found in the *Uperoleia rugosa* as well as in the very similar frog *Uperoleia marmorata*. The amount of the active principle varied between 400 and 1,200 μg/g dry skin. Also, *Taudactilus acutirostris* contains 15 to 200 μg/g dry skin of uperolein (26). According to preliminary data (Erspamer, *unpublished*) the *Uperoleia* skin contains another uperolein-like peptide, the isolation of which is in progress.

Phyllomedusin

A slightly different peptide with a shorter amino acid sequence, phyllomedusin, was isolated from methanol extracts of the Amazonian hylid frog *Phyllomedusa bicolor* (1,100 μg/g fresh skin) and found to be present (24) in several of the *Phyllomedusa* species (in μg/g dry skin: *Ph. dacnicolor*, 1,000–2,000; *Ph. helenae*, 250–800; *Ph. palliata*, 200–400; *Ph. trinitatus*, 60–200; *Ph. edentula*, 40–60; and *Ph. burmmeisteri*, 14–120).

Kassinin

Kassinin is a peptide isolated from African frogs *(Kassina senegalensis)*, where it occurs in concentrations varying from 70 to 250 $\mu g/g$ fresh skin; it has the longest amino acid sequence (12 amino acid residues) in this group and its synthesis has been described quite recently (71).

Eledoisin and Substance P

The group of tachykinins is usually considered to include two other peptides very similar in structure and pharmacological properties but of different origin: eledoisin and substance P.

Eledoisin was found in the posterior salivary glands of the Mediterranean octopods *Eledone moschata* and *Eledone aldrovandi* (two molluscan species belonging to the octopod Cephalopoda), which contain amounts of peptide varying from 20 to 150 $\mu g/g$ fresh tissue.

Substance P was described by von Euler and Gaddum in the mammalian brain and gastrointestinal tract as early as in 1931 (70) but its structure was elucidated approximately 40 years later. According to Erspamer (23), other, still different, tachykinins seem to occur in the skin of the South African frog *Hylambates maculatus.*

Structure-Activity Relationship

Table 1 shows the structures of the five peptides so far isolated from amphibian skin together with those of eledoisin and substance P that, although of nonamphibian origin, are added in parenthesis for the sake of completeness. The close structural relationship among these peptides is evident from this table and gives clues to their pharmacological similarities. Numerous synthetic analogs (especially of eledoisin and physalaemin-like compounds) have been synthetized and examined pharmacologically in order to establish the crucial part of the natural

TABLE 1. *Tachykinins*

Pyr-Ala-Asp-Pro-Asn-Lys-*Phe*-Tyr-*Gly-Leu-Met-NH₂*	Physalaemin
Pyr-Ala-Asp-Pro-Lys-Thr-*Phe*-Tyr-*Gly-Leu-Met-NH₂*	Lys⁵, Thr⁶-Physalaemin
Pyr-Pro-Asp-Pro-Asn-Ala-*Phe*-Tyr-*Gly-Leu-Met-NH₂*	Uperolein
Pyr-Asn-Pro-Asn-Arg-*Phe*-Ile-*Gly-Leu-Met-NH₂*	Phyllomedusin
Asp-Val-Pro-Lys-Ser-Asp-Glu-*Phe*-Val-*Gly-Leu-Met-NH₂*	Kassinin
(Pyr-Pro-Ser-Lys-Asp-Ala-*Phe*-Ile-*Gly-Leu-Met-NH₂*	Eledoisin)
(Arg-Pro-Lys-Pro-Gln-Gln-*Phe*-Phe-*Gly-Leu-Met-NH₂*	Substance P)

The amino acid residues common to the different peptides are in italics. In parentheses are shown the structures of two tachykinins of nonamphibian origin: eledoisin from octopods and substance P from mammals.

molecules and in the hope of dissociating the various activities of the peptides. Several conclusions have been drawn:

(a) The part of the tachykinin molecules essential for the maintenance of a conspicuous activity was the C-terminal hexapeptide, which showed highly hypotensive and spasmogenic effects and rather low sialagogue and edema-provoking activity.

(b) Whereas the amino acid residues in positions 4 or 6 (from the C-terminus) did not seem to be absolutely crucial for the maintenance of the biological activity, phenylalanine in position 5 (from the C-terminus) and the C-terminal tripeptide (-Gly-Leu-Met-NH$_2$) could not be changed without an enormous decline in activity.

(c) The C-terminal amide group could be substituted only by a nitrile group but not by other substituents.

(d) Changes of different amino acid residues in various positions yielded unpredictable results. Sometimes, the biological activity diminished or disappeared, and at other times it actually increased.

(e) Parallel bioassays showed that the activities of various synthetic analogs on the isolated guinea pig ileum correlated well with their abilities to depolarize the rat spinal motoneurons (73). This was not true concerning other parameters such as the hypotensive effect and the sialagogue action, and so forth (10). However, all of the attempts to obtain synthetic analogs more specific and perhaps with longer-lasting effects than those of the natural tachykinins so far have failed. It is of interest that the latest studies performed with the natural tachykinins under different experimental conditions (12,74,75) revealed that the N-terminal portion of these peptides, disregarded until now, may be important in determining substantial, qualitative differences.

Pharmacological Actions

The two main activities of tachykinins are those on vascular and extravascular smooth muscle and on exocrine glands. In addition, they possess a number of

TABLE 2. *Activities of tachykinins*

Action on extravascular smooth muscle	*Gastrointestinal tract*	
	Other areas	Urinary bladder
		Uterus
		Tracheal and bronchial muscle
Action on vascular smooth muscle	*Hypotensive effect*	
	(Hypertensive effect)	
	Increase in capillary permeability	
Action on exocrine glands	*Lacrimal glands*	
	Salivary glands	
	Pancreas	
Action on nervous system		

The most significant effects are in italic.

other pharmacological effects that, although less thoroughly and more recently investigated, appear of remarkable interest because they concern the nervous system and the biological role of substance P. Quantitative data are not available for Lys^5, Thr^6-physalaemin and very few data are available for kassinin, which was examined mostly as a purified extract. Most investigations concern physalaemin, eledoisin and, of course, substance P. However, a number of data are available also for phyllomedusin and uperolein. The spectrum of activities of these peptides is listed in Table 2.

Action on Extravascular Smooth Muscle

As already stated, the denomination *tachykinins* was first suggested for the promptness of the stimulant action on smooth muscle as opposed to another wide group of slow-acting peptides, the *bradykinins* (*bradus,* slow).

Gastrointestinal Tract

To date no gastrointestinal preparation was found to be insensitive to tachykinins; data available concern mainly experimental animals, since administration into humans is rather difficult because of the simultaneous hypotensive effect that parallels the effect on the gut or is even more prominent. For the same reason, most results in experimental animals concern *in vitro* rather than *in vivo* preparations.

In Vitro Experiments

Several preparations were used for the bioassay of tachykinins, among which the most common were the rabbit large intestine (kept in cold nutrient solution for 24–48 hr before use) and the guinea pig ileum; both preparations respond to concentrations of the different tachykinins, as low as 0.25 to 2 ng/ml. The action of tachykinins is usually a spasmogenic one, with a good dose-response relationship and a very rare tachyphylaxis found only for some peptides and some particular preparations. Also, rat duodenum and hen cecum, which are relaxed by bradykinins, are strongly contracted by tachykinins. The potency of the tachykinins exceeds by 10 to 100 times that of other nonpeptidic spasmogenic compounds (such as acetylcholine, 5-hydroxytryptamine, histamine, etc.). The bulk of the effects on gut motility concerns the contractions of the longitudinal muscle layers. Some recent data (Bertaccini, Molina, and Zappia, *unpublished*) showed, however, that the circular layer may be contracted also, although a dose 10 to 100 times higher was necessary and the responses appeared to be rather erratic in the guinea pig ileum. In rabbit duodenum, the response was more constant and consisted of the appearance of rhythmic contractions, with no increase in the basal tone. The inability of all kinds of inhibitors (anticholinergic, antihistaminics, antiserotonic, tetrodotoxin, etc.) to modify the spasmogenic effect of tachykinins seems to indicate a direct activity of these peptides. However, under particular experimental conditions (e.g., registering the increase in intraluminal pressure of the guinea pig ileum) atropine was shown to induce a partial inhibition of the effect of physalaemin, suggesting a partial interaction of the cholinergic system with this peptide (11). Moreover, Zséli et al. (75) showed that verapamil caused a complete block of the effect of all the different tachykinins on the longitudinal muscle of the guinea pig ileum. This suggested that these peptides act by interfering with the transport of Ca^{2+} ions. Again with the use of the guinea pig ileum, physalaemin was shown to potentiate contractions induced by acetylcholine, nicotine, 5-hydroxytryptamine, and by electrical stimulation, in concentrations (1.3×10^{-10} M) that had only a slight effect on the basal tone (29). The peptide was also shown to modify the longitudinal but not the circular response of the peristaltic reflex (31). On a "fatigued" preparation the peptide increased the slow longitudinal reflex, in contrast with the action of eledoisin. Even doses of physalaemin as high as 20 ng/ml were apparently unable to restore normal peristaltic activity previously inhibited by hexamethonium, procaine, morphine, or atropine. Comparative studies with all the tachykinins available and administered under the same experimental conditions are needed in order to assess their effect on the peristaltic reflex.

Recent experiments performed on strips of human gastrointestinal tract obtained from all the segments of the gastrointestinal tract from the stomach to the colon and removed during surgery showed that all the examined tachykinins were able to cause the appearance or reinforcement of rhythmic movements and an increase in the tone (74). The most sensitive tissue was the ileum (threshold stimulatory doses from 1 to 50 ng/ml for the different peptides), whereas

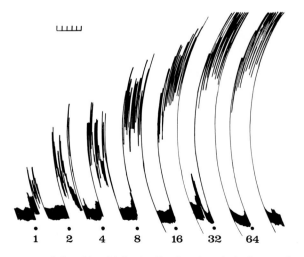

FIG. 1. Dose-response relationship obtained with physalaemin in human ileum (longitudinal muscle) *in vitro*. Doses are in ng/ml; time in minutes.

the least sensitive was the stomach (threshold doses from 10 to 300 ng/ml). The return to basal conditions after washing took a few minutes. Except for some cases in which tachyphylaxis was observed, a good dose-response relationship was usually found (Fig. 1). The common inhibitors did not affect the response to the different tachykinins whose stimulant action was blocked only by verapamil.

In the atonic rat anococcygeus muscle, eledoisin, in contrast to substance P (which had an inhibitory effect), produced dose-related contractions slow to develop but well maintained (32). This effect was abolished by phentolamine and was therefore considered an indirect sympathomimetic effect. Eledoisin (as well as substance P) was able to reduce the motor response to field stimulation of adrenergic nerves, whereas it was ineffective against contractions elicited by exogenous noradrenaline. Therefore, its inhibitory action is likely to be presynaptic.

In Vivo Experiments

Tachykinins were shown to stimulate gastrointestinal motility in all the animal species tested, although to various degrees, both in anesthetized and in conscious animals. These *in vivo* techniques allowed the evaluation not only of the potency of the peptides (intensity of effect) but also of the inactivation rate of the peptide in the blood, and/or of the binding capacity to the receptor sites (duration of the effects). An analysis of these two parameters allowed drawing some important conclusions on the problem of the structure/activity relationship of tachykinins. A recent study (12) concerning the spasmogenic effect of tachykinins on the stomach of the anesthetized rat revealed that eledoisin was the most potent peptide in terms of its threshold dose (from 0.1 to 1 μg/kg), that substance P was the least potent, and that phyllomedusin was by far the most effective as to the duration of the effect (Fig. 2). In the gastrointestinal tract of conscious dogs eledoisin and physalaemin showed a noticeable stimulatory effect on the electrical and mechanical activities: At low doses, the peptides produced an increase in frequency and duration of the interdigestive myoelectric complexes and an increase in coordinated mechanical activity; at high doses, the peptides caused the appearance of diffuse spike activity accompanied by intense local motor activity. Pacesetter potentials were not affected (14).

In the veterinary field Ormas et al. (47,48) reported that eledoisin administered intravenously (25–100 μg/kg) to anesthetized sheep stimulated the motility of the forestomachs and the small intestine, 10 to 30 times more effectively than substance P. Its action consisted of reinforcement of the tonic contractions and of an increase in the amplitude of phasic movements. When spontaneous movements were absent, the peptide caused the appearance of contractions with a good dose-response relationship. The action of eledoisin appeared promptly and lasted for 5 to 10 min, with a complete return to basal levels. Only dihydroergotamine caused a considerable reduction in the stimulatory effect of eledoisin on the duodenum and ileum, whereas propranolol caused a

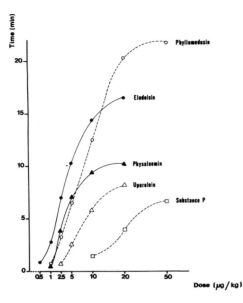

FIG. 2. Spasmogenic effect of different tachykinins on the stomach of the anesthetized rat. *Ordinate* duration of the effect (measured from the bulk of duodenal effluent). Mean values from four to eight experiments. (From reference 12.)

potentiation of the activity of the duodenum. The authors, taking into account the lack of activity of eledoisin on the cardiovascular system of ruminants, claim that the peptide may represent a new therapeutic agent for the treatment of forestomach atony that not infrequently occurs in ruminants.

Action on Salivary Glands and Pancreas

Tachykinins possess a unique, powerful stimulant activity on salivary and lacrimal secretion of dog, rat, hen, and man by a direct effect on secretory cells. Response of the salivary glands could be obtained not only by systemic administration but also by instillation of the peptides through the salivary duct. Recent experiments performed by intraarterial administration of physalaemin showed that the sensitivity of rat submaxillary gland is enormous (threshold stimulant dose $= 0.0015$ μg), and that of the parotid gland (0.062 μg) is somewhat smaller (67). In both dogs and rats physalaemin also markedly stimulated myoepithelial cells in the salivary ducts. In slices of rat parotid gland, eledoisin (like substance P) caused a rapid, dose-dependent increase in K^+ efflux and amylase release. The effect, which required the presence of Ca^{2+}, was independent of any effect on parotid cyclic AMP or cyclic GMP levels (56). In rat submandibular gland slices physalaemin and an eledoisin-related peptide were approximately equipotent in releasing K^+ (threshold dose $= 0.01$ μM) but they probably did not affect the same step of the secretory process as physalaemin since the activity of the latter required Ca^{2+} but that of the eledoisin did not (65).

Physalaemin and eledoisin were shown to exert a direct stimulatory activity

TABLE 3. *Results obtained from the parallel bioassay of different preparations*

Test preparation	Uperolein	Eledoisin	Phyllomedusin	Substance P
Rabbit large intestine	77(50–120)	58(30–80)	84(45–150)	50(30–75)
Guinea pig ileum	82(55–165)	75(30–120)	60(30–80)	54(50–60)
Guinea pig large intestine	76(70–95)	80(50–130)	53(35–75)	60(45–80)
Rat colon	80(50–100)	800(300–2,000)	105(50–250)	60(20–100)
Rat stomach	73(60–90)	120(90–135)	66(40–85)	58(50–65)
Rat salivary secretion	100	—	—	22(20–25)
Human stomach	200(180–225)	200(170–215)	300(275–315)	10(8–12)
Human duodenum	800(350–1,600)	500(300–650)	500(400–700)	—
Human ileum	80(50–130)	200(180–220)	150(100–170)	—
Human tenia coli	50(40–65)	500(300–600)	300(150–450)	25(20–35)

The activity of physalaemin was always considered = 100; that of the other tachykinins was expressed as percentage of this activity. Outside parenthesis, mean; within parenthesis, range; —, not tested.

on exocrine pancreas of dogs and cats. Although the threshold stimulatory doses for these tachykinins were relatively low (0.1 and 3 μg/kg, respectively) the effects obtained were by far less pronounced than those elicited by cholecystokinin (CCK) and secretin. In dispersed acinar cells from guinea pig pancreas physalaemin and eledoisin caused a fivefold increase in calcium outflux and a sevenfold increase in cellular cyclic GMP without altering cyclic AMP. They also caused a concentration-dependent two- to fivefold increase in amylase secretion and potentiated the effects of secretin and VIP but not those of CCK (68).

Investigations on central and peripheral nervous system concerned mainly substance P but these experiments are beyond the limit of this chapter. The reader interested in substance P may consult the two recent reviews by Bury and Mashford (13) and by Skrabanek and Powell (63).

Table 3 summarizes the main quantitative differences observed in the group of tachykinins in different *in vivo* and *in vitro* preparations. Very recent and still unpublished data (Falconieri-Erspamer et al., *personal communication*) were obtained with the new peptide kassinin, which was compared, in different *in vitro* and *in vivo* preparations, to physalaemin, whose activity was arbitrarily considered as 100. Relative activity of kassinin was as follows: on rat colon, 600 to 1,000; guinea pig ileum, 15 to 25; guinea pig gallbladder, 40 to 80; rabbit colon, 10 to 30; and rat salivary secretion, 6 to 7. These findings demonstrated also for kassinin the extreme variability in the potency of this new tachykinin in the various biological test preparations. The most important differences were the different mechanisms of actions, different receptors involved, and presence of tachyphylaxis. It is difficult at present to find a valid explanation for these discrepancies; however, the N-terminal part of these molecules may here play an important role. It also became obvious that results obtained with one tachykinin cannot be extrapolated to the other members of the peptide family.

Clinical Applications

No clinical applications of the pharmacological actions of eledoisin and physalaemin on the digestive tract have yet been reported.

CERULEINS

The importance of the cerulein group of peptides, and in particular of the prototype, cerulein, is connected with their close chemical and pharmacological similarity with some of the mammalian gastrointestinal hormones such as CCK and gastrin.

Occurrence and Distribution

The first member of the series is cerulein (ceruletide, Farmitalia) a decapeptide first isolated from methanol extracts of the skin of the Australian hylid frog *Litoria (Hyla) caerulea,* where it was found present in concentrations varying from 100 to 1,000 μg/g fresh tissue. The thick dorsal skin was found to contain an amount of active principle 8 to 10 times higher than the thin ventral skin. Fresh skin contained 20 to 40% more cerulein than dry skin. Authentic cerulein was found also in the skin of the South American leptodactylid frog *Leptodactylus pentadactylus labyrinthicus* and of the South African pipid frog *Xenopus laevis* (300 to 800 μg/g of fresh skin). In this frog cerulein was shown to originate from the granules of the cutaneous granular glands. Cerulein was reported to be present also in the skin of other Australian frogs (in *Litoria infrafrenata* and *Litoria moorei* up to 3,000 μg/g of dry skin) and in other South African frogs (in *Xenopus gilli* up to 1,500 μg/g of fresh skin).

The second member of the family is phyllocerulein, a nonapeptide found in the South American frogs *Phyllomedusa sauvagei* and *Phyllomedusa bicolor* (from 200 to 650 μg/g of fresh skin).

Finally, another peptide of similar structure (Asn^2, Leu^5-cerulein was isolated from the South African frog *Hylambates maculatus* (42).

The latest research on amphibian skin pointed out that the distribution of cerulein and its analogs is much broader than so far suspected; in fact, conspicuous amounts of cerulein-like peptides were traced in other amphibians from Papua New Guinea, Borneo, and the Philippines (*Nictimystes disrupta* and *Rana erythraea*).

Structure-Activity Relationship

The problem of the structure-activity relationship in this group of peptides is of crucial importance not only from a theoretical but also from a practical point of view, because of the already pointed out analogy between cerulein and the mammalian gastrointestinal hormones. The smallest fragment that still

TABLE 4. *Ceruleins*

Pyr-Gln-Asp-Pyr(SO₃H)-Thr-*Gly-Trp-Met-Asp-Phe-NH₂*	Cerulein
Pyr-Asn-Asp-Tyr(SO₃H)-Leu-*Gly-Trp-Met-Asp-Phe-NH₂*	Asn², Leu⁵-cerulein
Pyr-Glu-Tyr(SO₃H)-Thr-*Gly-Trp-Met-Asp-Phe-NH₂*	Phyllocerulein
[Asp-Tyr(SO₃H)-Met-*Gly-Trp-Met-Asp-Phe-NH₂*	Octa CCK-PZ][a]
[Tyr-(SO₃H)-*Gly-Trp-Met-Asp-Phe-NH₂*	Hexagastrin II][b]

Amino acid residues common to the different peptides in italics.
[a] C-terminal octapeptide of cholecystokinin (CCK).
[b] C-terminal hexapeptide of gastrin II.

retains the same spectrum of activity as that of gastrin is the C-terminal tetrapeptide. The smallest fragment retaining all of the activities of CCK is the C-terminal heptapeptide. These amino acid sequences are present in the three peptides occurring in amphibians, the only differences being that the methionyl residue in position 6 from the C-terminus in the CCK molecule is replaced by a threonyl residue in cerulein and phyllocerulein, and by leucyl residue in Asn², Leu⁵-cerulein (Table 4). The similarity between amphibian peptides and mammalian gastrointestinal hormones is even closer if we consider that CCK-33 and its recent variant, CCK-38, may represent precursors of the more active CCK-octapeptide (22,53) that seems to be predominant both in the gut and in the brain. It is now assumed that the major determinant for gastrin-like versus CCK-like activity is the sulfated tyrosyl residue in position 7 from the C-terminus in CCK and ceruleins and in position 6 in gastrin. It is thus no wonder that the ceruleins possess essentially CCK-like activity with little gastrin-like activity. The wide spectrum of activities and the obvious interest for gastrin, CCK, and cerulein prompted the investigators to synthetize hundreds of analogs in an attempt to find selective agonists and antagonists for specific functions. Although research in this direction was relatively fruitless, it allowed many general conclusions:

(a) The crucial part of the molecule that showed the whole spectrum of activity of cerulein (and CCK) is the C-terminal heptapeptide. Shorter fragments were found to display mainly gastrin-like activity. A certain degree of activity was found even in the C-terminal tripeptide and the dipeptide Asp-Phe-NH₂. In terms of threshold active doses, their potency was much lower than that of the parent substance. Their efficacy, however, in some smooth muscle preparations was almost the same as that of cerulein.

(b) In contrast with tachykinins, the N-terminal part of the cerulein molecule seems to be devoid of any particular importance. This is shown by data obtained with natural compounds (cerulein and phyllocerulein), as well as with several synthetic analogs. It must be pointed out, however, that studies directed to investigate not only quantitative but also qualitative differences are still lacking.

(c) The presence and the position of the tyrosyl-*O*-sulfate residue in relation to the C-terminal amino acid is of primary importance. Moving the tyrosyl-*O*-sulfate residue to the left by insertion of an amino acid residue or to the right by elimination of the threonyl or the threonyl and glycyl residues yields compounds that have no activity on smooth muscle but still retain a certain degree of gastrin-like activity. Desulfation or substitution of sulfate group with a phosphoric acid group yielded compounds with dramatically lower stimulatory activity on smooth muscle.

(d) The changes observed after substitution of the threonyl residue in the C-terminal heptapeptide of cerulein were largely dependent on the kind of substituent. Tryptophan, phenylalanine, glycine, and tyrosine gave compounds with lower activity, whereas methionine did not change the activity, and the more stable norleucyl residue had actually enhanced the potency of the compound.

(e) Experiments performed on the isolated mucosa of frog stomach using the "short circuit current" method showed that a prerequisite for activity in this test is the occurrence of the sulfated tyrosyl residue in position 7. This suggests that gastrins of lower vertebrate may be related chemically more closely to the ceruleins than to mammalian gastrins.

In conclusion, it has been noted that adequate modifications in the cerulein molecule may separate to a certain extent the different biological actions of this peptide (20), although no clear-cut dissociation has been so far obtained. Only two compounds were synthetized that appear to be less active than cerulein as stimulants but decidedly more potent as inhibitors of the gastric secretion induced by gastrin, even in experiments performed in humans (5). These are: Boc[1]-Tyr(SO₃H)-Thr-Gly-Trp-Nle-Asp-Phe-NH₂ and Tyr(SO₃H)-Trp-Met-Asp-Phe-NH₂. The data available so far are not sufficient to attribute a practical importance to these two peptides.

Many questions are still unresolved. The difficulties in the synthesis and scarce availability of sufficient amounts of the synthetic analogs have reduced the possibility of adequate studies. In most of the investigations of the pharmacological effects only the "potency" of the different compounds was evaluated, whereas the more important "efficacy" was rarely considered. Thus not only the study of the new compounds but also a more accurate study of the "old" peptides might give unsuspected results.

Pharmacological Activity

The pharmacological actions of the ceruleins, which resemble those of CCK and partly also those of gastrin, concern essentially the biliary system and the gastrointestinal tract. Other actions on different tissues, which do not belong to the subject of this volume, are not discussed in this chapter. They are listed in Table 5. Moreover, only the action of authentic cerulein, most extensively studied, is considered here, since that of the other peptides of the family did not show substantial differences from the prototype.

---

[1] Boc, *tert*-Butyloxycarbonyl

TABLE 5. *Activity of cerulein*

Action on smooth muscle	⌈ *Biliary system* | *Gastrointestinal tract* ⌊ Blood vessels
Action on exocrine glands	⌈ Stomach | *Pancreas* | Liver ⌊ *Brunner's glands*
Action on endocrine secretions	⌈ Insulin | Glucagon | Calcitonin ⌊ *Pancreatic peptide*
Miscellaneous activities	⌈ Inotropic and chronotropic effect on cat atria | Effect on the CNS | Trophic effects (pancreas, ⌊ stomach and duodenum)

The most remarkable effects are in italics.

Action on Smooth Muscle of the Biliary System

Cerulein exerts a potent spasmogenic effect on the gallbladder both *in vivo* and *in vitro* in all the species examined, including man.

In vivo studies showed that in man, guinea pig, rabbit, dog, cat, chicken, and sheep the threshold doses of cerulein were less than 1 ng kg^{-1} min^{-1} i.v. and less than 20 ng/kg s.c. Contractions began very soon and lasted from a few minutes to several hours according to the dose and the route of administration. In the dog doses of 1 to 2 μg/kg caused the complete disappearance of the gallbladder shadow on X-ray films. In man cerulein was very potent, but to avoid harmful side effects only relatively small doses were administered (1–2 ng kg^{-1} min^{-1} by i.v. infusion; 25–50 ng/kg by bolus injection; 0.1–0.75 μg/kg by s.c. or i.m. injection, and 0.5–1.5 μg/kg by nasal insufflation).

In vitro experiments showed that cerulein exerted its striking spasmogenic effect also on the isolated gallbladder (threshold dose often less than 0.1 ng/ml nutrient solution), with a good dose-response relationship and a constant lack of tachyphylaxis. The effect was resistant to atropine and tetrodotoxin, which suggested a direct activity of the peptide on the smooth muscle. Cerulein reduced the cyclic AMP levels in the gallbladder, but increased those in the sphincter of Oddi. In a recent report (28) the responses of guinea pig gallbladder to sulfated and nonsulfated cerulein were compared *in vivo* and *in vitro*. Tested *in vivo* sulfated cerulein was 75 times more potent than nonsulfated, whereas *in vitro* the difference was 150-fold. According to the authors, the differences in relative potencies may thus reflect not only chemical structure but also the method used for testing. Figures 3 and 4 exemplify the activity of cerulein in the guinea pig and in human gallbladder, respectively.

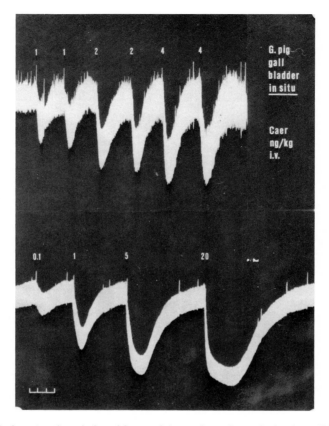

FIG. 3. Typical contractions induced by cerulein on the guinea pig *in situ* gallbladder. Note the good dose-response relationship in two different preparations (**top** and **bottom**). Time is in minutes.

The contracting effect on the gallbladder was accompanied, and in some cases actually preceded, by a relaxation of the choledocho-duodenal junction, which was particularly evident when the tone of the sphincter was elevated (either spontaneously or by premedication with morphine). When the tone was low, as in the isolated sphincter of the calf, cerulein actually exerted a contracting effect. As a consequence of the relaxation of the sphincter of Oddi, the choledochal resistance was lowered and bile flow increased in conscious dogs. Of all the peptides examined, cerulein was the most potent stimulant of the gallbladder contraction and the relaxant of the sphincter of Oddi. Only in the rabbit opposite effects of cerulein on the sphincter of Oddi were found, with a dose-related spasmogenic effect on the sphincter and a parallel increase in biliary pressure and a decrease in bile flow (58). This paradoxical effect, which was shown to be present also with CCK, probably reflects species differences and

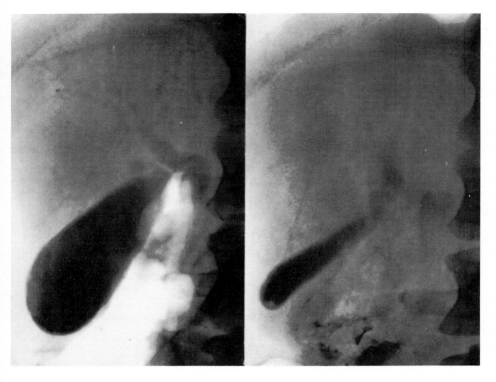

FIG. 4. Effect of cerulein (0.5 μg/kg i.m.) on human gallbladder. **Left:** Basal radiogram. **Right:** 30 min after administration of cerulein.

anatomical peculiarities of the rabbit sphincter of Oddi which, in contrast with other species, is functionally independent of the duodenal muscle.

Action on Smooth Muscle of the Gastrointestinal Tract

Also in the gastrointestinal tract cerulein displayed a combination of stimulatory and inhibitory actions, although the stimulatory were largely predominant.

Early *in vivo* experiments with cerulein demonstrated the striking spasmogenic effect of cerulein which, in the intact dog, caused vomiting and evacuation of the bowel both by intravenous and subcutaneous administration. In the anesthetized dog gut motility was increased, especially in the small bowel, with very small doses (1–5 ng/kg i.v.). In molar concentration cerulein was 2 to 1,000 times more active than all the other peptidic and nonpeptidic stimulatory materials. An example of the activity of cerulein on ileal motility was compared with that of physalaemin as shown in Fig. 5. Cerulein appeared to induce coordinated propulsion more than generalized muscular contractions. In the stomach the

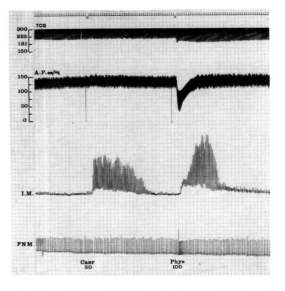

FIG. 5. From **top** to **bottom:** Time marks 10 sec; tachogram (TCG); arterial pressure in mm Hg (AP); ileal motility (IM) measured manometrically; pneumogram (PNM); cerulein (Caer.) and physalaemin (Phys.) administered intravenously in ng/kg in a dog of 16 kg.

peptide had different effects: in the denervated Heidenhain pouch of the anesthetized dog it caused the appearance or an increase of the tone and amplitude of the movements; in the stomach of the conscious dog it decreased the intragastric pressure and produced a significant inhibition of gastric motility. Rabbit and cat intestine were less sensitive to cerulein; rats appeared particularly sensitive at the gastroduodenal junction, which was strongly contracted by cerulein even with bolus injection of 2 to 5 ng/kg. This induced a considerable delay in gastric emptying, as observed quite recently in conscious rats by Scarpignato et al. (59). In the rat small intestine cerulein was shown to produce uniform distribution of contractions and acceleration of transit with doses of 1 and 10 $ng/kg^{-1}\ min^{-1}$, whereas it inhibited contractions and delayed transit at 1 μg $kg^{-1}\ min^{-1}$ (62). The sensitivity to atropine varied in the different species and it was maximal although not total in the dog and minimal or absent in rats and rabbits. Doses capable of affecting gastrointestinal motility were 20 to 40 times lower than those capable of inducing cardiovascular or respiratory changes, and this allowed a number of experiments to be performed in humans.

Studies performed by several groups of investigators by means of balloon methods, open tip tubes, by fluorography and cinematography or by simultaneous recording of myoelectric and mechanical activity confirmed results obtained in animals. A recent study performed on 16 normal subjects showed that the peptide exerted a dose-dependent, inhibitory effect on lower esophageal sphincter pressure (50). A marked inhibition of the motility in the body and the fundus of the stomach and also in the proximal part of the duodenum was also observed. Both motility index and basic electric rhythm (BER) frequency were reduced. Conversely, motility in the antrum and in the gut starting from the distal duodenum was strongly increased. This resulted in the increased propulsion in the gut and a reduced transit time from the stomach to the cecum, with doses of the peptide similar to those used in the study of the biliary tract. Recent studies (17) performed in patients submitted to total gastrectomy and esophago-jejuno-duodenal reconstruction showed that cerulein induced a dose-related motor activity in the transposed jejunal loops. Doses of the peptide were so low (0.25 ng kg^{-1} min^{-1}) as to be compared with doses of CCK released by a conventional fatty meal. This induced the authors to state that CCK has a physiological motor effect on the human jejunum. Cerulein also had a potent relaxing effect on the reticulum and omasum of conscious sheep.

Also, a striking atropine-resistant villokinetic activity was shown after intravenous infusion of cerulein (0.2–2 ng kg^{-1}), which stimulated the pump-like movements of the duodeno-jejunal villi of chicken, pigeon, and cat. Cerulein was also shown to antagonize the glucagon and PGE$_1$ depression of villous motility in the dog (36).

Recent and more accurate *in vitro* studies revealed that the peptide was indeed a very good stimulant of the gastrointestinal tract also *in vitro*. It had a stimulatory effect on all the different segments of the bowel in animals and in man except for human duodenum, which was relaxed. *In vitro* studies allowed a classic demonstration that cerulein (10^{-12} M) caused marked segmentation of the peristaltis in both small and large intestine of the guinea pig. It also caused a coordinated motor response in both muscle layers of the guinea pig and rabbit ileum, with an alternating contraction of the longitudinal and the circular muscle. The remarkable activity on the circular muscle was completely abolished by tetrodotoxin (40). Cerulein was shown to cause contraction of the lower esophageal sphincter (LES) of the opossum and this effect was increased by tetrodotoxin, suggesting a neural inhibitory component in the action of cerulein on the LES (Goyal and Rattan, *unpublished observations*). The *in vitro* studies demonstrated that cerulein, as well as other peptides of the gastrin and CCK family, acts predominantly by releasing acetylcholine from the Auerbach plexus. Only a very small percentage of the contracting activity was due to a direct effect on the smooth muscle (69). These data were recently confirmed by Fontaine et al. (30), who showed that cerulein in low concentration that had no contractile effects sensitized the guinea pig ileum to activities of various cholinergic and noncholinergic agonists. Higher concentrations in the presence of tetrodotoxin were inactive by themselves, but were also able to potentiate the effect of different agonists. In the circular muscle of the duodenum of the opossum, cerulein (like CCK) initiated periodic contractions, the amplitude of which was dose-related. This effect, which was not nerve-mediated, was not observed in the longitudinal muscle layer (6). If one extends these cerulein data to human gastrointestinal hormones, like gastrin and CCK, one may infer that these hormones participate in the complex neurohumoral control of gastrointestinal motility.

Action on Blood Vessels

Although cerulein possesses some generally hypotensive activity in most animal species, its local vasodilating effect, with increase in blood flow, on the stomach, pancreas, and liver is of certain interest. This was seen with doses that were at least 10 times lower than those causing systemic hypotension. The flow in the superior mesenteric artery was affected very slightly, if at all.

Action on Exocrine Secretions

Stomach

The action of cerulein on gastric secretion varies according to the animal species and the experimental conditions. In man and dogs, the peptide increases volume, acid, and pepsin in very low doses (ng/kg). However, the maximum effect is decidedly lower than that evoked by gastrin or histamine, so that cerulein may be considered as a partial agonist of gastric secretion. In other investigations it was found to act as a competitive antagonist of gastrin and pentagastrin, both in man and dogs, whereas it was completely ineffective when the hypersecretion was induced by histamine. Conversely, the peptide is a full agonist in cats and is also very effective in rats, chickens, and in some preparations *in vitro*. Here the amphibian stomachs were much more sensitive to cerulein than to every other stimulant. All these quantitative differences may suggest that different species may have their own species-specific hormone. This may in some instances be more closely related to cerulein than to human gastrin, which is used as a reference compound in most experiments. The secretion evoked by cerulein in humans, dogs, cats, and chickens was, although to different degrees, atropine-sensitive; in rats, pigeons, and in the isolated amphibian and guinea pig gastric mucosa, it was completely atropine-resistant. In the rat, cerulein caused also a remarkable increase in the secretion of intrinsic factor, being here on a molar basis 10,000 times more active than histamine. Also the activity of histidine decarboxylase in rat gastric mucosa was remarkably enhanced (up to 400% above basal levels) by cerulein. The same was true (to a much lesser degree) for the histamine methyltransferase activity (8).

Pancreas

Cerulein displayed a potent, atropine-resistant, stimulatory action on the exocrine pancreas, causing an increase in volume of pancreatic juice and protein output, with a negligible effect on bicarbonates. These effects were observed in man and in conscious and anesthetized dogs, cats, rats, rabbits, and chickens at doses similar to those affecting biliary and gut motility. Both in man and in the dog cerulein produced a remarkable potentiation of the effect of secretin and the bicarbonate response to VIP as well. Conversely the effect of cerulein appeared to be reduced in the dog after parenteral feeding for a period of 6 weeks (38). Unlike secretin, cerulein stimulated calcium secretion in the guinea pig and increased magnesium, calcium, and zinc concentrations in the pancreatic juice of the dog. In the rat, in contrast with man and dog, cerulein stimulated the flow of pancreatic juice more effectively than did secretin. However, fluid and enzyme secretion evoked by cerulein were rapidly abolished by reducing Ca^{2+} to near zero (51). It was recently demonstrated (61) that cerulein and similar secretagogues increase both ^{45}Ca influx and ^{45}Ca efflux by 60 to 100%, probably by changing the membrane permeability for Ca^{2+} rather than by releasing Ca^{2+} from intracellular stores. Apparently, secretion evoked by cerulein was less dependent on extracellular Ca^{2+} than that evoked by acetylcholine (7).

Cerulein was also shown to reduce considerably the acinar cell membrane potential and input resistance in both mouse and rat, probably through increasing its permeability to Na^+ and K^+. Cerulein was 7 and 70 times more active than CCK and gastrin, respectively (37). Experiments were recently performed (21,55) in an attempt to explain the mechanism of action of cerulein and synthetic analogs on the pancreas using tritiated cerulein, isolated acinar cells, and a purified pancreatic plasma membranes preparation. It was found that the binding of [^{3}H]cerulein to rat pancreatic plasma membranes was a specific time- and temperature-dependent reversible process. There was a good correlation between the K_m for adenylate cyclase activation by cerulein (and its synthetic analogs) and the corresponding apparent K_d for binding. All of these data suggest that the action of cerulein on pancreatic tissue directly or indirectly involves Ca^{2+} movements and changes in cyclic GMP and cyclic AMP levels.

In a histochemical study of the exocrine pancreas of the rat, De Carvalho-Brunet et al. (19) found that CCK caused a rapid degranulation of the exocrine cells followed by a progressive increase in the number of secretory granules and a subsequent, less evident phase of degranulation. In contrast, cerulein induced only a marked storage of secretory granules. These studies have a counterpart in the different behavior of the two peptides, after injection of [^{3}H]L-leucine, in regard to protein turnover. Since these studies show a noticeable difference between cerulein and CCK, which was not before described, they require confirmation.

A recent study (41) showed that the rate of amylase secretion reached the maximum values with low doses of cerulein, whereas the juice flow reached maximum at a 10 times larger dose. Cerulein plus secretin-induced stimulation in humans was strongly reduced by calcitonin. Cerulein injected subcutaneously into rats for 5 to 15 days produced significant dose- and time-dependent increases in pancreatic weight and contents of DNA, RNA, protein, amylase, trypsinogen, and chymotrypsinogen (64). These effects were potentiated by simultaneous treatment with secretin (25 μg/kg) and suggested that cerulein plus secretin exerted a trophic effect on the pancreas, involving both its acinar and ductal parts. Administration of high doses of cerulein to rats, both acutely and chronically, produced severe acinar cell damage with diffuse pancreatic fibrosis which, however, did not damage the endocrine pancreas (39).

Liver

The choleretic action of cerulein varied quantitatively and qualitatively in various species, whereas in the dog and in the goose cerulein had a pure hydrocholeretic effect; in chickens, rabbits, cats and pigeons it increased all the components of the bile; in the rat (18) it significantly increased bile flow and bicarbonate concentration and output, but decreased the concentration and output of bile acids.

Brunner's Glands

The early experiments showed the conspicuous stimulatory action of cerulein on these glands in the dog and in the cat.

Action on Endocrine Secretions

Cerulein in amounts similar to those active on exocrine pancreas stimulated also the pancreatic islets with consequent release of insulin and glucagon. According to the early experiments, the peptide (2 ng kg⁻¹ min⁻¹) produced in the dog a two- to fourfold increase in immunoreactive insulin (IRI) levels, being much more potent than CCK (Fig. 6), and a three- to fivefold increase in

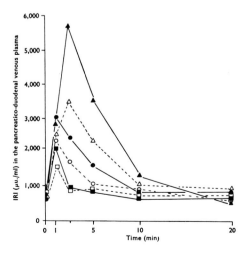

FIG. 6. Effects of rapid intravenous injection of cerulein *(continuous line)* and pancreozymin *(dotted line)* at the dose of 10 (■——■), 25 (●——●), and 50 (▲——▲) and 50 (□- - - -□), 100 (○- - - -○), and 200 ng/kg (△- - - -△), respectively, on immunoreactive insulin (IRI).

glucagon, in pancreaticoduodenal venous blood. More recent data (45) showed that higher doses of cerulein caused a prompt rise of insulin and a delayed increase of glucagon in the pancreatic vein of the dog, independent of blood glucose levels. Cerulein-induced glucagon secretion was not inhibited by an increased level of plasma insulin. Blood flow rate of the pancreatic vein increased noticeably after cerulein. Cerulein had also stimulated the isolated perfused dog pancreas, causing an enormous increase of glucagon in the presence of both low and high concentrations of glucose (3). The rat seemed to be much less sensitive than the dog. In man cerulein did not significantly change the plasma IRI; however, in some patients with insulinoma cerulein provoked a powerful insulin response.

All these data indicate that cerulein represents a potent stimulus for pancreatic hormones, although the mechanism remains to be clarified. The action of cerulein is at least partially atropine-sensitive and is reduced by high doses of atropine (60). In the rat chronic treatment with cerulein plus secretin did not change insulin or glucagon pancreatic contents, whereas it significantly increased content of somatostatin (72).

Cerulein was recently shown to act as a strong releaser of the pancreatic polypeptide (PP) in man and in the dog. The tremendous increase of PP in the dog under the effect of cerulein was paralleled by that of the GIP. The effect of cerulein is here atropine-resistant, but is inhibited by somatostatin (4). A similar and even more pronounced release of PP was observed in humans treated with intravenous cerulein (3). This was completely blocked by atropine (2). Since Taylor et al. (66) found that cerulein caused, in the dog, only an insignificant increase in serum PP concentration, this major discrepancy in results has to be clarified.

Another cerulein effect is the dose-related depression of food intake in the rabbit. On a molar basis, cerulein was here 2.2 times as effective as pure CCK. Since vagotomy did not abolish the satiety induced by the peptide, a sympathetic pathway could be involved (35). Cerulein also reversed the reduction of jejunal absorption of water, glucose, sodium, and potassium induced in the dog by secretin (33). In addition to the already mentioned trophic effect on pancreatic tissue, cerulein also showed a trophic effect on the stomach and the duodenum (23).

Clinical Applications

The use of cerulein in the radiological examination of biliary system and gastrointestinal tract was extensively reviewed by Orlandini et al. (46) and Bertaccini (9), who pointed out the usefulness of the peptide in diagnostic examination of more than 700 individuals. The promptness of its relaxant effect on the sphincter of Oddi associated with the contraction of the gallbladder represented a good alternative to the usual fatty meal. In the gastrointestinal tract, the decrease in the transit time of the contrast medium to 20 to 40 min from the duodenum to the cecum and the consequently good qualities of the radiograms of the whole small intestine were particularly appreciated. Our results were confirmed in a recent study performed on 33 individuals without disease and 22 symptomatic patients for the purpose of cholecystography. In all cases, excellent gallbladder contraction and visualization of the cystic and common ducts were obtained (57). The remarkable effect of cerulein in the radiological examination of the small bowel were confirmed on 106 patients by Novak (44), by several authors at the International Symposium on Gastrointestinal Hormones and Pathology of the Digestive System in Rome (1977), and at the Second International Symposium on Gastrointestinal Hormones in Beito, Norway (1978). The advantages of administration of cerulein to patients undergoing an intraoperative cholangiography included the abolition of false images, the avoidance of ebbing of the contrast medium into the Wirsung duct, the quick canalization of the intestine, and the easy evaluation of the anatomic and functional status of the sphincter of Oddi (15).

The early preliminary data concerning the usefulness of cerulein in the diagnosis of ulcer disease in which duodenal ulcer patients showed a maximum acid response to cerulein higher than control subjects were not substantiated by subsequent experiments; on the other hand, the value of cerulein (75 ng kg^{-1} hr^{-1} or 100 ng kg^{-1} hr^{-1}) in combination with secretin (1 CU kg^{-1} hr^{-1}) in the diagnosis of pancreatic diseases became well established (16,49,54,54b). The combination of the two peptides gave an excellent separation of the secretion of bicarbonate, lipase, and chymotrypsin between control groups and patients with chronic pancreatitis. Studies performed by cannulation of the Wirsung duct allowed a collection of the pure pancreatic juice without biliary or gastric contamination (27). The study of plasma cyclic AMP levels during infusion of secretin with cerulein for evaluation of the response of target tissues to hormone administration turned out to be more useful in evaluating hepatic than pancreatic impairment (1).

TABLE 6. *Therapeutic effect of cerulein in some pathological subjects*

Syndrome	Number of patients (Place of study)	Dose of cerulein and route of administration	No effect
Paralytic ileus	35 (Parma)	0.75 μg/kg i.m. (× 1–4 times)	5
	51 (Milan)	0.3 μg/kg i.m.	5
	178 (Munich)	0.5 μg/kg i.m.	8
	40 (Madrid)[a]		
	24 (Japan)	0.5 μg/kg i.m. (× 1)	2
	16 (Freiburg)	0.25 μg kg^{-1} hr^{-1} (× 2 hr)	4
Chronic fecal stasis	54 (Milan)	3 ng kg^{-1} min^{-1} (× 6 hr)	5
	30 (Milan)	0.75 μg/kg i.m. (× 1–2 times)	7
	6 (Bologna)	2–4 ng kg^{-1} min^{-1} (× 20 min)	
Megacolon (children)	14 (Parma)	3 ng kg^{-1} min^{-1} (× ½ hr)	4
Biliary colic	14 (Milan)	1 ng kg^{-1} min^{-1} (× 5 min)	1

[a] Data from ref. 43.
Quantitative data were not given.

Apart from the use of cerulein in diagnostics, a true therapeutic value of the peptide was shown in bowel hypomotility syndromes (adynamic ileus, chronic fecal stasis, megacolon, etc.) and surprisingly also in the treatment of biliary colics (52). Detailed data on cerulein effects obtained in these conditions are shown in Table 6.

In all the clinical studies performed with cerulein, harmful side effects were either absent or very moderate and appeared only in individuals treated with the maximum doses of the peptide (50–100 ng/kg by i.v. rapid injection; 5–6 ng kg^{-1} min^{-1} by i.v. infusion; 0.75–1 μg/kg by s.c. or i.m. injection). They consisted of dry mouth, nausea, flush, mild tachycardia, sweating, abdominal discomforts or cramps, and occasionally vomiting or diarrhea; they lasted only a few minutes and a full recovery always occurred.

SUMMARY

Tachykinins and ceruleins represent two distinct groups of peptides found in the amphibian skin that have their perfect counterpart in mammalian organisms.

Tachykinins, i.e., physalaemin, phyllomedusin, kassinin, uperolein (and eledoisin from octopods) resemble substance P of the mammalian organisms as to chemical structure and pharmacological activities. They are essentially vasoactive peptides inasmuch as they produce remarkable vasodilation in all vascular beds with consequent striking hypotensive effect. Moreover they stimulate, mainly in a direct way, extravascular smooth muscle and some exocrine secretions. They also have some activity on the central nervous system. All these different effects were manifest with exceedingly low doses (10^{-9}–10^{-12} g per kg under different experimental conditions).

Cerulein and its analogs (phyllocerulein and Asn^2, Leu^5-cerulein) present a striking similarity with the gastrointestinal hormone cholecystokinin-pancreozymin (CCK-P2). In addition, they have some gastrin-like effects as well. The activity of cerulein is mainly localized in the gastrointestinal tract and the biliary system. Predominant stimulatory effects have been noted both on the smooth muscle and on exocrine secretory systems of the stomach, pancreas, liver, and Brunner's glands, and on endocrine secretions (insulin, glucagon, calcitonin, pancreatic peptide). In addition, cerulein possesses other, less manifest actions on blood vessels, on isolated heart preparations, and on the CNS. Clinical applications of this peptide are of interest both in diagnosis (gallbladder motility tests, study of intestinal transit) and in therapeutics (treatment of paralytic ileus, chronic fecal stasis, and of biliary colics).

CONCLUSIONS AND PROJECTIONS FOR THE FUTURE

The importance of tachykinins and cerulein as pharmacological tools in the examination of smooth muscle contractility and of exocrine or endocrine glands function appears to be well established. The same is true for their clinical applications in diagnosis and therapy, especially in regard to cerulein. The recent findings suggest that the interpretation of the results obtained with cerulein can be applied to mammalian CCK, since no significant differences were so far observed between the two peptides. This is not true, however, in regard to transposition of the findings obtained with eledoisin and physalaemin to substance P, where an indiscriminate extrapolation of the data obtained with peptides of the same family could represent a significant source of errors.

The availability of these amphibian peptides in a pure, synthetic form allowed anticipation of the physiology of the mammalian peptides several years ahead of time. The conclusions that could be reached with the study of amphibian peptides appeared to be valid also for the mammalian analogs. Thus, the interest in the amphibian peptides largely surpasses that of simple pharmacologically active substances.

ACKNOWLEDGMENTS

Original work of the author was supported by a grant from the Consiglio Nazionale delle Richerche, Rome.

REFERENCES

1. Adler, M., Robberecht, P., Poitevin, M. G., and Christophe, J. (1978): Plasma cyclic AMP levels during a secretin-caerulein pancreatic function test in liver and pancreatic disease. *Gut,* 19:214–219.
2. Adrian, T. E., Besterman, H. S., Christofides, N. D., and Bloom, S. R. (1978): Interaction of gastrointestinal hormones and cholinergic innervation on the release of pancreatic polypeptide. *Scand. J. Gastroenterol. (Suppl. 49),* 13:1.
3. Adrian, T. E., Bloom, S. R., Besterman, H. S., and Bryant, M. G. (1978): PP-physiology and pathology. In: *Gut Hormones,* edited by S. R. Bloom, pp. 254–260. Churchill Livingstone, Edinburgh/London/New York.
4. Adrian, T. E., Bloom, S. R., Hermansen, K., and Iversen, J. (1978): Pancreatic polypeptide, glucagon and insulin secretion from the isolated perfused canine pancreas. *Diabetologia,* 14:413–417.
5. Agosti, A., Missale, G., and Bertaccini, G. (1976): Inhibitory effect of a caerulein-like peptide on human gastric secretion. *Eur. J. Pharmacol.,* 38:193–195.
6. Anuras, S., and Cooke, A. R. (1978): Effects of some gastrointestinal hormones on two muscle layers of duodenum. *Am. J. Physiol.,* 234:E60–E63.
7. Argent, B. E., Case, R. M., Greenwell, J. R., and Hirst, F. C. (1978): Differential effects of extracellular calcium on pancreatic amylase secretion stimulated by caerulein and acetylcholine. *Scand. J. Gastroenterol. (Suppl. 49),* 13:10.
8. Barth, H., Lorenz W., and Stenner, W. (1977): Alterations of histamine methyltransferase activity in guinea-pig stomach after feeding or application of gastric secretory stimulants. *Naunyn-Schmiedeberg's Arch. Pharmacol.,* 297:R43.
9. Bertaccini, G. (1973): Pharmacology and clinical use of caerulein. *In: Symposium on Gastrin and its Antagonists,* edited by J. Bory and G. Mozsik, pp. 47–66. Akadémiai Kiadò, Budapest.
10. Bertaccini, G. (1976): Active polypeptides of nonmammalian origin. *Pharmacol. Rev.,* 28:127–177.
11. Bertaccini, G. (1977): Action of substance P and some natural analogues on gastro-intestinal motility. In: *Abstracts of Joint Meeting of German and Italian Pharmacologists,* p. 95, Venice.
12. Bertaccini, G., and Coruzzi, G. (1977): Action of some natural peptides on the stomach of the anaesthetized rat. *Naunyn-Schmiedeberg's Arch. Pharmacol.,* 298:163–166.

13. Bury, R. W., and Mashford, M. L. (1977): Substance P: Its pharmacology and physiological roles. *Aust. J. Exp. Biol. Med. Sci.*, 55:671–735.
14. Caprilli, R., Frieri, G., Palla, R., and Broccardo, M. (1976): Effects of eledoisin on gastrointestinal electrical activity. In: *Abstracts Symposium on Physiology and Pharmacology of Smooth Muscle*, p. 12, Varna.
15. Caprino, A., and Salvatori, G. (1975): Impiego intraoperatorio del ceruletide nella chirurgia delle vie biliari. *Il Farmaco. Ed. Pr.*, 30:615–620.
16. Cavallini, G., Mirachian, R., Angelini, G., Vantini, I., Vaona, B., Bovo, P., Gelpi, F., Ederle, A., Dobrilla, G., and Scuro, L. A. (1978): The role of cerulein in tests of exocrine pancreatic function. *Scand. J. Gastroenterol.*, 13:3–15.
17. Corazziari, E., Tonelli, F., Pozzessere, C., Dani, S., Anzini, F., and Torsoli, A. (1976): The effects of graded doses of cerulein on human jejunal motor activity. *Rendic. Gastroenterol.*, 8:190–193.
18. Dangoumau, J., Balabaud, C., Bussiere-Leboe, U.F., Dallet-Duverge, F., and Noel, M. (1977): Influence de la pentagastrine, de la cholecystokinine et de la caeruleine sur la cholérese chez le rat. *J. Pharmacol.*, 8:197–204.
19. De Carvalho-Brunet, N., Dussourd d'Hunterland, L., and Tixier-Vidal, A. (1977): Comparison of cytological effects induced by pancreozymin and cerulein in exocrine and endocrine pancreas. In: *Hormonal Receptors in the Digestive Tract Physiology*, edited by S. Bonfils, P. Fromageot, and G. Rosselin, p. 99. North-Holland, Amsterdam/New York/Oxford.
20. De Castiglione, R. (1977): Structure-activity relationships in ceruletide-like peptides. In: *Hormonal Receptors in the Digestive Tract Physiology*, edited by S. Bonfils, P. Fromageot, and G. Rosselin, pp. 33–42. North Holland, Amsterdam/New York/Oxford.
21. Deschodt-Lanckman, M., Svoboda, M., Camus, J. C., and Robberecht, P. (1977): Regulation of the dissociation of ^{3}H caerulein from its pancreatic receptors: evidence for negative cooperativity. In: *Hormonal Receptors in the Digestive Tract Physiology*, edited by S. Bonfils, P. Fromageot, and G. Rosselin, pp. 325–326. North-Holland, Amsterdam/New York/Oxford.
22. Dockray, G. J. (1977): Immunoreactive component resembling cholecystokinin octapeptide in intestine. *Nature*, 270:359–361.
23. Erspamer, V. (1978): Correlations between active peptides of the amphibian skin and peptides of the avian and mammalian gut and brain. The gut-brain-skin triangle. In: *Abstracts of the 19th Congress of the Italian Pharmacological Society*, pp. 109–156. Ancona.
24. Erspamer, V., Falconieri Erspamer, G., and Linari, G. (1977): Occurrence of tachykinins (physalemin- or Substance P-like peptides) in the amphibian skin and their actions on smooth muscle. In: *Substance P*, edited by U.S. von Euler and B. Pernow, pp. 67–74. Raven Press, New York.
25. Erspamer, V., and Melchiorri, P. (1973): Active polypeptides of the amphibian skin and their synthetic analogues. *Pure Appl. Chem.*, 35:463–494.
26. Erspamer, V., Negri, L., Falconieri Erspamer, G., and Endean, R. (1975): Uperolein and other active peptides in the skin of the Australian leptodactylid frogs *Uperoleia* and *Taudactylus*. *Naunyn-Schmiedeberg's Arch. Pharmacol.*, 289:41–54.
27. Escourrou, J., Frexinos, J., and Ribet, A. (1978): Etude de la sécrétion pancréatique pure chez l'homme sous stimulation par sécrétine-céruléine. *Gastroenterol. Clin. Biol.*, 2:29–37.
28. Fara, J. W., and Erde, S. M. (1978): Comparison of *in vivo* and *in vitro* responses to sulfated and non-sulfated ceruletide. *Eur. J. Pharmacol.*, 47:359–363.
29. Fontaine, J., Famaey, J. P., and Reuse, J. (1977): Enhancement by physalaemin of the contractions induced by cholinomimetics in the guinea pig ileum. *J. Pharm. Pharmacol.*, 29:449–450.
30. Fontaine, J., Famaey, J., and Reuse, J. (1978): Sensitization by cerulein of guinea pig ileum to contractions by acetylcholine, histamine, 5-hydroxytryptamine and nicotine. *Naunyn-Schmiedeberg's Arch. Pharmacol.*, 302:51–54.
31. Fontaine, J., Van Neuten, J. M., and Reuse, J. (1978): The action of physalaemin on the peristaltic reflex of guinea pig isolated ileum. *J. Pharm. Pharmacol.*, 30:183–185.
32. Gillespie, J. S., and McKnight, A. T. (1978): The actions of some vasoactive polypeptides and their antagonists on the anococcygeus muscle. *Br. J. Pharmacol.*, 62:267–274.
33. Hirose, S., Yoshizaki, T., and Murata, I. (1978): Effects of secretin, pancreozymin and caerulein on jejunal absorption of glucose, water and electrolytes in the dog. In: *Abstracts of the 6th World Congress of Gastroenterology*, Madrid, p. 154.
34. Hotz, J., Goebel, H., and Ziegler, R. (1977): Calcitonin and exocrine pancreatic secretion in

man: Inhibition of enzymes stimulated by CCK-pancreozymin, caerulein, or calcium-no response to vagal stimulation. *Gut,* 18:615–622.

35. Houpt, T. R., Anika, S. M., and Wolff, N. C. (1978): Satiety effects of cholecystokinin and cerulein in rabbits. *Am. J. Physiol.,* 235:R23–R28.

36. Ihasz, M., Koiss, I., Nemeth, E'. P., Folly, G., and Papp, M. (1976): Action of cerulein, glucagon or prostaglandin E_1 on the motility of intestinal villi. *Pflügers Arch.,* 364:301–304.

37. Iwatsuki, N., Kato, K., and Nishiyama, A. (1977): The effects of gastrin and gastrin analogues on pancreatic acinar cell membrane potential and resistance. *Br. J. Pharmacol.,* 60:147–154.

38. Johnson, L. R., Schanbacher, L. M., Dudrick, S. J., and Copeland, E. M. (1977): Effect of long-term parenteral feeding on pancreatic secretion and serum secretin. *Am. J. Physiol.,* 233:E524–E529.

39. Kern, H. F., and Lampel, M. (1977): Target cell destruction *in vivo* by excessive doses of a pancreatic secretagogue. *Gastroenterology,* 72:A-7/817.

40. Lecchini, S., D'Angelo, L., Tonini, M., Perucca, E., Gatti, G., and Teggia Droghi, M. (1976): Effects of some autonomic drugs on the electrical activity of intestinal circular muscle. *Boll. Soc. Ital. Biol. Sper.,* 52:1158–1161.

41. Linari, G., and Baldieri Linari, M. (1977): The action of caerulein on the pancreatic secretion of the rat. *Il Farmaco. Ed. Pr.,* 32:611–616.

42. Montecucchi, P., Falconieri Erspamer, G., and Visser, J. (1977): Occurrence of Asn^2, Leu^5-cerulein in the skin of the African frog *Hylambates maculatus. Experientia,* 33:1138–1139.

43. Naveiro, M. C. (1978): Effects de la ceruleina sobre la motilidad intestinal y el ileo paralitico. In: *Abstracts of the 6th World Congress of Gastroenterology,* p. 200, Madrid.

44. Novak, D. (1977): Significance of caerulein in the roentgenology of small intestine. In: *Abstracts of the International Symposium on Gastrointestinal Hormones, Pathology of the Digestive System,* p. 66, Rome.

45. Ohneda, A., Horigome, K., Ishii, S., Kai, Y., and Chiba, M. (1978): Effect of cerulein upon insulin and glucagon secretion in dogs. *Horm. Metab. Res.,* 10:7–11.

46. Orlandini, I., Impicciatore, M., and Bertaccini, G. (1972): Diagnostica radiologica dell'apparato digerente sotto controllo farmacologico. In: *Abstracts of the 25th Congress S.I.R.M.N.,* pp. 1–101, Monticelli Terme.

47. Ormas, P., Beretta, C., Villalobos, S. J., Pompa, G., Andreini, G. C., Beretta, C., Jr., and Faustini, R. (1975: Some effects of eledoisin on ruminant's reticular, omasal, ruminal and aboma- sal smooth muscles *in vitro* and *in vivo. Pharm. Res. Commun.,* 7:527–534.

48. Ormas, P., Castelli, S., Beretta, C. M., Nilsson, I., Galbiati, A., Beretta, C., and Faustini, R. (1977): The effects of eledoisin on intestinal smooth muscle of ruminants. *Fol. Vet. Latina,* 7:252–257.

49. Otte, M., and Forell, M. M. (1978): Pancreas secretion after injection of ceruletide compared with the effect of cholecystokinin-pancreozymin (CCK). *Scand. J. Gastroenterol. (Suppl. 49),* 13:138.

50. Pandolfo, N., Bortolotti, M., Nebiacolombo, C., Sansone, G., and Mattioli, F. (1977): Action of cerulein on lower oesophageal sphincter pressure. In: *Abstracts of the International Symposium on Gastrointestinal Hormones, Pathology of the Digestive System,* p. 175, Rome.

51. Petersen, O. H., and Ueda, N. (1976): The importance of calcium for cerulein and secretin evoked fluid and enzyme secretion in the perfused rat pancreas. *J. Physiol.,* 263:223P–224P.

52. Praga, C., Santamaria, A., Lucani, G., and Muntorsi, W. (1978): Rapid relief of biliary colic with ceruletide. In: *Abstracts of the 6th World Congress of Gastroenterology,* p. 154, Madrid.

53. Rehfeld, J. F. (1978): Multiple molecular forms of cholecystokinin. In: *Gut Hormones,* edited by S. R. Bloom, pp. 213–218. Churchill Livingstone, Edinburgh/London/New York.

54a. Ribet, A., and Balas, D. (1977): Functional diagnoses of pancreatic disease. In: *Progress in Gastroenterology, Vol. III,* edited by G. B. J. Glass, pp. 895–912. Grune & Stratton, New York.

54b. Ribet, A., Tournut, R., Duffaut, M., and Vaysse, N. (1976): Use of cerulein with submaximal doses of secretin as a test of pancreatic function in man. *Gut,* 17:431–434.

55. Robberecht, P., Deschodt-Lanckman, M., Camus, J., Christophe, J., Morgat, J.-L., and Girma, J.-P. (1977): Specific binding and mode of action of cerulein on plasma membrane of rat pancreas. In: *Hormonal Receptors in the Digestive Tract Physiology,* edited by S. Bonfils, P. Fromageot, and G. Rosselin, pp. 261–274. North Holland, Amsterdam/New York/Oxford.

56. Rudich, L., and Butcher, F. R. (1976): Effect of substance P and eledoisin on K^+ efflux, amylase

release and cyclic nucleotide levels in slices of rat parotid gland. *Biochim. Biophys. Acta,* 444:704–711.

57. Sargent, E. N. (1977): Ceruletide in the radiologic examination of the gallbladder. In: *Abstracts of the International Symposium on Gastrointestinal Hormones, Pathology of the Digestive System,* pp. 63–64, Rome.

58. Sarles, J. C., Bidart, J. M., Devaux, M. A., Echinard, C., and Castagnini, A. (1976): Action of cholecystokinin and cerulein on the rabbit sphincter of Oddi. *Digestion,* 14:415–423.

59. Scarpignato, C., Capovilla, T., and Bertaccini, G. (1980): Evidence that cerulein delays gastric emptying in the rat. *Eur. J. Pharmacol. (in press).*

60. Scarpignato, C., and Costa, G. (1977): Ceruleina e secrezione insulinica: influenza del sistema nervoso autonomo. *Riv. Farmac. Ter.,* 8:161–169.

61. Schulz, I., Kondo, S., Sachs, G., and Milutinovic, S. (1977): The role of Ca^{++} in pancreatic enzyme secretion. In: *Hormonal Receptors in the Digestive Tract Physiology,* edited by S. Bonfils, P. Fromageot, and G. Rosselin, pp. 275–288. North Holland, Amsterdam/New York/Oxford.

62. Scott, L. D., and Summers, R. W. (1976): Correlation of contractions and transit in rat small intestine. *Am. J. Physiol.,* 230:132–137.

63. Skrabanek, P., and Powell, D. (1977): Substance P. *Ann. Res. Rev.,* 1:1–181, Eden Press, Canada.

64. Solomon, T. E., Petersen, H., and Grossman, M. I. (1978): Trophic effects of secretin on stomach and pancreas. *Scand. J. Gastroenterol. (Suppl. 49),* 13:182.

65. Spearman, T. N., and Pritchard, E. T. (1977): Potassium release from submandibular salivary gland *in vitro. Biochim. Biophys. Acta,* 466:198–207.

66. Taylor, I. L., Walsh, J. H., Carter, D. C., Wood, J., and Grossman, M. I. (1978): Effect of atropine and bethanechol on release of pancreatic polypeptide (PP) and gastrin by bombesin in dog. *Scand. J. Gastroenterol. (Suppl. 49),* 13:183.

67. Thulin, A. (1976): Secretory and motor effects in the submaxillary gland of the rat on intraarterial administration of some polypeptides and autonomic drugs. *Acta Physiol. Scand.,* 97:343–348.

68. Uhlemann, E. R., May, R. J., and Gardner, J. D. (1977): Effects of peptides from amphibian skin on amylase release from pancreatic acinar cells. *Clin. Res.,* 25:470A.

69. Vizi, S. E., Bertaccini, G., Impicciatore, M., and Knoll, J. (1973): Evidence that acetylcholine released by gastrin and related polypeptides contributes to their effect on gastrointestinal motility. *Gastroenterology,* 64:268–277.

70. Von Euler, U. S., and Gaddum, J. H. (1931): An unidentified depressor substance in certain tissue extracts. *J. Physiol. (Lond.),* 72:74–87.

71. Yajima, H., Sasaki, T., Ogawa, H., Fujii, N., Segawa, T., and Nakata, Y. (1978): Studies on peptides, LXXVI.[1,2] Synthesis of kassinin, a new frog skin peptide. *Chem. Pharm. Bull.,* 26:1231–1235.

72. Yamada, T., Solomon, T. E., Peterson, H., Levin, S. R., Walsh, J. H., and Grossman, M. I. (1978): Selective increase in pancreatic somatostatin content caused by glycentin and secretin plus cerulein. *Scand. J. Gastroenterol. (Suppl. 49),* 13:194.

73. Yanaihara, N., Yanaihara, C., Hirohashi, M., Sato, H., Iizuka, Y., Hashimoto, T., and Sakagami, M. (1977): Substance P analogs: Synthesis, and biological and immunological properties. In: *Substance P,* edited by U. S. Von Euler and B. Pernow, pp. 27–33. Raven Press, New York.

74. Zappia, L., Molina, E., Sianesi, M., and Bertaccini, G. (1978): Effects of natural analogues of substance P on the motility of human gastrointestinal tract *in vitro. J. Pharm. Pharmacol.,* 30:593–594.

75. Zseli, J., Molina, E., Zappia, L., and Bertaccini, G. (1977): Action of some natural polypeptides on the longitudinal muscle of the guinea pig ileum. *Eur. J. Pharmacol.,* 43:285–287.

Gastrointestinal Hormones, edited by
George B. Jerzy Glass.
Raven Press, New York © 1980.

Chapter 14

Peptides of the Amphibian Skin Active on the Gut. II. Bombesin-Like Peptides: Isolation, Structure, and Basic Functions

Vittorio Erspamer

Institute of Medical Pharmacology I, University of Rome Medical School, I-00100 Rome, Italy

In the preceding chapter *(this volume),* two major peptide families of the amphibian skin were thoroughly examined: the tachykinins and the ceruleins. This chapter discusses a third family, the bombesin-like peptides, which was chronologically the last to be identified. It has attracted particular attention because the prototype of this family, bombesin, was shown to display a number of potent direct and indirect actions on the gut (involving secretions and motility) and on the central nervous system (CNS). Moreover, bombesin has been the springboard for the discovery of new hormonal peptides, related to bombesin, in the gastrointestinal tract and brain of mammals and birds (27,30,31).

OCCURRENCE AND DISTRIBUTION

Eight peptides belonging to the bombesin family have so far been isolated in a pure form, and five of them have been synthesized and submitted to a thorough pharmacological study.

(I) Pyr-Gln-Arg-Leu-Gly-Asn-Gln-Trp-Ala-Val-Gly-His-Leu-Met-NH$_2$

(II) Pyr-Gly-Arg-Leu-Gly-Thr-Gln-Trp-Ala-Val-Gly-His-Leu-Met-NH$_2$

(III) Pyr————————Val-Pro-Gln-Trp-Ala-Val-Gly-His-Phe-Met-NH$_2$

(IV) Pyr————————Gln-Trp-Ala-Val-Gly-His-Phe-Met-NH$_2$

(V) Pyr————————Glu(OMe)-Trp-Ala-Val-Gly-His-Phe-Met-NH$_2$

(VI) Pyr————————Glu(OEt)-Trp-Ala-Val-Gly-His-Phe-Met-NH$_2$

(VII) Ser-Asp-Ala-Thr-Leu-Arg-Arg-Tyr-Asn-Gln-Trp-Ala-Thr-Gly-His-Phe-Met-NH$_2$

(VIII) X-Glx-Thr-Pro-Gln-Trp-Ala-Thr-Gly-His-Phe-Met-NH$_2$

Bombesin (I) is a tetradecapeptide obtained from methanol extracts of the skin of the two European discoglossid frogs, *Bombina bombina* and *Bombina variegata variegata,* where it is contained in amounts ranging from 200 to 700 μg/g fresh tissue (26). Authentic bombesin is also present in the skin of *Bombina orientalis.*

Alytesin (II) is also a tetradecapeptide, strictly related to bombesin, which is found in extracts of the skin of another European discoglossid frog, *Alytes obstetricans,* in amounts usually ranging from 600 to 1,300 μg/g wet skin, but sometimes as low as 50 μg/g when expressed in terms of bombesin (26).

Ranatensin (III) is an endecapeptide prepared from extracts of the skin of the American frog *Rana pipiens* (52). In our methanol extracts of dried skins of *Rana pipiens,* the content of ranatensin, assayed on the rat uterus preparation and expressed in terms of bombesin, ranged from 0.5 to 120 μg/g dry tissue.

The smallest natural bombesin-like peptides so far detected are represented by the nonapeptides litorin (IV), Glu(OMet)^2-litorin (V), and Glu(OEt)^2-litorin (VI). The first two have been isolated from skin extracts of the Australian frog *Litoria* (Hyla) *aurea,* and probably occur in other Australian *Litoria* species as well (1,2); Glu(OEt)^2-litorin has been recently isolated, together with litorin, from skin extracts of *Uperoleia rugosa* (53).

Finally, ranatensin-R (VII) and ranatensin-C (VIII) have been obtained from skin extracts of *Rana rugosa* and *Rana catesbeiana,* respectively (61,62).

Additional bombesin-like peptides have been traced in amphibians of Australia and Papua New Guinea belonging to the genera *Rana (R. daemeli, R. arfaki, R. krefti)* and *Pseudophryne (P. güntheri, P. bibroni, P. coriacea),* as well as in South American amphibians belonging to the genus *Phyllomedusa (Ph. sauvagei, Ph. rhodei).* The isolation of some of them is in progress.

ISOLATION AND PURIFICATION OF BOMBESIN

The purification and isolation of bombesin could be performed in essentially two steps:

(a) Alkaline alumina columns were loaded with crude skin extracts and eluted with descending concentrations of ethanol. The active material emerged in the 85–80% ethanol eluates.

(b) Sephadex G-10 columns were loaded with the above semipurified material and eluted with 0.01 M acetic acid. The active peptide emerging from these columns was generally pure enough to be used for sequential analysis. However, when needed, preparative paper electrophoresis was used as a final step in the purification procedure. At this point, the material presented on paper electrophoresis a single active spot that was negative to ninhydrin, but positive to the chlorine, Sakaguchi, Ehrlich, Pauly, and iodoplatinate reagents.

The sequence of bombesin was deduced by the results of total acid hydrolysis and by chemical (hydrazinolysis, dansylation) and enzymatic analysis (carboxypeptidases A and B, leucineaminopeptidase) of the fragments obtained by digestion with trypsin and chymotrypsin.

Bombesin was soon reproduced by synthesis at the Farmitalia Carlo Erba Research Laboratories, Milan. Purification of the other peptides of the bombesin family was carried out in a similar way. So far, in addition to bombesin, alytesin, litorin, Glu(OMe)^2-litorin, and ranatensin have been prepared by synthesis in different laboratories. Synthesis has always confirmed the structures suggested by analysis of the natural peptides.

PHARMACOLOGICAL EFFECTS ON THE GASTROINTESTINAL TRACT

Action on Gastric Acid Secretion. Release of Gastrin

Bombesin was found to be a potent stimulant of gastric acid secretion in gastric fistula dogs with Heidenhain pouches. The effect could be elicited not only by intravenous infusion of the polypeptide but also by subcutaneous injection. Rapid intravenous injection was considerably less effective (7).

The following pieces of evidence unequivocally demonstrate that the gastric secretagogue activity of bombesin is due to release of gastrin from the G cells of the antral mucosa (8,30,31,37):

(a) Gastric acid secretion was preceded and accompanied by an increase in plasma levels of immunoreactive gastrin. After intravenous infusion of bombesin, the increase in gastrin concentration was prompt, reached its maximum after approximately 30 min, and then, provided that the acid juice secreted in the main stomach was freely drained to the exterior, remained at a steady level throughout the duration of an experiment. After cessation of the bombesin infusion, plasma gastrin returned to basal levels in less than 1 hr.

From threshold infusion rates (0.05–0.1 μg kg^{-1}h^{-1}) up to the doses that produced optimum responses (1 μg kg^{-1}h^{-1}), there was a fair dose-response relationship. Peak increases of gastrin concentrations above plasma basal levels were of the order of 150 to 220 pg/ml (Fig. 1).

However, Miyata et al. (49) observed, at infusion rates of 2 μg kg^{-1}h^{-1}, an increase from basal 55 $\pm$ 6 to 531 $\pm$ pg/ml. No other known stimulus of gastrin release was more potent than bombesin. Peak acid responses to bombesin infusion were of the same magnitude as maximal responses to pentagastrin infusion.

(b) Antrectomy reduced the gastrin response to bombesin and the stimulation of acid gastric secretion by 85% to 90%. The same result was obtained after removal of the antral mucosa; regeneration of the mucosa gradually restored the response to bombesin.

(c) Blood collected from the gastroduodenal vein 30 min after the start of an intravenous infusion of bombesin (0.6 μg kg^{-1}h^{-1}) contained three times

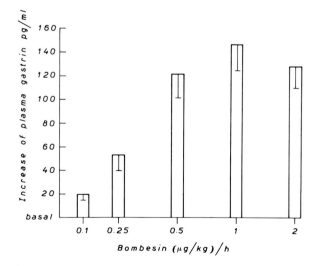

FIG. 1. Gastric fistula dogs. Peak increases in plasma gastrin levels, above basal levels, after intravenous infusion, for 60 min, of graded doses of bombesin. *Columns* represent the mean of two measurements in each of six dogs. *Vertical bars* show SEM. (From ref. 8, with permission.)

as much gastrin as that taken from a femoral artery (380 pg/ml vs. 135 pg/ml).

On the other hand, bombesin was found to be a powerful stimulant for release of gastrin from the isolated perfused canine antral mucosa also.

In dogs provided with antral pouches, acidification of the antrum caused a delay in gastrin release, or a temporary reduction of gastrin release stimulated by bombesin. Delay occurred when the acid was perfused throughout the period of bombesin infusion; temporary reduction occurred when the transition from neutral to acidified antrum was made during a bombesin infusion. The inhibitory effect of antral acidification, however, could be overcome by increasing either the duration or the rate of bombesin infusion. The effect of antral acidification on response to bombesin was the same for both innervated and denervated antral pouches.

Gastric acid secretion and gastrin release stimulated by bombesin were suppressed by duodenal acidification in the dog (51) but not in man (4). Bombesin in turn significantly inhibited the dog gastric acid secretion induced by pentagastrin, possibly via cholecystokinin (CCK) release.

When bombesin infusion in gastric fistula dogs provided with Heidenhain pouches was prolonged for 12 to 15 hr, at a rate of 0.6 μg kg^{-1}h^{-1}, at first the usual peak increase in plasma gastrin levels was observed, which lasted for approximately 2 hr. Then gastrin levels gradually declined to attain basal values after 10 hr. Food given at this time while continuing bombesin infusion no longer produced any significant change in plasma gastrin levels. It is conceivable that this is due to exhaustion of depletable gastrin stores in the G cells.

The gastrin response to bombesin was unaffected or moderately reduced by secretin (1.4–1.7 U kg^{-1}h^{-1}) and glucagon (3 mg kg^{-1}h^{-1}), but strongly inhibited by somatostatin and betanechol (100 μg kg^{-1}h^{-1}) (4,58).

However, it was conspicuously increased after truncal vagotomy. In fact, whereas bombesin infusion (1 μg kg^{-1}h^{-1}) prior to vagotomy caused a stepwise increase of gastrin levels from 49 $\pm$ 5 pg/ml to 184 $\pm$ 35 pg/ml, after vagotomy it produced a rise of gastrin levels from 80 $\pm$ 5 pg/ml to 200 $\pm$ 20 pg/ml at 5 min, and to a peak of 650 $\pm$ 70 pg/ml at 60 min. In the 2-hr observation period gastrin output was fourfold higher after than before vagotomy (56).

Following highly selective (fundic) vagotomy, results were similar, although less striking (35,36).

The potentiating effect of vagotomy on bombesin-stimulated gastrin release could be observed at intragastric pH levels of 4.5 and 2.5, indicating that it occurred, at least in part, because of a non-pH-dependent mechanism. It is suggested that the increased gastrin response to bombesin may be due not only to loss of acid inhibition but also to loss of inhibitory vagal effects on gastrin release (56,59).

It was found, however, (35) that despite the above ascertained differences in gastrin release, gastrin acid output following bombesin infusion was the same whether the fundus was denervated or innervated. This would mean that bombesin may stimulate gastric acid secretion by the release of an additional secreta-gogue that is not measured by the gastrin assay. In other words, the potent effect of bombesin on acid gastric secretion would be only in part attributable to gastrin release.

Although atropine did not affect gastrin release by bombesin, it did strongly inhibit gastric acid secretion, as expected. A somewhat less intense inhibitory effect on acid output was exhibited also by metiamide, a blocking agent for histamine H_2-receptors.

It would seem, from preliminary experiments, that gastrin-17 (G-17), the gastrin form that appears to be predominant in the G cells of the antral mucosa, is more promptly released than gastrin-34 (G-34), which is present mainly in extraantral tissue (30,34).

This last observation prompted Basso et al. (5) and Speranza et al. (57) to suggest a "bombesin test" for the diagnosis of retained antrum. Patients with retained antrum responded with a sharp increase in plasma gastrin levels to a bombesin infusion. If the antrum was completely removed, no response to bombe-sin was recorded.

The gastrin-releasing effect of bombesin was confirmed in man and cats. In man, the threshold infusion rate of bombesin was of the order of 0.15 μg kg^{-1}h^{-1}. Optimum stimulation unaccompanied by untoward side effects occurred with 0.6 μg kg^{-1}h^{-1}. Peak increases in plasma gastrin levels were significantly higher in females than in males.

Lezoche et al. (41) found that bombesin (2–8 ng kg^{-1}min^{-1}) conspicuously potentiated the food-stimulated gastrin release in man.

Cats were very sensitive to bombesin (threshold 0.02 μg kg^{-1}h^{-1}; maximum response 0.5 μg kg^{-1}h^{-1}), although increases in gastrin levels did not exceed 100 to 120 pg/ml. Secretin in this species sharply reduced not only the secreta-gogue effect but also the gastrin-releasing effect of bombesin.

Bombesin displayed a very poor stimulatory action, if any, on acid gastric secretion in the rat. In accordance with this observation, the gastrin-releasing effect of bombesin was also ambiguous, and subcutaneous doses of the polypep-tide as high as 500 μg/kg were required to raise plasma gastrin levels from 85 to 150 pg/ml. Subcutaneous doses of 50 to 200 μg/kg were ineffective (30).

In the chicken, bombesin stimulated gastric acid secretion at threshold doses of 0.2 to 0.3 μg kg^{-1}h^{-1}. The effect was inhibited by atropine and by acidification of the proventriculus, which supports the hypothesis that, also in the chicken, bombesin may increase acid through release of gastrin (42).

Action on Gallbladder Motility and Pancreatic Secretion. Release of Cholecystokinin

Strong evidence (28) suggests that bombesin also releases CCK from the duodenal mucosa in the dog. The intravenous infusion of bombesin elicited the following events:

(a) Contraction of the gallbladder in both anesthetized and conscious dogs. Response appeared after a latency period of 5 to 10 min, and after having gradually reached a maximum it persisted for some time after the infusion was discontinued. On the isolated dog gallbladder bombesin was virtually inactive (Fig. 2).

(b) Relaxation of the choledochoduodenal junction.

(c) Stimulation of the flow of pancreatic juice, again after a latency of approximately 10 min. The juice was poor in bicarbonate but rich in protein and enzymes. Amylase and trypsin concentrations rose by 200 to 300% (see also refs. 49 to 51).

The pancreatic response was dose-related only between 0.1 and 1 $\mu g\ kg^{-1}h^{-1}$. Increasing the infusion rate above this level did not increase protein output any further. Maximum output produced by infusion of porcine CCK or cerulein, however, was considerably higher than that caused by bombesin. One $\mu g\ kg^{-1}h^{-1}$ of bombesin produced approximately the same effect as 0.75 $\mu g\ kg^{-1}h^{-1}$ of CCK. Protein secretion stimulated by bombesin was enhanced by duodenal acidification (51).

Following removal in the dog of the antrum and small intestine, bombesin failed to show not only any change in the serum gastrin level but also any

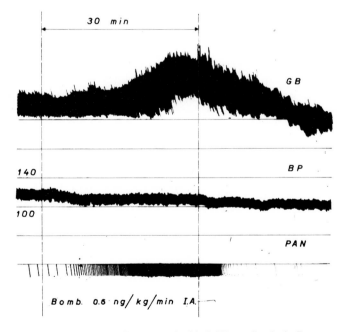

FIG. 2. Dog anesthetized with sodium pentobarbital (30 mg/kg i.v.). Response elicited by the infusion into the superior mesenteric artery of 0.5 ng $kg^{-1}min^{-1}$ bombesin for 30 min. From **top** to **bottom:** gallbladder motility (GB), systemic blood pressure (BP), and flow of pancreatic juice, in drops (PAN).

stimulation of the pancreatic secretion. Somatostatin, in turn, caused the inhibition of pancreatic protein secretion by bombesin, but failed to affect the response to CCK octapeptide (40).

Similarly, whereas infusion of bombesin in dog pancreas-duodenum preparations stimulated pancreatic enzyme secretion and, to a lesser degree, bicarbonate secretion, administration of the polypeptide was no longer effective after duodenectomy. However, when the functional unit of pancreas-duodenum was reconstructed, after duodenectomy, by a supporting animal in cross-perfusion, bombesin again stimulated pancreatic secretion (48).

Finally, the hypothesis that the effects of bombesin on the dog gallbladder and pancreas are mediated through the release of CCK appeared to be conclusively proved by the results of Fender et al. (34) and Miyata et al. (49). These authors found that bombesin released not only gastrin but also immunoreactive CCK, the levels of which in serum rose from 80 ± 10 pg/ml to 143 ± 9 pg/ml following 0.125 μg kg^{-1}h^{-1} bombesin, and to 412 ± 26 pg/ml after 2 μg kg^{-1}h^{-1} bombesin.

In another series of experiments by Miyata et al. (50), peak values of plasma immunoreactive CCK produced by doses of bombesin ranging from 0.125 to 1 μg kg^{-1}h^{-1} varied from 97 ± 24 to 602 ± 180 pg/ml. Release of CCK was dose dependent.

Bombesin caused stimulation of pancreatic secretion, and eventually gallbladder contraction, in all mammalian and avian species tested. However, the mechanism of action of the peptide cannot be generalized. The various species must be studied separately, and then it will be seen that in the guinea pig, rat, and mouse, bombesin seems to act on its target organs mostly directly, and not indirectly through release of CCK.

In man bombesin caused contraction of the gallbladder and striking stimulation of pancreatic enzyme secretion. Emptying of the gallbladder was seen at bombesin doses as low as 0.12 μg kg^{-1}h^{-1}, and 0.3 μg kg^{-1}h^{-1} elicited an effect close to that obtained with a fatty meal. Response began about 10 min after the infusion was started and sometimes progressed after the infusion had been discontinued (22). At a dose of 1 μg kg^{-1}h^{-1} bombesin caused a 9- to 10-fold increase of amylase and trypsin concentrations in the duodenal juice, and a 10- to 15-fold rise in total enzyme outputs, whereas bicarbonate concentration was unchanged (3). The mechanism of action of bombesin on the human gallbladder and pancreas has to be established, since no data are available on immunoreactive CCK levels in human plasma following bombesin administration. A CCK release seems most likely, however.

On the isolated guinea pig gallbladder, bombesin and litorin showed 1 to 4% of the action of cerulein, and as much as 5 to 20% of the action of cerulein on the in situ guinea pig gallbladder. On intravenous injection this effect was immediate and tachyphylaxis was apparently lacking (30).

As already stated, in vivo and in vitro studies carried out in the rat, mouse, and guinea pig strongly suggest that in these species a direct effect of bombesin on the pancreatic tissue is predominant. Again, studies on plasma-immunoreactive CCK are lacking.

In the intact anesthetized rat graded doses of bombesin or litorin produced graded increases of pancreatic juice flow and amylase or protein outputs. Threshold dose was approximately 0.3 to 0.6 μg kg^{-1}h^{-1}, and maximum response was obtained with 5 to 10 μg kg^{-1}h^{-1}. Increase in amylase output was not accompanied by changes in amylase concentration. Pancreatic stimulation was practically unaffected either by atropine or enterectomy. Cerulein was 2.5 to 10 times more active than bombesin (20,43).

Bombesin acted as a powerful stimulant of the amylase secretion also in rat and mouse pancreatic fragments. A fivefold increase in amylase output was induced on the average by 10^{-9} bombesin within 5 min and maintained for at least 30 min. Cyclic AMP content was not influenced. After addition of the peptide to isolated pancreatic acinar cells, there was a prompt fall of cellular ^{45}Ca due to enhancement of ^{45}Ca outflux. The adenylate cyclase activity of purified pancreatic plasma membranes was insensitive to bombesin (20,23,24).

The peptide caused depolarization of rat and mouse pancreatic cell membrane and reduction of membrane resistance; these effects were detectable at concentrations of approximately 30 pM, and were maximal at approximately 10 nM. In the higher dose range an electrical uncoupling of acinar cells within an acinus was observed, suggestive of a marked increase in junctional membrane resistance. These results were confirmed by microionophoretic peptide application on acinar cells of superfused segments of mouse pancreas. According to Iwatsuki and Petersen (38) and Petersen and Philpott (54), bombesin, CCK, cerulein, gastrin, and acetylcholine, although acting on different receptors, evoked the observed changes in electrical properties of acinar cell membrane through a common pathway.

Bombesin nonapeptide resembled CCK and acetylcholine also in its interaction with secretin: amylase secretion from rat pancreatic lobules *in vitro* elicited by bombesin nonapeptide was significantly potentiated by secretin (60).

Results obtained on the guinea pig pancreas were similar. In dispersed acinar cells bombesin and litorin increased outflux of ^{45}Ca, release of bound ^{45}Ca, initial ^{45}Ca uptake, accumulation of cyclic GMP, and release of amylase. These effects were atropine-resistant. Neither bombesin nor litorin altered cellular cyclic AMP or the increase caused by secretin or VIP. Bombesin and litorin were each approximately 10 times less potent and 85% as effective as cerulein in stimulating ^{45}Ca outflux. Threshold concentration was 5×10^{-10} M (44).

Strong and perhaps decisive support in favor of a direct action of bombesin-like peptides on the guinea pig acinar cells has been afforded by Jensen et al. (39), who found that bombesin and related peptides interacted with specific membrane receptors on the acinar cells, inhibiting binding of (^{125}I-4-tyrosyl)-bombesin. Acinar cells possessed approximately 5,000 receptors/cell and occupation of 25% of these receptors by bombesin-like peptides was sufficient to cause maximal changes in acinar cell function, including amylase secretion. Litorin was approximately 10% as active as bombesin in causing half-maximal inhibition of binding. Cerulein and CCK-octapeptide caused a 15 to 20% reduction of (^{125}I-4-tyrosyl)-bombesin binding only at concentrations above 0.1 M.

Bombesin strongly stimulated pancreatic secretion also in the chicken. By intravenous infusion the threshold dose was of the order of 0.45 to 0.9 μg kg^{-1}h^{-1}, and maximum effects were obtained with 3 to 4 μg kg^{-1}h^{-1}. At this dose level volume and bicarbonate outputs rose by about 2.5 times, whereas amylase and tryptic activities increased by 10 and 15 times, respectively. Because response to bombesin was not immediate but developed after a 15 min latency period and since it showed evidence of tachyphylaxis Linari et al. (43) suggested that it might be mediated, like in the dog, through release of CCK.

Action on Myoelectric and Mechanical Activity of the Gut

In conscious dogs provided with electrodes chronically implanted on the serosal surface of different gastrointestinal segments, bombesin infused for 30 min at a rate of 0.3 to 1 μg kg^{-1}h^{-1} produced a significant increase in the frequency of pacesetter potentials in antrum, duodenum, jejunum, and ileum. In the duodenum and jejunum, the increase in frequency showed linear correlation with the reduction of pacesetter potentials amplitude. The propagation velocity of

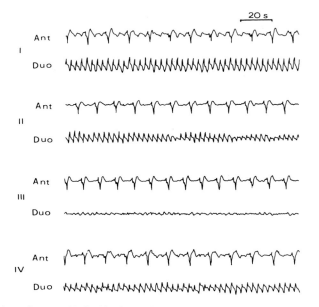

FIG. 3. Conscious dog provided with electrodes chronically implanted on the serosal surface of different gastrointestinal segments. Pacesetter potentials of the antrum (Ant) and the duodenum (Duo) before litorin administration (I), during an intravenous infusion of 10 ng kg^{-1}min^{-1} of litorin at 10 and 30 min of infusion, respectively (II and III), and 20 min after discontinuing litorin infusin (IV). (From ref. 25, with permission.)

the pacesetter potentials was approximately halved. At high infusion rates of bombesin disappearance of rhythmicity of contractions of the duodenum and upper jejunum was observed, with appearance of an irregular sequence of slow and small potentials (Fig. 3). This could be interpreted as due to the failure of coupling between relaxation oscillators over critical maximal frequencies. During recovery, electrical activity gradually returned toward the preinfusion pattern. Neither the C-terminal bombesin heptapeptide nor the octapeptide showed a significant effect on gastrointestinal myoelectric activity, whereas the effect of the nonapeptide and of litorin was 60 to 70% of that of bombesin (19).

In the conscious fasted dog, doses of bombesin of 2 to 5 ng $kg^{-1}min^{-1}$ resulted in termination of the interdigestive migrating complex within 2 min from the beginning of infusion (Fig. 4). After the infusion was discontinued, there was an increase in the frequency and propagation velocity of the interdigestive migrating complex (45).

The dog stomach responded to bombesin infusion (threshold 0.06 μg $kg^{-1}h^{-1}$) with contraction of the pylorus and the antrum accompanied by complete loss of basal motility and relaxation of the body and fundus, as shown by reduction of intragastric pressure. Somatostatin infusion did not affect the response to bombesin (9,12).

In man, administration of 0.6 μg $kg^{-1}h^{-1}$ of bombesin resulted in a brief increase followed by total inhibition of mechanical activity in the duodenum, whereas in the jejunum an immediate and almost total inhibition of mechanical activity was observed during the whole infusion period. Radiologically, there

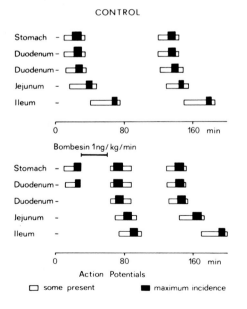

FIG. 4. Conscious fasted dogs provided with electrodes chronically implanted on the serosal surface of different gastrointestinal segments. Migration of the interdigestive complexes (action potentials) in the control animal and following intravenous infusion of 1 ng $kg^{-1}min^{-1}$ of bombesin for 30 min.

was a hypotonic dilatation of the duodenum but no evidence of change in jejunal tone. The pyloric antral region and the ileo-cecal valve were contracted. Motor hyperactivity and increased transit rate were observed in the postinfusional period. The bombesin nonapeptide was as potent as, or more potent than, bombesin itself. The rapid appearance and disappearance of the effects just after the beginning and the end of the peptide infusion suggest that bombesin acts directly on the intestinal smooth muscle. However, the postinfusional mechanical hyperactivity could be mediated by the release of CCK (10,21).

Action on Intestinal Absorption of Water and Electrolytes

Bombesin infused over a 60-min period at a rate of 0.6 μg kg^{-1}h^{-1} produced a 50% reduction of ^{3}H$_2$O, ^{24}Na, and chloride absorption by a perfused Thiry-Vella intestinal loop in the dog. A similar effect was observed in the mini-pig at an infusion rate of 1.8 μg kg^{-1}h^{-1}. At the same time there was a 40 to 60% increase in the bicarbonate excretion (Sopranzi and Improta, *in preparation*).

RELEASE AND RELEASE-INHIBITING EFFECTS OF BOMBESIN ON OTHER PEPTIDE HORMONES

Pancreatic Peptide (PP)

Bombesin is a very potent stimulant of PP release in the dog. A 2-hr infusion of 62 ng kg^{-1}h^{-1} of bombesin produced a mean increment in plasma PP concentration of 34 $\pm$ 20 pmoles/liter, and an infusion of 500 ng kg^{-1}h^{-1} caused an increment of 240 $\pm$ 92 pmoles/liter. Response to a meal in the same dogs over the same period of time was 170.6 $\pm$ 34 pmoles/liter. Atropine significantly inhibited bombesin-stimulated release of PP; bethanechol was ineffective (58). These results were confirmed in man (11).

Gastric Inhibitory Peptide (GIP)

Bombesin is a potent GIP releaser in the dog. Following intravenous infusion of 1 μg kg^{-1}h^{-1} of the peptide, immunoreactive GIP levels in plasma rose from 109 $\pm$ 12 to 544 $\pm$ 62 pg/ml at 60 min, and following 0.5 μg kg$^-$h^{-1} from a basal level of 139 $\pm$ 26 to 360 $\pm$ 39 pg/ml. Antral acidification did not significantly alter GIP release (6). These results were not confirmed in man (11).

Enteroglucagon

The intravenous infusion of 0.62, 2.5, and 10 pmoles kg^{-1}min$^-$ of bombesin for 30 min in five human volunteers caused a significant elevation of immunoreactive enteroglucagon plasma levels from 24 $\pm$ 4 to 36 $\pm$ 11, 42 $\pm$ 12, and 44 $\pm$ 4 pmoles/liter, respectively, at 20 min (11).

Motilin

Under the same conditions plasma levels of immunoreactive motilin rose from 12 ± 2 to 85 ± 27, 70 ± 18, and 50 ± 11 pmoles/liter, respectively, at 25 min (11). It may be seen that maximum release of motilin was produced by the lowest dose of bombesin.

Neurotensin

In man, plasma levels of immunoreactive neurotensin showed a twofold increase following bombesin infusion (11).

Glucagon

The statement by Fallucca et al. (33) that in man bombesin also causes an increase in plasma levels of immunoreactive glucagon was not confirmed by others (11). This may depend on the different specificity of the antisera used.

Vasoactive Intestinal Peptide (VIP)

In the dog, cat, and man, bombesin infusion inhibited the release of VIP, as shown by a fall of plasma VIP immunoreactivity levels (45).

Secretin

In the dog, secretin was not released by bombesin (47).

Insulin

Intravenous infusion of bombesin, up to 1 μg kg^{-1}h^{-1}, did not significantly change serum insulin levels (6).

Extraintestinal Hormonal Peptides

Bombesin and related peptides produced an activation of the renin-angiotensin system as well as erythropoietin release in the dog (32,47) while inhibiting TRH release in the rat (18).

It is at present impossible to have an idea of whether this astonishing array of releasing effects displayed by bombesin actually depends on a direct, specific action of the bombesin molecule on the different peptide cells or whether it is in part the indirect consequence of release or inhibition of release of a more limited number of primarily involved peptides.

CENTRAL EFFECTS

An important chapter in bombesin investigation was opened by Brown et al. (14–18), who found that bombesin and related peptides displayed in the rat CSN striking and important actions. The premise for these studies was the demonstration that bombesin-like peptides occurred not only in the amphibian skin, but also in the gastrointestinal mucosa of mammals and birds and in the CNS of mammals (see Chapter 29 by Melchiorri, pp. 717–729, *this volume*).

PHARMACOKINETICS

During a 60-min infusion of bombesin into human volunteers, at a rate of 4 and 8 ng kg^{-1}min^{1}, plasma concentrations of bombesin rose to a mean plateau of 0.77 and 1.5 ng/ml, respectively. The disappearance half-time on stopping the infusion was 5.25 min. The apparent distribution space was calculated to be 39.46 ml kg^{-1}, and the metabolic clearance rate was 5.21 ml kg^{-1}min^{-1} (44).

RELATIVE POTENCY OF BOMBESIN-LIKE PEPTIDES. STRUCTURE-ACTIVITY RELATIONSHIP

The five natural bombesin-like peptides occurring, in addition to bombesin, in amphibian skin and approximately 35 synthetic analogs have been compared with bombesin and/or litorin on a set of *in vitro* and *in vivo* preparations. This was done in order to determine the minimum length of the amino acid chain necessary for the appearance of bombesin activity, its minimum length for maximal activity, the key amino acid residues, and the possibility of dissociating the effects displayed on different target organs. This research may be considered only at its beginning but appears to be promising.

A few results are presented in Table 1. Other more numerous ones are discussed elsewhere (13,14,25,29).

Without entering into details, a few general conclusions may be stated:

(a) A minimum C-terminal sequence of seven amino acid residues was re-

TABLE 1. *Relative potency of bombesin-like peptides on a weight basis*

	Bombesin = 100			Litorin = 100
	Octapeptide[a]	Nonapeptide[a]	Litorin	Glu (OMe)²-Litorin
Rat large intestine	10–20	90–130	300–800	10–15
Guinea pig large intestine	1–10	100–120	200–500	5–15
Kitten small intestine	1–4	100–150	150–350	2–4
Guinea pig gallbladder *in situ*	=	100–125	200–250	5–10
Rat pancreas	=	90	35	=
Gastrin release (dog)	=	100	50	=
Gut myoelectric activity (dog)	10	75	50	=

Octapeptide and nonapeptide, C-terminal octa- and nonapeptide of bombesin; =, not investigated.

quired for the appearance of bombesin-like effects. The C-terminal hexapeptide was quite inactive, as were the N-terminal octa- and endecapeptides.

(b) Addition of the glutamine residue to the N-terminus of the heptapeptide produced a 5- to 20-fold increase of activity on all the smooth muscle preparations tested. Addition of an asparagine residue to the N-terminus of the octapeptide also produced a striking increase of activity in all the preparations tested. The C-terminal nonapeptide of bombesin was as active as, or even more active than, bombesin on all isolated smooth muscle preparations tested. In the *in vivo* test objects the nonapeptide had, on a weight basis, 50 to 150% of the activity of bombesin. No appreciable differences in activity could be seen between the nona- and the decapeptide, and between the deca- and the endecapeptide.

(c) Amino acid substitutions in the N-terminal moiety of the sequence were tolerated without appreciable losses of activity. This was not true for substitutions in the C-terminal moiety, which apparently contains the key amino acids of the molecule. For example, the presence of the L-tryptophan residue at position 8 and of a histidine residue at position 12 seemed necessary for the appearance of bombesin-like activity. L-Tryptophan could not be substituted for D-tryptophan. Similarly substitution of an alanine residue for the glycine residue at position 11 was accompanied by complete loss of activity.

(d) Litorin differed sharply from bombesin not only in the more rapid onset and disappearance of the effects, but also in its weak action on renin release in the dog, and PRL and GH secretion and thermoregulation in the rat. Glu(OMe)^2-litorin, in turn, differed markedly from litorin in its effects on isolated and *in situ* smooth muscle preparations.

(e) The pharmacological effects of alytesin, as tested so far, were exactly identical to those of bombesin. For ranatensin, the only comparative studies available concern thermoregulation and PRL and GH secretion in the rat, in which it was 10% and 2%, respectively, as active as bombesin (15).

These fragmentary and preliminary observations clearly demonstrate the feasibility of obtaining considerable quantitative changes in the spectrum of activity of bombesin-like peptides by suitable modifications in the length and composition of the amino acid sequence.

CONCLUSIONS AND PROJECTIONS FOR THE FUTURE

Three major peptide families of the amphibian skin have been discussed in this and in the preceding chapter of this volume: the tachykinins, the ceruleins, and the bombesin-like peptides. Other amphibian peptides active on the gut and having their counterpart in the mammalian gastrointestinal tract were not taken into consideration at the present time because their distribution in the amphibian skin has not yet been studied sufficiently and/or because their effects on the gastrointestinal tract are unknown.

We refer to xenopsin (Pyr-Gly-Lys-Arg-Pro-Trp-Ile-Leu), the counterpart, in the amphibian skin, of neurotensin, to immunoreactive VIP occurring in the skin of a few frogs, to thyrotropin-releasing hormone (Pyr-His-Pro-NH$_2$) contained, in large amounts, in the skin of *Bombina orientalis* and *Rana pipiens,* and finally to crinia-angiotensin II (Ala-Pro-Gly-Asp-Arg-Ile-Tyr-Val-His-Pro-Phe), an interesting counterpart of the plasma angiotensins II. It is certain that in the near future the number of members of the single families here described will increase and that other amphibian peptide families will join these already well established.

PROJECTIONS FOR THE FUTURE

At the present time the discovery of any new peptide in the amphibian skin is the incentive for the obligatory search of its counterpart in the mammalian intestine and brain. Vice versa, any intestinal and brain peptide must be checked for its duplicate in amphibian skin. The existence of a gut-brain-skin triangle is becoming a well established fact.

The chapter in this volume by P. Melchiorri (Chapter 30) illustrates how rewarding is the study of the amphibian skin peptides as an incentive for the search of new hormonal peptides in the gastrointestinal tract and brain in mammals.

Note added in proof: After preparation and submission of this manuscript two new peptide families have been definitely identified in the amphibian skin. The elucidation of their structure and the study of their pharmacological actions is in progress, and there are already sound reasons to believe that counterparts of these peptides occur in brain and intestine, where they appear to display striking effects.

ACKNOWLEDGMENT

Original research by the author and his co-workers quoted in this chapter has been supported throughout by grants from the Consiglio Nazionale delle Richerche, Rome.

REFERENCES

1. Anastasi, A., Erspamer, V., and Endean, R. (1975): Aminoacid composition and sequence of litorin, a bombesin-like nonapeptide from the skin of the Australian leptodactylid frog *Litoria aurea. Experientia,* 31:510.
2. Anastasi, A., Montecucchi, P., Angelucci, F., Erspamer, V., and Endean, R. (1977): Glu(OMe)^2-litorin, the second bombesin-like peptide occurring in methanol extracts of the skin of the Australian frog *Litoria aurea. Experientia,* 33:1289.
3. Basso, N., Giri, S., Improta, G., Lezoche, E., Melchiorri, P., Percoco, M., and Speranza, V. (1975): External pancreatic secretion after bombesin infusion in man. *Gut,* 16:994–998.
4. Basso, N., Giri, S., Lezoche, E., Materia, A., Melchiorri, P., and Speranza, V. (1976): Effect of secretin, glucagon and duodenal acidification on bombesin-induced hypergastrinemia in man. *Am. J. Gastroenterol.,* 66:44–451.
5. Basso, N., Lezoche, E., Giri, S., Percoco, M., and Speranza, V. (1977): Acid and gastrin levels after bombesin and calcium infusion in patients with incomplete antrectomy. *Am. J. Digest. Dis.,* 22:125–128.

6. Becker, H. D., Borger, H. W., Schafmayer, A., and Werner, M. (1978): Bombesin releases GIP in dogs. *Scand. J. Gastroenterol. (Suppl. 49)*, 13:14.
7. Bertaccini, G., Erspamer, V., and Impicciatore, M. (1973): The actions of bombesin on gastric secretions of the dog and the rat. *Br. J. Pharmacol.*, 49:437–44.
8. Bertaccini, G., Erspamer, V., Melchiorri, P., and Sopranzi, N. (1974): Gastrin release by bombesin in the dog. *Br. J. Pharmacol.*, 52:219–225.
9. Bertaccini, G., and Impicciatore, M. (1974): Action of bombesin on the motility of the stomach. *Rendic. Gastroenterol.*, 6:81–82.
10. Bertaccini, G., Impicciatore, M., Molina, E., and Zappia, L. (1974): Action of bombesin on human gastrointestinal motility. *Rendic. Gastroenterol.*, 6:45–51.
11. Bloom, S. R., Chatei, M. A., Christofides, N. D., Blackburn, A. M., Adrian, T. E., Lezoche, E., Basso, N., Carlei, F., and Speranza, V. (1979): Bombesin infusion in man, pharmacokinetics and effect on gastrointestinal and pancreatic hormonal peptides. *J. Endocrinol.*, 83:P51.
12. Broccardo, M. (1977): Effect of bombesin and GH-RIH on intragastric pressure in the dog. *Internat. Symposium Gastrointestinal Hormones and Pathol. Dig. System.* Rome, June 13–15. Abstr., p. 130.
13. Broccardo, M., Falconieri Erspamer, G., Melchiorri, P., Negri, L., and De Castiglione, R. (1975): Relative potency of bombesin-like peptides. *Br. J. Pharmacol.*, 55:221–227.
14. Brown, M., Rivier, J., Kobayashi, R., and Vale, W. (1978): Neurotensin-like and bombesin-like peptides: CNS distribution and actions. In *Gut Hormones,* edited by S. R. Bloom, pp. 550–558. Churchill Livingstone, Edinburgh/London/New York.
15. Brown, M., Rivier, J., and Vale, W. (1977): Bombesin: Potent effects on thermoregulation in the rat. *Science,* 196:998–999.
16. Brown, M., Rivier, J., and Vale, W. (1977): Actions of bombesin, thyrotropin releasing factor, prostaglandin E_2 and naloxone on thermoregulation in the rat. *Life Sci.,* 202:1681–1688.
17. Brown, M. R., Rivier, J., and Vale, W. (1977): Bombesin affects central nervous system to produce hyperglycemia in rats. *Life Sci.,* 21:1729–1734.
18. Brown, M. R., Rivier, J. E., Wolfe, A. I., and Vale, W. (1977): TRF and bombesin: Actions on thermoregulation and TSH secretion in rats. *Endocrinology,* 100:265A.
19. Caprilli, R., Melchiorri, P., Improta, G., Vernia, P., and Frieri, G. (1975): Effects of bombesin and bombesin-like peptides on gastrointestinal myoelectric activity. *Gastroenterology,* 68:1228–1235.
20. Christophe, J., Deschodt-Lanckman, M., Adler, M., and Robberecht, P. (1977): *In vitro* and *in vivo* effects of bombesin and bombesin-like peptides on the rat pancreas. Mechanism of action. In *Hormonal Receptors in the Digestive Tract Physiology.* INSERM Symp. No. 3, edited by S. Bonfils, P. Fromageot and G. Rosselin, pp. 247–260. North-Holland, Amsterdam/New York/Oxford.
21. Corazziari, E., Torsoli, A., Delle Fave, G. F., Melchiorri, P., and Habib, F. I. (1974): Effects of bombesin on the mechanical activity of the human duodenum and jejunum. *Rendic. Gastroenterol.,* 6:55–59.
22. Corazziari, E., Torsoli, A., Melchiorri, P., and Delle Fave, G. F. (1974): Effect of bombesin on human gallbladder emptying. *Rendic. Gastroenterol.,* 6:52–54.
23. Deschodt-Lanckman, M., Robberecht, P., De Neef, Ph., Labrie, F., and Christophe, J. (1975): *In vitro* interactions of gastrointestinal hormones on cyclic adenosine 3':5'-monophosphate levels and amylase output in the rat pancreas. *Gastroenterology,* 68:318–325.
24. Deschodt-Lanckman, P., Robberecht, P., De Neef, P., Lammers, M., and Christophe, J. (1976): *In vitro* action of bombesin and bombesin-like peptides on amylase secretion, calcium efflux and adenylate cyclase activity in the rat pancreas. *J. Clin. Invest.,* 58:891–898.
25. Endean, R., Erspamer, V., Falconieri Erspamer, G., Improta, G., Melchiorri, M., Negri, L., and Sopranzi, N. (1975): Parallel bioassay of bombesin and litorin, a bombesin-like peptide from the skin of *Litoria aurea. Br. J. Pharmacol.,* 55:213–219.
26. Erspamer, V., Falconieri Erspamer, G., Inselvini, M., and Negri, L. (1972): Occurrence of bombesin and alytesin in extracts of the skin of three European discoglossid frogs and pharmacological actions of bombesin on extravascular smooth muscle. *Br. J. Pharmacol.,* 45:333–348.
27. Erspamer, V., Falconieri Erspamer, G., Melchiorri, P., and Negri, L. (1979): Occurrence and polymorphism of bombesin-like peptides in the gastrointestinal tract of birds and mammals. *Gut,* 20 *(in press).*
28. Erspamer, V., Improta, G., Melchiorri, P., and Sopranzi, N. (1974): Evidence of cholecystokinin release by bombesin in the dog. *Br. J. Pharmacol.,* 52:227–232.

29. Erspamer, V., and Melchiorri, P. (1973): Active polypeptides of the amphibian skin and their synthetic analogues. *Pure Appl. Chem.*, 35:463–494.
30. Erspamer, V., and Melchiorri, P. (1975): Actions of bombesin on secretions and motility of the gastrointestinal tract. In: *Gastrointestinal Hormones*, edited by Thompson, pp. 575–589. University of Texas Press, Austin and London.
31. Erspamer, V., Melchiorri, P., Falconieri Erspamer, G., and Negri, L. (1978): Polypeptides of the amphibian skin active on the gut and their mammalian counterparts. In: *Gastrointestinal Hormones and Pathology of the Digestive System*, edited by M. Grossman, V. Speranza, N. Basso, and E. Lezoche, pp. 51–64. Plenum Press, New York and London.
32. Erspamer, V., Melchiorri, and Sopranzi, N. (1973): The action of bombesin on the kidney of the anaesthetized dog. *Br. J. Pharmacol.*, 48:438–455.
33. Fallucca, F., Delle Fave, G., Gambardella, S., Mirabella, C., De Magistris, L., and Carratù, R. (1978): Glucagon secretion induced by bombesin in man. In: *Gastrointestinal Hormones and Pathology of the Digestive System*, edited by M. Grossman, V. Speranza, N. Basso, and E. Lezoche, pp. 259–261. Plenum Press, New York and London.
34. Fender, H. R., Curtis, P. J., Rayford, Ph. L., and Thompson, J. C. (1976): Effect of bombesin on serum gastrin and cholecystokinin in dogs. *Surg. Forum*, 37:4141–4146.
35. Hirschowitz, B. I., and Gibson, R. G. (1978): Cholinergic stimulation and suppression of gastrin release in gastric fistula dogs. *Am. J. Physiol.*, 235:720–725.
36. Hirschowitz, B. I., and Gibson, R. G. (1979): Stimulation of gastrin release and gastric secretion: Effect of bombesin and a nonapeptide in fistula dogs with and without fundic vagotomy. *Digestion* 18:227–239.
37. Impicciatore, M., Debas, H., Walsh, J. H., Grossman, M. I., and Bertaccini, G. (1974): Release of gastrin and stimulation of acid secretion by bombesin in dog. *Rendic. Gastroenterol.*, 6:99–101.
38. Iwatsuki, N., and Peterson, O. H. (1978): *In vitro* action of bombesin on amylase secretion, membrane potentials and membrane resistance in rat and mouse acinar cells. Comparison with other secretagogues. *J. Clin. Invest.*, 61:41–46.
39. Jensen, R. T., Moody, T., Pert, C., Brown, M., Rivier, J. R., and Gardner, J. D. (1978): Interaction of bombesin and litorin with specific membrane receptors on pancreatic acinar cells. *Scand. J. Gastroenterol. (Suppl. 49)*, 13:94.
40. Konturek, S. J., Krol, R., and Tasler, J. (1976): Effect of bombesin and related peptides on the release and action of intestinal hormones on pancreatic secretion. *J. Physiol. (Lond.)*, 257:663–672.
41. Lezoche, E., Matarazzo, P. F., Vagni, V., Basso, N., and Speranza, V. (1978): Potentiation of food-stimulated gastrin by bombesin. *Gastroenterology*, 74:(Part 2)1132.
42. Linari, G., Baldieri, M., and Angelucci, L. (1975): The action of bombesin on gastric secretion of the chicken. *Eur. J. Pharmacol.*, 34:143–150.
43. Linari, G., Baldieri Linari, M., and Lutoslawska, G. (1977): The action of bombesin and litorin on pancreatic secretion of the rat. *Rendic. Gastroenterol.*, 9:178–184.
44. May, R. J., Conlon, T. P., Erspamer, V., and Gardner, J. D. (1978): Actions of peptides isolated from amphibian skin on pancreatic acinar cells. *Am. J. Physiol.*, 235:E112–E118.
45. Melchiorri, P. (1978): Bombesin and bombesin-like peptides of amphibian skin. In: *Gut Hormones*, edited by S. R. Bloom, pp. 534–540. Churchill Livingstone, Edinburgh/London/New York.
46. Melchiorri, P., Improta, G., and Sopranzi, N. (1975): Inibizione della secrezione di VIP da parte della bombesina nel cane, nel gatto e nell'uomo. *Rendic. Gastroenterol. (Suppl. 1)*, 7:57.
47. Melchiorri, P., Sopranzi, N., and Roseghini, M. (1976): Effects of bombesin on erythropoietin production in the anaesthetized dog. *Naunyn-Schmiedeberg's Arch. Pharmakol.*, 294:193–197.
48. Mennini, C., Basso, N., Minervini, S., Longo, R., Pallottini, P., Salemme, A., and Speranza, V. (1978): Meccanismo di azione della bombesina sulla secrezione pancreatica: perfusione di pancreas isolato di cane. *Policlinico (Sez. Chir.)*, 85:426–433.
49. Miyata, M., Guzman, S., Rayford, P. L., and Thompson, J. C. (1978): Effects of bombesin on release of gastrin, CCK, secretin and pancreatic exocrine secretion. *Gastroenterology*, 74:(Part 2)1137.
50. Miyata, M., (1979): Personal communication.
51. Miyata, M., Rayford, P. L., and Thompson, J. C. (1978): Influence of duodenal acidification on the secretion and hormonal release effects of bombesin. *Scand. J. Gastroenterol. (Suppl. 49)*, 13:123.

52. Nakajima, T., Tanimara, T., and Pisano, J. J. (1970): Isolation and structure of a new vasoactive polypeptide. *Fed. Proc.,* 29:282.
53. Nakajima, T., Yasuhara, T., Falconieri Erspamer, G., Negri, L., and Endean, R. (1979): Physalaemin- and bombesin-like peptides in the skin of the Australian leptodactylid frog *Uperoleia rugosa. Chem. Pharm. Bull. (in press).*
54. Petersen, O. H., and Philpott, H. G. (1979): Pancreatic acinar cells: Effects of microionophoretic caerulein and bombesin nonapeptide application on membrane potential and resistance. *J. Physiol. (Lond.),* 290:305–315.
55. Rivier, C., Rivier, J., and Vale, W. (1978): The effect of bombesin and related peptides on prolactin and growth hormone secretion in the rat. *Endocrinology,* 102:519–522.
56. Schaefmeyer, A., Teichmann, R. K., Swierczek, J. S., Rayford, P. L., and Thompson, J. C. (1978): Influence of vagus on mechanism for stimulation and inhibition of gastrin release. *Surgery,* 83:711–716.
57. Speranza, V., Basso, N., and Lezoche, E. (1978): Effect of bombesin and calcium on serum gastrin levels in patients with retained or excluded antral mucosa. In: *Gastrointestinal Hormones and Pathology of the Digestive System,* edited by M. Grossman, V. Speranza, L. Basso, and E. Lezoche, pp. 319–324. Plenum Press, New York and London.
58. Taylor, I. L., Walsh, J. H., Carter, D. C., Wood, J., and Grossman, M. I. (1978): Effect of atropine and bethanechol on release of pancreatic polypeptide (PP) and gastrin by bombesin in dog. *Scand. J. Gastroenterol. (Suppl. 49),* 13:183.
59. Thompson, J. C., Schaefmeyer, A., Guzman, S., and Rayford, P. L. (1978): Vagal influences in the stimulation and inhibition of gastrin release. *Scand. J. Gastroenterol. (Suppl. 49),* 13:185.
60. Wolpert, D. N., Mullican, Ch. I., and Salomon, T. E. (1979): Interaction of bombesin-nonapeptide and secretion on rat pancreas *in vitro. Gastroenterology (submitted).*
61. Yasuhara, T., Ishikawa, O., Nakajima, T., and Tachibana, S. (1974): The active substances on smooth muscle in the skin of *Rana rugosa. Proceed. 12th Symposium Peptide Chemistry,* edited by H. Yajima, p. 68. Protein Research Foundation, Osaka.
62. Yoshida, H., Takajima, T., Sakurai, K., and Fujita, Y. (1973): Isolation of biological active peptides from the skin of *Rana catasbeiana. Proceed. 11th Symposium Peptide Chemistry,* edited by H. Yajima, p. 116. Protein Research Foundation, Osaka.

Gastrointestinal Hormones, edited by
George B. Jerzy Glass.
Raven Press, New York © 1980.

Chapter 15

Somatostatin, Enkephalins, and Endorphins

Chester A. Meyers and David H. Coy

*Department of Medicine, Tulane University School of Medicine,
New Orleans, Louisiana 70112*

SOMATOSTATIN

Somatostatin is a cyclic tetradecapeptide that was isolated from mammalian hypothalami and named for its ability to inhibit growth hormone (GH) release from anterior pituitary cells. The hormone was soon found to have numerous actions on a variety of substances from diverse tissues, a finding that gained physiological significance when high concentrations of somatostatin-like immunoreactivity were demonstrated in those tissues. Remarkably, somatostatin is localized in the hypothalamus, pancreas, stomach, and brain, and it inhibits the release of GH, thyroid-stimulating hormone (TSH), insulin, glucagon, gastrin and gastric acid, secretin, and several other gut hormones. Even actions in the central nervous system (CNS) have been described. A hormone as versatile as somatostatin has important physiological implications and clinical potential that are being exploited by extensive structure-function studies that may, through the development of selective and long-acting synthetic analogs, lead to useful therapeutic agents for the treatment of diseases such as diabetes mellitus and acromegaly.

Several reviews on somatostatin have appeared (130,131,151).

ISOLATION AND STRUCTURE

The presence of a substance in ovine hypothalamic extracts that inhibits the basal release of immunoreactive pituitary growth hormone from rats *in vitro* was first demonstrated by Krulich et al. (77) and by Krulich and McCann (78). This observation was confirmed by the isolation of a peptide from sheep (16) and subsequently from pig (133) hypothalami that actively inhibited GH release *in vitro* and *in vivo*. The purification of the native hormone required extensive column chromatography and countercurrent distribution of fractions obtained from extracts of nearly one-half million ovine or porcine hypothalami. Fractions at various stages of purification were assayed for their ability to inhibit the release of radioimmunoassayable GH from enzymatically dispersed rat anterior pituitary cells in monolayer cultures (149). The ovine peptide was characterized by stepwise Edman degradation and mass spectroscopy, and found to be a cyclic tetradecapeptide with the amino acid sequence shown in Fig. 1 (16,24). The porcine material had the identical structure. The peptide was named somatostatin and was synthesized in several laboratories by a variety of solution and solid phase techniques (31,115,123,164). This provided the necessary quantities of material for extensive basic and clinical investigations. These studies were also facilitated by the development in our laboratory of a highly specific radioimmunoassay (RIA) for somatostatin (2).

Larger and more basic forms of somatostatin recently found in pig hypothalami are biologically and immunologically active, and may therefore represent precursors of somatostatin (132,133). High concentrations of somatostatin have also been found in extracts of pancreas, stomach, and duodenum along with two types of immunoreactive somatostatin (3), supporting observations that somatostatin has actions in several tissues.

H-Ala-Gly-Cys-Lys-Asn-Phe-Phe-Trp-Lys-Thr-Phe-Thr-Ser-Cys-Oh
 1   2   3   4   5   6   7   8   9   10   11   12   13   14

FIG. 1. Structure of somatostatin.

BIOLOGICAL ACTIONS OF SOMATOSTATIN

Pituitary

The availability of synthetic somatostatin resulted in numerous studies of its biological effects *in vitro* and *in vivo*. As mentioned, basal rat GH is inhibited by somatostatin *in vitro* from cultured pituitary cells and it was this assay that provided a basic tool during the isolation of the native hormone (16,133). Somatostatin also inhibits the stimulated secretion of GH *in vitro;* secretagogues used in these experiments included theophylline, derivatives of cyclic AMP, and prostaglandins (148). The GH release-inhibiting activity of somatostatin has now been confirmed by a variety of *in vivo* and *in vitro* assays in several species, including rats, dogs, sheep, baboons, and humans (10,59,130,135,151). In the *in vivo* models, somatostatin suppressed elevated plasma GH levels induced by such varied stimuli as barbiturates, L-DOPA, arginine, insulin, morphine, prostaglandin E_2, exercise, sleep, electrical stimulation of hypothalamus or amygdala, and catecholamines, including their infusion into the third ventricle (130,151).

Somatostatin also inhibits the release of pituitary TSH *in vitro* and *in vivo* (26,40,130,150,151). In normal man, the thyrotropin-releasing hormone (TRH)-induced secretion of TSH is inhibited by somatostatin, and the response is dose-dependent (26). Inhibition of spontaneous prolactin release by somatostatin has been observed *in vitro* (150), but appears not to be affected in normal individuals (60).

In addition to its presence in the hypothalamus, a physiological role of somatostatin in the regulation of GH and TSH secretion is supported by passive immunization studies in rats. Anti-somatostatin serum elevates basal GH levels and also prevents the stress-induced fall of GH in these animals (5,49). Similarly, somatostatin antiserum increases basal TSH levels and blocks the stress-induced decrease in TSH secretion. Anti-somatostatin also potentiates the TSH response to cold and TRH (4,5,49).

Somatostatin has been studied in a number of clinical situations involving pituitary tumors. It suppresses fasting GH levels in patients with acromegaly (10,59,168), but fails to inhibit GH induced by TRH or luteinizing hormone-releasing hormone (LH-RH) in such patients (53). Interestingly, elevated ACTH levels in patients with Nelson's syndrome, and in one patient with Cushing's disease, were suppressed by somatostatin infusion (145), whereas no effect on basal or insulin-hypoglycemia-induced corticotropin secretion was observed in normal subjects (59).

The reduced (linear) form of somatostatin (dihydrosomatostatin) is reported to be as active as the native oxidized (cyclic) form, suggesting that cyclization of the former occurs during the biological assays (151). Somatostatin acts directly on the pituitary to inhibit GH secretion, apparently without affecting its synthesis (60,151), but it has been reported to block TSH synthesis (150).

Pancreas

The first evidence that somatostatin affected the endocrine pancreas was the observation that it lowered plasma insulin and glucagon levels in humans and baboons (1,74,100). Further studies in several species have shown that both basal and stimulated glucagon and insulin are inhibited by a direct action on the respective A and B pancreatic islet cells (52,130). Somatostatin inhibits the release of insulin, glucagon, or both in response to virtually all of the widely diversified stimuli tested, including arginine, glucose, theophylline, isoproterenol, tolbutamide, calcium, epinephrine, gastric inhibitory polypeptide, and secretin (52,151).

With the development of a highly specific RIA for somatostatin (2), investigators looked for its presence in the tissues where biological activity had been observed. Luft et al. (89) were able to demonstrate somatostatin-like immunoreactivity (SLI) in rat and guinea pig pancreatic islets. Shortly afterward, immunocytochemical and histological studies revealed the localization of pancreatic somatostatin in D cells predominantly surrounding the well-known glucagon-containing A cells at the periphery of the islets (62,111). The suggestion of physiological control over insulin and glucagon secretion by somatostatin became more plausible with these findings, and a direct intra-islet, or "paracrine," regulatory system has been proposed (146,147).

Somatostatin inhibits the secretion of insulin or glucagon from pancreatic tumors (60,100), and may find use in the diagnosis of insulinomas, since tolbutamide-stimulated insulin secretion is not inhibited by somatostatin in these patients but is in normal subjects (88). Recently, two cases of "somatostatinoma" were reported (50,79). The patients had excessive somatostatin, low insulin, glucagon, and other hormone levels, and diabetes. In one patient, removal of the tumor resulted in remission of the diabetes (50).

Somatostatin also affects the exocrine pancreas by inhibiting pancreatic bicarbonate and protein secretion (13,75).

Stomach and Gut

The actions of somatostatin on the secretions of the alimentary tract are the subject of chapter 28 in this volume by Dr. Konturek and will not be covered here. Basically, somatostatin is present in D cells throughout the gastrointestinal mucosa (111) and in intestinal nerve fibers, and it inhibits the release of gastrin, gastric acid, pepsin, secretin, CCK-PZ, GIP, VIP, and motilin (130).

Central Nervous System

Somatostatin has a wide distribution in the brain and spinal cord, and evidence is accumulating that it has a variety of neurotropic actions, the significance of which is not yet clear. Although the hypothalamus has the greatest concentration of somatostatin, the largest amount seems to be in the cerebral cortex (23,76).

In mice treated with the monoamine oxidase inhibitor paragyline, somatostatin was found to increase their behavioral hyperactivity induced by a threshold dose of L-DOPA (DOPA potentiation test) (109). A smaller dose of somatostatin than of the common tricyclic antidepressants and antianxiety agents produced the effect, but other hypothalamic peptides (MIF-I, TRH) were much more potent than somatostatin in that system (68). Prange et al. described an amplification of pentobarbital-induced sedation and hypothermia in mice by somatostatin (112), and others reported that it increased the LD_{50} of strychnine (19). Decreases in the spontaneous firing of single neurons at several brain sites after microiontophoresis were also reported by Renaud et al. (113). Whereas these observations together suggest that somatostatin is a CNS depressant, the opposite is true of its effects on sleep and motor behavior. In rats, somatostatin caused an overall reduction in sleep, suppressing REM more than slow-wave sleep (114), and infusion of somatostatin into the cerebral ventricles caused excitation of circular running behavior (61). Paradoxical effects are observed between high and low doses of somatostatin in some CNS studies.

Recently, somatostatin has been reported to act within the CNS to prevent the rise in blood glucose following stress or intracisternal administration of the peptide bombesin (22).

Somatostatin has also been shown to affect smooth muscle tissue (e.g., guinea pig ileum, rabbit jejunum, rat vas deferens), apparently by inhibiting neuronal release of cholinergic and adrenergic transmitter substances (29,56,69,163). Several somatostatin analogs were also shown to inhibit contractions of the vas deferens (69).

STRUCTURE-FUNCTION STUDIES WITH SOMATOSTATIN ANALOGS

The broad spectrum of biological activities exhibited by somatostatin provides the potential for development of an attractive array of therapeutic agents that could be active against numerous diseases in several tissues. Yet it is precisely the multiple actions of somatostatin that limit its usefulness in treating a given disorder. Consequently, a major effort in the design of somatostatin analogs has been directed toward achieving more selective biological actions. Since somatostatin has a very short half-life in the blood (130), long-acting somatostatin analogs are also being sought to improve the therapeutic potential of this hormone. In order to reduce side effects, lower required doses, and promote dissociation of activities, analogs more potent than the parent compound have also been developed. It is hoped that combining those features that produce selective, prolonged, and enhanced activities will result in a unique arsenal of agents useful in treating such disorders as diabetes mellitus, acromegaly, insulinomas, glucagonomas, peptic ulcers, and acute pancreatitis.

Early structure-function studies on somatostatin began with systematic replacement of each amino acid by L-alanine (116). These analogs were compared with somatostatin for their ability to inhibit the release of GH, insulin, and glucagon. Ala²- and Ala⁵-somatostatin retained full biological potency. Most of the other alanyl analogs had negligible activity, but the changes in positions 4, 10, 12, and 13 caused a less drastic reduction in biological activity (116). This information provides the first glimpse at the side-chain groups that may be relatively more crucial to the proper functioning of the native hormone and those that are more tolerant to substitution.

Similarly, each amino acid in the somatostatin backbone was successively replaced by its D-isomer, yielding predominantly inactive, or modestly active, analogs (48,116). A striking exception was D-Trp⁸-somatostatin (117), which has been confirmed to be six to eight times as active as somatostatin in inhibiting GH, insulin, and glucagon release (32,117). As will be discussed later, D-Cys¹⁴-somatostatin was also interesting because it was selective for GH and glucagon inhibition (21,95). None of the D-amino acid-containing analogs were long-acting despite the blocking of specific enzyme (tryptic, chymotryptic) cleavage points. Since these first systematic studies, numerous somatostatin analogs have been synthesized and they represent several other design strategies including derivation of functional groups and the addition, deletion, or substitution of amino acids.

Efforts to increase the potency of analogs beyond that of somatostatin began with attempts to capitalize on the D-Trp⁸ modification mentioned earlier. Multiple substitutions brought limited success, since the effects were occasionally additive; [N-Tyr, D-Trp⁸]- and [D-Ala²-D-Trp⁸]-somatostatin were about 10 times more active than somatostatin in suppressing GH release *in vitro* (129). More dramatic results were obtained when we modified the tryptophyl indole nucleus by incorporating D- and L- halo-tryptophyl residues in position 8 of somatostatin. Whereas the D- and L- diastereomers of [5F-Trp⁸]-, [6F-Trp⁸]-, and [5Br-Trp⁸]-somatostatin were each more active than somatostatin in the *in vitro* GH assay, [D-5F-Trp⁸]- and [D-5Br-Trp⁸]-somatostatin were 25 and 30 times more active, respectively, in that assay (96,97). These are the most potent somatostatin analogs so far reported. They are also highly potent in rats *in vivo*, but not long-acting (Meyers et al., *unpublished observations*).

Selective biological actions have been observed for several somatostatin analogs. The first to be reported was des[Ala¹, Gly², Asn⁵]-somatostatin (46,125), which inhibits insulin and GH, but not glucagon release. Deletion of the Asn⁵ residue probably alone produced the effect, since deletion of the linear portion of the molecule (Ala¹-Gly²) has previously been shown to have no apparent effect on the biological activity of somatostatin peptides (18). Deletion of Asn⁵ in combination with the D-Trp⁸ modification resulted in a more potent insulin- and GH- specific analog (20). Recently, Lien and Garsky (83) reported that [D-Ala⁵, D-Trp⁸]-somatostatin features this same specificity of action, while exhibiting prolonged inhibiting activity (about 2 hr) when injected subcutaneously but not intravenously.

Analogs that specifically inhibit pituitary GH have also been found. Several cyclic, non-sulfur-containing analogs were reported to have no effect on insulin or glucagon release while retaining some GH-inhibiting activity, and one appeared long-acting at high doses (55,128). We tested several analogs modified at position 4 and found all but one to be less active than somatostatin in suppressing GH, insulin, and glucagon release. Phe^4-somatostatin was a potent selective inhibitor of GH release; it was twice as active as somatostatin in suppressing *in vitro* GH, but had less than 20% glucagon release-inhibiting activity and a negligible effect on insulin secretion (98,131). It should be noted that [D-5Br-Trp^8]-somatostatin may also find use as a selective GH inhibitor at certain doses, since it inhibits GH about 100 times more strongly than glucagon and does not affect insulin at all (Meyers et al., *unpublished observations*).

There is a need to find analogs that inhibit glucagon and GH without affecting insulin release, since these agents could be useful in treating certain types of diabetes. We (54,95) and others (21) observed this type of dissociated activity in rats with [D-Cys^{14}]-somatostatin and [D-Trp^8, D-Cys^{14}]-somatostatin. These results were reaffirmed in a perfused rat pancreas assay where we further reported that [Ala^2, D-Trp^8, D-Cys^{14}]-somatostatin and [pyro Gln, (Gly)$_2$,D-Trp^8]-somatostatin were also GH and glucagon-specific inhibitors (159). Whether any of these analogs are truly selective for the respective receptors must, however, await further testing, since these effects are apparently not observed at certain doses or in all assay systems (107). In any case, there is no evidence that these analogs are long-acting *in vivo*. Recently, [des(Ala^1,Gly^2)-His^{4,5}, D-Trp^8]-somatostatin was reported to be a selective inhibitor of GH and glucagon secretion at low doses, with prolonged action at higher doses where insulin suppression was also observed (127).

Results of systematic efforts to prepare somatostatin analogs with prolonged actions have so far been largely disappointing, but such studies have uncovered information about the importance of the disulfide bridge, other functional groups, and size of the ring in maintaining biological activity. Single or multiple D-amino acid substitutions in trypsin- and chymotrypsin- sensitive positions have not generally produced long-acting derivatives. It was mentioned earlier that [D-Ala^5, D-Trp^8]-somatostatin was long-acting when administered subcutaneously but not intravenously, indicating that it lacks resistance to enzymatic degradation and is instead slowly released following subcutaneous injection (83). Timed degradation studies by Marks et al. (91,93,94) showed that preferential cleavage of somatostatin occurred in the ring portion by endopeptidase activity, whereas the slow release of Ala and Cys argued against a major role for aminopeptidase and carboxypeptidase activity in the inactivation of somatostatin. In agreement with these findings, Ala and Gly are not required for biological activity, and various potent des[Ala^1,Gly^2]-N-acylated [Cys^3]-somatostatin analogs were not longer acting than somatostatin (18,47,48). In fact, an N^α-blocked somatostatin analog was shown to be cleaved internally by endopeptidase activity (91).

Nonreducible cyclic analogs, in which the sulfur atoms were replaced by carbon-carbon bonds, had high biological activity, and the descarboxy Cys^{14} derivative had a short protracted activity in suppressing stimulated gastric acid secretion (154). These studies reaffirmed the lack of an absolute requirement for the disulfide bridge in the expression of biological activity of somatostatin (124). The terminal carboxyl group was also not required (124,126,154), and it may have further been implicated in the prolonged action observed. Further studies of this region are warranted.

The 38-membered ring is also not a requirement for biological activity. The 35-membered [des Asn^5]-somatostatin analogs mentioned earlier were active, and one nonreducible cyclic analog with a 35-membered ring significantly suppressed plasma GH and was also long-acting at high doses (128). Recently, a cyclic somatostatin analog with only eight amino acids was said to retain some activity and was also long-acting (152). Similarly, we have prepared larger ring analogs (41 atoms in the ring) that were highly potent in suppressing GH *in vitro* and *in vivo* (35,96). Although one of these ([Cys^2, D-Ala^3,]-somatostatin) appeared long-acting in a preliminary test, we have obtained conflicting results and further tests are underway to resolve the discrepancy.

An ingenious study of bicyclic somatostatin analogs produced several potent derivatives and resulted in a proposed conformation of the ring portion of somatostatin at the receptor (153). The model is consistent with data obtained for the solution conformation proposed by Holladay and Puett (63,64), although other conformers which agree with those data are possible (118).

SUMMARY AND CONCLUSIONS

Somatostatin is among the most intriguing of the hypothalamic peptide hormones because of its presence and actions in widely distributed body tissues. In addition to regulating pituitary GH and TSH levels, its localization in pancreatic islet D cells, along with its ability to inhibit insulin and glucagon release, strongly support a physiological role for somatostatin in regulating nutrient metabolism. Somatostatin further inhibits the release of gastric acid and several gut hormones. There are a number of clinical possibilities for somatostatin, particularly in treating diabetes mellitus, acromegaly, and ulcer, but the molecule must be tailored to be selective and long-acting for its full therapeutic potential to be realized. This effort has been met with some success in several laboratories and hopefully will encourage further development of somatostatin analogs.

PROJECTIONS FOR THE FUTURE

Somatostatin has already had an impact on our understanding of the physiology of glucose metabolism and particularly on the role of glucagon. Progress in this area continues to be rapid as the interrelationships of insulin, glucagon, somatostatin, and the recently discovered islet hormone pancreatic polypeptide (PP) are explored. The unique actions of somatostatin in several tissues offer the opportunity for uncovering new insights into the mechanisms of receptor recognition and local control over hormone release.

The search for therapeutically useful analogs of somatostatin is in its infancy. As the properties of the molecule become more clearly defined with respect to the active conformation(s) and the relationships of various functional groups to biological activity in certain tissues, we can expect highly potent, selective, and long-acting analogs with valuable properties for treating specific disorders to emerge. Preliminary results suggest that we have produced the first analogs of somatostatin with antagonistic properties (Meyers, et al., *unpublished*), which in the future might be used to stimulate endogenous substances (e.g., insulin, GH) by specifically blocking the action of endogenous somatostatin. This could, for example, be advantageous in cases requiring GH replacement therapy since such treatment is expensive and limited, and the postulated growth hormone-releasing hormone has not yet been isolated.

THE ENKEPHALINS AND ENDORPHINS

ISOLATION

Investigations on the mode of action of the analgesic morphine alkaloids that used radioactively labeled materials led to the demonstration of the presence of stereospecific binding sites in the brains of several animal species, including man (106,137,140). It was then apparent that some endogenous substance, not corresponding to any known neurotransmitter or modulator, should exist that would be capable of binding to these receptors. Indeed, extracts of brain tissue were soon shown (66) to have inhibitory properties similar to the plant opiates on electrically stimulated contractions of the guinea pig ileum and mouse vas deferens and to compete for brain opiate receptors (102,142).

This work culminated in the isolation and sequencing by mass spectrometry (67) of a mixture of two pentapeptides from aqueous extracts of porcine brain that differed only by the presence of a methionine or leucine residue at their C-termini, there being approximately four times as much of the former. The two peptides were named methionine- and leucine-enkephalins and their amino acid sequences are illustrated in Fig. 2. Subsequently, the same two compounds were isolated from bovine brain (136), where they were present in the inverse ratio.

Almost immediately, it was recognized (14) that the pentapeptide sequence of Met-enkephalin was identical to the 61–65 residue of β-lipotropin (β-LPH), a 91-residue peptide originally isolated (80) from the pituitary and also containing the β-MSH sequence, although its primary biological function had remained obscure. Crude fractions with opiate activity had already been obtained (143)

H-Tyr-Gly-Gly-Phe-Leu-OH
1   5

Leucine-enkephalin

H-Tyr-Gly-Gly-Phe-Met-OH
1   5

Methionine-enkephalin

H-Tyr-Gly-Gly-Phe-Met-Thr-Ser-Glu-Lys-Ser-Gln-Thr-Pro-Leu-Val-Thr-OH
1   5   10   15

α-Endorphin

H-Tyr-Gly-Gly-Phe-Met-Thr-Ser-Glu-Lys-Ser-Gln-Thr-Pro-Leu-Val-Thr-Leu-OH
1   5   10   15

γ-Endorphin

H-Tyr-Gly-Gly-Phe-Met-Thr-Ser-Glu-Lys-Ser-Gln-Thr-Pro-Leu-Val-Thr-Leu-Phe-Lys-Asn-Ala-Ile-Lys-Asn-Ala-Tyr-Lys-Lys-Gly-Glu-OH
1   5   10   15   20   25   30

β$_h$-Endorphin

FIG. 2. Structures of the enkephalins and endorphins.

from the pituitary and hypothalamus and subsequently several very active C-terminal fragments of β-LPH were sequenced that were called endorphins. Two of these, α- and γ-endorphin (84), are 16- and 17-residue peptides representing positions 61–76 and 61–77 of β-LPH, respectively. The most potent, and perhaps most important, member of the series, is β-endorphin (14,81), which is the 61–91 C-terminal fragment of β-LPH. The α-, β-, and γ-nomenclature unfortunately represents their chronological order of discovery rather than the size of the fragment. Amino acid sequences are shown in Fig. 2 and all of the endorphins contain the Met-enkephalin pentapeptide sequence at their N-termini.

Recent evidence (90,119) suggests that β-LPH and ACTH form part of a 30,000 daltons MW precursor or protein present in the intermediate lobe of the pituitary. Both β-endorphin and ACTH are released simultaneously under stressful stimuli (58,101). It is not clear at present whether all of the opiate peptides actually function in situ. Certainly it appears that all of the Met-series can be formed by digestion of β-endorphin with brain homogenates (7) and since several of them are still found in fresh tissue extracts where manipulative degradation should be minimal (122), it is possible that their concentrations are regulated physiologically by specific enzymatic cleavages of β-endorphin and β-LPH.

BIOLOGICAL PROPERTIES OF THE ENKEPHALINS AND ENDORPHINS

Although, under suitable assay conditions, the enkephalins possess virtually all of the properties of the morphine opiates, their susceptibility to enzymatic destruction (36,41,70,92,99) and short duration of action makes their study difficult. Met- and Leu-enkephalins both bind to opiate receptors on brain membrane fractions with affinities comparable to morphine (27) when experiments are carried out at 0°C or in the presence of proteolytic enzyme inhibitors. In systems where enzymes are more active, such as the vas deferens and ileum assays, the peptides are less active than morphine. For induction of analgesia, very high doses of Met-enkephalin are required administered directly into the brain to produce very transient effects (9,25). Leu-enkephalin is even less active. As will be discussed later, a principal result of analog work on the pentapeptides has been the introduction of more stable compounds with high in vivo activity.

Some nonopioid CNS effects have been observed with the enkephalins and their analogs with comparatively minute peripheral doses. These include potentiation of the effects of DOPA (108), facilitation of learning (72), and reduction of passiveness (71) in the rat. With the localization of so many peptides, particularly gastrointestinal, in the CNS and, conversely, the demonstration (111) of enkephalin immunoreactivity in the gut, it is not surprising that the effects of opiates on gut and pancreatic processes are receiving considerable attention (see chapter 28 by Konturek, pp. 693–716).

β-Endorphin is less active (33) than Met-enkephalin in binding to brain membrane fractions and has about the same activity in the vas deferens bioassay (17). However, it is by far the most potent member of the family for inducing analgesia after intracerebroventricular injection (30,87). The reason for its high *in vivo* activity appears to be at least partly due to a considerable resistance to enzymatic attack at the critical N-terminus (6) and also at the C-terminus (51), both properties possibly being a function of the conformation of the molecule. This high stability is lost in shorter fragments such as α- and γ-endorphin, which exhibit far less *in vivo* activity, although *in vitro* they are more potent (17). Like morphine and the more active enkephalin and α- and γ-endorphin analogs, β-endorphin is a potent stimulator of GH and prolactin release (28, 37,42,43), by mechanisms probably involving hypothalamic factors.

The presence of so many LPH fragments suggests the possibility that each might have CNS functions peculiar to itself. Immunofluorescence techniques using antisera specific for β-endorphin have enabled (11,121) it to be localized in several areas of the brain, the hypothalamus, and the pituitary. Its presence, and the absence of enkephalins, in the pituitary, although absolute concentrations remain controversial (86), and release under stress (58,101) and in certain patients with endocrine disorders (138) suggest obscure peripheral as well as CNS functions. As with the enkephalins, behavioral effects, other than analgesia, have been observed with the endorphins (12,57,155) that appear to be different for each peptide. Favorable effects (73,156) have been reported in schizophrenic and depressed patients after treatment with β-endorphin. Estimates of potencies among opiate peptides and their analogs derived from release of GH and prolactin, from guinea pig ileum and mouse vas deferens bioassays, and from behavioral tests show considerable divergence that can best be explained by the presence of several receptor types (33,34,141) that may account for some of the above observations.

STRUCTURE-ACTIVITY STUDIES ON THE ENKEPHALINS AND ENDORPHINS

One possibility raised by the discovery of the opiate peptides was that they might have major therapeutic value as nonaddictive analgesics if problems caused by their short duration of action could be overcome by structural modification. Subsequent experiments revealed that both the enkephalins and the β-endorphins produce tolerance and physical dependence on prolonged administration (65,-144,162). The readily synthesized pentapeptide analogs, however, offer an ideal opportunity for mapping the requirements of receptor sites, elucidating specific peptidase susceptibility, and determining factors responsible for efficient passage into the brain. The possible presence of several receptor sites offers the opportunity of developing analgesic analogs with more specific affinities and fewer side effects and analogs with enhanced nonnarcotic CNS effects. Even β-endorphin and its analogs, which must be considered large and complex molecules from a synthetic viewpoint, can be made (33,82) in high yields and with great speed by solid-phase methodology.

Enkephalin Analogs

The many hundreds of Met- and Leu-enkephalin analogs that have been synthesized and tested have necessarily resulted in quite a comprehensive picture of the structural requirements for biological activity. It is now clear, and not surprising by analogy with general morphinoid structures, that tyrosine in position 1 of the opiate peptides is the active center and that its amino and hydroxyl group are the most important parts of the molecule. Any enzymatically stable modification of the tyrosine amine group that destroys basicity, such as acetylation (37), also destroys activity. Likewise, irreversible derivation (8) of the phenolic hydroxyl group also eliminates activity. Monomethylation (15) or dimethylation (8) of the amino group, which retains basicity, has no beneficial effects on opiate receptor affinity but increases *in vivo* activity, probably as a result of increased resistance to aminopeptidases. In contrast to N-allyl derivatives of morphine, such as naloxone, which are potent antagonists of opiate action, the N-allyl derivative (104) of a Met-enkephalin analog was devoid of inhibitory activity. At present no peptide antagonists have been reported. During our early screening of the pentapeptide molecule, we prepared a series of analogs in which L-amino acids were replaced by their D-isomers, of which [D-Tyr[1]]-Met-enkephalin was inactive.

In [D-Ala[2]]-Met-enkephalin, made independently by Pert et al. (105) and ourselves (160), one of the glycine residues was replaced by D-alanine to give one of the first analogs reported to have greatly increased activity. Both [D-Ala[2]]-Met-enkephalin and its amide gave (105,160) long-lasting analgesia when injected directly into the brain, in contrast with weak and transient activity produced by higher doses of Met-enkephalin. No increase in binding affinities was observed with these peptides, but they were found (103) to be considerably more resistant to enzymes in brain tissue homogenates than the natural peptides. Large D-amino acid substitutions in this position result in analogs with reduced binding affinity and *in vitro* activity; however, several of them have even higher *in vivo* analgesic activity and notable among these are analogs containing D-Met (139), D-Ser (134), and D-Thr (167) in position 2.

Replacement of the other Gly in position 3 by D-alanine results in almost complete loss of activity. Apart from an azaGly[3]-peptide (44), which appeared to have increased analgesic activity, all other substitutions so far reported for this position have given considerably reduced activities.

The bulk and lipophilic character of the phenylalanine side chain appear to be the most important factors in position 4. Replacements by a boron-containing amino acid, carboranylalanine (45), or hexahydrophenylalanine (44) are made with high retention of activity. [D-Ala[2], pentafluoro-Phe[4]]-Met-enkephalinamide

(38) was found to be over 10 times more effective than [D-Ala²]-Met-enkephalin-amide for inducing analgesia. As would be expected from this trend, the presence of a hydrophilic hydroxyl group on the benzene ring in [Tyr⁴]-Met-enkephalin (8) severely reduces biological activity. Position 4 is a conformationally important part of the chain, since [D-Phe⁴]-Met-enkephalin is almost devoid of activity. Conformational restrictions do not extend to [N-Me-Phe⁴]-Met-enkephalin (44), which has almost full activity.

Most amino acid substitutions for methionine or leucine in position 5 result in retention of quite high binding affinity and biological activity. As with the N-terminus, those alterations that impart some degree of stability toward enzymes such as proline (139), D-Leu (8), and D-Met give analogs with greatly improved *in vivo* activities, despite decreases in receptor affinity. Modifications to the carboxyl group have been numerous and almost always of value, including removal (38) and substitution by amide (27), ester (44), and alkylamide (37,44) groups.

Combinations of several beneficial changes in the same molecule have yielded some extremely active analogs (44,120,139), a number of which are active after peripheral injection of quite small amounts. Some analogs have been reported (44) to have very high analgesic activity with reduced side effects compared with morphine, whereas others (158) appear to have more severe side effects.

Endorphin Analogs

Since the extremely potent analgesic activity of β-endorphin appears to be due mainly to increased enzymatic stability at its termini produced by tertiary structure, it is not surprising that alterations made to the pentapeptides that increase the stability of the tyrosine residue do not have as great a beneficial effect on the large peptide. Thus, [D-Ala²]-β_h-endorphin (33,166) is only five times more active (161) than β_h-endorphin for inducing analgesia. Other large D-amino acids incorporated in position 2 gave considerable decreases in activity (165,166). [L-Ala²]-β-endorphin (165) was still 12% active for induction of analgesia, whereas the [L-Ala²]-enkephalins are virtually inactive. Modifications to position 5, such as incorporation of proline, D-Leu, or D-Met, which are effective in the enkephalins, reduce the activity of β-endorphin (165,166). [Leu⁵]-β-endorphin (33,85,165), a possible precursor for Leu-enkephalin, was only 20 to 30% as active as β-endorphin as an analgesic, but twice as active in the mouse vas deferens bioassay (33). As with the enkephalin analogs, a great difference in potencies has been observed (34) when endorphin analogs are compared for analgesic activity, GH and prolactin releasing effects, and effects on smooth muscle preparations that appear to be best explained in terms of receptor population heterogeneity. One analog, [des-Tyr¹]-γ-endorphin, lacks the opiate active center but possesses neuroleptic activity in the rat (39) suggesting that the endorphins carry more than one type of behavioral information and that, again, several types of receptors are involved in the expression of their activities. The des-

Tyr-peptide was effective when given to schizophrenics (157) who had previously been resistant to conventional neuroleptics.

SUMMARY AND CONCLUSIONS

Apart from Leu-enkephalin, the precursor for which remains to be identified, several peptides exist which bind to opiate receptor sites and whose sequences form parts of the β-LPH molecule. Both Leu- and Met-enkephalin and β-endorphin are discretely distributed in several brain areas; however, presumed differences in physiological function remain obscure. Leu- and Met-enkephalin, being rapidly degraded *in vivo,* exhibit weak opiate activity even after central injection but β-endorphin, which is relatively resistant to enzymatic attack, is the most potent analgesic agent of the family.

Numerous analogs of the pentapeptides have been prepared and comprehensive structure-activity relationships have been established. Analogs far more potent analgesics than the natural peptides are common. The problem of designing peptides that are able to cross the blood-brain barrier has been readily overcome since several analogs exist that are more active than morphine after intravenous injection. Whether any of these will assume therapeutic significance remains to be seen. Certainly, the initial hope of producing nonaddictive peptides has faded; however, the design of peptides with fewer adverse side effects than the morphinoids seems feasible.

PROJECTIONS FOR THE FUTURE

Several important questions remain to be answered in the opiate peptide field. Primary among these must be the reason for the existence of at least three peptides containing the same active center but exhibiting different physiological distributions. Perhaps the answer is related to the firm evidence that is accumulating that more than one type of opiate receptor is present and that ratios change according to the tissue area in question. This has considerable significance in the analog area, for it seems that specificity for a particular receptor might be built into a peptide. It has been demonstrated that the opiate peptides do possess CNS activities apart from analgesia, such as anti-depressant activity, which might be linked to a particular receptor population.

REFERENCES

1. Alberti, K. G. M. M., Christensen, S. E., Iversen, J., Seyer-Hansen, K., Christensen, N. J., Prange-Hansen, Aa., Lundbaek, K., and Orskov, H. (1973): Inhibition of insulin secretion by somatostatin. *Lancet,* ii:1299–1301.
2. Arimura, A., Sato, H., Coy, D. H., and Schally, A. V. (1975): Radioimmunoassay for GH-release inhibiting hormone. *Proc. Soc. Exp. Biol. Med.,* 148:784–789.
3. Arimura, A., Sato, H., Dupont, A., Nishi, N., and Schally, A. V. (1975): Somatostatin: Abundance of immunoreactive hormone in rat stomach and pancreas. *Science,* 189:1007–1009.
4. Arimura, A., and Schally, A. V. (1976): Increase in basal and thyrotropin-releasing hormone

(TRH)-stimulated secretion of thyrotropin (TSH) by passive immunization with antiserum to somatostatin in rats. *Endocrinology,* 98:1069–1072.

5. Arimura, A., Smith, W. D., and Schally, A. V. (1976): Blockade of the stress-induced decrease in blood GH by anti-somatostatin serum in rats. *Endocrinology,* 98:540–543.

6. Austen, B. M., and Smyth, D. G. (1977): The NH_2-terminus of C-fragment is resistant to the action of aminopeptidases. *Biochem. Biophys. Res. Commun.,* 76:477–482.

7. Austen, B. M., Smyth, D. G., and Snell, C. R. (1977): γ-Endorphin, α-endorphin, and Met-enkephalin are formed extracellularly from lipotropin C fragments. *Nature,* 269:619–621.

8. Bedell, C. R., Clark, R. B., Hardy, G. W., Lowe, L. A., Uratura, F. B., Vane, J. R., and Wilkinson, S. (1977): Structural requirements for opioid activity of analogues of the enkephalins. *Proc. B. Soc. (Lond.),* B197:249–265.

9. Beluzzi, J. D., Grant, N., Garsky, V., Sarantakis, D., Wise, C. D., and Stein, L. (1976): Analgesia induced in vivo by central administration of enkephalin in rat. *Nature,* 260:625–626.

10. Besser, G. M., Mortimer, C. H., Carr, D., Schally, A. V., Coy, D. H., Evered, D., Kastin, A. J., Tunbridge, W. M. G., Thorner, M. O., and Hall, R. (1974): Growth hormone-release inhibiting hormone in acromegaly. *Br. Med. J.,* 1:352–355.

11. Bloom, F., Battenburg, E., Rossier, J., Ling, N., and Guillemin, R. (1978): Neurons containing β-endorphin in rat brain exist separately from those containing enkephalin: immunocytochemical studies. *Proc. Natl. Acad. Sci. USA,* 75:1591–1595.

12. Bloom, F. E., Segal, D. S., Ling, N., and Guillemin, R. (1976): Endorphins: profound behavioral effects in rats suggest new etiological factors in mental illness. *Science,* 194:630–632.

13. Boden, G., Sivitz, M. C., Owen, O. E., Essa-Koumar, N., and Landor, J. H. (1975): Somatostatin suppresses secretin and pancreatic exocrine secretion. *Science,* 190:163–165.

14. Bradbury, A. F., Smyth, D. G., Snell, C. R., Birdsall, N. J. M., and Hulme, E. C. (1976): C-Fragment of lipotropin has a high affinity for brain opiate receptors. *Nature,* 260:793–795.

15. Bradbury, A. F., Smyth, D. G., Snell, C. R., Deakin, J. F. W., and Wendlandt, S. (1977): Comparison of the analgesic properties of lipotropin C-fragment and stabilized enkephalins in the rat. *Biochem. Biophys. Res. Commun.,* 74:748–754.

16. Brazeau, P., Vale, W., Burgus, R., Ling, N., Butcher, M., Rivier, J., and Guillemin, R. (1973): Hypothalamic peptide that inhibits the secretion of immunoreactive pituitary growth hormone. *Science,* 179:77–79.

17. Britton, D. R., Fertel, R., Coy, D. H., and Kastin, A. J. (1978): Effect of enkephalin and endorphin analogs on receptors in the mouse vas deferens. *Biochem. Pharmacol.,* 27:2275–2277.

18. Brown, M., Rivier, J., Vale, W., and Guillemin, R. (1975): Variability of the duration of inhibition of growth hormone release by $N\alpha$-acylated-des-[Ala^1-Gly^2]-H_2 somatostatin analogs. *Biochem. Biophys. Res. Commun.,* 65:752–756.

19. Brown, M., and Vale, W. (1975): Central nervous system effects of hypothalamic peptides. *Endocrinology,* 86:1333–1336.

20. Brown, M., Vale, W., and Rivier, J. (1977): Insulin selective somatostatin analogs. *Endocrinology (Suppl. 1),* 25:360A.

21. Brown, M., Rivier, J., and Vale, W. (1977): Somatostatin: analogs with selected biological activities. *Science,* 196:1467–1469.

22. Brown, M., Rivier, J., and Vale, W. (1978): Somatostatin: Central nervous system (CNS) action on glucoregulation. *Metabolism (Suppl. 1),* 27:1253–1256.

23. Brownstein, M., Arimura, A., Sato, H., Schally, A. V., and Kizer, J. S. (1975): The regional distribution of somatostatin in the rat brain. *Endocrinology,* 96:1456–1461.

24. Burgus, R., Ling, N., Butcher, M., and Guillemin, R. (1973): Primary structure of somatostatin, a hypothalamic peptide that inhibits the secretion of pituitary growth hormone. *Proc. Natl. Acad. Sci. USA,* 70:684–688.

25. Buscher, H. H., Hill, R., Römer, D., Cardinaux, F., Closse, A., Hauser, D., and Pless, J. (1976): Evidence for analgesic activity of enkephalin in the mouse. *Nature,* 261:423–425.

26. Carr, D., Gomez-Pan, A., Weightman, D. R., Roy, V. C. M., Hall, R., Besser, G. M., Thorner, M. O., McNeilly, A. S., Schally, A. V., Kastin, A. J., and Coy, D. H. (1975): Growth hormone-release inhibiting hormone: Actions on thyrotrophin and prolactin secretion after thyrotrophin-releasing hormone. *Br. Med. J.,* 3:67–69.

27. Chang, J. K., Fong, T. W. B., Pert, A., and Pert, C. B. (1976): Opiate receptor affinities

and behavioral effects of enkephalin: structure-activity relationship of ten synthetic peptide analogues. *Life Sci.*, 18:1473–1482.

28. Chihara, K., Arimura, A., Coy, D. H., and Schally, A. V. (1978): Studies on interaction of endorphins, substance P, and endogenous somatostatin in GH and prolactin release. *Endocrinology*, 102:281–290.

29. Cohen, M. L., Rosing, E., Wiley, K. S., and Slater, I. H. (1978): Somatostatin inhibits adrenergic and cholinergic neurotransmission in smooth muscle. *Life Sci.*, 23:1659–1664.

30. Cox, B. M., Goldstein, A., and Li, C. H. (1976): Opioid activity of a peptide, β-lipotropin-(61–91), derived from β-lipotropin. *Proc. Natl. Acad. Sci. USA*, 73:1821–1823.

31. Coy, D. H., Coy, E. J., Arimura, A., and Schally, A. V. (1973): Solid phase synthesis of growth hormone-release inhibiting factor. *Biochem. Biophys. Res. Commun.*, 54:1267–1273.

32. Coy, D. H., Coy, E. J., Meyers, C. A., Drouin, J., Ferland, L., Gomez-Pan, A., and Schally, A. V. (1976): Structure-function studies on somatostatin. *Endocrinology*, 98:305A.

33. Coy, D. H., Gill, P., Kastin, A. J., Dupont, A., Cusan, L., Labrie, F., Britton, D., and Fertel, R. (1977): Synthetic and biological studies on unmodified and modified fragments of human β-lipotropin with opioid activities. In: *Peptides: Proceedings of the Fifth American Peptide Symposium*, edited by M. Goodman and J. Meienhofer, pp. 107–110. J. Wiley and Sons, New York.

34. Coy, D. H., Kastin, A. J., and Plotnikoff, N. P. (1976): Études biologiques faites avec les encephalines, les endorphines et leurs analogues. *Ann. Anesthesiol. Fr.*, 5:373–378.

35. Coy, D. H., Meyers, C. A., Arimura, A., Schally, A. V., and Redding, T. W. (1978): Observations on the growth hormone, insulin, and glucagon release-inhibiting activities of somatostatin analogues. *Metabolism (Suppl. 1)*, 27:1407–1410.

36. Craves, F. B., Law, P. Y., Hunt, C. A., and Loh, H. H. (1978): The metabolic disposition of radiolabeled enkephalins *in vitro* and *in situ*. *J. Pharmacol. Exp. Ther.*, 206:492–506.

37. Cusan, L., Dupont, A., Kledzik, G. S., Labrie, F., Coy, D. H., and Schally, A. V. (1977): Potent prolactin and growth hormone releasing activity of more analogues of Met-enkephalin. *Nature*, 268:544–547.

38. Day, A. R., Carney, J. M., Rosecrans, J. A., Dewey, W. L., and Freer, R. J. (1978): Synthesis of two enzyme resistant enkephalin analogs possessing enhanced analgesic activity. *Res. Commun. Chem. Pathol. Pharmacol.*, 20:59–68.

39. de Wied, D., Bohus, B., van Ree, J. M., Kovacs, G. L., and Greven, H. M. (1978): Neuroleptic activity of [des-Tyr[1]]-γ-endorphin in rats. *Lancet*, i:1046.

40. Drouin, J., DeLéan, A., Rainville, D., Lachance, R., and Labrie, F. (1976): Characteristics of the interaction between thyrotropin-releasing hormone and somatostatin for thyrotropin and prolactin release. *Endocrinology*, 98:514–521.

41. Dupont, A., Cusan, L., Garon, M., Alvarado-Urbina, G., and Labrie, F. (1977): Extremely rapid degradation of [³H] methionine-enkephalin by various rat tissues *in vivo* and *in vitro*. *Life Sci.*, 21:907–914.

42. Dupont, A., Cusan, L., Garon, M., Labrie, F., and Li, C. H. (1977): β-endorphin: stimulation of growth hormone release in vivo. *Proc. Natl. Acad. Sci. USA*, 74:358–359.

43. Dupont, A., Cusan, L., Labrie, F., Coy, D. H., and Li, C. H. (1977): Stimulation of prolactin release in the rat by intraventricular injection of β-endorphin and methionine-enkephalin. *Biochem. Biophys. Res. Commun.*, 75:76–82.

44. Dutta, A. S., Gormley, J. J., Hayward, C. F., Morley, J. S., Shaw, J. S., Stacey, G. J., and Turnbull, M. T. (1977): Enkephalin analogues eliciting analgesia after intravenous injection. *Life Sci.*, 21:559–562.

45. Eberle, A., Leukart, O., Schiller, P., Fouchere, J. L., and Schwyzer, R. (1977): Hormone-receptor interactions: [4-carboranylalanine,5-leucine]-enkephalin as a structural probe for the opiate receptor. *FEBS Lett.*, 82:325–328.

46. Efendic, S., Luft, R., and Sievertsson, H. (1975): Relative effects of somatostatin and two somatostatin analogues on the release of insulin, glucagon and growth hormone. *FEBS Lett.*, 58:302–305.

47. Evered, D. C., Gomez-Pan, A., Tunbridge, W. M. G., Hall, R., Lind, T., Besser, G. M., Mortimer, C. H., Thorner, M. O., Schally, A. V., Kastin, A. J., and Coy, D. H. (1975): Analogues of growth-hormone release-inhibiting hormone. *Lancet*, i:1250.

48. Ferland, L., Labrie, F., Coy, D. H., Arimura, A., and Schally, A. V. (1976): Inhibition by six somatostatin analogs of plasma growth hormone levels stimulated by thiamylal and morphine in the rat. *Mol. Cell. Endocrinol.*, 4:79–88.

49. Ferland, L., Labrie, F., Jobin, M., Arimura, A., and Schally, A. V. (1976): Physiological role of somatostatin in the control of growth hormone and thyrotropin secretion. *Biochem. Biophys. Res. Commun.,* 68:149–156.
50. Ganda, O. P., Weir, G. C., Soeldner, J. S., Legg, M. A., Chick, W. L., Patel, Y. C., Ebeid, A. M., Gabbay, K. H., and Reichlin, S. (1977): "Somatostatinoma." A somatostatin containing tumor of the endocrine pancreas. *N. Engl. J. Med.,* 296:963–967.
51. Geisow, J. J., and Smyth, D. G. (1977): Lipotropin C-fragment has a COOH-terminal sequence with high intrinsic resistance to the action of exopeptidases. *Biochem. Biophys. Res. Commun.,* 75:625–629.
52. Gerich, J. E., Charles, M. A., and Grodsky, G. M. (1976): Regulation of pancreatic insulin and glucagon secretion. *Ann. Rev. Physiol.,* 38:353–388.
53. Giustina, G., Reschini, E., Peracchi, M., Cantalamessa, L., Cavagnini, F., Pinto, M., and Bulgheroni, P. (1974): Failure of somatostatin to suppress thyrotropin releasing factor and luteinizing hormone releasing factor-induced growth hormone release in acromegaly. *J. Clin. Endocrinol. Metab.,* 38:906–909.
54. Gordin, A., Meyers, C. A., Arimura, A., Coy, D. H., and Schally, A. V. (1977): An *in vivo* model for testing inhibition of arginine-induced insulin and glucagon release by somatostatin analogs. *Acta Endocrinol.,* 86:833–841.
55. Grant, N., Clark, D., Garsky, V., Juanakais, I., McGregor, W., and Sarantakis, D. (1976): Dissociation of somatostatin effects. Peptides inhibiting the release of growth hormone but not glucagon or insulin in rats. *Life Sci.,* 19:629–632.
56. Guillemin, R. (1976): Somatostatin inhibits the release of acetylcholine induced electrically in the myenteric plexus. *Endocrinology,* 99:1653–1654.
57. Guillemin, R., Ling, N., Burgus, R., and Bloom, F. (1977): Characterization of the endorphins, novel hypothalamic and neurohypophyseal peptides with opiate-like activity: evidence that they induce profound behavioral changes. *Psychoneuroendocrinology,* 2:59–62.
58. Guillemin, R., Vargo, T., Rossier, J., Minick, S., Ling, N., Rivier, C., Vale, W., and Bloom, F. (1977): β-Endorphin and adrenocorticotropin are secreted concomitantly by the pituitary gland. *Science,* 197:1367–1369.
59. Hall, R., Besser, G. M., Schally, A. V., Coy, D. H., Evered, D., Goldie, D. J., Kastin, A. J., McNeilly, A. S., Mortimer, C. H., Phenekos, C., Tunbridge, W. M. G., and Weightman, D. (1973): Actions of growth hormone-release inhibiting hormone in healthy men and in acromegaly. *Lancet,* ii:581–584.
60. Hall, R., and Gomez-Pan, A. (1976): The hypothalamic regulatory hormones and their clinical applications. *Adv. Clin. Chem.,* 18:173–212.
61. Havlicek, V., Rezek, M., and Friesen, H. (1976): Somatostatin and thyrotropin releasing hormone: Central effect on sleep and motor system. *Pharmacol. Biochem. Behav.,* 4:455–459.
62. Hökfelt, T., Efendic, S., Hellerstrom, C., Johansson, O., Luft, R., and Arimura, A. (1975): Cellular localization of somatostatin in endocrine-like cells and neurons of the rat with special references to the A_1-cells of the pancreatic islets and to the hypothalamus. *Acta Endocrinol. (Suppl. 200),* 80:5–41.
63. Holladay, L. A., and Puett, D. (1976): Somatostatin conformation: Evidence for a stable intramolecular structure from circular dichroism, diffusion, and sedimentation equilibrium. *Proc. Natl. Acad. Sci. USA,* 73:1199–1202.
64. Holladay, L. A., Rivier, J., and Puett, D. (1977): Conformational studies on somatostatin and analogues. *Biochemistry,* 16:4895–4900.
65. Hosobucki, Y., Meglio, M., Adams, J., and Li, C. H. (1977): β-Endorphin: development of tolerance and its reversal by 5-hydroxytryptophan in cats. *Proc. Natl. Acad. Sci. USA,* 74:4017–4019.
66. Hughes, J. (1975): Isolation of an endogenous compound from the brain with pharmacological properties similar to morphine. *Brain Res.,* 88:295–308.
67. Hughes, J., Smith, T. W., Kosterlitz, H. W., Fothergill, L. A., Morgan, B. A., and Morris, H. R. (1975): Identification of two related pentapeptides from the brain with potent opiate agonist activity. *Nature,* 253:577–579.
68. Kastin, A. J., Coy, D. H., Jacquet, Y., Schally, A. V., and Plotnikoff, N. P. (1978): CNS effects of somatostatin. *Metabolism (Suppl. 1),* 27:1247–1252.
69. Kastin, A. J., Coy, D. H., Schally, A. V., and Meyers, C. A. (1978): Activity of VIP, somatostatin and other peptides in the mouse vas deferens assay. *Pharmacol. Biochem. Behav.,* 9:673–676.

70. Kastin, A., Nissen, C., Schally, A. V., and Coy, D. H. (1976): Blood-brain barrier, half-time disappearance, and brain distribution for labeled enkephalin and a potent analog. *Brain Res. Bull.,* 1:583–589.
71. Kastin, A. J., Scollan, E. L., Ehrensing, R. H., Schally, A. V., and Coy, D. H. (1978): Enkephalin and other peptides reduce passiveness. *Pharmacol. Biochem. Behav.,* 9:515–519.
72. Kastin, A. J., Scollan, E. L., King, M. G., Schally, A. V., and Coy, D. H. (1976): Enkephalin and a potent analog facilitate maze performance after intraperitoneal administration in rats. *Pharmacol. Biochem. Behav.,* 5:691–695.
73. Kline, N. S., Li, C. H., Lehmann, H. E., Lajtha, A., Laski, E., and Cooper, T. (1977): β-Endorphin-induced changes in schizophrenic and depressed patients. *Arch. Gen. Psychiatry,* 34:1111–1113.
74. Koerker, D. J., Ruch, W., Chideckel, E., Palmer, J., Goodner, C. J., Ensinck, J., and Gale, C. C. (1974): Somatostatin: Hypothalamic inhibitor of the endocrine pancreas. *Science,* 184:482–484.
75. Konturek, S. J., Tasler, J., Obtulowicz, W., Coy, D. H., and Schally, A. V. (1976): Effect of growth hormone release-inhibiting factor on hormones stimulating exocrine pancreatic secretion. *J. Clin. Invest.,* 58:1–6.
76. Kronheim, S., Berelowitz, M., and Pimstone, B. L. (1976): A radioimmunoassay for growth hormone release-inhibiting hormone: Method and quantitative tissue distribution. *Clin. Endocrinol.,* 5:619–630.
77. Krulich, L., Dhariwal, A. P. S., and McCann, S. M. (1968): Stimulatory and inhibitory effects of purified hypothalamic extracts on growth hormone release from rat pituitary in vitro. *Endocrinology,* 83:783–790.
78. Krulich, L., and McCann, S. (1969): Effect of GH-releasing factor and GH-inhibiting factor on the release and concentration of GH in pituitaries incubated in vitro. *Endocrinology,* 85:319–324.
79. Larsson, L-I., Holst, J. J., Kuhl, C., Lundquist, G., Hirsch, M. A., Ingemansson, S., Lindkaer-Jensen, S., Rehfeld, J. F., and Schwartz, T. W. (1977): Pancreatic somatostatinoma, clinical features and physiological implications. *Lancet,* i:666–668.
80. Li, C. H. (1964): Lipotropin, a new active peptide from pituitary glands. *Nature,* 201:924–925.
81. Li, C. H., and Chung, D. (1976): Isolation and structure of an untriacontapeptide with opiate activity from camel pituitary glands. *Proc. Natl. Acad. Sci. USA,* 73:1145–1148.
82. Li, C. H., Yamashiro, D., Tseng, L., and Loh, H. H. (1977): Synthesis and analgesic activity of human β-endorphin. *J. Med. Chem.,* 20:325–328.
83. Lien, E. L., and Garsky, V. M. (1978): Prolonged suppression of insulin release by a somatostatin analog. *Endocrinology,* 103:81–85.
84. Ling, N., Burgus, R., and Guillemin, R. (1976): Isolation, primary structure, and synthesis of alpha-endorphin and gamma-endorphin, two peptides of hypothalamic-hypophyseal origin with morphinomimetic activity. *Proc. Natl. Acad. Sci. USA,* 73:3942–3946.
85. Ling, N., Minick, S., Lazarus, L., Rivier, J., and Guillemin, R. (1977): Structure-activity relationships of enkephalin and endorphin analogs. In: *Peptides: Proceedings of the Fifth American Peptide Symposium,* edited by M. Goodman and J. Meienhofer, pp. 96–99. John Wiley and Sons, New York.
86. Liotta, A. S., Suda, T., and Krieger, D. (1978): β-Lipotropin is the major opioid-like peptide of human pituitary and rat pars distalis: lack of significant β-endorphin. *Proc. Natl. Acad. Sci. USA,* 75:2950–2954.
87. Loh, H. H., Tseng, L. F., Wei, E., and Li, C. H. (1976): β-Endorphin is a potent analgesic agent. *Proc. Natl. Acad. Sci. USA,* 73:2895–2898.
88. Lorenzi, M., Gerich, J. E., Karam, J. H., and Forsham, P. H. (1975): Failure of somatostatin to inhibit tolbutamide-induced insulin secretion in patients with insulinomas: A possible diagnostic tool. *J. Clin. Endocrinol. Metab.,* 40:1121–1124.
89. Luft, R., Efendic, S., Hokfelt, T., Johansson, O., and Arimura, A. (1974): Immunohistochemical evidence for the localization of somatostatin-like immunoreactivity in a cell population of the pancreatic islets. *Med. Biol.,* 52:428–430.
90. Mains, R. E., Eipper, B. A., and Ling, N. (1977): Common precursor to corticotropins and endorphins. *Proc. Natl. Acad. Sci. USA,* 74:3014–3018.
91. Marks, N. (1977): Conversion and inactivation of neuropeptides. In: *Peptides in Neurobiology,* edited by H. Gainer, pp. 221–258. Plenum Press, New York.

92. Marks, N., Grynbaum, A., and Neidle, A. (1977): On the degradation of enkephalins and endorphins by rat and mouse brain extracts. *Biochem. Biophys. Res. Commun.*, 74:1552–1559.
93. Marks, N., and Stern, F. (1975): Inactivation of somatostatin (GH-RIH) and its analogs by crude and partially purified rat brain extracts. *FEBS Lett.*, 55:220–224.
94. Marks, N., Stern, F., and Benuck, M. (1976): Correlation between biological potency and biodegradation of a somatostatin analogue. *Nature*, 261:511–512.
95. Meyers, C. A., Arimura, A., Gordin, A., Fernandez-Durango, R., Coy, D. H., Schally, A. V., Drouin, J., Ferland, L., Beaulieu, M., and Labrie, F. (1977): Somatostatin analogs which inhibit glucagon and growth hormone more than insulin release. *Biochem. Biophys. Res. Commun.*, 74:630–636.
96. Meyers, C. A., and Coy, D. H. (1978): Superactive, selective, and long-acting somatostatin analogs. *Endocrinology*, 102:239A.
97. Meyers, C. A., Coy, D. H., Huang, W. Y., Schally, A. V., and Redding, T. W. (1978): Highly active position eight analogues of somatostatin and separation of peptide diastereomers by partition chromatography. *Biochemistry*, 17:2326–2331.
98. Meyers, C. A., Coy, D. H., Redding, T. W., Schally, A. V., and Arimura, A. (1980): Phe⁴-somatostatin; a selective inhibitor of growth hormone release. *Proc. Natl. Acad. Sci. USA. (in press).*
99. Miller, R. J., Chang, K. J., Cuatrecasas, P., and Wilkinson, S. (1977): The metabolic stability of the enkephalins. *Biochem. Biophys. Res. Commun.*, 74:1311–1317.
100. Mortimer, C. H., Carr, D., Lind, T., Bloom, S. R., Mallinson, C. N., Schally, A. V., Tunbridge, W. M. G., Yeomans, L., Coy, D. H., Kastin, A. J., Besser, G. M., and Hall, R. (1974): Effects of growth-hormone release-inhibiting hormone on circulating glucagon, insulin, and growth hormone in normal, diabetic, acromegalic, and hypopituitary patients. *Lancet*, i:697–701.
101. Nakao, K., Nakai, Y., Oki, S., Horii, K., and Imura, H. (1978): Presence of immunoreactive β-endorphin in normal human plasma—concomitant release of β-endorphin with adrenocorticotropin after metyrapone administration. *J. Clin. Invest.*, 62:1395–1398.
102. Pasternak, G. W., Goodman, R., and Snyder, S. H. (1975): An endogenous morphine-like factor in mammalian brain. *Life Sci.*, 16:1765–1769.
103. Pert, C. B., Bowie, D. L., Fong, B. T. W., and Chang, J. K. (1976): Synthetic analogues of Met-enkephalin which resist enzymatic destruction. In: *Opiates and Endogenous Opioid Peptides*, edited by H. W. Kosterlitz, pp. 79–86. Elsevier-North Holland Press, Amsterdam.
104. Pert, C. B., Bowie, D. L., Pert, A., Morell, J. L., and Gross, E. (1977): Agonist-antagonist properties of N-allyl-[D-Ala²]-Met-enkephalin. *Nature*, 269:73–75.
105. Pert, C. B., Pert, A., Chang, J., and Fong, B. (1976): [D-Ala²]-Met-enkephalinamide: a potent, long-lasting synthetic pentapeptide analgesic. *Science*, 194:330–332.
106. Pert, C. B., and Snyder, S. H. (1973): Opiate receptors: demonstration in nervous tissue. *Science*, 179:1011–1014.
107. Petrack, B., Czernik, A. J., Itterly, W., Ansell, J., and Chertock, H. (1978): Somatostatin analogs: selective inhibition of insulin but not glucagon secretion from the isolated perfused rat pancreas. *Diabetes (Suppl. 2)*, 27:264A.
108. Plotnikoff, N. P., Kastin, A. J., Coy, D. H., Christensen, C. W., Schally, A. V., and Spirtes, M. A. (1976): Neuropharmacological actions of enkephalin after systemic administration. *Life Sci.*, 19:1283–1288.
109. Plotnikoff, N. P., Kastin, A. J., and Schally, A. V. (1974): Growth hormone release-inhibiting hormone: Neuropharmacological studies. *Pharmacol. Biochem. Behav.*, 2:693–696.
110. Polak, J. M., Bloom, S. R., Sullivan, S. N., Facer, P., and Pearse, A. G. E. (1977): Enkephalin-like immunoreactivity in the human gastrointestinal tract. *Lancet*, i:972–974.
111. Polak, J. M., Pearse, A. G. E., Grimelius, L., Bloom, S. R., and Arimura, A. (1975): Growth-hormone release-inhibiting hormone in gastrointestinal and pancreatic D cells. *Lancet*, i:1220–1222.
112. Prange, A. J., Jr., Breese, G. R., Jahnke, G. D., Martin, B. R., Cooper, B. R., Cott, J. M., Wilson, I. C., Alltop, L. B., Lipton, M. A., Bissette, G., Nemeroff, C. B., and Loosen, P. T. (1975): Modification of pentobarbital effects by natural and synthetic polypeptides: Dissociation of brain and pituitary effects. *Life Sci.*, 16:1907–1914.
113. Renaud, L. P., Martin, J. B., and Brazeau, P. (1975): Depressant action of TRH, LH-RH and somatostatin on activity of central neurones. *Nature*, 225:233–235.
114. Rezek, M., Havlicek, V., Hughes, K. R., and Friesen, H. (1975): Cortical administration of

somatostatin (SRIF): Effect on sleep and motor behavior. *Pharmacol. Biochem. Behav.,* 5:73–77.

115. Rivier, J., Brazeau, P., Vale, W., Ling, N., Burgus, R., Gilon, C., Yardley, J., and Guillemin, R. (1973): Synthèse totale par phase solide d'un tétradécapeptide ayant les propriétés chimiques et biologiques de la somatostatine. *C.R. Acad. Sci. Paris,* 276:2737–2740.

116. Rivier, J., Brown, M., Rivier, C., Ling, N., and Vale, W. (1977): Hypothalamic hypophysiotropic hormones. In: *Peptides 1976,* edited by A. Loffet, pp. 427–451. Editions de L'Université de Bruxelles, Brussels.

117. Rivier, J., Brown, M., and Vale, W. (1975): D-Trp[8]-somatostatin: An analog of somatostatin more potent than the native molecule. *Biochem. Biophys. Res. Commun.,* 65:746–751.

118. Rivier, J., Brown, M., and Vale, W. (1976): Tyrosylated analogs of somatostatin. *J. Med. Chem.,* 19:1010–1013.

119. Roberts, J. L., and Herbert, E. (1977): Characterization of a common precursor to corticotropin and β-lipotropin: cell-free synthesis of the precursor and identification of corticotropin peptides in the molecule. *Proc. Natl. Acad. Sci. USA,* 74:4826–4830.

120. Roemer, D., Buescher, H. H., Hill, R. C., Pless, J., Bauer, W., Cardinaux, F., Closse, A., Hauser, D., and Huguenin, R. (1977): A synthetic enkephalin analogue with prolonged parenteral and oral analgesic activity. *Nature,* 268:547–549.

121. Rossier, J., Vargo, T. M., Minick, S., Ling, N., Bloom, F. E., and Guillemin, R. (1977): Regional dissociation of β-endorphin and enkephalin contents in rat brain and pituitary. *Proc. Natl. Acad. Sci. USA,* 74:5162–5165.

122. Rubinstein, M., Stein, S., Gerber, L. D., and Udenfriend, S. (1977): Isolation and characterization of the opioid peptides from rat pituitary: β-Lipotropin. *Proc. Natl. Acad. Sci. USA,* 74:3052–3055.

123. Sarantakis, D., and McKinley, W. A. (1973): Total synthesis of hypothalamic "Somatostatin." *Biochem. Biophys. Res. Commun.,* 54:234–238.

124. Sarantakis, D., McKinley, W. A., and Grant, N. H. (1973): The synthesis of biological activity of Ala[3,14]-somatostatin. *Biochem. Biophys. Res. Commun.,* 55:538–542.

125. Sarantakis, D., McKinley, W. A., Jaunakais, I., Clark, D., and Grant, N. H. (1976): Structure activity studies on somatostatin. *Clin. Endocrinol. (Suppl.),* 5:275–278.

126. Sarantakis, D., Teichman, J., Clark, D. E., and Lien, E. L. (1977): A bicyclo-somatostatin analog, highly specific for the inhibition of growth hormone release. *Biochem. Biophys. Res. Commun.,* 75:143–148.

127. Sarantakis, D., Teichman, J., Fenichel, R., and Lien, E. (1978): [des Ala[1], Gly[2]]-His[4,5] D-Trp[8]-somatostatin. A glucagon-specific and long-acting somatostatin analog. *FEBS Lett.,* 92:153–155.

128. Sarantakis, D., Teichman, J., Lien, E. L., and Fenichel, R. L. (1976): A novel undecapeptide, WY-40,770, with prolonged growth hormone release inhibiting activity. *Biochem. Biophys. Res. Commun.,* 73:336–342.

129. Schally, A. V., Coy, D. H., Arimura, A., Redding, T. W., Kastin, A. J., Vilchez-Martinez, J., Pedroza, E., Gordin, A., Meyers, C. A., Labrie, F., Hall, R., Reed, D., Gomez-Pan, A., and Besser, G. M. (1977): Hypothalamic regulatory hormones and their synthetic analogs. In: *Proc. 5th Int. Symp. Med. Chem.,* Paris, July 19–22. Elsevier-North Holland Press, Amsterdam *(in press).*

130. Schally, A. V., Coy, D. H., and Meyers, C. A. (1978): Hypothalamic regulatory hormones. *Ann. Rev. Biochem.,* 47:89–128.

131. Schally, A. V., Coy, D. H., Meyers, C. A., and Kastin, A. J. (1979): Hypothalamic peptide hormones: basic and clinical studies. In: *Hormonal Proteins and Peptides, Vol. 7,* edited by C. H. Li, pp. 1–54. Academic Press, New York.

132. Schally, A. V., Dupont, A., Arimura, A., Redding, T. W., and Linthicum, G. L. (1975): Isolation of porcine GH-release inhibiting hormone (GH-RIH): The existence of 3 forms of GH-RIH. *Fed. Proc.,* 34:584A.

133. Schally, A. V., Dupont, A., Arimura, A., Redding, T. W., Nishi, N., Linthicum, G. L., and Schlesinger, D. H. (1976): Isolation and structure of somatostatin from porcine hypothalami. *Biochemistry,* 15:509–514.

134. Shaw, J. S., and Turnbull, M. J. (1978): *In vitro* profile of some opioid pentapeptide analogues. *Eur. J. Pharmacol.,* 49:313–317.

135. Siler, T. M., Vandenberg, E., Yen, S. S. C., Brazeau, P., Vale, W., and Guillemin, R. (1973):

Inhibition of growth hormone release in humans by somatostatin. *J. Clin. Endocrinol. Metab.,* 37:632–634.

136. Simantov, R., and Snyder, S. H. (1976): Isolation and structure ·dentification of a morphine-like peptide 'Enkephalin' in bovine brain. *Life Sci.,* 18:781–788.

137. Simon, E. J., Hiller, J. M., and Edelman, I. (1973): Stereospecific binding of the potent narcotic analgesic [³H] etorphine to rat-brain homogenate. *Proc. Natl. Acad. Sci. USA,* 70:1947–1949.

138. Suda, T., Liotta, A. S., and Krieger, D. T. (1978): β-Endorphin is not detectable in plasma from normal human subjects. *Science,* 202:221–223.

139. Szekely, J. I., Ronai, A. Z., Dunai-Kovacs, Z., Miglecz, E., Berzetri, I., Bajusz, S., and Graf, L. (1977): [D-Met², Pro⁵]-enkephalinamide: a potent morphine-like analgesic. *Eur. J. Pharmacol.,* 43:293–294.

140. Terenius, J. (1973): Stereospecific interaction between narcotic analgesics and a synaptic plasma membrane fraction of rat cerebral cortex. *Acta Pharmacol. Toxicol.,* 32:317–320.

141. Terenius, L. (1977): Opioid peptides and opiates differ in receptor selectivity. *Psychoneuroendocrinology,* 2:53–58.

142. Terenius, L., and Wahlstrom, A. (1974): Inhibitors of narcotic receptor binding in brain extracts and cerebrospinal fluid. *Acta Pharmacol. Toxicol. (Suppl. 1),* 35:55.

143. Teschemacher, H., Opheim, K. E., Cox, B. M., and Goldstein, A. (1975): A peptide-like substance from pituitary that acts like morphine. 1. Isolation. *Life Sci.,* 16:1771–1776.

144. Tseng, L., Loh, H. H., and Li, C. H. (1977): Human β-Endorphin: Development of tolerance and behavioral activity in rats. *Biochem. Biophys. Res. Commun.,* 74:390–396.

145. Tyrrell, J. B., Lorenzi, M., Gerich, J. E., and Forsham, P. H. (1975): Inhibition of somatostatin of ACTH secretion in Nelson's syndrome. *J. Clin. Endocrinol. Metab.,* 40:1125–1127.

146. Unger, R. H., Dobbs, R. E., and Orci, L. (1978): Insulin, glucagon, and somatostatin secretion in the regulation of metabolism. *Ann. Rev. Physiol.,* 40:307–343.

147. Unger, R. H., and Orci, L. (1977): Hypothesis: The possible role of the pancreatic D-cell in the normal and diabetic states. *Diabetes,* 26:241–244.

148. Vale, W., Brazeau, P., Rivier, C., Brown, M., Boss, B., Rivier, J., Burgus, R., Ling, N., and Guillemin, R. (1975): Somatostatin. *Recent Prog. Horm. Res.,* 31:365–397.

149. Vale, W., Grant, G., Amoss, M., Blackwell, R., and Guillemin, R. (1972): Culture of enzymatically dispersed anterior pituitary cells: Functional validation of a method. *Endocrinology,* 91:562–572.

150. Vale, W., Rivier, C., Brazeau, P., and Guillemin, R. (1974): Effects of somatostatin on the secretion of thyrotropin and prolactin. *Endocrinology,* 95:968–977.

151. Vale, W., Rivier, C., and Brown, M. (1977): Regulatory peptides of the hypothalamus. *Ann. Rev. Physiol.,* 39:473–527.

152. Vale, W., Rivier, J., Ling, N., and Brown, M. (1978): Biologic and immunologic activities and applications of somatostatin analogs. *Metabolism (Suppl. 1),* 27:1391–1401.

153. Veber, D. F., Holly, F. W., Paleveda, W. J., Nutt, R. F., Bergstrand, S. J., Torchiana, M., Glitzer, M. S., Saperstein, R., and Hirschmann, R. (1978): Conformationally restricted bicyclic analogs of somatostatin. *Proc. Natl. Acad. Sci. USA,* 75:2636–2640.

154. Veber, D. F., Strachan, R. G., Bergstrand, S. J., Holly, F. W., Homnick, C. F., Hirschmann, R., Torchiana, M. L., and Saperstein, R. (1976): Nonreducible cyclic analogues of somatostatin. *J. Am. Chem. Soc.,* 98:2367–2369.

155. Veith, J. L., Sandman, C. A., Walker, J. M., Coy, D. H., and Kastin, A. J. (1978): Systemic administration of endorphins selectively alters open field behavior of rats. *Physiol. Behav.,* 20:539–542.

156. Verebey, K., Volavka, J., and Clouet, D. (1978): Endorphins in psychiatry. *Arch. Gen. Psychiatry,* 35:877–888.

157. Verhoeven, W. M. A., van Proog, H. M., Botter, P. A., Sunier, A., van Ree, J. M., and de Wied, D. (1978): [Des-Tyr¹]-γ-endorphin in schizophrenia. *Lancet,* i:1046–1047.

158. von Graffenfried, B., del Pozo, E., Krebs, E., Poldinger, W., Burmeister, P., and Kerp, L. (1978): Effects of the synthetic enkephalin analogue FK 33–824 in man. *Nature,* 272:729–730.

159. Voyles, N. R., Bhathena, S. J., Recant, L., Meyers, C. A., and Coy, D. H. (1979): Selective inhibition of glucagon and insulin secretion by somatostatin analogs. *Proc. Soc. Exp. Biol. Med.,* 160:76–79.

160. Walker, J. M., Berntson, G. G., Sandman, C. A., Coy, D. H., Schally, A. V., and Kastin,

A. J. (1977): An analog of enkephalin having prolonged opiate-like effects *in vivo. Science,* 196:85–87.

161. Walker, J. M., Sandman, C. A., Berntson, G. G., McGivern, R. F., Coy, D. H., and Kastin, A. J. (1977): Endorphin analogs with potent and long-lasting analgesic effects. *Pharmacol. Biochem. Behav.,* 7:543–548.

162. Wei, E., and Loh, E. (1976): Physical dependence on opiate-like peptides. *Science,* 193:1262–1263.

163. Williams, J. T., and North, R. A. (1978): Inhibition of firing of myenteric neurones by somatostatin. *Brain Res.,* 155:165–168.

164. Yamashiro, D., and Li, C. H. (1973): Synthesis of a peptide with full somatostatin activity. *Biochem. Biophys. Res. Commun.,* 54:882–887.

165. Yamashiro, D., Li, C. H., Tseng, L., and Loh, H. H. (1978): β-endorphin: synthesis and analgesic activity of several analogs modified in positions 2 and 5. *Int. J. Pept. Protein Res.,* 11:251–257.

166. Yamashiro, D., Tseng, L., Doneen, B. A., Loh, H. H., and Li, C. H. (1977): β-Endorphin: synthesis and morphine-like activity of analogs with D-amino acid residues in positions 1, 2, 4, and 5. *Int. J. Pept. Protein Res.,* 10:159–166.

167. Yamashiro, D., Tseng, L., and Li, C. H. (1977): [D-Thr^2, Th$_z^5$]- and [D-Met^2, Th$_2^5$]-enkephalinamides: Potent analgesics and intravenous injection. *Biochem. Biophys. Res. Commun.,* 78:1124–1129.

168. Yen, S. S. C., Siler, T. M., and DeVane, G. W. (1974): Effect of somatostatin in patients with acromegaly. Suppression of growth hormone, insulin and glucose levels. *N. Engl. J. Med.,* 290:935–938.

Gastrointestinal Hormones, edited by
George B. Jerzy Glass.
Raven Press, New York © 1980.

Chapter 16

Chymodenin: Between "Factor" and "Hormone"

Joel W. Adelson, Mary Elizabeth Nelbach, Ruth Chang,
Charles B. Glaser, and Gregory B. Yates

Institutes of Medical Sciences, 2200 Webster Street, San Francisco, California 94115

Chymodenin is a substance with an unusual (and controversial) biological activity: the stimulation of enzyme-specific secretion of chymotrypsinogen by the pancreas. Its effect appears restricted to chymotrypsinogen secretion, without parallel effect on the secretion of other digestive enzymes (3,4). Ongoing investigations of chymodenin's structure have clearly established its amino acid sequence homology with gastric inhibitory polypeptide (GIP) and with glucagon, and a radioimmunoassay (RIA) under development should allow determination of its presence or absence in serum. Whether or not chymodenin is a true gastrointestinal hormone remains a question that the next few years' work will likely resolve.

HISTORICAL BACKGROUND

During 1966 through 1968, Adelson and Ehrlich (1) found a contaminant in a crude preparation of cholecystokinin-pancreozymin (Boots Pancreozymin, Boots Pure Drug Co., England) that caused the release of enzymes from isolated pancreatic zymogen granules *in vitro.* The active factor at first was thought to be pancreozymin itself, and the activity against the zymogen granules was thought to be an *in vitro* model of pancreozymin's *in vivo* action on its target, the zymogen granule. In this model, pancreozymin would recognize and enter the pancreatic acinar cell, open the zymogen granule, and cause release of the granule contents into the pancreatic duct. Before long, however, it became clear in our laboratory that pancreozymin in pure form did not elicit the release of enzymes from zymogen granules; instead, one (or several) contaminant(s) in the crude preparation was responsible for the activity. In addition, it was demonstrated by many laboratories that peptide hormones do not generally enter cells. Thus, we reported in 1972 (2) a new interesting "factor" that caused enzyme release from pancreatic zymogen granules *in vitro* at low concentrations, and that this activity was destroyed by protease. We had little idea of what its biological role might be, but since the activity occurred in low concentrations, was unique, and originated in a hormone-containing mixture, it appeared worthy of further study.

PURIFICATION

Purification of the new "factor" was the next task, which was accomplished by standard chromatographic methods. The purification scheme has not yet been reported in detail. Chymodenin was purified from a side fraction obtained from Prof. Viktor Mutt's Gastrointestinal Hormone (GIH) Laboratory during their routine preparation of secretin, cholecystokinin-pancreozymin (CCK-PZ), and vasoactive intestinal polypeptide (VIP). Since the GIH Laboratory's method of producing these substances has varied somewhat over the years, the purification of chymodenin has necessarily been modified in response to these changes. In the original purifications, chymodenin's biological specific activity was used to guide its purification; later, relative purity was monitored by co-migration of pure chymodenin standards with intermediate mixtures in a high-resolution polyacrylamide gel electrophoresis system. The potential dangers of this approach were largely avoided through the use of stain countermigration techniques (5), which produced remarkably sharp and well-resolved electrophoretic bands.

At present, the purification of chymodenin is performed as follows: *A*cidic-*ME*thanol-*S*oluble *N*eutral pH *I*nsoluble material ("AMESNI"), obtained from the GIH Laboratory, Karolinska Institute, Stockholm, Sweden, is desalted on a column of Sephadex G-25. The peptide-protein fraction eluting at the void volume of this column is then applied to a column of sulfopropyl Sephadex SP-C25 in 0.05 M ammonium bicarbonate buffer, pH 7.5. After all ultraviolet-absorbing material that does not bind to the ion-exchange column in this buffer has been eluted, a shallow linear gradient of 0.05 M to 0.25 M ammonium bicarbonate, pH 7.5 to 8.0, is used to elute the remaining adsorbed material. Chymodenin routinely elutes from the column at 0.13 to 0.15 M ammonium bicarbonate, along with a number of other peptides. Variations in the composition of the AMESNI starting material produce a corresponding diversity of elution profiles at this stage of the purification, but useful qualitative similarities may be discerned. Samples of the collected fractions are then lyophilized and subjected to electrophoresis as outlined above. Chymodenin-containing fractions are identified by co-migration of authentic chymodenin in the same group of gels. These fractions are then pooled and lyophilized to remove the volatile ammonium bicarbonate salt.

Substantially pure chymodenin is obtained by column chromatography of the above material on carboxymethyl cellulose (CM-23, Whatman) in a shallower gradient of ammonium bicarbonate. The chymodenin elutes at about 0.13 M ammonium bicarbonate, pH 7.5, in a gradient run from 0.10 M to 0.20 M ammonium bicarbonate. The chymodenin-containing fractions at this stage of purification sometimes contain less than 5% peptide impurities, judged by gel electrophoresis. However, depending on the variability in the initial AMESNI starting material, this stage of purification may still result in about 10% inhomogeneity of the chymodenin-containing fractions.

Further purification is carried out either by gel filtration on Sephadex G-75 in 0.05 M acetic acid, or by equilibrium chromatography on QAE-Sephadex in a gradient of 0.01 M to 0.20 M sodium pyrophosphate, pH 8.55, where the chymodenin appears to run as an anion and to elute as a broad peak behind its more basic contaminants. The final product of the purification is lyophilized and stored at $-70°C$ as a powder. Laboratories wishing further details on purification are welcome to write to us.

PURITY AND GENERAL CHARACTERISTICS OF CHYMODENIN

Purity of the chymodenin preparation has been examined by a variety of criteria. (a) No dansyl-reactive contaminants are present, and since chymodenin contains a "blocked" N-terminal amino acid, the level of detection of peptide contaminants whose N-termini are not also blocked can be estimated as less than 1%. (b) A single C-terminus, isoleucine, is demonstrable after brief treatment with carboxypeptidase A. (c) No stainable contaminants can be detected in the counter-migration-of-dye disc gel electrophoresis system used in the purification procedure. (d) The number of tryptic peptides corresponds well to the molecular weight and content of lysine and arginine residues (see below). (e) A single peak is obtained on gel filtration on Sephadex G-75. (f) A single band that migrates very slowly is observed in polyacrylamide gels run at pH 9.5, pH 10, and pH 10.5; the peptide is cationic at pH 9.5 and very weakly anionic at pH 10. This suggests that the isoelectric pH of chymodenin is slightly below pH 10. No stainable contaminants of either cationic or anionic nature were detected at these pH levels. (g) A single band is observed in polyacrylamide gel electrophoresis in the presence of SDS and urea. Taken together, these criteria of homogeneity of the chymodenin preparation indicate that no single impurity is present at a level greater than 1%, and that the aggregate level of impurity is likely to be less than 5%.

CHARACTERIZATION OF CHYMODENIN

The molecular weight of chymodenin is in the range of 8,500 to 9,500 daltons. This is unusually high for a gastrointestinal hormone. The molecular weight has been estimated from migration on polyacrylamide gels in the presence of SDS and urea, analytical sedimentation equilibrium ultracentrifugation, amino acid composition, and sequencing of tryptic peptides.

Table 1 presents our current estimate of the amino acid composition of chymodenin. It is unusual in its observed content of four half-cystine residues, and is relatively rich in aromatic amino acids.

The N-terminal amino acid residue of chymodenin is blocked to dansylation, and it can be cleaved by pyrrolidone carboxylyl peptidase. This suggests that pyrrolidone carboxylic acid, or pyroglutamic acid, is at the N-terminus. There are two disulfide bridges, which have been identified by autoradiographs produced from tryptic maps of chymodenin that had been reduced by dithiothreitol and alkylated by ^{14}C-iodoacetic acid. The locations of the disulfide bridges have not yet been determined, although one disulfide appears to have one end located immediately adjacent to the blocked N-terminus. These data give a tentative view of the unusual configuration

$$
\begin{array}{c}
\text{S—} \\
| \\
\text{pyroGlu—Cys—Lys—}
\end{array}
$$

at the N-terminus. A portion of the amino acid sequence of the molecule has been partially elucidated by the dansyl Edman technique (10). It is of interest

TABLE 1. *Amino acid composition of chymodenin*

Amino acid	Residues/mole
Ala	6
Arg	6
Asx	9
½ Cys	3–4
Glx	8–9
Gly	4
His	1
Ile	3
Leu	3
Lys	5
Met	1
Phe	4
Ser	4
Thr	4
Trp	3
Tyr	3
Val	3
Number of residues/mole	74–76
Calculated molecular weight	~9,000

that the following region shows homology to the N-terminal region of the gluca-
gon-secretin family (8).

Chymodenin
peptide: -Asx-Asx-Arg-Arg⌐Ala-Glx-Gly-Thr-Phe⌐Pro -Gly-Lys -Ile ---
                           1   5
GIP: Tyr ⌐Ala-Glu-Gly-Thr-Phe⌐Ile -Ser -Asp-Tyr---
                           1   5
Glucagon: His -Ser ⌐Gln-Gly-Thr-Phe⌐Thr-Ser -Asp-Tyr---
                           1   5
Secretin: His -Ser -Asp⌐Gly-Thr-Phe⌐Thr-Ser -Glu-Leu---
                           1   5
VIP: His -Ser -Asp-Ala-Val ⌐Phe⌐Thr-Asp-Asn-Tyr---

The outlined region bears a pentapeptide sequence identical to one in GIP.
The region homologous to GIP occurs at the N-terminus of GIP. Chymodenin,
on the other hand, appears to extend further for an undetermined length toward
its N-terminus. In chymodenin, the region immediately adjacent to this homologous segment in the N-terminal direction contains the trypsin-sensitive sequence
Asx-Asx-Arg-Arg-. It is tempting to speculate that chymodenin might be cleaved
in this region under some physiological conditions, or that it might be a precursor
to one or more active peptides of smaller molecular weight.

RADIOIMMUNOASSAY OF CHYMODENIN

A specific radioimmunoassay (RIA) capable of detecting chymodenin at low
concentrations in serum and tissues is in the process of development (11). High-
titer antisera to purified chymodenin have been obtained from rabbits after
immunizing with multiple intradermal injections of hemocyanin-conjugated chymodenin emulsified with complete Freunds adjuvant. After three boosters, antiserum titers in the range of 1:25,000 to 1:100,000 have been found.

Methodology for labeling chymodenin with iodine-125 is still being improved.
Chymodenin has been labeled by the standard method of Greenwood et al.
(9), using the oxidizing agent chloramine-T. This has resulted in a labeled chymodenin of satisfactorily high specific radioactivity, but which rapidly loses
immunoreactivity during storage. An alternate method in which a water-insolu-
ble chloramide, 1,3,4,6-tetrachloro-3α,6α-diphenyl-glycoluril, was substituted
for chloramine-T in the reaction, improved the immunoreactivity and stability
of the labeled chymodenin somewhat, but still has not given a label of sufficient
stability for satisfactory routine RIA. However, such labeled chymodenin has
permitted the assay at this level of development to detect approximately 30
pg of chymodenin in a sample volume of 200 μl, as shown in Fig. 1.

The assay at this stage of development has been used to measure the cross-
reactivity of other gastrointestinal peptides that might be related to or suspected
contaminants in chymodenin: GIP, VIP, secretin, glucagon, CCK-PZ, and insu-

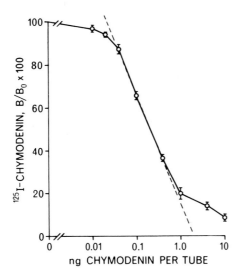

FIG. 1. RIA for chymodenin. Assay conditions are as described in ref 13. Each *horizontal* data bar gives the ratio of bound over total counts to the bound over total counts when no unlabeled chymodenin was added. Duplicate samples are shown; *circles* are the arithmetic average.

lin have shown only minimal cross-reactivity with chymodenin, at concentrations 10^3 to 10^4 times greater than chymodenin, as seen in Fig. 2.

Several attempts have been made to determine the presence of chymodenin in sera of fasted and fed rats. Whereas sera consistently show competition with labeled chymodenin in the assay, consistent with the presence of circulating chymodenin-like immunoreactivity, the potential presence of interfering sub-

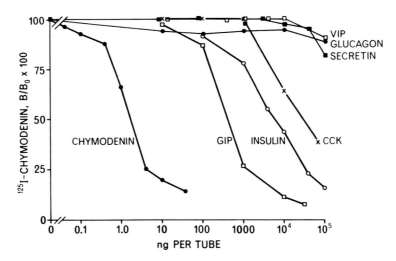

FIG. 2. RIA for chymodenin. Cross-reactivity in assay. Conditions as in Fig. 1 (VIP, secretin, and CCK were the generous gift of Prof. V. Mutt. GIP was purchased from the laboratory of J. C. Brown, Vancouver, Canada.)

stances in sera has thus far rendered equivocal any conclusion that chymodenin does circulate. Attempts are in progress to remove interfering substances, and to prepare chymodenin-free sera by affinity gel chromatography, to use as diluents in the assay.

For further improvement in the RIA for chymodenin, labeling by use of the method of Bolton and Hunter (6) has been carried out. This method avoids exposing chymodenin to any oxidizing conditions, which might be affecting the stability of the peptide, e.g., by oxidation of the methionine residue known to be present. In addition, instead of iodinating tyrosine residues, the Bolton-Hunter reagent couples to lysine residues, which may be located in a less sensitive region of the chymodenin molecule in terms of stability and immunoreactivity. The resulting labeled chymodenin has remained stable and useful for more than 3 months, in comparison with 1 to 2 weeks' useful lifetime for the chloramine-T labeled chymodenin. In order for the Bolton-Hunter-labeled chymodenin to be satisfactory, however, its specific radioactivity must be increased substantially, which will require development of a method to separate monoiodinated chymodenin from noniodinated chymodenin. This has proved difficult so far.

ACTIVITY OF CHYMODENIN

Although chymodenin was first purified on the basis of its ability to cause the lysis of zymogen granules *in vitro,* its primary known biological activity *in vivo* is to cause the rapid and dramatic secretion of pancreatic chymotrypsinogen, without concomitantly raising lipase activity (4). This is illustrated in Table 2A, where the *in situ* rabbit pancreas was exposed to 20 μg of chymodenin. A statistically significant ($p < 0.01$) threefold increase in chymotrypsinogen level was observed within 20 min. A smaller increase in total protein secretion was seen, corresponding to the protein increase expected if chymotrypsinogen secretion were being stimulated almost exclusively. Table 2B shows the similar effect of chymodenin *in vitro.* In Table 2C, with data from the same animals as shown in Table 2B, a surprising opposite enzyme-specific effect is shown. Here, lipase secretion dramatically increased relative to chymotrypsinogen and to total protein output, after stimulation of the *in vitro* pancreas preparation with methacholine chloride (4). Table 3 summarizes and contrasts the effects of chymodenin and of cholinergic stimulation by methacholine chloride on pancreatic secretion. These substances are capable of revealing an extraordinary enzyme-specific secretory capability of the pancreas.

The proposed activity of chymodenin is controversial; several publications have suggested that it is an impossible one (12,14), whereas others (13) have taken the existence of chymodenin as a proof of Pavlov's theory (7) that pancreatic enzymes should be secreted in nonparallel fashion. A balanced view might be that we do not understand the mechanism of action of chymodenin; that the exocytosis theory of cell secretion in its present form is difficult to reconcile with the activity of chymodenin; and that there is a variety of other,

TABLE 2. *Effect of chymodenin and methacholine chloride administration on secretion by the rabbit pancreas*

Experimental condition	Chymotrypsinogen	Protein	Lipase
A. Control	100 ± 10	100 ± 10	100 ± 20
Chymodenin	290 ± 70 ($p < 0.01$)	140 ± 14 ($p < 0.025$)	105 ± 15
B. Control	50 ± 10	90 ± 10	130 ± 50
Chymodenin	210 ± 60 ($p < 0.01$)	170 ± 30 ($p < 0.01$)	130 ± 100
C. Control	100	100	100
Methacholine	350 ± 50 ($p < 0.01$)	600 ± 60 ($p < 0.01$)	$2,700 \pm 700$ ($p < 0.01$)

A. Rabbit pancreas *in situ:* Dose was 20 µg chymodenin; mean output and SEM were normalized so that 100 equals the mean enzyme output for three 20-min periods following either saline (control) or chymodenin administration. The collection period after treatment was 20 min.

B. Rabbit pancreas *in vitro:* Dose was 20 µg of chymodenin in 100 ml bath; data were normalized so that 100 equals output ± SEM in the first of three 20-min pretreatment periods. Outputs are for the first of three 20-min posttreatment periods.

C. Rabbit pancreas *in vitro:* Paired data from pancreas preparations were normalized so that 100 equals output for 20-min collection period prior to treatment. Collection after treatment was for 40 min; data were then compared with pretreatment levels by a paired *t*-test.

All data in experiments A, B, and C are taken from ref. 4.

TABLE 3. *Qualitative comparison of the effects of chymodenin and of methacholine chloride treatment on pancreatic enzyme output* in vitro.

	Chymodenin	Methacholine
Chymotrypsinogen output	Major increase	Increase
Lipase output	No effect	Major increase
Total protein output	Minor increase	Major increase
Chymotrypsinogen/lipase ratio	Increase	Decrease

independent work supporting the observed phenomenon of nonparallel, enzyme-specific secretion (7). It does not seem impossible that chymodenin and exocytosis might coexist. Whatever the mechanism of action of chymodenin may be, the data are clear: the molecule increases chymotrypsinogen secretion without increasing lipase secretion, and with a minor increase in total protein secretion. This suggests, as Pavlov proposed originally, that the secretions of the digestive tract are rapidly modified to digest the actual food eaten, efficiently and without waste, rather than functioning without regard to the composition of substrate molecules in a particular meal. Chymodenin remains the first factor discovered, isolated, and characterized that is capable of mediating enzyme specific secretion in hormone-like fashion between gut and pancreas and thus between meal and digestion.

SUMMARY AND CONCLUSIONS

Chymodenin is a basic peptide purified to near homogeneity from porcine duodenum. It rapidly elicits the specific secretion of chymotrypsinogen from the rabbit pancreas *in vivo* and *in vitro*. Its molecular weight is approximately 9,000 daltons; the N-terminal amino acid residue appears to be a pyrrolidone carboxylyl group, and there are two disulfide bridges. One segment of chymodenin's sequence, at least, is homologous to GIP and glucagon. A RIA has been developed that is capable of detecting the peptide at low concentrations.

PROJECTIONS FOR THE FUTURE

In the future, further work will allow the complete elucidation of the amino acid sequence of chymodenin, and the possible activities of subfragments (active fragments). Because of its size and structure, there is a possibility that chymodenin may be a prohormone.

Further experiments, aided by the RIA, will be necessary to elucidate more exactly the role of chymodenin in digestive physiology. Questions of immediate interest include: What are basal levels of chymodenin in the circulation? What stimuli and digestive substrates elicit chymodenin release? At what levels does chymodenin appear in portal and systemic circulations and for how long? What specific tissues and cells contain chymodenin? What are the location and nature of cellular receptors for chymodenin?

The question remains open whether chymodenin may have other physiological activities besides the one studied. It is also of interest to speculate on the existence of other intestinal "factors" or "hormones" that might cause specific secretion of other digestive enzymes by the pancreas.

REFERENCES

1. Adelson, J. W., and Ehrlich, A. (1968): *In vitro* release of amylase from zymogen granules by factors from porcine duodenal mucosa. *Fed. Proc.,* 27: Abstr. 2005.
2. Adelson, J. W., and Ehrlich, A. (1972): The effect of porcine duodenal mucosa extract upon enzyme release from pancreatic zymogen granules *in vitro. Endocrinology,* 90:60–66.
3. Adelson, J. W., and Rothman, S. S. (1974): Selective pancreatic enzyme secretion due to a new peptide called chymodenin. *Science,* 183:1087–1089.
4. Adelson, J. W., and Rothman, S. S. (1975): Chymodenin, a duodenal peptide: Specific stimulation of chymotrypsinogen secretion. *Am. J. Physiol.,* 239:1680–1686.
5. Ahlroth, A., and Mutt, V. (1970): Polyacrylamide gel electrophoresis of polypeptides from the intestinal wall, with counter-migration of dye. *Anal. Biochem.,* 37:125–128.
6. Bolton, A. E., and Hunter, W. M. (1973): The labelling of proteins to high specific radioactivities by conjugation to a ^{125}I-containing acylating agent. *Biochem. J.,* 133:529–539.

7. Case, R. M. (1978): Synthesis, intracellular transport and discharge of exportable proteins in the pancreatic acinar cell and other cells. *Biol. Rev.,* 53:211–354.
8. Chang, R., Glaser, C. B., and Adelson, J. W. (1978): Structural studies on chymodenin, a hormone-like gastrointestinal peptide related to GIP and glucagon. *Scand. J. Gastroenterol. (Suppl. 49),* 13:36.
9. Greenwood, F. C., Hunter, W. M., and Glover, J. S. (1963): The preparation of ^{131}I-labelled human growth hormone of high specific radioactivity. *Biochem. J.,* 89:114–123.
10. Hartley, B. S. (1970): Strategy and tactics in protein chemistry. *Biochem. J.,* 119:805–822.
11. Nelbach, M. E., Yates, G. B., and Adelson, J. W. (1978): Radioimmunoassay of chymodenin, with a new ^{125}I-labeling method. *Scand. J. Gastroenterol. (Suppl. 49),* 13:133.
12. Palade, G. E. (1975): Intracellular aspects of the process of protein synthesis. *Science,* 189:347–358.
13. Rothman, S. S. (1977): The digestive enzymes of the pancreas: a mixture of inconstant proportions. *Ann. Rev. Physiol.,* 39:373–389.
14. Tartakoff, A. M., Jamieson, J. D., Scheele, G. A., and Palade, G. E. (1975): Studies on the pancreas of the guinea pig. *J. Biol. Chem.,* 250:2671–2677.

Gastrointestinal Hormones, edited by
George B. Jerzy Glass.
Raven Press, New York © 1980.

Chapter 17

Urogastrone: Isolation, Structure, and Basic Functions

H. Gregory

Imperial Chemical Industries Limited, Pharmaceuticals Division, Mereside, Alderley Park, Macclesfield, Cheshire, England

INTRODUCTION

As long ago as 1930, Sandweiss made the clinical observation that pregnancy caused improvement in the symptoms of duodenal ulceration. During pregnancy abundant amounts of hormones appeared in urine, and extracts of urine were therefore tested and shown to have beneficial effects on Mann-Williamson ulcers in dogs (35). In 1939 several workers reported that urine extracts could cause inhibition of gastric acid secretion and that this property extended to the urine of nonpregnant females and also males (8,14,17,32). The quantities of extracts found to be effective in protecting against ulceration in dogs were reported to be less than those required to inhibit gastric secretion (14), and this led to the suggestion that two independent factors existed in human urine.

One component was described with antiulcer properties, which promoted fibroblastic proliferation and epithelization of the mucosa and this was named anthelone (34). Beneficial effects were reported on experimental ulcers in a large number of dogs. Usually the human urine extracts were given parenterally, but considerable improvement was also described in a smaller number of Mann-Williamson dogs following oral treatment with extracts of pregnant mares' urine (36).

Anthelone was mainly studied by Sandweiss and co-workers (34–36), whereas Gray, Ivy, et al. (16–18) followed the inhibitor of acid secretion. These early studies showed that the latter was a more clearly definable property (5) and it subsequently received more attention. Because of a suggested relationship to the postulated duodenal hormone enterogastrone, the antisecretory agent was called urogastrone (16).

Considerable efforts were made to characterize the active agent, but although some biological and physical characterization was achieved, isolation of pure material had to await the arrival of new techniques. The original extracts were obtained by benzoic acid adsorption from urine (35); this process was modified somewhat by Gray et al. (18), but they considered their product not to be proteinaceous. Over 10 years later R. A. Gregory (25) obtained a much purer preparation that inhibited acid secretion in conscious gastric fistula dogs with amounts equivalent to 0.1 to 0.5 mg of urine, depending on the level of histamine used to evoke secretion. The product, a relatively specific inhibitor of acid secretion, was described as a combination of a low molecular weight protein and a yellow pigment.

Further advances were made in assay systems for rapid measurement using rats (33); additional evidence appeared for a protein structure (30), although some reports described urogastrone as a high molecular weight glycoprotein (4,31), and its existence was established beyond doubt.

ISOLATION

The earliest methods for processing urine were based on benzoic acid precipitation, some use was also made of ethanol and ammonium sulfate precipitation, and charcoal proved to be an effective adsorbent (25). For routine large-scale use, however, precipitation of the active material with tannic acid was found to be convenient (24). Volumes of approximately 400 liters daytime male urine were processed daily to give a solid, 20 to 30 mg/liter urine, which retained potency indefinitely when stored at −40°C. Subsequent studies showed that the process gave 50 to 70% recovery of the urogastrone, which amounted to approximately 30 μg/liter urine when measured by radioimmunoassay (RIA).

Inhibitory effects of urine extracts have been described in a number of species, and dogs with denervated fundic pouches, with histamine or pentagastrin as stimulant, were used to quantitate the gastric secretory response to purified fractions in our work. For routine, rapid testing of large numbers of fractions, rats with a simple stomach perfusion gave quick positive or negative evaluations.

The purification process constructed to give pure urogastrone contained 12 stages (Table 1). It was necessary to have a process that would routinely and reliably provide material of the same quality, so although the number of stages

TABLE 1. *The isolation of urogastrone*

Procedure	Yield	Potency[a] (μg/kg)	Recovery (%)
1. Precipitation with tannic acid and acid methanol extraction	80 g		100
2. Base ion-exchange resin and acetic acid elution	n.d.[b]		
3. Sephadex G-50 in ammonium hydrogen carbonate buffer	6.0 g	200	50[c]
4. Solvent extraction	n.d.		
5. Sephadex G-25 in acetic acid buffer	2.0 g	100	33
6. Carboxymethyl cellulose with ammonium acetate buffers	n.d.		
7. Biogel P6 in acetic acid buffer	140 mg	10	23
8. Carboxymethyl cellulose in sodium acetate buffers	n.d.		
9. Biogel P6 in ammonium acetate buffer	50 mg	4	20
10. Aminoethyl cellulose in ammonium acetate buffer	4 mg β, 4 mg γ	1	13
11. Carboxymethyl cellulose in sodium acetate buffers	n.d.		
12. Biogel P6 in ammonium acetate buffer	2.0 mg β, 2.0 mg γ	0.5	13

Reproduced from Gregory and Willshire (24).

[a] Expressed as approx. dose (μg/kg) for 50–70% inhibition of secretion in Heidenhain pouch dogs.

[b] n.d. samples were not weighed or assayed because of the presence of salts.

[c] Recovery from the crude starting material at stage 3 as determined by the rat assay was usually 25–50%—see discussion.

seemed large, the practice proved to be more efficient than trying to refine one particular stage and dispense with others. The individual stages used a number of different properties of urogastrone and could each be carried out reproducibly in a day. At a late stage in the isolation, active material was found in three regions of an aminoethyl cellulose column (stage 10, Table 1). Two of these led to separate pure entities, β and γ urogastrones, which had clearly different physical properties but the same biological potency (24).

The two urogastrones were each obtained in yields of less than 1 mg/1,000 liter urine; they were both acidic polypeptides and readily water soluble. Biological activity was retained after the peptides were kept in solutions pH 1 to 11 at 37°C for extended periods and also in solutions of strong organic acids such as trifluoroacetic acid. They were surprisingly resistant to degradation by mammalian proteolytic enzymes; treatment with trypsin or pepsin at 37°C for 12 hr left the molecule intact (20). Leucine aminopeptidase and both carboxypeptidases A and B failed to liberate significant quantities of amino acids from the ends of the molecules.

STRUCTURE

It was necessary to break the disulfide bonds in the urogastrones to enable clean enzymic digests to be prepared. Both S-carboxymethyl and S-carboxamidomethyl derivatives were made, and these had the same molecular size and amino acid composition as the parent molecules, thus indicating that they were single polypeptide chains. They were susceptible to a number of proteolytic enzymes, but trypsin, chymotrypsin, and thermolysin were particularly useful giving smaller peptide fragments that were each purified and their sequences established using the dansyl-Edman technique (18a). An enzyme isolated from the fungus *Armillaria mellea* had good specificity for bonds on the amino side of lysine, and this gave a good limited breakdown of the urogastrone derivatives; it would also liberate a six-residue peptide from the C-terminus of β-urogastrone. Partial acid hydrolysis gave additional peptide fragments, and with many small peptides from the different degradations, the overlapping sequences established the structure of β-urogastrone. As work progressed it became apparent that the γ-urogastrone had the same sequence apart from being one amino acid shorter (19).

The directions of the disulfide bonds were indicated from partial acid hydrolysates of the intact molecule. An important observation was that the disulfide bonds reformed from the open chain reduced compound to give a fully active urogastrone. The structure of β-urogastrone was found to be a single polypeptide chain of 53 residues with three internal disulfide bonds (Fig. 1) whereas γ urogastrone simply lacked the C-terminal arginine residue, and we have regarded urogastrone as a single entity for most purposes. These polypeptides were quite different from any other agent then known to affect gastrointestinal function (22).

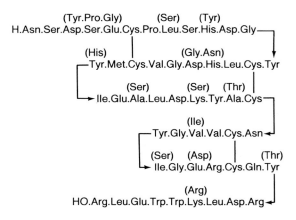

FIG. 1. Amino acid sequence of β-urogastrone. Residues altered in mouse epidermal growth factor are given in parentheses.

ACTION ON GASTRIC SECRETIONS

The inhibition of gastric acid secretion by crude urine preparations was, of course, well established, but this has been more clearly defined when using pure material. Parenteral administration of urogastrone to dogs with Heidenhain or Pavlov pouches, or with a gastric fistula, gave prompt and intense inhibition of induced secretion although the dose required depended on the level of stimulation. Thus, in Fig. 2, in which histamine was used to give about 70% of maximal acid output, the secretion was completely suppressed by urogastrone at 1 μg/ kg. The dose-response curve was steep, however, and under the same circumstances of stimulation 0.1 μg/kg gave little inhibition whereas at a lower level of agonist it was quite effective at that dose.

Urogastrone strongly suppresses acid secretion induced by the action of histamine and also the hormonal type of response to pentagastrin, the cholinergic stimulation of methacholine, or the physiological stimulus of a test meal in dogs (15). It is also effective in cats, monkeys, and rats, although the latter species is somewhat less sensitive. The dominant effect is on the volume of secretion. Acid concentration does fall slightly, pepsin concentration increases slightly and rises further as the levels of secretion rise toward the initial levels.

Doses as low as 0.25 μg/kg/hr i.v. gave inhibition of submaximal pentagastrin responses in man to the extent of 80%. Secretion stimulated by histamine or insulin was similarly suppressed without clinical side effects. Although acid and intrinsic factor outputs were reduced, pepsin output was less obviously affected but rose after completing the infusion of inhibitor (10). In patients

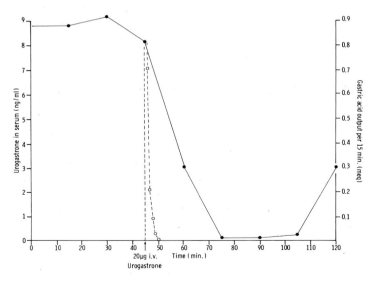

FIG. 2. Serum level of urogastrone in a Heidenhain pouch dog (20 kg) following intravenous injection and also the acid output with continuous histamine infusion. (From ref. 20.)

with Zollinger-Ellison syndrome the basal gastric secretion was reduced by 50 to 80% using the standard infusion of 0.25 μg/kg/hr (9). Acid concentration also decreased, but the production of intrinsic factor went up by 400% compared with a fall of some 25% in normal individuals, and this may be related to the doubling of plasma gastrin levels during the infusion. It was impressive that urogastrone still inhibited effectively in the presence of a substantial molar excess of the natural hormone agonist gastrin. The rise in gastrin levels from an autonomous source may be related to a reduced facility for binding at the parietal cell caused by urogastrone. Studies in ulcer patients confirmed the ability of urogastrone to suppress basal acid secretion; maximal secretion in response to pentagastrin was blocked to the extent of 50% by the standard 0.25 μg/kg/hr, and it remained equally effective after five daily infusions to these patients (29).

Earlier studies on the specificity of this peptide (25) have been confirmed and extended. Salivary, pancreatic, and bile secretions were not affected by doses several times greater than those affecting gastric secretion. It did not affect body temperature or blood pressure, nor did it have a primary effect in reducing stomach mucosal blood flow as a means of inhibiting secretion (15).

Clearly urogastrone, as an antagonist, was at least the equal of the natural agonist gastrin in similar blood concentration, but the mode of action was not obvious. To investigate this further, the action was studied on gastric mucosa *in vitro*. Pentagastrin-stimulated acid output from frog mucosa was reduced (15), as was the response to histamine from mammalian mucosa. Kitten mucosa *in vitro* gave a greater than twofold output of acid in response to 10^{-4} M histamine, and the effect was abolished by urogastrone at 10^{-6} M (20). However, urogastrone had little or no effect on histamine-induced responses of guinea pig atrium or ileum (E. L. Gerring, *personal communication*). Thus although the action appears to be at the mucosal level, it is not on histamine receptors.

RELATIONSHIP TO MOUSE EPIDERMAL GROWTH FACTOR

When urogastrone was characterized it was clearly different from known gastrointestinal peptides; however, a striking correlation with mouse epidermal growth factor (mEGF) emerged subsequently (Fig. 1). This peptide, which was present in male mouse submaxillary glands at over 0.1% of the wet weight, was also a polypeptide of 53 amino acid residues (37) with only 16 of these changed relative to urogastrone (19). The substitutions occur fairly evenly across the whole molecule, and 14 of them were compatible with single base changes in the triplet codons of the genetic code. Although urogastrone is rather more acidic than mEGF, predictably the changes would have little effect on the overall conformation of the two molecules (22).

Extensive investigations by Cohen and co-workers (7) have shown mEGF to be a powerful mitogen for epithelial cells. It caused proliferation in organ cultures and would, for example, cause regeneration of rabbit corneal epithelium *in vivo*. It also had the property of causing the eyes of newborn mice to open prematurely as a result of daily injections; urogastrone produced exactly the same effect at the same dose (19). Both peptides were equipotent in suppressing gastric acid secretion in rats and dogs under a number of circumstances. Preliminary physical data on a growth factor from human urine (6) were sufficiently close to urogastrone to make it probable that urogastrone is a human epidermal growth factor. Neither name is entirely appropriate to the particular molecule, but "urogastrone" has an established literature of over 30 years as a basis for its continued use.

ACTION ON CELLULAR PROCESSES

The effects of urogastrone and mEGF were compared on cultured human fibroblasts. DNA synthesis and α-aminobutyric acid uptake were stimulated to the same extent ($ED_{50} \sim 0.6$ ng/ml), and at submaximal concentrations the effects of the two peptides were additive but gave the same maximal effect. Urogastrone or mEGF competed similarly with either of the peptides labeled with ^{125}I, confirming that they shared a common site on the fibroblasts (27). Urogastrone and mEGF had such similar behavior in a number of systems that the much more readily available mouse peptide was often used routinely to study "urogastrone" actions in preliminary experiments. There is extensive literature on mEGF (2), but we will only comment here where it seems to be relevant to the gastrointestinal tract.

Studies with urogastrone have been extended to a number of experimentally prepared ulcer systems. In reserpine-induced ulcers in guinea pigs, infusions of urogastrone at 5 or 10 μg/kg/hr markedly inhibited the formation of gastric erosions, and acid and pepsin secretions were substantially reduced (20). In rats single acetic acid-induced duodenal ulcers showed a decrease of 50% compared with controls at a dose of 5 μg/kg/hr s.c.; mEGF gave a similar result (20).

Direct healing effects are not easily separated from the reduced acid secretion, but in rats mEGF at 50 μg/kg caused a 100% increase in ornithine and histidine decarboxylase activity in the stomach (P. B. Scholes, *personal communication*). mEGF also stimulated ornithine decarboxylase activity in the stomach and duodenum of neonatal mice (13). These two enzymes were associated with proliferating tissue and were also stimulated in mouse skin by the growth factor (1,40).

It is not known whether or not the immediate action on acid secretion and the more slowly observed mitogenic effects are manifestations of the same process. In the ZE patients the decrease in acid secretion was accompanied by an increase in intrinsic factor output; thus all parietal cell processes were not inhibited. All stimulants of acid secretion are blocked by urogastrone, and this could possibly be because the cell is switched to an alternative process. However, β- and γ-urogastrones and the 47-residue peptide, obtained by removing the C-terminal hexapeptide with *A. mellea* protease, were equipotent in inhibiting acid secretion, whereas the 47 amino acid unit had only 10% of the potency of the urogastrones in stimulating thymidine incorporation in human fibroblasts. This suggested different structural requirements for the two actions (28).

Membrane receptors on fibroblasts bind ^{125}I-labeled mEGF, and radioactivity is subsequently internalized and degraded (3). It is not known whether these events are part of the mitogenic process, but they would seem to be too slow to be involved in the very rapid onset of secretory inhibition. Growth factor receptors have been shown on many tissues—not as yet on the parietal cell, and on placental membranes the urogastrone receptor is probably a glycoprotein (38).

RADIOIMMUNOASSAY MEASUREMENTS

Antisera to urogastrone were raised directly in rabbits by immunizing with the peptide emulsified in Freund's complete adjuvant and subsequent boosting by small amounts of pure material. ^{125}I-labeled urogastrone was used to develop a RIA capable of measuring 5 pg peptide (21), and volumes of 1 to 2 μl human urine were thus assayed. The label was displaced only by mEGF at concentrations over 1,000-fold greater than human urogastrone, and no cross-reaction occurred with animal urines, other than primates, with volumes up to 50 μl. Thus, even though other species were known to have inhibitors in their urine, the metabolic fate of human urogastrone could be followed in them.

Within a few minutes of an intravenous injection of urogastrone, the blood level became undetectable and the half-life was of the order of 2 min (Fig. 2). This is much shorter than the half-life of peptides of comparable size such as insulin or the smaller 35-residue big gastrin. The biological effect was sustained for a much longer period in that complete inhibition of the histamine-induced secretion was obtained at 15 to 30 min and only began again 75 min postinjection, even though the secretagogue was infused continuously. Given subcutaneously, urogastrone was measurable in blood for a much longer period and the inhibitory effect was greatly prolonged even though the onset was still rapid (20). Interestingly, following the administration of an effective inhibitory dose the peak blood level was of the order 1 to 2 ng/ml. It was not perhaps realistic to make comparisons with the *in vitro* mitogenic concentrations (ED $\sim$ 0.6 ng/ml), but it was certainly not obvious whether either of the differing biological effects was of primary importance.

The dispersion of ^{125}I-labeled urogastrone in mice was followed by whole-body autoradiography. Radioactivity accumulated in the gastric mucosal region and gradually the stomach contents became labeled. However, this was subsequently found to be low molecular weight materal that may have derived from degradation at some site of action in the mucosa. It was also observed that radioactivity appeared rapidly in the bladder. The collection of urine by catheterization of female dogs confirmed that urogastrone appeared in the urine from

2 to 5 min after intravenous doses (11). The concentration in human urine is much higher than the total immunoreactivity in serum (21), which does not apply with hormones such as chorionic gonadotropin and suggests that rapid clearance from serum is an important facet of this peptide.

RIA measurements on normal males and females showed that daily outputs varied widely, 120 to 1,360 ng/kg/hr (21). Slightly higher values were noted for females. Levels did not appear to be clearly different in patients with duodenal ulcer, Sjorgren's disease, or psoriasis, nor were they particularly elevated in pregnancy urines although the numbers measured have been small. There was no meaningful variation discernible at different times of the menstrual cycle either.

Immunoreactivity measurements in serum across pregnancy did not vary appreciably, but changes could have been masked by there being more than one immunoreactive species, and it was also measurable in cord blood and amniotic fluid (39). Effects of mEGF on fetal development have been shown by infusion into one sheep fetus *in utero* for 10 days (days 115 to 125). The treated fetuses showed increased epithelial development, pulmonary maturation, and thyroid weight; thymus weights were reduced compared with those of the control fetuses, and there were major switches from fetal to adult hemoglobin—45% cf 10% in control (J. Robinson, *personal communication*).

ORIGIN OF UROGASTRONE

The availability of antibodies with good specificity enabled many human tissues to be examined by using a fluorescent localization technique (12). This showed immunoreactivity located only to submandibular glands and Brunner's glands of the duodenum (Fig. 3). Confirmation was obtained by using a peroxidase staining technique that identified granules in acinar cells and duct cells of the duodenal glands, but in addition stained material was present in the ducts of Brunner's glands, implying exocrine secretion (26).[1] Gel chromatography of saliva and gastric juice gave immunoreactivity at the same position as urogastrone, and furthermore these fractions also caused the incorporation of [³H] thymidine into cultured fibroblasts in a similar manner to urogastrone (23).[2] In blood the major portion of the immunoreactivity was of much greater molecular size than urogastrone (Fig. 4), but treatment with trypsin gave a fraction comparable in size to urogastrone, which again stimulated DNA synthesis.

---

[1] As pointed out earlier, urogastrone was named because of a possible relationship to a postulated duodenal hormone—enterogastrone (16). The latter has never been characterized, but the indications that urogastrone appeared as an exocrine secretion from Brunner's glands must give support to the earlier hypothesis.

[2] In 1949 it was found that human saliva could inhibit gastric secretion in animals (5a). The extract, called sialogastrone, appeared to be of higher molecular weight than urogastrone, but the preparation was of sufficiently low potency that a small amount of the potent inhibitor in the preparation could well account for the activity. However, this remains to be proved by correlating the inhibitory activity of sialogastrone preparations with the amounts of urogastrone detectable.

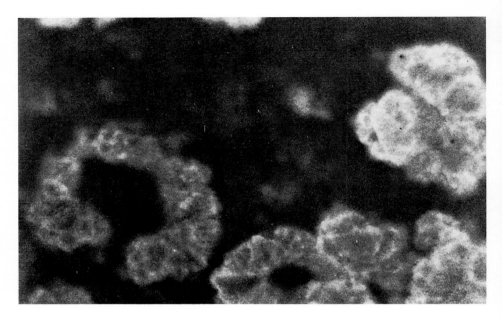

FIG. 3. Fluorescent labeling of Brunner's glands of the duodenum cut parallel to the mucosal surface using a specific anti-urogastrone serum. (Courtesy of Mr. J. Elder, Department of Surgery, Manchester University.)

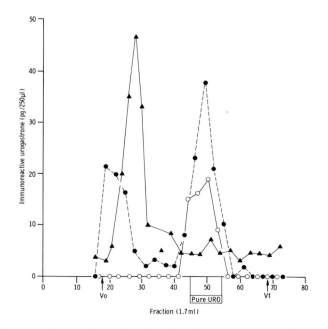

FIG. 4. Fractionation of serum (▲ — ▲), saliva (● — ●), and gastric juice (○ — ○) on a column of Sephadex G-200. Fractions at the same position as pure urogastrone also showed biological activity. (From ref. 23.)

It now seems that the early definition of an acid inhibitory factor and a healing agent in urine has been substantiated, but that both properties reside within a single molecule. The duodenal glands appear to form a major source of urogastrone, which raises the question again of a relationship to enterogastrone, and in addition to inhibiting gastric secretion, it may have a role in maintaining the integrity of the intestinal epithelium. It remains to be seen whether its mitogenic properties fulfill a physiological role at other sites in the body.

SUMMARY AND CONCLUSIONS

Urogastrone has been isolated in yields of about 1 μg/liter human urine (24) and the structure shown to consist of a single polypeptide chain of 53 amino acid residues with three internal disulfide bonds (22). A second molecular species was isolated that lacked the C-terminal arginine residue. Urogastrone was shown to be a powerful and specific inhibitor of gastric acid secretion against any stimulant used and in a number of different species (15). In human volunteers or patients with Zollinger-Ellison syndrome (9) acid secretion was inhibited by doses as low as 0.25 μg/kg.

Urogastrone was shown to be closely related to mouse epidermal growth factor, and the two molecules shared the properties of inhibiting acid secretion and causing cell and tissue proliferation (19). The second property might be contributory to the healing of experimental ulcers. The earliest studies with urine extracts suggested the separate existence of antisecretory and antiulcer agents, but it subsequently appeared that both properties reside within the same molecule.

Based on the localization of immunoreactive material, submaxillary glands and dominantly Brunner's glands appeared to be the source in the human (12,26). Furthermore, immunoreactive material with biological activity on cultured fibroblasts has been identified in saliva and gastric juice (23).

PROJECTIONS FOR THE FUTURE

Urogastrone is perhaps too large to allow for ready synthesis by the conventional techniques that exist at present. However, if the promise of protein production by genetic manipulation methods continues to progress, then large amounts of pure urogastrone may be obtainable. This would allow for detailed studies on the healing of ulcers of the gastrointestinal tract, but it may also allow for the realization of the potential to promote healing of epithelial wounds in other parts of the body.

REFERENCES

1. Blosse, P. T., Fenton, E. L., Henningsson., Kahlson, G., and Rosengren, E. (1974): Activation of decarboxylases of histidine and ornithine in young mice after injection of epidermal growth factor. *Experientia,* 30:22–23.

2. Carpenter, G. (1978): The regulation of cell proliferation: Advances in the biology of action of epidermal growth factor. *J. Invest. Dermatol.*, 71:283–288.
3. Carpenter, G., and Cohen, S. (1976): ^{125}I-labelled human epidermal growth. Binding, internalisation and degradation in human fibroblasts. *J. Cell. Biol.*, 71:159–171.
4. Carrea, G., Cassellato, M. M., Manera, E., Pastra, P., and Lugaro, G. (1973): Purification of a human urinary glycoprotein with gastric antisecretory activity. *Biochim. Biophys. Acta*, 295:274–282.
5. Code, C. F. (1951): The inhibition of gastric secretion: A review. *Pharmacol. Rev.*, 3:59–78.
5a. Code, C. F., Ratke, H. V., Livermore, G. R., and Lundberg, W. (1949): Occurrence of gastric secretary inhibitor activity in fresh gastric and salivary mucin. *Fed. Proc.*, 8:26–27.
6. Cohen, S., and Carpenter, G. (1975): Human epidermal growth factor: Isolation and chemical and biological properties. *Proc. Natl. Acad. Sci. U.S.A.*, 72:1317–1321.
7. Cohen, S., and Savage, C. R., Jr. (1974): Recent studies on the chemistry and biology of epidermal growth factor. *Recent. Prog. Horm. Res.*, 30:551–574.
8. Culmer, C. U., Atkinson, A. J., and Ivy, A. C. (1939): Depression of gastric secretion by the anterior pituitary-like fraction of pregnancy urine. *Endocrinology*, 24:631–637.
9. Elder, J. B., Ganguli, P. C., Gillespie, I. E., Delamore, I. E., and Gregory, H. (1975): Effect of urogastrone in the Zollinger-Ellison syndrome. *Lancet*, 1:424–433.
10. Elder, J. B., Ganguli, P. C., Gillespie, I. E., Gerring, E. L., and Gregory, H. (1975): Effect of urogastrone on gastric secretion and plasma gastrin levels in normal subjects. *Gut*, 16:887–893.
11. Elder, J. B., Kiff, E. S., and Gregory, H. (1978): Half-life of urogastrone in conscious dogs. *Gut*, 19:A436.
12. Elder, J. B., Williams, G., Lacey, E., and Gregory, H. (1978): Cellular localisation of human urogastrone/epidermal growth factor. *Nature*, 271:466–467.
13. Feldman, E. J., Aures, D., and Grossman, M. I. (1978): Effect of epidermal growth factor in intestinal mucosal ornithine decarboxylase activity. *Gastroenterology*, 74:1033.
14. Friedman, M. H. F., Recknagel, R. O., Sandweiss, D. J., and Patterson, T. L. (1939): Inhibitory effect of urine extracts on gastric secretion. *Proc. Soc. Exp. Biol. Med.*, 41:509–511.
15. Gerring, E. L., Bower, J. M., and Gregory, H. (1974): Urogastrone: A potential drug in the treatment of duodenal ulcer. In: *Chronic Duodenal Ulcer*, edited by C. Wastell, pp. 171–180. Butterworths, London.
16. Gray, J. S., Culmer, C. U., Wieczorowski, E., and Adkinson, J. L. (1940): Preparation of pyrogen free urogastrone. *Proc. Soc. Exp. Biol. Med.*, 46:691–693.
17. Gray, J. S., Wieczorowski, E., and Ivy, A. C. (1940): Inhibition of gastric secretion by extracts of normal male urine. *Science*, 89:489–490.
18. Gray, J. S., Wieczorowski, E., Wells, J. A., and Harris, S. (1942): Preparation and properties of urogastrone. *Endocrinology*, 30:129–134.
18a. Gray, W. R. (1967): Sequential degradation plus dansylation. *Meth. Enzymol.*, 2:469–475.
19. Gregory, H. (1975): Isolation and structure of urogastrone and its relationship to epidermal growth factor. *Nature*, 257:325–327.
20. Gregory, H., Bower, J. M., and Willshire, I. R. (1972): Urogastrone and epidermal growth. In: *Growth Factors*, edited by K. W. Kastrup and J. H. Nielsen, pp. 75–84. Pergamon Press, Oxford.
21. Gregory, H., Holmes, J. E., and Willshire, I. R. (1977): Urogastrone levels in the urine of normal adult humans. *J. Clin. Endocrinol. Metab.*, 45:668–672.
22. Gregory, H., and Preston, B. M. (1977): The primary structure of human urogastrone. *Int. J. Pept. Protein Res.*, 9:107–118.
23. Gregory, H., Walsh, S. W., and Hopkins, C. R. (1979): The identification of urogastrone in serum, saliva and gastric juice. *Gastroenterology*, 77:313–318.
24. Gregory, H., and Willshire, I. R. (1975): The isolation of the urogastrones—Inhibitors of gastric acid secretion from human urine. *Hoppe Seylers Z. Physiol. Chem.*, 356:1765–1774.
25. Gregory, R. A. (1955): A new method for the preparation of urogastrone. *J. Physiol. (Lond.)*, 129:528–546.
26. Heitz, Ph. U., Kasper, M., Van Noorden, S., Polak, J. M., Gregory, H., and Pearse, A. G. E. (1978): Immunohistochemical localisation of urogastrone to human duodenal and submandibular glands. *Gut*, 19:408–413.
27. Hollenberg, M. D., and Gregory, H. (1977): Human urogastrone and mouse epidermal growth factor share a common receptor site in cultured human fibroblasts. *Life Sci.*, 20:267–274.

28. Hollenberg, M. D., and Gregory, H. (1978): Urogastrone—EGF: Receptor binding and activities of derivatives. Abstracts, 2nd Pan American Association of Biochemical Societies Congress, Caracas, Venezuela, 3.

28a. Kobayashi, M., and Yamamoto, M. (1969): Studies on the inhibitory substances of gastric secretion. Extraction and separation of sialogastrone from human saliva. *J. Pharm. Soc. Japan.,* 89:222–229.

29. Koffman, C. G., Elder, J. B., Ganguli, P. C., Gillespie, I. E., Gregory, H., and Geary, G. (1977): The effect of urogastrone on gastric secretion and serum gastrin concentration in duodenal ulcer patients. *Gastroenterology,* 72:1082.

30. Mongar, J. L., and Rosenoer, V. M. (1962): The preparation of urogastrone. *J. Physiol. (Lond.),* 162:163–172.

31. Morimoto, T., and Yamamoto, M. (1962): Studies of inhibitory substances of gastric secretion. I. Isolation of urogastrone from human primary pregnancy and non-pregnancy urine. *J. Pharm. Soc. Japan,* 89:215–221.

32. Necheles, H., Hanke, N. E., and Fantl, E. (1939): Preparation and assay of the inhibitor of gastric secretion and motility from normal human urine. *Proc. Soc. Exp. Biol. Med.,* 42:618–619.

33. Rosenoer, V. M., and Schild, H. O. (1962): The assay of urogastrone. *J. Physiol. (Lond.),* 162:155–162.

34. Sandweiss, D. J. (1943): The immunising effect of the anti-ulcer factor in normal human urine (anthelone) against the experimental gastrojejunal (peptic) ulcer in dogs. *Gastroenterology,* 1:965–969.

35. Sandweiss, D. J., Saltzstein, N. C., and Farbman, A. A. (1938): Prevention or healing of experimental ulcer in M-W dogs with anterior pituitary-like hormone (Antuitrin S). *Am. J. Dig. Dis.,* 5:24–30.

36. Sandweiss, D. J., Scheinberg, S. R., and Salzstein, H. C. (1954): The effect of pregnant mare's urine extract (Uroanthelone-Kutrol) and a placental extract on M-W ulcers in dogs. *Gastroenterology,* 27:411–416.

37. Savage, C. R., Jr., Inagami, T., and Cohen, S. (1972): The primary structure of epidermal growth factor. *J. Biol. Chem.,* 247:7612–7621.

38. Sayhoun, N., Hock, R. A., and Hollenberg, M. D. (1978): Insulin and epidermal growth factor—Urogastrone: Affinity cross linking to specific binding sites in rat liver membranes. *Proc. Natl. Acad. Sci. U.S.A.,* 75:1675–1679.

39. Scott, I. V., Bardsley, W. G., Gregory, H., and Tindall, V. R. (1979): Human placental diamine oxidase concentration and urogastrone: A possible role in polyamine metabolism and fetal growth control. In: *Proceedings of the 8th International Symposium on Clinical Enzymology,* edited by A. Burlina and S. Galzigna. Piccini Medical Books, Padua and London *(in press).*

40. Stasny, M., and Cohen, S. (1970): Epidermal growth factor IV. The induction of ornithine decarboxylase. *Biochim. Biophys. Acta,* 204:578–589.

Synthesis, Heterogeneity and Receptor Interactions of the Gastrointestinal Hormones and Peptides

Gastrointestinal Hormones, edited by
George B. Jerzy Glass.
Raven Press, New York © 1980.

Chapter 18

Synthesis of Gastrointestinal Hormones

Miklos Bodanszky and Joseph Z. Kwei

Department of Chemistry, Case Western Reserve University, Cleveland, Ohio 44106

INTRODUCTION

The gastrointestinal hormones can be classified according to structure, function, and synthesis. We have chosen to group the hormones that have been the object of active synthetic efforts according to their sequence into the following classes: the gastrin family (Fig. 1), the secretin family (Fig. 2), and motilin (Fig. 3), which thus far does not belong to any particular group. The gastrin family consists of cholecystokinin-pancreozymin (CCK-PZ) and the gastrins. The secretin family contains secretin, vasoactive intestinal peptide (VIP), and gastric inhibitory polypeptide (GIP). Although, in a broad sense, glucagon (35), substance P (33), and cerulein (32) are gastrointestinal hormones, they were originally isolated from areas other than the gastrointestinal tract. For the sake of completeness, these substances are discussed briefly, as is somatostatin.

Relatively few of the known intestinal peptides have been synthesized. This

CCK-PZ   Lys-Ala-Pro-Ser-Gly-Arg-Val-Ser-Met-Ile-Lys-Asn-Leu-Gln-Ser-Leu-
G-34   Pyr-Leu-Gly-Pro-Gln-Gly-His-Pro-Ser-Leu-Val-Ala-Asp-Pro-Ser-Lys-Lys-

CCK-PZ   -Asp-Pro-Ser-His-Arg-Ile-Ser-Asp-Arg-Asp-Tyr*-Met-Gly-Trp-Met-Asp-Phe-NH$_2$
G-34   -Gln-Gly-Pro-Trp-Leu-Glu-Glu-Glu-Glu-Ala-Tyr*-Gly-Trp-Met-Asp-Phe-NH$_2$
Cerulein   Pyr-Gln-Asp-Tyr*-Thr-Gly-Trp-Met-Asp-Phe-NH$_2$

Tyr* denotes a sulfate ester of tyrosine; it is absent in gastrin. I. CCK-PZ is a porcine peptide; G-34 is the sequence in humans.

FIG. 1. Gastrin family. Areas of homology are underlined.

	1	2	3	4	5	6	7	8	9	10	11	12	13	14
Secretin	His-	Ser-	Asp-	Gly-	Thr-	Phe-	Thr-	Ser-	Glu-	Leu-	Ser-	Arg-	Leu-	Arg-
VIP	His-	Ser-	Asp-	Ala-	Val-	Phe-	Thr-	Asp-	Asn-	Tyr-	Thr-	Arg-	Leu-	Arg-
Glucagon	His-	Ser-	Gln-	Gly-	Thr-	Phe-	Thr-	Ser-	Asp-	Tyr-	Ser-	Lys-	Tyr-	Leu-
GIP	Tyr-	Ala-	Glu-	Gly-	Thr-	Phe-	Ile-	Ser-	Asp-	Tyr-	Ser-	Ile-	Ala-	Met-

	15	16	17	18	19	20	21	22	23	24	25	26	27	28	29
Secretin	Asp-	Ser-	Ala-	Arg-	Leu-	Gln-	Arg-	Leu-	Leu-	Gln-	Gly-	Leu-	Val-	NH_2	
VIP	Lys-	Gln-	Met-	Ala-	Val-	Lys-	Lys-	Tyr-	Leu-	Asn-	Ser-	Ile-	Leu-	Asn-	NH_2
Glucagon	Asp-	Ser-	Arg-	Arg-	Ala-	Gln-	Asp-	Phe-	Val-	Gln-	Trp-	Leu-	Met-	Asn-	Thr
GIP	Asp-	Lys-	Ile-	Arg-	Gln-	Gln-	Asp-	Phe-	Val-	Asn-	Trp-	Leu-	Leu-	Ala-	Gln

	30	31	32	33	34	35	36	37	38	39	40	41	42	43
GIP	Gln-	Lys-	Gly-	Lys-	Lys-	Ser-	Asp-	Trp-	Lys-	His-	Asn-	Ile-	Thr-	Gln

FIG. 2. Secretin family (porcine sequences).

1	2	3	4	5	6	7	8	9	10	11
Phe-	Val-	Pro-	Ile-	Phe-	Thr-	Tyr-	Gly-	Glu-	Leu-	Gln-

12	13	14	15	16	17	18	19	20	21	22
Arg-	Met-	Gln-	Glu-	Lys-	Glu-	Arg-	Asn-	Lys-	Gly-	Gln

FIG. 3. Sequence of porcine motilin.

might be due to the difficulties both of isolation and of synthesis. In the following sections dealing with the individual hormones, we attempt to point out the principal aims of synthesizing gastrointestinal hormones: the proof of their structures, the determination of structure-activity relationships, and the production of substances potentially useful to medicine.

GASTRINS

In 1905, Edkins (31) announced that extracts of antral mucosa stimulated gastric secretion of acid and hypothesized the presence of a substance he named gastrin. This discovery was questioned by several investigators until 1964, when pure gastrin was isolated from hog antral mucosa by Gregory and Tracy (37). The substance isolated was shown actually to consist of two distinct 17-peptides designated as gastrins I and II. Their structures were determined by H. Gregory et al. (36) and demonstrated to be different only in that gastrin I has tyrosine in position 12, whereas tyrosine-*O*-sulfate occurs in the same position in gastrin II (Fig. 4a). It is interesting to note that the gastrins, hormones that stimulate acid secretion, are extremely acidic peptides: not less than five glutamyl residues

                                    R
                                    |
a: Pyr-Gly-Pro-Trp-Met-Glu-Glu-Ala-Glu-Glu-Ala-Tyr-Gly-Trp-Met-Asp-Phe-NH₂

b: Pyr-Leu-Gly-Pro-Gln-Gly-His-Pro-Ser-Leu-Val-Ala-Asp-Pro-Ser-Lys-Lys-
    Gln-Gly-Pro-Trp-Leu-Glu-Glu-Glu-Glu-Glu-Ala-Tyr-Gly-Trp-Met-Asp-Phe-NH₂
                                                  |
                                                  R
c: Leu-Glu-Glu-Glu-Glu-Glu-Ala-Tyr-Gly-Trp-Met-Asp-Phe-NH₂
                |
                R

FIG. 4. a. Gastrin. **b.** Big gastrin. **c.** Mini-gastrin. R = —H or —SO₃.

occur in the 17-peptide of gastrin I, and gastrin II has also the additional acidic group of the sulfuric acid half-ester.

A synthesis of gastrins I and II was desirable to confirm the structure of the two peptides. Anderson et al. (2) proceeded to do this by segment condensation (Fig. 5). The three segments containing residues 1–5, 6–13, and 14–17 (S₁₋₅, S₆₋₁₃, S₁₄₋₁₇) of the sequence were prepared through conventional stepwise routes. The γ-carboxyl groups of the glutamyl residues were protected by the tertiary-butyl group, readily removable on treatment with trifluoroacetic acid. The α-carboxyl group at the C-terminus of each segment was protected in the form of methyl ester which, before coupling, was removed by saponification with sodium hydroxide. Segments S₁₋₅ and S₆₋₁₃ were linked by the azide method (30), and then the resultant peptide S₁₋₁₃ was coupled to segment S₁₄₋₁₇ through its diphenylphosphoric acid mixed anhydride (29). The complete peptide chain

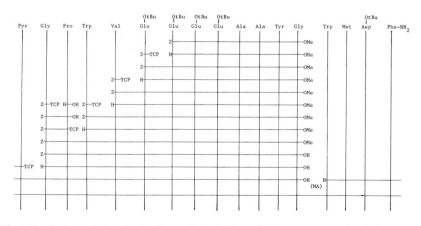

FIG. 5. Synthetic route leading to the protected 17-peptide hormone, gastrin. Z, benzyloxycarbonyl; OtBu, t-butyl ester; TCP, trichlorophenyl ester; Pyr, pyroglutamic acid; MA, mixed anhydride coupling.

was then deprotected by acidolysis, and the product purified by gel-filtration chromatography on Sephadex G-25 and then by gradient elution from a column of aminoethylcellulose. After this purification the synthetic product was identical to gastrin I in all physical characteristics and was fully active when injected into test animals. Starting with the synthetic gastrin I, gastrin II was prepared by sulfation of the tyrosine residue. It, too, exhibited all the characteristic features of the corresponding natural hormone.

Recently, other forms of gastrin have been found in extracts of human gastrinomas. Of these, one also has been identified in plasma and tissues by Yalow and Berson (79) and named "big gastrin." This was isolated from gastrinoma extracts and its amino acid sequence has been determined by Gregory and Tracy (38). "Big gastrin" is built of 34 amino acid residues (Fig. 4b) and contains the sequence of gastrin and hence also of mini-gastrin (39) (Fig. 4c). Recently, the laboratories of E. Wünsch and G. W. Kenner (28) collaborated in the synthesis of human big gastrin by a segment condensation of segments S_{1-20} and S_{21-34}. Independently, Wünsch and co-workers also synthesized the entire 34-peptide hormone through the condensation of five segments (77). Still larger forms of gastrin have been detected in the blood and tissues (66,80), but have not yet been chemically or biologically characterized.

CHOLECYSTOKININ-PANCREOZYMIN

Ivy and Oldberg (44) described cholecystokinin, an intestinal hormone that stimulates the contraction of the gall bladder, in 1928. Subsequently, in 1943 Harper and Raper (41) reported that pancreozymin, also a gut hormone, stimulates the release of pancreatic enzymes. It was not until 21 years later that in their work toward the final isolation of these hormones, Jorpes et al. (48) demonstrated that a single compound elicited both biological responses. Structural studies showed cholecystokinin-pancreozymin to be a peptide with 33 amino acid residues (Fig. 6a). A variant of CCK which has an additional 6-peptide of the sequence Tyr-Ile-Gln-Gln-Ala-Arg at its N-terminus (56) has also been described (Fig. 6b) by Mutt (56).

The synthesis of cholecystokinin-pancreozymin (CCK-PZ) has not yet been accomplished. However, it was feasible to prepare portions of the molecule

```
       1              5                   10                    15
a:  Lys-Ala-Pro-Ser-Gly-Arg-Val-Ser-Met-Ile-Lys-Asn-Leu-Gln-Ser-Leu-Asp-

        20                  25                        30          33
    Pro-Ser-His-Arg-Ile-Ser-Asp-Arg-Asp-Tyr(SO₃H)-Met-Gly-Trp-Met-Asp-Phe-NH₂
```

b: Tyr-Ile-Gln-Gln-Ala-Arg —— | CCK-PZ$_{1-33}$ |

FIG. 6. **a.** Sequence of cholecystokinin-pancreozymin. **b.** N-terminal 6-peptide sequence of the CCK-PZ variant.

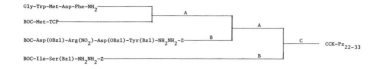

FIG. 7. The synthetic scheme leading to the biologically active C-terminal 12-peptide of cholecystokinin. A, trifluoroacetic acid; B, H_2/Pd; C, SO_3, pyridine; Z, Benzyloxycarbonyl; Bzl, Benzyl; TCP, Trichlorophenyl ester.

that exhibited full biological activity. Ondetti and co-workers (63) have synthesized a 12-peptide (Fig. 7) with the C-terminal sequence of CCK-PZ that has the biological properties of the entire hormone. The similarly potent C-terminal 8-peptide amide is now available for diagnostic purposes. Additional segments of the molecule of CCK-PZ have also been prepared (11,50,65). The complete 33-residue sequence of CCK-PZ, but without the sulfated tyrosine residue, has been synthesized by Yajima and co-workers (78). The same sequence was assembled on a solid support by Lindeberg and Ragnarsson (52). However, it showed very little activity. This demonstrates the importance of the sulfate ester on the tyrosyl residue at position 27. Also, when the tyrosine sulfate of the bioactive 7-peptide, Boc-Tyr(SO_3)-Met-Gly-Trp-Met-Asp-Phe-NH_2, was replaced by serine sulfate, the new analog had only weak hormonal activity (16). A similar substitution with ϵ-hydroxynorleucine sulfate, which has a side chain similar in length to that of tyrosine sulfate, produced (Fig. 8) a potent analog (14). Replacement of the sulfate group with phosphate was studied on the closely

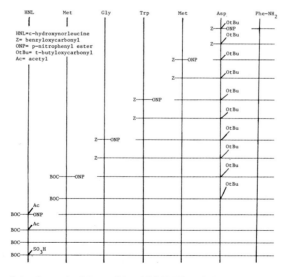

FIG. 8. Synthesis of the C-terminal 7-peptide of CCK-PZ, with hydroxynorleucine sulfate replacing tyrosine sulfate.

related peptide cerulein, which has biological activities similar to those of CCK-PZ (1). A major difficulty in the synthesis of CCK is caused by the tyrosine-*O*-sulfate residue. The sulfate ester group either has to be introduced early and maintained during the synthetic procedures, or else introduced at its conclusion. Yet, the sulfate ester moiety is acid-sensitive, ruling out repeated deprotections with strong acids, and cannot be selectively introduced in the presence of unprotected serine residues by simple chemical means.

CERULEIN

Cerulein was isolated from the skin of amphibians (la), and was subsequently found to have an effect on the gastrointestinal tract. Inspection of its amino acid sequence (Fig. 1) (la) reveals obvious resemblances to the gastrin family.

The 10-peptide corresponding to the sequence of cerulein was synthesized (6a) through a segment condensation scheme in solution. Segments S_{1-4} and S_{5-10} were coupled by the azide method, and then the tyrosine in position 3 was sulfated. After deprotection, the peptide showed identical electrophoretic and chromatographic qualities and possessed the same biological activity as natural cerulein.

SECRETIN

The gastrointestinal hormone secretin was discovered in 1902 by Bayliss and Starling (3a). It was approximately 60 years, however, until the pure peptide was isolated (46), and its structure (Fig. 2) elucidated (47,57,58).

The first synthesis of porcine secretin by Bodanszky and associates (18,20) was based on the stepwise strategy (9) by lengthening the chain with the nitrophenyl esters (8,19) according to the pattern of the first stepwise synthesis of oxytocin (12). A characteristic feature of this approach is the use of excess acylating agents during the chain-lengthening process in order to suppress intramolecular side reactions and to carry the individual acylation reactions to completion.

The synthesis started with the formation of the terminal amide bond of L-valine (Fig. 9). Benzyloxycarbonyl-L-valine *p*-nitrophenyl ester was ammono-

$$
\begin{array}{ccccccccccccc}
\text{Z} & \text{BZl} & \text{OBzl} & & \text{Bzl} & & \text{Bzl} & \text{Bzl} & \text{OBzl} & & \text{Bzl} & \text{NO}_2 & & \text{NO}_2 \\
\text{Z-His-} & \text{Ser-} & \text{Asp} & \text{-Gly-} & \text{Thr-} & \text{Phe-} & \text{Thr-} & \text{Ser-} & \text{Glu} & \text{-Leu-} & \text{Ser-} & \text{Arg} & \text{-Leu-} & \text{Arg-} \\
1 & 2 & 3 & 4 & 5 & 6 & 7 & 8 & 9 & 10 & 11 & 12 & 13 & 14
\end{array}
$$

$$
\begin{array}{ccccccccccccc}
\text{OBzl} & \text{Bzl} & & \text{NO}_2 & & & \text{NO}_2 \\
\text{Asp} & \text{-Ser-} & \text{Ala-} & \text{Arg} & \text{-Leu-} & \text{Gln-} & \text{Arg} & \text{-Leu-} & \text{Leu-} & \text{Gln-} & \text{Gly-} & \text{Leu-} & \text{Val-NH}_2 \\
15 & 16 & 17 & 18 & 19 & 20 & 21 & 22 & 23 & 24 & 25 & 26 & 27
\end{array}
$$

FIG. 9. Protected 27-peptide amide with the sequence of porcine secretin synthesized by the stepwise method. Z, benzyloxycarbonyl; Bzl, benzyl; NO₂, nitro.

lyzed, the hydrobromide of the free amine was produced by removal of the benzyloxycarbonyl protecting group (5) with hydrobromic acid in glacial acetic acid (4), and then the chain was progressively lengthened by acylation with benzyloxycarbonyl-amino acid p-nitrophenyl esters until the C-terminal 6-peptide amide Leu-Leu-Gln-Gly-Leu-Val-NH$_2$ (S$_{22-27}$) was obtained.

The next amino acid to be added was arginine, and this was incorporated in the form of benzyloxycarbonyl-L-nitroarginine-2,4 dinitrophenyl ester (17). Nitroarginine was chosen because the nitro group can be removed under mild conditions by catalytic hydrogenation (6). Similarly, all other protecting groups for amino acid side chains having functional groups were selected so that they could be removed in a single operation by hydrogenolysis at the end of the synthesis. Thus, the hydroxyl groups of L-serine, and the side chain carboxyl groups of glutamic acid and aspartic acid were all protected by the benzyl group.

The synthesis was continued in the same fashion until the protected 11-peptide amide corresponding to sequence 17–27 was secured. At this point, because of the desire to keep the nitro-protecting group of arginine intact by avoiding hydrogenation, and because treatment with hydrobromic acid in acetic acid causes partial O-acetylation of serine residues, the t-butyloxycarbonyl amino-protecting group (27,53) was chosen and used. This allowed the deprotection of amino groups with trifluoroacetic acid, a reagent that leaves the O-benzyl protecting group of serine intact. In this manner, the synthesis was continued until the protected 27-peptide[1] encompassing the entire sequence of secretin was secured.

While all the protected intermediates were isolated in analytically pure form simply by washing with organic solvents, a more extensive purification of the protected peptides took place at two points in the synthesis. The protected 11-peptide with sequence 17–27 was crystallized from methanol, and the blocked C-terminal 14-peptide (S$_{14-27}$) was purified by countercurrent distribution in a system of butanol-pyridine-acetic acid-water. An attempt at purification by countercurrent distribution in the above system led to partial inactivation of the completed 27-peptide. Hence, after the deprotection, the crude material was purified by the procedure used in the isolation of natural secretin from pork intestines (46): countercurrent distribution in a butanol-phosphate buffer system followed by adsorption on and elution from alginic acid. The purified material was indistinguishable from natural secretin in all respects including full biological activity.

A comparison of the ORD-CD spectra (7) of natural and synthetic secretin demonstrated that their secondary and tertiary structures were also identical.

Soon after the stepwise synthesis of secretin, its preparation through a segment

---

[1] The expressions 2-peptide, 3-peptide, etc. instead of dipeptide, tripeptide, etc. were proposed by one of us (M.B.) at the Fifth American Peptide Symposium (LaJolla, California, June, 1977).

condensation was also achieved in the same laboratory (62). Segments containing residues 1–4, 5–9, 9–13, and 14–27 were synthesized by the stepwise method as before. These segments were then combined according to the pattern shown in Fig. 2. The azide method of carboxyl activation (30) [with the Medzihradszky modification (54)] was applied in order to keep racemization of the C-terminal amino acid of the individual segments at a minimum. In order to ensure complete utilization of the more valuable longer segments, the protected and activated carboxyl components were used in considerable excess. The intermediates and the final product were purified by countercurrent distribution and ion exchange chromatography to give once again a synthetic secretin preparation in homogeneous form.

Subsequently additional syntheses of secretin and its analogs have been reported. Wünsch and co-workers carried out a synthesis of secretin (76) by segment condensation. An alternative synthesis of the hormone has been reported more recently by Jäger et al. (45). A synthesis on an insoluble support (55) has been described by Hemmasi and Bayer (42). Finally, a stepwise synthesis through the same protected intermediates as used in the first synthesis of secretin, but with the exclusive use of the mixed anhydride method for coupling, has been performed by Van Zon and Beyerman (74). Syntheses of several analogs of secretin have contributed to a picture of the structure-activity relationships.

A study of synthetic analogs of the C-terminal 23-peptide, which in itself has intrinsic secretin-like activity, shed some light on the forces that determine the architecture of the molecule (34). Substitution of the 15-aspartic acid residue in secretin by lysine, which occupies that position in VIP, resulted in an analog that has less secretin and more VIP-like activities (15).

GLUCAGON

Pancreatic glucagon, in conjunction with insulin, has the important role of governing glycogenolysis in the liver. Recently, glucagon or a peptide closely resembling it was also detected in the intestines where other substances possessing glucagon-like immunoreactivity are present as well (20b,52b,72).

The amino acid sequence of porcine glucagon (Fig. 2) has been known since 1957 (52a). It was not until 10 years later, however, that Wünsch et al. achieved a total synthesis of glucagon (74a,75a,75b) by condensation of segments. The synthetic hormone preparation showed full biological activity when tested in animals, and was also indistinguishable from natural samples by radioimmunoassay (2a).

Other syntheses of porcine glucagon include one by segment condensation completed by Fujino et al. (35a), as well as a segment condensation on a polymeric support performed by the Synthetic Protein Research Group of the China Biochemical Institute (72a). More recently, the amino acid sequence for duck glucagon (71a) has been determined, and its synthesis completed (61a).

GASTRIC INHIBITORY POLYPEPTIDE

A peptide which inhibits gastric acid secretion was isolated from porcine intestines in 1970 by Brown, Mutt, and Pederson (25), and was named gastric inhibitory polypeptide (GIP). It consists of 43 amino acid residues in a single chain (Fig. 2) (22). As it can be readily seen in Fig. 2, a major N-terminal portion of GIP in a number of positions contains the same amino acid residues as glucagon and secretin (20b) in the corresponding positions.

To date, several partial sequences of GIP have been synthesized (26,51,60) and a total synthesis was reported by Ogawa et al. (61). This latter synthesis

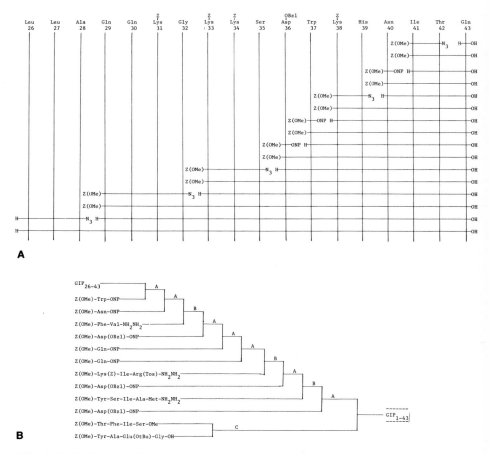

FIG. 10.A. Synthesis of the protected 18-peptide GIP$_{26-43}$. Z(OMe), 4-methoxy-benzyloxycarbonyl; Z, benzyloxycarbonyl; ONP, *p*-nitrophenyl ester; Bzl, benzyl. **10.B.** Total synthesis of the 43-peptide GIP. Z(OMe), 4-methoxy-benzyloxycarbonyl; OtBu, *t*-butyl ester; ONP, *p*-nitrophenyl ester; Tos, tosyl; Bzl, benzyl. A-ONP, TFA; B-Azide, TFA; C-TFA, DCC + HOBT, NH$_2$NH$_2$, D-Azide, HF.

of GIP was started with the C-terminal 18-peptide (50), and proceeded by the addition of segments as shown in Figs. 10a and b. Coupling of segments was performed by the azide method (43), in order to avoid racemization. Because of difficulties in preparing peptide hydrazides containing asparagine, tryptophan, aspartic acid, glutamic acid, and glutamine, these residues were introduced in a stepwise manner by the nitrophenyl ester method (12). The protected 43-peptide was then deblocked with cold hydrofluoric acid (69) and purified extensively by chromatographic procedures. The synthetic GIP, when tested for suppression of gastric acid secretion and insulin release, showed activities of the gastric inhibitory polypeptide from hog intestines.

VASOACTIVE INTESTINAL PEPTIDE

A vasoactive intestinal peptide (VIP) was isolated (67) in 1970 from hog intestines by Said and Mutt. It has been found (64,68) to cause vasodilation, enhanced myocardial contractibility, and relaxation of smooth muscle. Its amino acid sequence was determined (59) and the 28-peptide (Fig. 2) was seen to be closely related to secretin, glucagon, and GIP.

So far there is only one report (13) on the total synthesis of porcine VIP, and a preliminary one (10) on chicken VIP, which differs from the porcine peptide in positions 11, 13, 26, and 28. In preparing pork VIP, the stepwise strategy of building a peptide chain from its C-terminal residue by the addition of a single amino acid at a time proved to be difficult because of the insolubility of the C-terminal protected intermediates. Consequently, segments corresponding to sequences 1–6, 7–13, 14–17, and 18–28 were prepared stepwise and combined by the azide method (Fig. 11). The benzyloxycarbonyl group was used for the protection of the amino function in the side chain of lysine residues, and the carboxyl group in side chains containing carboxyl components were protected with the benzyl group. Before coupling, these side chain carboxyl

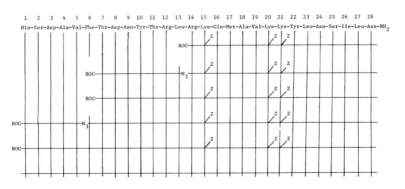

FIG. 11. Synthesis of the 28-peptide hormone VIP. BOC, *t*-butyloxycarbonyl; Z, benzyloxycarbonyl; N_3, azide.

groups were deprotected by hydrogenation. On completion of the 28-residue peptide chain, the benzyloxycarbonyl protecting groups on the side chains of lysine residues and the *t*-butyloxycarbonyl group attached to the N-terminal histidine were removed by prolonged acidolysis with trifluoroacetic acid. After purification by countercurrent distribution, the free 28-peptide gave the expected amino acid analysis, electrophoretic mobility, and biological activity comparable to that of VIP. In addition, comparisons of fragments from enzyme degradations of both natural and synthetic VIP showed no differences, and hence the synthesis corroborated the sequence (Fig. 2) of porcine VIP.

MOTILIN

In 1934, Thomas and co-workers (73) demonstrated increased gastric motor activity and accelerated gastric emptying when gastric contents were withdrawn before reaching the duodenum. A similar observation was made by Brown et al. (23) when the duodenum of the dog was made alkaline, and this led them to hypothesize the presence of a substance they named motilin, which was later isolated (24) and shown to be a 22-peptide (Fig. 3) having a stimulatory effect on stomach motor activity and pepsin secretion. The sequence of porcine motilin was determined (21), but later revised (70) to account for certain anomalous results.

The total synthesis of motilin has been reported by Kai et al. (49). The synthetic route to motilin (Fig. 12) involved the stepwise synthesis of segments corresponding to S_{1-5}, S_{6-8}, S_{10-13}, and S_{14-22}. These segments were coupled by the Honzl-Rudinger modification of the azide method (43). The side chains of glutamic acid residues were blocked with the benzyl group, whereas those of lysine residues were protected as the benzyloxycarbonyl derivative. The guanidino group in the side chain of arginine was also protected; the tosyl group was used here. Final deprotection was effected by a treatment of the completed 22-peptide with hydrofluoric acid. After purification by chromatography, biological assay

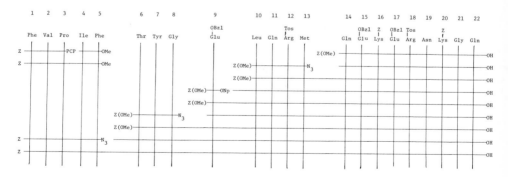

FIG. 12. Synthetic route to the protected 22-peptide motilin. ONp, *p*-nitrophenyl ester; Z(OMe), 4-methoxy-benzyloxycarbonyl; Bzl, benzyl; Tos, tosyl; Z, benzyloxycarbonyl.

showed that the synthetic porcine motilin had the characteristic activity of the natural hormone.

Two analogs having sequences corresponding to the originally proposed sequence of motilin have been prepared by Wünsch and co-workers (75). Also, these synthetic analogs contained either norleucine or leucine in position 13 of motilin, instead of methionine. The preparative route involved the condensation of six segments with sequences corresponding to S_{1-5}, S_{6-8}, S_{9-11}, S_{12-13}, S_{14-17}, and S_{18-22}. After deprotection by acidolysis and subsequent purification, both analogs exhibited the full biological activities of motilin. The 8-L-Ala-motilin and the 8-D-Ala-motilin analogs have been prepared by Shinagawa et al. (71). In comparison with synthetic motilin, the 8-D-Ala-motilin analog showed increased potency, whereas 8-L-Ala-motilin was less potent.

SUBSTANCE P

Substance P was first discovered in intestinal tissues by Euler and Gaddum in 1931 (33), and was shown to cause powerful contractions of the jejunum when injected into rabbits. However, it was not isolated in pure form until recently (27b). Once its amino acid sequence was determined (Fig. 13) (27c), it became possible to synthesize the 11-peptide hormone. This was accomplished by a solid-phase procedure (73a). Comparisons of the synthetic preparation of substance P with its natural counterpart demonstrated equal biological activities and identical physical properties.

Since then, substance P has been prepared in several laboratories employing solid-phase techniques (25a,34a), conventional methods (4a,77a), and through intermediates anchored to a soluble polymer (3).

SOMATOSTATIN

Somatostatin was secured from ovine hypothalamic extracts (20a), and found to inhibit the release of growth hormone, and also the secretion of glucagon and insulin (35b). Its amino acid sequence (Fig. 13b) was determined by mass spectrometry (52a) and then verified through the synthesis of somatostatin by Rivier et al. (66a). Somatostatin was also synthesized by Coy et al. (29a). Both syntheses started from the C-terminal end and proceeded stepwise by the addition of single amino acids to the polymerbound intermediates. Synthetic somatostatin was fully active in studies by radioimmunoassay and in inhibiting the production of growth hormone.

a. Arg-Pro-Lys-Pro-Gln-Gln-Phe-Phe-Gly-Leu-Met-NH$_2$

b. Ala-Gly-Cys-Lys-Asn-Phe-Phe-Trp-Lys-Thr-Phe-Thr-Ser-Cys-OH

FIG. 13. a. Amino acid sequence of substance P. **b.** Amino acid sequence of somatostatin.

Analogs of somatostatin that inhibit glucagon or insulin release to varying degrees have been prepared (27a,55a,55b), and are potentially useful in treating certain disorders such as acromegaly and diabetes mellitus.

CONCLUSIONS AND PROJECTIONS FOR THE FUTURE

We hope that the brief sections dealing with syntheses of gastrointestinal hormones demonstrated the usefulness of peptide synthesis in establishing the correctness of amino acid sequences determined by degradation and the research potential of synthetic analogs in the exploration of structure-biological activity relationships. Such analogs are perhaps the most effective probes in the study of hormone-receptor interaction. Also, the synthetic approach, at least in some cases, can provide medicine with diagnostic tools. For instance, the sulfated C-terminal of CCK: octapeptide L-aspartyl-L-tyrosyl(O-sulfate)-L-methionyl-gly-cyl-L-tryptophyl-L-methionyl-L-aspartyl-L-phenylalanine   amide   (sinkalide, known under the trade name Kinevac, Squibb) is now applied in the radiological examination of the gall bladder. It is very likely that peptide synthesis will continue to produce diagnostic materials and eventually therapeutic compounds as well. This has been the case with peptide hormones not directly related to the gastrointestinal tract, e.g., oxytocin, vasopressin, or corticotropin. Thus, if a gastrointestinal hormone would gain significance as a therapeutic agent, synthesis may be the most efficient approach for its production in commercial amounts.

Hence, we can be confident that the role of synthesis in the area of peptide hormones will continue to increase.

SOURCES OF SYNTHETIC PREPARATIONS OF GASTROINTESTINAL HORMONES

Information concerning the availability of synthetic hormones is generally as scarce as the materials themselves. Small amounts of the synthetic preparations are often available from the laboratories where they were prepared. These sources, however, are easily exhausted. Although research supply houses could be a somewhat better source for these peptides, they too may not always be in a position to replenish their stocks of materials. Therefore, the sources listed here are possibly valid only for a given period of time.

Secretin
    Research Plus Laboratories, Inc.
    P. O. Box 571
    Denville, New Jersey 07834

Secretin
    Bachem, Inc.
    3132 Kashiwa St.
    Torrance, California 90505

Kinevac® - C-terminal 8-peptide of cholecystokinin (sulfated)
E. R. Squibb and Sons, Inc.
Box 4000
Princeton, New Jersey 08540

Gastrin, Secretin
Boehringer Mannheim Biochemicals
7941 Castleway Drive
P. O. Box 50816
Indianapolis, Indiana 46250

15-Leucine-Gastrin I
Beckman Instruments
Bioproducts Department
1117 California Ave.
Palo Alto, California 94304

Secretin, VIP, C-terminal 8-peptide of CCK (non-sulfated)
Peninsula Laboratories Inc.
P. O. Box 1111
San Carlos, California 94070

Cerulein (ceruletide, diethylammonium salt)
Adria Laboratories, Inc.
1105 Market St.
Wilmington, Delaware 19899
(distributors for Farmitalia, Inc., Italy)

Pentagastrin (Peptavlone)
Ayerst Laboratories
685 Third Ave.
New York, New York 10017

Secretin (natural and synthetic), CCK and its variant, VIP
The Gastrointestinal Hormone Resource
National Institute of Arthritis, Metabolism and Digestive Diseases
Dr. George Kitzes
Westwood Building, Room 603
Bethesda, Maryland 20016[1]

A comprehensive survey of sources of supply of gastrointestinal hormones and related peptides has been published by Grossman (40).

---

[1] For GIH secretin or CCK-PZ (Karolinska Institutet, Stockholm) for human use under his IND, apply to Armand Littman, M.D., V.A. Hospital, Hines, Ill., or directly to FDA, Washington, D.C. General distributor: AB Kabi Diagnostica, S-110, 87 Stockholm, Sweden.

REFERENCES

1. Anastasi, A., Bernardi, L., Bertaccini, G., Bosisio, G., DeCastiglione, R., Erspamer, V., Goffredo, O., and Impicciatore, M. (1968): Synthetic peptides related to caerulein. *Experientia,* 24:771–773.

1a. Anastasi, A., Erspamer, V., and Endean, R. (1967): Isolation and structure of caerulein, an active decapeptide from the skin of Hyla caerulea. *Experientia,* 23(9):699–700.

2. Anderson, J. C., Barton, M. A., Gregory, R. A., Hardy, P. M., Kenner, G. W., MacLeod, J. K., Preston, J., and Sheppard, R. C. (1964): Synthesis of gastrin. *Nature,* 204:933–934.

2a. Assan, G. R., Drouet, G., Rosselin, G., Wünsch, E., and Schroeder, E. (1969): Etude radio-immunologique de glucagons natural et synthetique et de peptides synthetiques apparentés. *Pathol. Biol. (Paris),* 17:757–762.

3. Bayer, E., and Mutter, M. (1974): Synthese des biologisch aktiven Undecapeptids Substanz P nach der Flüssig-Phasen Method. *Chem. Ber.,* 107:1344–1352.

3a. Bayliss, W., and Starling, E. H. (1902): The mechanism of pancreatic secretion. *J. Physiol. (Lond.),* 28:325–353.

4. Ben-Ishai, D., and Berger, A. (1952): Cleavage of N-carbobenzoxy groups by dry hydrogen bromide and hydrogen chloride. *J. Org. Chem.,* 17:1564–1570.

4a. Bergmann, J., Bienert, M., Wiedrich, H., Mehlis, B., and Oehme, P. (1974): Uber den Einfluss der Kettenlänge bei C-terminalen Sequenzen der Substanz P - in Vergleich mit analogen Physalaemin und Eledoisin-Peptiden-auf die Wirksamkeit am Meerschweinchen-Ileum. *Experientia,* 30:401–403.

5. Bergmann, M., and Zervas, L. (1932): A general process for the synthesis of peptides. *Ber. Deutsch Chem. Ges.,* 65:1192–1201.

6. Bergmann, M., Zervas, L., and Rinke, H. (1934): New process for synthesis of peptides of arginine. *Z. Physiol. Chem.,* 224:40–44.

6a. Bernardi, L., Bosisio, G., DeCastiglione, R., and Goffredo, O. (1967): Synthesis of caerulein. *Experientia,* 23(9):700–702.

7. Bodanszky, A., Ondetti, M. A., Mutt, V., and Bodanszky, M. (1969): Synthesis of secretin IV. Secondary structure in a miniature protein. *J. Am. Chem. Soc.,* 91:944–949.

8. Bodanszky, M. (1955): Synthesis of peptides by aminolysis of nitrophenyl esters. *Nature,* 175:685.

9. Bodanszky, M. (1960): Stepwise synthesis of peptides by the nitrophenyl ester method. *Ann. NY Acad. Sci.,* 88:655–664.

10. Bodanszky, M., Bodanszky, A., and Said, S. I. (1978): Synthesis of the avian vasoactive intestinal peptide (VIP). *Fed. Proc.* 37(6), 3071.

11. Bodanszky, M., Chaturvedi, N., Hudson, D., and Itoh, M. (1972): Cholecystokinin-pancreozymin. I. The synthesis of peptides corresponding to the N-terminal sequence. *J. Org. Chem.,* 37:2303–2307.

12. Bodanszky, M., and DuVigneaud, V. (1959): A method of synthesis of long peptide chains using a synthesis of oxytocin as an example. *J. Am. Chem. Soc.,* 81:5688–5691.

13. Bodanszky, M., Klausner, Y. S., Lin, C. Y., Mutt, V., and Said, S. I. (1974): Synthesis of the vasoactive intestinal peptide (VIP). *J. Am. Chem. Soc.,* 96:4973–4978.

14. Bodanszky, M., Martinez, J., Priestley, G. P., Gardner, J. D., and Mutt, V. (1978): Cholecystokinin (pancreozymin). 4. Synthesis and properties of a biologically active analogue of the C-terminal 7-peptide with ε-hydroxynorleucine sulfate replacing tyrosine sulfate. *J. Med. Chem.,* 21:1030–1035.

15. Bodanszky, M., Natarajan, S., Gardner, J., Makhlouf, G. M., and Said, S. I. (1978): Synthesis and some pharmacological properties of the 23-peptide 15-lysine-secretin-(5-27). Special role of the residue in position 15 in biological activity of the vasoactive intestinal polypeptide. *J. Med. Chem.,* 21:1171–1173.

16. Bodanszky, M., Natarajan, S., Hahne, W., and Gardner, J. D. (1977): Cholecystokinin (pancreozymin). 3. Synthesis and properties of an analogue of the C-terminal heptapeptide with serine sulfate replacing tyrosine sulfate. *J. Med. Chem.,* 20:1947–1950.

17. Bodanszky, M., and Ondetti, M. A. (1966): On active esters of benzyloxycarbonylnitroarginine. *Chem. Ind. (Lond.),* 26–27.

18. Bodanszky, M., Ondetti, M. A., Levine, S. D., and Williams, N. J. (1967): Synthesis of secretin II. The stepwise approach. *J. Am. Chem. Soc.,* 89:6753–6757.

19. Bodanszky, M., and Sheehan, J. T. (1964): Active esters and resins in peptide synthesis. *Chem. Ind. (Lond.)*, 1423–1424.
20. Bodanszky, M., and Williams, N. J. (1967): Synthesis of Secretin I. The protected tetradecapeptide corresponding to sequence 14–27. *J. Am. Chem. Soc.*, 89:685–689.
20a. Brazeau, P., Vale, W., Burgus, R., Ling, N., Butcher, M., Rivier, J., and Guillemin, R. (1973): Hypothalamic polypeptide that inhibits the secretion of immunoreactive pituitary growth hormone. *Science*, 179:77–79.
20b. Bromer, W. W., Sinn, L. G., and Behrens, O. K. (1957): The amino acid sequence of glucagon. V. Location of amide groups, acid degradation studies and summary of sequential evidence. *J. Am. Chem. Soc.*, 79:2807–2810.
21. Brown, J. C., Cook, M. A., and Dryburgh, J. R. (1973): Motilin, a gastric motor activity stimulating polypeptide: The complete amino acid sequence. *Can. J. Biochem.*, 51:533–537.
22. Brown, J. C., and Dryburgh, J. R. (1971): A gastric inhibitory polypeptide II: The complete amino acid sequence. *Can. J. Biochem.*, 49:867–872.
23. Brown, J. C., Johnson, L. P., and Magee, D. F. (1966): Effect of duodenal alkalinization on gastric motility. *Gastroenterology*, 50:333–339.
24. Brown, J. C., Mutt, V., and Dryburgh, J. R. (1971): The further purification of motilin, a gastric motor activity stimulating polypeptide from the mucosa of the small intestine of hogs. *Can. J. Physiol. Pharmacol.*, 49:399–405.
25. Brown, J. C., Mutt, V., and Pederson, R. A. (1970): Further purification of a polypeptide demonstrating enterogastrone activity. *J. Physiol. (Lond.)*, 209:57–64.
25a. Bury, R. W., and Mashford, M. L. (1976): Biological activity of C-terminal partial sequences of substance P. *J. Med. Chem.*, 19:854–856.
26. Camble, R. (1972): In: *Chemistry and Biology of Peptides*, edited by J. Meienhofer. Ann Arbor Science Pub., Ann Arbor, Michigan.
27. Carpino, L. A. (1957): Oxidative reactions of hydrazines. II. Isophthalimides. New protective groups on nitrogen. *J. Am. Chem. Soc.*, 79:98–101.
27a. Chang, C. D., and Meienhofer, J. (1978): Solid-phase synthesis using mild base cleavage of Nα-fluorenylmethyloxycarbonylamino acids, exemplified by a synthesis of dihydrosomatostatin. *Int. J. Pept. Protein Res.*, 11:246–249.
27b. Chang, M. M., and Leeman, S. E. (1970): Isolation of a sialogogic peptide from bovine hypothalamic tissue and its characterization as substance P. *J. Biol. Chem.*, 245:4784–4790.
27c. Chang, M. M., Leeman, S. E., and Niall, H. D. (1971): Amino acid sequence of substance P. *Nature (New Biol.)*, 232:86–87.
28. Chaudhury, A. M., Kenner, G. W., Moore, S., Ramage, R., Richards, P. M., Thorp, W. D., Moroder, L., Wendlberger, G., and Wünsch, E. (1976): Synthesis of human big gastrin-I. *Proceedings of the 14th European Peptide Symposium*, pp. 257–261.
29. Cosmatos, A., Photaki, I., and Zervas, L. (1961): Peptidsynthesen über N-Phosphorylaminosäure-phosphorsaure-anhydride. *Chem. Ber.*, 94:2644–2655.
29a. Coy, D. H., Coy, E. J., Arimura, A., and Schally, A. (1973): Solid phase synthesis of growth hormone-release inhibiting factor. *Biochem. Biophys. Res. Commun.*, 54:1267–1273.
30. Curtius, T. (1902): Synthetische versuche mit hippurazid. *Ber. Deutsch Chem. Ges.*, 35:3226–3228.
31. Edkins, J. S. (1905): On the chemical mechanism of gastric secretion. *Proc. Roy. Soc. Lond. (Biol.)*, 76:376.
32. Erspamer, V., Roseghini, M., Endean, R., and Anastasi, A. (1966): Biogenic amines and active polypeptides in the skin of Australian amphibians. *Nature*, 212:204.
33. Euler, von U. S., and Gaddam, J. H. (1931): An unidentified depressor substance in certain tissue extracts. *J. Physiol. (Lond.)*, 72:74–87.
34. Fink, M. L., and Bodanszky, M. (1976): Secretin. VI. Simultaneous "in situ" syntheses of three analogues of the C-terminal tricosapeptide and a study of their conformation. *J. Am. Chem. Soc.*, 98:974–977.
34a. Fisher, G. H., Humphries, J., Folkers, K., and Pernow, B. (1974): Synthesis and some biological activities of Substance P. *J. Med. Chem.*, 17:843–846.
35. Foa, P. P. (1975): The metabolic role of pancreatic glucagon, of enteroglucagon, and of other glucagon-like immunoreactive materials in health and disease. *Diabetes Mellitus*, 4:23–27.
35a. Fujino, M., Wakimasu, M., Shinagawa, S., Kitada, C., and Yajima, H. (1978): Synthesis of the nonacosapeptide corresponding to mammalian glucagon. *Chem. Pharm. Bull. (Tokyo)*, 26(2):539–548.

35b. Gerich, J. E., Lorenzi, M., Schneider, V., Karam, H. H., Rivier, J., Guillemin, R., and Forsham, P. (1974): Effects of somatostatin on plasma glucose and glucagon levels in human diabetes mellitus. *N. Engl. J. Med.*, 291:544–547.

36. Gregory, H., Hardy, P. M., Jones, D. S., Kenner, G. W., and Sheppard, R. C. (1964): The antral hormone gastrin. *Nature*, 204:931–933.

37. Gregory, R. A., and Tracy, H. J. (1964): The constitution and properties of two gastrins extracted from hog antral mucosa. *Gut*, 5:103–117.

38. Gregory, R. A., and Tracy, H. J. (1972): Isolation of two "big gastrins" from Zollinger-Ellison tumour tissue. *Lancet*, ii:797–799.

39. Gregory, R. A., and Tracy, H. J. (1974): Isolation of two minigastrins from Zollinger-Ellison tumour tissue. *Gut*, 15:683–685.

40. Grossman, M. I. (1976): Sources of supply of gastrointestinal hormones and related peptides. *Gastroenterology*, 71:166–168.

41. Harper, A. A., and Raper, M. S. (1943): Pancreozymin, a stimulant of the secretion of pancreatic enzymes in extracts of the small intestine. *J. Physiol. (Lond.)*, 102:115–125.

42. Hemmasi, B., and Bayer, E. (1977): The solid phase synthesis of porcine secretin with full biological activity. *Int. J. Pept. Protein Res.*, 9:63–70.

43. Honzl, J., and Rudinger, J. (1961): Amino-acids and peptides. XXXIII. Nitrosyl chloride and butyl nitrite as reagents in peptide synthesis by the azide method: suppression of amide formation. *Coll. Czech. Commun.*, 26:2333–2344.

44. Ivy, A. C., and Oldberg, E. (1928): A hormone mechanism for gall-bladder contraction. *Am. J. Physiol.*, 86:599–613.

45. Jäger, G., König, W., Wissmann, H., and Geiger, R. (1974): Beitrag zur Synthese des Sekretins. *Chem. Ber.*, 107:215–231.

46. Jorpes, J. E., and Mutt, V. (1961): On the biological activity and amino acid composition of secretin. *Acta Chem. Scand.*, 15:1790–1791.

47. Jorpes, J. E., Mutt, V., Magnusson, S., and Steele, B. B. (1962): Amino acid composition and N-terminal amino acid sequence of porcine secretin. *Biochem. Biophys. Res. Commun.*, 9:275–279.

48. Jorpes, J. E., Mutt, V., and Toczko, K. (1964): Further purification of cholecystokinin and pancreozymin. *Acta Chem. Scand.*, 18:2408–2410.

49. Kai, Y., Kawatani, H., Yajima, H., and Itoh, Z. (1975): Studies on peptides. LV. Total synthesis of porcine motilin, a gastric motor activity stimulating polypeptide. *Chem. Pharm. Bull. (Tokyo)*, 23(10):2346–2352.

50. Klausner, Y. S., and Bodanszky, M. (1977): Cholecystokinin-Pancreozymin. 2. Synthesis of a protected heptapeptide hydrazide corresponding to sequence 17–23. *J. Org. Chem.*, 42:147–152.

51. Kovacs, K., Petres, J. K., Wendlberger, G., and Wünsch, E. (1973): Zur Synthese von gastric inhibitory polypeptide (GIP). I. *Z. Physiol. Chem.*, 354:890–893.

52. Lindeberg, G., and Ragnarsson, U. (1977): *Unpublished results*.

52a. Ling, N., Burgus, R., Rivier, J., Vale, W., and Brazeau, P. (1973): The use of mass spectrometry in deducing the sequence of somatostatin -a hypothalamic polypeptide that inhibits the secretion of growth hormone. *Biochem. Biophys. Res. Commun.*, 50:127–133.

52b. Makman, M. H., and Sutherland, E. W. (1964): Use of adenylcyclase for assay of glucagon in human gastrointestinal tract and pancreas. *Endocrinology*, 75:127–134.

53. McKay, F. C., and Albertson, N. F. (1957): New amine-masking groups for peptide synthesis. *J. Am. Chem. Soc.*, 79:4686–4690.

54. Medzihradszky, K. (1960): Über die Ermittlung der Bindungsart von Aminodicarbonsäuren in Polypeptiden. *Chimia*, 14:375.

55. Merrifield, R. B. (1963): Solid phase peptide synthesis. I. The synthesis of a tetrapeptide. *J. Am. Chem. Soc.*, 85:2149–2154.

55a. Meyers, C., Arimura, A., Gordin, A., Fernandez-Durango, R., Coy, D. H., Schally, A. V., Drouin, J., Ferland, L., Beaulieu, M., and Labrie, F. (1977): Somatostatin analogs which inhibit glucagon and growth hormone more than insulin release. *Biochem. Biophys. Res. Commun.*, 74:630–636.

55b. Meyers, C., Coy, D. H., Huang, W. Y., Schally, A. V., and Redding, T. (1978): Highly active position eight analogues of somatostatin and separation of peptide diastereomers by partition chromatography. *Biochemistry*, 17:2326–2331.

56. Mutt, V. (1976): Further investigations on intestinal hormonal polypeptides. *Clin. Endocrinol. (Oxf.) (Suppl.),* 5:175s–183s.
57. Mutt, V., and Jorpes, J. E. (1967): Contemporary developments in the biochemistry of the gastrointestinal hormones. *Rec. Prog. Horm. Res.,* 23:483–495.
58. Mutt, V., Magnusson, S., Jorpes, J. E., and Dahl, E. (1968): Structure of porcine secretin. I. Degradation with trypsin and thrombin. Sequence of the tryptic peptides. The C-terminal residue. *Biochemistry,* 4:2358.
59. Mutt, V., and Said, S. I. (1974): Structure of the porcine vasoactive intestinal octacosapeptide. *Eur. J. Biochem.,* 42:581–589.
60. Ogawa, H., Kubota, M., and Yajima, H. (1976): Studies on peptides. LXII. Synthesis of the protected octadecapeptide corresponding to positions 26 through 43 of porcine gastric inhibitory polypeptide (GIP). *Chem. Pharm. Bull. (Tokyo),* 24(10):2428–2434.
61. Ogawa, H., Kubota, M., Yajima, H., Tobo, T., Fujimura, M., Henmi, K., Torizuka, K., Adachi, H., Imura, H., and Taminato, T. (1976): Studies on peptides. LXIV. Synthesis of the tritetracontapeptide corresponding to the entire amino acid sequence of porcine gastric inhibitory polypeptide (GIP). *Chem. Pharm. Bull. (Tokyo),* 24(10):2447–2456.
61a. Ogawa, H., Sugiura, M., Yajima, H., Sakurai, H., and Tsuda, K. (1978): Studies on peptides. LXXVII. Synthesis of the nonacosapeptide corresponding to the entire amino acid sequence of avian glucagon (duck). *Chem. Pharm. Bull. (Tokyo),* 26(5):1549–1557.
62. Ondetti, M. A., Narayanan, V. L., von Salta, M., Sheehan, J. T., Sabo, E. F., and Bodanszky, M. (1968): The synthesis of secretin. III. The fragment-condensation approach. *J. Am. Chem. Soc.,* 90:4711–4716.
63. Ondetti, M. A., Pluscĕč, J., Sabo, E. F., Sheehan, J. T., and Williams, N. J. (1970): Synthesis of cholecystokinin-pancreozymin. I. The C-terminal dodecapeptide. *J. Am. Chem. Soc.,* 92:195–199.
64. Piper, P. J., Said, S. I., and Vane, J. R. (1970): Effects on smooth muscle preparations of unidentified vasoactive peptides from intestine and lung. *Nature,* 225:1144–1146.
65. Polak, J. M., Pearse, A. G. E., Szelke, M., Bloom, S. R., Hudson, D., Facer, P., Buchan, A. M. J., Bryant, M. G., Christophodes, N., and MacIntyre, I. (1977): Specific immunostaining of CCK cells by use of synthetic fragment antisera. *Experientia,* 33:762–763.
66. Rehfeld, J. F., Stadil, F., and Vikelsoe, J. (1974): Immunoreactive gastrin components in human serum. *Gut,* 15:102–111.
66a. Rivier, J., Brazeau, P., Vale, W., Ling, N., Burgus, R., Gilon, C., Yardley, J., and Guillemin, R. (1973): Synthése totale par phase solide d'un tétradecapeptide ayant les propriétés chimiques et biologiques de la somatostatine. *C. R. Acad. Sci. (D) (Paris),* 276:2737–2743.
67. Said, S. I., and Mutt, V. (1970): Polypeptide with broad biological activity: isolation from small intestine. *Science,* 169:1217–1218.
68. Said, S. I., and Mutt, V. (1972): Isolation from porcine-intestinal wall of a vasoactive octacosapeptide related to secretin and to glucagon. *Eur. J. Biochem.,* 28:199–204.
69. Sakakibara, S., Shimonishi, Y., Kishida, Y., Okada, M., and Sugihara, H. (1967): Use of anhydrous hydrogen fluoride in peptide synthesis. I. Behavior of various protective groups in anhydrous hydrogen fluoride. *Bull. Chem. Soc. Jpn.,* 40:2164–2167.
70. Schubert, H., and Brown, J. F. (1974): Correction to the amino acid sequence of porcine motilin. *Can. J. Biochem.,* 52:7–8.
71. Shinagawa, S., Fujino, M., Yajima, H., Segawa, T., and Okuma, Y. (1978): Synthesis and biological activity of 8-L-Ala-motilin and 8-D-Ala-motilin. *Chem. Pharm. Bull. (Tokyo),* 26(3):880–884.
71a. Sundby, F., Frandsen, S. K., Thomsen, J., Kristianien, K., and Brunfeldt, K. (1972): Crystallization and amino acid sequence of duck glucagon. *FEBS Lett.,* 26(1):289–293.
72. Sutherland, E. W., and DeDuve, C. (1948): Origin and distribution of hyperglycemic-glycogenolytic factor of pancreas. *J. Biol. Chem.,* 175:663–674.
72a. Synthetic Protein Research Group, China Biochemical Institute (1975), *Acta Biochim. Biophys. Sinica* 7:119; c.f. Ogawa et al. (1978): Studies on peptides. LXXVII. Synthesis of the nonacosapeptide corresponding to the entire amino acid sequence of avian glucagon (duck). *Chem. Pharm. Bull. (Tokyo),* 26(5):1549–1557.
73. Thomas, J. E., Crider, J. O., and Mogan, C. J. (1934): A study of reflexes involving the pyloric sphincter and antrum and their role in gastric evacuation. *Am. J. Physiol.,* 108:683–800.
73a. Tregear, G., Niall, H. D., Potts, J. T., Leeman, S. E., and Chang, M. M. (1971): Synthesis of substance P. *Nature [New Biol.],* 232:87–89.

74. van Zon, A., and Beyerman, H. C. (1976): Synthesis of the gastrointestinal peptide hormone secretin by repetitive excess mixed anhydride (REMA) method. *Helv. Chim. Acta,* 59:1112–1126.

74a. Wünsch, E. (1967): Die totale Synthese des Pankreas-Hormons Glucagon. *Z. Naturforsch. (B),* 22:1269–1276.

75. Wünsch, E., Jaeger, E., Knof, S., Scharf, R., and Thamm, P. (1976): Zur Synthese von Motilin, III. Reindurstellung and Charakterisierung von [13-norleucine]Motilin und [13-Leucin]Motilin. *Z. Physiol. Chem.,* 347:467–476.

75a. Wünsch, E., Jaeger, E., and Scharf, R. (1968): Zur Synthese des Glucagon, XIX. Reindarstellung des synthetischen Glucagons. *Chem. Ber.,* 101:3664–3670.

75b. Wünsch, E., and Wendlberger, G. (1968): Zur Synthese des Glucagons, XVIII, Carstellung der Gesamtsequenz. *Chem. Ber.,* 101:3659–3663.

76. Wünsch, E., and Wendlberger, G. (1972): Zur Synthese des Secretins V. Darstellung der Gesamtsequenz. *Chem. Ber.,* 105:2508–2514.

77. Wünsch, E., Wendlberger, G., Hallett, A., Jaeger, E., Knof, S., Moroder, L., Scharf, R., Schmidt, I., Thamm, R., and Wilschowitz, L. (1977): Zur Totalsynthese des Human-Big-Gastrins I and seines 32-Leucin-Analogons. *Z. Naturforsch.[C]* 32:495–506.

77a. Yajima, H., Kitagawa, K., and Segawa, T. (1973): Studies on peptides. XXXVIII. Structure-activity correlations in substance P. *Chem. Pharm. Bull. (Tokyo),* 21:2500–2506.

78. Yajima, H., Mori, Y., Koyama, K., Tohe, T., Setoyama, M., Adachi, H., Kanno, T., and Saito, A. (1972): Synthesis of the tritetracontapeptide amide corresponding to the entire amino acid sequence of the desulfated form of porcine cholecystokinin-pancreozymin (CCK-PZ). *Chem. Pharm. Bull. (Tokyo),* 24(11):2794–2802.

79. Yalow, R. S., and Berson, S. A. (1970): Radioimmunoassay of gastrin. *Gastroenterology,* 58:608–615.

80. Yalow, R. S., and Wu, N. (1973): Additional studies on the nature of big gastrin. *Gastroenterology,* 65:19–27.

Gastrointestinal Hormones, edited by
George B. Jerzy Glass.
Raven Press, New York © 1980.

Chapter 19

Heterogeneity of Gastrointestinal Hormones

Jens F. Rehfeld

Institute of Medical Biochemistry, University of Aarhus, Aarhus, Denmark

INTRODUCTION

Like other proteins, peptide hormones are heterogenous, i.e., they exist in the same species in different molecular forms. Gastrointestinal hormones are no exception to the rule of heterogeneity, although this feature has been recognized only after some hesitation.

This chapter takes into account the number and nature of the various molecular forms of gastrointestinal hormones as they are recognized at present. The biological and clinical implications of the heterogeneity are then reviewed. This is preceded by an outline of the general aspects and definition of heterogeneity. A short discussion of the methods employed in the study of heterogeneity is also appropriate because many of the molecular forms of gut hormones are defined by the methods through which they have been discovered.

GENERAL ASPECTS AND DEFINITIONS

Molecular heterogeneity is a feature of all mammalian proteins and polypeptides, that so far has been studied in this respect. By heterogeneity is meant that a protein exists in a number of molecular forms having different covalent structures in the same species. The difference may vary from derivatization of a single amino acid residue to a gross variation in the molecular size and conformation. Although the gross heterogeneities are readily discernible by available physicochemical techniques, subtle variations may still exist that cannot currently be detected by any known method.

The existence of heterogeneity of proteins has been recognized for several decades. Thus, subfractionation of human albumin into various molecular forms was reported as early as in 1947 (28). As discussed in a following section, molecular heterogeneity is generated by a multiplicity of biochemical mechanisms, some of which are understood rather poorly. The number of different molecular forms of a protein or polypeptide in one mammalian species is probably large. As to the order of magnitude, it has been suspected that "ten is too small and a thousand might be excessive" (17). To conceive the degree and nature of the molecular heterogeneity, it is essential to distinguish "microheterogeneity" from "macroheterogeneity." The term microheterogeneity in connection with proteins was introduced 26 years ago (10). In the following discussion microheterogeneity is defined as derivatization or substitution of a single amino acid residue in the protein. In contrast, macroheterogeneity refers to variations in the protein or polypeptide chain length by two or more amino acids (53).

METHODS IN THE STUDY OF GUT HORMONE HETEROGENEITY

Materials and Extractions

Biological fluids such as plasma, serum, urine, and cerebrospinal fluid (CSF) are well suited for heterogeneity studies. Tissue extracts of any kind may also be studied. It is, however, important to realize that different molecular forms extracted from the same source may not only differ in size but also in respect to charge and solubility under various physicochemical conditions. Consequently, it may be necessary to use several different procedures to extract all the molecular forms of a given hormone. An example of this problem has been our recent

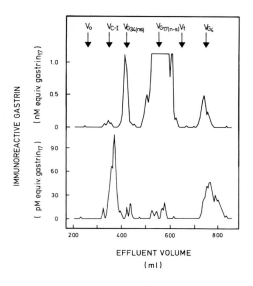

FIG. 1. Gel chromatography on Sephadex G-50 superfine columns of gastrin in extracts of porcine antral mucosa. **Top:** The component pattern by extraction in boiling water at pH 6.6. **Bottom:** The component pattern by extraction acid pH using 0.5 M acetic acid. The elutions were monitored by the same COOH-terminal specific gastrin assay.

experience with cholecystokinin (CCK) and gastrin. By extraction of the jejunal mucosa at neutral pH essentially only small-molecular forms (CCK-8 and CCK-4) were released from the tissue, whereas extraction at low pH released the large-molecular forms of CCK (13,50). Similarly, by extraction of antral mucosa with boiling water (pH 6.6) all of the five main components of gastrin were released. At acid pH, however, only the largest component, I, and the smallest component, V, were released (Fig. 1). Hence, evaluation of the true molecular pattern in a tissue requires variations in the conditions of extraction (pH, salt, temperature, degree of hydrophobicity), with due attention given at each step to degradation or modification of the structure of the hormones.

Separation of the Different Molecular Forms

Gel chromatography has so far been the preferred fractionation technique. Sephadex chromatography is simple and gentle. Moreover, the Sephadex G-50 gel has a fractionation range appropriate for screening of the molecular heterogeneity of most gastrointestinal hormones. Gel filtration techniques to be utilized vary from crude separation into a few fractions, similar to desalting (small columns, rapid flow rate, large sample size) to high-resolution chromatography into many hundred fractions (large and long columns, moderate flow rate, minimal sample size, superfine gel beads). The latter type of gel chromatography, which also contains elements of ion-exchange chromatography and hydrophobic interaction, obviously allows a very high degree of separation and information (Fig. 2).

For some studies fractionation into a few known components may be sufficient (e.g., separation of "big" from "little" GIP, or gastrin-34 from gastrin-17 in

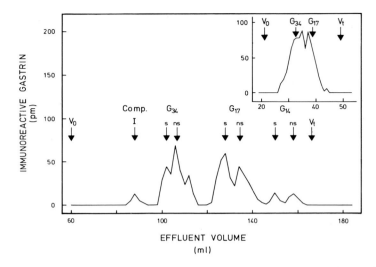

FIG. 2. Gel chromatography of immunoreactive gastrin in one serum sample from a Zollinger-Ellison patient, LB. **Upper right:** The elution pattern from a small Sephadex G-50 fine column (50 × 1 cm), eluted with 0.02 M veronal buffer, pH 8.4, containing 0.1% albumin. Fractions of 1.0 ml were collected at a flow rate of 6 ml/hr at 4°C. **Larger diagram:** The elution pattern from a long Sephadex G-50 superfine column (200 × 1 cm), eluted with 0.1 M sodium phosphate buffer, pH 7.5. Fractions of 2.0 ml were collected at a flow rate of 4 ml/hr at 4°C. Since aliquots from the same serum sample were applied to both columns, and since the effluents were monitored by the same radioimmunoassay the two elution diagrams can be compared. While the small column using fine Sephadex quality provides a separation into only two components (G-34- and G-17-like), the longer column with superfine Sephadex quality separates not only the four main components, but also sulfated and nonsulfated gastrins.

serum). When the degree of heterogeneity is unknown, however, and the existence of new molecular forms is under study, crude gel chromatography is inappropriate. Several fractionation techniques are required for this purpose. Most laboratories are, or should be, able to perform high-resolution gel chromatography, ion-exchange chromatography, and disc-gel electrophoresis. Discovery of new molecular forms needs confirmation by rechromatography, affinity chromatography, chromatography in 8 M urea or 6 M guanidine hydrochloride, and cleavage with various proteolytic enzymes. The new finding should ultimately result in purification and elucidation of the structure of the new component.

The necessity of applying more than one fractionation technique (and more than one assay) for monitoring has been illustrated recently by the discovery of new molecular forms of vasoactive intestinal polypeptide (VIP). Earlier studies based on gel chromatography indicated that only one form of VIP was present in the tissue (2,34). Ion-exchange chromatography revealed several forms (11), however. Also CCK-33 and CCK-39 elute in the same position even if high-resolution gel chromatography is used (50). However, cation-exchange cellulose chromatography produced excellent separation of the two forms (43).

Monitoring of Fractionations

Fractionations can be monitored by bio- and immunoassays. Bioassays are necessary for purification of a hormone that is defined only by its biological activity. In addition, bioassays are useful in the subsequent characterization of new molecular forms of a hormone. In other situations, however, bioassays are inappropriate because of their poor sensitivity, lack of specificity, time consuming performance, and high cost in comparison with immunoassays. Thus, when the first molecular form of a hormone is purified, sensitive and well-characterized radioimmunoassays (RIAs) can be developed and used for further exploration of the heterogeneity. The RIAs, however, require critical evaluation before they can be applied to heterogeneity studies. Thus, it is necessary because of the great homology of gastrointestinal hormones to know which part of the amino acid sequence of the hormone the assay will measure. For instance, assays specific for the COOH-terminal sequence of gastrin will also measure CCK because the antibody binding site can bind a peptide sequence of four to six amino acid residues, and the pentapeptide sequence common for gastrin and CCK is highly immunogenic. Also, cross-reactivity between secretin, glucagon, GIP, and VIP may be encountered due to their sequence homology. Other problems may arise if an assay is specific for either the NH_2- or COOH-terminus of the peptide. Here the terminals may not be available for antibody binding in the extended precursor molecules. Another, although less common problem, arises if the antibody requires the entire antigen for binding, and, hence, recognizes neither a larger nor a smaller molecular form of the hormone. Such antiserum was fortuitously produced against gastrin (15). It is useful for many purposes except for heterogeneity studies. If such antisera were common, the recognition of heterogenity would have been greatly delayed.

The optimal tool for monitoring heterogeneity studies is sequence-specific RIA. That is a range of assays, which are specific for different sequences of the primary hormonal antigen. This assay system was originally developed for the parathyroid hormone (68). We have now developed similar systems for CCK-33 and gastrin-17 (51), and they have proved highly useful. In this context the high degree of specificity of an antibody binding site has to be emphasized. The binding site not only recognizes a given peptide sequence but it is also sensitive to subtle modifications of a single amino residue. Thus, amidation or methylation of one residue may influence the detection of the peptide by the assay (Fig. 3). Due to this degree of specificity, sequence-specific RIAs, which cover the majority of a hormonal sequence, have now been accepted as a versatile, fast, and elegant tool in structural studies of phylogenesis, biosynthesis, tissue localization, and conformation in peptide synthesis.

In addition to the proper immunological specificity problems of homologous hormones and related molecular variants, significant problems have emerged in evaluation of the apparent immunoreactivity eluted in the void volume of gel columns. As mentioned before, Sephadex G-50 columns have a fractionation

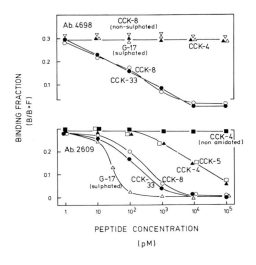

FIG. 3. Significance of microheterogeneity (modification of amino acid residues) for antibody binding. **Top:** The displacement of ^{125}I-CCK-33 from an antiserum (4698) specific for sequence 25–30 of CCK-33 by congeners and modified CCKs. **Bottom:** The displacement of ^{125}I-gastrin-17 from an antiserum (2609) specific for sequence 14–17 of gastrin-17 by congeners and modified gastrins and CCKs.

range appropriate for most gastrointestinal hormones in that it covers proteins and peptides of a molecular weight between 30,000 and 1,500, provided the molecules are globular. Thus all globular molecules having molecular masses above 30,000 daltons are eluted in the void volume. Samples with low concentrations of the hormones such as normal serum and some tissue extracts contain much protein, which elutes in the void volume. Some of these proteins, e.g., albumin and immunoglobulins, may, in an unspecific way, interfere with the antigen-antibody reaction of the RIA, and thus erroneously appear as a large hormonal form. This has recently been proven true for the so-called "big big" gastrin (57) and "big big" pancreatic polypeptide (PP) (67). Immunoglobulins may also, however, interfere in a specific way with the RIA and cause erroneous results. Thus, the "big plasma glucagon" (75) has recently been demonstrated to be due to cross-reaction in glucagon RIAs with IgG molecules, which in their Fc-fragment (C_H3-domain) contain sequences partly identical with the midsequence of pancreatic glucagon (66). Although the cross-reaction of IgG with glucagon may be weak on a molar basis, it becomes highly significant in plasma due to the high concentration of IgG (66).

Irrespective of the explanation for the apparent "immunoreactivity" in the void volume of chromatography columns, the phenomenon requires careful investigation and interpretation, not in the least because true macromolecular forms may exist. However, they would appear under circumstances different from those under which the artifactual macromolecules so far have been described, e.g., as very early biosynthetic precursor molecules (9,24).

Biosynthesis

Since the molecular heterogeneity of peptides reflects posttranslational covalent modifications of the ribosomal product, studies of the biosynthesis will give valuable information on the heterogeneity of hormones. Crucial information has already been obtained by investigation of the ribosomal synthesis of insulin and parathyroid hormone (9,24,70). Direct pulse-chase studies of the biosynthesis of gastrointestinal hormones have been reported only for CCK in tissue of the brain (56). Indirect information about the biosynthetic relationships can, however, be obtained by comparison of the molecular forms of a hormone in the tissue and the circulation. Existence of large molecular forms that are not secreted suggests that they are precursors. This was recently found to be true for the gastrins in the cat, where components I and II ("big gastrin") were present only intracellularly (62).

HETEROGENEITY OF THE INDIVIDUAL HORMONES

The Gastrin Family

The gastrin family includes gastrin and CCK. Met-enkephalin, motilin, and somatotropin may be considered as more distant relatives in the family (53). The identity of the biologically active COOH-terminal pentapeptide sequence of gastrin and CCK suggests a common ancestry for these two hormones, evidence for which has recently been discovered (36).

Gastrin

Gastrin circulates as four main components in man, pig (46,61), and dog (14) (Fig. 2). Four corresponding components have been isolated from extracts of antral mucosa and gastrinomas. The amino acid sequence of three molecular forms is known (20–22). Component I (46) has a molecular size (Stokes' radius) of 22 Å. Component II ["big gastrin" (77,78)] corresponds to the tetratriaconta-peptide amide, gastrin-34 (22). Component III corresponds to the well-known heptadecapeptide amide, gastrin-17 (20), and component IV to the tetradecapep-tide, gastrin-14 or "minigastrin" (21). In addition to these forms, a fragment corresponding to the NH_2-terminal tridecapeptide of gastrin-17 has been found in serum from Zollinger-Ellison patients (16). This fragment was recently demon-strated also in serum of normal subjects (57). Its presence supports the notion that a small peptide resembling the COOH-terminal tetrapeptide amide of gastrin may also exist. Recently we have actually found large amounts of this tetrapeptide amide in the antrum (55), duodenum, and jejunum (50).

It has been claimed that a major part of gastrin in the blood and tissue is a macromolecule called "big big" gastrin (79,80). This immunoreactivity appears, however, as previously mentioned, to be due to the protein interference in the RIA (57). However, some large tumors produce true macromolecular forms of gastrin (19,57,80). Their putative role as early intracellular biosynthetic pre-cursors (57) remains to be studied.

The heterogeneity of gastrin is even more complex than just described. By high-resolution gel chromatography (60) and anion-exchange chromatography

(19) each of the four main components in the blood and tissue has been demonstrated to be not merely, as first assumed, a paired sulfated and nonsulfated variant. Each of the components I and II circulates in six forms (60) and each of the components III and IV in four forms (19,60). Similar degree of heterogeneity also emerges for other proteins and peptide hormones like insulin (69). It is known that for gastrin, insulin, and other hormones large differences in size of the various molecular forms (macroheterogeneity) usually are accompanied by significant differences in their biological potency (76). However, microheterogeneity is equally important. For instance, removal of sulfate groups (30) or deamidation of the COOH-terminus (40) reduces the activity of CCK and gastrin dramatically. Consequently, microheterogeneity deserves as much attention as the macroheterogeneity of gastrointestinal hormones.

Cholecystokinin

The molecular heterogeneity of CCK in blood has not yet been described due to great problems in the development of RIA for CCK and its application to measurements in plasma or serum. Recently, however, sequence-specific CCK assays were developed (51), which allowed characterization of CCK in intestinal extracts (50). Extracts of both porcine and human jejunum contained five main components of CCK (Fig. 4), in analogy with the five main components of gastrin: component I, M. W. approximately 15,000; component II, corresponding in size to CCK-33; component III, corresponding to CCK-12; component IV, corresponding to the COOH-terminal octapeptide; and a fifth component, which corresponds to the COOH-tetrapeptide common to both gastrin and CCK (Fig. 4). Like gastrin, CCK is also present in the central and peripheral nerves (37). CCK is, however, present in the central nervous system in considerably larger amounts than gastrin (50,52). Neuronal CCK is also heterogenous (12,42,50), and the gel chromatography monitored by sequence-specific assays yields components similar to the jejunal forms of the CCK. These predominantly consist of smaller components IV and V (37,50). Similarly to gastrin, the phenomenon of microheterogeneity applies to CCK as well.

Motilin

Extensive studies on motilin heterogeneity have not yet been reported. Brown and Dryburgh (4) have recently described, however, the identification of two immunoreactive peaks of motilin obtained by cation-exchange chromatography of intestinal extracts. They suggested that the first peak contained glutamic acid in its sequence, whereas the second peak contained glutamine instead, an example of microheterogeneity.

Enkephalin

Immunoreactive enkephalin has been demonstrated in the antral and duodenal gastrin cells (45). Since these also contain immunoreactive ACTH (31,32), and

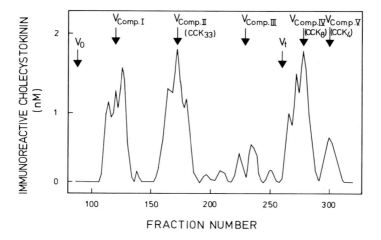

FIG. 4. Gel chromatography of immunoreactive CCKs in human jejunal mucosa. A boiled and acidified extract was applied to a Sephadex G-50 superfine column (200 × 2.5 cm) eluted with 0.25 M ammonium bicarbonate, pH 8.2. Fractions of 3.0 ml were collected at a flow rate of 20 ml/hr at 4°C. The effluent was monitored with a radioimmunoassay specific for the COOH-terminal sequence of CCK-33.

since met-enkephalin and ACTH are derived from the same large precursor (38), it is possible that gastrin cells, in addition to the different molecular forms of gastrin, also synthetize different peptides containing the small met-enkephalin molecule within their sequence. Such peptides might include β-LPH and the α-, β-, and γ-endorphins. Whether gastrin is present in the large 31 K precursor of ACTH and β-LPH (38) remains to be established.

The Secretin Family

The secretin family includes glucagon, VIP, and GIP in addition to secretin. The amphibian skin peptide bombesin also displays a slight structural similarity with VIP. The sequence analysis of the recently discovered mammalian bombesin will determine the degree of homology between VIP and bombesin. In addition, somatostatin displays some similarity with the members of the secretin family. In analogy with the members of the gastrin family, the structural similarity among the members of the secretin family also suggests a common ancestry.

Secretin

The existence of several molecular forms of secretin in plasma and duodenal extracts has been described in an abstract form (3,39). Other groups using gel filtration have found only one molecular form (65,71). In view of the general problems in evaluation of molecular heterogeneity, extensive studies are necessary before the question of secretin heterogeneity will be settled.

Glucagon

Since Sutherland and de Duve, in 1948, detected a hyperglycemic factor in the canine gastric mucosa (72), the existence of glucagon-like substances in the gut has been considered. Immunochemical and chemical studies in recent years have revealed a considerable heterogeneity of gut glucagons (26,41,73). A large molecular form with a M.W. of 11,000 has been purified, and its structure partly analyzed (29). (See Chapter 12 by F. Sundby and A. J. Moody, pp. 307–314, *this volume.*) Due to its content of 100 amino acids the name glicentin has been proposed (*gli:* glucagon-like-immunoreactants; *cent:* 100). A form with a M.W. of approximately 9,000 constitutes a large fraction of the gut glucagon. Also, small amounts of a component similar or possibly identical to the pancreatic glucagon (M.W., 3,500) have been found in porcine duodenum (64) and in large amounts in canine gastric mucosa (35,64). Finally, a smaller fragment (M.W., 2,500) has also been found in duodenal extracts (26,64). A still larger heterogeneity of each of the main components of glucagon has been suspected (26,41), but this requires further exploration.

Vasoactive Intestinal Polypeptide

VIP is present in large amounts in nerves throughout the gastrointestinal tract, most abundantly in the colon (2,34). The nerves in the genitourinary tract (33) and the central nervous system also contain large amounts of VIP (7,34,63). The extracts from the gut and brain contain only one immunoreactive peak on gel chromatography (7,34), but ion-exchange chromatography has revealed a considerable heterogeneity of VIP in some of the assays (11). Different molecular forms of VIP are now under investigation.

Gastric Inhibitory Polypeptide

Like other members of the family, GIP is also heterogenous. Both serum (6) and extracts of the proximal gut (5) contain at least three distinct immunoreactive peaks by gel chromatography. The peak in the void volume appears to be due to protein interference (5). The structural and functional characteristics of the "big" GIP will probably be reported soon.

Other Gut Hormones

In addition to the hormones just described, recent RIA and cytochemistry studies have disclosed a number of hormonal substances in the gut that were first recognized as brain peptides, presumably having transmitter functions. Investigations of the heterogeneity of these hormones are still sparse, but so far at least two different molecular forms of gastrointestinal substance P (44), somatostatin (1), and neurotensin (8) have been described. Using sequence-specific

RIAs to monitor different extracts of antral mucosa for somatostatin, we have recently found considerably more than two molecular forms of somatostatin. Of these forms some were larger than the tetradecapeptide somatostatin, and one form was smaller *(unpublished studies)*.

BIOCHEMICAL GENERATION OF DIFFERENT MOLECULAR FORMS OF GUT HORMONES

Information concerning the biochemical processes that determine the heterogeneity of gastrointestinal hormones is as yet limited, despite the efforts directed toward their elucidation. By combining the available information on the chemistry of the various forms of gut hormones with known facts about the biosynthesis of other polypeptide hormones (9,24,70), the following concept is plausible:

The peptide hormones are synthesized on polyribosomes into a single, long polypeptide chain. After translation, this chain is subjected to two distinct types of covalent modifications. The first is the cleavage of certain peptide bonds by proteolytic enzymes, some of which are trypsin- and carboxypeptidase B-like. This type of modification determines the macroheterogeneity of the peptide molecules ("big" and "small" molecular forms). The second type is the covalent derivatization of the single amino acid residues, a process suggested to influence the microheterogeneity. Well known examples of the latter are the synthesis of tyrosine-*O*-sulfate and the COOH-terminal amidation of phenylalanine, valine, and asparagine. Recently, 140 other examples of posttranslational derivatizations of the 20 amino acids have been assembled (74).

The foregoing concept raises a number of questions, the most important of which are: (a) Where do the covalent modifications take place? (b) What determines the specificity of the modification processes? (c) What is the relationship of any given modification to a specific biological activity? As long as these questions remain unanswered, no scientist working in the area of gut endocrinology shall be unemployed in the coming decade.

IMPLICATIONS OF HETEROGENEITY OF GUT HORMONES FOR ASSAY METHODOLOGY

Sensitive RIAs for gut hormones have greatly advanced our knowledge about the normal and pathological functions of the gastrointestinal tract. Moreover, these RIAs have proved indispensable for diagnosis of endocrine tumors of the gut and the pancreas. In order to obtain reliable results it is, however, necessary to evaluate the specificity of each assay in regard to the different molecular forms of a particular hormone.

As previously discussed (48,49), RIAs are usually developed against a single molecular form of the hormone. And so, essentially all of the gastrin assays have been established with antisera against gastrin-17, using ^{125}I-labeled gastrin-17 and unlabeled gastrin-17 as standards (49). Some assays are specific

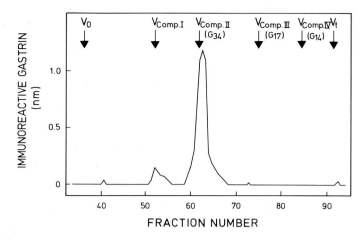

FIG. 5. Gel chromatography of immunoreactive gastrins in serum from a Zollinger-Ellison patient. The serum sample was applied to a long Sephadex-50 superfine column as described in the legend to Fig. 1. Note that only large molecular forms of gastrin were eluted.

exclusively for gastrin-17 (15) and others measure the four main gastrin components with equimolar potency (47). Most of the assays, however, measure the larger forms of gastrin with varying potency, which is lower than that of gastrin-17. Some of the assays are also sensitive to microheterogeneity such as sulfation (25,51) and deamidation (40). The specificity of the antibody against different molecular forms of a particular hormone can be tested in two ways. Either different pure forms of the hormone can be measured, or, if the purified forms are not available (only a few are at present) an enzymatic procedure that cleaves the large molecular forms to smaller ones can be used (49).

The importance of evaluating the specificity of the assay for the different molecular forms is illustrated by a case of a Zollinger-Ellison syndrome, in whom gastrin components I and II constituted almost all gastrin (Fig. 5). The serum samples were analyzed by a laboratory where gastrin assays were used that measured mainly "little gastrin." The case was misdiagnosed until the serum sample was sent to another laboratory, which was equipped for various types of gastrin assays.

IMPLICATIONS OF HETEROGENEITY OF HORMONES FOR GASTROINTESTINAL PHYSIOLOGY

The physiology of gut hormones is complex because of their pronounced interactions. Each of the hormones interacts with the other hormones and the adrenergic, cholinergic, and peptidergic nerves, as well as with the different molecular forms of the same hormone. Since the different molecular forms may have different biological potencies (76), the response to a hormone depends on the molecular pattern of the circulating hormone (for review, see ref. 23). A valid picture of release pattern and hormonal activity requires careful study of the release, transport, and action of each of the hormonal forms, alone and in combination with the interacting substances.

IMPLICATIONS OF HETEROGENEITY OF HORMONES FOR CLINICAL GASTROENTEROLOGY

The secretion of different molecular forms of a hormone may be of diagnostic significance if the pattern of components changes in a pathognomonic way. Such a pattern has been observed in insulinomas in regard to the ratio of proinsulin to insulin. A large percentage of proinsulin in the serum supports the diagnosis of an insulinoma (18). Similar unambiguity of the component patterns for the diagnosis has not as yet been demonstrated in the sera of patients with gut hormone-producing tumors. On the contrary, the individual component patterns of the gastrinoma patients vary greatly (59), and the molecular heterogeneity of gut hormones has not yet proved useful for diagnostic purposes.

The fact that endocrine cells of the gut release several, and not a single, molecular forms of a hormone may be of pathogenetic significance if forms with relatively low biological activity are released in abnormally large amounts. These forms may occupy the receptors for the molecular forms of high potency, and thus cause deficiency syndromes. Only few gastrointestinal diseases have been investigated in this respect. It appears likely that reactive hypoglycemia is caused by such a mechanism (54). Here, the excess of gut glucagons, bound to hepatic glucagon receptors (27), may inhibit the postprandial glycogenolysis and consequently induce reactive hypoglycemia.

Whether similar mechanisms play a role in other gastrointestinal diseases remains to be seen. A prerequisite for such studies is the further exploration of the heterogeneous nature of gut hormones.

SUMMARY AND PROJECTIONS FOR THE FUTURE

Molecular heterogeneity is a fundamental characteristic of proteins including plasma proteins, enzymes, and also polypeptide hormones. Heterogeneity reflects basic mechanisms of ribosomal biosynthesis, posttranslational and postsecretory cleavage, and amino acid modification. All gastrointestinal hormones are heterogenous, but the degree of heterogeneity reported for the individual gut hormone has varied. The most extensively studied gut hormone, gastrin, has displayed a high degree of heterogeneity. Similar degrees will probably emerge for the rest of the gastrointestinal hormones after they have been studied in greater detail. According to the extent of the molecular difference a distinction between macro- and microheterogeneity is proposed. *Macroheterogeneity* indicates a variation in peptide chain length of two or more amino acids. *Microheterogeneity* indicates derivatizations or substitutions in a single amino acid residue. The molecular heterogeneity has serious implications for the extraction, measurement, and evaluation of the action of the individual hormone. Thus, extraction of all molecular forms of a hormone requires several different procedures. Measurement of hormones in biological fluids requires careful evaluation of the specificity of the hormone assay. Understanding of the biology and pathophysiology of gut hormones requires clarification of their molecular heterogeneity.

REFERENCES

1. Arimura, A., Sato, H., Dupont, H., Nishi, N., and Schally, A. V. (1975): Somatostatin: Abundance of immunoreactivity in rat stomach and pancreas. *Science,* 198:1007–1009.
2. Bloom, S. R., and Polak, J. M. (1975): The role of VIP in pancreatic cholera. In: *Gastrointestinal Hormones,* edited by J. C. Thompson, pp. 635–642. University of Texas Press, Austin.
3. Boden, G., Murphy, N. S., and Silver, E. (1975): "Big" secretin. *Clin. Res.,* 23:245 (Abstr.).
4. Brown, J. C., and Dryburgh, J. R. (1978): Isolation of motilin. In: *Gut Hormones,* edited by S. R. Bloom, pp. 327–331. Churchill Livingstone, Edinburgh/London/New York.
5. Brown, J. C., Dryburgh, J. R., Frost, J. L., Otte, S. R., and Pederson, R. A. (1978): Properties and actions of GIP. In: *Gut Hormones,* edited by S. R. Bloom, pp. 277–282. Churchill Livingstone, Edinburgh/London/New York.
6. Brown, J. C., Dryburgh, J. R., Ross, S. A., and Dupre, J. (1975): Identification and actions of gastric inhibitory polypeptide. *Res. Progr. Horm. Res.,* 31:487–532.
7. Bryant, M. G., Bloom, S. R., Polak, J. M., Albuquerque, R. H., Modlin, I., and Pearse, A. G. E. (1976): Possible dual role for vasoactive intestinal peptide as gastrointestinal hormone and neurotransmitter substance. *Lancet,* i:991–993.
8. Carraway, R., and Leeman, S. E. (1976): Characterization of radioimmunoassayable neurotensin in the rat. Its differential distribution in the central nervous system, small intestine and stomach. *J. Biol. Chem.,* 251:7045–7052.
9. Chan, S. D., Keim, P., and Steiner, D. F. (1976): Cell-free synthesis of rat pre-proinsulins: Characterization and partial amino acid sequence determination. *Proc. Natl. Acad. Sci. USA,* 73:1964–1968.
10. Colvin, J. R., Smith, D. B., and Cook, V. H. (1954): The microheterogeneity of proteins. *Chem. Rev.,* 54:687–711.
11. Dimaline, R., and Dockray, G. J. (1978): Multiple immunoreactive forms of vasoactive intestinal peptide in human colonic mucosa. *Gastroenterology,* 75:387–392.
12. Dockray, G. J. (1976): Immunochemical evidence of cholecystokinin-like peptides in brain. *Nature,* 264:568–570.
13. Dockray, G. J. (1977): Immunoreactive component in small intestine resembling the COOH-terminal octapeptide of cholecystokinin. *Nature,* 270:359–361.
14. Dockray, G. J., Debas, H. T., Walsh, J. H., and Grossman, M. M. (1975): Molecular forms of gastrin in antral mucosa and serum of dogs. *Proc. Soc. Exp. Biol. Med.,* 149:550–554.
15. Dockray, G. J., and Taylor, I. L. (1976): Heptadecapeptide gastrin: measurement in blood by specific radioimmunoassay. *Gastroenterology,* 71:971–977.
16. Dockray, G. J., and Walsh, J. F. (1975): Amino terminal gastrin fragment in serum of Zollinger-Ellison syndrome patients. *Gastroenterology,* 68:222–230.
17. Foster, J. F. (1977): Some aspects of the structure and conformational properties of serum albumin. In: *Albumin Structure, Function and Uses,* edited by V. M. Rosenoer, M. Oratz, and M. A. Rotschild, pp. 53–84. Pergamon Press, Oxford/New York/Toronto/Paris/Sidney/Frankfurt.
18. Gorden, P., Sherman, B., and Roth, J. (1971): Proinsulin-like component of circulating insulin in the basal state and in patients and hamsters with islet-cell tumors. *J. Clin. Invest.,* 50:2113–2120.
19. Gregory, R. A. (1976): Heterogeneity of the gastrins in blood and tissue. In: *Polypeptide Hormones: Molecular and Cellular Aspects,* edited by R. Porter and D. W. Fitzsimons, pp. 251–261. Elsevier-North Holland, Amsterdam/Oxford/New York.
20. Gregory, R. A., and Tracy, H. J. (1964): The constitution and properties of two gastrins extracted from hog antral mucosa. *Gut,* 5:103–117.

21. Gregory, R. A., and Tracy, H. J. (1974): Isolation of two minigastrins from Zollinger-Ellison tumor tissue. *Gut*, 15:683–685.
22. Gregory, R. A., and Tracy, H. J. (1975): The chemistry of the gastrins: Some recent advances. In: *Gastrointestinal Hormones*, edited by J. C. Thompson, pp. 13–24. University of Texas Press, Austin.
23. Grossman, M. I. (1979): Neural and hormonal regulation of gastrointestinal function: An overview. *Annu. Rev. Physiol. (in press).*
24. Habener, J., Potts, J. T., Jr., and Rich, A. (1976): Preproparathyroid hormone: Evidence for an early biosynthesis precursor of proparathyroid hormone. *J. Biol. Chem.*, 251:3893–3899.
25. Hansky, J., Soveny, C., and Korman, M. G. (1974): Studies with two gastrin antisera of different specificity for gastrins I and II. *Digestion*, 10:97–107.
26. Holst, J. J. (1977): Extraction, gel filtration pattern, and receptor binding of porcine gastrointestinal glucagon-like immunoreactivity. *Diabetologia*, 13:159–169.
27. Holst, J. J., and Rehfeld, J. F. (1975): Human circulating gut glucagon: binding to liver cell plasma membranes. In: *Gastrointestinal Hormones*, edited by J. C. Thompson, pp. 529–536. University of Texas Press, Austin.
28. Hughes, W. L., Jr. (1947): An albumin fraction isolated from human plasma as a crystalline mercuric salt. *J. Am. Chem. Soc.*, 69:1836–1837.
29. Jacobsen, H., Demandt, A., Moody, A. J., and Sundby, F. (1977): Sequence analysis of porcine gut GLI-I. *Biochim. Biophys. Acta*, 493:452–459.
30. Johnson, L. R., Stening, G. F., and Grossman, M. I. (1970): Effect of sulfation on the gastrointestinal actions of caerulein. *Gastroenterology*, 58:208–212.
31. Larsson, L.-I. (1977): Corticotropin-like peptides in central nerves and in endocrine cells of gut and pancreas. *Lancet*, ii:1321–1323.
32. Larsson, L.-I. (1978): Distribution of ACTH-like immunoreactivity in rat brain and gastrointestinal tract. *Histochemistry*, 55:225–233.
33. Larsson, L.-I., Fahrenkrug, J., and Schaffalitzky de Muckadell, O. B. (1977): Vasoactive intestinal polypeptide occurs in nerves of the female genitourinary tract. *Science*, 197:1374–1375.
34. Larsson, L.-I., Fahrenkrug, J., Schaffalitzky de Muckadell, O. B., Sundler, F., Håkanson, R., and Rehfeld, J. F. (1976): Localization of vasoactive intestinal polypeptide (VIP) to central and peripheral neurons. *Proc. Natl. Acad. Sci. USA*, 73:3197–3200.
35. Larsson, L.-I., Holst, J. J., Håkanson, R., and Sundler, F. (1975): Distribution and properties of glucagon immunoreactivity in the digestive tract of various mammals: an immunohistochemical and immunochemical study. *Histochemistry*, 44:281–290.
36. Larsson, L.-I., and Rehfeld, J. F. (1977): Evidence of a common evolutionary origin of gastrin and cholecystokinin. *Nature*, 269:335–338.
37. Larsson, L.-I., and Rehfeld, J. F. (1979): Localization and molecular heterogeneity of cholecystokinin in the central and peripheral nervous system. *Brain Res.*, 165:201–218.
38. Mains, R. E., Eipper, B. A., and Ling, N. (1977): Common precursor to corticotropins and endorphins. *Proc. Natl. Acad. Sci. USA*, 74:3014–3018.
39. Mason, J. C., Murphy, R. F., and Buchanan, K. D. (1977): Characterization of secretin-like peptides from tissue and plasma extracts using immunoaffinity chromatography. *Gut*, 18: A 982 (Abstr.).
40. McGuigan, J. E., and Thomas, H. F. (1972): Physiological and immunological studies with desamidogastrin. *Gastroenterology*, 62:553–558.
41. Moody, A. J. (1972): Gastrointestinal glucagon-like immunoreactivity. In: *Glucagon: Molecular Physiology, Clinical and Therapeutic Implications*, edited by P. J. Lefebvre and R. H. Unger, pp. 319–341. Pergamon Press, Oxford.
42. Muller, J. E., Straus, E., and Yalow, R. S. (1977): Cholecystokinin and its COOH-terminal octapeptide in pig brain. *Proc. Natl. Acad. Sci. USA*, 74:3065–3068.
43. Mutt, V. (1976): Further investigations on intestinal hormonal polypeptides. *Clin. Endocrinol. (Suppl.)*, 5:175s–183s.
44. Nilsson, G., and Brodin, E. (1977): Tissue distribution of substance-P-like immunoreactivity in dog, cat, rat and mouse. In: *Substance P*, edited by U. S. von Euler and B. Pernow, pp. 49–54. Raven Press, New York.
45. Polak, J., Sullivan, S. N., Bloom, S. R., Facer, P., and Pearse, A. G. E. (1977): Enkephalin-like immunoreactivity in human gastrointestinal tract. *Lancet*, i:972–974.
46. Rehfeld, J. F. (1972): Three components of gastrin in serum. Gel filtration studies on the molecular size of immunoreactive serum gastrin. *Biochim. Biophys. Acta (Amst.)*, 285:364–372.

47. Rehfeld, J. F. (1976): Disturbed islet-cell function related to endogenous gastrin release. *J. Clin. Invest.*, 58:41–49.
48. Rehfeld, J. F. (1978): Problems in the technology of radioimmunoassays for gut hormones. In: *Gut Hormones*, edited by S. R. Bloom, pp. 145–148. Churchill Livingstone, Edinburgh/London/New York.
49. Rehfeld, J. F. (1978): Radioimmunoassay of gastrin. In: *Gut Hormones*, edited by S. R. Bloom, pp. 145–148. Churchill Livingstone, Edinburgh/London/New York.
50. Rehfeld, J. F. (1978): Immunochemical studies on cholecystokinin II. Distribution and molecular heterogeneity in the central nervous system and small intestine of man and hog. *J. Biol. Chem.*, 252:4022–4030.
51. Rehfeld, J. F. (1978): Immunochemical studies on cholecystokinin. I. Development of sequence-specific radioimmunoassays for porcine triacontratriapeptide cholecystokinin. *J. Biol. Chem.*, 253:4016–4021.
52. Rehfeld, J. F. (1978): Localization of gastrin to neuro- and adenohypophysis. *Nature*, 271:771–773.
53. Rehfeld, J. F. (1979): Gastrointestinal Hormones. In: *Gastrointestinal Physiology III*, edited by R. K. Crane, pp. 291–321. University Park Press, Baltimore.
54. Rehfeld, J. F., Heding, L. G., and Holst, J. (1973): Increased gut glucagon release as pathogenetic factor in reactive hypoglycemia. *Lancet*, i:116–118.
55. Rehfeld, J. F., and Larsson, L.-I. (1979): The predominating antral gastrin and intestinal cholecystokinin resembles the common COOH-terminal tetrapeptide amide. In: *Gastrins and the Vagus*, edited by J. F. Rehfeld and E. Amdrup, pp. 85–94. Academic Press, London.
56. Rehfeld, J. F., Larsson, L.-I., Goltermann, N., Emson, P. C., and Lee, C. M. (1979): Gastrins and cholecystokinins in the central and peripheral nervous system. *Fed. Proc.*, 38:2325–2329.
57. Rehfeld, J. F., Schwartz, T. W., and Stadil, F. (1977): Immunochemical studies on macromolecular gastrins. Evidence that "big big" in blood and mucosa are artifacts—but truly present in some large gastrinomas. *Gastroenterology*, 73:469–477.
58. Rehfeld, J. F., and Stadil, F. (1972): Big gastrins in the Zollinger-Ellison syndrome. *Lancet*, ii:1200–1201.
59. Rehfeld, J. F., and Stadil, F. (1973): Gel filtration studies on immunoreactive gastrin in serum from Zollinger-Ellison patients. *Gut*, 14:369–373.
60. Rehfeld, J. F., Stadil, F., Malmström, J., and Miyata, M. (1975): Gastrin heterogeneity in serum and tissue. A progress report. In: *Gastrointestinal Hormones*, edited by J. C. Thompson, pp. 43–58. University of Texas Press, Austin.
61. Rehfeld, J. F., Stadil, F., and Vikelsoe, J. (1974): Immunoreactive gastrin components in human serum. *Gut*, 15:102–111.
62. Rehfeld, J. F., and Uvnäs-Wallensten, K. (1978): Gastrins in cat and dog: Evidence for a biosynthetic relationship between the large molecular forms of gastrin and heptadecapeptide gastrin. *J. Physiol. (Lond.)*, 283:379–396.
63. Said, S. I., and Rosenberg, R. (1976): Vasoactive intestinal polypeptide: Abundant immunoreactivity in neural cell lines and normal nervous tissues. *Science*, 192:907–909.
64. Sasaki, H., Rubalcava, B., Baetens, D., Blazgues, E., Srikant, C. B., Orci, L., and Unger, R. H. (1975): Identification of glucagon in the gastrointestinal tract. *J. Clin. Invest.*, 56:135–145.
65. Schaffalitzky de Muckadell, O. B., and Fahrenkrug, J. (1978): Secretion pattern of secretin in man: Regulation by gastric acid. *Gut*, 19:812–818.
66. Schenck, H. V., and Grubb, A. O. (1980): Glucagon immunoreactivity in purified human immunoglobulins. *J. Clin. Invest. (in press)*.
67. Schwartz, T. W. (1980): True and artifactual heterogeneity of pancreatic polypeptide in plasma. *Clin. Chim. Acta (in press)*.
68. Segre, G. V., Tregear, G. W., and Potts, J. T., Jr. (1975): Development and application of sequence-specific radioimmunoassays for analysis of the metabolism of parathyroid hormone. *Methods Enzymol.*, 37 (B):38–66.
69. Steiner, D. F. (1976): Discussion of heterogeneity of the gastrins. In: *Polypeptide Hormones: Molecular and Cellular Aspects*, edited by R. Porter and D. W. Fitzsimons. Elsevier-North Holland, Amsterdam/Oxford/New York.
70. Steiner, D. F., Cunningham, D. D., Spigelman, L., and Aten, B. (1967): Insulin biosynthesis: Evidence for a precursor. *Science*, 157:697–700.

71. Straus, E., and Yalow, R. S. (1978): Immunoreactive secretin in gastrointestinal mucosa of several mammalian species. *Gastroenterology*, 75:401–404.
72. Sutherland, E. W., and de Duve, C. (1948): Origin and distribution of the hyperglycemic—glycogenolytic factor of the pancreas. *J. Biol. Chem.*, 175:663–674.
73. Unger, R. H., Ketterer, H., and Eisentraut, A. M. (1966): Distribution of immunoassayable glucagon in gastrointestinal tissues. *Metabolism*, 15:865–876.
74. Uy, R., and Wold, F. (1977): Posttranslational covalent modification of proteins. *Science*, 198:890–896.
75. Valverde, I., Villanueva, M. L., Lozano, I., and Marco, J. (1974): Presence of glucagon immunoreactivity in the globulin fraction of human plasma ("big plasma glucagon"). *J. Clin. Endocrinol. Metab.*, 39:1020–1028.
76. Walsh, J. H. (1975): Biological activity and disappearance rates of big, little and mini-gastrins in dog and man. In: *Gastrointestinal Hormones*, edited by J. C. Thompson. pp. 75–83. University of Texas Press, Austin.
77. Yalow, R. S., and Berson, S. A. (1970): Size and charge distinctions between endogenous human plasma gastrin in peripheral blood and heptadecapeptide gastrins. *Gastroenterology*, 58:609–615.
78. Yalow, R. S., and Berson, S. A. (1971): Further studies on the nature of immunoreactive gastrin in human plasma. *Gastroenterology*, 60:203–214.
79. Yalow, R. S., and Berson, S. A. (1972): And now, "big big" gastrin. *Biochem. Biophys. Res. Commun.*, 48:391–395.
80. Yalow, R. S., and Wu, N. (1973): Additional studies on the nature of big big gastrin. *Gastroenterology*, 65:19–22.

Gastrointestinal Hormones, edited by
George B. Jerzy Glass.
Raven Press, New York © 1980.

Chapter 20

Gastrointestinal Hormone-Receptor Interactions in the Pancreas

J. Christophe, M. Svoboda, P. Calderon-Attas, M. Lambert,
M. C. Vandermeers-Piret, A. Vandermeers, M. Deschodt-
Lanckman, and P. Robberecht

*Department of Biochemistry and Nutrition, Medical School, Université Libre de Bruxelles,
B-1000 Brussels, Belgium*

List of abbreviations: Cyclic AMP, adenosine $3':5'$-monophosphate; cyclic GMP, guanosine $3':5'$-monophosphate; Gpp(NH)p = p(NH)ppG, guanosine $5'$-(β,γ-imido) triphosphate; EDTA, ethylenediamine tetraacetic acid; EGTA, ethyleneglycol-bis-(2-amino-ethylether)-N,N,N',N'-tetraacetic acid; CDR, calcium-dependent protein regulator or calmodulin; PZ = CCK, = CCK-PZ, cholecystokinin-pancreozymin; OC-PZ = CCK-OP, C-terminal octapeptide of pancreozymin-cholecystokinin; VIP, vasoactive intestinal peptide; D_{50} = concentration required to exert half-maximal response (hormone binding, activation, etc . . .).

Code number of enzymes mentioned in the text: Cyclic nucleotide phosphodiesterase or $3':5'$-cyclic GMP and $3':5'$-cyclic AMP $5'$-nucleotidohydrolase (EC 3.1.4.17); guanylate cyclase or GTP pyrophosphate-lyase (cyclizing) (EC 4.6.1.2), adenylate cyclase or ATP pyrophosphate-lyase (cyclizing) (EC 4.6.1.1); NTPase or nonspecific nucleoside triphosphatase (EC 3.6.1-); cyclic AMP-dependent protein kinase (EC 2.7.1.37).

INTRODUCTION

In this chapter we do not attempt to present a comprehensive review of the field. Excellent reviews on pancreatic exocrine metabolism (11,98) as well as volumes and collections of papers delivered at international congresses on gastrointestinal hormones (4,6,13,21,26,41,91) have been published recently. Our emphasis lies primarily on the mode of action of pancreozymin (CCK-PZ) and secretin on rat and guinea pig pancreatic acinar cells, with limited examination of stimulations by bombesin, muscarinic agents, and vasoactive intestinal peptide (VIP), and only incidental coverage of the effects of other hormones and neuroendocrine agents susceptible to act on the exocrine pancreas.

The pancreas is a heterocellular epithelium, with the acinar cell as the major cell type contained therein. Most of the results of experiments performed *in vivo* or *in vitro* in the isolated organ, on tissue fragments and lobules, and on pancreatic extracts are therefore attributable to acinar cells. In this context, the data presently available on isolated acinar cells (1) and on preparations of dispersed acini free of duct system and islets (49) reinforce the value of previous data on the whole organ or total extracts.

POSTULATED ACTION OF TWO GROUPS OF SECRETORY AGENTS IN PANCREATIC ACINAR CELLS

Pancreatic emiocytosis in response to secretagogues requires energy and calcium for the fusion-fission of the zymogen granule membrane with the apical plasmalemma (11). The tentative scheme in Fig. 1 proposes a working model for hormone-receptor interactions in pancreatic acinar cells. This model implies

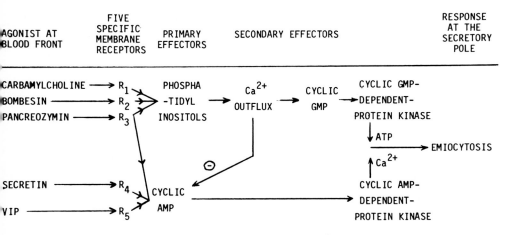

FIG. 1. Postulated action of two groups of secretory agents on pancreatic acinar cells.

that two partly independent chains of events between stimulus and secretion can implement the same final response.

In the major pathway, a group of secretagogues including pancreozymin, bombesin (a tetradecapeptide), or acetylcholine provokes the emiocytosis of zymogen granules through increased phosphatidylinositol turnover, an elevation of free cytosolic calcium, and the activation of guanylate cyclase. The short-lived rise in cyclic GMP allows a prolonged secretory response through the activation of a cyclic GMP-dependent protein kinase (48,94) and a sustained phosphorylation of proteins directly involved in emiocytosis.

In the second sequence of events, the scheme suggests that the binding of secretin and VIP results in the activation of adenylate cyclase in pancreatic plasma membranes, the elevation of cyclic AMP, and the stimulation of cyclic AMP protein kinase activity (22,48,64), which in turn leads to the secretion of hydrolases. This second class of hormones does not influence the phosphatidylinositol turnover, calcium movements, and cyclic GMP levels.

Both pathways do interact beyond the receptor level by influencing the adenylate cyclase system: (a) The specific occupancy of pancreozymin receptors can independently stimulate the same catalytic subunit in pancreatic plasma membranes as that stimulated by secretin. (b) However, a second interaction is observed in intact acinar cells where those calcium movements elicited by pancreozymin in turn appear to inhibit the adenylate cyclase system. Whatever the mechanism, pancreozymin and secretin, when used in conjunction, allow supramaximal rates of protein secretion, i.e., potentiation.

EFFECTS OF SECRETORY AGENTS ON LIPID METABOLISM IN THE EXOCRINE PANCREAS

When used at their optimal concentration secretagogues influencing calcium movements, i.e., pancreozymin, bombesin, and carbamylcholine, rapidly induce a wide range of effects on lipid metabolism in rat pancreas. Some of these might be related to or might alter the secretory response.

The lipolytic effect developing in response to these secretagogues is relatively calcium-dependent, and consists of the release of diglycerides and free fatty acids (Calderon-Attas et al., *unpublished data*). It is conceivable that the secretagogues activate calcium-dependent phospholipases. In addition, the malonic acid pathway of lipogenesis is inhibited, whereas the elongation of polyenoic fatty acids is unaltered. This preservation of the metabolism of polyenoic fatty acids during emiocytosis might be of importance in the renewal of membrane phospholipids. It should be noted that the lipolytic effects and the accompanying 25% fall in ATP levels observed with the first class of secretagogues are not encountered with secretin concentrations that allow similar hypersecretion. These effects are therefore not essential for stimulus-secretion coupling.

The stimulation of the turnover of phosphatidylinositols may have a more direct bearing on stimulus-secretion coupling (Calderon et al., ref. 10 and *unpublished data*). The sustained turnover of phosphatidylinositols includes an increased breakdown into free inositol and phosphatidic acids (44). This allows the release of free fatty acids after further catabolism. If one compares the increased incorporation of various radioactive precursors into phosphatidylinositols that may contribute to the turnover, it appears that inositol is incorporated relatively less. This implies the reutilization of endogenous inositol that is released through breakdown.

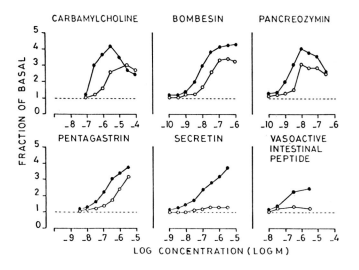

FIG. 2. Dose-effect relationship of six secretory agents on stimulation of amylase secretion (●—●) and phosphatidylinositol labeling with [1-¹⁴C] acetate (○—○). Rat pancreas fragments were incubated for 60 min with 0.5 mM [1-¹⁴C] acetate. Amylase secretion was determined on aliquots of incubation medium and phosphatidylinositol labeling was determined after lipid separation by thin-layer chromatography. Results are expressed in fraction of control values. (From Calderon-Attas et al., *unpublished data*.)

The derivatives of cyclic GMP induce amylase hypersecretion without the phosphatidylinositol effect. This suggests that the latter effect has to precede any mediation of cyclic GMP. Two observations indicate that this is not a consequence of Ca^{2+} movements: (a) The phosphatidylinositol effect is less dependent on extracellular Ca^{2+} than amylase hypersecretion provoked by carbamylcholine and pancreozymin. (b) The divalent ionophore A-23187, in the presence of Ca^{2+}, induces amylase hypersecretion but only a very low stimulation of phosphatidylinositol labeling. Dose-response curves of phosphatidylinositol labeling are observed at higher agonist concentrations when compared with dose-response curves of amylase hypersecretion (Fig. 2). Such a dose relationship may suggest that the phosphatidylinositol effect contributes to the amplification of a signal in response to secretagogues implementing calcium movements. There is no direct evidence, however, that the phosphatidylinositol effect is located at the cell membrane (29) and that it results from a local interaction of agonists with their receptors prior to calcium movements, as proposed by Michell [reviewed by Case (11)]. It remains therefore to be demonstrated whether the phosphatidylinositol effect is an intermediate process preceding the induced changes in calcium movements or whether this effect evolves in parallel and yields consequences unknown as yet. An increased turnover of phosphatidylinositols has been documented not only in secretory tissues such as pancreas (44) and parotid glands but also in smooth muscle and nervous system. This, together with the lack of phosphatidylinositol effect in the rat pancreas in the presence of secretin, clearly indicates that this effect is not related to emiocytosis *per se*.

INTRA- AND EXTRACELLULAR CALCIUM

In the exocrine rat, mouse, and guinea pig pancreas, the calcium needed initially to promote emiocytosis of hydrolases, in response to pancreozymin, bombesin, or cholinergic stimulation, is released from reserves in the cell membranes (12,25,28,34,39,65,71,84,86) (Fig. 3). The stimulation of ^{45}Ca outflux from dispersed acinar cells preloaded with ^{45}Ca is observed within 1 min and subsides after 5 to 10 min (Fig. 4). After that period, adding fresh pancreozymin, bombesin, or carbamylcholine fails to stimulate ^{45}Ca outflux in cells previously exposed to one of these secretagogues (34,39). This may reflect a secondary redistribution of calcium with free cellular ^{45}Ca accumulation that masks a persistent and specific effect of the secretagogue on membrane-bound ^{45}Ca (86). Indeed, when the stimulation is prolonged, cytosolic calcium seems to originate in the extracellular medium since this calcium is required to maintain a maximal response (2,11,12,68,74). Thus, bidirectional calcium movements are observed through the blood front of acinar cells. Pancreatic plasma membranes contain a (Mg, Ca) nucleoside triphosphatase (NTPase) of high activity and low specificity whose physiological role is not clear since it does not appear to be the target of secretagogues (56). Therefore, a direct interaction (through phosphatidylinositol turnover?) of the receptors for these secretagogues with membranous vectorial Ca^{2+} pumps has yet to be documented.

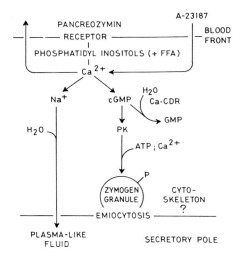

FIG. 3. Tentative localization of calcium movements and role of cyclic GMP (cGMP) in pancreatic acinar cells submitted to pancreozymin or the ionophore A-23187.

The relationship between calcium movements and cell membrane potential is actively explored (46,47,68,69). Pancreozymin, bombesin, and acetylcholine evoke an identical and reversible depolarization of the plasma membrane of acinar cells within 0.2 to 0.3 sec. They also increase the plasma membrane ion conductance, and provoke the electrical uncoupling of neighboring acinar cells. An analysis of the ionic dependence of these electrical events suggests that one of the responses to calcium movements is a reduction in the resistance for Na^+ followed by the sustained passive intracellular influx of Na^+ and Cl^-. This is accompanied by influx of water and allows the secretion by acinar cells of a plasma-like fluid. It is independent of emiocytosis but is required to dissolve the hydrolases. The electrical uncoupling mediated by Ca^{2+} movements suggests

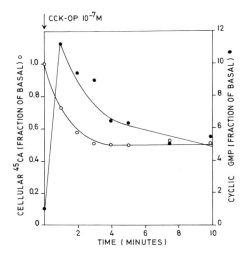

FIG. 4. Effects of OC-PZ on cellular ^{45}Ca and cyclic GMP in dispersed guinea pig pancreatic acinar cells. In cells preincubated for 40 min with 0.5 mM ^{45}Ca, basal cellular ^{45}Ca was determined, 10^{-7} M OC-PZ was added (↓), and cellular ^{45}Ca was determined during a 10-min incubation (○). In cells preincubated for 40 min without ^{45}Ca, samples were taken to determine basal cyclic GMP, 10^{-7} M OC-PZ was added (↓), and cyclic GMP was determined during a 10-min incubation (●). Results for cellular ^{45}Ca and cyclic GMP were expressed as the fraction of the amount determined in basal samples. (From ref. 25.)

a decreased contact of acinar cells at gap junctions. This should not be confused with a concurrent increase in the permeability of tight junctions between adjacent acinar cells that also takes place, and that may facilitate *in vivo* movements of fluids through intercellular spaces (J.J.H.H.M. de Pont, *personal communication*).

Finally, since a sharp decrease in amylase secretion in response to secretin is also observed in the presence of EGTA, and since secretin does not influence calcium fluxes, one may infer that calcium is not an exclusive "second" messenger of the first pathway, and may also act at other sites of the secretory process (Figs. 1 and 3).

THE CYCLIC GMP SYSTEM

A peak in pancreatic cyclic GMP levels is observed after the intravenous administration of pancreozymin and pilocarpine in rats (78). *In vitro,* secretagogues of the first group increase the concentration of cyclic GMP in dispersed acinar cells and pancreatic lobules (25,42,49,66). Increases are observed as fast as 15 to 30 sec, are maximal after 1 to 2 min, and return progressively to prestimulatory values whereas the hypersecretion persists. There is good agreement between the time-course of cyclic GMP levels and ^{45}Ca outflux (Fig. 4). There is also a good agreement between dose-response curves of peak cyclic GMP levels and ^{45}Ca outflux (Fig. 5). The increase in cyclic GMP is not attributable to a decrease in cellular calcium *per se,* since EGTA does not increase cellular cyclic GMP. The ionophore A-23187 can short-circuit the natural secretagogues and stimulate cyclic GMP levels even when dispersed acinar cells are incubated with EGTA (25). This suggests that, under conditions where calcium outflux only is possible, the sequence of the initial steps in the mechanism of action of the calcium ionophore and of pancreozymin, bombesin, or acetylcholine, is the mobilization of intracellular calcium followed by increased cyclic GMP (Fig. 3). The evidence collected in other tissues tempts one to suggest that the soluble and/or particulate forms of guanylate cyclase are activated by a rise in cytosolic calcium and the sequestration of membranous Ca^{2+}, respectively (85). The free fatty acids liberated during the phospholipid effect might also contribute to the stimulation of guanylate cyclase(s).

The transient elevation of the cyclic GMP concentration in response to pancreozymin, bombesin, and carbamylcholine might conceivably result from a sequential stimulation of guanylate cyclase and the soluble low Km cyclic GMP phosphodiesterase, the latter enzyme acting in the presence of cytosolic Ca^{2+} and the calcium-dependent regulator (CDR), also called calmodulin.

Thus, the role of cyclic GMP in stimulus-secretion coupling appears to be relatively well documented. In this respect, it is of interest to note that a twofold stimulation over basal amylase secretion from rat pancreatic fragments is evoked by two derivatives of cyclic GMP (8-bromo-cyclic GMP and N^2-monobutyryl cyclic GMP) when offered at a 1 mM concentration. This is not accompanied

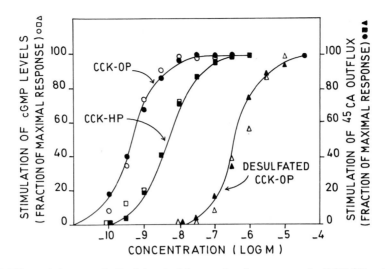

FIG. 5. Effect of three synthetic C-terminal fragments of pancreozymin (CCK-OP = OC-PZ) ● ○; C-terminal heptapeptide of pancreozymin = CCK-HP □ ■; and desulfated OC-PZ (CCK-OP) △ ▲ on A/ cyclic GMP peaks *(open symbols)* and B/ ^{45}Ca outflux *(closed symbols)* in dispersed guinea pig pancreatic acinar cells. **A:** Cells were preincubated for 5 min and cyclic GMP was determined after 2 min of incubation in the presence of the added peptides. (Results are expressed as the fraction of stimulation of cyclic GMP produced by 10^{-6} M CCK-OP.) **B:** To determine ^{45}Ca outflux from cells preincubated for 40 min with 0.5 mM ^{45}Ca; 5 mM EDTA was added with or without the indicated agent. ^{45}Ca outflux was calculated as the fraction of cellular radioactivity lost from the cells after 5 min. Results are expressed as the fraction of stimulation of ^{45}Ca outflux produced by 10^{-6} M CCK-OP. (From ref. 25.)

by a phospholipid effect [(11,40) and Calderon-Attas et al., *unpublished data*].

More than one molecular form of soluble cyclic nucleotide phosphodiesterase has been documented in mammalian tissues including the rat pancreas (50,79, 83,93) on the basis of kinetic and chromatographic evidence. The soluble supernatant fraction of rat pancreas homogenate subjected to gel filtration on Sephadex G-200 in the presence of EGTA reveals three peaks with cyclic nucleotide phosphodiesterase activity and one peak of CDR (Fig. 6 and ref. 93). The activity of the third phosphodiesterase fraction with cyclic GMP as substrate (Km_{app} of 2 μM) is specifically stimulated three- to fivefold by CDR in the presence of Ca^{2+}. CDR is a heat-stable acidic protein that possesses four divalent cation binding sites, two or three of them having a high affinity for Ca^{2+} (62, 95,96). On binding of Ca^{2+} there is a change in conformation of CDR and Ca^{2+}-CDR then associates with cyclic GMP phosphodiesterase to form the activated Ca^{2+}-CDR enzyme complex.

The average concentration of CDR in rat pancreas is 5 μM, i.e., a concentration similar to that in liver (93). Such a concentration is in a 30-fold excess over the concentration required for half-maximal activation of low Km_{app} cyclic GMP phosphodiesterase in the pancreatic cytosol and might account for a large proportion of the total cytosolic Ca^{2+} binding activity. Since CDR requires only micromolar levels of free Ca^{2+} to induce phosphodiesterase activation,

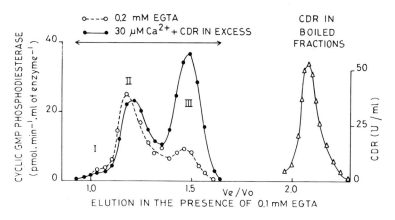

FIG. 6. Partial purification of three cyclic nucleotide phosphodiesterases and of CDR from rat pancreas by gel filtration on Sephadex G-200. Rat pancreases were homogenized in 10 mM Tris-HCl buffer (pH 7.5) containing 1 mM MgCl₂, 2 mM 2-mercaptoethanol, and 0.2 mM EGTA. The 105,000 × *g* supernatant was eluted by 20 mM Tris-HCl buffer (pH 7.5) containing 0.1 M NaCl, 1 mM MgCl₂, 0.1 mM EGTA, and 0.1 mM dithiothreitol. Phosphodiesterase activity was assayed using 0.4 μM cyclic GMP in the presence of 0.2 mM EGTA (○---○) or of 30 μM Ca²⁺ and a large excess of purified bovine pancreas CDR (●—●). Rat pancreas CDR (△—△) was monitored in aliquots of fractions that had been boiled for 1 min. (From refs. 92,93.)

variations in free Ca^{2+} concentration in the 10^{-7} M to 10^{-6} M range might regulate those mechanisms depending on the presence of CDR. CDR appears simply to enhance the sensitivity to Ca^{2+} and by so doing provides a link between Ca^{2+} and cyclic GMP metabolism in stimulus-secretion coupling, by returning the elevated cyclic GMP to the prestimulated level. Other roles for Ca^{2+}-CDR might include the phosphorylation of the actomyosin complex (Fig. 3). Bundles of actin filaments are present in pancreatic acinar cells (11,87). The existence of a tropomyosin-troponin-like system regulating the Ca^{2+} sensitivity of contractility and ATPase activity of pancreatic actomyosin (27) is not ruled out because tropomyosin-like material (36) and actomyosin (Vandermeers et al., *unpublished data*) have been separated from the pancreas.

The transient elevation in cyclic GMP is apparently sufficient to stimulate a labile cyclic GMP-dependent protein kinase (48,94), which allows the phosphorylation of proteins directly involved in stimulus-secretion coupling. This might include, among others, specific proteins in the membranes of zymogen granules (53,54,55), and the cytoskeleton.

PANCREOZYMIN RECEPTORS

Binding-Secretion Relationship for Pancreozymin Analogs

The binding of [³H] cerulein (a stable, biologically active labeled analog of pancreozymin; see Table 1) to semipurified rat pancreatic plasma membranes and to isolated rat pancreatic acinar cells is time- and temperature-dependent.

TABLE 1. *Amino acid sequences in three families of peptides stimulating pancreatic acinar cells*

	Bombesin	<Glu-Gln-Arg-Leu-Gly-Asn-Gln-Trp-Ala-Val-Gly-His-Leu-Met-NH$_2$

◆ PZ

$$\overset{\text{SO}_3\text{H}}{|}$$
R$_1{}^a$-Arg-Asp-Tyr-Met-Gly-Trp-Met-Asp-Phe-NH$_2$

● OC-PZ

$$\overset{\text{SO}_3\text{H}}{|}$$
Asp-Tyr-Met-Gly-Trp-Met-Asp-Phe-NH$_2$

△ Cerulein

$$\overset{\text{SO}_3\text{H}}{|}\quad\overset{\text{Nps}^c}{|}$$
<Glu^b-Gln-Asp-Tyr-Thr-Gly-Trp-Met-Asp-Phe-NH$_2$

▽ Nps^c-Cerulein

$$\overset{\text{SO}_3\text{H}}{|}$$
<Glu^b-Gln-Asp-Tyr-Thr-Gly-Trp-Met-Asp-Phe-NH$_2$

+ [Boc$^d{}_3$,Nle^8]Cerulein-(3–10)-octapeptide

$$\overset{\text{SO}_3\text{H}}{|}$$
Boc^d-Tyr-Thr-Gly-Trp-*Nle*-Asp-Phe-NH$_2$

0 [Tyr(SO$_3$H)^6]Cerulein-(6–10)-pentapeptide — Tyr-Trp-Met-Asp-Phe-NH$_2$

◇ Desulfated OC-PZ — Asp-Tyr-Met-Gly-Trp-Met-Asp-Phe-NH$_2$

□ Desulfated cerulein — <Glu^b-Gln-Asp-Tyr-Thr-Gly-Trp-Met-Asp-Phe-NH$_2$

■ Human gastrin I (desulfated) — R$_2{}^e$-Glu-Glu-Glu-Ala-Tyr-Gly-Trp-Met-Asp-Phe-NH$_2$

▽ Heptagastrin I(11–17)-heptapeptide(desulfated) — Ala-Tyr-Gly-Trp-Met-Asp-Phe-NH$_2$

▲ Pentagastrin — Boc-βAla-Trp-Met-Asp-Phe-NH$_2$

	1	2	3	4	5	6	7	8	9	10	11	12	13	14
VIP	His	Ser	Asp	Ala	Val	Phe	Thr	Asp	Asn	Tyr	Thr	Arg	Leu	Arg
Secretin	His	Ser	Asp	Gly	Thr	Phe	Thr	Ser	Glu	Leu	Ser	Arg	Leu	Arg

	15	16	17	18	19	20	21	22	23	24	25	26	27	28
VIP (end)	-Lys	Gln	Met	Ala	Val	Lys	Lys	Tyr	Leu	Asn	Ser	Ile	-Leu	Asn-NH$_2$
Secretin (end)	-Asp	Ser	Ala	Arg	Leu	Gln	Arg	Leu	Leu	Gln	Gly	Leu	Val-NH$_2$	

The abbreviated denomination and the symbol utilized in Fig. 7 are mentioned before each formulation.
[a] R$_1$ in PZ[33], (Lys-Ala-Pro-Ser-Gly-Arg-Val-Ser-Met-Ile-Lys-Asn-Leu-Gln-Ser-Leu-Asp-Pro-Ser-His-Arg-Ile-Ser-Asp-)
[b] <Glu, pyroglutamyl residue.
[c] Nps, O-nitrophenylsulfenyl.
[d] Boc, t-butoxycarbonyl.
[e] R$_2$ in human gastrin I (17). [<Glu-Gly-Pro-Trp-Leu-Glu-Glu-Glu-].

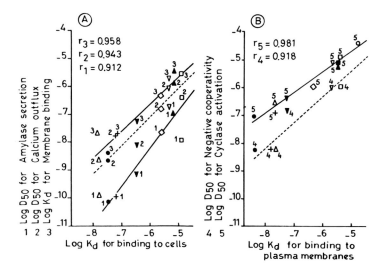

FIG. 7. Apparent affinities of various pancreozymin analogs for [³H] cerulein binding sites (Kd) and concentrations required for biological activities (D₅₀). The Kd for binding are derived from binding displacement experiments, considering that each analog was a competitive inhibitor of [³H] cerulein for binding sites. **A:** Correlation of the D₅₀ for amylase secretion (1), of D₅₀ for calcium outflux (2), and of Kd for binding to plasma membranes (3) to the Kd for binding to pancreatic acinar cells of cerulein and seven pancreozymin analogs. **B:** Correlation of the D₅₀ for negative cooperativity (4) and of the D₅₀ for adenylate cyclase activation (5) to the Kd for binding to pancreatic plasma membranes of cerulein and nine pancreozymin analogs. The linear correlation coefficient between each couple of parameters is indicated. Symbols are the same as those in Table 1. (From ref. 81.)

It is also saturable, specific, and reversible (24,31,81). In general, the biological potencies of pancreozymin analogs on a series of parameters (Table 1) are proportional to their capacity to inhibit the binding of [³H] cerulein (Fig. 7). The respective parameters include calcium outflux and cyclic GMP elevation in isolated acinar cells, adenylate cyclase activity in pancreatic plasma membranes, and amylase hypersecretion from pancreatic fragments. This can be interpreted as a reflection of the affinity with which the various peptides interact with hormone receptors. The conclusion is that the C-terminal tetrapeptide of pancreozymin is sufficient for binding and for evoking the entire spectrum of biological activities. The presence of a tyrosyl sulfated residue in position 7 (from the C-terminal end) increases the affinity for the peptide substantially, and is also necessary for full efficiency of the adenylate cyclase activation (Fig. 8).

Presence of Pancreozymin Two-State Receptors in Pancreatic Plasma Membranes and of Spare Receptors Linked to a Two-Effector System: Calcium Ionophore and Adenylate Cyclase

The curvilinearity of Scatchard plots of [³H] cerulein binding (24,31) indicates either the presence of more than one class of binding receptors and/or the

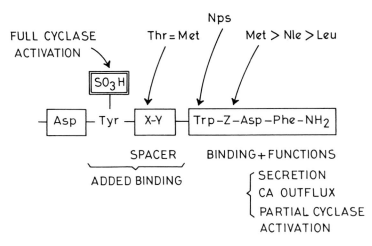

FIG. 8. Structural requirements for the binding and biological activities of pancreozymin-like peptides.

presence of only one class of receptors with peptide affinity dependent on the degree of site occupancy. Since an excess of unlabeled cerulein induces an increase of the dissociation rate of bound [3H] cerulein (31), the dissociation kinetics support experimentally the existence of negative cooperativity. These results are consistent with the presence of a single homogeneous class of receptors existing in two states, one showing high affinity-slow dissociation, and the other low affinity-fast dissociation. The relative proportions of sites in each state depend on the degree of occupancy of the binding sites by the peptide. Such a negative cooperativity might arise from site-to-site interactions inducing a conformational change of cerulein receptors (30). It might also derive from a variable affinity of mobile receptors for effector(s) at the surface of fluid and mosaic membranes (81). More specifically, the affinity for effector(s) would be greater if the receptor were occupied by pancreozymin-like peptides. Mathematical models are available that "explain" the effect of partial hormone agonists behaving as antagonists toward better agonists, the apparent existence of spare receptors, and negative cooperativity, with the assumption that reversible aggregation of components is taking place in plasma membranes (81).

The main question remains the determination of physiological relevance of binding data. Indeed, the concentrations of pancreozymin and cerulein analogs required for half-maximal amylase secretion are approximately ten times lower than the corresponding D_{50} for Ca^{2+} outflux and 30 to 300 times lower than the corresponding Kd_{app} for binding and Km_{app} for adenylate cyclase activation (Fig. 7). These variable degrees of correlation between the directly measured binding and physiological responses suggest the amplification of the signal by nonlinearly coupled steps between binding (stimulus) and secretion. At least two interpretations are conceivable, which are not self-exclusive:

(a) The tracer concentration of [^{3}H] cerulein used is high enough to cause a transition to a low-affinity state for pancreozymin receptors. Negative cooperativity may already be induced by a fractional occupation of the pancreozymin binding sites (30).

(b) The maximum secretory response observed at low receptor occupancy reflects the existence of numerous "spare" receptors on the pancreatic cell surface. The occupancy of a limited number of the available binding sites in the high affinity state would suffice for initiating Ca^{2+} movements and maximal secretion. At high pancreozymin concentration spare receptors in a low affinity state, if occupied by pancreozymin, could undergo a locking interaction with the catalytic subunit of adenylate cyclase. This would not generate any further increase in the secretory response, in addition to that resulting from the first effector system that controls Ca^{2+} movements. It is feasible that additional receptors could, on binding pancreozymin, associate themselves with pinocytotic, storage, and degrading sites.

To conclude, a high number of pancreozymin receptors allows negative cooperativity, i.e., high sensitivity to low concentrations of pancreozymin. This is of interest, since a paracrine secretion of pancreozymin cannot occur in the pancreas *in vivo,* which is at variance with the probable local secretion of pancreozymin-like peptides taking place at the surface of neurons in brain cortex. If classic hormone secretion is playing a major role in the pancreas, then a high sensitivity of target acinar cells to pancreozymin and the potentiation of this hormone by secretin might be of great importance (see below).

Switching-Off Mechanisms for Inactivating Signals from the Pancreozymin Family

The estimation of protein output in pancreatic juice collected from the Wirsung's duct by cannulation under duodenoscopy indicates that the half-life for the decay of the stimulatory effects of a bolus intravenous injection of pancreozymin *in vivo* is 80 sec on an average in man (76). Such a short duration may result from rapid extra- or intracellular hormone degradation, a secondary hormonal release from binding sites on target cells, and/or intracellular switch-off mechanisms.

In rats, the proportion of pancreozymin binding sites existing in the low-affinity state depends not only on the degree of site occupancy (negative cooperativity) but also on the intracellular concentration of guanyl nucleotides. The addition of an excess of unlabeled peptide results in a faster release of bound [^{3}H] cerulein from intact acinar cells (24) as compared with pancreatic plasma membranes (31); this may be due to the presence of intracellular GTP in the first preparation. Indeed, GTP, Gpp(NH)p, and GDP increase the rate of dissociation of pancreozymin-like peptides from pancreatic plasma membranes (25,35). Therefore, the control of pancreozymin binding may include the concentration

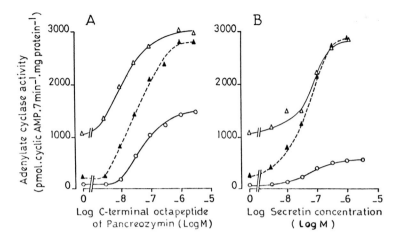

FIG. 9. Dose-response curves of adenylate cyclase activity stimulated by C-terminal octapeptide of pancreozymin **(A)** or secretin **(B)**. Rat pancreatic plasma membranes were incubated for 7 min at 37°C in the presence of increasing concentrations of peptide in the adenylate cyclase medium (—○—) or in the same medium enriched with 10 μM GTP (---▲---) or 10 μM Gpp(NH)p (—△—). (From ref. 89.)

of GTP at the internal face of plasma membranes. Since most of the *in vitro* effects of GTP are maximal at 10 μM (Fig. 9 and ref. 89), intracellular GTP compartmentation may be of importance in regulating GTP levels at proper sites during the activation and deactivation processes.

RECEPTORS FOR SECRETIN AND VASOACTIVE INTESTINAL PEPTIDE (VIP)

Secretin and vasoactive intestinal peptide (VIP), but not the parent hormone, glucagon, stimulate the secretion of hydrolases and increase the cyclic AMP concentration in rat and guinea pig pancreas. Secretin and VIP also activate adenylate cyclase in pancreatic plasma membranes (51,88). In addition, cyclic AMP derivatives moderately stimulate protein secretion from rat (3), mouse (52), and rabbit (73) pancreas, and theophylline potentiates the stimulatory effect of submaximal concentrations of secretin.

Existence of Two Functionally Distinct Classes of Receptors with Overlapping Affinities for Secretin and VIP in Dispersed Guinea Pig Pancreatic Acinar Cells

A Scatchard plot of ¹²⁵I-VIP binding at steady state is curvilinear with an upward concavity. The curve can be fitted into two straight lines. This does not indicate negative cooperativity since there is no acceleration of dissociation

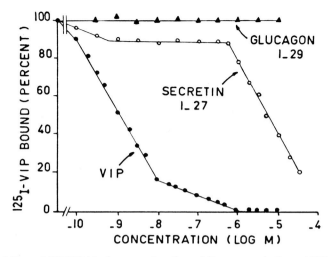

FIG. 10. Inhibition of ^{125}I-VIP binding as a function of the concentration of VIP (●), secretin (○), and glucagon (▲). Dispersed guinea pig acinar cells were incubated for 10 min at 37°C with 2.6×10^{-11} M ^{125}I-VIP plus the indicated peptides. Binding of ^{125}I-VIP was expressed as the percent of radioactivity specifically bound in the absence of nonradioactive peptide. (From ref. 23.)

of bound ^{125}I-VIP by unlabeled VIP (23). The data are consistent with the presence of two distinct classes of VIP-binding sites. It has been calculated that there are 9,000 high-affinity sites for VIP per cell and that half of these sites are occupied at a concentration of 7×10^{-10} M. In addition, 135,000 low affinity binding sites are 50% occupied at a VIP concentration of 8×10^{-8} M.

Secretin inhibits binding of ^{125}I-VIP to pancreatic acinar cells (Fig. 10). A low 10^{-9} M concentration of secretin produces a small but reproducible decrease in binding. At concentrations of secretin above 5×10^{-7} M, inhibition of ^{125}I-VIP binding is more pronounced. This indicates that the high-affinity VIP binding sites have a low affinity for secretin whereas those with a low affinity for VIP have a high affinity for secretin. The parent hormone glucagon does not inhibit binding of ^{125}I-VIP to pancreatic acinar cells (Fig. 10). Data based on the binding of ^{125}I-secretin and ^{125}I-VIP to cat pancreatic plasma membranes also suggest the coexistence of secretin-preferring and VIP-preferring receptors (67).

Structural Requirements for VIP and Secretin Binding to Dispersed Guinea Pig Acinar Cells

The difference between the relative affinities of VIP and secretin for the high-affinity VIP binding sites is primarily due to the N-terminal moiety of these hormones (23). The comparison of the amino acid sequences in the N-terminal moieties of VIP and secretin shows two differences in the charge distribution:

a negative charge in position 8 rather than in 9 and, more conspicuously, a reversal of charge in position 15 (Table 1). The C-terminal moiety of VIP and secretin contains five to six hydrophobic amino acids that might enhance the binding potency of both hormones through hydrophobic forces (5).

Structural Requirements for VIP- and Secretin-Stimulation of Cyclic AMP Levels in Dispersed Guinea Pig Acinar Cells

The most significant observation favoring the existence of two classes of VIP binding sites is the good agreement between the concentration producing half-maximal inhibition of ^{125}I-VIP binding by the acinar pancreatic cells and that provoking half-maximal stimulation of cyclic AMP levels in the same system (75). The interaction of VIP with its high-affinity receptors produces a three-fold increase in cyclic AMP, whereas the interaction of VIP with its low-affinity receptors produces a sixfold increase in cyclic AMP. In contrast with VIP, the dose-response curve showing a maximum tenfold increase in cyclic AMP concentration in response to secretin expresses interaction of this peptide with a single class of high-affinity secretin receptors, which occurs with half-maximal stimulation at a low 2×10^{-10} M secretin concentration. Given that the maximal adenylate cyclase activation of either VIP or secretin is obtained when the hormone considered is saturating all its corresponding high-affinity binding sites, it follows that the lower capacity of high-affinity VIP receptors as compared with high-affinity secretin receptors in inducing adenylate cyclase activation is due to a smaller number of receptors of the first class in guinea pig pancreatic acinar cells.

The intrinsic hormone activity of secretin and VIP appears to reside in the extended N-terminal part of the molecule, inasmuch as secretin (1–14) [but not secretin(5–27)] is capable of increasing cyclic AMP concentration (75). The preservation of the same His-Ser-Asp sequence in the amino-terminal part and of the hydrophobic phenylalanine residue in position 6 (Table 1) emphasizes the functional importance of this area in both hormones. The fact that activation is possible with secretin(1–14) indicates that the N-terminal moiety contains an amino acid sequence allowing minimal binding in addition to chemical excitation.

In conclusion, three functional regions may be distinguished in the structure of both VIP and secretin. The N-terminal extremity(1–4) portion is essential for adenylate cyclase activation. The next (5–14) portion is necessary for minimal binding. Specific binding ability of each hormone is enhanced by position 15 and the C-terminal hydrophobic portion of the molecule. Thus the entire amino acid sequence is of importance for optimal potency of both hormones.

INTERACTIONS OF SECRETIN AND VIP WITH PANCREOZYMIN

One of the major effects of secretin on pancreatic acinar cells might be to modulate the action of pancreozymin. The increase in the plasma levels of secretin and pancreozymin following a meal is induced by acid and by digested fat and protein acting on endocrine cells in the upper intestine. The genuine hormonal status of both peptides is rendered more evident when one considers their synergistic action on pancreatic acinar cells. Indeed, when pancreozymin and secretin are administered in combination, i.e., when a hormone that increases cyclic GMP and a hormone that increases cyclic AMP are used together, the resulting hypersecretion of hydrolases from rat pancreatic fragments and dispersed guinea pig pancreatic acinar cells is greater than that obtained with one hormone only (33,40). This potentiation is also demonstrated *in vivo* in man (99), rat (37), cat (7,97), and the dog (43). Whether VIP acts as a physiological hormonal agent able to interact with pancreozymin is doubtful. The relatively high concentration of VIP in nerves running through the exocrine tissue might, however, allow a local release of VIP from peptidergic neurons (see below). It remains to be seen whether the primary physiological action of secretin and VIP on the pancreatic acinar cells of a number of species is limited to the potentiation of pancreozymin-induced secretion or involves unexplored as yet biological responses.

At a molecular level, gastrointestinal hormone interactions are illustrated by the fact that three types of hormonal receptors (for secretin, VIP, and pancreozymin) can activate adenylate cyclase in rat pancreatic plasma membranes and that their coupling is competitive rather than additive (51,88). In the fragments of rat pancreas, however, only high concentrations of pancreozymin analogs promote a limited increase in cyclic AMP concentration. When pancreozymin is administered in pair with secretin, however, the rise in cyclic AMP in response to secretin is moderately but significantly inhibited (33). It is tempting to hypothesize that a rise in cytosolic calcium induced by pancreozymin in intact acinar cells might account for its inhibitory effects on adenylate cyclase.

ROLE OF GUANYL NUCLEOTIDES IN HORMONE-EFFECTOR COUPLING IN PANCREATIC PLASMA MEMBRANES

Guanyl Nucleotide Binding Sites Facilitate a Collision Coupling of Floating Hormone Receptors with Adenylate Cyclase

We know already that pancreatic plasma membranes have specific binding sites for pancreozymin, secretin, and VIP. Each gastrointestinal hormone stimulates a membrane adenylate cyclase system but these activations are not additive (88,89). Thus, distinct hormone receptors, when occupied, are coupled to a common class of catalytic units. This is consistent with the concept of uncoupled hormone receptors and catalytic units migrating independently in the plane of the plasma membrane but responding to gastrointestinal hormones with a reversible locking interaction that activates the cyclase (61,72). The HRE complex dissociates rapidly after activation so that R and E* are no longer coupled in the activated state E*. This model requires the existence of the free activated catalytic subunit E* and resembles the *collision coupling* mechanism recently developed by Tolkovsky and Levitzki (92) for turkey erythrocyte membranes.

As in other eukaryotic systems (59,61,63,70,72), hormones are positive activators of the enzyme activity stimulated by the two guanine nucleotides Gpp(NH)p and GTP. Gpp(NH)p is a stable analog of GTP where the terminal POP group of GTP is replaced by a PNP group that cannot be hydrolyzed by a GTPase. The hormone actions are limited to an acceleration of the binding and release of guanyl nucleotides to and from the guanyl nucleotide regulatory sites (17).

Hormone-Stimulated GTPase Activity as a Switch-Off Mechanism

Gpp(NH)p is a better activator than GTP and allows a quasi-irreversible activation of adenylate cyclase (Fig. 9). This finding raises the question of the role of GTP hydrolysis in the adenylate cyclase system (16,60). Experiments following the method of Cassel and Selinger (16,18,19) allow the detection of two GTPase activities in rat pancreatic plasma membranes: one, with high affinity for GTP (Km_{app} 0.1–0.2 μM) (57) and a second, with a lower affinity that corresponds to the NTPase activity (56). Dose-response curves for specific GTPase stimulation with hormones and hormone analogs are shown in Fig. 11. OC-PZ is the most potent activator: a stimulation occurs at a concentration as low as 10^{-10} M. [Boc^3, Nle^8] cerulein-(3-10)-octapeptide and cerulein, two full agonists of OC-PZ vis-à-vis adenylate cyclase [81], produce the same maximal effect on GTPase activity but their potency is approximately 10 times lower.

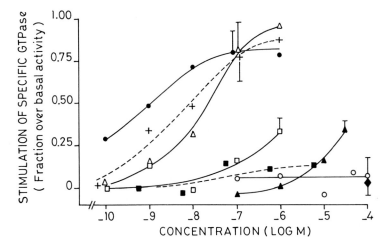

FIG. 11. Dose-effect relationship of hormones and hormone analogs on the specific GTPase activity. Pancreatic plasma membranes were incubated for 6 min at pH 7.4 with 0.25 or 30 μM GTP. Each increment over specific basal value is the mean of 2 to 5 separate experiments (*vertical bars* indicate SEM values in the latter case). ●—●, OC-PZ; +---+, [Boc^3,Nle^8]-cerulein-(3-10)-octapeptide; △—△, cerulein; □—□, secretin; ■--■, VIP; ▲—▲, pentagastrin; ○—○, [$Tyr(SO_3H)^6$] cerulein-(3-10)-octapeptide; ◆, carbamylcholine.

Pentagastrin, a weak and partial agonist of OC-PZ on pancreatic adenylate cyclase [81], produces a 30% increase in specific GTPase activity at the highest concentration tested. With secretin, lesser stimulation of specific GTPase is observed than that with OC-PZ, but it is likely that secretin, when tested under the conditions required for the assay of the specific GTPase, cannot saturate this enzyme with its substrate, precluding therefore maximal stimulation (Fig. 9 and ref. 89).

Regulatory Cycle of Pancreatic Adenylate Cyclase

Recent data obtained in our laboratory on the pancreas (89,90) corroborate those obtained on liver (72) and suggest that adenylate cyclase and hormone receptors are separate molecules, each associated with a distinct guanyl nucleotide regulatory site (G_2 and G_1, respectively). They imply that the OC-PZ stimulated GTPase activity is associated with the nucleotide site G_2 and can modulate the activity of adenylate cyclase. If data on turkey erythrocytes (20) apply to the pancreas, then gastrointestinal hormones accelerate the release of GDP from site G_1 which becomes available for GTP or Gpp(NH)p.

In this model oscillating between active (E^*) and inactive (E) states, the two functionally distinct guanyl nucleotide regulatory sites G_1 and G_2 act synergistically with the hormone. The first regulatory site G_1 is associated with hormone receptors. It not only allows the coupling with the effector system but also facilitiates the hormonal release. The second guanyl nucleotide regulatory site G_2 contains GDP in the inactive state. The coupling with the hormone-receptor-G_1 system accelerates the exchange between GDP and GTP at site G_2. This allows the activation of adenylate cyclase that does not require any more the permanent coupling of the hormone-receptor-G_1 system with the G_2-cyclase moiety of the complex. Furthermore, the G_2 site is endowed with a specific GTPase activity. The stimulation of the hydrolysis of GTP by this indirectly stimulated hormone activity leads to the occupation of G_2 by GDP, and subsequently provides a turning-off mechanism for hormone stimulation when fresh hormone and GTP are no longer available.

Thus, the regulatory cycle (14,15,17,18,19) of adenylate cyclase activation in pancreatic plasma membranes can be tentatively formulated as follows: (a) When G_2 is operating in the presence of Gpp(NH)p (Fig. 12A) the hormone permits a permanent activation of the cyclase since Gpp(NH)p cannot be hydrolyzed by the GTPase subunit. (b) In the simultaneous presence of GTP and hormone, GDP is rapidly released from G_2 and there results a higher accessibility of G_2 to GTP, so that the activation of adenylate cyclase is stimulated (Fig. 12). The GTPase in G_2 is also saturated by this local influx of substrate and works at maximal capacity. The constant arrival of GTP in G_2, replacing GDP, is, however, rapid enough to maintain the adenylate cyclase fully active. In this model, the indirect hormone stimulation of GTPase activity reflects an increased concentration of G_2 sites occupied by GTP.

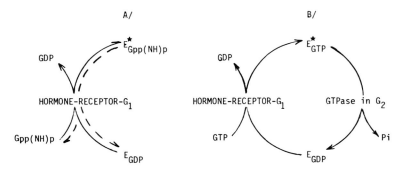

FIG. 12. The regulatory GTPase cycle of rat pancreatic adenylate cyclase. **A:** Persistent activation attained with hormone and Gpp(NH)p used in combination. The GTPase cannot hydrolyze the guanyl nucleotide. **B:** The GTPase acting on GTP is indirectly stimulated by the hormone. In this scheme the GTPase is part of site G_2 closely connected to E. Site G_1 operates in conjunction with the hormone-receptor complex.

CONCLUSIONS AND RELEVANCE OF THE PANCREATIC GASTROINTESTINAL HORMONE-RECEPTOR INTERACTIONS TO THE FIELD OF NEUROENDOCRINOLOGY PROJECTIONS FOR THE FUTURE

This chapter outlines a first group of secretagogues provoking a transient calcium outflux and cyclic GMP elevation in pancreatic acinar cells. This group includes carbamylcholine and bombesin, and also pancreozymin, which additionally activates adenylate cyclase in pancreatic plasma membranes. An increased turnover of phosphatidylinositols might contribute to the amplification of a signal implementing calcium movements and finally lead to protein phosphorylation and emiocytosis. A second group of secretagogues is represented by secretin and VIP, which elevate cyclic AMP levels in intact pancreatic cells with resulting activation of cyclic AMP-dependent protein kinase(s).

Methodological and conceptual advances have rapidly expanded our knowledge in the field of gut endocrinology during the last decade. Work in progress has established the existence in pancreatic acinar cells of specific receptors for bombesin (49), insulin (H. Billich et al.), and muscarinic cholinergic agents (G. Poirier et al.). I. Schulz recently made duct cells available in reasonable yield by counterflow centrifugation and has undertaken the direct exploration of their hormone-receptor interactions.

Much interest is presently evoked by finding pancreozymin, VIP, bombesin, and somatostatin both in the gut and in peripheral or central neurons (4). Gut brain peptides may act in any or all of three ways: endocrine, paracrine, or as neurotransmitters. Pancreozymin and secretin originating from mucosal endocrine cells are typically released into the general circulation, as evidenced by increased blood levels after a meal. Somatostatin, which is present in pancreatic D cells and inhibits the increase in pancreatic cyclic AMP caused by secretin (80) might act by paracrine mechanism, i.e., exert its action as a local tissue hormone. VIP and bombesin are distributed not only in endocrine cells but also, and perhaps predominantly, in peptidergic nerves including those running through the exocrine pancreas (8,9,58). Here, recent neuroendocrinology concepts suggest that VIP and bombesin are released as neurotransmitters from peptidergic neurons. In brain extracts gastrointestinal peptides are also actively investigated. In our laboratory, bioassays, including radioreceptor assays, of pancreatic acinar cells and pancreatic plasma membranes, have been utilized to explore the problem (82). In the rat brain, OC-PZ and a minor peak of biologically active rat pancreozymin have been identified [Deschodt-Lanckman et al., *unpublished data*] and the histochemical localization of pancreozymin-like peptides has been determined (45). VIP receptors are also present in the brain whose biochemical role appears to consist of the stimulation of adenylate cyclase (32,38,77).

ACKNOWLEDGMENTS

Experimental work from the author's laboratory reported in this chapter was aided by Grant 20,403 from the Fonds de la Recherche Scientifique Médicale (Belgium) and Grant RO-1AM-17010 from the National Institutes of Health (U.S.A.).

REFERENCES

1. Amsterdam, A., and Jamieson, J. D. (1974): Studies on dispersed pancreatic exocrine cells I and II. *J. Cell Biol.,* 63:1037–1056 and 1057–1073.
2. Argent, B. E., Case, R. M., and Scratchard, T. (1973): Amylase secretion by the perfused cat pancreas in relation to the secretion of calcium and other electrolytes and as influenced by the external ionic environment. *J. Physiol. (Lond.),* 230:575–593.
3. Bauduin, H., Rochus, L., Vincent, D., and Dumont, J. E. (1971): Role of cyclic 3′,5′-AMP in the action of physiological secretagogues on the metabolism of rat pancreas in vitro. *Biochim. Biophys. Acta,* 252:171–183.
4. Bloom, S. R. (Ed.) (1978): *Gut Hormones,* 664 pp. Churchill Livingstone, Edinburgh.
5. Bodanszky, M., Klausner, Y. S., and Said, S. I. (1973): Biological activities of synthetic peptides corresponding to fragments of and to the entire sequence of the vasoactive intestinal peptide. *Proc. Natl. Acad. Sci. USA,* 70:382–384.
6. Bonfils, S., Fromageot, P., and Rosselin, G. (Eds.) (1977): *Hormonal Receptors in Digestive Physiology: Inserm Symposium 3,* 514 pp. North-Holland Publishing Company, Amsterdam.
7. Brown, J. C., Harper, A. A., and Scatchard, T. (1967): Potentiation of secretin stimulation of the pancreas. *J. Physiol. (Lond.),* 190:519–530.
8. Bryant, M. G., Bloom, S. R., Polak, J. M., Albuquerque, R. H., Modlin, I., and Pearse, A. G. E. (1976): Possible dual role for vasoactive intestinal peptide as gastrointestinal hormone and neurotransmitter substance. *Lancet,* i:991–993.
9. Buffa, R., Capella, C., Solcia, E., Frigerio, B., and Said, S. I. (1977): Vasoactive intestinal peptide (VIP) cells in the pancreas and gastrointestinal mucosa. An immunohistochemical and ultrastructural study. *Histochemistry,* 50:217–227.
10. Calderon, P., Furnelle, J., and Christophe, J. (1977): Accelerated synthesis de novo of phosphati-

dylinositols in the rat exocrine pancreas is not necessarily associated with enzymatic hypersecretion. Secretin and vasoactive intestinal peptide (VIP) stimulate amylase output *in vitro* without favouring this synthesis. *Arch. Int. Physiol. Biochem.*, 85:388–389.

11. Case, M. (1978): Synthesis, intracellular transport, and discharge of exportable proteins in the pancreatic acinar cell and other cells. *Biol. Rev.*, 53:211–354.

12. Case, R. M., and Clausen, T. (1973): The relationship between calcium exchange and enzyme secretion in the isolated rat pancreas. *J. Physiol. (Lond.)*, 235:75–102.

13. Case, R. M., and Goebell, H. (Eds.) (1976): *Stimulus-Secretion Coupling in the Gastrointestinal Tract,* 437 pp. MTP Press, Lancaster.

14. Cassel, D., Levkovitz, H., and Selinger, Z. (1977): The regulatory GTPase cycle of turkey erythrocyte adenylate cyclase. *J. Cycl. Nucl. Res.*, 3:393–406.

15. Cassel, D., and Pfeuffer, T. (1978): Mechanism of cholera toxin action: Covalent modification of the guanyl nucleotide-binding protein of the adenylate cyclase system. *Proc. Natl. Acad. Sci. USA*, 75:2669–2673.

16. Cassel, D., and Selinger, Z. (1976): Catecholamine-stimulated GTPase activity in turkey erythrocyte membranes. *Biochim. Biophys. Acta,* 452:538–551.

17. Cassel, D., and Selinger, Z. (1977): Catecholamine-induced release of [³H]-Gpp(NH)p from turkey eythrocyte adenylate cyclase. *J. Cycl. Nucl. Res.*, 3:11–12.

18. Cassel, D., and Selinger, Z. (1977): Activation of turkey erythrocyte adenylate cyclase and blocking of the catecholamine-stimulated GTPase by guanosine 5'-(γ-thio)triphosphate. *Biochem. Biophys. Res. Commun.*, 77:868–873.

19. Cassel, D., and Selinger, Z. (1977): Mechanism of adenylate cyclase activation by cholera toxin: Inhibition of GTP hydrolysis at the regulatory site. *Proc. Natl. Acad. Sci. USA*, 74:3307–3311.

20. Cassel, D., and Selinger, Z. (1978): Mechanism of adenylate cyclase activation through the β-adrenergic receptor: Catecholamine-induced displacement of bound GDP by GTP. *Proc. Natl. Acad. Sci. USA*, 75:4155–4159.

21. Ceccarelli, B., Meldolesi, J., and Clementi, F. (Eds.) (1974): *Cytopharmacology of Secretion, Advances in Cytopharmacology, Vol. 2,* 388 pp. Raven Press, New York.

22. Cenatiempo, Y., Mangeat, P., and Marchis-Mouren, G. (1975): Purification and properties of cyclic AMP dependent and independent protein kinases from rat pancreas. *Biochimie,* 57:865–873.

23. Christophe, J. P., Conlon, T. P., and Gardner, J. D. (1976): Interaction of porcine vasoactive intestinal peptide with dispersed pancreatic acinar cells from the guinea pig: Binding of radioiodinated peptide. *J. Biol. Chem.*, 251:4629–4634.

24. Christophe, J., De Neef, P., Deschodt-Lanckman, M., and Robberecht, P. (1978): The interaction of caerulein with the rat pancreas. II. Specific binding of [³H] caerulein on dispersed acinar cells. *Eur. J. Biochem.*, 91:31–38.

25. Christophe, J. P., Frandsen, E. K., Conlon, T. P., Krishna, G., and Gardner, J. D. (1976): Action of cholecystokinin, cholinergic agents and A-32187 on accumulation of guanosine 3':5'-monophosphate in dispersed guinea pig pancreatic acinar cells. *J. Biol. Chem.*, 251:4640–4645.

26. Christophe, J., Robberecht, P., and Deschodt-Lanckman, M. (1977): Hormone-receptor interactions in the gastrointestinal tract: The pancreatic acinar cell as a model target in gut endocrinology. In: *Progress in Gastroenterology,* edited by G. B. J. Glass, pp. 241–284. Grune & Stratton, New York.

27. Clarke, M., and Spudich, J. A. (1977): Nonmuscle contractile proteins: The role of actin and myosin in cell motility and shape determination. *Ann. Rev. Biochem.*, 46:797–822.

28. Clemente, F., and Meldolesi, J. (1975): Calcium and pancreatic secretion. I. Distribution of calcium and magnesium in the acinar cells of the guinea pig pancreas. *J. Cell Biol.*, 65:88–102.

29. De Camilli, P., and Meldolesi, J. (1974): Subcellular distribution of the PI effect in the pancreas of the guinea pig. *Life Sci.*, 15:711–721.

30. De Meyts, P., Bianco, A. R., and Roth, J. (1976): Site-site interactions among insulin receptors. Characterization of the negative cooperativity. *J. Biol. Chem.*, 251:1877–1888.

31. Deschodt-Lanckman, M., Robberecht, P., Camus, J., and Christophe, J. (1978): The interaction of caerulein with the rat pancreas. I. Specific binding of [³H] caerulein on plasma membranes and evidence for negative cooperativity. *Eur. J. Biochem.*, 91:21–29.

32. Deschodt-Lanckman, M., Robberecht, P., and Christophe, J. (1977): Characterization of VIP-sensitive adenylate cyclase in guinea pig brain. *FEBS Lett.*, 83:76–80.

33. Deschodt-Lanckman, M., Robberecht, P., De Neef, P., Labrie, F., and Christophe, J. (1975):

In vitro interactions of gastrointestinal hormones on cyclic adenosine 3':5':monophosphate levels and amylase output in the rat pancreas. *Gastroenterology,* 68:318–325.

34. Deschodt-Lanckman, M., Robberecht, P., De Neef, P., Lammens, M., and Christophe, J. (1976): *In vitro* action of bombesin and bombesin-like peptides on amylase secretion, calcium outflux and adenylate cyclase activity in the rat pancreas. A comparison with other secretagogues. *J. Clin. Invest.,* 58:891–898.

35. Deschodt-Lanckman, M., Svoboda, M., Camus, J. C., and Robberecht, P. (1977): Regulation of the dissociation of [³H] caerulein from its pancreatic receptors: evidence for negative cooperativity. In: *Hormonal Receptors in Digestive Tract Physiology,* edited by S. Bonfils, P. Fromageot, and G. Rosselin, pp. 325–326. Elsevier/North-Holland, Amsterdam.

36. Fine, R. E., and Blitz, A. L. (1975): A chemical comparison of tropomyosins from muscle and non-muscle tissues. *J. Mol. Biol.,* 95:447–454.

37. Fölsch, U. R., and Wormsley, K. G. (1973): Pancreatic enzyme response to secretin and cholecystokinin-pancreozymin in the rat. *J. Physiol. (Lond.),* 234:79–94.

38. Fuxe, K., Hökfelt, T., Said, S., and Mutt, V. (1977): Vasoactive intestinal polypeptide and the nervous system: immunochemical evidence for localisation in central and peripheral neurons, particularly intracortical neurons of the cerebral cortex. *Neurosci. Lett.,* 5:241–246.

39. Gardner, J. D., Conlon, T. P., Klaeveman, H. L., Adams, T. D., and Ondetti, M. A. (1975): Action of cholecystokinin and cholinergic agents on calcium transport in isolated pancreatic acinar cells. *J. Clin. Invest.,* 56:366–375.

40. Gardner, J. D., and Jackson, M. J. (1977): Regulation of amylase release from dispersed pancreatic acinar cells. *J. Physiol. (Lond.),* 270:439–454.

41. Glass, G. B. J. (Ed.) (1977): *Progress in Gastroenterology, Vol. III,* 1052 pp. Grune & Stratton, New York.

42. Haymovits, A., and Scheele, G. A. (1976): Cellular cyclic nucleotides and enzyme secretion in the pancreatic acinar cells. *Proc. Natl. Acad. Sci. USA,* 73:156–160.

43. Henriksen, F. W., and Worning, H. (1967): The interaction of secretin and pancreozymin on the external pancreatic secretion in dogs. *Acta Physiol. Scand.,* 70:241–249.

44. Hokin-Neaverson, M., Sadeghian, K., and Majumda, A. L. (1975): Inositol is the water-soluble product of acetylcholine-stimulated breakdown of phosphatidylinositol in mouse pancreas. *Biochem. Biophys. Res. Commun.,* 67:1537–1544.

45. Innis, R. B., Corrêa, F. M. A., Uhl, G. R., Schneider, B., and Snyder, S. H. (1979): Cholecystokinin octapeptide-like immunoreactivity: histochemical localization in rat brain. *Proc. Natl. Acad. Sci. USA,* 76:521–525.

46. Iwatsuki, N., and Petersen, O. H. (1977): Pancreatic acinar cells: The acetylcholine equilibrium potential and its ionic dependency. *J. Physiol. (Lond.),* 269:735–751.

47. Iwatsuki, N., and Petersen, O. H. (1978): *In vitro* action of bombesin on amylase secretion, membrane potential and membrane resistance in rat and mouse pancreatic acinar cells. A comparison with other secretagogues. *J. Clin. Invest.,* 61:41–46.

48. Jensen, R. T., and Gardner, J. D. (1978): Cyclic nucleotide-dependent protein kinase activity in acinar cells from guinea pig pancreas. *Gastroenterology,* 75:806–817.

49. Jensen, R. T., Moody, T., Pert, C., Rivier, J. E., and Gardner, J. D. (1978): Interaction of bombesin and litorin with specific membrane receptors on pancreatic acinar cells. *Proc. Natl. Acad. Sci. USA,* 75:6139–6143.

50. Kakuichi, S., Yamazaki, R., Teshima, Y., Uenishi, K., and Miyamoto, E. (1975): Multiple cyclic nucleotide phosphodiesterase activities from rat tissues and occurrence of a calcium-plus-magnesium-ion-dependent phosphodiesterase and its protein activator. *Biochem. J.,* 146:109–120.

51. Kempen, H. J. M., De Pont, J. J. H. H. M., and Bonting, S. L. (1974): Rat pancreas adenylate cyclase. II. Inactivation and protection of its hormone receptor sites. *Biochem. Biophys. Acta,* 370:573–584.

52. Kulka, R. G., and Sternlicht, E. (1968): Enzyme secretion in mouse pancreas mediated by adenosine 3'-5'-cyclic phosphate and inhibited by adenosine-3'-phosphate. *Proc. Natl. Acad. Sci. USA,* 61:1123–1128.

53. Lambert, M., Camus, J., and Christophe, J. (1973): Pancreozymin and caerulein stimulate *in vitro* protein phosphorylation in the rat pancreas. *Biochem. Biophys. Res. Commun.,* 52:935–942.

54. Lambert, M., Camus, J., and Christophe, J. (1974): Phosphorylation of protein components of isolated zymogen granule membranes from the rat pancreas. *FEBS Lett.,* 49:228–232.

55. Lambert, M., Camus, J., and Christophe, J. (1975): Phosphorylation in vitro of proteins in the rat pancreas and parotids of rats: Effects of hormonal secretagogues and cyclic nucleotides. *Biochem. Pharmacol.*, 24:1755–1758.
56. Lambert, M., and Christophe, J. (1978): Characterization of (Mg,Ca)-ATPase activity in rat pancreatic plasma membranes. *Eur. J. Biochem.*, 91:485–492.
57. Lambert, M., Svoboda, M., and Christophe, J. (1979): Hormone-stimulated GTPase activity in rat pancreatic plasma membranes. *FEBS Lett.*, 99:303–307.
58. Larsson, L. I., Fahrenkrug, J., Schaffalitzky de Muckadell, O., Sundler, F., Håkanson, R., and Rehfeld, J. F. (1976): Localization of vasoactive intestinal polypeptide (VIP) to central and peripheral neurons. *Proc. Natl. Acad. Sci. USA*, 73:3197–3200.
59. Lefkowitz, R. J., and Caron, M. G. (1975): Characteristics of 5'-guanylyl imidodiphosphate-activated adenylate cyclase. *J. Biol. Chem.*, 250:4418–4422.
60. Levinson, S. L., and Blume, A. J. (1977): Altered guanine nucleotide hydrolysis as basis for increased adenylate cyclase activity after cholera toxin treatment. *J. Biol. Chem.*, 252:3766–3774.
61. Levitzki, A. (1977): The role of GTP in the activation of adenylate cyclase. *Biochem. Biophys. Res. Commun.*, 74:1154–1159.
62. Lin, Y. M., Liu, Y. P., and Cheung, W. Y. (1974): Cyclic 3':5'-nucleotide phosphodiesterase. Purification, characterization, and active form of the protein activator from bovine brain. *J. Biol. Chem.*, 249:4943–4954.
63. Londos, C., Salomon, Y., Lin, M. C., Harwood, J. P., Schramm, M., Wolff, J., and Rodbell, M. (1974): 5'-Guanylylimidodiphosphate, a potent activator of adenylate systems in eukaryotic cells. *Proc. Natl. Acad. Sci. USA*, 71:3087–3090.
64. Mangeat, P. H., Chahinian, H., and Marchis-Mouren, G. J. (1978): Characterization of the cyclic AMP-dependent protein kinase from rat pancreas, further purification of the catalytic subunit, substrate specificity, effect of the pancreatic heat stable inhibitor. *Biochimie*, 60:777–785.
65. Matthews, E. K., Petersen, O. H., and Williams, J. A. (1973): Pancreatic acinar cells: Acetylcholine-induced membrane depolarization, calcium efflux and amylase release. *J. Physiol. (Lond.)*, 234:689–701.
66. May, R. J., Conlon, T. P., Erspamer, V., and Gardner, J. D. (1978): Actions of peptides isolated from amphibian skin on pancreatic acinar cells. *Am. J. Physiol.*, 235:E112–E118.
67. Milutinovic, S., Schulz, I., and Rosselin, G. (1976): The interaction of secretin with pancreatic membranes. *Biochim. Biophys. Acta*, 436:113–127.
68. Petersen, O. H. (1976): Electrophysiology of mammalian gland cells. *Physiol. Rev.*, 56:535–577.
69. Petersen, O. H., and Ueda, N. (1977): Secretion of fluid and amylase in the perfused rat pancreas. *J. Physiol.*, 264:819–835.
70. Pfeuffer, T., and Helmreich, E. J. M. (1975): Activation of pigeon erythrocyte membrane adenylate cyclase by guanylnucleotide analogues and separation of a nucleotide binding protein. *J. Biol. Chem.*, 250:867–876.
71. Poulsen, J. H., and Williams, J. A. (1977): Effects of the calcium ionophore A 23187 on pancreatic acinar cell membrane potentials and amylase release. *J. Physiol. (Lond.)*, 264:323–339.
72. Rendell, M. S., Rodbell, M., and Berman, M. (1977): Activation of hepatic adenylate cyclase by guanyl nucleotides. *J. Biol. Chem.*, 252:7909–7912.
73. Ridderstap, A. S., and Bonting, S. L. (1969): Cyclic AMP and enzyme secretion by the isolated rabbit pancreas. *Pflüger's Arch. Ges. Physiol.*, 313:62–70.
74. Robberecht, P., and Christophe, J. (1971): Secretion of hydrolases by perfused fragments of rat pancreas: Effect of calcium. *Am. J. Physiol.*, 220:911–917.
75. Robberecht, P., Conlon, T. P., and Gardner, J. D. (1976): Interaction of porcine vasoactive intestinal peptide with dispersed pancreatic acinar cells from the guinea pig: Structural requirements for effects of vasoactive intestinal peptide and secretin on cellular adenosine 3':5'-monophosphate. *J. Biol. Chem.*, 251:4635–4639.
76. Robberecht, P., Cremer, M., Vandermeers, A., Vandermeers-Piret, M. C., Cotton, P., De Neef, P., and Christophe, J. (1975): Pancreatic secretion of total protein and of three hydrolases collected in healthy subjects via duodenoscopic cannulation. *Gastroenterology*, 69:374–379.
77. Robberecht, P., De Neef, P., Lammens, M., Deschodt-Lanckman, M., and Christophe, J. (1978):

Specific binding of vasoactive intestinal peptide to brain membranes from the guinea pig. *Eur. J. Biochem.,* 90:147–154.

78. Robberecht, P., Deschodt-Lanckman, M., De Neef, P., Borgeat, P., and Christophe, J. (1974): *In vivo* effects of pancreozymin, secretin, vasoactive intestinal polypeptide and pilocarpine on the level of cyclic AMP and cyclic GMP in the rat pancreas. *FEBS Lett.,* 43:139–143.
79. Robberecht, P., Deschodt-Lanckman, M., De Neef, P., and Christophe, J. (1974): Hydrolysis of cyclic adenosine and guanosine 3',5'-monophosphates by rat pancreas. *Eur. J. Biochem.,* 41:585–591.
80. Robberecht, P., Deschodt-Lanckman, M., De Neef, P., and Christophe, J. (1975): Effects of somatostatin on pancreatic exocrine function. *Biochem. Biophys. Res. Commun.,* 67:315–323.
81. Robberecht, P., Deschodt-Lanckman, M., Morgat, J.-L., and Christophe, J. (1978): The interaction of caerulein with the rat pancreas. III. Structural requirements for *in vitro* binding of caerulein-like peptides and its relationship to increased calcium outflux, adenylate cyclase activation, and secretion. *Eur. J. Biochem.,* 91:39–48.
82. Robberecht, P., Deschodt-Lanckman, M., and Vanderhaeghen, J. J. (1978): Demonstration of biological activity of brain gastrin-like peptidic material in the human: Its relationship with the COOH-terminal octapeptide of cholecystokinin. *Proc. Natl. Acad. Sci. USA,* 75:524–528.
83. Rutten, W. J., Schoot, B. M., de Pont, J. J. H. H. M., and Bonting, S. L. (1973): Adenosine 3',5'-monophosphate phosphodiesterase in rat pancreas. *Biochim. Biophys. Acta,* 315:384–393.
84. Schreurs, V. V. A. M., Swarts, H. G. P., de Pont, J. J. H. H. M., and Bonting S. L. (1975): Role of calcium in exocrine pancreatic secretion. I. Calcium movements in the rabbit pancreas. *Biochim. Biophys. Acta,* 404:257–267.
85. Schultz, G., Hardman, J. G., Schultz, K., Baird, C. E., and Sutherland, E. W. (1973): The importance of calcium ions for the regulation of guanosine 3':5'-cyclic monophosphate levels. *Proc. Natl. Acad. Sci. USA,* 70:3889–3893.
86. Shelby, H. T., Gross, L. P., Lichty, P., and Gardner, J. D. (1976): Action of cholecystokinin and cholinergic agents on membrane-bound calcium in dispersed pancreatic acinar cells. *J. Clin. Invest.,* 58:1482–1493.
87. Stock, C., Launay, J. F., and Bauduin, H. (1977): About the implication of the microfilamentous and microtubular system in the secretory cycle of the pancreatic acinar cell. In: *Hormonal Receptors in Digestive Tract Physiology,* edited by S. Bonfils, P. Fromageot, and G. Rosselin, pp. 199. North-Holland, Amsterdam.
88. Svoboda, M., Robberecht, P., Camus, J., Deschodt-Lanckman, M., and Christophe, J. (1976): Subcellular distribution and response to gastrointestinal hormones of adenylate cyclase in the rat pancreas. Partial purification of a stable plasma membrane preparation. *Eur. J. Biochem.,* 69:185–193.
89. Svoboda, M., Robberecht, P., Camus, J., Deschodt-Lanckman, M., and Christophe, J. (1978): Association of binding sites for guanine nucleotides with adenylate cyclase activation in rat pancreatic plasma membranes. Interaction of gastrointestinal hormones. *Eur. J. Biochem.,* 83:287–297.
90. Svoboda, M., Robberecht, P., and Christophe, J. (1978): Deactivation of persistently activated pancreatic adenylate cyclase. Evidence of uncoupling of hormone receptors and enzyme effector in the persistently activated state, and of the presence of two guanyl nucleotide regulatory sites. *FEBS Lett.,* 92:351–356.
91. Thompson, J. C. (Ed.) (1975): *Symposium Gastrointestinal Hormones,* University of Texas Press, 666 pp. Austin and London.
92. Tolkovsky, A., and Levitzki, A. (1978): Mode of coupling between the β-adrenergic receptor and adenylate cyclase in turkey erythrocytes. *Biochemistry,* 17:3795–3810.
93. Vandermeers, A., Vandermeers-Piret, M. C., Rathé, J., Kutzner, R., Delforge, A., and Christophe, J. (1977): A calcium-dependent protein activator of guanosine 3':5'-monophosphate phosphodiesterase in bovine and rat pancreas. Isolation, properties and levels *in vivo. Eur. J. Biochem.,* 81:379–386.
94. Van Leemput-Coutrez, M., Camus, J., and Christophe, J. (1973): Cyclic nucleotide-dependent protein kinases of the rat pancreas. *Biochem. Biophys. Res. Commun.,* 54:182–190.
95. Wang, J. H., Teo, T. S., Ho, H. C., and Stevens, F. C. (1975): Bovine heart protein activator of cyclic nucleotide phosphodiesterase. *Adv. Cycl. Nucl. Res.,* 5:179–194.
96. Watterson, D. M., Harrelson, W. G., Keller, P. M., Sharief, F., and Vanaman, T. C. (1976): Structural similarities between the Ca^{2+}-dependent regulatory proteins of 3':5'-cyclic nucleotide phosphodiesterase and actomyosin ATPase. *J. Biol. Chem.,* 251:4501–4513.

97. Way, L. W., and Grossman, M. I. (1970): Pancreatic stimulation by duodenal acid and exogenous hormones in conscious cats. *Am. J. Physiol.,* 219:449–454.
98. Webster, P. D. III, Black, O., Jr., Mainz, D. L., and Singh, M. (1977): Pancreatic acinar cell metabolism and function. *Gastroenterology,* 73:1434–1449.
99. Wormsley, K. G. (1969): A comparison of the response to secretin, pancreozymin and a combination of these hormones in man. *Scand. J. Gastroenterol.,* 4:413–417.

Gastrointestinal Hormones, edited by
George B. Jerzy Glass.
Raven Press, New York © 1980.

Chapter 21

Hormone Receptor Control of Electrolyte Secretion in the Gastrointestinal Tract

Miguel J. M. Lewin

Unité de Recherches de Gastroentérologie, INSERM U.10, Hopital Bichat, 75877 Paris Cedex 18, France

INTRODUCTION

This chapter summarizes the recent developments relating to the characterization of hormone receptors in the stomach and the intestine. It concentrates only on those receptors that are assumed to be involved in the control of ion (and water) transport. Emphasis is placed on biochemical studies providing evidence for the existence of these receptors in the gastrointestinal tract, the documentation of their structural requirement, the nature of their intracellular effectors, and their possible interrelationship. Other information on hormonal control of gastrointestinal ion transport is found in various chapters of this volume. Gastrin and histamine receptors in the gastric mucosa have been recently reviewed (87).

GENERAL MECHANICS AND CELLULAR ASPECTS
OF TRANSPORT CONTROL

Cellular Sites of Electrolyte Transport

In the stomach, the so-called "acid secretion" is strongly suggested to originate in a single cell type, the parietal cell, which is highly specialized in mammals (40,57,61). This does not imply, however, that the parietal cell is necessarily the only common target for all stimuli that act on gastric acid secretion, since some stimuli may well exert their effects by causing the release of second mediators from other cell types. Thus, it has been suggested rather early that gastrin might indirectly stimulate gastric secretion via histamine release from storage cells (28). This still remains a moot question (87).

In contrast with the situation in the stomach, the nature of the cell(s) responsible for electrolyte transport in the intestine is not precisely known. From the data presently available it seems not even possible to answer the question as to whether or not there are separate cells for absorption and secretion. Circumstantial evidence has been presented for a primary role of the crypt cells of the gland of Lieberkühn in intestinal electrolyte secretion. However, the possibility that mature villous cells also participate in the secretion cannot be ruled out. The conversion from a secretory to an absorptive capacity during the course of cell maturation has been suggested (42). In this respect uncertainties remain regarding the final target(s) of hormonal stimuli acting on ion transport in the intestine. The possibility can always be raised that the observed secretory response in the intestine is the net result of two processes associated with two different cell types.

Membrane Transport Mechanisms

The membrane mechanisms responsible for ion transport by the gastric and intestinal epithelium have been recently reviewed (42,132).

In the stomach, electrolyte secretion mainly consists of concentrated HCl. This is a highly energetic process that involves a specific H^+-K^+ dependent ATPase and, possibly, an ATP-driven Cl^- transport mechanism (130,144). At the serosal side, Cl^- entry into and OH^- exit off the parietal cell are mediated by a neutral $Cl^- \leftrightarrows HCO_3^-$ interchange; a neutral NaCl symport is also suggested that is indirectly coupled to a Na^+-K^+ dependent ATPase (36,39).

In contrast with stomach, the primary function of intestine is absorption, not secretion. The occurrence of a net hydroelectrolytic secretion is, however, evident under pathological conditions featuring severe diarrhea (113). Accordingly, it is now generally accepted that the intestine is capable, under "normal" physiological conditions, of active secretion of water and salt, mainly NaCl and HCO_3^-. The importance of this secretion and its functional significance have been discussed in a previous review (96). Intestinal secretion (as well as intestinal absorption) of electrolytes is primarily dependent on the activity of a Na^+-K^+ dependent ATPase that regulates the overall transepithelial transport of Na^+. In addition, this has been suggested to involve a neutral NaCl symport and a $Cl^- \leftrightarrows HCO_3^-$ interchange similar in nature to that occurring in the stomach. Furthermore, it would involve independent Cl^- and Na^+ channels permitting diffusional movements of these ions across the basal membrane of the enterocytes (41,42,43,56,96,114,139).

The fundic gastric epithelium has been shown to be of a "tight" type with only minor paracellular route for ions and water movements (132). In contrast, intestine has a "leaky" epithelium that offers paracellular shunt pathways of low resistance across the intercellular junctions. This makes it possible for an electrochemical feedback to operate between the intestinal serosal and mucosal layers (positively and negatively charged, respectively) that favor partial reentry into the intestinal lumen of absorbed Na^+ with accompanying water (41). The presence of a low resistance paracellular pathway in the intestine may furthermore account for the occurrence of a large filtration flow across the epithelium in response to changes in plasma colloid oncotic pressure and hydrostatic pressure in the capillary bed (96). Thus, intestinal secretion and intestinal absorption appear to be two closely linked processes. The net secretion may result from inhibition of absorption mechanisms as well as from stimulation of secretion mechanisms.

These observations may have interesting implications regarding the intracellular mediators of hormone activation of gastrointestinal ion transport. In both the stomach and the intestine, ATP appears to be the necessary substrate for the ATPase- and the ATP-driven ion pumps. ATP may therefore be considered as a final common mediator for the stimuli coupling metabolic energy to the transport processes. Since gastrointestinal ion transport also involves passive interchange and diffusion processes, it may be assumed to be controlled further by factors affecting membrane permeability. Among these factors, Ca^{2+} has been suggested to have a special importance (35,68,120,131). This cation also participates in the maintenance of the intercellular junction (94) that was just suggested to play a prominent role in paracellular transport by the intestine. Furthermore, Ca^{2+} has been implicated in the membrane fusion processes that have been claimed to occur, upon stimulation of gastric acid secretion, in order to make possible the incorporation of the H^+-pump into the apical membrane of the parietal cell (40,57,61,131).

The Peptide Hormone Receptor Concept: Present-Day Status

All gastrointestinal hormones identified so far are peptidic in nature. They are, therefore, suggested to produce their effects, as other peptide hormones, by activating appropriate receptors located on the basal membrane of the secretory cells. According to current evidence, peptide hormone receptor interaction is assumed to successively involve (a) the selective recognition of the hormone by the receptor and their mutual binding, (b) the activation of a complementary effector unit with production of an intracellular "second messenger" at the inner face of the cell membrane, and finally (c) the interaction of the second messenger(s) with the cellular machinery that delivers the final "hormone response" (27).

The first step is controlled by a "recognition unit" that faces the outside of the cell and possesses structural congruence with the hormone "active site." The structural demands of this recognition unit are, therefore, determinants of the specificity of the hormone signal. These demands account for the interactions that may be obverved between various gastrointestinal hormones of the same family. It is known, however, that binding to the "recognition unit" is not synonymous with activation of the receptor. This activation requires the presence of a "functional structure" in the active site of the hormone as a counterpart of a "functional site" present in the recognition unit (87). Thus, two structurally related hormones, showing the same affinity for binding to the receptor, may, once bound, differ in their ability to promote the biological response, which is, e.g. the case of gastrin and CCK in man (see p. 486).

The second step of peptide hormone receptor interaction could proceed in two alternative modes. Either the recognition unit on the cell and the effector unit on the hormone are firmly associated *(permanent coupling)*, or, once bound, the "hormone recognition unit complex" associates with the "effector moiety" to form a "transient ternary complex" [*collision coupling* (125)]. In the latter case, the recognition and/or the effector units are presumed not to be fixed but are thought to float in the cellular membrane in order to meet each other. Such a scheme applies to most of the membrane hormone receptors investigated so far, where the role of the effector unit is fulfilled by the well documented adenylate cyclase. The latter enzyme is known to hydrolyse ATP to produce the "secondary messenger" cyclic AMP, which in turn is degraded by a phosphodiesterase. In the case of gastrointestinal hormones, different messengers (hence different transduction mechanisms) have also been considered, e.g., cyclic GMP and Ca^{2+} ions. It is also conceivable that a unique hormone receptor interaction can involve two parallel second messengers that are different in nature (11,42, 69,87,132).

The third and last step may actually include a series of cascade events that offer multiple possibilities for secondary interactions (47). In contrast with the case of the pancreatic acinar cell (see Chapter 20 by J. Christophe et al., pp.

451–476, *this volume*), the nature of these events in the parietal cell and the enterocyte is not firmly documented.

According to the comments made above, it may be speculated that the final step of hormone action on parietal cells and enterocytes should result in the activation of the cellular metabolism, with production of ATP as a substrate for the ion pumps. Coupling between membrane effectors and cellular metabolism is generally assumed to involve mobile enzyme systems such as cyclic AMP-dependent protein kinases. These enzyme systems could be also required for the phosphorylation of membrane transport components. Calcium, the putative role of which was outlined above, is suggested to be released from the cellular stores, either directly (as a consequence of hormone-receptor interaction, at the membrane level), or indirectly (via, e.g., cyclic AMP mediation) (42,132).

Recent studies on liver hormone receptors have provided evidence for the occurrence of two additional "regulatory units" that complement the above model: one controls the conformation of the recognition site, whereas the other controls the activity of the catalytic moiety. These units are thought to possess binding sites for guanylnucleotides, especially guanosine triphosphate (GTP), which is assumed to be the natural effector. This is hydrolyzed to guanosine diphosphate (GDP) by a GTPase that, in doing so, terminates the hormonal signal, presumably by shifting the receptor recognition unit to a "closed" conformation no longer accessible to the hormone (26,71,79,111,152). Such a mechanism may be assumed to also occur in the case of gastrointestinal receptors. It could account for the observation that the nonhydrolyzable GTP analogs such as guanosyl-5'-(β,γ-imino)triphosphate [Gpp(NH)p] may induce a permanently active state of the receptor. It also explains the remarkable action of substances that block GTPase activity, such as cholera enterotoxin (Fig. 1) (64,70,83,91,96,117).

Methodological Approaches

Ideally, proof of hormone receptor control of gastrointestinal epithelial transport would involve demonstration of the three successive steps that were outlined above, with an evidence for a cause-effect relationship. In practice, however, studies in this area have taken two separate directions.

The "Forward" or "Direct" Approach

In the "forward" or "direct" approach, the investigations concentrate on the binding of radiolabeled hormones to the putative receptor recognition sites on the epithelial cell membrane. This appears to be the most valid method for defining the specificity of hormone action and for studying direct interaction between parent hormones and structurally related peptides with either agonist

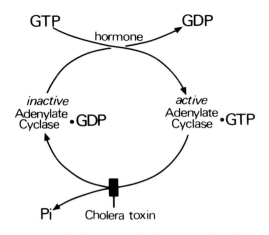

FIG. 1. Suggested mechanism for hormone stimulation of adenylate cyclase systems. This model is based on the assumption that adenylate cyclase occurs in two states depending on the presence of GTP (active state) or GDP (inactive state) at the regulatory unit. Binding of the hormone to the recognition unit facilitates the displacement of bound GDP by free GTP. The subsequent hydrolysis of GTP at the regulatory site is assumed to revert the system to the inactive state. The permanent activation of all the adenylate cyclase systems by cholera toxin may be simply explained by an inhibitory effect on the GTPase that results in the blockade of the system in the activated state. (From ref. 26.)

or antagonist effects. Such an approach, however, raises two crucial problems: (a) the preparation of radiolabeled hormones with acceptably high levels of radioactivity without altering their chemical structure or biological activity; and (b) the determination of what is "specific" versus "nonspecific" in the bindings observed. The first problem poses questions that have been recently dealt with elsewhere (47,100,153). The second relates to the multiplicity of possible artifacts in evaluating the so called "specific binding." These are due to (a) binding that is not actually relevant to the cell studied but refers to a different biological or even nonbiological material, (b) binding that involves a portion of the hormone molecule that does not include the active site, and (c) binding to specific receptor sites that because of qualitative or quantitative considerations are likely to be pharmacological rather than physiological in nature. Here, critical information is provided by quantitative approaches to the binding reaction. Kinetic and stochiometric analyses of the reaction, according to mathematical models described elsewhere (87), make it possible to estimate the apparent affinity and the maximum binding capacity of the putative receptor sites. This allows useful comparisons with predictions from physiological studies. However, since investigations of the binding are generally carried out *in vitro,* receptors with presumably physiological status may be evidenced that cannot function *in vivo,* because in this situation the hormone is not available at the target cell level, or the receptor sites are not accessible to the hormone.

The Alternative "Backward" or "Indirect" Approach

In the alternative "backward" or "indirect" approach, investigators attempt to characterize the receptor from the correlations between the hormonal concentration and biological response. When the biological response under consideration refers to the ultimate transport step, e.g., water or ion output, this approach leads to a definition of the receptor that is purely operational. For example, the mathematical analysis of the dose-response curves according to the Michaelis-Menten enzymatic model allows speculations as to the occurrence and the putative interaction properties of gastric receptors for the hormones of the other members of the gastrin family (87,92). From the studies in which the biological response under consideration is a more primary event, e.g., change in intracellular cyclic AMP level or activation of adenylate cyclase, the characterization of the receptor will be substantiated also on biochemical grounds. Using this approach, one is unable however, to detect those receptors that have unidentified effectors. Also, an ambiguity may appear if a unique effector is shared by different receptors or if interactions may occur between different "second messengers."

Tissue Preparations

Since parietal cells are not the only mucosal cells contained in the stomach, they are concentrated in the fundic area together with pepsin and mucus secreting cells, and with some endocrine cells as well. That they only account for 20 to 30% of the total cell population of the fundic mucosa presents a major difficulty when one attempts to draw specific conclusions from the *in vivo* and *in vitro* studies dealing with the entire tissue preparations. Uncertainties arise from possible cellular interactions. Furthermore, the reliable correlations between biochemical determinations and specific parietal cell activity are frustrated by the heterocellular nature of the samples. In these respects "pure" preparations of isolated and "normally responsive" parietal cells would represent a very convenient model. Accordingly, several investigators tried to develop methods for gastric cells isolation and sorting (7,8,15,55,84,85,129,142). Recent studies on gastrin receptor have already taken advantage of the availability of enriched parietal cell populations (143).

The study of electrolyte transport in the intestine is even more complicated, because the techniques for isolation of cell populations have not yet reached a high level of sophistication. Besides the principal "enterocytes" that line the luminal "brush border" the intestinal mucosa contains also other cell types with distinct functional characteristics. These include zymogen cells in the Brunner's gland of the duodenum, Paneth cells in the crypts of Lieberkühn, and a large population of goblet cells containing mucus. Up to the present, most investigations concerned with intestinal transport pertained to the studies of unidirectional fluxes and short-circuit-currents carried out mostly on *in vitro* preparations of entire tissue, such as "chambered" mucosa (42). These approaches, by their nature, are unable, however, to provide specific information relevant to the cellular level. Recently, suspensions of isolated intestinal mucosal cells have been successfully prepared and hormone-receptor studies have been carried on these preparations (76,77,95). However, a better separation of the isolated intestinal mucosal cells remains an unresolved problem.

In addition to the intact isolated cell preparations, subcellular fractions are also of interest in the study of gastrointestinal receptors. The use of centrifugation techniques and of specific membrane markers has permitted the preparation from homogenates of the whole epithelium of purified plasma membrane fractions, containing receptors (88,89). Using these preparations, however, one is left with the problem of cell specificity, since the purified membranes originate from various cell types contained in the tissue.

The advantages and disadvantages of various tissue preparations in the study of hormone binding have recently been reviewed (47). From a practical standpoint, the dispersed intact cell preparations offer a number of advantages over tissue fragments; of these the better reproducibility and reduction of hormone trapping by extra-cellular spaces are most significant. As compared with membrane fragments, intact isolated cells are more easily filtered and more rapidly centrifuged during separation of the free from the bound hormone. The use of intact isolated cells also makes possible the correlation of hormone binding with successive post-membrane-binding events, up to the stage of the full cellular response. However, hormone interactions that occur *in vivo* may not necessarily be detected with isolated cell preparations, because the procedure used in isolating and maintaining the cell *in vitro* may result in alterations of receptors or of cellular metabolism. It is also possible that hormone receptors in the isolated cells are no longer compartmentalized in the basolateral membranes, because of the dissolution of the tight junctions. As a consequence, the various structures of the hormone receptors may become dispersed all over the cell membrane and this may result in a striking alteration of the efficiency of hormone-target cell interaction.

GUT HORMONES ACTIVE ON GASTROINTESTINAL ION TRANSPORT

Molecular Forms and Structure-Activity Relationships

Most of the presently known gut hormones may be grouped into two families on the basis of structural similarities that also reflect similarities in function. The gastrin family consists of the gastrins and the cholecystokinins (CCKs), including, in a broader sense, the structurally related amphibian peptides such as cerulein and phyllocerulein. The secretin family consists of secretin, glucagon from pancreatic origin, and glucagon-like immunoreactive materials from gut (GLIs), vasoactive intestinal polypeptide (VIP), and gastric inhibitory peptide

(GIP). To this family may be also related the amphibian peptide bombesin and the bombesin-like substances recently detected by radioimmunoassay (RIA) in the gastrointestinal tract.

In addition to these two families, gut hormones also include the so-called "brain-gut" peptides. This group refers to those peptides that were originally described in the brain but have been subsequently found also in the stomach and the intestine as well. These peptides include neurotensin, substance P, opioids, and somatostatin.

Detailed information on all these hormone peptides is found in various chapters of this volume. For each of them, there exists a number of molecular forms of different size or with slight changes in amino acid composition. The reasons for this heterogeneity are discussed in Chapter 19 by J. F. Rehfeld et al. (pp. 433–449, *this volume*). For the present discussion, this heterogeneity implies that each individual hormonal action on electrolyte transport may actually involve a variety of homologous peptides with possible difference in potency.

The Gastrin Family

The information on the antral hormone, gastrin, has been worked out in much detail (33,52,151) (see also Chapter 6 by G. Nilsson, pp. 127–168, *this volume*). Gastrin is well known to play a crucial role as stimulant of gastric acid secretion in physiological as well as pathological conditions (17). The role of gastrin in intestinal ion transport appears to be much less important. It has been reported that gastrin reduces net absorption of water and electrolyte in the small intestine, possibly by depressing the glucose dependent Na^+ absorption (96,97).

All the peptides possessing gastrin-like activity have been found to have the C-terminal sequence Trp-Met-Asp-PheNH$_2$. Therefore, this tetradecapeptide amide has been suggested to represent the minimal fragment for the biological activity, i.e., the "active unit" (103). The N-terminal fragment, however, is very likely to play some complementary role in the activity of gastrins, perhaps because it facilitates the conforming of the C-terminal fragment to an efficient ternary structure (112). Thus, the naturally occurring gastrin heptadecapeptide is apparently much more potent (although equally efficient) than the synthetic analog, pentagastrin, of shorter length (87). In the CCK-like peptide, the minimal fragment for typical biological effects is represented by the C-terminal heptadecapeptide (see Chapter 7 by V. Mutt, pp. 169–222, *this volume*).

CCKs have been shown to be powerful pharmacological stimulants of gastric acid secretion. In man they competitively inhibit the action of the gastrins, and therefore are suggested to behave as partial agonists of the gastrin receptor (18). In the intestine the actions of CCKs are not so clearly established. Purified CCK was reported to produce a decrease in net absorption (or an increase in net secretion) of water, Na^+, and Cl^- by the human jejunum (93), but in animal studies, results are controversial (96).

Such similarities between the effects of CCK-like peptides and those reported for gastrin-like peptides, on both gastric and intestinal targets, may easily be accounted for by the similarities that can be observed in their respective chemical structures. In effect, the minimum active unit for CCK-like activity includes that for gastrin-like activity. CCKs and gastrins have also a similar tyrosine residue at position 6 (gastrins) or 7 (CCKs) counting from the carboxyl terminus. However, this residue is always sulfated in CCKs, whereas in gastrins it may be sulfated (gastrin I) or not (gastrin II). In mammals, it is apparent that the sulfated tyrosine residue plays no significant role in the activity of gastrin-like peptides, since gastrin I and gastrin II are equipotent agonists of gastric acid secretion (1,102). In contrast, gastrin II is 10 to 30 times more potent than gastrin I in its action on the pancreatic target, and desulfation results in a marked loss of their biological activity on this target with reversion to gastrin-like activity (66). An increase in gastric acid secretory potency on sulfation has been recently reported, in the cat, for gastrin-like peptides of shorter length (M. W. below 1,520 daltons). This, however, most likely reflects an increase in their resistance to degradation (60).

From these observations it appears, therefore, that the receptors for gastrins and those for CCKs are very similar but possibly not identical in nature. It is not known if the interaction between CCKs and gastrins observed under pharmacological conditions reflects interactions that may actually occur *in vivo* (54).

The Secretin Family

In the secretin family, structural similarities between homologous peptides are less evident than in the gastrin family. Furthermore, the residues required for biological activity do not appear to be concentrated in the form of a unique amino acid sequence, but rather are dispersed all over the length of the molecule (13,118,123). This feature stresses the major role that the stereo-conformation may play in the binding to their receptors of the peptides related to the secretin family (16,63).

With the exception of bombesin, all the members of the secretion family possess the property of inhibiting gastric acid secretion (87). They have, however, a stimulatory effect on intestinal net electrolyte secretion (96).

High doses of secretin were reported to inhibit pentagastrin-stimulated acid secretion in the dog, as well as in man. This inhibition, however, appears to be noncompetitive in nature (18,65). It is unlikely, therefore, that secretion and gastrin may interact on a common receptor, an assumption that is consistent with the apparent lack of structural similarities between these two peptides. It cannot be ruled out, however, that these peptides could relate to receptors differing only in their recognition units ("two-site hypothesis") (53). On the other hand, it is doubtful whether secretin-gastrin interaction has any physiological importance with respect to the minute amount of secretin released after a meal (110,135). The effect of secretin on intestinal secretory functions remains obscure.

In man, purified porcine secretin has been shown to inhibit the absorption (or increase the secretion) of water, sodium, and chloride by the jejunum in a manner that resembles that of CCK from a qualitative as well as a quantitative point of view (59,101). However, studies looking for an effect of secretin on intestinal transport of water and ions have been generally negative in *in vitro* animal preparations at the isolated segments of jejunum, ileum, or colon. It has been, therefore, suggested that the effects observed *in vivo* could be only secondary to the stimulatory action of secretin on bilioduodeno-pancreatic secretions (96).

Pancreatic glucagon has been reported to inhibit basal gastric acid secretion, as well as that stimulated by a variety of pharmacological and physiological stimulants including gastrins. It was also reported to reduce the net absorption (or increase the net secretion) of water and electrolytes in the human and dog intestine *in vivo* (13,87,96) (see also Chapter 27 by T.-M. Lin, pp. 639–692, *this volume*). It is uncertain whether or not these effects are secondary to the action of glucagon on blood sugar levels and on mucosal blood flow. The occurrence of a glucagon receptor on the parietal cell and the enterocyte is therefore an interesting possibility that deserves further investigations.

Much effort has been devoted to the purification of the so called GLIs from the stomach and the intestine (99). However, the molecular structures of these candidate hormones, are still only partially known (62,98). The putative physiological role of GLIs in the control of electrolye transport is discussed in Chapter 12 by F. Sundby and A. V. Moody, pp. 307–314, *this volume*.

Isolation, structure, and basic functions of GIP are detailed in Chapter 8 by J. C. Brown et al., pp. 223–232, *this volume*. GIP has been shown to exert a strong inhibitory effect on gastric acid secretion stimulated by histamine, pentagastrin, or hypoglycemia and a stimulatory effect on hydroelectrolytic secretion of the small intestine *in vivo* (58,108). It is not presently known, however, whether these effects are due to the presence of GIP receptors on the gastric and intestinal secretory cells, or are secondary to the insulinotropic-glucagonotropic action that GIP exerts on endocrine pancreas (20,109).

VIP has both a glucagon-like activity inducing hyperglycemia and a secretin-like activity stimulating pancreatic bicarbonate secretion. In addition, like GIP, VIP stimulates insulin release and inhibits pentagastrin- as well as histamine-stimulated gastric acid secretion (74,133) (see Chapter 10 by S. Said, pp. 245–274, *this volume*). In the dog intestine, relatively small doses of exogenous VIP have been shown to stimulate the hydroelectrolytic secretion of the small bowel in particular of the jejunum (6), as well as of the colon (119). In the rat, this stimulation was shown to be inhibited by high doses (10^{-5} M) of somatostatin (25). In *in vitro* preparations of "chambered" fragments of ileal mucosa from rabbit and man, VIP was shown to increase the short circuit current and to reverse the absorption of sodium chloride to a net secretion (140). VIP has furthermore been implicated in the WDHA (pancreatic cholera) syndrome (12). All these observations strongly argue for a crucial role of VIP in the control of intestinal electrolytic secretion. This is furthermore supported by biochemical studies discussed below.

The "Brain Gut" Hormones

Not all of the peptides of the "brain gut" hormones are of equal interest in regard to the control of gastrointestinal electrolyte transport.

Substance P most likely plays no direct role in this transport (116). The opiate-like enkephalins present in many parts of the brain and found also in antral and duodenal G cells (115) display structural identities with a portion of the C-terminal sequence of gastrin-like peptides (123). However, they do not contain the active unit of the gastrin family. Their effects on gastrointestinal secretions are controversial, and have been suggested to result at least in part, from a primary action on the central nervous system (CNS) (73). Because of the lack of relevant *in vitro* studies, the occurrence of epithelial opiate receptors on gastrointestinal secretory cells remains an open question.

The tridecapeptide neurotensin is widely distributed in the CNS, but it is present, in larger amounts, in the stomach and especially in the intestine (24). It has been shown to have a large spectrum of pharmacological actions including the inhibiting effect on canine gastric acid secretion stimulated by pentagastrin, but not by histamine (4,22). There is no evidence, however, for a direct action of neurotensin on the parietal cell or on the enterocyte.

The tetradecapeptide somatostatin, or growth hormone-release inhibiting factor (GH-RIF) was initially discovered in hypothalamic tissue and subsequently found also in the synaptosomes of the brain cortex (37). Outside of the CNS, immunoreactive somatostatin is found in the largest amount in the digestive tract. This, in addition to the pancreas, contains the highest concentration and the major portion of somatostatin of the entire body (5). The nature of the biologically active residues in the somatostatin molecule is only partially known and the structure-activity relationship of synthetic analogs is the subject of intensive investigations (149). Apart from its effect on growth hormone release, somatostatin was shown to inhibit the release of various gastrointestinal hormones, especially gastrin (106). In addition, somatostatin has been shown to inhibit competitively gastric acid secretion stimulated by pentagastrin (21,128), an observation which strongly supports the occurrence of somatostatin receptors on the parietal cell (see below). In view of this effect on gastric acid secretion, somatostatin may be expected to act on intestinal electrolyte secretion as well. This has not yet been documented, however.

Tissue Localization and Mode of Release

Most of the peptides just mentioned are found both in neurons and endocrine cells (145).

Endocrine cells of the gastroenteropancreatic (GEP) system (44) have been extensively investigated by electron microscopy and cytochemical as well as immunocytochemical methods (see Chapter 1 by E. Solcia et al., pp. 1–18, *this volume*). Their distribution along the intestinal tract has been recently reviewed (14). As is true also for other typical endocrine cells, they are characterized by the presence of secretory granules that accumulate at the basal pole. This feature is consistent with hormonal release into the bloodstream. A particular characteristic of these cells, however, is the fact that they are of an "open type," i.e., their apical membrane is exposed to the gastrointestinal lumen, making possible their direct activation by stimuli coming from food or endogenous secretions (45). In this way a number of feedback mechanisms and hormone interactions may operate under physiological conditions that may not be evidenced in *in vitro* studies; in the well known example of the autoregulation of gastric secretion by acid gastrin stimulates acid production, which in turn inhibits gastrin release from antral G cells and releases secretin from the duodenum. Another interesting feature of some gut endocrine cells is their location in a relative proximity to their corresponding target cell. For instance, D cells containing somatostatin are found in the fundic glands of the stomach together with the parietal cells. This observation had led to the suggestion that these cells might release their hormone content directly to the receptors of the neighboring parietal cells. The occurrence of this so called "paracrine" secretion appears plausible for those hormones that are very short-lived in blood, as is the case for somatostatin (14). It should be noted that paracrine secretion could result in extremely high concentration of hormone at the receptors, a condition that is intentionally avoided in current *in vitro* investigations.

The possible occurrence of a "luminal" secretion has been also suggested to account for the fact that large amounts of hormones can be found in the gastric juice (146). It is, however, unlikely that the luminally secreted hormones can reenter the epithelial layer to interact with the receptors on the basal membrane of the secretory cells.

In addition to endocrine cells, an increasing number of gut hormones has been found to be located also in peripheral and/or central neurons (34). The presence of CCK-like immunoreactive material has been reported in the brain as well as in the small intestine (30,31,122,127). Gastrin (mostly in the heptadecapeptide form) has been demonstrated in the neuro- and adeno-hypophysis (121) and in the abdominal portion of the vagus nerves of cat, dogs, and man (147,148). VIP has been detected within the brain as well as in gastrointestinal nerve fibers, especially abundantly in the intestine (9,10,50,80,134). These findings, in connection with the existence of the brain gut hormones mentioned above, have led to the reexamination of current views based on separate humoral and nervous controls of gastrointestinal secretory function. It has become clear that a crucial role in the control is played by the so-called "peptidergic" nerves that release hormones acting as neurotransmitters (23,51,136,147). This new look may have implications of considerable importance in the general understanding of the gastrointestinal physiology (see Chapter 2 by J. M. Polak and

S. B. Bloom, pp. 19–52, *this volume*). As to the control of electrolyte secretion, the fact that various active neuropeptides can be selectively released in proximity of the secretory cells appears to cause some confusion in regard to the problem of mediators' interactions. This important factor has not yet been considered in the *in vitro* receptor studies.

Ontogenic and Evolutionary Aspects

The acronym "APUD" cells has been earlier proposed for the GEP endocrine cells to account for their common ability to accumulate and decarboxylate amine precursors, such as 5-hydroxytryptophan. It had been suggested that APUD cells derive from a common ancestral cell of a "neural origin, perhaps coming from the neural crest" (107). It is now recognized that they are derived from neuroendocrine programmed cells of ectoblastic origin (82). These evolutionary aspects are consistent with the unity of the nervous and endocrine control of gastrointestinal secretions.

The comparative studies have provided a genetic basis for the remarkable similarities between structurally related hormones. They have shown that the peptides of the gastrin family and those of the secretin family are each very likely to be derived from a common ancestor gene. Thus, gastrin/CCK-like peptides occur in the oldest vertebrate groups and analogous peptides such as cerulein are found in the skin of our amphibian ancestors. Similarly, peptides of the secretin/glucagon family have been evidenced in all species studied, and their common ancestral molecule is thought to be more than 200 million years old (32,81). These evolutionary aspects are of significance in the understanding of hormone receptor control of gastrointestinal secretory functions. They provide an explanation for the close structure-activity relationship that has been established over the years of evolution between gastrointestinal hormones and their receptors according to the evolutionary trends. It is conceivable also that the genetic mutation that resulted in a change of the hormone structure could have favored the emergence of a new hormonal target. Thus, the divergence in molecular structure of gastrointestinal hormones could have been the reflection of the evolution of the digestive tract itself. Accordingly, two hormone peptides of the same family (i.e., of the same ancestral origin) do not necessarily relate to identical receptors. This appears to be the case with gastrins and CCKs, which have diverged over the years to assume the control of different organs.

Following on previous studies on β-adrenergic receptor (138) it has been suggested in a recent report that VIP receptors from a cell line derived from a human colon carcinoma can be successfully coupled with the adenylate cyclase system of the Friend erythroleukemia cells to form an active hybrid (78). This supports the view that receptor recognition units and effector systems originating from various tissues might actually be compatible with each other. It further suggests that different hormone receptors in the gastrointestinal tract might have evolved from a common ancestor by mutations at the recognition site (78).

BIOCHEMICAL EVIDENCE FOR HORMONE RECEPTORS IN THE GASTROINTESTINAL TRACT

In this section studies are reviewed that deal with direct biochemical investigations along the lines discussed above. To date, there are only three types of receptors that have been documented directly—gastric receptors for gastrin and somatostatin and intestinal receptors for VIP. Even in these three instances, the criteria for establishing the significance of the receptors as biological entities in the gastrointestinal tract have been fulfilled only partially.

Gastric Receptors for Gastrin

Evidence for gastrin receptors in the fundic gastric mucosa has been gathered by studying the effects of gastrin and related peptides on mucosal adenylate cyclase and guanylate cyclase activity. Here, the results reported are confusing, however, because of apparent species differences and uncertainties as to whether or not biochemical changes in gastric mucosal homogenate are specifically representative of the parietal cells activity (87). Thus, whereas gastric adenylate cyclase in the Necturus and frog were shown to be stimulated by pentagastrin (104), in rat, guinea pig, and dog similar *in vitro* studies consistently produced negative results, with only one exception (88). In man, the effect of pentagastrin on the production of the gastric mucosal cyclic AMP was not consistent. Similarly, the potentiation of the pentagastrin stimulatory effect on gastric acid by caffeine, an inhibitor of the phosphodiesterase, was not consistent (69). Also, the possible role of cyclic GMP in mediation of acid secretion has been supported only by the increase in cyclic GMP content of gastric juice in response to pentagastrin (2).

In contrast with the reported effects of CCKs on the isolated gastric cells (see Chapter 20 by J. Christophe et al., pp. 451–476, *this volume*), gastrin does not produce any evident change in calcium movements in the isolated gastric cells but has been reported (7) to stimulate K^+ uptake by the guinea pig gastric cells inconsistently.

A forward approach to the characterization of gastric gastrin receptors has been attempted using ^3H gastrin and ^{125}I-gastrin. ^3H-gastrin used in these studies was prepared from human synthetic gastrin I (GI-17) that retained full biological activity of the native hormone. This was shown to bind to purified plasma membrane and isolated cells from rat fundic mucosa (88). Native gastrin competed with tritiated gastrin, a finding that supports the specificity of the binding (Table 1). Scatchard analysis of the results suggested the occurrence of a single class of binding sites, with an apparent equilibrium constant of $K = 0.5 \ 10^{-8}$

TABLE 1. *Competition between native and tritiated gastrin for binding to gastric plasma membranes from rat fundic mucosa*

| Total gastrin concentration (M) | | Bound gastrin (moles/mg protein) |
Native	Tritiated	
0	0.9×10^{-8}	20.2×10^{-14}
0	1.8×10^{-8}	29.5×10^{-14}
0.9×10^{-8}	0.9×10^{-8}	12.1×10^{-14}

From ref. 86.

moles/liter at pH 7.4 and 20°C, and a maximum binding capacity of $N = 0.4$ pmoles.mg^{-1} membrane protein (89). This corresponds to about 10,000 to 15,000 binding sites per cell. Using preparative centrifugation techniques, it has been also shown that these binding sites are specifically located on the parietal cells (143) (Fig. 2). In other studies using ^{125}I-labeled gastrin analogs gastrin binding sites have been demonstrated in crude subcellular fractions prepared from rat fundic mucosa, and furthermore a number of arguments have been provided supporting the specificity of these sites (19,67). Among these arguments is the fact that gastrin binding had been competitively inhibited by pentagastrin, CCK, and cerulein, but not by secretin (67). This was in agreement with the expected behavior of gastrin receptors.

Admittedly all these findings, however, are not sufficient to demonstrate the physiological significance of the gastrin receptors in the stomach. Yet the participation of the ^{3}H-gastrin binding sites on the cells in the mechanism of gastric acid stimulation by gastrin is strongly supported by studies with NPS-gastrin. This analog of gastrin (nitrophenylsulfenyl-14-tryptophan GI-17) was shown to compete with a similar affinity in the rat for binding with ^{3}H-gastrin, whereas it quantitatively inhibited the stimulation of gastric acid secretion by gastrin (90).

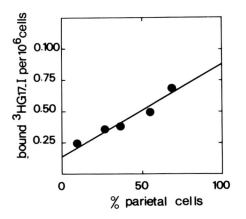

FIG. 2. Binding of tritiated gastrin (^{3}H-human non sulfated heptadecapeptide GI-17) to isolated gastric cells from rat fundus as a function of enrichment of cell suspensions in parietal cells. Results are in 10^{-13} moles per million cells; 30 min incubation at 22°C, pH 7.4. This figure suggests strongly that the gastric gastrin binding sites evidenced in previous studies (86) are mainly, if not exclusively, associated with the parietal cells. (From ref. 143.)

If the gastrin binding sites described in the above studies are actually involved in acid secretion, their specific location on the parietal cell is of a special interest. It suggests that gastrin acts directly on the parietal cell rather than as a second mediator via the release of histamine. The possibility that histamine could be released or synthetized within the parietal cell cannot, however, be ruled out (89).

The foregoing studies are concerned with a more thorough characterization and purification of the gastrin receptors. They are expected to better explain the complex interactions that occur in the control of gastric acid secretion between gastrin and other gut hormones as well as between gastrin and histamine or carbamylcholine. In preliminary studies, cimetidine and metiamide, two antagonists of the histamine H_2 receptors, were reported not to affect gastrin binding (19,89). The drawing of safe conclusions from these studies must await, however, evidence for the preservation of histamine receptors in the preparation used (86). Also, the better understanding of these interactions will be obtained when further studies will reveal the nature of the missing links between membrane receptor occupancy and the activation of the secretory mechanisms.

Gastric Receptors for Somatostatin

No evidence has been provided, so far, for a stimulatory or inhibitory effect of somatostatin on adenylate or guanylate cyclase or on calcium transport in the gastric parietal cells.

A direct evidence for specific binding of ^{125}I-Tyr$_1$-somatostatin to isolated rat parietal cells has been recently submitted (124). In these studies two classes of binding sites were evidenced in the crude isolated gastric cell populations. Studies performed with purified preparations showed that sites with an apparent K_D of 4.5 10^{-9} M were specifically associated with the parietal cells whereas sites with an apparently higher affinity ($K_D = 0.85\ 10^{-10}$ M) were associated with gastric cells of smaller size, possibly chief cells. Furthermore, the time course of somatostatin binding to parietal cells showed an apparent lag period that might suggest that the sites associated with parietal cells are intracellularly located. This is supported also by previous observations documenting the possible existence of an intracellular somatostatin binding protein in various tissues, including gastric mucosa (105). Contrary to these observations, however, somatostatin binding to parietal cells manifested reversibility, as is the case for somatostatin binding to pituitary cells in culture (137). Also, somatostatin binding to the gastric cells, so far, was not associated with any biological signal and its physiological relevance therefore remains an open question. Furthermore, this binding was found not to be affected by the presence of gastrin or pentagastrin. This suggests that the peptides of the gastrin family are not recognized by somatostatin "receptors" (Fig. 3). Thus far, interaction of somatostatin with the gastrin receptors has not yet been documented.

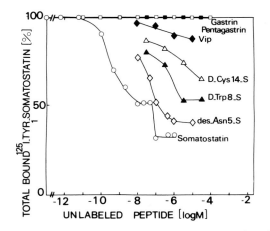

FIG. 3. Inhibition of ^{125}I-Tyr$_1$-somatostatin binding to isolated rat gastric cells by various unlabeled peptides. Results are expressed as percent of total radioactivity bound in the absence of added unlabeled peptides. Thus, it may be appreciated that "unspecific" binding (i.e., in the presence of 10^{-6} M native somatostatin) accounts for 30% of the total counts (nonpurified cell populations). The biphasic pattern of ^{125}I-Tyr$_1$-somatostatin binding inhibition by native somatostatin is consistent with the occurrence of at least two classes of binding sites (corresponding to parietal and nonparietal cell receptors). Analogs of somatostatin compete for binding with varying degrees of potency. VIP has a very little effect. Gastrin and pentagastrin are apparently uneffective even in very high concentrations. (From ref. 124.)

Intestinal Receptors for VIP

In line with the stipulated mechanism (see p. 493) for the action of cholera toxin on the enterocyte, cyclic AMP has been shown to be implicated as cellular mediator of intestinal electrolyte secretion. In the ileum, net secretion could be the consequence of a decrease in electrolyte absorption due to an inhibitory effect of cyclic AMP on the neutral NaCl symport. In the colon, electrogenic chloride secretion would result from changes in membrane permeability, secondary to mobilization of calcium from cellular stores (42).

VIP has been reported to stimulate adenylate cyclase activity in various homogenates and membrane preparations from intestinal mucosa (3,46,72,140,150). This is in agreement with previous results on the effect of VIP noted on membranes from the liver and fat (29). Furthermore, VIP has been recently reported to stimulate cyclic AMP accumulation in isolated enterocytes in concentrations as low as 10^{-10} M (76). Secretin also stimulated cyclic AMP production but with a potency 120 times lower. Glucagon failed to produce the stimulation, even at 10^{-5} M. Similarly, other gut hormones including CCK, gastrin, and somatostatin failed to produce stimulation as well. Consistent with these observations are studies that have shown specific binding of ^{125}I-labeled VIP to enterocytes (75,118). This occurred in both rat and human, and on various intestinal cell preparations from duodenum to rectum (77). Quantitative analysis of this binding suggested the existence of two independent classes of receptor sites: "high affinity" sites ($K_D = 1.6 \times 10^{-9}$ M, 140,000 sites per cell), and "low" affinity sites ($K_D = 7.4 \times 10^{-8}$ M, 1,100.000 sites per cell) (118). Because of the heterogeneity of the preparations used, it cannot presently be decided whether or not both these classes of sites are associated with a single type. This is however indirectly supported by the fact that VIP binding displayed a similar pattern in the various preparations used. Secretin antagonized VIP binding to the enterocytes with a 70 times lower affinity, however. Glucagon and GIP were uneffective at 10^{-5} and 10^{-7} M, respectively. Furthermore, the results obtained with various secretin analogs emphasized the crucial importance that the NH_2-terminal portion of VIP has in the binding of this hormone to its intestinal receptors (118) and in part in the activation of its catalytic moiety (76) (Fig. 4).

These observations are apparently consistent with previous studies providing evidence for ^{125}I-VIP binding to liver, fat tissue, and pancreatic acinar cells (29,48,49,126). It is apparent, however, that VIP receptors predominate in the intestine, whereas secretin and glucagon receptors predominate in pancreas and liver, respectively (76). This would be consistent with the presumed hierarchy of function of VIP, secretin, and glucagon in the above tissues. Furthermore, in contrast with the results on pancreas, where two separate receptors for VIP and secretin appear to be present (48,49,126) the dose-response curves of cyclic AMP to VIP or secretin are monophasic, which suggests that secretin effect on the enterocyte is mediated through the VIP receptors (76).

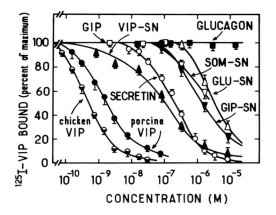

FIG. 4. Inhibition of ^{125}I-VIP binding to isolated intestinal epithelial cells from rat by various peptides structurally related to VIP (2 hr incubation at 15°C). Chicken VIP is about seven times more affine than porcine VIP, suggesting a possible role in the binding of threonine residues in position 28 (Asn-NH_2 and Tr-NH_2, respectively). Secretin competes with VIP for binding but with a 70 times lower affinity. Glucagon and GIP are seen to have no effect on VIP binding. VIP-SN, SOM-SN, Glu-SN, and GIP-SN represent hybrid molecules obtained by changes in the NH_2-terminal pentapeptide sequence of secretin. Enhancement of affinity that is observed by these changes suggests strongly that the hydrophobic residues at the NH_2-terminal hexapeptide sequence of the VIP molecule should play an important role in the binding to the VIP receptor. (From ref. 118.)

In conclusion, these findings strongly support the occurrence of functional VIP receptors on the enterocytes. However, evidence for the implication of these receptors in the regulation of intestinal electrolyte transport has not yet been provided. It should be also noted that recent studies have suggested a stimulating effect of VIP on human gastric mucosal adenylate cyclase (141). However, gastric binding sites for VIP have not so far been documented.

CONCLUSIONS

In recent years significant progress has been achieved in the characterization of hormone receptors in the gastrointestinal tract. This progress has been mainly made possible by the successful development of suitable methods for isolating gastric and intestinal epithelial cells, as well as by the improvement of nondamaging methods for the radiolabeling of peptidic hormones. Progress in the results of investigation on hormone receptors in the gastrointestinal tract is also greatly indebted to the advances in our general understanding of hormone receptor interaction phenomena that have come about from studies carried out in other tissues, chiefly the liver and the pancreas.

An important stimulus in this field of research has been the discovery of new gut hormones implicated in the control of electrolyte transport, especially somatostatin and VIP.

The evidence has been provided for somatostatin binding sites on isolated gastric cells and for VIP binding sites on isolated enterocytes and their derived membranes. Furthermore, the gastrin binding sites that had been previously evidenced in gastric membranes have been shown to be specifically associated with the parietal cells. These sites appear to fulfill the classic criteria of saturability, reversibility and specificity that are generally assumed to be inherent features of receptor recognition units. Furthermore, their kinetic parameters, i.e., measurable affinity and maximum binding capacity, lay in the "physiological range."

Gastrin receptors in the stomach have been suggested to be implicated in the stimulation of gastric acid secretion on the basis of similarities observed between *in vitro* and *in vivo* studies. However, the nature of the intracellular effector of gastrin receptors is still a matter of controversy. Gastric receptors sites for somatostatin have not yet been associated with the triggering of any biological signal. Intestinal receptors for VIP have the most firm basis. Their occupancy is strongly suggested to initiate the production of cyclic AMP as the intracellular "second messenger." *In vitro* studies have not been yet able, however, to provide evidence for the implication of these VIP receptors or enterocyte in the electrolyte transport.

PROJECTIONS FOR THE FUTURE

Although receptors for gastrin, VIP and, to a lesser extent, somatostatin, are becoming to be recognized as biochemical entities, further studies are required to better assess their physiological implication in the control of gastrointestinal secretory functions. Since the suitable experimental tools are now available, one may anticipate that new receptors will be soon detected for a number of peptide hormones that, in addition to gastrin, VIP, and somatostatin, are suspected to play a role in gastrointestinal ion transport. A more thorough characterization of gastrointestinal receptors in regard to their structural requirements, intracellular messengers, their precise cellular, and subcellular location and functional interrelationship appear to be the most fruitful areas of research on gastrointestinal hormones for the future.

ACKNOWLEDGMENTS

I am very grateful to Pr. John Landor and Ms. Fabienne Pamart, Annick Soumarmon, and Françoise Grelac for their excellent assistance in the preparation of the manuscript. This work was partially supported by INSERM grant no. 7479106.

REFERENCES

1. Amer, M. S. (1969): Studies with cholecystokinin. II. Cholecystokinetic potency of porcine gastrins I and II and related peptides in three systems. *Endocrinology,* 84:1277–1281.
2. Amer, M. S. (1974): Cyclic GMP and gastric acid secretion. *Am. J. Dig. Dis.,* 19:71–74.
3. Amiranoff, B., Laburthe, M., Dupont, C., and Rosselin, G. (1978): Characterization of vasoactive intestinal peptide sensitive adenylate cyclase in rat intestinal epithelial membrane. *Biochim. Biophys. Acta,* 544:474–481.
4. Anderson, S., Chang, D., Folkers, K., and Rossel, S. (1976): Inhibition of gastric acid secretion in dogs by neurotensin. *Life Sci.,* 19:367–370.
5. Arimura, A., Coy, D. H., Chihara, M., Fernandez-Durango, F., Samols, E., Chihara, K., Meyers, C. A., and Schally, A. V. (1978): Somatostatin. In: *Gut Hormones,* edited by S. R. Bloom, pp. 437–445. Churchill Livingstone, Edinburgh.
6. Barbezat, G. O. (1973): Stimulation of intestinal secretion by polypeptide hormones. *Scand. J. Gastroenterol. (Suppl. 22),* 8:3–21.
7. Batzri, S., and Gardner, J. D. (1978): Potassium transport in dispersed mucosal cells from guinea pig stomach. *Biochim. Biophys. Acta,* 508:328–338.
8. Berglindh, T., and Obrink, K. J. (1976): A method for preparing isolated glands from the rabbit gastric mucosa. *Acta Physiol. Scand.,* 96:150–159.
9. Besson, J., Laburthe, M., Bataille, D., Dupont, C., and Rosselin, G. (1978): Vasoactive intestinal peptide (VIP): Tissue distribution in the rat as measured by radioimmunoassay and by radioreceptor assay. *Acta Endocrinol.,* 87:799–810.
10. Besson, J., Rotsztejn, W., Laburthe, M., Epelbaum, J., Beaudet, A., Kordon, C., and Rosselin, G. (1979): Vasoactive intestinal peptide (VIP): Brain distribution, subcellular localization and effect of deafferentation of the hypothalamus in male rats. *Brain Res.,* 165:79–85.
11. Bieck, P. R. (1976): The role of cyclic nucleotides in gastric acid secretion. In: *Stimulus-Secretion Coupling in the Gastrointestinal Tract,* edited by R. M. Case and H. Goebell. pp. 129–146. MTP, Lancaster.
12. Bloom, S. R. (1978): Vasoactive intestinal peptide, the major mediator of the WDHA (pancreatic cholera) syndrome: Value of measurement in diagnosis and treatment. *Am. J. Dig. Dis.,* 23:373–376.
13. Bloom, S. R., and Polak, J. M. (1977): The new peptide hormones of the gut. In: *Progress in Gastroenterology, Vol. III,* edited by G. B. J. Glass, pp. 109–151. Grune & Stratton, New York.
14. Bloom, S. R., and Polak, J. M. (1978): Gut hormone overview. In: *Gut Hormones,* edited by S. R. Bloom, pp. 3–18. Churchill Livingstone, Edinburgh.

15. Blum, A. L., Shah, G. T., Wiebelhaus, B. D., Brennan, F. T., Helander, H. F., Ceballos, R., and Sachs, G. (1971): Pronase method for isolation of viable cells from Necturus gastric mucosa. *Gastroenterology*, 61:189–200.

16. Bodanszky, M. (1979): Synthetic analogs in the study of hormone receptor interactions. In: *Hormone Receptors in Digestion and Nutrition*, edited by G. Rosselin, P. Fromageot and S. Bonfils, pp. 15–24. Elsevier/North Holland, Amsterdam.

17. Bonfils, S., Dubrasquet, M., Accary, J. P., Girodet, J., and Mignon, M. (1978): Bioassay vs. gastrin radioimmunoassay in the Zollinger-Ellison syndrome. In: *Gut Hormones*, edited by S. R. Bloom, pp. 158–162. Churchill Livingstone, Edinburgh.

18. Brooks, F. P., and Grossman, M. I. (1970): Effect of secretin and cholecystokinin on pentagastrin stimulated gastric secretion in man. *Gastroenterology*, 59:114–119.

19. Brown, J., and Gallagher, N. D. (1978): A specific gastrin receptor site in the rat stomach. *Biochim. Biophys. Acta*, 538:42–49.

20. Brown, J. C., Dryburgh, J. R., Frost, J. L., Otte, S. C., and Pederson, R. A. (1978): Properties and actions of GIP. In: *Gut Hormones*, edited by S. R. Bloom, pp. 277–282. Churchill Livingstone, Edinburgh.

21. Brown, M. P., Coy, D. H., Gomez-Pan, A., Hirst, B. H., Hunter, M., Meyers, C., Reed, J. D., Schally, A. V., and Shaw, B. (1978): Structure-activity relationships of eighteen somatostatin analogues on gastric secretion. *J. Physiol. (Lond.)*, 277:1–14.

22. Brown, M. P., Rivier, J., Kobayashi, R., and Vale, W. (1978): Neurotensin-like and bombesin-like peptides: CNS distribution and actions. In: *Gut Hormones*, edited by S. R. Bloom, pp. 550–558. Churchill Livingstone, Edinburgh.

23. Bryant, M. G., Bloom, S. R., Polak, J. M., Albuquerque, R. H., Modlin, I., and Pearse, A. G. E. (1976): Possible dual role for vasoactive intestinal peptide as gastrointestinal hormone and neurotransmitter substance. *Lancet*, i:991.

24. Carraway, R., and Leeman, S. E. (1976): Characterization of radioimmunoassayable neurotensin in the rat. Its differential distribution in the central nervous system, small intestine, and stomach. *J. Biol. Chem.*, 251:7045–7052.

25. Carter, R. F., Bitar, K. N., Zfass, A. M., and Makhlouf, G. M. (1978): Inhibition of VIP stimulated intestinal secretion and cyclic AMP production by somatostatin in the rat. *Gastroenterology*, 74:726–730.

26. Cassel, D., and Selinger, Z. (1978): Mechanism of adenylate cyclase activation through the β-adrenergic receptor: catecholamine-induced displacement of bound GDP by GTP. *Proc. Natl. Acad. Sci. USA*, 75:4155–4159.

27. Catt, K. J., and Dufau, M. L. (1977): Peptide hormone receptors. *Annu. Rev. Physiol.*, 39:529–557.

28. Code, C. F. (1956): Histamine and gastric secretion. In: *Ciba Foundation Symposium on Histamine*, edited by G. E. W. Walstemholme and C. H. O'Connor, pp. 189–219. Little Brown, Boston.

29. Desbuquois, M., Laudat, M. H., and Laudat, P. L. (1973): Vasoactive intestinal polypeptide and glucagon stimulation of adenylate cyclase via distinct receptors in liver and fat cell membranes. *Biochem. Biophys. Res. Commun.*, 53:1187.

30. Dockray, G. J. (1976): Immunocytochemical evidence of cholecystokinin-like peptides in brain. *Nature*, 264:568–570.

31. Dockray, G. J. (1977): Immunoreactive component in small intestine resembling the COOH terminal octapeptide of cholecystokinin. *Nature*, 270:359.

32. Dockray, G. J. (1977): Molecular evolution of gut hormones: application of comparative studies on the regulation of digestion. *Gastroenterology*, 72:344–358.

33. Dockray, G. J. (1978): Gastrin overview. In: *Gut Hormones*, edited by S. R. Bloom, pp. 129–139. Churchill Livingstone, Edinburgh.

34. Dockray, G. J., Vaillant, C., Hutchison, J., Dimaline, R., and Gregory, R. A. (1979): Characterization of molecular forms of cholecystokinin (CCK), vasoactive intestinal peptide (VIP) and bombesin-like immunoreactivity (BLI) in nerves and endocrine cells. In: *Hormone Receptors in Digestion and Nutrition*, edited by G. Rosselin, P. Fromageot, and S. Bonfils, pp. 501–511. Elsevier/North Holland, Amsterdam.

35. Douglas, W. W. (1976): The role of calcium. In: *Stimulus Secretion Coupling in the Gastrointestinal Tract*, edited by R. M. Case and H. Goebell, pp. 17–48. MTP, Lancaster.

36. Durbin, R. P. (1977): Chloride transport and acid secretion in stomach. *Gastroenterology*, 73:927–930.

37. Epelbaum, J., Brazeau, P., Tsang, D., Brawer, J., and Martin, J. B. (1977): Subcellular distribution of radio immunoassayable somatostatin in rat brain. *Brain Res.*, 126:309–323.
38. Evans, E. M., Wrigglesworth, J. M., Burdett, K., and Pover, W. F. R. (1971): Studies on epithelial cells isolated from guinea pig small intestine. *J. Cell Biol.*, 51:452–464.
39. Forte, J. G., and Lee, H. C. (1977): Gastric adenosine triphosphatases: a review of their possible role in HCl secretion. *Gastroenterology*, 73:921–926.
40. Forte, T. M., Machen, T. E., and Forte, J. G. (1977): Ultrastructure changes in oxyntic cells associated with secretory functions: A membrane-recycling hypothesis. *Gastroenterology*, 73:941–954.
41. Frizzel, R. A., Field, M., and Schultz, S. G. (1979): Sodium coupled chloride transport by epithelial tissues. *Am. J. Physiol.*, 326(1):F1–F8.
42. Frizzel, R. A., and Schultz, S. G. (1979): Models of electrolyte absorption and secretion by gastrointestinal epithelia. *Int. Rev. Physiol.*, 19:205–225.
43. Fromm, D., Dibala, R. P., and Sullivan, H. W. (1975): Ion transport by rabbit jejunum *in vivo*. *Am. J. Physiol.*, 228:160–165.
44. Fujita, T., and Kobayashi, S. (1978): Paraneuronal cells in the GEP endocrine system. In: *Gut Hormones*, edited by S. R. Bloom, pp. 414–422. Churchill Livingstone, Edinburgh.
45. Fujita, T., and Yanatori, Y. (1976): Intestinal endocrine cell reception of luminal stimuli. In: *Endocrine Gut and Pancreas*, edited by T. Fujita, pp. 237–243. Elsevier, Amsterdam.
46. Gaginella, T. S., Phillips, S. F., Dozois, R. R., and Go, V. L. W. (1978): Stimulation of adenylate cyclase in homogenates of isolated intestinal epithelial cells from hamsters. Effects of gastrointestinal hormones, prostaglandins, and deoxycholic and ricinoleic acids. *Gastroenterology*, 74:11–15.
47. Gardner, J. D. (1979): Receptors for gastrointestinal hormones. *Gastroenterology*, 76:202–214.
48. Gardner, J. D., Conlon, T. P., Fink, M. L., and Bodanszky, M. (1976): Interaction of peptides related to secretin with hormone receptors on pancreatic acinar cells. *Gastroenterology*, 71:965–970.
49. Gardner, J. D., Long, B. W., Uhlemann, E. R., and Peikin, S. R. (1978): Membrane receptors for VIP and secretin. In: *Gut Hormones*, edited by S. R. Bloom, pp. 92–96. Churchill Livingstone, Edinburgh.
50. Giachetti, A., Said, S. I., Reynolds, R. C., and Koniges, F. C. (1977): Vasoactive intestinal polypeptide in brain: localization in and release from isolated nerve terminals. *Proc. Natl. Acad. Sci. USA*, 74:3424–3428.
51. Glowinski, J. (1979): Criteria to identify peptides as neurotransmitters. In: *Hormone Receptors in Digestion and Nutrition*, edited by G. Rosselin, P. Fromageot and S. Bonfils. Elsevier/North Holland, Amsterdam.
52. Gregory, R. A., and Tracy, H. J. (1975): The chemistry of the gastrins: some recent advances. In: *Gastrointestinal Hormones*, edited by J. C. Thompson, pp. 13–24. University of Texas Press, Austin.
53. Grossman, M. I. (1970): Hypothesis: gastrin, cholecystokinin and secretin act at one receptor. *Lancet*, i:1088–1089.
54. Grossman, M. I. (1977): Physiological effects of gastrointestinal hormones. *Fed. Proc.*, 36:1930.
55. Haffen, K., Lewin, M. J. M., and Robberecht, P. (1979): Intérêt du modèle de cellules isolées du pancréas exocrine, de l'estomac et de l'intestin grêle pour la recherche en gastroentérologie. *Gastroenterol. Clin. Biol.*, 3:267–281.
56. Hawker, P. C., Mashiter, K. E., and Tunberg, L. A. (1978): Mechanisms of transport of Na, Cl, and K in the human colon. *Gastroenterology*, 74:1241–1247.
57. Helander, H. F. (1976): Stereological changes in rat parietal cells after vagotomy and antrectomy. *Gastroenterology*, 71:1010–1018.
58. Helman, C. A., and Barbezat, G. O. (1977): The effect of gastric inhibitory polypeptide on human jejunal water and electrolyte transport. *Gastroenterology*, 72:376–379.
59. Hicks, T., and Turnberg, L. A. (1973): The influence of secretin on ion transport in the human jejunum. *Gut*, 14:485–490.
60. Hirst, B. H., Smeaton, L. A., Shaw, B., Blair, E. L., and De Castiglione, R. (1979): Gastric acid secretory potency of sulphated and non sulphated gastrin- and CCK-PZ-like peptides in the cat. In: *Hormone Receptors in Digestion and Nutrition*, edited by G. Rosselin, P. Fromageot, and S. Bonfils, pp. 413–418. Elsevier/North Holland, Amsterdam.
61. Ito, S., and Schofield, G. C. (1978): Ultrastructural changes in mouse parietal cells after high H^+ secretion. *Acta Physiol. Scand. (Spec. Suppl.)*, 25–34.

62. Jacobsen, H., Demandt, A., Moody, A. J., and Sundby, F. (1977): Sequence analysis of porcine gut GLI-1. *Biochim. Biophys. Acta,* 493:452.
63. Jaeger, E., Filippi, B., Knof, S., Moroder, L., and Wünsch, E. (1979): Circular dichroism studies on secretin and some analogues with different biological activities. In: *Hormone Receptors in Digestion and Nutrition,* edited by G. Rosselin, P. Fromageot and S. Bonfils, pp. 25–32. Elsevier/North Holland, Amsterdam.
64. Johnson, G. L., Kaslow, H. R., and Bourne, H. R. (1978): Reconstitution of cholera toxin-activated adenylate cyclase. *Proc. Natl. Acad. Sci. USA,* 75:3113–3117.
65. Johnson, L. R., and Grossman, M. I. (1971): Intestinal hormones as inhibitors of gastric secretion. *Gastroenterology,* 60:120–144.
66. Johnson, L. R., Stening, G. F., and Grossman, M. I. (1970): Effect of sulfation on the gastrointestinal actions of caerulein. *Gastroenterology,* 58:208–216.
67. Johnson, L. R., Takeuchi, K., and Speir, G. L. (1979): Mucosal gastrin receptor. In: *Hormone Receptors in Digestion and Nutrition,* edited by G. Rosselin, P. Fromageot, and S. Bonfils, pp. 401–412. Elsevier/North Holland, Amsterdam.
68. Kasbekar, D. K., and Chugani, H. (1976): Role of calcium ion in in vitro acid secretion. In: *Gastric Hydrogen Ion Secretion, Vol. III,* edited by D. K. Kasbekar, G. Sachs, and W. S. Rehm, pp. 187–211. M. Dekker, New York.
69. Kimberg, D. V. (1974): Cyclic nucleotides and their role in gastrointestinal secretion. *Gastroenterology,* 67:1023–1064.
70. Kimberg, D. V., Field, M., Gershon, E., and Henderson, A. (1974): Effects of prostaglandins and cholera enterotoxin on intestinal mucosal cyclic AMP accumulation. Evidence against an essential role for prostaglandins in the action of toxin. *J. Clin. Invest.,* 53:974–979.
71. Kimura, N., and Nagata, N. (1977): The requirement of guanine nucleotides for glucagon stimulation of adenylate cyclase in rat liver plasma membranes. *J. Biol. Chem.,* 252:3829–3835.
72. Klaeveman, H. L., Conlon, T. P., Levy, A. G., and Gardner, J. D. (1975): Effect of gastrointestinal hormones on adenylate cyclase activity in human jejunal mucosa. *Gastroenterology,* 68:667–675.
73. Konturek, S. J., Pawlik, W., Tasler, J., Thor, P., Walus, K., Krol, R., Jaworek, J., and Schally, A. V. (1978): Effects of enkephalin on the gastrointestinal tract. In: *Gut Hormones,* edited by S. R. Bloom, pp. 507–512. Churchill Livingstone, Edinburgh.
74. Konturek, S. J., Thor, P., Dembinski, A., and Krol, R. (1975): Vasoactive intestinal peptide: comparison with secretin for potency and spectrum of biological action. In: *Gastrointestinal Hormones,* edited by J. C. Thompson, pp. 611–633. University of Texas Press, Austin.
75. Laburthe, M., Besson, J., Hui Bon Hoa, D., and Rosselin, G. (1977): Récepteurs du peptide intestinal vasoactif (VIP) dans les entérocytes: liaison spécifique et stimulation de l'AMP cyclique. *C. R. Acad. Sci. (Paris),* 284:D2139–D2142.
76. Laburthe, M., Prieto, J. C., Amiranoff, B., Dupont, C., Hui Bon Hoa, D., and Rosselin, G. (1979): Interaction of vasoactive intestinal peptide with isolated intestinal epithelial cells from rat. II. Characterization and structural requirements of the stimulatory effect of VIP on adenosine $3':5'$-monophosphate production. *Eur. J. Biochem.,* 96:239–248.
77. Laburthe, M., Prieto, J. C., Amiranoff, B., Hui Bon Hoa, D., Broer, Y., and Rosselin, G. (1979): Vasoactive intestinal peptide (VIP) receptors in intestinal epithelial cells: Distribution throughout the intestinal tract in rat. In: *Hormone Receptors in Digestion and Nutrition,* edited by G. Rosselin, P. Fromageot, and S. Bonfils, pp. 241–254. Elsevier/North Holland, Amsterdam.
78. Laburthe, M., Rosselin, G., Rousset, M., Zweibaum, A., Korner, M., Selinger, Z., and Schramm, M. (1979): Transfer of the hormone receptor for vaso-intestinal peptide to an adenylate cyclase system in another cell. *FEBS Lett.,* 98:41–43.
79. Lad, P. M., Welton, A. F., and Rodbell, M. (1977): Evidence for distinct guanine nucleotide sites in the regulation of the glucagon receptor and of adenylate cyclase activity. *J. Biol. Chem.,* 252:5942–5946.
80. Larsson, L. I., Fahrenkrug, J., Schaffalitzky de Muckadell, O., Sundler, F., Hakanson, R., and Rehfeld, J. F. (1976): Localization of vasoactive intestinal polypeptide (VIP) to central and peripheral neurons. *Proc. Natl. Acad. Sci. USA,* 73:3197–3200.
81. Larsson, L. I., and Rehfeld, J. F. (1977): Evidence of a common evolutionary origin of gastrin and cholecystokinin. *Nature,* 269:335–338.
82. Le Douarin, N. (1979): Les migrations des cellules dans l'embryon. *La Recherche,* 10:137–146.

83. Levinson, S. L., and Blume, A. J. (1977): Altered guanine nucleotide hydrolysis as basis for increased adenylate cyclase activity after cholera toxin treatment. *J. Biol. Chem.*, 252:3766–3774.

84. Lewin, M., Cheret, A. M., Soumarmon, A., and Girodet, J. (1974): Méthode pour l'isolement et le tri des cellules de la muqueuse fundique de rat. *Biol. Gastroenterol. (Paris)*, 7:139–144.

85. Lewin, M., Cheret, A. M., Soumarmon, A., Girodet, J., Ghesquier, D., Grelac, F., and Bonfils, S. (1976): Isolated cells and highly enriched population of parietal cells from rat mucosa for the study of H^+ secretion mechanisms. In: *Stimulus Secretion Coupling in the GI Tract*, edited by R. M. Case and H. Goebell, pp. 371–375. MTP, Lancaster.

86. Lewin, M. J. M., Grelac, F., Cheret, A. M., René, E., and Bonfils, S. (1979): Demonstration and characterization of histamine H_2-receptor on isolated guinea pig gastric cell. In: *Hormone Receptors in Digestion and Nutrition*, edited by G. Rosselin, P. Fromageot, and S. Bonfils, pp. 383–390. Elsevier/North Holland, Amsterdam.

87. Lewin, M. J. M., and Soumarmon, A. (1977): Receptors for gastrin and histamine in gastric mucosa. In: *Progress in Gastroenterology*, Vol. III, edited by B. G. J. Glass, pp. 203–240. Grune & Stratton, New York.

88. Lewin, M., Soumarmon, A., Bali, J. P., Bonfils, S., Girma, J. P., Morgat, J. L., and Fromageot, P. (1976): Interaction of ^3H synthetic human gastrin I with rat gastric plasma membranes. Evidence for the existence of biologically reactive gastrin receptor sites. *FEBS Lett.*, 66:168–172.

89. Lewin, M., Soumarmon, A., and Bonfils, S. (1977): Gastrin receptor sites in rat gastric mucosa. In: *Hormonal Receptors in Digestive Tract Physiology*, edited by S. Bonfils, P. Fromageot, and G. Rosselin, pp. 379–387. Elsevier/North Holland, Amsterdam.

90. Lewin, M., Soumarmon, A., Morgat, J. L., and Bonfils, S. (1977): Characterization of gastrin receptor sites in rat gastric mucosa. *Gastroenterology*, 72:A8/818.

91. Londos, C., Lin, M. C., Welton, A. F., Lad, P. M., and Rodbell, M. (1977): Reversible activation of hepatic adenylate cyclase by guanyl-5'-y1-(α,βmethylene)diphosphonate and guanyl-5'-y1 imidodiphosphate. *J. Biol. Chem.*, 252:5180–5182.

92. Makhlouf, G. M. (1973): Dose-response curves to gastric secretory stimulants in man. In: *International Encyclopedia of Pharmacology and Therapeutics*, edited by P. Holton, pp. 173–194. Pergamon Press, Oxford.

93. Matuchansky, C., Huet, P. M., and Mary, J. Y. (1972): Effect of cholecystokinin and metoclopramide on jejunal movements of water and electrolytes and on transit time of luminal fluid in man. *Eur. J. Clin. Invest.*, 2:169–175.

94. Meldolesi, J., De Camilli, P., and Brenna, A. (1977): The topology of plasma membrane in pancreatic acinar cells. In: *Hormonal Receptors in Digestive Tract Physiology*, edited by S. Bonfils, P. Fromageot, and G. Rosselin, pp. 203–212. Elsevier/North Holland, Amsterdam.

95. Mitjavila, M. T., Mitjavila, S., and Derache, R. (1972): Measurement of cell breakdown during incubation of isolated epithelial cells from rat intestine and new definition of respiratory coefficient. *Biol. Gastroenterol. (Paris)*, 5:273–280.

96. Modigliani, R., Bernier, J. J., Matuchansky, C., and Rambaud, J. C. (1977): Intestinal water and electrolyte transport in man under the effect of exogenous hormones of the gut and prostaglandins in patients with endocrine tumors of the pancreas. In: *Progress in Gastroenterology*, Vol. III, edited by G. B. J. Glass, pp. 285–319. Grune & Stratton, New York.

97. Modigliani, R., Mary, J. Y., and Bernier, J. J. (1976): Effects of synthetic human gastrin I on movements water, electrolytes, and glucose across the human small intestine. *Gastroenterology*, 71:978–984.

98. Moody, A. J., Frandsen, E. K., Jacobsen, H., and Sundby, F. (1979): Speculations on the structure and function of gut GLIs. In: *Hormone Receptors in Digestion and Nutrition*, edited by G. Rosselin, P. Fromageot, and S. Bonfils, pp. 55–68. Elsevier/North Holland, Amsterdam.

99. Moody, A. J., Jacobsen, H., and Sundby, F. (1978): Gastric glucagon and gut glucagon-like immunoreactants. In: *Gut Hormones*, edited by S. R. Bloom, pp. 369–378. Churchill Livingstone, Edinburgh.

100. Morgat, J. L., Girma, J. P., and Fromageot, P. (1977): Tritium labelling of peptidic hormones. In: *Hormonal Receptors in Digestive Tract Physiology*, edited by S. Bonfils, P. Fromageot, and C. Rosselin, pp. 43–51. Elsevier/North Holland, Amsterdam.

101. Moritz, M., Finkelstein, G., and Meshkinpour, H. (1973): Effect of secretin and cholecystokinin on the transport of electrolyte and water in human jejunum. *Gastroenterology*, 64:76–80.

102. Morley, J. S. (1971): Gastrin and related peptides. In: *Structure-Activity Relationships of Protein*

and Polypeptide Hormones, edited by M. Margoulies and F. C. Greenwood, pp. 11–17. Excerpta Medica, Amsterdam.

103. Morley, J. S. (1977): Information about peptide hormone receptors from structure activity studies. In: *Hormonal Receptors in Digestive Tract Physiology,* edited by S. Bonfils, P. Fromageot, and G. Rosselin, pp. 3–12. Elsevier/North Holland, Amsterdam.

104. Nakajima, S., Hirschowitz, B. I., and Sachs, G. (1971): Studies on adenylate cyclase in Necturus gastric mucosa. *Arch. Biochem. Biophys.,* 143:123–126.

105. Ogawa, N., Thompson, T., Friesen, H. G., Martin, J. B., and Brazeau, P. (1977): Properties of soluble somatostatin-binding protein. *Biochem. J.,* 165:269–277.

106. Pearse, A. G. E., Polak, J. M., and Bloom, S. R. (1977): The newer gut hormones. Cellular sources, physiology, pathology and clinical aspects. *Gastroenterology,* 72:746–761.

107. Pearse, A. G. E., and Takor Takor, T. (1976): Neuroendocrine embryology and the APUD concept. *Clin. Endocrinol (Suppl.),* 5:229s–244s.

108. Pederson, R. A., and Brown, J. C. (1972): Inhibition of histamine, pentagastrin and insulin-stimulated canine gastric secretion by pure "gastric inhibitory polypeptide." *Gastroenterology,* 62:393–399.

109. Pederson, R. A., Schubert, H. E., and Brown, J. C. (1975): The insulinotropic action of gastric inhibitory polypeptide. *Can. J. Physiol. Pharmacol.,* 53:217–223.

110. Pelletier, M. J., Chayvialle, J. A. P., and Minaire, Y. (1978): Uneven and transient secretin release after a liquid test meal. *Gastroenterology,* 75:1124–1132.

111. Pfeuffer, T. (1977): GTP-binding proteins in membranes and the control of adenylate cyclase activity. *J. Biol. Chem.,* 252:7224–7234.

112. Pham Van Chuong, P., Penke, B., de Castiglione, R., and Fromageot, P. (1979): Conformational study of gastrin C-terminal peptides by circular dichroism. In: *Hormone Receptors in Digestion and Nutrition,* edited by G. Rosselin, P. Fromageot, and S. Bonfils, pp. 33–44. Elsevier/North Holland, Amsterdam.

113. Phillips, S. F., and Gaginella, T. S. (1977): Intestinal secretion as a mechanism in diarrheal disease. In: *Progress in Gastroenterology, Vol. III,* edited by G. B. J. Glass, pp. 481–504. Grune & Stratton, New York.

114. Podesta, R. B., and Mettrick, D. F. (1977): HCO_3^- and H^+ secretion in rat ileum *in vivo. Am. J. Physiol.,* 1:E574–E579.

115. Polak, J. M., Sullivan, S. N., Bloom, S. R., Facer, P., and Pearse, A. G. E. (1977): Enkephalin-like immunoreactivity in human gastrointestinal tract. *Lancet,* i:972.

116. Powell, D., Cannon, D., Skrabanek, P., and Kirrane, J. (1978): The pathophysiology of substance P in man. In: *Gut Hormones,* edited by S. R. Bloom, pp. 524–529. Churchill Livingstone, Edinburgh.

117. Powell, D. W., Farris, R. K., and Carbonetto, S. T. (1974): Theophylline, cyclic AMP, choleragen and electrolyte transport by rabbit ileum. *Am. J. Physiol.,* 227:1428–1435.

118. Prieto, J. C., Laburthe, M., and Rosselin, G. (1979): Interaction of vasoactive intestinal peptide with isolated intestinal epithelial cells from rat. I. Characterization, quantitative aspects and structural requirements of binding sites. *Eur. J. Biochem.,* 96:229–237.

119. Racusen, L. C., and Binder, H. J. (1977): Alteration of large intestinal electrolyte transport by vasoactive intestinal polypeptide in the rat. *Gastroenterology,* 73:790–796.

120. Rasmussen, H., Jensen, P., and Goodman, D. B. P. (1976): Interaction between calcium and cyclic nucleotides in control of secretion. In: *Stimulus Secretion Coupling in the Gastrointestinal Tract,* edited by R. M. Case and H. Goebell, pp. 33–47. MTP, Lancaster.

121. Rehfeld, J. F. (1978): Dual localization of true gastrins in neuro- and adeno-hypophysis. *Nature,* 271:771–773.

122. Rehfeld, J. F. (1978): Immunochemical studies on cholecystokinin. II. Distribution and molecular heterogeneity in the central nervous system and small intestine of man and hog. *J. Biol. Chem.,* 253:4022.

123. Rehfeld, J. F. (1979): Gastrointestinal hormones. *Int. Rev. Physiol.,* 19:291–321.

124. Reyl, F., Silve, C., and Lewin, M. J. M. (1979): Somatostatin receptors on isolated gastric cells. In: *Hormone Receptors in Digestion and Nutrition,* edited by G. Rosselin, P. Fromageot, and S. Bonfils, pp. 391–400. Elsevier/North Holland, Amsterdam.

125. Rimon, G., Hanski, E., Braun, S., and Levitzki, A. (1978): Mode of coupling between hormone receptors and adenylate cyclase elucidated by modulation of membrane fluidity. *Nature,* 276:394–396.

126. Robberecht, P., Deschodt-Lanckman, M., Dehaye, J. P., and Christophe, J. (1978): Secretin-VIP interactions. In: *Gut Hormones,* edited by S. R. Bloom, pp. 97–103. Churchill Livingstone, Edinburgh.

127. Robberecht, P., Deschodt-Lanckman, M., and Vanderhaeghen, J. J. (1978): Demonstration of biological activity of brain gastrin-like peptidic material in the human: Its relationship with the COOH-terminal octapeptide of cholecystokinin. *Proc. Natl. Acad. Sci. USA,* 75:524–528.

128. Robein, M. J., de la Mare, M. C., Dubrasquet, J. M., and Bonfils, S. (1979): Utilization of the perfused stomach in anaesthetized rats to study the inhibitory effect of somatostatin in gastric acid secretion. *Agents Actions (In press).*

129. Romrell, L. J., Coope, M. R., Munro, D. R., and Ito, S. (1975): Isolation and separation of highly enriched fractions of viable mouse gastric parietal cells by velocity sedimentation. *J. Cell Biol.,* 65:428–438.

130. Sachs, G., Chang, H. H., Rabon, E., Schackman, R., Lewin, M., and Saccomani, G. (1976): A non electrogenic H^+ pump in plasma membrane of hog stomach. *J. Biol. Chem.,* 251:7690–7698.

131. Sachs, G., Rabon, E., Hung, H., Schackman, R., Sarau, H. M., and Saccomani, G. (1977): An H^+ pump and fusion model in stomach. In: *Hormonal Receptors in Digestive Tract Physiology,* edited by S. Bonfils, P. Fromageot, and G. Rosselin, pp. 347–360. Elsevier/North Holland, Amsterdam.

132. Sachs, G., Spenney, J. G., and Lewin, M. (1978): H^+ transport: Regulation and mechanism in gastric mucosa and membrane vesicles. *Physiol. Rev.,* 58:106–173.

133. Said, S. I. (1978): VIP overview. In: *Gut Hormones,* edited by S. R. Bloom, pp. 465–469. Churchill Livingstone, Edinburgh.

134. Said, S. I., and Rosenberg, R. N. (1976): Vasoactive intestinal polypeptide: Abundant immunoreactivity in neural cell lines and normal nervous tissue. *Science,* 192:907–908.

135. Schaffalitzky de Muckadell, O. B., and Fahrenkrug, J. (1978): Secretion pattern of secretin in man: regulation by gastric acid. *Gut,* 19:812.

136. Schaffalitzky de Muckadell, O. B., Fahrenkrug, J., and Holst, J. J. (1977): Release of vasoactive intestinal polypeptide (VIP) by electric stimulation of the vagal nerves. *Gastroenterology,* 72:373–375.

137. Schonbrunn, A., and Tashjian, A. H., Jr. (1978): Characterization of functional receptors for somatostatin in rat pituitary cells in culture. *J. Biol. Chem.,* 253:6473–6483.

138. Schramm, M., Orly, J., Eimerl, S., and Korner, M. (1977): Coupling of hormone receptors to adenylate cyclase of different cells by cell fusion. *Nature,* 268:310–313.

139. Schultz, S. G. (1977): Sodium-coupled solute transport by small intestine: a status report. *Am. J. Physiol.,* 2:249–254.

140. Schwartz, J. C., Kimberg, D. V., Sheerin, H. E., Field, M., and Said, S. I. (1974): Vasoactive intestinal peptide stimulation of adenylate cyclase and active electrolyte secretion in intestinal mucosa. *J. Clin. Invest.,* 54:536–544.

141. Simon, B., and Kather H. (1979): Human gastric mucosal adenylate cyclase. Modulation of enzyme activity by histamine, vasoactive intestine peptide and prostaglandins. In: *Hormone Receptors in Digestion and Nutrition,* edited by G. Rosselin, P. Fromageot, and S. Bonfils, pp. 419–429. Elsevier/North Holland, Amsterdam.

142. Soll, A. H. (1978): The actions of secretagogues on oxygen uptake by isolated mammalian parietal cells. *J. Clin. Invest.,* 61:370–380.

143. Soumarmon, A., Cheret, A. M., and Lewin, M. J. M. (1977): Localization of gastrin receptors in intact isolated and separated rat fundic cells. *Gastroenterology,* 73:900–903.

144. Soumarmon, A., and Racker, E. (1978): Chloride transport in gastric cells and microsomes. In: *Frontiers of Biological Energetics,* Vol. I, edited by P. L. Dutton, J. Leigh, and A. Scarpa, pp. 555–562. Academic Press, New York.

145. Sundler, F., Alumets, J., and Hakanson, R. (1978): Peptides in the gut with a dual distribution in nerves and endocrine cells. In: *Gut Hormones,* edited by S. R. Bloom, pp. 406–413. Churchill Livingstone, Edinburgh.

146. Uvnäs-Wallensten, K. (1977): Occurrence of gastrin in gastric juice in antral secretion and in antral perfusates of cats. *Acta Physiol. Scand.,* 96:19.

147. Uvnäs-Wallensten, K., and Effendic, S. (1979): Release of gastrin and insulin by electrical

vagal stimulation and sulphonuric drugs from endocrine cells and nerves in the cat. In: *Hormone Receptors in Digestion and Nutrition,* edited by G. Rosselin, P. Fromageot, and S. Bonfils, pp. 493–500. Elsevier/North Holland, Amsterdam.

148. Uvnäs-Wallensten, K., Rehfeld, J. F., Larsson, L. I., and Uvnäs, B. (1977): Heptadecapeptide gastrin in the vagal nerve. *Proc. Natl. Acad. Sci. USA,* 74:5707–5710.

149. Veber, D. F., Holly, F. W., Paleveda, W. J., Nutt, R. F., Bergstrand, S. J., Torchiana, M., Glitzer, M. S., Saperstein, R., and Hirschmann, R. (1978): Conformationally restricted bicyclic analogs of somatostatin. *Proc. Natl. Acad. Sci. USA,* 75:2636–2640.

150. Waldman, D. B., Gardner, J. D., Zfass, A. M., and Makhlouf, G. M. (1977): Effects of vasoactive intestinal peptide, secretin and related peptides on rat colonic transport and adenylate cyclase activity. *Gastroenterology,* 73:518–523.

151. Walsh, J. H., and Grossman, M. I. (1975): Gastrin. *N. Engl. J. Med.,* 292:1324–1334 and 1377–1384.

152. Welton, A. F., Lad, P. M., Newby, A. C., Yamamura, H., Nicosia, S., and Rodbell, M. (1977): Solubilization and separation of the glucagon receptor and adenylate cyclase in guanine nucleotide-sensitive states. *J. Biol. Chem.,* 252:5947–5950.

153. Wunsch, E. (1979): Peptide factors: definition of purity. In: *Hormone Receptors in Digestion and Nutrition,* edited by G. Rosselin, P. Fromageot, and S. Bonfils, pp. 115–125. Elsevier/North Holland, Amsterdam.

Effects of Gastrointestinal Hormones and Peptides on Gastrointestinal Tract

Gastrointestinal Hormones, edited by
George B. Jerzy Glass.
Raven Press, New York © 1980.

Chapter 22

Effect of Gastrointestinal Hormones on Growth of Gastrointestinal Tissue

Leonard R. Johnson

Department of Physiology, University of Texas Medical School, Houston, Texas 77025

INTRODUCTION

During the past 5 years much of the renewed interest in gastrointestinal hormones developed from observations demonstrating that the members of this group of peptides regulate growth of digestive tract tissue, may have important actions outside the gastrointestinal tract, are released from nerves in some cases, and regulate the release of other hormones—insulin in particular. This represents a clear departure from the classic concept of the actions of the gastrointestinal hormones. Their obvious actions, the actions that led to their discoveries and the actions for which they are named, are their dramatic effects on motility and secretion of the digestive tract.

The other hormones are primarily regarded as regulators of metabolism or the secretion of hormones. The classic actions of the gastrointestinal hormones and the notion that they were confined to the mucosa of the gastrointestinal tract placed them solely in the realm of digestive physiology and outside the realm of endocrinology in general.

This spurious division has, however, come to an end, and the major interest in this field now concerns the role of gastrointestinal peptides in carbohydrate metabolism, hormone release, growth of gut mucosa and the pancreas, and neural transmission. The purpose of this chapter is to summarize the information available concerning the effects of the gastrointestinal hormones on growth and to set that information in perspective with normal physiology.

The first presumptive evidence that gastrointestinal hormones influence growth is found in a number of studies describing the long-term effects of antrectomy on the remaining oxyntic gland mucosa. Lees and Grandjean (44) biopsied the gastric mucosal remnant in 33 healthy postantrectomy patients. One of these was considered normal and 22 exhibited moderate to complete atrophy. In another study 56 patients, 81.5% of whom had normal preoperative gastric mucosal biopsies, underwent partial gastrectomy for duodenal ulcer (21). Twelve months later 70.4% had varying degrees of atrophic gastritis, and the thickness of the parietal cell layer had decreased from a mean of 0.71 mm preoperatively to 0.51 mm. These results cannot be explained on the basis of disuse hypotrophy, for vagotomy and antrectomy both decrease acid by about 60% yet mucosal atrophy does not occur after vagotomy (55). The decrease in acid secretion after antrectomy in man can be partially prevented by infusing pentagastrin continuously during the first week after antrectomy (61). This finding indicates that exogenous gastrin prevents mucosal atrophy in man following antrectomy.

The opposite picture, mucosal hyperplasia, occurs in patients having hypergastrinemia due to the so-called Zollinger-Ellison syndrome (23). Gastric mucosal hyperplasia with an increased parietal cell count are characteristic of this disease (15). Clinically, therefore, the overproduction of gastrin is associated with gastrointestinal mucosal growth and the lack of the hormone with mucosal atrophy.

These observations could be explained if gastrin were a trophic hormone and led us to examine the effect of pentagastrin on protein synthesis (31). Rats were divided into three groups and injected with saline, pentagastrin, or histamine. Doses of pentagastrin ranged from threshold to supermaximal for gastric acid secretion. The animals were killed 90 min after a single injection and homogenates of various tissues incubated with [^{14}C]leucine. A dose of pentagastrin, submaximal for acid secretion, caused a 60 to 100% stimulation of protein synthesis in oxyntic glandular mucosa and a 300% stimulation in duodenal mucosa (31). There was no stimulation of protein synthesis in either liver or skeletal muscle. Histamine had no effect on protein synthesis in any of the tissues examined. The stimulation of leucine incorporation was related to the dose of pentagastrin in a typical sigmoid manner. From this study we concluded that: (a) gastrin stimulates protein synthesis, (b) this effect is specific to certain tissues of the digestive tract, and (c) the effect is independent of secretory phenomena. In addition, we hypothesized that gastrin was a trophic hormone and regulated the growth of gastrointestinal tract mucosa (31).

The above conclusions have been supported by numerous studies, and gastrin has been shown to stimulate most of the metabolic responses associated with growth (30).

TROPHIC EFFECTS OF EXOGENOUS GI HORMONES

Gastrin

Chronic *in vivo* administration of pharmacological amounts of pentagastrin causes oxyntic gland hyperplasia with increased mucosal height and volume and parietal cell mass (7). The peptic cell population increased approximately 20%, but this was not statistically significant. Crean et al. (7) attributed these results to either increased acid secretion or a direct effect of pentagastrin.

Most investigators have examined one or more of the metabolic processes associated with growth rather than actually determining increases in cell numbers. The obvious advantages to this are that the biochemical changes occur rapidly after single or only a few injections of hormone and that the assay methods are less time consuming. The biochemical processes regulated by trophic hormones include increased amino acid uptake, stimulation of protein, RNA, and DNA synthesis, and decreased protein catabolism. Collectively this reaction to a growth-stimulating substance is called the pleiotypic response. Stimulation of RNA, protein, and DNA synthesis have all been shown to occur with gastrin (28). In rats treated repeatedly with gastrin for at least 48 hr the increases in tissue content of protein and nucleic acids become significant (28).

As mentioned earlier, pentagastrin stimulates the *in vitro* incorporation of leucine into protein of gastric and duodenal mucosa (31). Synthetic human gastrin also caused a significant stimulation of *in vivo* protein synthesis in both duodenal and gastric mucosa (30). This study was the first to examine the trophic effects of a pure circulating form of gastrin.

Protein synthesized under the stimulation of pentagastrin appears to be confined to the gastric mucosal cells rather than secreted. Enochs and Johnson (17) injected rats with pentagastrin or saline and incubated pieces of oxyntic gland mucosa in tissue culture medium containing labeled amino acid. Over a period of time labeled protein appeared in both mucosa and the medium. However, the amounts appearing in the medium were the same for both groups of rats whereas there was considerable stimulation of the synthesis of protein in the tissue (17). Sutton and Donaldson (72) supported this finding by demonstrating that the *in vitro* addition of pentagastrin to isolated gastric mucosa maintained by organ culture increased the overall incorporation of [^{14}C]leucine into gastric mucosal protein. Acetylcholine, cholecystokinin (CCK), secretin, and pentagastrin all stimulated the secretion of macromolecular protein, but only pentagastrin increased synthesis of tissue protein (72). Sutton and Donaldson interpreted their findings as confirming the trophic effect of pentagastrin.

Tissue cultures of gastric mucosal epithelial cells exposed to pentagastrin accumulated protein much more rapidly than their counterparts exposed to saline or histamine (57). Five days after culture flasks were inoculated with equal amounts of identical cells, those treated with pentagastrin contained twice as much protein as the saline or histamine controls.

Three injections of 250 μg/kg of pentagastrin resulted in a significant stimulation of RNA synthesis in both duodenal and gastric mucosa (5). RNA synthesis was measured by following the incorporation of [^{14}C]orotic acid into RNA. Gastrin did not stimulate RNA synthesis in the liver. Pentagastrin prevents the decrease in RNA and DNA content of fundic and duodenal mucosa in antrectomized animals (32). Chronic administration of pentagastrin increases the total amount of pancreatic RNA in both normal (53) and hypophysectomized (54) rats. This effect appears to be restricted to the acinar cells. Duodenal and gastric RNA synthesis appears to peak 2 to 3 hr after a single injection of pentagastrin (17).

In order to prove that an agent stimulates growth, one must demonstrate an increased number of cells after exposure to the agent. Increased DNA synthesis and tissue content of DNA are biochemical indicators of equal significance. Protein and RNA synthesis and content also increase during growth; however, these parameters can increase at times (hypertrophy) when cell numbers are not increasing. Ideally one must be able to demonstrate an increase in total DNA content to ensure that a measured increase in DNA synthesis is not being matched by an increase in cell turnover. This is not possible in short-term experiments, since it takes at least 48 hr for DNA to accumulate sufficiently to show a statistically significant increase. The best approach has proven to be a combination of short- and long-term experiments whereby different doses, tissues, and agents can be rapidly screened for trophic effects by measuring DNA synthesis. Once optimal conditions are established, a chronic study can be done to demonstrate a significant accumulation of DNA. In a long-term study a steady state has usually been reached and the incorporation of [^{3}H]thymidine into DNA expressed per micrograms DNA will be no different from control.

Willems et al. (78) found stimulation of the uptake of [^{3}H]thymidine into canine gastric mucosa after a 4-hr infusion of porcine gastrin. Thymidine uptake was significantly stimulated at 12 hr after gastrin infusion and peaked at 16 hr. Also using autoradiography we have demonstrated that pentagastrin stimulates the uptake of [^{3}H]thymidine into nuclei of cultured duodenal cells (47).

In neither of the above studies was it possible to distinguish between bound thymidine and thymidine actually incorporated into DNA. There is little doubt, however, that incorporation occurred because thymidine uptake was followed by increased cell division in both studies (47,78). Assessment of DNA synthesis by measuring the incorporation of [^{3}H]thymidine into DNA isolated from gastrointestinal mucosa has proven that gastrin stimulates the formation of DNA (34,35).

We injected rats with 250 μg/kg of pentagastrin or an equivalent volume of saline and killed them at various times after injection (35). Small pieces from the oxyntic gland area, duodenum, ileum, and liver were removed and incubated for 30 min in tissue culture medium containing [^{3}H]thymidine. The DNA was extracted and the incorporation of thymidine determined. Pentagastrin had no effect on DNA synthesis in the liver. In all other tissues maximal stimulation occurred 16 hr after injection of hormone. In this particular study incorporation of thymidine in pentagastrin-injected animals was 275% of control for the stomach, 300% for the duodenum, and 480% for the ileum. In another series of studies histamine (20 mg/kg) had no effect on DNA synthesis. If pentagastrin is administered over a 48-hr period as six equally spaced injections, one is able to detect significant increases in total DNA and RNA as well as in DNA synthesis (35).

These effects of gastrin on parameters related to growth are essentially identical to those that have been described for growth hormone, androgens, and estrogens (26,74,80).

Most experiments involving the trophic effects of exogenous gastrin have utilized the synthetic analog pentagastrin. Gastrin was originally isolated by Gregory and co-workers (24) from porcine antral mucosa as the heptadecapeptide now referred to as G-17 or "little gastrin." Subsequently Yalow and Berson (83) found that the major circulating form of gastrin was a 34 amino acid peptide (G-34), which they named "big gastrin." Qualitatively the actions of pentagastrin, G-17, and G-34 in mammalian systems have proven to be identical although their potencies differ (75). The results of a study designed to compare the trophic activity of the circulating gastrins with that of pentagastrin were not unexpected (37). Those results were in general agreement with the structure-activity relationships of the gastrin molecules as determined for their stimulation of acid secretion. The maximal effects of G-34 II, G-17 I, G-17 II, and pentagastrin on DNA synthesis and DNA accumulation in duodenal and oxyntic gland mucosa were equal. Peak stimulation occurred with 6.75 nmoles/kg G-34 II, 13.5 nmoles/kg G-17 I and G-17 II, and with 32.5 nmoles/kg of pentagastrin. From this study we concluded that (a) the naturally occurring gastrins possess trophic activity, (b) sulfation has no effect on trophic activity, and (c) G-17 and G-34 are at least as effective in stimulating growth as they are in stimulating gastric acid secretion (37).

Gastrin appears to be a trophic hormone for the oxyntic gland mucosa and the mucosa of the entire small and large intestines. The trophic effects of gastrin on the oxyntic gland and duodenal mucosa have been documented previously in this chapter. Using similar studies, investigators also have shown that gastrin stimulates DNA synthesis and increases DNA, RNA, and protein content of ileal (35) and proximal large bowel mucosa (38). Gastrin does not appear to stimulate growth of gut smooth muscle (30).

The most notable exceptions to the trophic action of gastrin are the mucosae of the antrum and esophagus (29). It is not surprising that gastrin stimulates growth of the two tissues, oxyntic gland and duodenal mucosa, proximal and distal to the antrum without affecting the antrum itself. Regulation of antral growth by gastrin would be in opposition to the general concepts of endocrine physiology, for this tissue is the origin of most physiologically released gastrin. Thyroxine, cortisol, androgens, and estrogens regulate metabolism and growth in a number of tissues, but not in their glands of origin. The growth of the thyroid, adrenals, and sex glands is regulated by pituitary peptide hormones. Endocrine cells of the antrum proliferate during periods of chronic stimulation for the release of gastrin. Antrocolic transposition resulted in significant increases in enterochromaffin cells (43,46) and gastrin cells (46). Lichtenberger et al. (48) have demonstrated that fasting reduces both antral and serum gastrin content. Both were increased by feeding. In general, stimulation of gastrin release results in higher levels of antral gastrin.

There have been no trophic effects described for gastrin in any tissue outside the gastrointestinal tract except for the pancreas. Those that have been examined include liver (31,34,35,54), skeletal muscle (31), kidneys (39,54), spleen (39,54), and testes (39).

As in the case of most fields of study involving acute biochemical experiments, the standard animal employed for the investigation of the trophic effects of gastrin has been the rat. Most of the experiments described in the preceding discussion have utilized this animal. Gastrin stimulates thymidine uptake and increases the mitotic index in the dog (78). Physiologic serum levels of gastrin have also been shown to stimulate DNA synthesis of the canine Heidenhain pouch as well as the normally innervated stomach (67). Most evidence that gastrin has trophic effects in man has been indirect, stemming in large part from observations of mucosal hyperplasia in patients with hypergastrinemia (15,58). These studies plus those showing mucosal atrophy in patients having undergone antrectomy provide presumptive evidence that growth of human gastrointestinal mucosa is regulated by gastrin. It is obvious that direct studies are necessary before the physiological significance of the trophic action of gastrin can be established in man.

Cholecystokinin (CCK)

Cholecystokinin (CCK) is structurally and functionally related to gastrin. The active C-terminal tetrapeptide amide of gastrin is duplicated in CCK. The major structural difference that dictates whether a peptide of the CCK-gastrin family has a gastrin-like or CCK-like pattern of activity is the position of the tyrosyl residue and whether or not it is sulfated. Qualitatively the actions of gastrin and CCK are identical, but gastrin has high affinity for receptors stimulating acid secretion and low affinity for those involved in gallbladder contraction and pancreatic enzyme secretion. The opposite pattern prevails for peptides more closely related to CCK. Owing to the overlapping activity patterns and the tendency for CCK to have a higher affinity for tissues located more distally in the digestive tract, it seemed likely that CCK would have trophic influences on the pancreas and small intestine.

Most studies involving the trophic action of CCK have been conducted on the pancreas and are covered in a later section of this chapter together with the actions of all the gut hormones on pancreatic growth. The effects of CCK on growth of oxyntic gland and duodenal mucosa have been examined in only one study that I am aware of (36). Low doses of CCK octapeptide (CCK–OP) causing a small but significant increase in pancreatic DNA synthesis had no stimulatory effect on mucosa of the oxyntic gland area or duodenum of the same animals. DNA content of the pancreas was also increased, indicating that the increase in synthesis was not matched by an increase in turnover. At higher doses of CCK–OP there was a slight increase in duodenal DNA synthesis and content that was of borderline statistical significance. Further increasing the dose of CCK–OP inhibited the trophic effect of pentagastrin in both the stomach and the duodenum. We concluded that although CCK is probably a physiologically important regulator of growth of the exocrine pancreas, it is unlikely that it exerts a trophic influence on either the stomach or duodenum (36).

Secretin

There have been relatively few studies involving the trophic action of secretin on the mucosa of the gastrointestinal tract. In general, secretin appears to inhibit the trophic actions of gastrin and to have no antitrophic activity of its own. In one study rats having gastric cannulas were injected three times daily for 2 weeks with pentagastrin, secretin, pentagastrin plus secretin, or saline (69). Basal and maximal acid outputs were measured before, during, and after the injection period. Parietal cell mass was determined at the end of the study. Pentagastrin injection led to a 90% increase in maximal acid output. This increase failed to occur in the rats receiving secretin in addition to pentagastrin. The parietal cell population increased by 70% in the gastrin-injected rats. This too was prevented by secretin. The animals receiving only secretin had slightly lower secretory capacities and parietal cell counts than the saline-injected controls (69).

Secretin has been shown to inhibit the gastrin stimulation of DNA synthesis and accumulation in mucosa of the oxyntic gland area of the stomach, the duodenum (35), and the colon (38). The effects of secretin do not depend on its ability to inhibit gastrin-stimulated acid secretion, since metiamide, a potent inhibitor of acid secretion, had no significant effect on the trophic response to gastrin (35). Pansu et al. (63) found that secretin prevented the peaks in the labeling and mitotic indices in the circadian rhythm of rat jejunal mucosa. Pentagastrin, on the other hand, prevented the nadirs. These authors concluded that secretin and gastrin act as trophic factors for intestinal mucosa producing opposite effects on cell proliferation (63).

The remaining question is whether secretin has antitrophic activity of its own or whether it acts solely by inhibiting the growth-promoting effects of gastrin. Considering the profound inhibition of gastrin's trophic activity caused by secretin, it is entirely possible that these antitrophic effects were due to the inhibition of endogenous gastrin. Because it is almost impossible to remove all sources of gastrin surgically, this point will best be settled by studying the metabolic effects of secretin on *in vitro* systems involving cell or organ culture.

Other GI Peptides

The trophic effects of two additional members of the secretin family, vasoactive intestinal peptide (VIP) and glucagon, have been examined in mucosa of the oxyntic gland and proximal colon (29). Like secretin, VIP had no effect on DNA synthesis when given by itself and inhibited the stimulation caused by gastrin. Glucagon, however, stimulated DNA synthesis at several doses. The maximal effect of glucagon equaled about 50% of the increase caused by pentagastrin in the same experiments. Glucagon produced no inhibition of the trophic action of gastrin. There is no evidence supporting a physiological role for either VIP or glucagon in the regulation of mucosal growth.

Effects of GI Peptides on Pancreatic Growth

The pancreas was formerly considered to be a stable organ not possessing growth and regenerative capabilities (42). This conclusion was based on low numbers of mitotic indices (62) and autoradiographic data (42). However, numerous other studies indicated that the pancreas was capable of growth and regeneration. Fitzgerald et al. (18,19,45) demonstrated pancreatic regeneration after surgical resection of 50% of the gland or following the cessation of ethionine administration. Both hypertrophy and hyperplasia have been described in rats and chickens fed uncooked soybeans (2,6). It was then shown that soybeans contained a trypsin inhibitor, and that inhibition of tryptic activity in the duodenum augmented pancreatic secretion. It was also suggested that the hypersecretion led to increased pancreatic growth (2). Green and Lyman (22) have postulated that trypsin inhibition acts by binding trypsin and chymotrypsin and thus preventing their feedback inhibition of CCK release from endocrine cells of the duodenal mucosa.

Rothman and Wells (66) in 1967 first described the effects of CCK on pancreatic size and weight. The increases in weight were presumed to be due to increased synthesis of pancreatic enzymes and total enzyme content of the gland. Mayston and Barrowman (53) found that chronic injection of pentagastrin resulted in pancreatic hypertrophy but not hyperplasia. Mainz et al. (50) were actually the first to show that a gastrointestinal hormone increased pancreatic DNA, thus stimulating the growth of the organ. They elegantly demonstrated that CCK, but not bethanechol, also a secretagogue, increased DNA content of the pancreas and stimulated DNA synthesis. This study proved that trophic effects of pancreatic secretagogues were not necessarily tied to their secretory properties. Similar data had been provided for the trophic effect of gastrin on oxyntic gland mucosa (31). CCK, however, has also been shown to dramatically increase the enzymatic secretory capacity of the pancreas (65). In that study chronic treatment with pentagastrin or secretin appeared to have no effect on pancreatic enzyme and bicarbonate responses to CCK and secretin.

To my knowledge, there are only two papers reporting effects of chronic secretin treatment on the pancreas. Petersen et al. (65) injected rats with 100 unit/kg secretin three times a day for 15 days and found a 9% increase in pancreatic weight. Secretin treatment decreased the sensitivity of the pancreas to secretin without altering the maximal bicarbonate response. In a second study by the same group Solomon et al. (68) showed that secretin significantly increased pancreatic weight and content of RNA and lipase after 15 days treatment. We found that secretin increased pancreatic RNA significantly after 7 days, but also significantly increased DNA content and stimulated DNA synthesis (13). From our data we concluded that secretin stimulates pancreatic hyperplasia as well as hypertrophy.

The effects of the combination of secretin and cerulein are dramatic (13,68). Pancreatic weight and total pancreatic RNA and DNA content were all significantly greater than could be explained by simple addition of the individual effects of the peptides. This finding of potentiation was supported by results with DNA synthesis (13). This indicates that the noncompetitive augmentation of DNA and RNA content by secretin and cerulein, which must be expressed per whole pancreas to be evident, is indeed due to the interactions of these agents on the cell division process. This potentiation of growth appears to be identical to the enhanced secretory effects of secretin and CCK when they are administered jointly (56), and suggests that the interaction of these peptides is physiologically important in regulating pancreatic growth as well.

The administration of large doses of pentagastrin (2 mg/100 g body wt/day) over a 2-week period resulted in pancreatic acinar cell hypertrophy (53). Hypertrophy was accompanied by a decrease in the specific activities of pancreatic enzymes, which was a result of increased protein and RNA content of the tissue. There was no increase in pancreatic DNA; thus the RNA:DNA ratio increased significantly. Chronic histamine administration had no similar effects on the pancreas. Mayston and Barrowman (53) concluded that gastrin was a trophic hormone for the pancreas and that this tissue should be added to the others shown to be under its influence. Actually the results of this study do not suggest a growth-stimulating effect on the pancreas, for DNA did not increase and acinar cell hyperplasia did not occur, only hypertrophy. In a more recent study, however, the same authors have demonstrated both pancreatic hypertrophy and hyperplasia in hypophysectomized animals treated with pentagastrin (54). The deleterious results of hypophysectomy were prevented not only in the pancreas but also in the stomach and duodenum. Pentagastrin did not stimulate growth of the liver, kidneys, or adrenal glands of the hypophysectomized rats (54).

We have recently demonstrated that gastrin stimulates DNA synthesis (13) and confirmed the findings of others that it increases pancreatic RNA, DNA, and protein content. Unexpectedly, we also found that secretin, even though it stimulated pancreatic growth by itself and augmented the effect of CCK, inhibited the effect of gastrin. Since gastrin and CCK are structurally related, the different effects of secretin on the pancreatic trophic responses to these two agents may indicate that the receptors for the trophic effects of gastrin and CCK in the pancreas are different and that secretin interacts in a different manner with these two receptors.

Taken together, the dramatic action of gut hormones on pancreatic growth opens up an interesting and important new field of investigation.

MECHANISMS OF THE TROPHIC EFFECT OF GASTRIN

A number of basic questions can be asked about the mechanism of action of any hormone. First, is the metabolic effect in question a direct result of a secondary process stimulated by the hormone—gastric acid secretion in the case of gastrin? Second, is the effect in question due to a direct action of the hormone or due to another factor whose synthesis and release are stimulated by the hormone? Third, what are the basic biochemical events leading to the observed effect of the hormone?

Independence of the Trophic and Secretory Effects of Gastrin

Many experiments involving the trophic action of gastrin have included a group of histamine-injected animals to control for acid secretion. The results of these studies have been unanimous in that metabolic actions of gastrin were not duplicated by histamine. These experiments have demonstrated gastrin stimulation of parietal cell hyperplasia (7), pancreatic hyperplasia (53), gastric and duodenal protein synthesis (31), gastric and duodenal RNA synthesis (5), DNA synthesis and growth of cultured duodenal cells (47), and gastric, duodenal, and ileal DNA synthesis (34,35).

The studies listed above were done on rats, and histamine is an extremely poor secretagogue when compared with gastrin in the rat (27). Therefore, it can be argued that these experiments are not really effective controls for the effects of acid secretion. For this reason the study by Willems et al. (78) using the dog is especially significant. They infused either gastrin or histamine over a period of 4 hr in doses producing nearly identical acid outputs. Thymidine uptake into gastric mucosal cells and cell division were significantly stimulated in the animals receiving gastrin. There was no stimulation in any histamine-infused dog.

Further evidence that the trophic actions of gastrin are independent of secretory effects is provided by a study in which DNA synthesis in response to pentagastrin was studied in the presence of inhibitors of gastric acid secretion (35). Metiamide, a histamine H_2-receptor antagonist that also inhibits gastrin-stimulated acid secretion, was administered in combination with pentagastrin in a dose shown to block acid secretion almost completely. In this experiment pentagastrin alone caused a 40% stimulation of DNA synthesis in the oxyntic gland mucosa and an 80% increase in duodenal mucosa. These values were not significantly altered when metiamide was administered with pentagastrin.

From the foregoing discussion it is also obvious that gastrin stimulates growth in numerous parts of the digestive tract that do not secrete acid. Other areas, such as the lower small intestinal mucosa, colonic mucosa, and the pancreas are never exposed to acid. Yet doses of gastrin trophic for the mucosa of the oxyntic gland are trophic for these tissues as well. Secretin, which inhibits the trophic action of gastrin in the oxyntic gland area, is just as potent an inhibitor in small and large bowel mucosa. As one body of data these studies provide overwhelming evidence that the growth response to gastrin is unrelated to its secretory effects.

Gastrin Stimulates Growth Directly

The best evidence that a hormone is acting directly on its target cells is to be able to demonstrate its effects by exposing tissue to the hormone *in vitro*. Such a demonstration, of course, does not eliminate the possibility that a second messenger, such as one of the cyclic nucleotides, is involved in stimulating processes within the cell. It does, however, mean that the hormone is not causing the synthesis and/or release of a second agent that is transported by the blood to react with receptors on the target cells. Growth hormone and somatomedin offer the best examples of this second type of process (10,11). Stimulation of sulfate uptake and protein synthesis in cartilage are widely recognized effects of growth hormone. These effects cannot be produced by adding growth hormone directly to cartilage *in vitro*. Plasma from normal rats added to cartilage from hypophysectomized rats, however, stimulates sulfate and amino acid incorporation (11). Recently this "sulfation factor" contained in normal plasma has been identified as a peptide whose synthesis in the liver is dependent on growth hormone. This substance has been named somatomedin and is responsible for many, and perhaps most, of the effects of growth hormone (10).

There are several studies demonstrating trophic actions of gastrin *in vitro*. Miller et al. (57) found that pentagastrin at a concentration of 500 ng/ml maintained tissue cultures of rat and human oxyntic gland mucosa. Saline-treated cultures contained primarily fibroblasts whereas epithelial cells with junctional complexes predominated in the gastrin-inoculated flasks. At confluency the mitotic activity of the pentagastrin-treated culture was more than twice that of controls. Gastrin-treated cultures contained twice the amount of protein when compared with control cultures started at the same time with identical inocula (57). Using organ cultures of oxyntic gland mucosa, Sutton and Donaldson (72) showed that although most secretagogues stimulated pepsinogen synthesis, only gastrin was capable of stimulating the synthesis of structural protein.

Lichtenberger et al. (47) examined the effects of pentagastrin on duodenal cells growing in tissue culture. After cultures of adult rat duodenal cells were established, the contents of half the flasks were exposed to pentagastrin and half to saline once daily. After 3 months the pentagastrin-treated cultures contained approximately 90% epithelial cells and 10% fibroblasts, whereas the control cultures constituted an epithelial cell-fibroblast admixture of about 50% each. Epithelial cells appeared quite similar in structure to crypt cells, although a positive identification was not made. However, because gastrin-stimulated cultures of gastric mucosal cells also contained poorly differentiated cells, this evidence suggests that the trophic effect of gastrin is on generative cells in the mitotic locus and not on secretory cells. Pentagastrin-treated cultures had a faster doubling time, 19.5 hr compared with 31.5 hr for saline-treated controls. This was attributed in part to the greater percentage of cells in the proliferative population in the hormone-treated cultures, 73% in comparison with the controls' 36%. This latter measurement was arrived at by autoradiographic determination of [^{3}H]thymidine incorporation into DNA.

The results of these *in vitro* studies employing organ and tissue culture techniques are proof that the trophic action of gastrin is due to a direct interaction of the hormone with receptors on its target cells, and not to a secondary factor released or synthesized by gastrin.

Biochemical Mechanism

Following the binding of a peptide hormone to its receptor, a chain of events begins that leads to the overt manifestation of hormone action. Whether the binding of gastrin stimulates the production of a second messenger is unknown. The earliest response related to growth following the administration of gastrin is a significant increase in mRNA (17). Significant increases in mRNA occur 30 to 60 min after gastrin treatment. By 2 to 3 hr all other species of RNA are also significantly increased (17). Majumdar and Goltermann (51) found a 100% increase in the number of gastric mucosal polysomes 1 hr after the injection of pentagastrin in fasted rats. This observation supports the findings of Enochs and Johnson (17) that stimulation of mRNA production is one of the earliest events associated with the trophic action of gastrin. Protein synthesis began to increase 2 to 4 hr after gastrin injection and peaked at 6 hr (17). In organ cultures of gastric mucosa protein synthesis was increased 7 hr after gastrin treatment (72). Inhibition of mRNA synthesis with actinomycin-D prevented the gastrin-induced stimulation of protein synthesis (17). Sixteen hours after gastrin injection DNA synthesis is maximally elevated in the gastric mucosa of both the rat (17) and dog (78). The mitotic index in canine gastric mucosa is increased fivefold at 20 and 24 hr (78).

This picture of the biochemical events following the injection of gastrin is consistent with the known mechanisms of action of other trophic hormones. Korner (40) has shown that hypophysectomized animals have a deficiency in the formation of polyribosomes that can be corrected by addition of polyuridine, indicating a decreased availability of mRNA. The addition of growth hormone resulted in a initial stimulation of mRNA followed by increases in all types of RNA and the stimulation of protein synthesis (41). Subsequent experiments indicated that growth hormone facilitated the formation of DNA-RNA polymerase complex and hence RNA synthesis (64).

The next step in elucidating the mechanism by which gastrin stimulates the biochemical responses leading to growth would be identification of the receptor involved in the response. Ideally one would then proceed to correlate receptor binding with some aspect of the trophic response.

PHYSIOLOGICAL SIGNIFICANCE

Exogenous Gastrin and Endogenous Serum Gastrin Levels

In a recent study Ryan et al. (67) tested whether exogenous gastrin, at a dose that increased serum gastrin levels the same amount as a meat meal, would stimulate DNA synthesis in dog oxyntic gland mucosa. After a 24-hr fast either saline, histamine (24 μg/kg-hr), or G-17 II (160 ng/kg-hr) was infused into conscious dogs for 4 hr. The doses of histamine and gastrin used elicited one-half maximal gastric acid secretion in the same dogs. At various times before, during, and after infusion, mucosal biopsies were taken from both the vagally denervated pouches and the gastric remnant. Gastrin caused a significant (three-to fivefold) increase in DNA synthesis 16 and 20 hr after the start of infusion when compared with zero time or saline and histamine at the same time. Feeding a meat meal to the same dogs produced similar increases in DNA synthesis. Serum gastrin levels in response to gastrin infusion and the meat meal were not statistically different. The authors concluded that the trophic effect of gastrin was a physiological action of the hormone (67).

Antrectomy

The classic method for proving that a tissue is dependent on a particular hormone for its growth and integrity is to remove the source of the hormone and observe atrophy or cessation of growth in the target tissues, and then to supply the hormone exogenously and reverse the changes brought on by extirpation of the endocrine cells. These studies are difficult in the case of the gastrointestinal hormones, since the endocrine-producing cells are not contained in a discrete gland. Instead they are scattered throughout a large area of mucosa, and total removal of the sites of production of a particular hormone is almost impossible without severely compromising the health of the animal.

In a recent study rats were either antrectomized to remove the primary source of gastrin or subjected to a sham operation (12). Three weeks after surgery half the antrectomized rats were injected with pentagastrin (250 μg/kg) four times per day for a total of 7 days. Antrectomy lowered serum gastrin levels to one-third normal. DNA synthesis and RNA and DNA content were significantly reduced in all tissues where gastrin is known to exert a trophic effect (pancreas and mucosa of the oxyntic gland area, duodenum, and colon), but not in the liver or kidney. In each case pentagastrin treatment of the antrectomized rats prevented the decrease. These results indicate that endogenous gastrin has an important role in the regulation of the growth of these tissues and support previous studies on the oxyntic and duodenal mucosa in which serum gastrin was not measured (32,52).

Similar data exist in man showing that the decrease in acid secretory capacity after antrectomy is significantly less if the patients are given pentagastrin after surgery (61). Mucosal atrophy of the gastric remnant after antrectomy in man has been discussed previously (21,44).

Association Between Gastrin Levels and Growth

Evidence that the trophic actions of gastrin are physiologically significant comes from examining growth of the gastrointestinal tract after natural alteration of serum and antral gastrin levels. There are a number of times when gastrin levels change dramatically due to developmental and physiological events. It is possible to exaggerate and prolong these changes without resorting to surgery.

Starvation is known to cause profound changes in small intestinal structure and function. Villus and crypt height in the rat are diminished after 3 to 6 days of starvation (1,49), and mucosal RNA, DNA, and protein are markedly decreased after 3 to 6 days of starvation (48,70). These decreases are significantly greater than the loss of body weight. During 3 days of starvation rat antral gastrin levels dropped from 32 μg/g of wet weight to 5 μg/g of wet weight, and serum gastrin concentration decreased from 330 pg/ml to 70 pg/ml (48). In these same animals intestinal DNA, RNA, and protein content decreased significantly compared with body weight. Specific lactase and maltase activity increased. Animals injected with pentagastrin during the period of starvation showed significantly smaller changes than the starved saline-injected control rats (48).

Ingestion of a meal is followed by increases in DNA synthesis and in the mitotic index of canine fundic mucosa (79). This pattern can be reproduced by a 4-hr infusion of gastrin (78), suggesting that gastrin might be one of the factors responsible for postprandial cell renewal.

Although the studies mentioned above implicate decreased gastrin levels as a cause of the profound deleterious effects that short periods of starvation have on the gut, interpretation of these studies is made difficult by the inability to separate the metabolic changes associated with starvation from those caused purely by the absence of food from the gut. Our laboratory has used the intravenously alimented rat as a model to study gut structure and function in the well-nourished animal whose gastrointestinal tract has gone unexposed to food and the stimuli arising from its ingestion and presence. Several findings from these studies are of special significance. First, the parenterally fed animals often gained weight and always remained in positive nitrogen balance (4). Second, tissue to body weight ratios for oxyntic gland area, small intestine, and pancreas were significantly decreased in the parenterally fed animals, whereas the weights of other organs were unaffected (33,39). Third, specific and total activities of the different disaccharidase enzymes were only a fraction of those found in the orally fed controls (4,39). Fourth, the parenterally fed animals were nearly depleted of antral gastrin (33,39). Fifth, these results could not be completely explained on the basis of food intake, dietary constitutents, enzyme induction, or the absence of luminally derived nutrition in the parenterally fed animals.

In the latest of these studies one group of parenterally nourished animals received a continuous infusion of 6.0 μg/kg/hr pentagastrin, a dose considerably less than the D_{50} for acid secretion in this species (39). The animals were killed approximately 2 weeks later and compared with parenterally fed rats that had received either histamine or nothing in addition to the intravenous diet. Serum as well as antral gastrin concentrations decreased significantly in all groups of parenterally fed animals. Weights of the oxyntic gland area, small intestine, and pancreas decreased significantly in all parenterally fed rats except those receiving gastrin. Gastrin completely prevented the decrease in disaccharidase activity normally associated with total parenteral nutrition. These data were interpreted to indicate that the oral ingestion of food and its presence in the gastrointestinal tract are necessary to maintain endogenous gastrin levels, and that the trophic action of endogenous gastrin is essential for the day to day maintenance of the structural and functional integrity of the gut (39).

Viewed as one body of evidence, the parallelism between serum and antral gastrin levels and growth of gastrointestinal tract tissue is striking. In each instance decreased endogenous gastrin levels were associated with decreased growth, and the addition of exogenous gastrin was able to significantly increase growth toward normal levels. In the study involving parenterally fed animals the dose of gastrin infused was well below the limit considered to be physiological. Since the effects of exogenous gastrin in this study were dramatic (39), it may indicate that the continuing presence of a low level of the hormone is more effective in stimulating growth than periodic extreme fluctuations in hormone concentration. In summary, the evidence in favor of the trophic action of gastrin being a physiological action is strong, perhaps as strong as for any other action of a gastrointestinal hormone.

CONCLUSIONS AND PROJECTIONS FOR THE FUTURE

Although the gut is the largest endocrine organ in the body, gastrointestional hormones have traditionally been considered in the realm of digestive rather than endocrine physiology. The fact that they have now been shown to stimulate growth of gastrointestinal tract tissues as well as secretion and motility makes it imperative that gastrointestinal hormones be included in any serious treatment of the regulation of metabolism by endocrine substances.

It is also becoming obvious that the gastrointestinal hormones physiologically influence and are influenced by the other endocrines. Glucagon inhibits the release of endogenous gastrin. All three gastrointestinal hormones stimulate insulin release, and gastric inhibitory peptide (GIP) may prove to be the "incretin" responsible for the rapid clearing of glucose seen during oral glucose tolerance tests. CCK has been shown to stimulate glucagon release, and both CCK and gastrin stimulate calcitonin release (25). Clinically, hyperplasia of antral gastrin cells (G cells) and increased antral gastrin content have been demonstrated in patients with primary hyperparathyroidism and acromegaly (8). Creutzfeldt et al. (8) interpreted these findings as indicating that serum calcium and growth hormone may have a trophic action on the G cells. However, a study by the same laboratory was unable to confirm their previous findings (9).

The secretion and/or synthesis of trophic hormones outside the gastrointestinal tract, and growth of the glands that contain them are dependent on the pituitary. There is presumptive evidence that the pituitary, and growth hormone in particular, may exert a similar regulation on gastrin and the antrum. Chronic injections of gastrin prevent atrophy of the pancreas, duodenum, and oxyntic gland mucosa following hypophysectomy, without affecting other tissues or body weight (54). Mayston and Barrowman (54) concluded from their study that some of the effects of the pituitary on the gastrointestinal tract may be mediated by influences on the endocrine cells of the gut. Enochs and Johnson (16) then hypothesized that growth hormone was necessary for normal serum gastrin levels. We measured serum and antral gastrin levels in hypophysectomized, hypophysectomized plus growth hormone injected, and sham-operated pair-fed rats. Fasted hypophysectomized rats had less than 50% of the normal serum gastrin levels. Feeding increased serum gastrin significantly in the sham-operated animals without altering levels in the hypophysectomized rats. Growth hormone maintained serum gastrin at normal values in both fed and fasted hypophysectomized rats (16).

These studies offer strong support for the idea that the gut hormones are part of a single interrelated system of endocrine agents. Furthermore, a case can be made that the most important actions of the gastrointestinal hormones for survival of the species are their metabolic ones, not their digestive ones.

Motility is largely under neural control. Secretion is in part regulated by direct effects of contact with food and by nerves. The hormonal components of secretory regulation can be eliminated without compromising the physiology of the individual. The integrity of the epithelial cells themselves, however, is necessary for both secretion and absorption and the life of the individual.

There are a number of clinical implications of the trophic actions of the gut hormones in addition to those already discussed, Zollinger-Ellison syndrome and antrectomy. Patients with pernicious anemia have abnormally high circulating levels of gastrin and atrophy of the oxyntic gland mucosa. This apparent anomaly to the trophic action of gastrin could be explained in several ways. There are causes of endocrine disease in addition to under- or overproduction of hormones. Two of these are end organ or receptor insensitivity and the production of biologically inactive hormones. These have never been investigated for any of the gut hormones. Patients with pernicious anemia often have high titers of parietal cell antibodies and have a greatly increased risk of developing gastric carcinoma. Therefore, these areas could prove to be fruitful subjects of investigation.

Following the resection of one part of the small intestine, in many species including man, the remaining intestinal mucosa undergoes both structural (20,59) and functional (14,76) changes, including small bowel dilation, villus enlargement, epithelial cell hyperplasia, increased cell migration rate, and increased absorptive capacity. Although most investigators suggest that changes in local nutrition or exposure to bile and pancreatic juice account for some or all of the hyperplasia involved, it is obvious that other, nongradient, mechanisms must also be in operation. Gastric hypersecretion with hyperplasia of gastric epithelial cells occurs after partial gut resection (81). Distal small bowel resection causes hyperplasia of the proximal small bowel mucosa (60), and removal of the colon results in hyperplasia of the ileum (82). It is obvious that none of these findings can be accounted for by a gradient-oriented mechanism. Interestingly enough, hypergastrinemia has been found in four patients with short bowel syndrome (71), in dogs after intestinal resection (77), and in rats following intestinal resection but not bypass (3). It is obvious that gastrin may account for some of the growth response after resection. Gastrin is the only known trophic agent whose level is increased under these conditions. Evidence suggests that other specific mechanisms exist but they have not been identified.

It is interesting to speculate about the role of gastrin in ulcer formation. A normal gastric mucosa is the manifestation of balance between the forces acting to destroy the lining of the stomach and those acting to maintain or rebuild it. Theoretically, an ulcer can develop if either regeneration decreases or destruction increases sufficiently to result in an imbalance. The destructive factors have been thoroughly studied—acid, pepsin, aspirin, bile, alcohol, and a host of other events labeled as stress—but we know little about alterations in regenerative forces that could lead to ulcer formation or, for that matter, prevention.

We recently tested the hypothesis that the trophic action of gastrin is important in maintaining the resistance of the gastric mucosa to stress ulcers (73). Stress ulcer formation was examined in the following groups of 18 rats each: (a) chow fed controls, (b) those fed an isocaloric amount of a liquid diet, and (c) those on a liquid diet plus pentagastrin injections (250 μg/kg, 3 times per day). The diet regimen lasted 10 days, and injections of saline, pentagastrin, or histamine occurred over the last 7 days prior to water immersion stress. Six rats from each group were killed prior to (zero time) and after 4 and 20 hr of stress. Serum gastrin and oxyntic gland DNA synthesis were significantly lower before stress in all liquid-fed rats compared with chow-fed controls. At this time the ulcer index was zero in all groups. DNA synthesis decreased and the ulcer index increased progressively in all groups with exposure to stress. After 4 hr stress the ulcer index was 3.8 in the group receiving pentagastrin compared with 14.1 and 10.7 in the animals receiving liquid diet alone or with histamine injections, respectively. During stress, DNA synthesis in the group receiving pentagastrin decreased significantly less than in all other groups. There was a significant correlation $r = 0.782$ ($p < 0.01$) between ulcer index and the decrease in DNA synthesis. We concluded that rats fed liquid diets to lower endogenous gastrin levels are more susceptible to restraint-induced stress ulcers, and that exogenous pentagastrin increased the resistance of these animals to ulceration. The susceptibility of all groups of animals to stress ulceration was directly correlated with decreases in DNA synthesis (73).

In conclusion, it is obvious that the trophic and metabolic effects of gastrointestinal hormones are among their most important, if not the most important, actions. The implications of these findings are many and provide areas of investigation related to both basic physiology and clinical medicine.

REFERENCES

1. Altmann, G. G. (1972): Influence of starvation and refeeding on mucosal size and epithelial renewal in the rat small intestine. *Am. J. Anat.,* 133:391–400.
2. Booth, A. N., Robbins, D. J., Ribelin, W. E., and DeEds, F. (1960): Effect of raw soybean meal and amino acids on pancreatic hypertrophy in rats. *Proc. Soc. Exp. Biol. Med.,* 104:681–684.
3. Bowen, J. C., Paddack, G. L., Bush, J. C., Wilson, R. J., and Johnson, L. R. (1978): Diverse gastric responses to small intestinal resection and bypass in rats. *Surgery,* 83:402–405.
4. Castro, G. A., Copeland, E. M., Dudrick, S. J., and Johnson, L. R. (1975): Intestinal disaccharidase and peroxidase activity in parenterally nourished rats. *J. Nutr.,* 105:776–781.
5. Chandler, A. M., and Johnson, L. R. (1972): Pentagastrin stimulated incorporation of ^{14}C-orotic acid into RNA of gastric and duodenal mucosa. *Proc. Soc. Exp. Biol. Med.,* 141:110–113.
6. Chernick, S. S., Lepkovsky, S., and Chaikoff, I. L. (1948): A dietary factor regulating the enzyme content of the pancreas: Changes induced in size and proteolytic activity of the chick pancreas by the ingestion of raw soybean meal. *Am. J. Physiol.,* 155:33–41.
7. Crean, G. P., Marshall, M. W., and Rumsey, R. D. E. (1969): Parietal cell hyperplasia induced by the administration of pentagastrin (ICI 50,123) to rats. *Gastroenterology,* 57:147–156.
8. Creutzfeldt, W., Arnold, R., and Creutzfeldt, C. (1971): Gastrin and G-cells in the antral mucosa of patients with pernicious anemia, acromegaly, and hyperparathyroidism and in a Zollinger Ellison tumour of the pancreas. *Eur. J. Clin. Invest.,* 1:461–479.
9. Creutzfeldt, W., Creutzfeldt, C., and Arnold, R. (1974): Gastrin-producing cells. In: *Endocrinol-*

ogy of the Gut, edited by W. Y. Chey and F. P. Brooks, pp. 35–62. Charles B. Slack, Thorofare, N.J.

10. Daughaday, W. H. (1974): The adenohypophysis. In: *Textbook of Endocrinology,* edited by R. H. Williams, pp. 31–79. W. B. Saunders Co., Philadelphia.

11. Daughaday, W. H., and Garland, J. T. (1972): The sulfation factor hypothesis: Recent observations. In: *Growth and Growth Hormone,* edited by A. Pecile and E. E. Muller, pp. 168–179. Excerpta Medica, Amsterdam.

12. Dembinski, A. B., and Johnson, L. R. (1979): Growth of pancreas and gastrointestinal mucosa in antrectomized and gastrin treated rats. *Endocrinology,* 105:769–773.

13. Dembinski, A. B., and Johnson, L. R. (1980): Stimulation of pancreatic growth by secretin and caerulein. *Endocrinology,* 106:323–328.

14. Dowling, R. H., and Booth, C. C. (1967): Structural and functional changes following small intestinal resection in the rat. *Clin. Sci.,* 32:139–149.

15. Ellison, E. H., and Wilson, S. D. (1967): Further observations on factors influencing the symptomatology manifest by patients with Zollinger-Ellison syndrome. In: *Gastric Secretion,* edited by T. K. Shnitka, J. A. L. Gilbert, and R. C. Harrison, pp. 363–369. Pergamon, New York.

16. Enochs, M. R., and Johnson, L. R. (1976): Effect of hypophysectomy and growth hormone on serum and antral gastrin levels in the rat. *Gastroenterology,* 70:727–732.

17. Enochs, M. R., and Johnson, L. R. (1977): Changes in protein and nucleic acid synthesis in rat gastric mucosa after pentagastrin. *Am. J. Physiol.,* 232:E223–E228.

18. Fitzgerald, P. J., Herman, L., Carol, B., Rogue, A., Marsh, W. H., Rosenstock, L., Richards, C., and Perl, D. (1968): Pancreatic acinar cell regeneration. I. Cytologic cytochemical and pancreatic weight changes. *Am. J. Pathol.,* 52:983–1011.

19. Fitzgerald, P. J., Vinijchaikul, K., Carol, B., and Rosenstock, L. (1968): Pancreatic acinar cell regeneration. III. DNA synthesis of pancreas nuclei as indicated by thymidine-H^3 autoradiography. *Am. J. Pathol.,* 52:1039–1065.

20. Flint, J. M. (1912): The effect of extensive resection of the small intestine. *Johns Hopkins Med. J.,* 23:127–131.

21. Gjurldsen, S. T., Myren, J., and Fretheim, B. (1968): Alterations of gastric mucosa following a graded partial gastrectomy. *Scand. J. Gastroenterol.,* 3:465–470.

22. Green, G. M., and Lyman, R. L. (1972): Feedback regulation of pancreatic enzyme secretion as a mechanism for trypsin inhibitor-induced hypersecretion in rats. *Proc. Soc. Exp. Biol. Med.,* 140:6–12.

23. Gregory, R. A., Grossman, M. I., Tracy, H. J., and Bentley, P. H. (1967): Nature of the gastric secretagogue in Zollinger-Ellison tumors. *Lancet,* 2:543–544.

24. Gregory, R. A., and Tracy, H. J. (1964): The contribution and properties of two gastrins extracted from hog antral mucosa. I. The isolation of two gastrins from hog antral mucosa. *Gut,* 5:103–114.

25. Grossman, M. I. (1974): Gastrointestinal hormones: Spectrum of actions and structure-activity relations. In: *Endocrinology of the Gut,* edited by W. Y. Chey and F. P. Brooks, pp. 65–75. Charles B. Slack, Thorofare, N.J.

26. Jensen, E. V., and DeSombre, E. R. (1972): Estrogens and progestins. In: *Biochemical Actions of Hormones, Vol. III,* edited by G. Litwack, pp. 215–256. Academic Press, New York.

27. Johnson, L. R. (1971): The control of gastric secretion: No room for histamine? *Gastroenterology,* 61:106–118.

28. Johnson, L. R. (1976): The trophic action of gastrointestinal hormones. *Gastroenterology,* 70:278–288.

29. Johnson, L. R. (1977): New aspects of the trophic action of gastrointestinal hormones. *Gastroenterology,* 72:788–792.

30. Johnson, L. R., Aures, D., and Hakanson, R. (1969): Effect of gastrin on the *in vivo* incorporation of [^{14}C]leucine into protein of the digestive tract. *Proc. Soc. Exp. Biol. Med.,* 132:996–998.

31. Johnson, L. R., Aures, D., and Yuen, L. (1969): Pentagastrin induced stimulation of the *in vitro* incorporation of [^{14}C]leucine into protein of the gastrointestinal tract. *Am. J. Physiol.,* 217:251–254.

32. Johnson, L. R., and Chandler, A. M. (1973): RNA and DNA of gastric and duodenal mucosa in antrectomized and gastrin-treated rats. *Am. J. Physiol.,* 224:937–940.

33. Johnson, L. R., Copeland, E. M., Dudrick, S. J., Lichtenberger, L. M., and Castro, G. A. (1975): Structural and hormonal alterations in the gastrointestinal tract of parenterally fed rats. *Gastroenterology,* 68:1177–1183.

34. Johnson, L. R., and Guthrie, P. D. (1974): Mucosal DNA synthesis: A short term index of the trophic action of gastrin. *Gastroenterology,* 67:453–459.
35. Johnson, L. R., and Guthrie, P. D. (1974): Secretin inhibition of gastrin-stimulated deoxyribonucleic acid synthesis. *Gastroenterology,* 67:601–606.
36. Johnson, L. R., and Guthrie, P. D. (1976): Effect of cholecystokinin and 16,16-dimethyl PGE_2 on RNA and DNA of gastric and duodenal mucosa. *Gastroenterology,* 70:59–65.
37. Johnson, L. R., and Guthrie, P. D. (1978): Stimulation of DNA synthesis by big and little gastrin (G-34 and G-17). *Gastroenterology,* 71:599–602.
38. Johnson, L. R., and Guthrie, P. D. (1978): Effect of secretin on colonic DNA synthesis. *Proc. Soc. Exp. Biol. Med.,* 158:521–523.
39. Johnson, L. R., Lichtenberger, L. M., Copeland, E. M., Dudrick, S. J., and Castro, G. A. (1975): Action of gastrin on gastrointestinal structure and function. *Gastroenterology,* 68:1184–1192.
40. Korner, A. (1963): Growth hormone control of messenger RNA synthesis. *Biochem. Biophys. Res. Commun.,* 13:386–389.
41. Korner, A. (1964): Regulation of the rate of synthesis of messenger RNA by growth hormone. *Biochem. J.,* 92:449–456.
42. Leblond, C. P., and Walker, B. E. (1956): Renewal of cell populations. *Physiol. Rev.,* 36:255–276.
43. Lechago, J., and Benscome, S. A. (1973): The endocrine cells of the upper gut mucosa in dogs with transplantation of the pyloric antrum to the colon. *Z. Zellforsch. Mikrosk. Anat.,* 146:237–242.
44. Lees, F., and Grandjean, L. C. (1968): The gastric and jejunal mucosae in healthy patients with partial gastrectomy. *Arch. Intern. Med.,* 101:9437–9451.
45. Lehv, M., and Fitzgerald, P. J. (1968): Pancreatic cell regeneration. IV. Regeneration after surgical resection. *Am. J. Pathol.,* 53:513–535.
46. Lehy, T., Voillemot, N., Dubrasquet, M., and Dufougeray, F. (1975): Gastrin cell hyperplasia in rats with chronic antral stimulation. *Gastroenterology,* 68:71–82.
47. Lichtenberger, L. M., Miller, L. R., Erwin, D. N., and Johnson, L. R. (1973): The effect of pentagastrin on adult rat duodenal cells in culture. *Gastroenterology,* 65:242–251.
48. Lichtenberger, L. M., Welsh, J. D., and Johnson, L. R. (1975): Relationship between the changes in gastrin levels and intestinal properties in the starved rat. *Am. J. Dig. Dis.,* 21:33–38.
49. McNeil, L. K., and Hamilton, J. R. (1971): The effect of fasting on disaccharidase activity in the rat small intestine. *Pediatrics,* 47:65–72.
50. Mainz, D. L., Black, O., and Webster, P. D. (1973): Hormonal control of pancreatic growth. *J. Clin. Invest.,* 52:2300–2304.
51. Majumdar, A. P. N., and Goltermann, N. (1977): Effects of fasting and pentagastrin on protein synthesis by isolated gastric mucosal ribosomes in a cell-free system. *Gastroenterology,* 73:1060–1064.
52. Martin, F., Macleod, I. B., and Sircus, W. (1970): Effects of antrectomy on the fundic mucosa of the rat. *Gastroenterology,* 59:437–444.
53. Mayston, P. D., and Barrowman, J. A. (1971): The influence of chronic administration of pentagastrin on the rat pancreas. *Q. J. Exp. Physiol.,* 56:113–122.
54. Mayston, P. D., and Barrowman, J. A. (1973): Influence of chronic administration of pentagastrin on the pancreas in hypophysectomized rats. *Gastroenterology,* 64:391–399.
55. Melrose, A. G., Russell, R. I., and Dick, A. (1964): Gastric mucosal structure and function after vagotomy. *Gut,* 5:546–549.
56. Meyer, J. H., Spingola, L. J., and Grossman, M. I. (1971): Endogenous cholecystokinin potentiates exogenous secretin on pancreas of dog. *Am. J. Physiol.,* 221:742–747.
57. Miller, L. R., Jacobson, E. D., and Johnson, L. R. (1973): Effect of pentagastrin on gastric mucosal cells grown in tissue culture. *Gastroenterology,* 64:254–267.
58. Neuberger, P. H., Lewin, M., deRecherche, C., and Bonfils, S. (1972): Parietal and chief cell populations in four cases of the Zollinger-Ellison syndrome. *Gastroenterology,* 63:937–942.
59. Nygaard, K. (1967): Resection of the small intestine in rats. III. Morphological changes in the intestinal tract. *Acta Chir. Scand.,* 133:233–248.
60. Nygaard, K. (1974): Small bowel resection and by-pass. In: *Intestinal Adaptation,* edited by R. H. Dowling and E. O. Riecken, pp. 47–59. F. K. Schauttauer Verlag, Stuttgart.
61. Olbe, L. (1974): Differences between human and animal gastric acid secretion. In: *Syllabus for AGA Postgraduate Course on Peptic Ulcer Disease,* San Francisco.

62. Opie, E. L. (1932): Cytology of the pancreas. In: *Special Cytology, Ed. 2, Vol. I, Sect. X,* edited by E. V. Cowdry, pp. 375–389. Paul B. Hoelser, New York.
63. Pansu, D., Berard, A., Dechelette, M. A., and Lambert, R. (1974): Influence of secretin and pentagastrin on the circadian rhythm of cell proliferation in the intestinal mucosa of rats. *Digestion,* 11:266–274.
64. Pegg, A. E., and Korner, A. (1965): Growth hormone action on rat liver RNA polymerase. *Nature,* 205:904–905.
65. Petersen, H., Solomon, T., and Grossman, M. I. (1978): Effect of chronic pentagastrin, cholecystokinin and secretin on pancreas of rats. *Am. J. Physiol.,* 234:E286–E293.
66. Rothman, S. S., and Wells, H. (1967): Enhancement of pancreatic enzyme synthesis by pancreozymin. *Am. J. Physiol.,* 213:215–218.
67. Ryan, G. P., Copeland, E. M., and Johnson, L. R. (1978): Effects of gastrin and vagal denervation on DNA synthesis in canine fundic mucosa. *Am. J. Physiol.,* 235:E32–E36.
68. Solomon, T. E., Petersen, H., Elashoff, J., and Grossman, M. I. (1978): Interaction of caerulein and secretin on pancreatic size and composition in rat. *Am. J. Physiol.,* 235:E714–E719.
69. Stanley, M. D., Coalson, R. E., Grossman, M. I., and Johnson, L. R. (1972): Influence of secretin and pentagastrin on acid secretion and parietal cell number in rats. *Gastroenterology,* 63:264–269.
70. Steiner, M., Bouges, H. R., Freedman, L. S., and Gray, S. J. (1968): Effect of starvation on the tissue composition of the small intestine in the rat. *Am. J. Physiol.,* 215:75–77.
71. Straus, E., Gerson, C. D., and Yalow, R. D. (1974): Hypersecretion of gastrin associated with the short bowel syndrome. *Gastroenterology,* 66:175–180.
72. Sutton, D. R., and Donaldson, R. M. (1975): Synthesis and secretion of protein and pepsinogen by rabbit gastric mucosa in organ culture. *Gastroenterology,* 69:166–174.
73. Takeuchi, K., and Johnson, L. R. (1979): Pentagastrin protects against stress ulceration in rats. *Gastroenterology,* 76:327–334.
74. Tomkins, G. M., and Gelehrter, T. D. (1972): The present status of genetic regulation by hormones. In: *Biochemical Actions of Hormones, Vol. II,* edited by G. Litwack, pp. 1–20. Academic Press, New York.
75. Walsh, J. H., and Grossman, M. I. (1975): Gastrin. *New Engl. J. Med.,* 292:1324–1332, 1377–1384.
76. Weser, E., and Hernandez, M. H. (1971): Studies of small bowel adaptation after intestinal resection in the rat. *Gastroenterology,* 60:69–75.
77. Wickborn, G., Landor, J. H., Bushkin, F. L., and McGuigan, J. E. (1975): Changes in canine gastric acid output and serum gastrin levels following massive small intestinal resection. *Gastroenterology,* 69:448–452.
78. Willems, G., Vansteenkiste, Y., and Limbosch, J. M. (1972): Stimulating effect of gastrin on cell proliferation kinetics in canine fundic mucosa. *Gastroenterology,* 62:583–589.
79. Willems, G., Vansteenkiste, Y., and Smets, P. L. (1971): Effects of food ingestion on the cell proliferation kinetics in the fundic mucosa. *Gastroenterology,* 61:323–327.
80. Williams-Ashman, H. G., and Reddi, A. M. (1972): Androgenic regulation of tissue growth and function. In: *Biochemical Actions of Hormones, Vol. II,* edited by G. Litwack, pp. 257–294. Academic Press, New York.
81. Winborn, W. B., Seelig, L. L., Nakayama, H., and Weser, E. (1974): Hyperplasia of gastric glands after small bowel resection in the rat. *Gastroenterology,* 66:384–395.
82. Wright, H. K., Poskitt, T., and Cleveland, J. C. (1969): The effect of total colectomy on morphology and absorptive capacity of the ileum in the rat. *J. Surg. Res.,* 9:301–307.
83. Yalow, R. S., and Berson, S. A. (1970): Size and charge distinctions between endogenous human plasma gastrin in peripheral blood and heptadecapeptide gastrins. *Gastroenterology,* 58:609–615.

Gastrointestinal Hormones, edited by
George B. Jerzy Glass.
Raven Press, New York © 1980.

Chapter 23

Gastrointestinal Hormones and Gastric Secretion

Stanislaw J. Konturek

Institute of Physiology, Medical Academy, 31531 Krakow, Poland

INTRODUCTION

Gastric secretion of hydrochloric acid and pepsin depends on the mass and functional capacity of respective secretory elements in the gastric mucosa and the action of various hormonal and nervous stimulants and inhibitors. The rate of secretion and the composition of gastric juice show profound alterations in response to physiological stimuli such as meal, which may affect the secretory activity of gastric glands either directly by luminal contents or indirectly through gastrointestinal hormones and other chemical messengers delivered to the secretory cells by endocrine, paracrine, or neurocrine pathways. Increased knowledge of gastric physiology has clearly shown that a number of hormonal peptides present both in the endocrine-paracrine cells and in the nerves of the digestive system are involved in the control of acid and pepsin secretion both under basal conditions and during postprandial states. There is a striking degree of interdependence between these hormones and the autonomic nervous system in the control of the secretory activity of the gastric glands.

This chapter reviews our current knowledge of the hormonal control of human gastric secretion. The data obtained for animals will be referred to only for those aspects of gastric secretion for which no information on humans is available.

STRUCTURAL BASIS OF EXOCRINE AND ENDOCRINE GASTRIC SECRETION

Gastric mucosa is divided into three regions related to three different types of glands: the cardiac, oxyntic, and pyloric. The total surface area of the human gastric mucosa is approximately 800 cm². The cardiac gland area occupies the first few millimeters immediately below the gastroesophageal junction and contains tubular, highly branched glands consisting of mucous cells and a few oxyntic and peptic cells. It secretes alkaline mucus and a small amount of electrolytes. It is unknown whether it has any specific endocrine function.

The oxyntic gland area comprises 75 to 80% of the total gastric mucosal area and occupies the fundus and the body of the stomach. The oxyntic glands, which number approximately 35 million, are straight or slightly coiled tubules, closely packed and opening into the gastric pits. They contain numerous mucous cells interspersed with oxyntic (parietal) cells in the midportion of the gland. There are approximately 1 billion oxyntic cells, which comprise approximately 35% of the volume of the oxyntic mucosa (44). They have a remarkably large number of mitochondria corresponding with the high oxygen and energy demands for the production of highly concentrated hydrochloric acid. In addition to acid, they secrete water and intrinsic factor discharged into the gland lumen through a composite network of intracellular canaliculi starting at the cell base and opening after a tortuous course into the apical cell surface. These intracellular canaliculi are lined with microvilli and are surrounded by the cytoplasm with numerous tubulovesicular structures. The oxyntic cells undergo a very dramatic morphological transformation during stimulation: the tubulovesicles coalesce and become transformed into the microvillous membrane (40). The acid secretory apparatus is apparently housed in the membranes of the tubulovesicular and secretory canaliculi and the morphological transformation observed during stimulation serves to increase the luminal secretory surface (30). At present the characteristic features of oxyntic cells can be conveniently examined in isolated cell preparations obtained by dispersing the gastric cells, using sequential exposure to collagenase and EDTA. The response of the cells to stimulation can be determined by monitoring the consumption of oxygen, the uptake of ^{14}C-aminopyrine, and the morphological transformation (115–117).

The peptic cells comprise approximately 25% of the volume of oxyntic mucosa (44) and are also present in small number in cardiac, pyloric, and upper duodenal mucosae. They show numerous large granules that are located mainly in the apical portion of the cytoplasm and contain pepsinogens. It has been demonstrated by immunochemical studies (108,109) that there are five types of pepsinogen-producing cells. Two of these, the peptic and mucous neck cells, present in the oxyntic glands, have been shown to contain pepsinogen fractions termed group I pepsinogens (PGI) and group II pepsinogens (PGII), whereas the mucous cells of cardiac glands, pyloric glands, and Brunner's glands contain only PGII. Pepsinogens are secreted into the gastric lumen and are also released into the blood, where they can be determined by immunochemical methods (110).

The pyloric gland area constitutes the lower 20% of the gastric mucosa (44) and contains pyloric glands, which are simple branched tubular glands composed of mucous cells, very few oxyntic cells, and endocrine cells. It secretes alkaline mucus and some electrolytes such as calcium phosphate, sodium, and potassium bicarbonates and chloride.

A variety of endocrine cells are present in the gastric mucosa, usually scattered between the basement membrane and the exocrine cells (113,114). In many cases the endocrine cells have microvillous borders exposed to the lumen so they can respond to chemicals in the stomach content. They are characterized by the presence of granules often situated at the cell base that store the peptide products. Each cell type has typical granules that can be described in terms of diameter, density, and appearance. Most of the cells appear to contain a single peptide hormone but some contain two distinct peptides and also biogenic amines (97). Many of these cells were identified earlier by their affinity to silver stains (enterochromaffin, argentaffin, argyrophil). Pearse (91) suggested that all cells producing peptide hormone are derived from neuroectoderm and show common biochemical features. Several types of endocrine cells have been identified by immunocytochemistry in the oxyntic and pyloric gland area, including the G cells responsible for the production of gastrin, EC_1 (enterochromaffin cells) for substance P, EC_2 cells for motilin, EC_3 cells for enkephalin, D cells for somatostatin, D_1 cells for vasoactive intestinal peptide (VIP) and bombesin, P cells for neuropeptides (?), and ECL cells for histamine and serotonin. For more information on this subject, see Chapter 1 by E. Solcia et al., pp. 1–18, *this volume.*

The hormonal peptides released by the endocrine cells can be delivered to the target cells either by way of the blood (endocrine path) or by diffusion through the intercellular fluid to act directly on the adjacent cells (paracrine path). Recently, it has been shown that certain peptide hormones, such as VIP, somatostatin, endorphin, substance P, bombesin, and gastrin are also present in the nerves and ganglia of the gastric and intestinal wall (47). It has been speculated that these peptides may be released locally by nervous stimulation to produce the effects on the adjacent tissues (neurocrine path). See also Chapter 2 by J. M. Polak and S. R. Bloom, pp. 19–52, *this volume.*

The gland cells of the gastric mucosa are continuously renewed. Cells on the surface of the gastric mucosa are constantly replaced by a desquamation and migration of new cells from the base of the pits to the surface. The undifferentiated, immature neck cells of the glands appear to represent the "mother cells" that are the precursors of the mucous cells as well as of oxyntic and peptic cells (130). The turnover of surface epithelium cells ranges from 2 to 6 days and that of oxyntic and chief cells is much slower. This process appears to be under hormonal control. In experimental animals, the prolonged administration of gastrin causes increased synthesis of protein, DNA, and RNA by gastric mucosa accompanied by an increase in the maximal acid secretory capacity (17,53). Similar gastric mucosal hypertrophy can be observed in patients with Zollinger-Ellison syndrome and this has been attributed to hypergastrinemia found in this condition. Secretin counteracts the mucosal hyperplasia induced by gastrin. For more information on this subject, see Chapter 22 by L. R. Johnson, pp. 507–526, *this volume.*

SECRETION OF HYDROCHLORIC ACID

Hydrochloric acid is secreted into the gastric lumen by the oxyntic cells. The primary secretion of these cells, as it appears in the intracellular canaliculi, has a very high concentration of acid, reaching approximately 170 mM, which is more than three million times greater than in the blood or tissues. The secretory process requires two major intracellular steps: production and active transport of hydrogen ions, both of which consume energy and oxygen.

The energy is generated in the oxyntic cells mainly by aerobic metabolism and involves the production of high energy phosphate bonds. Oxygen consumption is tightly linked to the secretion of acid and more than one hydrogen ion is secreted per oxygen molecule (41). There are conflicting studies on the source of substrate pool but probably both fatty acids and glucose are metabolized to yield the products involved in acid secretion (42,107), namely the hydrogen ion itself, ATP, carbon dioxide, and the hydroxyl radical. The source of the hydrogen ions for the secretion of acid and the means of the delivery of metabolic energy to the hydrogen-ion pump are not known but two major theories have been proposed in this regard. According to the redox theory, the hydrogen ions are directly generated from the oxidation-reduction process and delivered to the secretory surface via the electron transport system. The ATP theory suggests that ATP generated from the substrate metabolism provides the necessary energy via a specialized ATPase. Gastric mucosa contains several ATPases but a specialized K^+-stimulated ATPase appears to represent an integral part of the acid secretory mechanism. This ATPase was recently found in the vesicles isolated from the tubulovesicles of the oxyntic cells and shown to be capable of concentrating acid in the presence of exogenous ATP (29).

There is much uncertainty about the effect of physiological stimuli such as gastrin or histamine on the metabolic processes. It appears that the redox changes in the oxyntic cells occur almost immediately after the onset of stimulation and much earlier than the actual secretion of acid commences. This observation, combined with an increase in oxygen consumption, indicates that the primary effect of gastric secretagogue is mobilizing substrates in the oxyntic cells (41).

The concentration of hydrogen ion in the gastric juice is a function of the rate of secretion. As the rate of secretion increases, the hydrogen ion concentration rises and the sodium concentration falls, whereas the potassium and chloride concentrations remain within a fairly narrow range (45,121).

HORMONAL RECEPTORS ON OXYNTIC CELLS AND INTERACTIONS BETWEEN SECRETAGOGUES

The oxyntic cells *in vivo* are exposed to the action of a variety of endogenous hormonal stimulants and inhibitors delivered to them through endocrine, paracrine, or neurocrine pathways. At least three types of secretagogues are known to play a physiological role in the activation of the oxyntic cells, namely gastrin, histamine, and acetylcholine. There is a marked interaction and interdependence between these secretagogues, which have been demonstrated both *in vivo* in the intact stomach and *in vitro* in the isolated oxyntic cell preparation (117). The most convincing evidence *in vivo* was obtained using H_2-receptor antagonists such as metiamide or cimetidine, which were found to inhibit gastric acid response not only to histamine but also to gastrin and cholinergic stimulants (36). Similarly, anticholinergic drugs inhibit acid response not only to cholinergic stimulus but also to gastrin and histamine (80). In the same manner, vagotomy and antrectomy, used in the surgical therapy of peptic ulcer disease, decrease the acid response to all modes of stimulation, including gastrin, histamine, and food (5,80).

The interactions between secretagogues were also observed in the isolated oxyntic cell preparation in which the response to stimulation was determined by monitoring the consumption of oxygen, the uptake of ^{14}C-aminopyrine, and the morphological transformation (115,117). Through use of these indirect indices of oxyntic cell activity, it was found that gastrin, histamine, and acetylcholine each directly stimulates the oxyntic cells. The response to each of these secretagogues was rather weak but the combination of two or three of them resulted in a potentiating interaction. When all three secretagogues were added together, each at a concentration that produced threshold stimulation, a marked three-way potentiation was observed (116,117). Basal isolated oxyntic cell activity was not affected by H_2-blockers and anticholinergics which, however, were specific inhibitors of histaminic or cholinergic stimulation, respectively. Thus, the response to cholinergic stimulus was blocked by atropine but not by H_2-receptor antagonist, the response to histamine was abolished by H_2-blocker but not atropine, and the response to gastrin was not blocked by either inhibitor. When the effects of these inhibitors were tested against combinations of stimulants that produced potentiated responses, the inhibitors retained their respective specificities against related stimulants but displayed an apparent cross-specificity to unrelated stimulants by interfering with the potentiating interactions between secretagogues (117). Thus, the isolated oxyntic cells may serve as a model to study the interactions between various secretagogues. This phenomenon seems to occur also *in vivo* in the intact stomach, where oxyntic cells are exposed to histamine and acethylcholine released locally and gastrin delivered by the endocrine pathway. Since the amounts of these endogenous stimulants acting on the oxyntic cells may vary under various physiological conditions, it is no surprise to find that the potentiating interactions may be of variable magnitude. In fact, gastrin appears to contribute relatively little to the potentiating interaction and is a rather weak direct stimulant of oxyntic cells (116). Gastrin also seems to be an intrinsically weak direct stimulant *in vivo* because H_2-blocker is capable of completely suppressing meal or gastrin-induced gastric acid secretion (62). The weak stimulatory effect of gastrin is, however, greatly potentiated by either histamine or acetylcholine and this potentiation can be abolished by cimetidine or atropine, respectively. These data suggest that the oxyntic cells possess separate and specific receptors for gastrin, histamine, and acetylcholine and that *in vivo* they are under sufficient effects of endogenous secretagogues to support potentiating interaction (Fig. 1).

Critical to the concept of secretagogue interaction should be the demonstration of cellular localization of gastric receptors on the same oxyntic cells. Although no direct biochemical evidence is presently available as to the localization of gastric receptors, attempts have been made to identify and characterize the binding sites for gastric secretagogues. Gastrin binding sites have been demonstrated in preparations of isolated oxyntic cells and in partially purified gastric

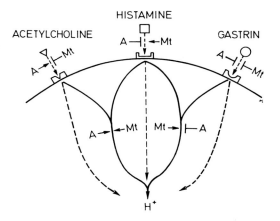

FIG. 1. A working model for the actions and interactions of secretagogues of the isolated parietal cell. The *dashed lines* represent independent actions of secretagogues and the *solid lines* represent interactions. Sites at which atropine (A) and metiamide (Mt) are respectively inhibitory (→) and at which these agents are not inhibitory (⊣) are indicated. (From ref. 116.)

plasma membranes. Radiolabeled gastrin and its derivatives were shown to bind specifically to mucosal membrane preparations from the oxyntic and duodenal but not antral mucosa of the rat (82a,120a). This gastric binding was found to be competitively inhibited by cholecystokinin, caerulein and pentagastrin, the peptides possessing a common C-terminal tetrapeptide. Fasting decreased the binding capacity of gastrin receptor and refeeding brought the receptor level back to control range, suggesting that this receptor exhibit an autoregulation by endogenous gastrin. The formation of gastrin-binding site complex was concomitant with the activation of the adenyl cyclase (in membrane preparation) and with the accumulation of cyclic AMP (in isolated oxyntic cell preparation). Biochemical evidence for separate histamine or acetylcholine receptors is less firm. The existence of histamine H_2-receptors is based mainly on the indirect pharmacophysiological studies. Attempts to demonstrate histamine-receptor complex have been unsuccessful so far, perhaps because the reaction between histamine and receptors occurs at a high turnover rate or because the affinity of histamine to proper receptor sites is basically different from that of gastrin. No reports on cellular fixation of the radiolabeled histamine have yet been presented.

The interdependence among gastric secretagogues has been explained by another theory proposing that histamine is a final common mediator for all secretagogues of gastric secretion ("mediator" hypothesis). According to this theory, championed by Code (16) and Black (9), gastrin and acetylcholine release histamine in gastric mucosa and the oxyntic cells have functional receptors only for histamine. Direct studies of the release of histamine by gastrin or cholinergic agents have given, however, inconclusive results in most species tested. Only in rats was it shown conclusively that gastrin and feeding result in the induction of histidine decarboxylase and in the potential availability of histamine (4,56). The crucial evidence for this theory would be a demonstration that all types of gastric secretagogues release histamine in oxyntic mucosa in amounts sufficient to activate the oxyntic cells and that these cells either possess receptors only for histamine but not for other secretagogues, or that receptors for gastrin and histamine are localized on separate subcellular structures of the same cells. The evidence available at present indicates that histamine is generated by oxyntic mucosa and that it does play an important role in the activation of oxyntic cells, mainly by sensitizing these cells to other stimuli ("permissive" theory) (35).

STIMULUS-SECRETION COUPLING

Since the discovery of mediation of hormone activation by cyclic AMP, attempts have been made to implicate the cyclic nucleotides as possible mediators of secretagogues exciting the oxyntic cells. In spite of several contradictory reports in this regard, there is a considerable body of evidence to suggest that the stimulatory effect of histamine (but not of gastrin or acetylcholine) on gastric secretion is mediated by cyclic AMP (21,49). It was shown that the oxyntic mucosa contains histamine-sensitive adenylate cyclase that can be competitively blocked by H_2-receptor antagonists (21). This histamine-sensitive adenylate cyclase was found in the oxyntic mucosa of several species and localized in acid-producing cells. In the dispersed gastric mucosal cell preparation histamine (but not gastrin or acetylcholine) caused an increase in the production of cyclic AMP (118). With progressive enrichment of the parietal cells, a highly significant correlation was found between the oxyntic cell content and the histamine-induced rise in cyclic AMP production, indicating that the oxyntic cells are, in fact, responsible for the histamine effect.

It is of interest that secretin and prostaglandins (PGs), which inhibit gastric acid secretion, were also shown to increase mucosal production of cyclic AMP (49,122). These effects were observed, however, mainly in unenriched mucosal cell preparations. Through use of a cell separation technique, they were found primarily in cells other than oxyntic cells, mainly in the mucous cells (118). Furthermore, the effects of histamine on cyclic AMP production, oxygen consumption, or aminopyrine uptake occurred at the dose range that should be considered as physiological, whereas the effects of secretin or PGs were demonstrated only at very high, unphysiological doses of these agents (6).

The mechanism by which cyclic AMP formed in response to histamine could activate the acid secretory process is unknown. It is assumed that cyclic AMP leads to the activation of protein kinase, which in turn directly and reversibly phosphorylates specific protein involved in the active transport of hydrogen ions.

There are no solid candidates for the intracellular mediation of gastrin or acetylcholine but recent studies in intact animals suggest that cyclic GMP may be implicated in the stimulus-secretion coupling of these secretagogues (49).

GASTROINTESTINAL HORMONES AND THE STIMULATORY
MECHANISMS OF GASTRIC ACID SECRETION

The regulation of gastric acid secretion is one of the most complex physiological processes in the body. Classically, gastric secretion is divided into the interdigestive and the digestive periods; the latter can be further subdivided into three phases according to the site at which the stimuli act: the cephalic, gastric, and intestinal phases. In the past, the cephalic phase was equated with nervous excitation and the gastric and intestinal phases with hormonal stimulation. It is now widely thought that all three phases have the same dual nervous and hormonal components, which potentiate each other. The vagus and gastrin are strikingly interdependent in stimulating gastric acid secretion.

GASTRIN

Gastrin is one of the three "old" hormones (gastrin, secretin, and cholecystokinin) discovered some decades ago (22) but isolated chemically, identified, and synthesized only in the last decade. It is a major factor responsible for the stimulation of gastric acid secretion under various physiological conditions. A detailed discussion of gastrin is given in a separate chapter of this volume. Here, only the role of gastrin in the control of human gastric secretion is considered.

Chemistry and Distribution of Gastrin

Like other hormonal peptides, gastrin exists in several molecular forms of different size, charge, and biological activity (102,126,133). The largest quantities of gastrin are found in the antral mucosa, which contains 5 to 25 μg of hormone per gram of fresh tissue, an amount sufficient to stimulate acid secretion at half maximal rate for about 10 hr. The gastrin content in the proximal duodenum is about 10% that of the antrum (84). The two major forms of gastrin are big gastrin, G-34, and little gastrin, G-17, both existing as the pairs of nonsulfated and sulfated peptides. The smaller forms, known as minigastrin, G-14, and tetragastrin, G-4, have also been detected in small amounts in the antral mucosa. Approximately 90% of antral mucosal gastrin is composed of little gastrin, whereas approximately 50% of duodenal gastrin consists of big gastrin. It is generally assumed that all gastrin components may originally be synthesized in the G cells in the form of big gastrin and subsequently converted to the shorter molecules. The significance of the sulfation of gastrin components is not clear, as there is no biological difference between the sulfated and the nonsulfated forms. The biologically active region of all gastrin components appears to be the carboxyl-terminal region of the molecule (Table 1).

The relative contribution of various gastrin components to the total gastrin

TABLE 1. *Gastrin family of peptides*

	Gastrin peptides			Cholecystokinin peptides			Motilin	Met-Enkephalin
	G-34	G-17	G-14	CCK-V	CCK	Cerulein		
Residues	34	17	14	39	33	10	22	5
Molecular weight (I)	3,839	2,098	1,833	—	—	—	2,698	794
(II)	3,919	2,178	1,913	4,678	3,918	1,352	—	—
39				Tyr				
38				Ile				
37				Gln				
36				Gln				
35				Ala				
34	Glp			Arg				
33	Leu			Lys	Lys			
32	Gly			Ala	Ala			
31	Pro			Pro	Pro			
30	Gln			Ser	Ser			
29	Gly			Gly	Gly			
28	His			Arg	Arg			
27	Pro			Val	Val			
26	Ser			Ser	Ser			
25	Leu			Met	Met			
24	Val			Ile	Ile			
23	Ala			Lys	Lys			
22	Asp			Asn	Asn		Phe	
21	Pro			Leu	Leu		Val	
20	Ser			Gln	Gln		Pro	
19	Lys			Ser	Ser		Ile	
18	Lys			Leu	Leu		Phe	
17	Gln	Glp		Asp	Asp		Thr	
16	Gly	Gly		Pro	Pro		Tyr	
15	Pro	Pro		Ser	Ser		Gly	
14	Trp	Trp	Trp	His	His		Gln	
13	Leu	Leu	Leu	Arg	Arg		Leu	
12	Glu	Glu	Glu	Ile	Ile		Gln	

Glu	Glu	Glu	Ser	Ser	Glp	Arg		11
Glu	Glu	Glu	Asp	Asp	Gln	Met		10
Glu	Glu	Glu	Arg	Arg	Gln	Gln		9
Glu	Glu	Glu	Asp	Asp	Asp	Glu		8
Ala	Ala	Ala	Tyr-SO_3H	Tyr-SO_3H	Tyr-SO_3H	Lys		7
Tyr-R	Tyr-R	Tyr-R	Met	Met	Thr	Glu		6
Gly	Gly	Gly	Gly	Gly	Gly	Arg	Met	5
Trp	Trp	Trp	Trp	Trp	Trp	Asn	Phe	4
Met	Met	Met	Met	Met	Met	Lys	Gly	3
Asp	Asp	Asp	Asp	Asp	Asp	Gly	Gly	2
Phe-NH_2	Phe-NH_2	Phe-NH_2	Phe-NH_2	Phe-NH_2	Phe-NH_2	Gln	Tyr-NH_2	1

R = H (gastrin -I); R = SO_3H (gastrin -II); Met-Enkephalin = Methionine-enkephalin.

content in the plasma may vary in different physiological and pathological conditions (126). In healthy subjects the most abundant component of plasma gastrin in the interdigestive period was thought to be big, big gastrin (BBG), the major source of which was believed to be the jejunal mucosa (134). In fact, BBG was reported to be the only major circulating gastrin component after antrectomy and gastrojejunostomy. More recently, the existence of BBG as a "true" gastrin component has been questioned and the immunoreactivity corresponding to BBG has been attributed to the unspecific protein interference in the radioimmunoassay (RIA) (101). The other gastrin components of fasting plasma gastrin are present in small amounts insufficient for accurate identification. After meals, G-17 is the most abundant form immediately following food intake and then G-34 becomes the most abundant (approximately 70% of total gastrin) during prolonged release of gastrin in the postprandial period. Most of the hypergastrinemias (pernicious anemia, gastrinoma) examined so far are characterized by the abundance of G-34, smaller amounts of G-17, and little or no G-14 or BBG. Because of the heterogeneity of circulating gastrin and the differences in the biological activity of each gastrin component, the total gastrin concentration in plasma determined by RIA is only a crude index of hormone bioactivity. This explains the relatively poor correlation between the plasma gastrin level and gastric acid secretion encountered in various physiological conditions (126).

Release and Physiological Actions of Gastrin

Gastrin is produced, stored, and released by endocrine G cells in the pyloric and upper duodenal mucosa. Using mucosal biopsy and analyzing specimens obtained from corpus, antrum, duodenum, and jejunum of normal and duodenal ulcer patients, Malmstrom et al. (84) found a steep gradient of gastrin concentration distally from the pylorus. As compared with the antral mucosa, the concentration of gastrin in the proximal duodenum, the distal duodenum, and jejunum was 10, 1, and 0.5%, respectively. No major differences were found between normal subjects and duodenal ulcer patients. The presence of gastrin in the duodenum is probably responsible for the marked postprandial increase in plasma gastrin observed in patients with previous antrectomy and gastroduodenostomy (120).

All mechanisms of gastrin release appear to operate through chemicals that act directly on the G cells. These chemicals can reach the G cells by blood, by diffusion from the neighboring paracrine cells, or from the nerve terminals and by direct action from the gastric contents. Blood-borne chemicals that have been shown to release gastrin are calcium and magnesium ions, epinephrine, growth hormone, and bombesin. It is unknown which of these substances contribute to the gastrin release under physiological conditions but hypergastrinemia in patients with gastrinoma combined with hyperparathyroidism can be attributed, at least in part, to raised calcium blood levels, and in patients with pheochromocytoma to epinephrine (126). Bombesin released by the intestinal D_1

cells or locally from the peptidergic nerves may serve as a releaser of antral gastrin, particularly during the intestinal phase of gastric secretion (48,94). Growth hormone in combination with other pituitary hormones (prolactin, ACTH, and corticosteroids) is capable of reducing cellular atrophy of gastric mucosa and of restoring gastrin release by the antral G cells in hypophysecto-mized rats (23a).

Gastrin has been shown to affect all basic functions of the digestive system, including secretion, motility, absorption, visceral circulation, and also the growth and structure of the digestive organs. The physiological effects of this hormone are, however, limited to the stimulation of acid secretion and perhaps to the growth of the acid-secreting mucosa of the stomach. Acute administration of gastrin leads to increased DNA, RNA, and protein synthesis. Prolonged adminis-tration results in hyperplasia of the oxyntic gland region of the stomach (17,53). For more information on this subject, see Chapter 22 by L. R. Johnson; pp. 507–526, *this volume.*

Vagus and Gastrin in Control of Acid Secretion

It is well established that vagal activation stimulates acid secretion and gastrin release as well. It was thought previously that vagal release of gastrin is mediated by acetylcholine released from the preganglionic and postganglionic nerve end-ings and acting directly on the G cells (34). Cephalic phase stimuli act solely through vagal efferents, whereas gastric distention such as occurs during the gastric phase may act through both vago-vagal reflexes and local intramural reflexes.

Apparently, vagal release of gastrin in man is less important in acid response to vagal excitation than in other species (e.g., dogs) (Fig.2). In man, acid response to sham-feeding is only slightly decreased after the resection of the antrum and duodenal bulb, the main sites of gastrin production (57). Sham-feeding produces little or no increase in the plasma gastrin level (57,86), although it evokes acid secretion amounting to about 50% of the maximal response to pentagastrin. In fact, it was found that only duodenal ulcer patients show an increase in acid and gastrin response to sham-feeding, but normal subjects respond only with increased acid secretion and no increase in gastrin (86). Recently, Richardson et al. (103) found that neither sham-feeding nor distention of the stomach with saline caused an increase in serum gastrin but that the two acting together did (Fig. 3). It is noteworthy that atropine, particularly when used in small doses, produces an enhancement rather than an inhibition of gastrin release in response to many stimuli, including sham-feeding (27). In addition, vagal gastrin release cannot be mimicked by cholinergic agents, which cause little or no stimulation of acid secretion in man (105). These findings remain in disagreement with the previous concept of cholinergic release of gastrin (34) during vagal excitation and suggest that it is noncholinergic. Since bombesin releases gastrin by an atropine-resistant mechanism (48) and since it is present

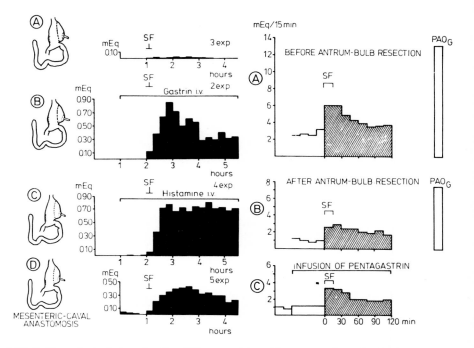

FIG. 2. The effect of sham-feeding (SF) on gastric acid response from the Pavlov pouch in dogs with resected antrum and duodenal bulb without **(A)** and with intravenous infusion of gastrin **(B)**, histamine **(C)** and mesenteric-caval anastomosis **(D) (left)**; the effect of sham-feeding on four duodenal ulcer patients before **(A)** and after antrum-bulb resection **(B)** and intravenous infusion of pentagastrin **(C) (right)**. PAO_G, mean peak acid responses to pentagastrin. (From ref. 57.)

in some neuronal axons (94), it may play the role of mediator in vagal release of gastrin. In addition, gastrin was found recently in the vagal nerves (124), suggesting that vagally released gastrin may originate directly from the vagal nerves themselves.

The cephalic phase stimulation can be mimicked by agents that reduce blood glucose level or interfere with glucose metabolism. These include insulin, tolbutamide, and 2-deoxyglucose. These substances produce a marked rise in gastric acid secretion amounting to the maximal response to pentagastrin. These glucopenic agents also induce a significant release of gastrin. Atropine or vagotomy abolishes the acid response to glucopenic agents but has little or no effect on the gastrin release (119), so it is apparently neither vagal nor cholinergic. It would appear that other noncholinergic mechanisms, perhaps adrenergic (15), mediate the release.

Although the predominating effect of vagal activation is the stimulation of gastric secretion and gastrin release, there is an increasing body of evidence suggesting that actually it also produces an inhibition. Vagal inhibition of acid

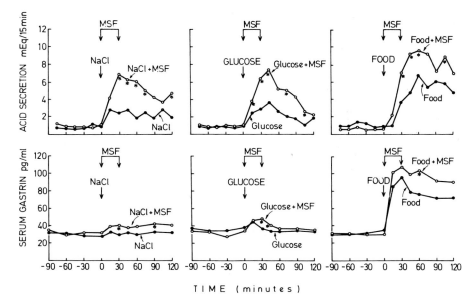

FIG. 3. Acid secretion **(top)** and serum gastrin concentration **(bottom)** in nine normal subjects in the basal state and after 600 ml NaCl, glucose, or homogenized food was infused into the stomach. Each experiment was performed with and without modified sham-feeding (MSF). *Asterisks* indicate statistically significant difference ($p < 0.05$) by paired t test between each stimulus alone and with modified sham-feeding. (From ref. 103.)

secretion has been demonstrated in dogs (112) and the name "vagogastrone" (37) has been proposed for the hypothetical hormone mediating vagal inhibitory effects. Since VIP was shown to be released by vagal stimuli and to inhibit gastric secretion (25), it could play the role of vagogastrone.

In the case of man, no direct evidence was presented for the existence of vagal inhibitory influence on acid secretion but several findings suggest that gastrin release may be under the inhibitory action of vagus. Vagotomies of all types including proximal gastric vagotomy (119) were found to increase serum gastrin level, presumably because this procedure decreases the release of an inhibitor of gastrin release. Similarly, atropine markedly increases gastrin response to sham-feeding (27) and to a meal (128) and this also may be considered as evidence for cholinergic inhibition of gastrin release.

In summary, gastric acid secretion and gastrin release in response to vagal activation results from the interplay of stimulation and inhibition; the mediators of these processes have not yet been determined.

Role of Gastrin in Chemical Stimulation of Acid Secretion

Food present in the stomach constitutes a natural and most potent stimulus of gastric acid secretion by virtue of its chemical and mechanical properties.

Recently, a method has been developed to measure gastric acid secretion in the presence of food in the intact stomach (28). This method, known as "intragastric titration," permits continuous monitoring of acid secretion in response to various meals introduced into the stomach. Through use of this method, it was found that the only chemicals present in food that stimulate acid secretion are amino acids and peptides (104). Undigested protein does not stimulate, but following light peptic digestion it is transformed into a potent stimulant. Peptic digests may stimulate acid secretion in at least four ways: (a) by releasing gastrin from the antral and intestinal G cells; (b) by the elevation of the gastric content pH by buffering the secreted acid and thus facilitating the release of gastrin; (c) by direct action on the oxyntic glands; and (d) by acting on the intestinal mucosa to activate the intestinal stimulatory mechanisms.

There is little doubt that the principal mechanism of gastric acid stimulation by amino acids and peptides is the release of gastrin. Most of the amino acids bathing the pyloric gland area stimulate gastrin release and gastric acid secretion (75). An amino acid mixture stimulates gastrin release and increases acid secretion to approximately 50% of pentagastrin-induced maximum (104). Individual amino acids introduced into the stomach vary in their potency of stimulating acid secretion, the most effective being phenylalanine, tryptophan, aspartic acid, leucine, and cysteine. Of these, only phenylalanine, tryptophan, and cysteine cause a signficant release of gastrin (14). This release may be mediated by direct action of chemicals on the G cells, and the luminal microvillous border of these cells seems well suited to receive such chemical stimuli. Atropine increases, rather than inhibits, gastrin release by chemicals, indicating that this release is either noncholinergic or cholinergic but atropine-resistant.

The fact that certain amino acids bathing gastric mucosa stimulate acid secretion without elevating serum gastrin indicates that an additional mechanism may be involved. In fact, the application of certain amino acids directly to the fundic mucosa in Heidenhain pouch dogs results in an increase in acid secretion without any change in plasma gastrin level (78). The most effective stimulant appears to be histidine, presumably due to the transformation into histamine in the gastric mucosa. In addition, some amino acids such as histidine, phenylalanine, and glycine are effective stimulants of gastric secretion after intravenous administration, suggesting direct action on the oxyntic cells without mediation of gastrointestinal hormones (69,77).

A slight increase in serum gastrin level has been observed after carbohydrate or fat meals but acid secretion was actually inhibited by these dietary constituents (104). This again indicates that proteins are the only food products that both release gastrin and stimulate acid secretion (Fig. 4).

Food in the stomach stimulates acid secretion also through the distention of the gastric wall, which is accompanied by the release of little or no gastrin. Selective fundic distention was reported to stimulate acid secretion in man to approximately 50% of maximal response to pentagastrin (39). Antral distention was ineffective in gastric acid stimulation in normal subjects but did elicit a

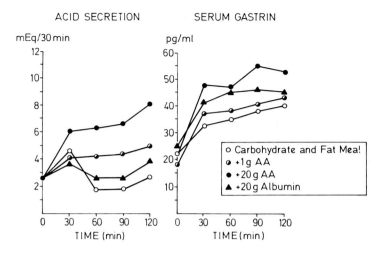

FIG. 4. Pattern of acid secretion and serum gastrin response after meals containing carbohydrate and fat plus various amounts of amino acids or albumin. Test meal volume was 500 ml; osmolarity was 480 mOsm/kg. Basal acid secretion and fasting serum gastrin concentration are indicated. Mean results in eight normal subjects are shown. (From ref. 104.)

secretory response in patients with duodenal ulcer, particularly in those with active disease (6). Acid secretion in response to gastric distention, unlike that in response to chemical stimulation, was found to be markedly depressed by vagotomy and atropine (38). This finding, together with the observation that gastric distention does not affect gastrin release, indicates that acid response to distention stimulus is mediated by cholinergic reflexes, both "long" vago-vagal and "short" intramural directly activating the oxyntic glands.

ENTERO-OXYNTIN

The upper portion of the small intestine is an important source of hormonal stimulation of gastric acid secretion in man (70) and in laboratory animals (74). The introduction of peptide or amino acid meal into the duodenum results in an increase of acid secretion amounting to approximately 30 to 40% of the maximal response to pentagastrin (Fig. 5).

The mechanism of gastric acid stimulation by the intestinal meal has not been elucidated (60). Although gastrin was found in the upper duodenal mucosa, release of this hormone by the intestinal meal is slight in the dog (68) and negligible in man (70). This indicates that antral-type gastrin from the duodenum accounts for only a small part (if any) of acid secretion during the intestinal phase. It seems that the major factor responsible for the intestinal phase stimulation is an as yet unidentified hormone, named "entero-oxyntin" (an enteric substance that stimulates oxyntic cells) (37). This substance has not yet been isolated and chemically characterized but it appears to be markedly inactivated

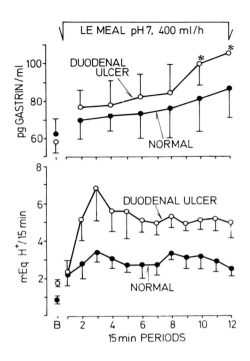

FIG. 5. Effect of duodenal instillation of 10% liver extract meal at 400 ml/hr on gastric acid and serum gastrin in healthy subjects and in duodenal ulcer patients. Mean (± SEM) of 10 tests on each of 10 subjects. (From ref. 70.)

by the liver, differing in this respect from gastrin and cholecystokinin. This is supported by the finding that the intestinal phase of acid secretion is greatly enhanced by shunting portal blood around the liver (90). The postshunt gastric hypersecretion is not accompanied by any change in postprandial serum gastrin level, indicating that gastrin is not responsible for this hypersecretion.

Another characteristic feature of entero-oxyntin is its marked potentiating effect on gastrin or histamine-induced gastric secretion (19). This criterion has been proposed to distinguish the hormone of the intestinal phase from nonspecific stimulators. Recently, several attempts have been made to isolate the active principle responsible for the intestinal phase of gastric secretion and for the portacaval shunt-related gastric hypersecretion, but its chemical nature has not been revealed (87,89).

The mediation by intestinal hormones of intestinal phase stimulation does not exclude the possibility that some products of protein digestion may stimulate the oxyntic glands after absorption from the gut. As shown in dogs (74) and in man (69), an amino acid mixture given intravenously produces gastric acid secretion similar to that obtained when an identical solution is given intraintestinally. This, of course, should not be interpreted as indicating that intestinal amino acids stimulate gastric secretion solely after being absorbed from the gut, because most of them are probably taken up from the circulation during passage through the liver (82). The fact that amino acids given intraportally are less potent stimulants of acid secretion than when given systemically and that serum gastrin is not changed during amino acid-induced gastric secretion suggests that they may act directly on the oxyntic cells without mediation of gastrointestinal hormones. Since amino acids given intravenously do not potentiate the gastric response to exogenous stimulants such as gastrin or histamine (69), it is unlikely that they could serve as an entero-oxyntin type mediator of the intestinal phase of gastric secretion.

CHOLECYSTOKININ (CCK)

The test meals (amino acids, peptides, liver extract, and food) used to induce the intestinal phase of gastric secretion are also potent releasers of cholecystokinin (CCK). This hormone is structurally related to gastrin and belongs to the "gastrin family" of peptides. It exists in the endocrine I cells of the intestine in several molecular forms representing various peptides ranging from the large variant form of CCK to C-terminal octapeptide (88). Another peptide with CCK-like activity has been isolated from the skin of certain frogs and named caerulein (1). Like gastrin, CCK is also present in central and peripheral nerves (20).

CCK and its C-terminal hepta- and octa-peptide fragments stimulate acid secretion in addition to many other actions such as stimulation of pancreatic enzyme secretion or gallbladder contraction. They are partial agonists of acid secretion in man (10,65) and in dogs (55) but full agonists in other species (cat, rat). They probably activate the same receptors on the parietal cells as gastrin does, but in those species in which they are partial agonists (10,65) with a weak efficacy (man, dog) they may stimulate gastric secretion when given alone or with small doses of exogenous gastrin, but competitively inhibit the response to high doses of gastrin. Through use of bioassay and immunoassay, it was shown (85,123) that circulating levels of CCK are greatly increased after the meal but to date no study has been performed to determine the possible role of this hormone in the intestinal phase of gastric secretion. Way et al. (129) observed that intestinal meals in dogs with removed antra potentiated the effect of exogenous CCK on Heidenhain pouch secretion in dogs. This suggests that CCK stimulates different receptors than entero-oxyntin stimulates and, therefore, has a different type of molecular structure. See also Chapter 7 by V. Mutt, pp. 169–222, *this volume.*

MOTILIN AND ENKEPHALIN

Motilin and enkephalin may be considered as more distant members of the gastrin family peptides (Table 1).

Motilin is a weak stimulant of basal acid secretion in dogs but it inhibits stimulation of acid secretion induced by pentagastrin, histamine, and food (64). The action of motilin on gastric secretion is independent of antral pH and of serum gastrin level. It is unknown whether motilin is involved in the physiological stimulation of gastric secretion.

Enkephalins are peptides with opiate-like activity that have been recently demonstrated by immunocytochemistry and RIA in the endocrine-paracrine type cells of the gastrointestinal mucosa and the pancreas as well as in the nerves of the digestive system (99). They show powerful actions on gastrointestinal motility. In addition, they stimulate gastric acid secretion and increase the gastric mucosal blood flow without affecting serum gastrin levels (72,73). The biological effects of enkephalin are presented in Chapter 15 by C. A. Meyers and D. H. Coy, pp. 363–386, *this volume*.

GASTRIC AND INTESTINAL BOMBESIN-LIKE PEPTIDE

Recently, McDonald et al. (87) reported that the extracts obtained from nonantral gastric tissue and the gut are capable of releasing gastrin from the antral G cells and of stimulating gastric acid secretion. Previous studies with peptone meal introduced into the fundic gland area or into the gut suggested that there may be a gastric and intestinal factor capable of stimulating gastric secretion *via* releasing antral gastrin (60,74). After the isolation from the frog skin of bombesin, a tetradecapeptide with a powerful stimulatory effect on gastrin release and gastric secretion (24,48), attempts were made to identify similar hormonal substances in the gastrointestinal tract. In fact, Polak et al. (94,95) succeeded in the demonstration of the presence of bombesin-like immunoreactivity in endocrine D_1 cells and in nerves of the digestive system. The discovery of a peptide with biological actions similar to bombesin (87) suggests that this factor may be the mammalian counterpart of amphibian bombesin (see Chapter 29 by P. Melchiorri, pp. 717–726, and Chapter 43I by T. J. McDonald, pp. 972–977).

GASTROINTESTINAL HORMONES AND THE INHIBITORY MECHANISMS OF GASTRIC ACID SECRETION

The observation that secretion of gastric acid is markedly increased after the ingestion of food and virtually abolished during the interdigestive period formed a basis for the concept that gastric secretion depends on the interplay of stimulatory and inhibitory influences arising from the stomach and the intestines. Through interactions between nervous and hormonal stimuli, gastric secretion is controlled by complex feedback mechanisms (59). The known initiators of inhibition are acid in the stomach and duodenum, fat or hypertonic solutions in the duodenum, and hyperglycemia.

ANTRAL AND FUNDIC FEEDBACK INHIBITION OF GASTRIC SECRETION. ROLE OF GASTRONE AND SOMATOSTATIN

Woodward et al. (131) found that bathing the antral mucosa with acid suppressed gastrin release and gastric acid secretion. Lowering gastric pH from

5.5 to 1.0 completely suppressed gastrin release in response to an amino acid or peptone meal and resulted in a marked inhibition of acid secretion. The inhibition was reported to be more pronounced in normal subjects than in duodenal ulcer patients (127) but this was not confirmed by other studies (63). This inhibition probably occurs under physiological conditions, as after a mixed meal intragastric content reaches a pH level of about 2 to 3; that is enough to suppress gastrin release and to inhibit gastric acid secretion (Fig. 6).

Suppression of gastrin release is the only recognized mechanism by which acid bathing the pyloric gland area inhibits acid secretion (59). It is unknown, however, whether acid directly suppresses the G cells or whether it releases an inhibitor of gastrin release from the antral mucosa. The observation that acid bathing the antral mucosa counteracts all modes of gastrin release including that induced by acetylcholine, which is assumed to release gastrin by direct activation of G cells, has been taken as evidence that acid operates by direct suppression of the activity of G cells (34).

In the past, some workers postulated that acid in the pyloric gland area caused release of an antral inhibitory hormone ("antral chalone") that suppresses the activity of the oxyntic cells (37). Despite the many ingenious attempts to

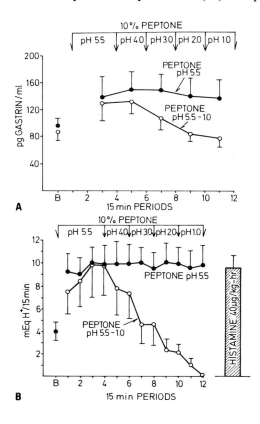

FIG. 6. Serum gastrin **(A)** and gastric acid response **(B)** to a peptone meal at pH levels varying from 5.5 to 1.0 or at constant pH 5.5. For comparison the maximal acid response to histamine is presented. Mean (± SEM) of six tests on each of six duodenal ulcer patients. (From ref. 61.)

elucidate the physiological role of this hormone, the question of its existence is still unanswered.

Gastrone and Somatostatin

Another candidate for the active principle released by antral acidification is gastrone (37), an inhibitor substance present in the achlorhydric gastric juice of pernicious anemia patients. (For further information, see Chapter 42 by G. B. J. Glass, pp. 929–969, *this volume.*) Gastrone has been identified by immunocytochemistry in antral mucosa (30a) and found to be an inhibitor of acid secretion, but it has not been isolated and chemically characterized. The final evidence that it is involved in the physiological mechanisms controlling gastric secretion is still to be obtained and its relationship to other inhibitory substances found in saliva (sialogastrone) and in the urine (urogastrone) remains to be established. The latter has been recently isolated from urine and chemically characterized (31). It is a linear peptide containing 53 amino acid residues, of which 37 occupy positions identical to those in the epidermal growth factor, isolated from the submaxillary salivary glands of male mice. Both peptides inhibit gastric acid secretion (23,31) and also increase the rate of cell proliferation (106). A RIA has been developed for human urogastrone and the plasma level of this peptide was found to increase in pregnancy. This may contribute to the decreased incidence of peptic ulcer disease during pregnancy. Urogastrone could promote healing of ulcer by inhibition of acid secretion and by stimulation of epithelial cell proliferation in the gastroduodenal mucosa. For more detailed information see Chapter 17 by H. Gregory, pp. 397–411, *this volume.*

Somatostatin

The problem of antral inhibitory hormone has recently been revived with the discovery of somatostatin immunoreactivity in the endocrine cells and nerves in the vicinity of the G cells in the pyloric gland area and in the oxyntic gland area (46,98). Somatostatin is a potent inhibitor of gastrin release and of gastric acid secretion induced by a meal and exogenous stimulants acting directly on the oxyntic cells. Recently, Schusdziarra et al. (111) reported that immunoreactive somatostatin is released under basal conditions into the blood draining the stomach and the pancreas and that gastric or duodenal acidification results in a marked rise in the plasma level of somatostatin. This suggests that somatostatin may be involved in the antral and duodenal inhibitory mechanisms but further studies are needed to determine the physiological role of this peptide in antral and duodenal feedback inhibition of gastric secretion. For more details on this subject see Chapter 15 by C. A. Meyers and D. H. Coy, pp. 363–386, *this volume.*

It is of interest that an amino acid or peptone meal stimulates acid secretion when directly bathing the oxyntic gland area (78). This stimulation is gastrin-independent but pH-sensitive. Decreasing the pH of the meal tends to lead to a fall of acid secretion in a pH-dependent manner. This finding, together with the observation that the acidification of canine oxyntic mucosa increases the level of immunoreactive somatostatin in the venous outflow from the fundic portion of the stomach (111), suggests that somatostatin may be a mediator of the inhibitory mechanism of acid secretion arising from the oxyntic mucosa as well. This inhibition of gastric acid secretion by direct acidification of the fundic mucosa was found so far only in the Heidenhain pouch dog (78) and it has not yet been examined in man.

DUODENAL FEEDBACK INHIBITION OF GASTRIC ACID SECRETION. ROLE OF SECRETIN

Instillation of large amounts of acid into the duodenum inhibits both gastrin and histamine-stimulated gastric acid secretion in the dog (66,76) and man (58,132). The kinetics of this inhibition are competitive and can be reproduced by large doses of exogenous secretin (7,8). Although gastric inhibition by acid in the canine duodenum is probably of considerable physiological interest, the physiological significance of acid in the human duodenum in the inhibition of gastric secretion has not yet been established. It has been reported that duodenal acidification in man inhibits gastrin-induced gastric acid secretion only when acidification is severe and prolonged (132) (Fig. 7).

Secretin

The principal humoral mechanism of gastric inhibition by duodenal acidification is the release of secretin from the endocrine S cells present in the duodenal mucosa. Secretin, a 27-amino acid linear peptide, structurally resembles three

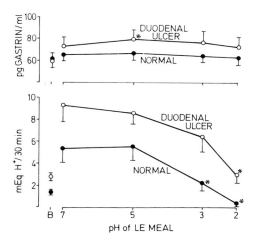

FIG. 7. Gastric acid and serum gastrin responses to a liver extract meal adjusted to pH levels varying from 7 to 2 and instilled into the duodenum in 10 duodenal ulcer patients. (From ref. 70.)

other relatives of this peptide family [glucagon, VIP, and gastric inhibitory peptide (GIP)] and shares with them a similar action on the stomach, namely inhibition of acid secretion and suppression of gastrin release (Table 2). Although exogenous secretin does inhibit gastrin, histamine, and food-induced acid se-

TABLE 2. *The secretin-glucagon family of peptides*

	GIP	Glucagon	Secretin	VIP
Amino acid residues	43	29	27	28
Molecular weight	5,104	3,484	3,055	3,326
	Tyr	His	—	—
	Ala	Ser	—	—
	Glu	Gln	Asp	—
	Gly	—	—	Ala
	Thr	—	—	Val
	Phe	—	—	—
	Ile	Thr	—	—
	Ser	—	—	Asp
	Asp	—	Glu	Asn
	Tyr	—	Leu	Tyr
	Ser	—	—	Thr
	Ile	Lys	Arg	—
	Ala	Tyr	Leu	—
	Met	Leu	Arg	—
	Asp	—	—	Lys
	Lys	Ser	—	Gln
	Ile	Arg	Ala	Met
	Arg	—	—	Ala
	Gln	Ala	Leu	Val
	Gln	—	—	Lys
	Asp	—	Arg	Lys
	Phe	—	Leu	Tyr
	Val	—	Leu	—
	Asn	Gln	—	Asn
	Trp	—	Gly	Ser
	Leu	—	—	Ile
	Leu	Met	Val-NH$_2$	Leu
	Ala	Asp		Asn-NH$_2$
	Gln	Thr		
	Gln			
	Lys			
	Gly			
	Lys			
	Lys			
	Ser			
	Asp			
	Trp			
	Lys			
	His			
	Asn			
	Ile			
	Thr			
	Gln			

(—) Indicates amino acid residue identical to preceding column.

cretion (7,61), it seems unlikely that it is the only mediator of gastric inhibition by duodenal acidification (55). In dogs, the strongest inhibition triggered by acid is confined to the duodenal bulb, which has been thought to release a special inhibitory hormone named bulbogastrone (2) (see Chapter 41 by G. Nilsson, pp. 911–928, *this volume*). In addition, gastric inhibition by bulbar acidification was shown to be effective only in the fully innervated duodenal bulb (67), suggesting that the inhibition is mediated, at least in part, by a neural reflex activated by acid in the bulb. Acidification of the postbulbar duodenum below pH 4.5 (the pH threshold for secretin release in the dog) releases enough secretin to inhibit gastric secretion so that this inhibition appears to be secretin-dependent (76). In humans, the pH threshold for secretin release was found to be between pH 2 and 3 (26). Such a low pH threshold can be achieved under physiological conditions only in the duodenal bulb and the amount of secretin release from this area is certainly not sufficient to account for the observed gastric secretory inhibition. It is possible that the neural reflex inhibition is also involved, since it has been shown that vagotomy (truncal, selective, or highly selective) abolishes the gastric inhibition evoked by duodenal acidification in man (50). Whatever the significance of secretin in gastric acid inhibition in man, there does not appear to be any difference between the normals and duodenal ulcer patients in the release of endogenous secretin in response to exogenous hormone (18) (Fig. 8).

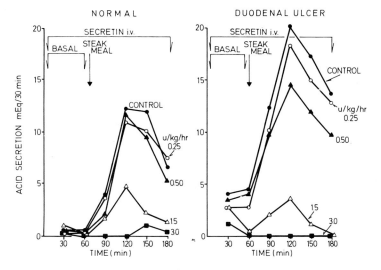

FIG. 8. The effect of control saline infusion or secretin in doses of 0.25, 0.5, 1.5, and 3.0 μg/kg-hr on food stimulated acid secretion when secretin infusion was begun 1 hr before injection of the meal into the stomach in seven normal subjects and seven duodenal ulcer patients. (From ref. 18.)

INHIBITION OF GASTRIC ACID SECRETION BY FAT AND HYPERTONIC SOLUTIONS IN THE DUODENUM. ROLE OF CCK, GIP, AND VIP

Fat introduced into the duodenum in an absorbable form inhibits gastric secretion. This inhibition is effective against gastrin-, histamine-, and food-induced acid secretion (55) and can be demonstrated in both healthy subjects and in duodenal ulcer patients (33).

The mechanism by which fat inhibits acid secretion is not fully understood but gut hormones are involved, at least in part (71,100). A neural inhibitory reflex similar to that triggered by acid in the duodenal bulb has also been proposed as the mode of action of fat in the duodenum, since the inhibition was reported less pronounced after vagotomy (51). However, the vagus may interact with inhibitory hormones at the level of the oxyntic cells or may facilitate the release of these hormones from the gastrointestinal tract.

Cholecystokinin (CCK)

A number of studies have been undertaken to identify the hormones that are released by fat and involved in gastric acid inhibition. It is now well established that fat releases CCK from the intestinal mucosa but there is little doubt that this hormone cannot be solely responsible for inhibition, since fat induces suppression of histamine-stimulated acid secretion that cannot be reproduced by CCK or secretin regardless of the dose used (54).

Gastric Inhibitory Peptide (GIP)

Fat also releases GIP from the intestinal endocrine-type K cells (12,13). GIP is a linear 43-amino acid peptide that inhibits gastric acid secretion in the dog during stimulation by pentagastrin, histamine, insulin, or food (93). Maximal inhibition was found to be produced by doses that caused blood concentrations similar to those found after ingestion of a mixed meal. Large doses of GIP also inhibited gastrin release in dogs (125). Recently, GIP was also demonstrated to inhibit pentagastrin or meal-induced gastric secretion in man, but doses used increased serum GIP levels two- to fivefold higher than those measured after ingestion of a mixed meal (3). Although GIP appears to satisfy most completely the criteria for being an "enterogastrone" described by Kosaka and Lim (81), further studies are needed to determine how much of the inhibition of acid secretion by fat can be accounted for by release of GIP. For more information see Chapter 8 by J. C. Brown et al., pp. 223–232, *this volume.*

Vasoactive Intestinal Peptide (VIP)

VIP is another candidate for the agent that is released by fat and inhibits gastric secretion. VIP contains 28 amino acid residues and is present both in the endocrine H cells in the gastrointestinal mucosa and also in nerve fibers of the myenteric plexus. It is a potent inhibitor of pentagastrin and histamine-stimulated gastric secretion (79). It suppresses food-stimulated gastric secretion and gastrin release. If VIP is released by fat in sufficient amounts, it might also be considered as an enterogastrone controlling gastric secretion when fatty meal is present in the gut. For more information see Chapter 10 by S. I. Said, pp. 245–274, *this volume.*

Hypertonic Solutions

Hypertonic solutions instilled into the duodenum inhibit gastric secretion (66) but neither the mechanism of this effect nor the extent to which it operates under physiological conditions is known. Since the inhibition persisted after the denervation and transplantation of the fundic pouches in dogs, it was concluded that it is hormonal in nature. In the case of hypertonic glucose in the duodenum, at least two mechanisms are involved; one is hyperglycemia, which inhibits gastric secretion by central suppression of vagal activity (83), and the other is GIP, which is released by glucose in the gut and affects gastric secretion (71).

PEPSIN SECRETION

Synthesis and Release of Pepsinogens

Pepsins are the chief proteolytic enzymes in the gastric juice playing an important role in the digestive processes. They are stored in an inactive form as pepsinogens in five types of cells described at the beginning of this chapter. The granules containing pepsinogens accumulate in the resting cells and induce a negative feedback mechanism to slow down new synthesis (43). In the unstimulated state, small amounts of pepsinogens are released all the time into the gastric lumen, in part because synthesis is continuous and "overflow secretion" occurs when the peptic cells are filled with granules. Pepsin may be present in appreciable amounts in the basal gastric juice, even in the absence of other constituents such as hydrochloric acid. Basal secretion usually contains several times more pepsin when compared with acid than the histamine- or gastrin-stimulated juice (43).

The general pattern of pepsinogen secretion after stimulation shows an initially high rate of secretion due to release of pepsinogens from preformed granules. This is followed by a prolonged plateau of increased secretion at a lower level, which represents the release of both stored and newly synthesized protein. The rate of depletion of all zymogen granules from peptic cells depends on the strength and duration of the stimulus and requires several hours on the average (43).

In the presence of acid, pepsinogens are converted autocatalytically to pepsins by the cleavage of several small basic peptides. Pepsins are active at acid pH and are irreversibly inactivated at neutral or slightly alkaline pH.

Pepsinogens and pepsins are a heterogenous group of proenzyme and enzyme proteins that can be subdivided by chemical and immunological methods (108,109). Through use of agar gel electrophoresis, eight proteolytic fractions have been found in human gastric mucosa, of which seven were inactivated by alkali and called pepsinogens 1 to 7; one fraction was alkali-stable and called slow moving protease (SMP). The seven pepsinogen fractions could be further subdivided into two immunologically unrelated groups: group I pepsinogens (PGI), which included pepsinogens 1 to 5, and group II pepsinogens (PGII), which included pepsinogens 6 and 7. By immunofluorescent studies, both PGI and PGII have been localized in the same granules of the peptic cells and mucous neck cells in the oxyntic gland mucosa. In addition, PGIIs were also found in the mucous cells of cardiac, pyloric, and duodenal (Brunner's) glands. Thus, the peptic cell population is heterogenous and the amount of PGI and PGII secreted into the gastric juice depends on the rate of their synthesis and release from the cells. Although both types of immunoreactive pepsinogens are stored in the same granules of the peptic cells, it is possible that the ratio of PGI and PGII secreted may vary with different stimulants. Strong stimulants of pepsinogen secretion, such as cholinergic agents, have no effect on pepsinogen secretion from the pyloric glands and Brunner's glands. The ingestion of food, on the other hand, has been reported to stimulate pepsinogen secretion by Brunner's glands but not by pyloric glands.

Role of Gastrointestinal Hormones in Pepsinogen Secretion

The basal secretion of pepsin is continuous but relatively small. The strongest stimulants of pepsin secretion include feeding and cholinergic stimulation induced by central vagal excitation (sham-feeding, insulin hypoglycemia) or local cholinergic stimulation by gastric distention or stable choline esters. Increased pepsin secretion by cholinergic stimulation is mediated by acetylcholine released in the vicinity of the peptic cells and by circulating gastrin, and these act synergistically (43,108).

Gastrin and Related Peptides

Gastrin and related peptides, such as pentagastrin, strongly stimulate pepsin secretion. The peak rates of pepsin secretion achieved by gastrin-like peptides are similar to those obtained with histamine and range from two to four times basal secretion (59). Since gastrin release occurs under basal conditions and markedly increases during all three phases of the digestive period, it is reasonable to assume that postprandial pepsin secretion is, at least in part, due to the stimulation of peptic cells by gastrin. Hypercalcemia induced by intravenous calcium infusion also causes pepsin secretion, probably due to the release of gastrin and direct stimulation of peptic cells by calcium ions (108).

Other members of the "gastrin family" of peptides such as CCK, (54,55), motilin (64), and enkephalin (73) also stimulate pepsin secretion when acting alone. This stimulation may result in part from direct action of these hormonal peptides on the peptic cells and in part may be a consequence of mucosal acidification, which was shown to increase pepsin secretion by a local cholinergic reflex (52).

Secretin

Secretin inhibits basal and gastrin-induced acid secretion and is a strong stimulant of pepsin secretion, whether released endogenously by duodenal acidification or given exogenously (11). Other relatives of the "secretin family" of peptides (VIP, GIP, glucagon) inhibit pepsin secretion (61a,59,79).

Trace amounts of pepsinogen can be detected by RIA in the serum and have been used as an estimate of the secretory capacity of the peptic cells (110). It is not known whether pepsinogen found in the blood is actively secreted by the peptic cells or is derived from the degenerating peptic cells. Samloff and co-workers (110) showed that there is a good correlation between maximal acid secretion and serum PGI level. Serum PGI level is significantly higher in duodenal ulcer patients than in healthy subjects and decreases markedly after vagotomy, suggesting that the secretion of PGI remains under the tonic influence of vagal nerves. No information is available concerning whether gastrointestinal hormones affect the release of pepsinogen into the circulation.

CONCLUSIONS AND PROJECTIONS FOR THE FUTURE

The physiological mechanisms controlling gastric acid and pepsin secretion are complex and poorly understood. The stomach is now recognized not only as an important exocrine gland but also as the major endocrine organ, with a large mass of endocrine tissue and high degree of complexity in the interactions between various gastrointestinal hormones and interrelationships between gut hormones and the autonomic nervous system. The dispersion of the distinctive endocrine-paracrine cells between the oxyntic glands and the presence of some hormones in the nerves suggest an important role of the local hormone release in the regulation of gastric secretion. At present, various new peptide hormones such as bombesin, somatostatin, and enkephalin have been found in the gastric mucosa, but their physiological role remains unresolved because of the difficulties in investigating their paracrine or neurocrine release and actions. There is still a long list of hypothetical hormones and hormone candidates such as enterooxyntin, gastrone, bulbogastrone, and vagogastrone that have been postulated to affect gastric secretion, but neither their chemical nature nor the modes of release and actions have so far been determined. These will surely attract the attention of research workers in the near future.

There is good evidence that vagal nerves have not only stimulatory but also inhibitory effects on gastric secretory functions. Future research should reveal the mechanism of the suppressive vagal action on gastric secretion and gastrin release under various physiological conditions. Recent findings that some vagal nerves contain gastrin and other hormones, and that these hormones may be released during vagal excitation, open a new field for study of the neurohormonal interactions and their physiological importance.

Some encouraging advances in our understanding of the control of gastric secretory processes have been gained from recent studies on the cellular secretory mechanisms. The isolated oxyntic cell model may be found useful in investigating the interdependence and interactions among gastric hormonal stimulants and inhibitors that has fascinated physiologists for several decades. Further studies are necessary to characterize various hormonal receptors on the oxyntic and pepsin secreting cells, to elucidate the mechanisms of their activation, and to determine the intracellular mediators involved in acid and pepsin secretory processes.

REFERENCES

1. Anastasi, A. V., Erspamer, V., and Endean, R. (1967): Isolation and structure of caerulein, an active decapeptide from the skin of Hyla caerulea. *Experientia,* 23:699–700.
2. Andersson, S. (1975): Bulbogastrone. In: *Gastrointestinal Hormones,* edited by J. C. Thompson, pp. 552–562. University of Texas Press, Austin.
3. Arnold, R., Ebert, R., Creutzfeldt, W., Becker, H. D., and Börger, H. (1978): Inhibition of gastric acid secretion by gastric inhibitory polypeptide (GIP) in man. *Scand. J. Gastroenterol. (Suppl.),* 13:11.
4. Beaven, M. A. (1978): Histamine: a reassessment of its role in physiological and pathological processes. *Prog. Allergy, (in press).*
5. Bergegårdh, S., Broman, G., Knutson, U., Palmer, L., and Olbe, L. (1976): Gastric acid responses to graded i.v. infusions of pentagastrin and histalog in peptic ulcer patients before and after antrum-bulb resection. *Scand. J. Gastroenterol.,* 11:337–346.
6. Bergegårdh, S., Nilsson, G., and Olbe, L. (1976): The effect of antral distension on acid secretion and plasma gastrin in duodenal ulcer patients. *Scand. J. Gastroenterol.,* 11:475–479.
7. Berstad, A., and Petersen, H. (1970): Dose-response relationship of the effect of secretin on acid and pepsin secretion in man. *Scand. J. Gastroenterol.,* 5:647–654.
8. Berstad, A., and Petersen, H. (1972): Effect of duodenal acidification on the gastric secretory response to pentagastrin in man. *Digestion,* 6:193–199.
9. Black, J. W., Duncan, W. A. M., Durant, C. J., Ganellin, C. R., and Parsons, E. M. (1972): Definition and antagonism of histamine H_2-receptors. *Nature,* 236:385–390.
10. Brooks, A. M., Agosti, A., Bertaccini, G., and Grossman, M. I. (1970): Inhibition of gastric acid secretion in man by peptide analogues of cholecystokinin. *N. Eng. J. Med.,* 282:535–538.
11. Brooks, A. M., Isenberg, J., and Grossman, M. I. (1969): The effect of secretin, glucagon, and duodenal acidification on pepsin secretion in man. *Gastroenterology,* 57:159–162.
12. Brown, J. C., Dryburgh, J. R., Frost, J. L., Otte, S. C., and Pederson, R. A. (1978): Properties and actions of GIP. In: *Gut Hormones,* edited by S. R. Bloom, pp. 277–282. Churchill Livingstone, Edinburgh.
13. Brown, J. C., Dryburgh, J. R., Moccia, P., and Pederson, R. A. (1975): The current status of GIP. In: *Gastrointestinal Hormones,* edited by J. C. Thompson, pp. 537–547. University of Texas Press, Austin.

14. Byrne, W. J., Christie, D. L., Ament, M. E., and Walsh, J. H. (1979): Acid secretory response in man to 18 individual amino acids. *Clin. Res. (Abstr.), (in press).*
15. Christensen, K. C., and Stadil, F. (1976): On the beta-adrenergic contribution to the gastric acid and gastrin responses to hypoglycaemia in man. *Scand. J. Gastroenterol. (Suppl.),* 37:81–86.
16. Code, C. F. (1965): Histamine and gastric secretion; a later look, 1955–1965. *Fed. Proc.,* 24:1311–1321.
17. Crean, G. P., Marshall, M. W., and Rumsey, R. D. E. (1969): Parietal cell hyperplasia induced by the administration of pentagastrin (ICI 50, 123) to rats. *Gastroenterology,* 57:147–155.
18. Dalton, M. D., Eisenstein, A. M., Walsh, J. H., and Fordtran, J. S. (1976): Effect of secretin on gastric function in normal subjects and in patients with duodenal ulcer. *Gastroenterology,* 71:24–29.
19. Debas, H. T., Slaff, G. F., and Grossman, M. I. (1975): Intestinal phase of gastric acid secretion: augmentation of maximal response of Heidenhain pouch to gastrin and histamine. *Gastroenterology,* 68:691–698.
20. Dockray, G. J. (1976): Immunochemical evidence of cholecystokinin-like peptides in brain. *Nature,* 264:568–570.
21. Dousa, T. P., and Dozois, R. R. (1977): Interrelations between histamine, prostaglandins and cyclic AMP in gastric secretion: a hypothesis. *Gastroenterology,* 73:904–912.
22. Edkins, J. S. (1906): The chemical mechanism of gastric secretion. *J. Physiol. (Lond.),* 34:183–185.
23. Elder, J. B., Ganguli, P. C., Guillespie, I. E., and Gregory, H. (1974): Initial observations on the inhibitory action of urogastrone on gastric secretory responses in man. *Gut,* 15:337–341.
23a. Enoch, M. R., and Johnson, L. R. (1977): Hormonal regulation of gastrointestinal growth; biochemical and physiological aspects. In: *Progress in Gastroenterology,* Vol. III, edited by G. B. J. Glass, pp. 3–28. Grune and Stratton, New York.
24. Erspamer, V., and Melchiorri, P. (1975): Actions of bombesin on secretions and motility of the gastrointestinal tract. In: *Gastrointestinal Hormones,* edited by J. C. Thompson, pp. 575–589. University of Texas Press, Austin.
25. Fahrenkrug, J., Schaffalitzky de Muckadell, O. B., and Holst, J. J. (1978): Nervous release of VIP. In: *Gut Hormones,* edited by S. R. Bloom, pp. 488–491. Churchill Livingstone, Edinburgh.
26. Fahrenkrug, J., Schaffalitzky de Muckadell, O. B., and Rune, S. J. (1978): pH Threshold for release of secretin in normal subjects and in patients with duodenal ulcer and patients with chronic pancreatitis. *Scand. J. Gastroenterol.,* 13:177–186.
27. Feldman, J., Richardson, C. T., Taylor, I. L., and Walsh, J. H. (1979): Effect of atropine on vagal release of gastrin and pancreatic polypeptide. *J. Clin. Invest.,* 63:294–298.
28. Fordtran, J. S., and Walsh, J. H. (1973): Gastric acid secretion rate and buffer content of the stomach after eating: results in normal subjects and in patients with duodenal ulcer. *J. Clin. Invest.,* 52:645–657.
29. Forte, J. G., and Lee, H. C. (1977): Gastric ATPases: a review of their possible role in HC1 secretion. *Gastroenterology,* 73:921–926.
30. Forte, T. M., Machen, T. E., and Forte, J. G. (1977): Ultrastructural changes in oxyntic cells associated secretory function: a membrane recycling hypothesis. *Gastroenterology,* 73:941–955.
30a. Glass, G. B. J., Balanzo, J. T., and Rosenthal, W. S. (1973): Cellular localization of gastrone in gastrointestinal mucosa by immunofluorescence. *Am. J. Dig. Dis.,* 18:279–288.
31. Gregory, H. (1975): Isolation and structure of urogastrone and its relationship to epidermal growth factor. *Nature,* 257:325–328.
32. Gregory, R. A., and Tracy, H. J. (1975): The chemistry of the gastrins. Some recent advances. In: *Gastrointestinal Hormones,* edited by J. C. Thompson, pp. 13–24. University of Texas Press, Austin.
33. Gross, R. A., Isenberg, J. I., Hogan, D., and Samloff, I. M. (1978): Effect of fat on meal-stimulated duodenal acid load, duodenal pepsin load and serum gastrin in duodenal ulcer and normal subjects. *Gastroenterology,* 75:357–362.
34. Grossman, M. I. (1976): Neural and hormonal stimulation of gastric secretion of acid. In: *Handbook of Physiology,* Alimentary Canal, Vol. II, edited by C. F. Code, pp. 835–863, American Physiological Society, Washington, D.C.

35. Grossman, M. I. (1978): Control of gastric secretion. In: *Gastrointestinal Disease,* edited by M. H. Sleisenger and J. S. Fordtran, pp. 640–659, Saunders, Philadelphia.
36. Grossman, M. I., and Konturek, S. J. (1974): Inhibition of acid secretion by metiamide, a histamine antagonist acting on H_2-receptors. *Gastroenterology,* 66:517–521.
37. Grossman, M. I., et al. (1974): Candidate hormones of the gut. *Gastroenterology,* 67:730–755.
38. Grötzinger, U., Bergehardh, S., and Olbe, L. (1977): The effect of fundic distention on gastric acid secretion in duodenal ulcer patients. *Gut,* 18:105–110.
40. Helander, H. F., and Hirschowitz, B. I. (1974): Quantitative ultrastructural studies on inhibited and partly stimulated gastric parietal cells. *Gastroenterology,* 67:447–452.
41. Hersey, S. J. (1974): Interactions between oxidative metabolism and acid secretion in gastric mucosa. *Biochim. Biophys. Acta,* 344:157–203.
42. Hersey, S. J. (1977): Metabolic changes associated with gastric stimulation. *Gastroenterology,* 73:914–919.
43. Hirschowitz, B. I. (1967): Secretion of pepsinogen. In: *Handbook of Physiology, Alimentary Canal,* Vol. II, edited by C. F. Code, pp. 889–918. American Physiological Society, Washington, D. C.
44. Hogben, C. A. M., Kent, T. H., Woodward, P. A., and Sill, A. J. (1974): Quantitative histology of the gastric mucosa: man, dog, cat, guinea pig, and frog. *Gastroenterology,* 67:1143–1154.
45. Hollander, F. (1952): Gastric secretion of electrolytes. *Fed. Proc.,* 11:706.
46. Hökfelt, T., Efendic, S., and Hellerstrom, C. (1975): Cellular localization of somatostatin in endocrine-like cells and neurons of the rat with special reference to the A_1 cells of the pancreatic islets and the hypothalamus. *Acta Endocrinol. (Suppl.),* 80:5–40.
47. Hökfelt, T., Schultzberg, M., Johansson, O., Ljungdahl, A., Elfvin, L., Elde, R., Terenius, L., Nilsson, G., Said, S., and Goldstein, M. (1978): Central and peripheral peptide producing neurons. In: *Gut Hormones,* edited by S. R. Bloom, pp. 423–433. Churchill Livingstone, Edinburgh.
48. Impicciatore, M., Debas, H., Walsh, J. H., Grossman, M. I. and Bertaccini, G. (1974): Release of gastrin and stimulation of acid secretion by bombesin in dog. *Rendiconti,* 6:99–101.
49. Jacobson, E. D., and Thompson, W. J. (1976): Cyclic AMP and gastric secretion: the illusive second messenger. *Adv. Cyclic Nucleotide Res.,* 7:199–224.
50. Johnson, D., and Duthie, H. L. (1965): Inhibition of gastric secretion in human stomach. *Lancet,* ii:1032–1036.
51. Johnson, D., and Duthie, H. L. (1969): Effect of fat in the duodenum on gastric acid secretion before and after vagotomy in man. *Scand. J. Gastroenterol.,* 4:561–567.
52. Johnson, L. R. (1972): Regulation of pepsin secretion by topical acid in the stomach. *Gastroenterology,* 62:33–38.
53. Johnson, L. R. (1976): Progress in Gastroenterology: The trophic action of gastrointestinal hormones. *Gastroenterology,* 70:278–288.
54. Johnson, L. R., and Grossman, M. I. (1969): Effect of fat, secretin and cholecystokinin on histamine stimulated gastric secretion. *Am. J. Physiol.,* 216:1176–1179.
55. Johnson, L. R., and Grossman, M. I. (1972): Intestinal hormones as inhibitors of gastric secretion. *Gastroenterology,* 60:120–144.
56. Kahlson, G., and Rosengren, E. (1968): New approaches to the physiology of histamine. *Physiol. Rev.,* 48:155–196.
57. Knutson, U., Olbe, L., and Ganguli, P. D. (1974): Gastric acid and plasma gastrin responses to sham feeding in duodenal ulcer patients before and after resection of antrum and duodenal bulb. *Scand. J. Gastroenterol.,* 9:351–356.
58. Konturek, S. J. (1970): Effect of secretin and jejunal acidification on gastric and pancreatic secretion in man. *Gut,* 11:158–162.
59. Konturek, S. J. (1974): Gastric secretion. In: *Gastrointestinal Physiology,* edited by E. D. Jacobson, pp. 227–264. Physiology Series One, MPT International Review of Science. University Park Press, Baltimore.
60. Konturek, S. J. (1977): Intestinal mechanisms regulating gastric secretion. In: *Progress in Gastroenterology,* edited by G. B. J. Glass, pp. 395–437. Grune and Stratton, New York.
61. Konturek, S. J., Biernat, J., and Grzelec, T. (1973): Inhibition by secretin of the gastric acid responses to meals and to pentagastrin in duodenal ulcer patients. *Gut,* 14:842–849.

61a. Konturek, S. J., Biernat, J., Kwiecien, N., and Oleksy, J. (1975): Effect of glucagon on meal-induced gastric secretion in man. *Gastroenterology,* 68:448–454.

62. Konturek, S. J., Biernat, J., and Oleksy, J. (1974): Effect of metiamide, a histamine H_2-receptor antagonist, on gastric response to histamine, pentagastrin, insulin, and peptone meal in man. *Am. J. Dig. Dis.,* 19:609–616.

63. Konturek, S. J., Biernat, J., and Oleksy, J. (1974): Serum gastrin and gastric acid responses to meals at various pH levels in man. *Gut,* 15:526–530.

64. Konturek, S. J., Dembinski, A., Krol, R., and Wünsch, E. (1976): Effects of motilin on gastric and pancreatic secretion in dogs. *Scand. J. Gastroenterol. (Suppl.),* 11:57–61.

65. Konturek, S. J., and Gabrys, B. (1970): Effect of caerulein on histamine and pentagastrin-induced gastric secretion in man. *Am. J. Dig. Dis.,* 15:791–795.

66. Konturek, S. J., and Grossman, M. I. (1965): Effect of perfusion of intestinal loops with acid, fat and dextrose on gastric secretion. *Gastroenterology,* 49:481–489.

67. Konturek, S. J., and Johnson, L. R. (1979): Evidence for an enterogastric reflex for the inhibition of acid secretion. *Gastroenterology,* 61:667–674.

68. Konturek, S. J., Kaess, H., Kwiecien, N., Radecki, T., Dorner, M., and Tackentrupp, U. (1976): Characteristics of intestinal phase of gastric secretion. *Am. J. Physiol.,* 230:325–340.

69. Konturek, S. J., Kwiecien, N., Obtulowicz, W., Mikos, E., Sito, E., and Oleksy, J. (1978): Comparison of intraduodenal and intravenous administration of amino acids on gastric secretion in healthy subjects and patients with duodenal ulcer. *Gut,* 19:859–864.

70. Konturek, S. J., Kwiecien, N., Obtulowicz, W., Sito, E., and Oleksy, J. (1978): Intestinal phase of gastric secretion in patients with duodenal ulcer. *Gut,* 19:321–326.

71. Konturek, S. J., Kwiecien, N., Radecki, T., Erlbert, R., Finke, V., and Creutzfeldt, W. (1978): Effect of fat and glucose on serum gastrin and gastric inhibitory polypeptide (GIP) and gastric acid responses to gastric and intestinal meals. *Scand. J. Gastroenterol., (Suppl.),* 13:100.

72. Konturek, S. J., Pawlik, W., Walus, K., Tasler, J., Coy, D. H., and Schally, A. V. (1978): The influence of enkephalin on gastric and pancreatic secretion in dog. *Scand. J. Gastroenterol., (Suppl.),* 13:101.

73. Konturek, S. J., Pawlik, W., Walus, K., Coy, D. H., and Schally, A. V. (1978): Methionine-enkephalin stimulates gastric secretion and gastric mucosal blood flow. *Proc. Soc. Exptl. Biol. Med.,* 158:156–160.

74. Konturek, S. J., Radecki, T., and Kwiecien, N. (1978): Stimuli for intestinal phase of gastric secretion in dogs. *Am. J. Physiol.,* 234:E64–E69.

75. Konturek, S. J., Tasler, J., Cieszkowski, M., Dobrzanska, M., and Wünsch, E. (1977): Stimulation of gastrin release and gastric secretion by amino acids bathing pyloric gland area. *Am. J. Physiol.,* 233:E170–E174.

76. Konturek, S. J., Tasler, J., and Obtulowicz, W. (1971): Duodenal mechanisms for inhibition of gastric secretion in dog. *Am. J. Physiol.,* 200:918–921.

77. Konturek, S. J., Tasler, J., Cieszkowski, M., and Jaworek, J. (1978): Comparison of intravenous amino acids in the stimulation of gastric secretion. *Gastroenterology,* 75:817–824.

78. Konturek, S. J., Tasler, J., Obtulowicz, W., and Cieszkowski, M. (1976): Comparison of amino acids bathing the oxyntic gland area in the stimulation of gastric secretion. *Gastroenterology,* 70:66–69.

79. Konturek, S. J., Thor, P., Dembinski, A., and Krol, R. (1975): Vasoactive intestinal peptide: Comparison with secretin for potency and spectrum of biological action. In: *Gastrointestinal Hormones,* edited by J. C. Thompson, pp. 611–633. University of Texas Press, Austin.

80. Konturek, S. J., Wysocki, A., and Oleksy, J. (1968): Effect of medical and surgical vagotomy on gastric response to graded doses of pentagastrin and histamine. *Gastroenterology,* 54:392–400.

81. Kosaka, T., and Lim, R. K. S. (1930): Demonstration of the humoral agent in fat inhibition of gastric secretion. *Proc. Soc. Exp. Biol. Med.,* 27:890–896.

82. Landor, J. H., Beloni, A., and Mariano, E. C. (1977): Some properties shared by amino acids and entero-oxyntin. *Gastroenterology,* 72:A62/1085.

82a. Lewin, M. J. M., Soumarmon, A., and Bonfils, S. (1977): Receptors for gastrin and histamine in gastric mucosa. In *Progress in Gastroenterology,* Vol. III, edited by G. B. J. Glass, pp. 203–240. Grune and Stratton, New York.

83. MacGregor, I. L., Deveney, C., Way, L. W., and Meyer, J. H. (1976): The effect of acute hyperglycemia on meal-stimulated gastric, biliary, and pancreatic secretion, and serum gastrin. *Gastroenterology,* 70:197–202.

84. Malmstrom, J., Stadil, F., and Rehfeld, J. F. (1976): Gastrins in tissue. Concentration and component pattern in gastric duodenal and jejunal mucosa of normal human subjects and patients with duodenal ulcer. *Gastroenterology,* 70:697–703.
85. Marshall, C. E. (1976): Automated biological assay of cholecystokinin. Med. Biol. *Engineering* 10:327–329.
86. Mayer, G., Arnold, R., Feurle, G., Fuchs, K., Ketterer, H., Track, N. S., and Creutzfeldt, W. (1974): Influence of feeding and sham feeding upon serum gastrin and gastric acid secretion in control subjects and duodenal ulcer patients. *Scand. J. Gastroenterol.,* 9:703–710.
87. McDonald, T. J., Nilsson, G., Vagne, M., Ghatei, M., Bloom, S. R., and Mutt, V. (1978): A gastrin releasing peptide from the porcine nonantral tissue. *Gut,* 19:767–774.
88. Mutt, V. (1976): Further investigations on intestinal hormonal polypeptides. *Clin. Endocrinol. (Suppl.),* 5:176s–183s.
89. Orloff, M. J., Guillemin, R. C. L., and Nakaji, N. T. (1976): Isolation of the hormone responsible for the intestinal phase of gastric secretion. *Symposium on Hormones and Ulcer,* Los Angeles.
90. Orloff, M. F., Villar-Valdes, H., Abott, A. G., and Rosen, H. (1970): Site of origin of the hormone responsible for gastric hypersecretion associated with portacaval shunt. *Surgery,* 68:202–208.
91. Pearse, A. G. E. (1977): The diffuse neuroendocrine system and the APUD concept: Related "endocrine" peptides in brain, intestine, pituitary, placenta, and anuran cutaneous glands. *Med. Biol.,* 55:115–125.
92. Pearse, A. G. E., Polak, J., and Bloom, R. S. (1977): The newer gut hormones: cellular sources, physiology, pathology and clinical aspects. *Gastroenterology,* 22:746–761.
93. Pederson, R. A., and Brown, J. C. (1972): Inhibition of histamine-, pentagastrin- and insulin-stimulated canine gastric secretion by pure gastric inhibitory polypeptide. *Gastroenterology,* 62:393–400.
94. Polak, J. M., and Bloom, S. R. (1978): Peptidergic innervation of the gastrointestinal tract. In: *Gastrointestinal Hormones and Pathology of the Digestive System,* edited by M. Grossman, V. Speranza, N. Basso and E. Lezoche, pp. 27–49. Plenum Press, New York.
95. Polak, J. M., and Bloom, S. R. (1978): The endocrine background. In: *Scientific Foundations in Gastroenterology,* edited by W. Sircus and A. N. Smith. Williams Heineman Med. Book, Edinburgh.
96. Polak, J. M., Bloom, S. R., Hobbs, S., Solcia, E., and Pearse, A. G. E. (1976): Distribution of a bombesin-like peptide in human gastrointestinal tract. *Lancet,* i:1109–1110.
97. Polak, J. M., Facer, P., Pearse, A. G. E., and Jaffe, B. M. (1978): Amine and peptide in the same APUD cell demonstrated by immunocytochemistry. *Scand. J. Gastroenterol., (Suppl.),* 13:147.
98. Polak, J. M., Pearse, A. G. E., Grimelius, L., Bloom, S. R., and Arimura, A. (1975): Growth-hormone release inhibiting hormone (GH-RIH) in gastrointestinal and pancreatic D cells. *Lancet,* i:1220–1222.
99. Polak, J. M., Sullivan, S. N., Bloom, S. R., Facer, P., and Pearse, A. G. E. (1977): Enkephalin-like immunoreactivity in the human gastrointestinal tract. *Lancet,* i:972–974.
100. Rayford, P. L., Konturek, S. J., and Thompson, J. C. (1978): Effect of duodenal fat on plasma levels of gastrin and secretion and on gastric acid responses to gastric and intestinal meals in dogs. *Gastroenterology,* 75:773–777.
101. Rehfeld, J. F., Schwartz, T. W., and Stadil, F. (1977): Immunochemical studies on macromolecular gastrins. Evidence that "big big" in blood and mucosa are artifacts—but truly present in some large gastrinomas. *Gastroenterology,* 73:469–477.
102. Rehfeld, J. F., Stadil, F., Malmstrom, J., and Miyata, M. (1975): Gastrin heterogeneity in serum and in tissues: A progress report. In: *Gastrointestinal Hormones,* edited by J. C. Thompson, pp. 43–58. University of Texas Press, Austin.
103. Richardson, C. T., Walsh, J. H., Cooper, K. A., Feldman, M., and Fordtran, J. S. (1977): Studies on the role of cephalic-vagal stimulation in the acid secretory response to eating in normal human subjects. *J. Clin. Invest.,* 60:435–441.
104. Richardson, C. T., Walsh, J. H., Hicks, M. I., and Fordtran, J. S. (1976): Studies on the mechanisms of food-stimulated gastric acid secretion in normal human subjects. *J. Clin. Invest.,* 58:623–631.
105. Roland, M., Berstad, A., and Liavag, I. (1975): Effect of carbacholine and urecholine on pentagastrin-stimulated gastric secretion in healthy subjects. *Scand. J. Gastroenterol.,* 10:357–362.

106. Rose, S. P., Prus, R. M., and Herschman, H. R. (1975): Initiation of 3T3 fibroblast cell division by epidermal growth factor. *J. Cell Physiol.,* 86:593–598.
106a. Rosenthal, W. S., Balanzo, J. T., and Glass, G. B. J. (1973): Antibody to gastrone endogenous inhibitor of gastric secretion. *Am. J. Dig. Dis.,* 18:349–359.
107. Sachs, G., Chang, H., Rabon, E., Shackman, R., Sarau, H. M., and Saccomani, G. (1977): Metabolic and membrane aspects of gastric H^+ transport. *Gastroenterology,* 73:931–940.
108. Samloff, I. M. (1971): Pepsinogens, pepsins and pepsin inhibitors. *Gastroenterology,* 60:586–604.
109. Samloff, I. M., and Liebman, W. M. (1973): Cellular localization of the group II pepsinogens in the human stomach and duodenum by immunofluorescence. *Gastroenterology,* 65:36–42.
110. Samloff, I. M., Secrist, D. M., and Passaro, E., Jr. (1975): A study of the relationship between serum group I pepsinogen levels and gastric acid secretion. *Gastroenterology,* 69:1196–1200.
111. Schusdziarra, V., Harris, V., Conlon, J. M., Arimura, A., and Unger, R. (1978): Pancreatic and gastric somatostatin release in response to intragastric and intraduodenal nutrients and HC1 in the dog. *J. Clin. Invest.,* 62:509–518.
112. Sjodin, L. (1975): Inhibition of gastrin-stimulated canine acid secretion by sham-feeding. *Scand. J. Gastroenterol.,* 10:73–80.
113. Solcia, E., Capella, C., Buffa, R., Trigerio, B., Usellini, L., and Fontana, P. (1978): Endocrine cells of the gut and related growth: Recent development and classification. In: *Gut Hormones,* edited by S. R. Bloom, pp. 77–81, Churchill Livingstone, Edinburgh.
114. Solcia, E., Polak, J. M., and Pearse, A. G. E. (1978): Lusanne 1977 classification of gastroenteropancraetic endocrine cells. In: *Gut Hormones,* edited by S. R. Bloom, pp. 40–48, Churchill Livingstone, Edinburgh.
115. Soll, A. H. (1978): The actions of secretagogues on oxygen uptake by isolated mammalian parietal cells. *J. Clin. Invest.,* 61:370–380.
116. Soll, A. H. (1978): The interactions of histamine with gastrin and carbamylcholine on oxygen uptake by isolated mammalian parietal cells. *J. Clin. Invest.,* 61:381–389.
117. Soll, A. H., and Grossman, M. I. (1978): Cellular mechanisms in acid secretion. *Ann. Rev. Med.,* 28:495–507.
118. Soll, A. H., and Wollin, A. (1977): The effects of histamine, prostaglandin E_2, and secretin on cyclic AMP in separated canine fundic mucosal cells. *Gastroenterology,* 72:116 *(Abstr.).*
119. Stadil, F., and Rehfeld, J. F. (1974): Gastrin response to insulin after selective, highly selective, and truncal vagotomy. *Gastroenterology,* 66:7–15.
120. Stern, D. H., and Walsh, J. H. (1973): Gastrin release in postoperative ulcer patients. Evidence for release of duodenal gastrin. *Gastroenterology,* 64:363–369.
120a. Takeuchi, K., Speir, G. R., and Johnson, L. R. (1979): Mucosal gastrin receptor. I. Assay standardization and fulfillment of receptor criteria. *Am. J. Physiol.,* 273:E284–E295.
121. Teorell, R. (1947): Electrolyte diffusion in relation to the acidity regulation of the gastric juice. *Gastroenterology,* 9:425–430.
122. Thompson, W. J., Chang, L. K., Rosenfeld, G. C., and Jacobson, E. D. (1977): Activation of rat gastric mucosal adenylyl cyclase by secretory inhibitors. *Gastroenterology,* 72:251–254.
123. Thompson, J. C., Fender, H. R., Ramus, N. I., Villar, H. V., and Rayford, P. L. (1975): Cholecystokinin metabolism in man and dogs. *Ann. Surg.,* 182:496.
124. Uvnäs-Wallenstein, K., Rehfeld, J. F., Larsson, L. I., and Uvnäs, B. (1977): Heptadecapeptide gastrin in the vagal nerve. *Proc. Natl. Acad. Sci. USA,* 74:5707–5710.
125. Villar, H. V., Fender, H. R., Rayford, P. L., and Thompson, J. C. (1976): Suppression of gastrin release by gastric inhibitory polypeptide (GIP) and vasoactive intestinal polypeptide (VIP). *Ann. J. Surg.,* 184:97–102.
126. Walsh, J. H., and Grossman, M. I. (1975): Gastrin. *N. Engl. J. Med.,* 292:1324–1334, 1377–1384.
127. Walsh, J. H., Richardson, C. T., and Fordtran, J. S. (1975): pH-dependence of acid secretion and gastric release in normal and ulcer subjects. *J. Clin. Invest.,* 55:462–468.
128. Walsh, J. H., Yalow, R. S., and Berson, S. A. (1971): The effect of atropine on plasma gastrin response to feeding. *Gastroenterology,* 60:16–21.
129. Way, L. W., Cairns, D. W., and Deveney, C. W. (1975): The intestinal phase of gastric secretion: A pharmacological profile of enterooxyntin. *Surgery,* 77:841–849.
130. Willems, G. (1973): Control of cell proliferation and differentiation in the normal stomach. *Rendiconti,* 5:196–210.

131. Woodward, E. R., Lyon, E. S., Landor, J., and Dragstedt, L. R. (1954): The physiology of the gastric antrum. *Gastroenterology,* 27:766–785.
132. Wormsley, K. G. (1970): Response to duodenal acidification in man. II. Effects on the gastric secretory response to pentagastrin. *Scand. J. Gastroenterol.,* 5:207–215.
133. Yalow, R. S. (1975): Heterogeneity of peptide hormones with relation to gastrin. In: *Gastrointestinal Hormones,* edited by J. C. Thompson, pp. 25–41. University of Texas Press, Austin.
134. Yalow, R. S., and Wu, N. (1973): Additional studies on the nature of big big gastrin. *Gastroenterology,* 65:19–27.

Gastrointestinal Hormones, edited by
George B. Jerzy Glass.
Raven Press, New York © 1980.

Chapter 24

Gastrointestinal Hormones and Pancreatic, Biliary, and Intestinal Secretions

William Y. Chey

The Isaac Gordon Center for Digestive Diseases and Nutrition, The Genesee Hospital, and University of Rochester School of Medicine and Dentistry, Rochester, New York 55901

I. Gastrointestinal Hormones and Pancreatic Secretion

With the discovery of secretin (4) and cholecystokinin (41)-pancreozymin (36) (CCK-PZ), exocrine pancreatic secretion was thought to depend mainly on the release of these hormones from the upper small intestinal mucosa. More recent evidence suggests that the whole length of the gastrointestinal tract, from the body of the stomach to the colon, and the pancreas, may affect exocrine pancreatic secretion by neuroendocrine mechanisms.

INFLUENCE OF THE VAGUS

It has been well recognized that stimulation of the efferent vagus fibers increases pancreatic secretion in laboratory animals. In the pig, vagal stimulation produces large amounts of water, bicarbonate, and enzymes. Interestingly, the electrolyte secretion is atropine resistant (39). Vagal stimulation produces a moderate amount of pancreatic juice in dog (12) and in cat also (50). In the latter two animal species, however, the increased enzyme output is a more prominent effect of vagal stimulation (12,50) that is prevented by atropine. This is elicited partly by a direct cholinergic effect on the acinar cells of the pancreas and partly by the release of antral gastrin. In this regard, sham feeding in the dog elicited an increased protein secretion that was prevented by acidification of an innervated antral pouch and was suggested to depend on the vagal release of gastrin (67).

As a meal reached the stomach, chemical and mechanical stimulation of the antrum produced a humorally mediated increase in pancreatic enzyme secretion. The existence of a gastric phase of pancreatic secretion has been demonstrated in man (81) and in the dog (65,80).

EFFECTS OF GUT HORMONES ON PANCREATIC SECRETION

The pancreatic secretory response during digestion depends on the release of gut hormones from the antrum and the small intestinal mucosa by acid and products of carbohydrate, protein, and fat digestion (Table 1).

Gastrin

Gastrin and gastrin analogs have been shown to stimulate pancreatic enzyme secretion (32,78). The dose of gastrin that had been used, however, falls in the pharmacological range.

Secretin and Cholecystokinin-Pancreozymin (CCK-PZ)

The major part of the pancreatic secretion during digestion depends on the release of endogenous secretin and CCK-PZ from the upper small intestine. Endogenous secretin is mainly released by gastric acid delivered into the proximal duodenum (15,42,71). The pH threshold for the release of secretin in dog has been shown to be 4.5 (60,77). Below the threshold pH, the pancreatic bicarbonate secretion was a function of the rate of entry of titratable acid into the intestine.

TABLE 1. *Gut hormones or peptides that influence pancreatic secretion*

Stimulants	Inhibitors
Secretin (1,20)	Glucagon (58)
Gastrin (11,12)	Somatostatin (62,63)
CCK-PZ (2,3,20)	Pancreatic polypeptide (64–70)
VIP (51,52,52a,57)	Met-enkephalin (72)
Chymodenin (55,56)	Anti-cholecystokinin peptide (73)

The pancreatic secretory response was also a function of the length of small intestine that underwent acidification. When the pH was below 3.0, the bicarbonate secretion was independent of the pH of the acid entering the intestine (67). During normal digestion, however, only a limited length of the proximal duodenum appears to be frequently exposed to acidic pH (6,15,42,71). It has recently become clear that significant amounts of endogenous secretin is released to elevate plasma immunoreactive secretin in man (15,66,71) and in dog (Fig. 1) (42). The amount of secretin that reaches circulation is estimated to be in a range of 0.06 to 0.25 clinical units/kg-hr (42). Certainly this small amount of secretin alone could not account for the volume of the pancreatic juice produced by the meal, although secretin classically stimulates production of pancreatic juice rich in bicarbonate (35).

It has recently been shown that plasma secretin concentration increases significantly by intraduodenal infusion of ox bile in man (64) or the infusion of micellar solution of fatty acids in physiological amounts in the dog (27). It has been suggested by Meyer and Soals (58) that a secretin-like humoral substance may be responsible for pancreatic secretion stimulated by fatty acids in dogs. Although oral ethanol ingestion has been reported to produce prompt and significant increases in peripheral plasma secretin level (74), several other groups failed to observe the increase in plasma secretin concentration within 20 min after ethanol ingestion in human (28,44) or dog (44,52). A prompt rise in the plasma secretin level in either man or dog could not be confirmed by Chey et al. either *(unpublished data)*. A significant increase in the secretin levels that was observed 60 min after alcohol ingestion in dog (52) was not likely due to a direct effect of alcohol but, rather to a secondary phenomenon. It is well known that ethanol stimulates gastric secretion of acid in dog (14). Thus, gastric acid delivered to the duodenum is likely to be the stimulant for endogenous secretin release (14).

Nevertheless, the main stimulant of endogenous secretin release during di-

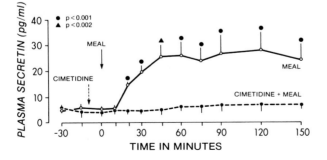

FIG. 1. Plasma secretin concentrations in fasting and postprandial state in three dogs. Each point represents a mean ± SE of six experiments (2 expts./dog). The meal consisted of 150 g of cooked ground beef, two slices of bread, and 100 ml of milk. The *solid circle* represents the plasma secretin values determined before and after cimetidine 150 mg given intravenously. (From ref. 42.)

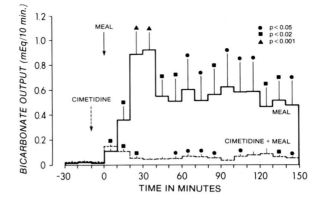

FIG. 2. Effect of cimetidine given intravenously in a dose of 150 mg on pancreatic secretion of bicarbonate in four dogs. Each point represents a mean ± SE of eight experiments (2 expts./dog). (From ref. 42.)

gestion appears to be acid that is delivered to the proximal duodenum (15,42, 66,71). In dogs, a marked suppression of gastric acid secretion by intravenous cimetidine not only produces a marked inhibition of pancreatic secretion (Fig. 2), but it also abolished a significant postprandial rise in plasma secretin levels in dogs (Fig. 1) (42). Similar observations were made in man either by neutralizing gastric acid with sodium bicarbonate (Fig. 3) (15) or by suppression of acid secretion (71).

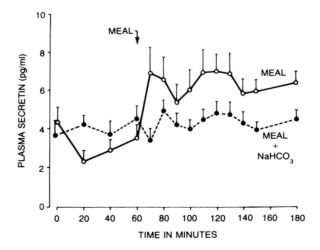

FIG. 3. Plasma secretin concentration in nine healthy subjects in fasting and postprandial states. Each subject ate 60 g of cooked ground beef, two slices of bread, 150 ml of coffee, and 120 ml of orange juice. The *solid circle* represents a mean ± SE while intragastric pH was maintained above 5.5. (From ref. 15.)

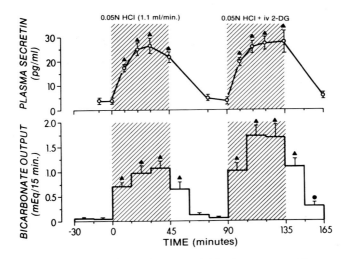

FIG. 4. Plasma secretin concentration and pancreatic bicarbonate output in response to intra-duodenal infusion of 0.05 N HCl infusion and 2-deoxyglucose administration (100 mg/kg-hr) in four dogs with pancreatic fistula. Each value represents a mean ± SE of eight experiments (2 expts./dog). ▲, $p < 0.001$; ●, $p < 0.05$. (From ref. 12.)

Although the release of endogenous secretin by acid does not appear to be influenced by the vagus nerve (12,79) or atropine (12), the action of secretin on the pancreas to produce pancreatic juice appears to be modulated by the vagus or cholinergic nerve (Figs. 4 through 6) (12). It has been shown that vagotomy or atropine significantly reduces the effect of secretin on pancreatic secretion. Thus, the vagus or cholinergic nerve plays an important role on the action of endogenous secretin on the pancreas, although the vagus nerve itself produces a moderate amount of pancreatic secretion without influencing the plasma level of secretin (12).

The product of fat digestion, peptones, and L-isomers of amino acids resulting from protein digestion classically release CCK-PZ (26,31,41,57). Among the amino acids, phenylalanine, valine, methionine, and tryptophan are highly effective in stimulating pancreatic enzyme secretion in man (31); whereas only phenyl-alanine and tryptophan have a similar effect in the dog (57). It has been shown that the pancreatic enzymes' secretory response to intestinal infusion of fatty acid depends on the chain length of fatty acids, fatty acid loads, and the length of the intestine exposed (55). Long-chain fatty acids were found to be more potent than medium- or short-chain fatty acids. Calcium-ion perfused intra-duodenally in a physiological concentration stimulates pancreatic enzyme se-cretion and also produces gallbladder contractions in a dose-related fashion, achieving responses comparable to those produced by exogenous CCK-PZ (40). Since 1926, bile has also been known to stimulate pancreatic secretion in the dog (56); and, more recently, the intraduodenal infusion of bile salts has been

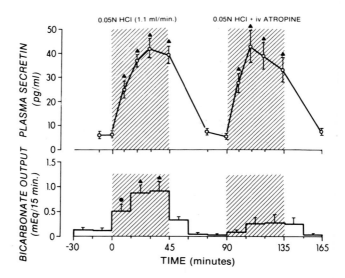

FIG. 5. Plasma secretin concentration and pancreatic bicarbonate secretion in response to intraduodenal infusion of 0.05 *N* HCl alone and a combination of 0.05 *N* HCl infusion and atropine administration in four pancreatic fistula dogs. Each value represents a mean ± SE of eight experiments (2 expts./dog). ▲, $p < 0.001$; ●, $p < 0.01$. (From ref. 12.)

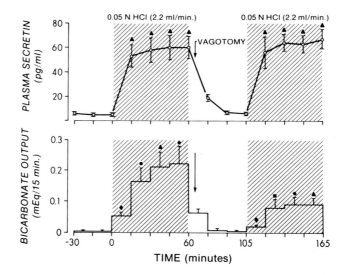

FIG. 6. Plasma secretin concentration and pancreatic bicarbonate output in response to intraduodenal infusion of 0.05 *N* HCl at a rate of 2.2 ml/min before and after cervical vagotomy in eight vagotomized dogs. Each value represents a mean ± SE of eight experiments. ▲, $p < 0.001$; ◆, $p < 0.002$; ●, $p < 0.01$; ■, $p < 0.02$. (From ref. 12.)

shown to stimulate pancreatic secretion—particularly enzymes (30,55,83). Although acid in the duodenum is a potent stimulant of secretin release, it is also a weak stimulant for CCK-PZ (3).

Recently it has been found that CCK-PZ exists in significant amounts in not only the intestinal mucosa but also in the brain tissue (22,70,73). Using a region-specific antisera against CCK-PZ-33, the cerebral CCK-PZ was found to consist of three small molecular forms: (a) a minor fraction corresponding to tricontatriapeptide; (b) a large fraction corresponding to the COOH-terminal octapeptide of CCK-PZ-33; and (c) a small immunoreactive component corresponding to the COOH-terminal tetrapeptide of CCK-PZ-33. In the intestinal mucosa extracts (70), five molecular forms were found: (a) the largest molecular forms were found in positions similar to those of pro-insulin and gastrin component I (69); (b) the second largest forms similar to those of CCK-PZ-33 and CCK-PZ-39 (63); (c) molecular forms smaller than CCK-PZ-33 corresponding to the COOH-terminal dodecapeptide of CCK-PZ-33; (d) the majority of the CCK-immunoreactivity corresponding to COOH-terminal octapeptide of CCK; and (e) two peptides corresponding to each half of the COOH-terminal octapeptide (23,70). High concentrations of these CCK-PZs were found in the upper small intestine as well as in the brain (69). Because of several problems—including heterogeneity, nonequivalence of biological activity, and immunoreactivity of the different CCK-PZs and potential cross-reactivity of gastrins—the development of a specific, highly sensitive, and reliable radioimmunoassay of CCK-PZ has been difficult. A successful immunoassay will allow us to determine which one of these CCK-PZs predominates in the circulation to affect the physiological phenomena of the digestive tract. Nevertheless, CCK-PZ-like immunoreactivity has been reported to rise in the plasma after a meal (37,68). Until a reliable immunoassay of CCK-PZ will be available, it will be difficult to assess a possible role of the vagus or cholinergic nerve in the endogenous release of CCK-PZ or its effect on the action of CCK-PZ under physiological conditions.

Interaction Between Secretin and CCK-PZ

It is well recognized that pure CCK-PZ primarily stimulates pancreatic enzyme secretion, but CCK-PZ on its own does not produce significant amounts of water and bicarbonate, nor can secretin alone, in the amount secreted during digestion, produce a comparable amount of pancreatic juice to that which is produced after a meal. Undoubtedly, the combined actions of the two hormones and the vagus or cholinergic nerve are needed. Meyer et al. (59) have shown that endogenous CCK can potentiate the primary effect of secretin in a small amount (Fig. 7). Moreover, Grossman and Konturek (33) have found that when dogs are given a liquid liver extract meal with pH constantly adjusted to 5.0, there was very little bicarbonate secretion from the pancreas. As a small dose of exogenous secretin, 0.25 unit/kg-hr, was infused with the meal, pH 5.0, pancreatic secretion of bicarbonate was comparable to that achieved by the

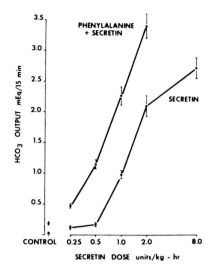

FIG. 7. Pancreatic bicarbonate responses to secretin alone or secretin plus 3.2 mmoles/15 min of phenylalanine (eight observations in four dogs). The responses to 8 U/kg-hr of secretin alone were obtained in separate experiments (four observations in four dogs). (From ref. 59.)

meal itself. This dose of secretin was necessary to produce pancreatic bicarbonate secretion by a meat meal in dogs (42). By the same token, exogenous secretin was necessary to achieve maximum protein output from the pancreas that is stimulated by a meat meal (33). The importance of endogenous secretin in the circulation on exocrine pancreatic secretion produced by a meat meal was shown by another approach. When endogenous secretin in the circulation was bound in dogs by a specific rabbit anti-secretin serum, pancreatic bicarbonate output during digestion drastically decreased to only 20% of that produced by the meal (Fig. 8) (13). Protein output also decreased to 60% as a result of

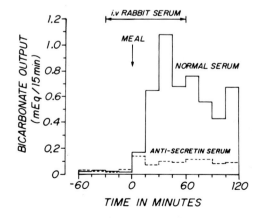

FIG. 8. Effects of normal rabbit serum *(solid line)* and anti-secretin serum *(dotted line)* on the concentration and output of pancreatic bicarbonate in a dog with pancreatic fistula.

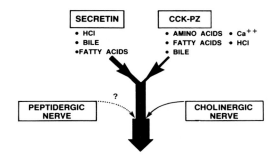

FIG. 9. Roles of secretin, CCK-PZ, cholinergic nerve, and peptidergic nerve on external pancreatic secretion. This concept applies to man and dog only.

a drastic decrease in pancreatic flow. It was also possible, based on this observation (13), that secretin was needed for pancreatic secretion of protein comparable to that achieved by a meal alone. This non-secretin component of pancreatic bicarbonate secretion must be accounted for by other factors including CCK-PZ (20), vasoactive intestinal polypeptide (48,54), and the vagus nerve or cholinergic nerve (12). It has been well established that vagotomy drastically decreases pancreatic secretion (49,84). Vagotomy or atropinization produce a significant decrease in the pancreatic bicarbonate secretion stimulated by exogenous secretin in a physiological range (12). On the basis of the available information, interaction between secretin and CCK-PZ and the interplay between these gut hormones and the cholinergic nerve appear to be essential for pancreatic secretion during digestion (Fig. 9).

Chymodenin and Vasoactive Intestinal Polypeptide (VIP)

Another new hormonal candidate, chymodenin (1), was isolated from hog duodenal mucosa and found to produce a dramatic increase in the secretion of chymotrypsinogen with only a moderate effect on the other pancreatic enzyme secretions. The molecular size of this peptide is estimated to be about 9,000 (11).

VIP in a pharmacological dose range was shown to stimulate pancreatic secretion of bicarbonate in dog (48,54), in cat (45), and in man (24). Compared with the pancreatic stimulatory potencies of secretin, the maximal bicarbonate response to VIP was about 17% of the response to secretin in dog (54), whereas in cat VIP is a full agonist of the pancreatic bicarbonate secretion. Possible physiological roles of VIP and chymodenin on the exocrine pancreatic secretion, however, will require further investigations.

Hormones or Peptides that Inhibit Exocrine Pancreatic Secretion

There are at least five known hormones or peptides that inhibit external pancreatic secretion (Table 1). These include pancreatic glucagon, somatostatin, pancreatic polypeptide, met-enkephalin, and anti-cholecystokinin peptide. Pancreatic glucagon was shown to inhibit pancreatic secretion of bicarbonate and enzymes stimulated by secretin and CCK-PZ (25). It is reasonable to assume that gastric glucagon (62) may have similar inhibitory action. Somatostatin is probably the most potent inhibitor among the known peptides that inhibit exocrine pancreatic secretion stimulated by either secretin or duodenal acidification in dog (46). Similarly, in man somatostatin significantly inhibits exocrine pancreatic secretion stimulated by CCK-PZ (19) or secretin or duodenal acidification (34). One of the inhibitory mechanisms of somatostatin on exocrine pancreatic secretion is its suppressive action on the release of endogenous secretin in dog (5) and in man (Fig. 10) (34). In addition, somatostatin inhibits release of endogenous gastrin and gastrin-stimulated acid secretion (18). The decrease in acid load delivered in the duodenum by endogenous somatostatin may result in further inhibition of pancreatic secretion. Another new hormone candidate, pancreatic polypeptide (PP) (10,43) has been shown to rise in the plasma during digestion

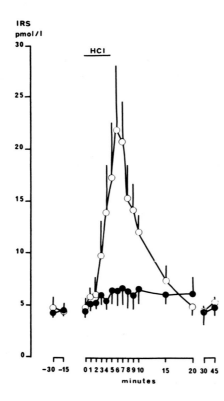

FIG. 10. Plasma immunoreactive secretin concentration before and after duodenal acidification in man with 40 ml 100 mmoles/liter HCl over a 5-min period. *Open symbols,* without somatostatin infusion; *closed symbols,* with a constant infusion of somatostatin (500 μg/hr). Mean $\pm$ SE, $n = 5$. (From ref. 34.)

in man (2,29,72) and in dog (51,76). It has recently been found in dogs that the dose of bovine PP that achieved the plasma levels of PP comparable to, or even lower than that observed during digestion, significantly inhibited pancreatic secretion. The observation suggests strongly that PP may well be a hormone that plays an important role in the regulation of pancreatic secretion. The endogenous PP release is markedly diminished by truncal vagotomy or atropine in man (72) or in dog (75). The plasma PP level is increased by insulin-induced hypoglycemia, but this increase is abolished by vagotomy or hexamethonium or atropine (72), indicating an important role of the vagus on the release of PP. Besides glucagon, somatostatin and PP, met-enkephalin (47), and anti-cholecystokinin peptide (21) are known to inhibit pancreatic secretion. Interestingly, met-enkephalin has an inhibitory action on endogenous secretin release by a meal or duodenal acidification (47). Anti-cholecystokinin peptide found in the colon inhibits specifically the pancreatic enzyme secretion stimulated by CCK-PZ. Among these inhibitory peptides, PP and somatostatin appear to have a physiological role on pancreatic secretion.

CELLULAR MECHANISMS CONTROLLING PANCREATIC SECRETION

Pancreatic secretion of water and electrolytes is believed to occur in the centroacinar and ductular cells under the influence of secretin (35). The vagus nerve also appears to stimulate pancreatic secretion independent of release of endogenous secretin in dog (12) and in pig (39,53). Based on the study in anesthetized cat, it has been suggested that secretin stimulates these cells by increasing adenyl cyclase with a consequent increase in the intracellular conversion of ATP to cyclic AMP in the pancreas (7). Cyclic AMP then stimulates the secretory mechanism of water and electrolytes (8). Approximately 95% of the pancreatic bicarbonate is derived from the extracellular fluid. It has been proposed that the bicarbonate secretion takes place as the result of a primary alteration in the secretory cell membrane permeability with the exchange of external sodium ion for internal hydrogen ions. The hydrogen ions increase the production of carbon dioxide from circulating bicarbonate. The carbon dioxide diffuses into the cells when it combines with water to form carbonic acid, a process assisted by carbonic anhydrase and is finally secreted as bicarbonate (9).

Pancreatic secretion of enzymes occurs in the acinar cells. Cholinergic nerves, CCK-PZ, secretin, and VIP appear to participate in the secretory mechanism according to recent works using guinea pig acinar cell preparations (16,17). Two partly independent chains of events between stimulus and secretion can lead to the same final response. In the major pathway, acetylcholine, CCK-PZ, or bombesin provoke increased secretion of enzymes through increased phosphatidylinositol turnover and free fatty acid release, an elevation of free cytosolic calcium, and the activiation of guanylate cyclase. The transient rise in cyclic GMP allows a prolonged secretory response through the activation of a cyclic GMP-dependent protein kinase and a sustained phosphorylation of protein directly involved in emiocytosis. In another pathway of events, increased enzyme secretion occurred in the acinar cell preparation of rat and guinea pig. The receptor binding of secretin and VIP leads to prolonged elevation of cyclic AMP and the activation of cyclic AMP-dependent kinases. This process does not require calcium on the turnover of phosphatidylinositols. Both pathways are slower to interact. When secretin and CCK-PZ are administered simultaneously, the resulting hypersecretion of enzymes is shown to be greater than that obtained with only one hormone (16). This potentiation has been observed in *in vivo* studies with man (38) and dog (59,82). Whether or not secretin or VIP has a similar role in the acinar cells of other species, such as dog or human, is not known.

The preparation of isolated pancreatic centro-acinar and ductular cells has not been available for the direct exploration of the actions of the known gut hormones such as secretin and CCK-PZ or neurohormones. The future research in this area will uncover many fascinating intracellular mechanisms for a better understanding of pancreatic secretion. It is highly desirable that similar studies should be carried out in dog and human pancreas to determine the roles of secretin, CCK-PZ, VIP, and gastrin on the cellular mechanisms of external pancreatic secretion. The observations made on the guinea pig's pancreatic cell preparation might not necessarily correspond to the events that occur in dogs or humans.

REFERENCES

1. Adelson, J. W., and Rothman, S. S. (1975): Chymodenin, a duodenal peptide: Specific stimulation of chymotrypsinogen secretion. *Am. J. Physiol.,* 229:1680–1686.
2. Adrian, T. E., Bloom, S. R., Bryant, M. G., Polak, J. M., Heitz, P. H., and Barnes, A. J. (1976): Distribution and release of human pancreatic polypeptide. *Gut,* 17:940–944.
3. Barbezat, G. O., and Grossman, M. I. (1975): Release of cholecystokinin by acid. *Proc. Soc. Exp. Biol.,* 148:463–467.
4. Bayliss, V. M., and Starling, E. H. (1902): The mechanism of pancreatic secretion. *J. Physiol.,* 28:325–353.
5. Boden, G., Sivitz, M. C., Own, O. E., Essa-Koumar, N., and Landor, J. H. (1975): Somatostatin suppresses secretin and pancreatic exocrine secretion. *Science,* 190:163–165.
6. Brooks, A. M., and Grossman, M. I. (1970): Postprandial pH and neutralizing capacity of the proximal duodenum in dog. *Gastroenterology,* 59:85–89.
7. Case, R. M., Johnson, M., Scatchard, T., and Sherratt, H. S. A. (1972): Influence of respiration and respiratory sinus arrhythmia on aortic regurgitation. *J. Physiol.,* 223:668–672.
8. Case, R. M., and Scatchard, T. (1972): Heterogeneity of 3',5'-phosphodiesterase. *J. Physiol.,* 223:649–650.
9. Case, R. M., Scatchard, T., and Wynne, R. D. A. (1970): The origin and secretion of pancreatic juice bicarbonate. *J. Physiol.,* 210:1–15.
10. Chance, R. E., and Jones, W. E. (1974): Polypeptide from bovine, ovine, human and porcine pancrease. *US Patent Office* 3, 842:063.
11. Chang, R., Glaser, C. B., and Adelson, J. W. (1978): Structural studies on chymodenin, a hormone-like gastrointestinal polypeptide related to GIP and glucagon. *Scand. J. Gastroenterol. (Suppl 49),* 13:36.
12. Chey, W. Y., Kim, M. S., and Lee, K. Y. (1979): Influence of the vagus nerve on release and action of secretin in dog. *J. Physiol.,* 293:435–446.

13. Chey, W. Y., Kim, M. S., Lee, K. Y., and Chang, T. M. (1978): A physiological role of secretin in postprandial state. *Scand. J. Gastroenterol. (Suppl. 49)*, 13:40.
14. Chey, W. Y., Kosay, S., and Lorber, S. H. (1972): Effects of chronic administration of ethanol on gastric secretion in dogs. *Am. J. Dig. Dis.*, 17:153–159.
15. Chey, W. Y., Lee, Y. H., Hendricks, J. G., Rhodes, R. A., and Tai, H. H. (1978): Plasma secretin concentrations in fasting and postprandial state in man. *Am. J. Dig. Dis.*, 231:981–988.
16. Christophe, J., Calderon, P., Svoboda, M., Deschodt-Lanckman, M., and Robberecht, P. (1978): A working model of stimulus-secretin coupling in pancreatic acinar cells. In *Gut Hormones*, edited by S. R. Bloom, pp. 104–111. Churchill Livingstone, Edinburgh/London/New York.
17. Christophe, J., Robberecht, P., and Deschodt-Lanckman, M. (1977): Hormone receptor interactions in the gastrointestinal tract: The pancreatic acinar cells as a model target in gut endocrinology. In *Progress in Gastroenterology*, edited by G. B. J. Glass, pp. 241–284. Grume & Stratton, New York.
18. Creutzfeldt, W., and Arnold, R. (1979): Somatostatin and the stomach: Exocrine and endocrine aspects. *Metabolism (Suppl. 1)*, 27:1309–1315.
19. Creutzfeldt, W., Lankisch, P. G., and Folsch, U. R. (1975): Hemmung der Secretin und Cholezystokinin-Pankreozimin-induzierten Saft und Enzymsekretion des Pankreas und der Gallblasenkontraktion bein Menschen durch Somatostatin. *Dtsch. Med. Woschenschr.*, 100:1135–1138.
20. Debas, H. T., and Grossman, M. I. (1973): Pure cholecystokinin: Pancreatic protein and bicarbonate response. *Digestion*, 9:469–481.
21. Demol, P., Langier, R., and Sarles, H. (1978): Control of pancreatic secretion by ileum and colon. In *Gut Hormones*, edited by S. R. Bloom, pp. 314–317. Churchill Livingstone, Edinburgh/London/New York.
22. Dockray, G. J. (1976): Immunochemical evidence of cholecystokinin-like peptides in the brain. *Nature*, 264:568–570.
23. Dockray, G. J. (1977): Immunoreactive component resembling cholecystokinin octapeptide in intestine. *Nature*, 270:359–361.
24. Domschke, S., Domschke, W., Rosch, W., Konturek, S. J., Sprugel, W., Mitznegg, P., Wunsch, E., and Demling, L. (1977): Vasoactive intestinal polypeptide: A secretin-like partial agonist for pancreatic secretion in man. *Gastroenterology*, 74:478–480.
25. Dyck, W. P., Texter, E. C. Jr., and Lasater, J. M. (1970): Influence of glucagon on pancreatic exocrine secretion in man. *Gastroenterology*, 58:532–539.
26. Ertan, A., Brooks, F. P., Ostrow, J. D., Arvan, D. A., William, C. N., and Cerda, J. J. (1971): Effect of jejunal amino acid perfusion and exogenous cholecystokinin on the exocrine pancreatic and biliary secretion in man. *Gastroenterology*, 61:686–692.
27. Fahrenkrug, J., and Schaffalitzky de Muckadell, O. B. (1977): Plasma secretin concentration in man: effect of intraduodenal glucose, fat, amino acids, ethanol, HCl on ingestion of a meal. *Eur. J. Clin. Invest.*, 7:201–203.
28. Faichney, A., Chey, W. Y., and Kim, M. S. (1979): Release of endogenous secretin by sodium oleate in dog. *Clin. Res.*, 27:266A.
29. Floyd, J. C., Fajans, S. S., and Pek, S. (1976): Regulation in healthy subjects of the secretion of human pancreatic polypeptide, a newly recognized pancreatic islet polypeptide. *Rec. Prog. Horm. Res.*, 32:146–158.
30. Forell, M. M., Otte, M., Kohl, H. J., Lehnert, P., and Stahlheber, H. P. (1971): The influence of bile salts on pancreatic secretion in man. *Scand. J. Gastroenterol.*, 6:261–265.
31. Go, V. L. W., Hoffmann, A. F., and Summerskill, W. H. G. (1970): Pancreozymin bioassay in man based on pancreatic enzyme secretion: Potency of specific amino acids and other digestive products. *J. Clin. Invest.*, 49:1558–1564.
32. Gregory, R. A., and Tracy, H. J. (1964): The constituents and properties of two gastrins extracted from hog antral mucosa. *Gut*, 5:103–117.
33. Grossman, M. I., and Konturek, S. J. (1974): Gastric acid does drive pancreatic bicarbonate secretion. *Scand. J. Gastroenterol.*, 9:299–302.
34. Hanssen, L. E., Hanssen, K. F., and Myren, J. (1977): Inhibition of secretin release and pancreatic bicarbonate secretion by somatostatin infusion in man. *Scand. J. Gastroenterol.*, 12:391–394.
35. Harper, A. A. (1967): Hormonal control of pancreatic secretion. In *Handbook of Physiology, Section 6, Alimentary Canal, Vol. II, Secretion*, edited by C. F. Code, pp. 969–995. Williams & Wilkins, Baltimore, Maryland.

36. Harper, A. A., and Raper, H. S. (1943): Pancreozymin, a stimulant of the secretion of pancreatic enzymes in extracts of the small intestine. *J. Physiol.,* 102:115–125.
37. Harvey, R. F. (1978): Pathology of cholecystokinin in man. In *Gut Hormones,* edited by S. R. Bloom, pp. 219–223. Churchill Livingstone, Edinburgh/London/New York.
38. Henriksen, F. W., and Worming, H. (1967): The interaction of secretin and pancreozymin on the external pancreatic secretion in dogs. *Acta Physiol. Scand.,* 70:241–249.
39. Hickson, J. C. D. (1943): The secretion of pancreatic juice in response to stimulation of pancreatic enzymes in extracts of the small intestine. *J. Physiol.,* 102:115–125.
40. Holtemuller, K. H., Malagelada, J. R., McCall, J. T., and Go, V. L. W. (1976): Pancreatic, gallbladder and gastric responses to intraduodenal calcium perfusion in man. *Gastroenterology,* 70:693–696.
41. Ivy, A. C., and Oldberg, E. (1928): A hormone mechanism for gallbladder contraction and evulation. *Am. J. Physiol.,* 86:599–613.
42. Kim, M. S., Lee, K. Y., and Chey, W. Y. (1979): Plasma immunoreactive secretin concentration in fasting and postprandial state in dog. *Clin. Res.,* 26:321A; *Am. J. Physiol.,* 236:E539–E544.
43. Kimmel, J. R., Hayden, L. J., and Pollock, H. G. (1975): Isolation and characterization of a new pancreatic polypeptide hormone. *J. Biol. Chem.,* 250:9369–9376.
44. Kolts, B. E., Sekine, T., McDonald, A. P., Snyder, S. T., and Woodward, E. R. (1977): Absence of a secretin response to ethanol ingestion in human and canine subjects. *Clin. Res.,* 25:313A.
45. Konturek, S. J., Pucher, A., and Radecki, T. (1976): Comparison of vasoactive intestinal peptide and secretin in stimulation of pancreatic secretion. *J. Physiol.,* 255:497–509.
46. Konturek, S. J., Tasler, J., Obfulowicz, W., Coy, D. H., and Schally, A. V. (1976): Effect of growth hormone-release inhibiting hormone on hormone stimulating exocrine pancreatic secretion. *J. Clin. Invest.,* 58:1–6.
47. Konturek, S. J., Tasler, J., Schally, A. V., and Chey, W. Y. (1979): Enkephalin inhibits the release and action of secretin on pancreatic secretion (Abstr.). *Gastroenterology,* 76:1174.
48. Konturek, S. J., Thor, P., Dembinski, A., and Ryszard, K. (1975): Vasoactive intestinal peptide: Comparison with secretin for potency and spectrum of physiologic action. In *Gastrointestinal Hormones,* edited by J. C. Thompson, pp. 611–633. University of Texas Press, Austin, Texas.
49. Lenninger, S. G., Magee, D. F., and White, T. T. (1965): Effect of gastric, extragastric and truncal vagotomy on the external secretion of the pancreas in dog. *Ann. Surg.,* 162:1057–1062.
50. Lenninger, S., and Ohlin, P. (1971): The flow of juice from the pancreatic gland of the cat in response to vagal stimulation. *J. Physiol.,* 216:303–318.
51. Lin, T. M., Chance, R. E., Evans, D. C., Spray, G. F., Bloodquist, W. E., Warrick, M. W. (1978): Bovine pancreatic peptide: Plasma concentration and action on pancreatic secretion and gut motility. *Reported at Second International Symposium on Gastrointestinal Hormones,* August 30–September 2, Beito, Norway.
52. Llanos, O. L., Swiergzek, J. S., Teichman, R. K., Rayford, P. L., and Thompson, J. C. (1977): Effect of alcohol on the release of secretin and pancreatic secretion. *Surgery,* 81:661–667.
53. Magee, D. F., and White, T. T. (1965): Influence of vagal stimulation on secretion of pancreatic juice in the pig. *Ann. Surg.,* 161:605–607.
54. Maklouf, G. M., and Said, S. I. (1975): The effect of vasoactive intestinal peptide (VIP) on digestive and hormonal function. In *Gastrointestinal Hormones,* edited by J. C. Thompson, pp. 599–610. University of Texas Press, Austin, Texas.
55. Malagelada, J. R., Dimagno, E. P., Summerskill, W. H. G., and Go, V. L. W. (1976): Regulation of pancreatic and gallbladder functions by fatty acids and bile acids in man. *J. Clin. Invest.,* 58:493–499.
56. Mellanby, J. (1926): The secretion of pancreatic juice. *J. Physiol.,* 61:419–435.
57. Meyer, J. H. (1975): Release of secretin and cholecystokinin. In *Gastrointestinal Hormones,* edited by J. C. Thompson, pp. 475–489. University of Texas Press, Austin, Texas.
58. Meyer, J. H., and Jones, R. S. (1974): Canine pancreatic responses to intestinally perfused fat and products of fat digestion. *Am. J. Physiol.,* 1178–1187.
59. Meyer, J. H., Spingola, L. J., and Grossman, M. I. (1971): Endogenous cholecystokinin potentiates exogenous secretin on pancreas of the dog. *Am. J. Physiol.,* 221:742–747.
60. Meyer, J. H., Way, L. W., and Grossman, M. I. (1970): Pancreatic bicarbonate responses to various acids in the duodenum of dog. *Am. J. Physiol.,* 219:964–970.
61. Moody, A. S., Jacobsen, H., and Sundby, F. (1978): Gastric glucagon and gut glucagon-like immunoreactants. In *Gut Hormones,* edited by S. R. Bloom, pp. 369–378. Churchill Livingstone, Edinburgh/London/New York.

62. Munoz-Barragan, L., Blazquez, E., Patton, G. S., Dobbs, R. E., and Unger, R. H. (1976): Gastric A-cell function in normal dogs. *Am. J. Physiol.,* 231:1057–1061.
63. Mutt, V. (1976): Further investigations on intestinal hormonal polypeptides. *Clin. Endocrinol* 5:183s–197s.
64. Osnes, M., Hanssen, L. E., Flaten, O., and Myren, J. (1978): Exocrine pancreatic secretin and immunoreactive secretin (IRS) release after intraduodenal instillation of bile in man. *Gut,* 19:180–184.
65. Passaro, E. P., Jr., and Grossman, M. I. (1963): Influence of vagal innervation on response to gastrin and histamine. *Surg. Forum,* 14:310–311.
66. Pelletier, M. J., Chayvialle, J. A. P., and Minaire, Y. (1978): Uneven and transient secretin in man: Regulation by gastric acid. *Gut,* 19:812–819.
67. Preshaw, R. M., Cooke, A. R., and Grossman, M. I. (1966): Sham feeding and pancreatic secretion in the dog. *Gastroenterology,* 50:171–178.
68. Rayford, P. L., Schafmayer, A., Teichmann, R. K., and Thompson, J. C. (1978): Cholecystokinin radioimmunoassay. In *Gut Hormones,* edited by S. R. Bloom, pp. 208–212. Churchill Livingstone, Edinburgh/London/New York.
69. Rehfeld, J. F. (1972): Three components of gastrin in human serum. Gel filtration studies on the molecular size of immunoreactive serum gastrin. *Biochem. Biophys. Acta,* 285:364–372.
70. Rehfeld, J. F. (1976): Immunochemical studies on cholecystokinin. II. Distribution and molecular heterogeneity in the central nervous system and small intestine of man and dog. *J. Biol. Chem.,* 253:568–570.
71. Schaffalitzky de Muckadell, O. B., and Fahrenkrug, J. (1978): Secretion pattern of secretin in man: regulation by gastric acid. *Gut,* 19:812–819.
72. Schwartz, T. W., Stadil, F., Chance, R. E., Rehfeld, J. G., Larsson, L.-I., and Moon, N. (1976): Pancreatic polypeptide response to food in duodenal ulcer patients before and after vagotomy. *Lancet,* i:1102–1105.
73. Straus, E., Muller, J. E., Choi, H. S., Paronetto, F., and Yalow, R. (1977): Immunochemical localization in rabbit brain of a peptide resembling the COOH-terminal octapeptide of cholecystokinin. *Proc. Natl. Acad. Sci. USA,* 74:3033–3034.
74. Straus, E., Urback, H. J., and Yalow, R. S. (1975): Alcohol-stimulated secretion of immunoreactive secretin. *N. Eng. J. Med.,* 293:1031–1032.
75. Taylor, I. L., Impicciatore, M., and Walsh, J. H. (1977): Effect of atropine and vagotomy on the pancreatic polypeptide response to a meal. *Gastroenterology,* 72:1139.
76. Taylor, I. L., Solomon, T. E., Walsh, J. H., and Grossman, M. I. (1978): Studies on the metabolism and biologic activity of pancreatic polypeptide (PP). *Scand. J. Gastroenterol. (Suppl. 49),* 13:182.
77. Thomas, J. E., and Crider, J. (1940): A quantitative study of acid in the intestine as a stimulus for the pancreas. *Am. J. Physiol.,* 131:394–396.
78. Valenzuela, J. E., Walsh, J. H., and Isenberg, J. I. (1976): Effect of gastrin on pancreatic enzyme secretion and gallbladder emptying in man. *Gastroenterology,* 71:409–411.
79. Ward, A. S., and Bloom, S. R. (1975): Effect of vagotomy on secretin release in man. *Gut,* 16:951–956.
80. White, T. T., Lundh, G., and Magee, D. F. (1960): Evidence for the existence of gastropancreatic reflex. *Am. J. Physiol.,* 198:725–728.
81. White, T. T., McAlexander, R. A., and Magee, D. F. (1962): Gastropancreatic reflex after various gastric operations. *Surg. Forum,* 13:266–268.
82. Wormsley, K. G. (1969): A comparison of the response to secretin, pancreozymin, and a combination of these hormones in man. *Scand. J. Gastroenterol.,* 4:413–417.
83. Wormsley, K. G. (1970): Stimulation of pancreatic secretion by intraduodenal infusion of bile-salts. *Lancet,* ii:586–588.
84. Wormsley, K. G. (1972): The effect of vagotomy on the human pancreatic response to direct and indirect stimulation. *Scand. J. Gastroenterol.,* 7:85–91.

II. Gastrointestinal Hormones and Bile Secretion

Hormonal regulation of bile secretion appears to affect mainly the bile acid-independent canalicular and ductular or duct secretions.

Several hormones influence the canalicular bile secretion. While thyroxine (13), insulin (5), glucagon (4,9,17,18), vasopressin (22), and cortisol (15) stimulate bile secretion, estrogen (12,19) inhibits secretion of bile.

Bile secretion from the ductules and ducts is mainly affected by several known gut hormones or peptides. Secretin increases the volume and bicarbonate concentration of bile in both animal species (7,10,20,21,23) and man (2,25). In dogs, endogenous secretin released by duodenal acidification was also reported to stimulate bile secretion (21). Secretin (10) characteristically stimulates bile secretion rich in bicarbonate and chloride but does not affect bile acid secretion. Secretin does not appear to stimulate canalicular bile secretion since erythritol and mannitol clearance rates remain unchanged by secretin (1,26). Although the mechanism of secretin-induced choleresis has not been clearly understood, it has been suggested that secretin-induced bile secretion involves carbonic anhydrase (25) and possible roles for the Na^+-K^+-dependent ATPase and active Na^+ transport as the driving force (3). The increase in biliary cyclic AMP concentrations in response to exogenous secretin parallel with the increases in bile flow and bicarbonate concentrations suggest that cyclic AMP may be a possible mediator for bile production (14). A similar choleretic effect was produced by vasoactive intestinal polypeptide (16,24) and glucagon (4,9,17,18). The gastrin group of the gut hormone family—gastrin, CCK-PZ, and cerulein—are also known to stimulate bile secretion (11). The stimulating potency of these peptides on ductule and duct secretion of water and electrolytes decreases in the following order: cerulein, CCK-PZ, and gastrin (6,11). There is only one known peptide that inhibits spontaneous bile secretion in anesthetized dogs. Substance P (8) given in doses of 1.0 ng/kg-min or higher decreases bile flow and biliary output of sodium and amylase.

Although bile secretion is affected by these hormones or peptides, the physiological role of each individual hormone or peptide will have to await further investigations using a physiological dose of each hormone or endogenous hormones that are released in more physiologically designed experiments.

REFERENCES

1. Boyer, J. L., and Bloomer, J. R. (1973): Canalicular bile secretion in man. *J. Clin. Invest.,* 52:11a.
2. Boyer, J. L., and Bloomer, J. R. (1974): Canalicular bile secretion in man. Studies utilizing the biliary clearance of [^{14}C] mannitol. *J. Clin. Invest.,* 54:773–781.
3. Chenderovitch, J. (1972): Secretory function of the rabbit common bile duct. *Am. J. Physiol.,* 223:695–706.
4. Dyck, W. P., and Janowitz, H. D. (1971): Effects of glucagon on hepatic bile secretion in man. *Gastroenterology,* 60:400–404.

5. Fritz, M. E., and Brooks, F. P. (1963): Control of bile flow in the cholecystectomized dog *Am. J. Physiol.*, 204:825–828.
6. Gardiner, B. N., and Small, D. M. (1976): Simulataneous measurement of the pancreatic and biliary response to CCK and secretin. *Gastroenterology*, 70:403–47.
7. Hardison, W. G., and Norman, J. C. (1967): Effects of bile salt and secretion upon bile flow from the isolate perfused pig liver. *Gastroenterology*, 53:412–417.
8. Holm, I., Thulin, L., and Hellgren, M. (1978): Anticholinergic effect of substance P in anesthetized dogs. *Acta Physiol. Scand.*, 102:274–280.
9. Jones, R. S., Geist, R. E., and Hall, A. D. (1971): The choleretic effects of glucagon and secretin in the dog. *Gastroenterology*, 60:64–68.
10. Jones, R. S., and Grossman, M. I. (1969): Choleretic effects of secretin and histamine in the dog. *Am. J. Physiol.*, 217:532–535.
11. Jones, R. S., and Grossman, M. I. (1970): Choleretic effects of cholecystokinin, gastrin II, and cerulein in the dog. *Am. J. Physiol.*, 219:1014–1018.
12. Kreek, M. J., Peterson, R. E., Sleisinger, M. H., and Jeffries, G. H. (1967): Influence of ethinyl estradiol-induced cholestasis on bile flow and biliary excretion of estradiol and bromosulfophthalein by the rat. *J. Clin. Invest.*, 46:1080.
13. Layden, T. J., and Boyer, J. L. (1976): The effects of thyroid hormone on bile salt-independent bile flow and Na^+-K^+-ATPase activity in liver plasma membranes enriched in bile canaliculi. *J. Clin. Invest.*, 57:1009–1018.
14. Levine, R. A., and Hall, R. C. (1976): Cyclic AMP in secretin choleresis, evidence for a regulatory role in man and baboons but not in dogs. *Gastroenterology*, 70:537–544.
15. Macarol, V., Morris, T. Q., Baker, K. J., and Bradley, S. E. (1970): Hydrocortisone choleresis in the dog. *J. Clin. Invest.*, 49:1714–1723.
16. Makhlouf, G. M., Said, S. I., and Yau, W. M. (1974): Interplay of vasoactive intestinal peptide (VIP) and synthetic VIP fragments with secretin, octapeptide of cholecystokinin (Octa-CCK) on pancreatic and biliary secretion. *Gastroenterology*, 66:737.
17. Morris, T. Q. (1972): Choleretic responses to cyclic AMP and theophylline in the dog. *Gastroenterology*, 62:187.
18. Morris, T. Q., Sardi, F. F., and Bradley, S. E. (1967): Character of glucagon-induced choleresis. *Fed. Proc.*, 26:774.
19. Mueller, M. N., and Kappas, A. (1964): Estrogen pharmacology. 1. The influence of estradiol and estriol on hepatic disposal of sulfobromophthalein (BSP) in man. *J. Clin. Invest.*, 43:1905–1914.
20. Pissidis, A. G., Bombeck, C. T., Merchant, F., and Nyhus, L. M. (1969): Hormonal regulation of bile secretion: A study in the isolate, perfused liver. *Surgery*, 66:1075–1084.
21. Preisig, R., Cooper, H. L., and Wheeler, H. O. (1962): The relationship between taurocholate secretion rate and bile production in the unanesthetized dog during cholinergic blockade and during secretin administration. *J. Clin. Invest.*, 41:1152–1162.
22. Preisig, R., Strebel, H., Egger, G., and Macarol., V. (1972): Effects of vasopressin on hepatocytic and ductal bile formation in the dog. *Experientia*, 28:1436–1437.
23. Soloway, R. D., Clark, M. L., Powell, K. M., Senior, J. R., and Brooks, F. P. (1972): Effects of secretin and bile salt in infusions on canine bile composition and flow. *Am. J. Physiol.*, 222:681–686.
24. Thulin, L., and Hellgren, M. (1976): Choleretic effect of vasoactive intestinal peptide. *Acta Chir. Scand.*, 142:235–237.
25. Waitman, A. M., Dyck, W. P., and Janowitz, H. D. (1969): Effects of secretin and acetazolamide on the volume and electrolyte composition of hepatic bile in man. *Gastroenterology*, 56:286–294.
26. Wheeler, H. O., Ross, E. D., and Bradley, S. E. (1968): Canalicular bile production in dogs. *Am. J. Physiol.*, 214:866–874.

III. Gastrointestinal Hormones and Intestinal Secretion

Intestinal secretion is the net result of absorption and secretion that occur concurrently in the intestinal lumen. As early as 1935, Nasset et al. (17) reported that intestinal mucosal extracts of dog or pig stimulated intestinal secretion in dog and called the humoral substance "enterocrinin." The actions on the intestinal secretion of several pure hormones or gut peptides have been studied in recent years. In dogs with a Thiry-Vella loop of the jejunum or ileum, the volume and electrolyte composition of the secretion from the loops were measured in response to intravenous administration of glucagon, pentagastrin, vasoactive intestinal polypeptide (VIP), gastric inhibitory polypeptide (GIP), pure synthetic porcine secretin, and the octapeptide of CCK-PZ (CCK-OP) (2). Glucagon, pentagastrin, VIP, and GIP stimulated intestinal secretion, whereas synthetic secretin and CCK-OP failed to stimulate secretion. The responses to glucagon and pentagastrin were dose-related in both jejunum and ileum whereas the response to GIP was dose-related in the jejunum only. In man, synthetic human gastrin I (G-17-1) in varying doses did not stimulate secretion of water and electrolytes but it depressed the glucose-induced sodium absorption when gastrin was given in a dose of 0.5 μg/kg-hr or greater (15). Secretin (10), CCK-PZ (16), and glucagon (11) were also studied in man. All three of these hormones were shown to be capable of inducing a net intestinal secretion. The newest gut hormone, GIP, has also been shown to inhibit water absorption in man (8,9). During GIP infusion, the net water, Na, K, and HCO_3 absorption was significantly reduced and chloride flux was switched from absorption to secretion (9). The dose of GIP capable of influencing water absorption, 1 μg/kg-hr, is probably within a physiological dose range. In addition to these hormones, prostaglandins and serotonin are known to stimulate intestinal secretion of water and electrolytes also. Prostaglandins E_1, E_2, and $F_{2\alpha}$ stimulate intestinal secretion of water and electrolytes, both in experimental animals and in man (14). Serotonin is another agent that inhibits small intestinal absorption of water and electrolytes in rabbits (12). More recently, it has been found that serotonin (3) stimulates ileal secretion and decreases mid-jejunal absorption of water and electrolytes but does not affect water absorption in the proximal jejunum or colon. Beside these gut hormones there are hormones that affect intestinal secretion. Thyrocalcitonin provokes small intestinal secretion of water and electrolytes in rabbit (13) and in man (7). Antidiuretic hormone was also shown to affect the small intestine by either increased secretion of water and salt or direct interference with the active sodium transport mechanism in man (19).

In the colon, glucagon was found to stimulate secretion of water and electrolytes in dog (2), whereas synthetic secretin and pentagastrin did not. Neither glucagon nor pentagastrin alone was capable of inducing diarrhea in dog. When a combination of these two hormones or CCK-OP and pentagastrin was given intravenously in large doses, diarrhea occurred in dogs (2). In rat and rabbit, it was shown that prostaglandins invariably produced diarrhea but VIP, GIP, secretin, and motilin failed to produce diarrhea (20). Pure natural porcine VIP in doses up to 4.0 mg/kg-hr for 4 hr failed to produce diarrhea both in rat and rabbit (20). It has recently been found that glucagon produces diarrhea regularly in rat also (Chey et al., *unpublished data*).

Both prostaglandins (1) and VIP (18) are potent stimulants of the adenylate cyclase-cyclic AMP system, which is probably responsible for the intestinal secretion of water and electrolytes induced by the two agents. The cellular mechanism of stimulating intestinal secretion by other gut hormones is not known at present.

Brush border enzyme secretion from the small intestinal mucosa was shown to be stimulated by gut hormones also. Secretin and CCK-PZ given intravenously as a bolus resulted in a marked increase in intestinal alkaline phosphatase in dog (4) and in man (6). These two hormones increased secretion of disaccharidases also, i.e., sucrase, maltase, and lactase in dogs (5).

In spite of numerous observations studying the effects of these gut hormones on the intestinal secretion, their physiological roles will have to await future investigations. The dosages of these hormones used in the investigations were mostly in the pharmacological range.

REFERENCES

1. Al-Awqati, Q., and Greenough, W. B. III. (1972): Prostaglandins inhibit intestinal sodium transport. *Nature,* 238:26–30.
2. Barbezat, G. O. (1973): Stimulation of intestinal secretion by polypeptide hormones. *Scand. J. Gastroenterol.,* 8(22):1–21.
3. Donowitz, M., Charney, A. N., and Heffernan, J. M. (1977): Effect of serotonin treatment on intestinal transport in the rabbit. *Am. J. Physiol.,* 232:E85–E94.
4. Dyck, W. P. (1973): Hormonal control in intestinal alkaline phosphatase secretion in the dog. *Gastroenterology,* 65:445–450.
5. Dyck, W. P. (1974): Hormonal stimulation of intestinal disaccharidase release in the dog. *Gastroenterology,* 66:533–538.
6. Dyck, W. P., Martin, G. A., and Ratliff, C. R. (1973): Influence of secretion and cholecystokinin on intestinal alkaline phosphatase secretion. *Gastroenterology,* 64:599–602.
7. Gray, T. K., Bieberdorf, F. A., and Fordtran, J. S. (1973): Thyrocalcitonin and the jejunal absorption of calcium, water and electrolytes in normal subjects. *J. Clin. Invest.,* 52:3084–3088.
8. Helman, C. A., and Barbezat, G. O. (1976): Effect of gastric inhibitory polypeptide on jejunal water and electrolyte transport in man. *Lancet,* i:1129.
9. Helman, C. A., and Barbezat, G. O. (1977): Effect of gastric inhibitory polypeptide on human jejunal water and electrolyte transport. *Gastroenterology,* 72:376–379.
10. Hicks, T., and Turnberg, L. A. (1972): The influence of secretin on ion transport in the human jejunum. *Gut,* 14:485–490.
11. Hicks, T., and Turnberg, L. A. (1974): Influence of glucagon on the human jejunum. *Gastroenterology,* 67:1114–1118.
12. Kisloff, B., and Moor, E. W. (1976): Effect of serotonin on water and electrolyte transport in the in vivo rabbit small intestine. *Gastroenterology,* 71:1033–1038.
13. Kisloff, B., and Moor, E. W. (1977): Effects of intravenous calcitonin on water, electrolytes and calcium movement across in vivo rabbit jejunum and ileum. *Gastroenterology,* 72:462–468.
14. Matuchansky, C., and Bernier, J. J. (1976): Prostaglandins and ions transported in the human

intestine. A current survey. In *Intestinal Ion Transport*, edited by J. W. L. Robinson, pp. 355–368. MTP Press, Lancaster.

15. Modigliani, R., Mary, J. Y., and Bernier, J. J. (1976): Effects of synthetic human gastrin I on movements of water, electrolytes and glucose across the human small intestine. *Gastroenterology,* 71:978–984.

16. Moritz, M., Finkelstein, G., Meshkinpour, H., and Moor, E. (1973): Effect of secretin and cholecystokinin on the transport of electrolytes and water in human jejunum. *Gastroenterology,* 64:76–80.

17. Nassett, E. S., Pierce, H. B., and Murlin, J. R. (1935): Proof of a hormonal control of intestinal secretion. *Am. J. Physiol.,* 111:145–158.

18. Schwartz, C. J., Kimberg, D. V., Sheerin, H. E., Field, M., and Said, S. I. (1974): Vasoactive intestinal peptide stimulation of adenylate cyclase and active electrolyte secretion in intestinal mucosa. *J. Clin. Invest.,* 54:536–544.

19. Soergel, K. H., Whalen, G. E., Harris, J. A., and Geenen, J. E. (1968): Effect of antidiuretic hormone on human small intestinal water and solute transport. *J. Clin. Invest.,* 47:1071–1082.

20. Tai, H. H., Chey, W. Y., Escoffery, R. G., and Hendricks, J. (1976): Diarrheic factors in nonislet cell tumor of the pancreas. *Clin. Res.,* 24:292A.

SUMMARIES AND CONCLUSIONS

Pancreatic Secretion

Hormones and/or hormonal candidates released from the gut and pancreas play important physiological roles in external pancreatic secretion. Secretin is a well-established physiological hormone to stimulate pancreatic secretion of water and bicarbonate, whereas CCK-PZ is the hormone that stimulates pancreatic secretion of enzymes. The latter appears to augment the action of secretin, particularly in postprandial state. VIP is a partial agonist of pancreatic secretion of bicarbonate in man and dog, whereas it is a full agonist in cat. Chymodenine is a peptide that stimulates secretion of chymotrypsinogen in rabbit. Whether or not the effects of exogenous VIP and chymodenine on the pancreas are physiological are not known.

There are at least five known hormones or hormone candidates that inhibit the external pancreatic secretion. They are pancreatic glucagon, somatostatin, pancreatic polypeptide, met-enkephalin, and anti-cholecystokinin peptide. Among these, the actions of somatostatin and pancreatic polypeptide appear to be physiological ones.

The vagus nerve plays important roles by stimulating pancreatic secretion of water, bicarbonate, and enzymes, by modulating action of secretin in the pancreas, and by affecting release of endogenous pancreatic polypeptide.

Bile Secretion

Bile ductular and ductal secretion, rich in bicarbonate, is stimulated by secretin, glucagon, VIP, gastrin, CCK-PZ, and cerulein. Among these, the action of secretin is probably physiological.

Intestinal Secretion

Several gut hormones and/or gut hormone candidates were shown to affect the small intestine or colon by either stimulating secretion of water and electrolytes or by suppressing the active absorption of water and electrolytes. In dogs, the small intestinal secretion of water and electrolytes has been stimulated by glucagon, pentagastrin, VIP, GIP, and prostaglandins, and in man by secretin, CCK-PZ, glucagon, GIP, and prostaglandins. Both secretin and CCK-PZ were shown to stimulate intestinal secretion of brush border enzymes. Among these hormones, prostaglandins and VIP are known to activate the adenylate cyclase-cyclic AMP system to produce intestinal secretion of water and electrolytes. Only one hormone, glucagon, is known to stimulate colonic secretion of water and electrolytes in the dog. Whether the actions of these hormones are physiological or not will be answered by future investigations.

PROJECTIONS FOR THE FUTURE

Pancreatic Secretion

There are several hormones or gut peptides that are known to stimulate or inhibit external pancreatic secretion. Both secretin and CCK-PZ have come to be considered unquestionably as hormones that play important physiological roles in the production of pancreatic juice. However, further research is needed to produce the highly sensitive and specific immunoassay which will provide us with a better understanding of the physiological roles of CCK-PZ.

The assessment of the physiological and pathophysiological roles on pancreatic secretion of other hormones or hormone candidates such as chymodenin, pancreatic polypeptide, glucagon, glucagon-like immunoreactants (61), anti-cholecystokinin peptide, and neuro-endocrine peptides including VIP, somatostatin, and enkephalin, will require many more years of extensive research. Furthermore, careful observations on the actions of the cholinergic, sympathetic, and peptidergic nervous systems and the interactions between these systems and gut hormones on the external pancreatic secretion will undoubtedly add new knowledge on the physiological mechanisms of the exocrine pancreas.

Lastly, future investigations should include studies on the intracellular regulatory mechanism of the pancreas controlled by gut peptides and neuro-peptides, using human and/or canine pancreas, from which most of the current knowledge of the physiology and pathophysiology of the exocrine pancreas has been derived. In order to assess the intracellular secretory mechanism of water and electrolytes from the pancreas, the specific secretory cell preparations that primarily contribute to the secretion of water and electrolytes will have to be developed. Such preparations have not yet been available.

Bile Secretion

Although bile ductular and ductal secretion is stimulated by several exogenous gut hormones, it is not known whether or not their action on bile secretion is physiological. More studies are forthcoming to determine the physiological regulation of gut hormones on bile secretion. More studies are to be done on the secretory mechanisms induced by these gut hormones in the future. Substance P is the only known peptide that inhibits bile ductal secretion. More of such hormones will probably be discovered in the future and their physiological role will be classified.

Intestinal Secretion

Several gut hormones or neuropeptides are shown to affect intestinal secretion. Most of the observations were made in experimental animals by intravenous administration of these peptides. The physiological significance of each of these peptides will have to be clarified by better designed experiments, using exogenous hormones in physiological doses or endogenous hormones. The study is to be expanded further to clinical investigation. The mechanisms of actions of these peptides have been poorly understood. Except for that of VIP and prostaglandins, the secretory mechanisms produced by other gut hormones are virtually unknown. There will be exciting studies in the future to investigate the mechanisms of action of these hormones on the intestinal mucosal cells.

As new hormonal candidates will be discovered, it is possible that hormonal agents, other than VIP and prostaglandins responsible for the mechanism of severe secretory diarrhea associated with APUDOMA, will be known to improve the early diagnosis and successful treatment of water diarrhea syndrome.

Gastrointestinal Hormones, edited by
George B. Jerzy Glass.
Raven Press, New York © 1980.

Chapter 25

Gastrointestinal Hormones and Motor Function of the Gastrointestinal Tract

Hans Ruppin and Wolfram Domschke

Department of Medicine, University of Erlangen-Nürnberg, Erlangen, West Germany

INTRODUCTION

Problems in the Elucidation of the Physiological Role of Gastrointestinal Hormones in the Regulation of Motor Activity of the Gut

Impurity of Hormones

Only recently have synthetic preparations become available for systematic investigations. A variety of controversial results observed with gastrointestinal hormones are undoubtedly due to impurities in natural tissue extracts. This holds true especially for cholecystokinin (CCK).

Lack of Reliable Hormone Assays

The decision whether or not a given motor response to the exogenous gastrointestinal hormone reflects the physiological action of the endogenous polypeptide depends critically on the knowledge of the plasma level of the substance during its parenteral administration in comparison with the plasma concentration of the endogenous product released in response to an appropriate physiological stimulus. However, with the exception of gastrin, reproducible values of fasting and postprandial hormone levels have not been obtained until recently, and some, like CCK, still cannot be assayed with confidence.

Species-Specific Differences

Hormones may have direct (muscular) and/or indirect (neurally mediated) actions on smooth muscle motor activity and these may vary from species to species in different sections of the gut and in different (circular or longitudinal) muscle layers.

The physiological significance of most effects of gastrointestinal hormones on gut motor function has, therefore, been seriously questioned (39).

PEPTIDES PREDOMINANTLY STIMULATING GASTROINTESTINAL MOTOR ACTIVITY

Gastrin

Studies with gastrin on gastrointestinal motor activity have been performed in a variety of mammals, including man. Natural hog GII, synthetic preparations of little gastrin (G17) and big gastrin (G34) and C-terminal pentapeptide (PG) and tetrapeptide (TG) have been used. At proper dosage, effects can be obtained at nearly every level of the gastrointestinal tract but most of these are clearly pharmacological. Table 1 summarizes the actions of gastrin and its analogs on gastrointestinal motor activity.

Stomach

Isolated muscle strips of human (2), canine (28,74), cat, guinea pig, and hamster (72) fundus or antrum are contracted by natural and synthetic G17 (4.8×10^{-12}–2.0×10^{-9} M), PG (5×10^{-12} M), and TG. On a molar basis, PG is the most potent of all gastrin analogs tested (72,74). Antral strips respond predominantly by an increment in frequency as well as in amplitude of phasic contractions, whereas the effects on fundus preparations are mainly represented

TABLE 1. *Gastrin: effects on motility*

	In vitro	In vivo		References
		Pharmacological	Physiological	
Stomach, isolated strips, motility, man, dog, cat, hamster, guinea pig	↑			2,28,71,74
Stomach pouch, motility, guinea pig, dog	↑	↑	↑	33,35,80,106
Intact antrum, motility, man		↑		97,72
Innervated fundic pouch, tension, dog		↓		80,125
Gastric emptying, fluid, dog		↓		19,20,26,107
Gastric emptying, fluid, man		↓		45
Gastric emptying, solids, man		↓		41,69
Intestinal strips, motility, man, animals	O			2,97
Intact small intestine, motility, man		↑		72,97
Interdigestive migrating complex, presence, dog		↓		65,122,127
Interdigestive migrating complex, presence, man		↓		43
Colon strips, motility, man, rat, cat	↑			2,97
Sigmoid colon, electrical activity, man		↑		98,100,112
Gallbladder pouch, motility, dog		↑		116
Gallbladder strips, motility, guinea pig, salmon	↑			119,133
Bile duct strips, motility, man, dog	↑			113

O, no effect; ↑, increase; ↓, decrease.

by an elevation of the muscular tone. The patterns of motor responses to gastrin of *in vitro* pouch preparations of guinea pig antrum and corpus (33,35), *in vivo* canine antral pouches (80,106), or of intact human antrum (71,97) are similar to those of isolated strips. Gastrin and its analogs exert their effects partly via postganglionic cholinergic fibers, i.e., through the release of acetylcholine (62,74,106,120), and partly via direct interaction with muscle cell receptors (2,62,74,97,106). In contrast with their stimulatory action on cholinergic nerves, and smooth muscle cell membranes of the stomach, high intravenous doses of the polypeptides (PG: 1.3×10^{-9}–2×10^{-8} moles/kg-hr; Gastrin: 4.8×10^{-11}–1.6×10^{-9} moles/kg-hr) delay gastric emptying of fluid in man (45) and dog (19,20,26) and of solid food in man (41,66). This apparent contradiction has been partly resolved by the demonstration of the dose-dependent relaxing effect of PG (8×10^{-11}–1.6×10^{-9} moles/kg-hr) on the distended innervated fundic pouch of the dog with a subsequent fall in transmural pouch pressure (80,125).

Denervation of the pouch causes a shift of the dose-response curve to the right by one order of magnitude, indicating a decrease in the sensitivity of the pouch to the inhibitory action of PG (80). Thus, part of the enhancing action of gastrin on receptive relaxation of proximal canine stomach is supposedly mediated via afferent or efferent inhibitory vagal fibers (53). Neither distal antrectomy (26) nor diversion of duodenal contents (19) will influence the rate or pattern of emptying induced by PG. Also, the slowing of gastric evacuation is independent of duodenal acidification in response to the increased amount of acid secreted into and emptied from the stomach (19,26,45).

It has been clearly shown that the driving force behind the emptying of liquids is represented by the pressure gradient between stomach and duodenum (107). Consequently, the delay in the emptying of fluid induced by exogenous gastrin is best explained through depression of transmural fundic tone. In contrast, emptying of solids has been suggested to be governed by antral peristaltic activity (27,65,124) which, in turn, is stimulated by gastrin in both man (71,97) and dog (19,80,106). In addition, gastrin has been shown not to contract the pylorus in humans (29).

These considerations are less conclusive with respect to the inhibiting effect of the polypeptides on the emptying of solid food in man (41,69). In evaluating the role of antral motility on emptying of solids, plastic spheres have been used as substituents for solid food (27). However, unlike plastic spheres, digestible solids are liquefied prior to their entry into the upper small intestine (70). Moreover, by raising the frequency of the antral pacesetter potential (and, thus, of rhythmic antral peristalsis) the discharge of plastic spheres from the stomach will be enhanced, in contrast with that of digestible solids, which remains unchanged (44). Once chemically digested and mechanically triturated, solid food would pass into the liquid phase and be dependent on intragastric pressure and, predominantly, on the caloric density of the meal (46). Whereas high plasma concentrations of gastrin delay stomach emptying, physiological doses of the hormone eliciting one-half maximal gastric acid secretion (D_{50}) have been shown not to affect stomach emptying of liquids (20,107).

Small Intestine

In vitro, high local concentrations of natural hog GII (9.5×10^{-10}–4.8×10^{-9} M) do not contract small intestinal muscle strips of various rodents, cat, or pigeon (97); nor do GI and GII (2.4×10^{-8}–4.8×10^{-8} M) or PG (4.8×10^{-7}–10^{-5} M) affect strips of human duodenum, jejunum, and ileum (71). By using pressure-sensitive telemetering capsules, gastrin and PG have been found ineffective in stimulating ileal peristaltic activity when administered at doses that are submaximal for gastric acid secretion (18), whereas supramaximal doses of the polypeptides induce jejunal and ileal contractions (97). In the dog, feeding and intravenous infusion of large doses of PG (8×10^{-9} moles/kg-hr) have been shown to interrupt cyclically recurring interdigestive migrating myoelectric complexes (IMCs) of stomach and small intestine (67,122). Whereas feeding abolishes migrating complexes at all levels of the gut and increases the total incidence of action potentials in jejunum and ileum (131), intravenous infusion of a physiological dose of PG (D_{50}) neither interferes consistently with the IMC nor increases the absolute incidence of action potentials (127). Similarly, in man, D_{50} of PG is ineffective with respect to disruption of the fasting pattern of intestinal motor activity (43). Consequently, endogenous gastrin is unlikely to be of physiological significance for the regulation of postprandial small bowel motility unless subthreshold plasma concentrations of the hormones will potentiate the effects of other polypeptides having greater capacity for stimulation of intestinal motor activity, like CCK (127) or glucagon (128).

Large Intestine

Strips from the circular and longitudinal muscle coats of human ascending colon (2) and from descending colon of the rat and cat (97) contract on addition of gastrin (5×10^{-5} M and 10^{-4} M, respectively). Since colonic motility increases within a few minutes following a meal, resulting in an urge to defecate, gastrin has been considered one of several agents that might function as humoral mediator of the so-called gastrocolic reflex (112). However, *in vivo* studies in man employing pressure-sensitive telemetering capsules (71) or miniature balloons (18) and using intravenous bolus injections rather than continuous infusions of gastrin or PG have yielded contradictory results. The controversy regarding the role of gastrin in controlling colonic motility has been explained on the basis of the observation that PG (2.9×10^{-6} moles/kg-hr) stimulates human sigmoid motor activity only when a slow wave frequency of 3 cycles/min is present but not at the faster electrical rhythm of 6 to 9 cycles/min (112). By simultaneously recording myoelectric activity and intraluminal pressure and using bipolar silver-silver chloride clip electrodes and continuously perfused open-tip catheters, relatively small doses of synthetic GI (5×10^{-11}–10^{-10} moles/ kg-hr) that raised plasma gastrin concentrations to the postprandial level of the endogenous hormone were found to increase the incidence of rectal and rectosigmoidal action potentials and the number and amplitude of intraluminal pressure waves (98,100). The slow postprandial increment in endogenous plasma gastrin concentration, however, does not coincide with the rapid response of colonic motor activity to a meal (100). The question whether gastrin or any other gastrointestinal hormone takes part in the colonic response to eating cannot be answered until the kinetics of their postprandial release and their possible interactions at neural and muscular receptor sites have been further evaluated.

Gallbladder and Bile Ducts

In guinea pig and dog, purified porcine GI, GII, and PG act as weak cholecystokinetic stimulants (116,133) that exert their action directly on gallbladder muscle, as do the approximately thousand times more potent polypeptides CCK and cerulein (133). Also, muscular strips from extrahepatic bile ducts of dog and man respond to high local concentrations of gastrin (113). These actions of gastrin and its analogs are truly pharmacological and their investigation is of purely phylogenetic interest (119). For additional information on gastrin, see Chapter 6 by G. Nilsson, pp. 127–168, *this volume.*

Cholecystokinin (CCK)

CCK and its C-terminal octapeptide (OP-CCK) have been most extensively used in studying the effects of gut hormones on gastrointestinal motor functions.

TABLE 2. *Cholecystokinin: effects on motility*

	In vitro	In vivo		References
		Pharmacological	Physiological	
Antral strips, motility, dog	↑			28
Stomach strips, motility, man	↑			9
Stomach pouch, motility, guinea pig	↑			34,36
Stomach pouch, motility, dog		↓		3,7,111
Intact stomach, motility, man		↓		22,55
Gastric emptying, liquids, dog			↓	20,107
Gastric emptying, liquids, man		↓		12,103
Small intestine, strips, motility, guinea pig	↑			90
Small intestine, motility, dog	↑	↑		85,90,104
Proximal duodenum, motility, man		O		31,79
Distal duodenum, jejunum, motility, man		↑		24,31,40
Jejunum, electrical activity, dog			↑ ?	76,127
Interdigestive migrating complex, presence, dog		↓		76,127
Intestinal transit time, man		↓		42,60,66,83
Rectosigmoid colon, motility, man		↓		23,99
Gallbladder strips, motility, guinea pig	↑			133
Gallbladder pouch, motility, dog		↑		116
Intact gallbladder, motility, guinea pig, dog		↑		90
Intact gallbladder, motility, man		↑	↑ ?	109

O, no effect; ↑, increase; ↓, decrease.

The motility patterns induced by CCK and gastrin along the entire gastrointestinal and biliary tract resemble each other to the degree of similarity of their C-terminal heptapeptide amino acid sequences (56,81,119,133). The motor effects of CCK are summarized in Table 2.

Stomach

In the guinea pig, basic tension and amplitude of contractions of isolated antral and fundic pouch preparations are increased by 20% pure CCK at concentrations of 0.1 to 0.75 U/ml (34,36). Analogous contractile effects can be observed on human fundic and antral muscle strips (9). Certain natural preparations of CCK have been shown to be contaminated with motilin, a potent stimulant of gastric and small intestinal smooth muscles, and, when freed from the contaminant by further purification, to inhibit rather than to stimulate *in vivo* gastric pouch motility in the dog (3,7). Additional observations suggest, however, that, *in vitro,* CCK itself may contract stomach smooth muscles of guinea pig and dog: Synthetic motilin is ineffective with respect to guinea pig (105) and canine (54) alimentary tract muscle strip preparations and synthetic OP-CCK (4.5 × 10^{-9} M) will enhance frequency and amplitude of canine antral circular muscle directly via muscular receptors shared by synthetic gastrin (28).

In contrast with these *in vitro* experiments, however, CCK has been found to inhibit spontaneous contractions and/or to decrease basic tension of the innervated antral (111) or denervated fundic (3,7) pouch of the dog and of intact human stomach (22,55). The latter observations are consistent with the ability of exogenous CCK and OP-CCK to delay gastric emptying of liquids in both dogs (20,107) and human subjects (12,103). Since the pylorus contracts on intravenous administration of submaximal doses of CCK (30,68,77), the effect on stomach evacuation has also been attributed to CCK-induced pyloric closure. However, the role of the antropyloric region in the regulation of gastric emptying has been the subject of extensive investigation, as outlined in the section on gastrin. It is now generally accepted that the rate of gastric emptying of liquid food is determined by intragastric pressure (107), and, thus, delayed by receptive relaxation of the fundus, while being independent from the diameter of the pylorus (101).

In the dog, inhibition of gastric emptying has been suggested as a physiological function of endogenous CCK (20,107).

Small Intestine

The effects of CCK and OP-CCK on small bowel motility have received much attention, especially with respect to intestinal transit time, which has been and is still of considerable clinical interest.

Muscle strips from guinea pig ileum respond to high concentrations of natural CCK (0.4 U/ml) and OP-CCK (10^{-8} M) with increased phasic contractions

(90). In the dog, intravenous injections of 0.1 to 1.0 U/kg or μg/kg of the two peptides, respectively, are sufficient to stimulate duodenal and jejunal motor activity for periods up to 15 min (85,90). Nevertheless, threshold concentrations of CCK and OP-CCK necessary to activate intestinal muscles are two to ten times higher than those for appropriate preparations of gallbladder (90).

In both longitudinal strips of guinea pig ileum and circular muscle of the isolated and perfused jejunum of the dog, the action of CCK is mediated through the release of acetylcholine from postganglionic cholinergic nerves and its interaction with nonnicotinic muscular receptors (104,120). In man, proximal duodenal myoelectric and mechanical activity is not significantly influenced by intravenous boluses of 1 U/kg of CCK (31,79), whereas distal duodenum (40) and proximal jejunum (24,31,40) are fairly sensitive to the polypeptide administered intravenously by either continuous infusion or single injection.

During fasting, exogenous CCK at physiological dosage (D_{50}) increases the incidence of electrical spikes and the duration of irregular activity (phase II of the IMC) in duodenum and jejunum (76,127) but has relatively little effect in terminal ileum (127). At higher dosage ($> D_{50}$), OP-CCK interrupts phase III of the IMC (76), whereas pure CCK abolishes the progression of phase III along proximal but not distal small intestine (127).

In contrast with the interference with migrating activity in the fasted state, CCK speeds the intestinal transit of a barium meal (42,60,83). In 10 healthy subjects 2.4×10^{-11} moles/kg-hr of OP-CCK decreased the time necessary for intestinal passage of barium sulfate by 85% on the average (42). In a group of six subjects without intestinal disease, graded doses of the drug (4.4–17.5 $\times 10^{-12}$ moles/kg) accelerated small bowel transit of contrast medium by 38 to 85%, respectively (60). Also, in patients with celiac sprue or with granulomatous enterocolitis, a considerable reduction of transit time (from 180–300 to 3–9 min and from 120–300 to 3–30 min, respectively) was observed when 50 to 100 Ivy dog units of Vitrum CCK were administered intravenously (83).

In man, during small bowel perfusion of isotonic sugar-free solutions, mean transit time of a dye bolus through a 35-cm long jejunal perfusion segment could be reduced by 61% when CCK (6 IDU/kg-hr) was infused intravenously. This increase in flow velocity may be explained partly by a decrease in lumenal diameter by 40% or more and partly by the stimulation of net fluid secretion into small bowel lumen (68). The association of small bowel hypermotility with (electrogenic) intestinal secretion has also been suggested to occur in the interdigestive state (85). It may be one of several mechanisms responsible for the watery diarrhea in certain neuroendocrine tumors with intestinal hormone hyperproduction.

Large Intestine

The colon of both man (23,100) and cat (99) is sensitive to low doses of OP-CCK. In man, myoelectric and mechanical activity of rectum and sigmoid colon is stimulated by 4.4 to 35×10^{-12} moles/kg-hr of the peptide, and the response to 9×10^{-12} moles/kg-hr is similar to that following a 1,000 calorie meal (100). Previously, manometric studies in distal human colon had demonstrated that purified CCK dose dependently (0.5–2 U/kg-hr) increased sigmoidal but not rectal motor activity (23). The possible implication of endogenous CCK in the response of the colon to eating awaits further elucidation.

Gallbladder and Bile Ducts

The concept of hormonal control of gallbladder muscle contraction was first suggested by Ivy and Goldberg (51) in 1928 and fully developed by a number of subsequent studies (1,56,81,90,102,110,113,114,116,119,133).

In conscious dogs with fistulas of the gallbladder, relative cholecystokinetic potencies versus natural porcine CCK of the structurally related C-terminal TG and PG, GI, GII, and cerulein are 1/143, 1/143, 1/23, 1/21, and 1/16, respectively, when referred to molar concentrations (116). OP-CCK is even more potent than Vitrum CCK in contracting isolated strips and *in situ* preparations of guinea pig gallbladder and canine gallbladder *in vivo* (90). The half-maximal contractile response of guinea pig gallbladder strips can be elicited by molar concentrations of OP-CCK ten and five times smaller than those of 10% pure CCK and cerulein, respectively (133). Canine and human common bile duct specimens mounted along their longitudinal axis respond to high local concentrations of CCK (0.001–0.1 U/ml) with regular phasic contractions superimposed on increments in basic tone (113). Emptying of the bile is the result of a number of successive events starting out with a progressive increase in tension of gallbladder wall followed by intermittent opening of the sphincter-like cholecysto-cystic junction, phasic contractions of the common bile duct along its axis and, finally, active opening and closing of the choledocho-duodenal sphincter with periodical discharge of bile into the duodenum (114). The intravenous injection of graded doses of OP-CCK results in the reduction of gallbladder size by a maximum of 44% as measured on X-ray film (110), whereas a 77% or greater reduction was observed after a fatty meal or following continuous intravenous infusion of cerulein (11). These differences are undoubtedly due to the short half-life of the polypeptide owing to which the effect of an intravenous bolus of the substance is limited to no longer than a few minutes. The administration of single cholecystokinetic polypeptides probably does not reflect the physiological situation following a meal, since, in the dog, subthreshold doses of secretin have been found to potentiate the effect of CCK on gallbladder function (102). Unlike small intestine of guinea pig (120) and dog (104) and similarly to canine antral circular muscle (28), the gallbladder responds to the direct action of CCK at receptor sites residing on or in the muscle cell itself (1,133).

Motilin

13-Methionine motilin (METM), a relatively recently discovered gastrointestinal polypeptide, is structurally unrelated to gastrin or any other polypeptide hormone or candidate hormone known so far (4,5). Its physiological role in gastrointestinal motor function during fasting and after eating has not been yet definitely clarified. However, the association of METM and of its synthetic analog, 13-norleucine motilin (NLEM), with the interdigestive migrating myo-electric or motor complex (IMC) in the dog (47,130) and man (64,118) has been established.

Stomach and Small Intestine

Purified hog METM (7.2×10^{-10} moles/kg, i.v.) strongly stimulates motor activity of vagally and sympathetically denervated canine fundic or antral pouches (6). Furthermore, graded doses ($1.4–23 \times 10^{-11}$ moles) of NLEM produce linearly related increases in integrated intraluminal pressure and in total electrical spike activity of the isolated vascular-perfused stomach and duodenum of the dog when given into the arterial supply of the preparation (38). In striking contrast to the *in vivo* or *ex vivo* preparations, isolated strips of various parts of canine alimentary tract do not respond to concentrations up to 3.6×10^{-7} M of METM (54). Similarly, strips of guinea pig and rat gastrointestinal tract are insensitive to 1.8×10^{-7} M of NLEM (105). Isolated strips of rabbit and

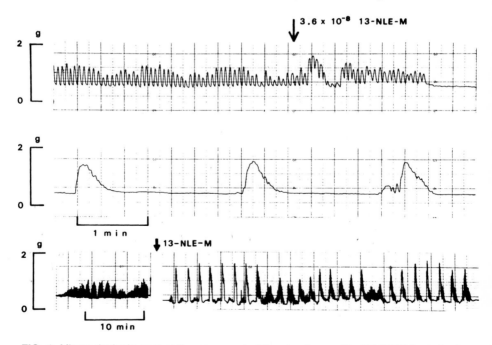

FIG. 1. Minute-rhythmic contractile response to 13-norleucine motilin (13-NLE-M) of circular muscle strip of rabbit duodenum. Vertical scales on the left indicate basic tension and amplitude of contractions in grams. The strip was mounted in an organ bath containing isotonic Hepes-Krebs solution at 37°C and gassed with 100% O_2. Concentration of 13-NLE-M in M (moles/liter).

human stomach and small intestine, however, are highly sensitive to NLEM, threshold concentrations being between 10^{-9} and 10^{-7} M (105). In both rabbit duodenum and human stomach, the site of action of NLEM proved to be directly on or in the muscle cell itself and not on intrinsic nervous receptors (96,105). The only naturally occurring antagonist for motilin known so far, at least in the rabbit, appears to be the vasoactive intestinal polypeptide (VIP) (108).

Isolated circular strips of duodenal muscle respond to NLEM (3.6×10^{-8} M) in the form of strong minute-rhythmic contractions (Fig. 1) that can be abolished and prevented by low pressure or high concentrations of ouabain (93). The minute-rhythmic contractions are preceded by analogous minute-rhythmic bursts of action potentials superimposed on periods of membrane depolarization (89). The effect of NLEM on rabbit duodenum can be blocked by the calcium antagonist verapamil (105). This is known to prevent the calcium influx into guinea pig *taenia coli* muscle cells during K-induced contracture (69). No such intracellular accumulation of calcium, however, can be seen during the minute-rhythmic response induced by NLEM (92). This might be the result of unidirectional transmembrane calcium fluxes alternating between inward and outward directions that is associated with rhythmically alternating contractions and relaxations.

In striking contrast with the localized effects of METM and NLEM on strips, isolated organs or pouch preparations, the intact gastrointestinal tract of fasted dog and man responds to motilin with premature IMCs (47,64,118,130). Figure 2 shows an original record of NLEM-induced IMC from normal human small

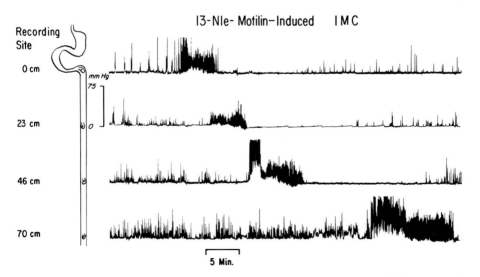

FIG. 2. Migrating interdigestive small intestinal motor complex (IMC) recorded in a normal male by continuously perfused (0.1 ml/min) open-tipped catheters placed at regular intervals from proximal to distal jejunum. The vertical scale of the left indicates the amplitude of pressure waves in mm Hg. IMC started 20 min following the start of intravenous infusion of 13-norleucine motilin (13-NLE-Motilin) at the rate of 0.4 μg/kg-hr.

intestine. Although the exact origin of the cyclically recurring bursts of strong regular contractions (phase III of the IMC) in stomach and small intestine is unknown, its propagation along the entire small intestine is undoubtedly under nonvagal extrinsic nervous control (10,123). The integrated response of canine alimentary canal to synthetic MET can be abolished by subcutaneous atropine (0.1 mg/kg) or intravenous hexamethonium (13 mg/kg-10 min) but not by truncal vagotomy (82), suggesting a postganglionic cholinergic path for the polypeptide. Whereas exogenous motilin is the only substance known to trigger migrating interdigestive contractions, the role of the endogenous peptide in the generation of the IMC is still a matter of controversy: In both dog (49,59) and man (63,117), fasting plasma motilin concentration is subject to cyclic variations. This bears a fixed association with the cycles of interdigestive motor activity in the dog (49,59) and also in some human subjects (117), but not in all individual studies (63). Feeding (49,59), intravenous atropine (59), duodenal drainage (48), or intraduodenal infusion of nutrients (48) have all been reported to simultaneously abolish plasma motilin fluctuations and IMCs in the dog. In contrast, intravenous infusions of PG (48), synthetic human GI (59), or OP-CCK (59) interrupt the IMC and switch the gut toward digestive motor activity but do not interfere with waxing and waning of endogenous plasma motilin levels. Furthermore, diametrically opposed results can be obtained with duodenal acidification in man. Whereas some subjects appear to respond to intraduodenal infusion (5 ml/min) of 0.1 N HCL with periods of regular contractions resembling the duodenal IMC but without concomitant release of endogenous motilin (61), in others, a 50-ml intraluminal bolus and continuous infusion (5 ml/min) of 0.1 N HCL disrupt the IMC but are followed by a sustained increment in plasma motilin (88). These and other conflicting observations do not yet allow a decision to be reached on the physiological role of motilin in the interdigestive state. Natural, highly purified secretin has been reported to prevent the IMC in the dog at relatively low rates of intravenous infusion (75). In man, synthetic secretin significantly decreases endogenous plasma motilin concentration at similar rates of intravenous administration (73). The interference of secretin with the intrinsic clock that regulates cyclic motor activity during fasting could be interpreted as being either mediated through or responsible for the decay in radioimmunoassayable plasma motilin. However, facing the profound discrepancies between man and dog with respect to the *in vitro* effects and the mechanism of endogenous release of motilin (25), the above hypothesis might easily become disproved by future investigations.

The interdigestive motor activity in man is characterized by minute-rhythmic bursts of action potentials (32) and contractions (94) occurring largely during phase II of the IMC. NLEM has been shown to stimulate minute-rhythmic membrane depolarizations (89) and contractions (93) of duodenal circular muscle. Whether such minute-rhythmic electrical and mechanical events during fasting are also due to endogenous motilin deserves further investigation.

NLEM at doses of 3.6×10^{-11} to 1.4×10^{-10} moles/kg-hr dose dependently delays gastric emptying in man of hypertonic D-mannitol buffered at pH 3.0 (91), whereas METM (9×10^{-11}–7.2×10^{-10} moles/kg-hr) enhances emptying of normal saline in the dog (21) and of the ^{129}Cs-labeled solid meal in man (15). The controversial results observed with liquid meals might be due to differences in species or methods used in these studies (21,91). In any event, the enhancing effect of METM on the delivery of saline and "solid food" from stomach to duodenum is not likely to be the result of propulsive (migrating) motor activity. It has been clearly shown that feeding and intragastric instillation of saline interrupt the IMC in both dog (17,47,50) and man (87), and that METM is ineffective in disrupting the digestive pattern of motor activity (47,50). Gastric emptying of liquids and of digestible food is controlled mainly by intragastric pressure and not by gastric peristalsis (44,107). It is, therefore, conceivable but not yet proven that METM in the digestive state, in which it is without effect on gastrointestinal peristalsis, increases intragastric pressure by elevating the muscular tone of the fundus.

NLEM (1.4×10^{-10} moles/kg-hr) accelerates the transit of barium sulfate through the human small bowel by 50% on the average (95). In contrast, flow velocity estimated from dilution curves of nonabsorbable marker substances in jejunal or ileal perfusion segments is not significantly influenced by this peptide (94). However, flow rates in the jejunum are substantially increased by NLEM, probably through the stimulation of intestinal fluid secretion (94). The enhancing effect of NLEM on the movement of viscous contrast medium might, therefore, be simply the result of a decrease in viscosity of the barium sulfate suspension following dilution by water added to the intestinal lumen.

Large Intestine

The colon appears to be relatively insensitive to NLEM: Isolated strips of *taenia coli* of rat, guinea pig, and rabbit colon and circular strips of descending colon of rat, guinea pig, and man, as well as of human sigmoid colon and rectum, do not contract on addition of NLEM at concentrations up to 3.6×10^{-6} M. Human *taenia coli* is sensitive to 1.8×10^{-6} M and circular strips of rabbit descending colon to 7.2×10^{-9} M of the polypeptide (105). To our knowledge, no studies with motilin on intact colon of any species have been reported so far.

Gallbladder

There is no structural relationship between CCK and motilin. It is, therefore, not unexpected that, *in vitro,* NLEM does not stimulate gallbladder motor activity (105). We do not know of any study where METM was tested on the motor function of the biliary tract.

PEPTIDES PREDOMINANTLY INHIBITING GASTROINTESTINAL MOTOR ACTIVITY

Secretin

A physiological significance of secretin for digestive tract motility has not been yet established. The pattern of inhibitory actions of secretin may however, delineate a pathway by which structurally related polypeptides like glucagon and other unidentified substances could interfere physiologically with interdigestive motor activity. The effects of secretin on motility are summarized in Table 3.

Stomach

Natural and synthetic secretin (1.6×10^{-7} M) decrease number and amplitude of spontaneous phasic contractions of human fundic and antral strips and lower basic tension of strips from human fundus (9). In the dog, synthetic secretin

TABLE 3. *Secretin: effects on motility*

	In vitro	In vivo		References
		Pharmacological	Physiological	
Stomach strips, motility, man	↓			9
Intact stomach, motility, man		↑ ↓		22,55
Intact stomach, motility, dog		↓		13,16
Innervated antral pouch, motility, dog		↓		111
Denervated antral pouch, motility, dog		O		13
Gastric emptying, fluid, man		↓		12,115
Gastric emptying, fluid, dog		↓		16
Small intestine, motility, man		↓		24,40
Small intestine, digestive electrical activity, dog		O		75
Interdigestive migrating complex, presence, dog		↓		75,127
Rectosigmoid colon, motility, man		↓; O		14,23,98
Gallbladder strips, motility, dog, man	↑			113
Gallbladder pouch, spontaneous motility, dog		O		102
Gallbladder pouch, CCK-stimulated motility, dog		↑	↑ ?	102
Bile duct strips, motility, dog	↑			113

O, no effect; ↑, increase; ↓, decrease

$(1.5 \times 10^{-8}$ M) depresses the response of antral circular muscle to the stimulating actions of gastrin or OP-CCK, whereas it is ineffective with respect to spontaneous tone and contractions (55). In man, minor, mostly biphasic changes of intragastric pressure, characterized by an initial increase and subsequent decrease of the latter, have been observed following intravenous administration of Vitrum secretin $(8 \times 10^{-9}$ moles/kg-hr). To the contrary, Boots or Jorpes secretin $(1.6 \times 10^{-7}$ moles/kg) given as single intravenous boluses promptly and significantly diminished spontaneous and urecholine-stimulated antral contractions as measured by continuously perfused open-tip catheters (22). The inhibitory effect of secretin on gastric motility has also been confirmed for the intact stomach and the innervated antral pouch of the dog (111). Denervated fundic pouches, however, do not respond to secretin (13).

In man, gastric emptying of normal saline and distilled water can be delayed by relatively small doses of this hormone administered by single injection (8×10^{-12} moles/kg) (12) or continuous infusion (10^{-11}–10^{-10} moles/kg-hr) (115). In comparison, the dog appears to be quite insensitive to secretin with respect to gastric evacuation of fluid, since approximately thousand times higher dosage is necessary for a significant inhibition of gastric evacuation (16). Pyloric sphincter tone in man has been reported to increase in response to infusion of secretin at a rate of 1 U/kg-hr (29). However, as earlier discussed in detail in the section on gastrin, the rate of gastric emptying of fluid is solely dependent on intragastric pressure (101,107).

Small Intestine

In humans spontaneous or CCK-stimulated duodenal and jejunal motor activity is almost abolished by secretin given at the rate of 1.6×10^{-10} moles/kg-hr (40), whereas smaller doses of the hormone prove insufficient (24). This would indicate that the stomach is more sensitive (115) than small intestine to the inhibitory action of secretin. The following observations are consistent with this conclusion: In the dog, the onset of phase III of the IMC in the stomach can be prevented by as little as 4×10^{-11} moles/kg-hr of secretin (75). A four times larger dose of this hormone, however, is without effect on propagation of the IMC once it reaches the upper small intestine (75). These differences in sensitivity toward secretin between stomach and small intestine during fasting might reflect different mechanisms controlling the initiation of the IMC in the stomach and its migration along the small bowel. In contrast, the postprandial pattern and the frequency of small intestinal myoelectric spikes remain unaffected by secretin at doses that interfere with interdigestive motor activity (75).

Large Intestine

Controversial results have been obtained with secretin in studies on human rectosigmoidal motility. In a group of 10 subjects, secretin attenuated the amplitude and decreased the number of pressure waves per time unit, its threshold dose being about 8×10^{-11} moles/kg-hr (23). Twice that dose inhibited motor activity of sigmoid colon stimulated by CCK (23). In contrast, at 10 cm above the anus, secretin did not alter motility of human rectum (23). Also, in another group of 12 subjects, bolus injections of secretin (0.16×10^{-7} moles/kg) caused no change in the incidence of electrical spikes measured by silver-silver chloride clip electrode in either rectum or rectosigmoid colon (98). Food-induced sigmoid contractions may be suppressed by 3.3×10^{-10} moles/kg-hr of secretin preceded by its single bolus of 0.8×10^{-10} moles/kg (14). Differences in sensitivity to secretin of the various sections of the distal 25 cm of large intestine may have contributed to these contradictory results.

Gallbladder and Bile Ducts

Secretin alone does not stimulate gallbladder contraction in the dog at even unphysiologically high doses (102). However, a medium dose (1.6×10^{-10} moles/kg-hr) of the peptide given as background infusion augments the cholecystokinetic potency of CCK (102). Moreover, endogenous secretin released by duodenal acidification in response to PG-stimulated acid secretion similarly enhances gallbladder contraction elicited by CCK. In contrast, the cholecystokinetic effect of low doses of PG can be abolished by diversion of gastric acid from duodenum (102). *In vitro,* high local concentrations of Boots secretin (0.07–0.3 U/ml) bring about immediate contractions of full-thickness strips of canine gallbladder as well as delayed increments in tension of longitudinal muscles of common bile ducts (113). These observations, made *in vitro,* are unlikely to be of physiological significance. However, secretin might be involved in the regulation of postprandial gallbladder motility by potentiation of the action of CCK when present at even low and by themselves inefficient concentrations. For additional information on secretin, see Chapter 5 by V. Mutt, pp. 85–126, *this volume.*

Glucagon

Only a small number of studies has been published regarding the effects of glucagon on gastrointestinal motility. The results obtained are controversial and do not allow for final conclusions with respect to the role of glucagon in gastrointestinal motor function. However, some recent observations suggest that glucagon might be even more likely than CCK in mediating postprandial motor activity of canine small intestine.

Stomach

As early as 1955, Stunkard et al. reported that pancreatic glucagon infused intravenously at a rate of 9.2×10^{-9} moles/kg-hr immediately abolished "hunger contractions" of the stomach in normal human individuals that were associated with long-lasting increments in blood glucose concentration and disappearance of subjective hunger sensations (109). In conscious and anesthetized dogs, intravenous boluses of 1.4 to 28×10^{-9} moles/kg of glucagon also inhibited prostigmin-stimulated gastric contractions and wall tension measured by small inflated balloons (78). In contrast, spontaneous contractions and basic tension of strips from antrum and body of human stomach were not altered by glucagon at concentrations as great as 2.9×10^{-7} M (9).

Small Intestine

In man, glucagon given 5 to 7 days following laparotomy as single bolus injections into peripheral venous or portal blood caused inhibition of intrajejunal pressure and phasic jejunal contractions (58). In "chronic dogs," prepared with serosally implanted electrodes, intravenous injections of glucagon (2.8×10^{-7} moles) reduced duodenal myoelectric activity, whereas the recordings obtained from jejunum and ileum remained unchanged (132). However, when administered by continuous intravenous infusion ($3.6–14 \times 10^{-8}$ moles/hr), glucagon would interrupt the IMC and generate strong irregular spike activity at all levels of canine small intestine (Fig. 3) (128,132). As discussed in a previous section, secretin inhibits the IMC in dog as well (75). Since glucagon shares

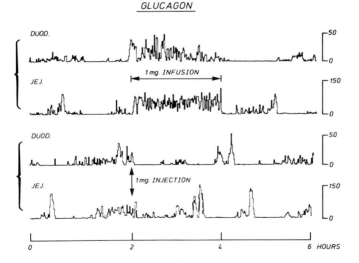

FIG. 3. Histogram of spike activity in the duodenum of two dogs. Vertical scales on the right indicate the number of spike per minute. Both dogs received an intravenous infusion of physiological saline for 6 hr. In one dog **(above)**, 1 mg of glucagon was infused over 2 hr as shown. In the other dog **(below)** a rapid intravenous injection of 1 mg of glucagon was given at 2 hr as shown. It should be noted that the injection has inhibited a duodenal migrating motor complex 1 hr after the injection, although the complex is clearly seen in the jejunum. (From ref. 129, with permission.)

part of its amino acid sequence with secretin (121), a common mechanism for both the hormones might be considered with respect to inhibition of cyclic interdigestive activity. However, the peptides differ in that secretin would inhibit rather than stimulate action potential incidence when infused intravenously at constant rates (75,127). Conversely, CCK, at physiological doses, disrupts the IMC and increases duodenal but not jejunal or ileal myoelectric activity, and gastrin neither interferes with the IMC nor alters total incidence of spikes at infusion rates considered to be in the physiological range (127).

These observations prompted Wingate (128) to conclude that if any single hormone should be responsible for switching the gut from the interdigestive to the digestive pattern of motor activity in response to feeding, glucagon would be the candidate of choice (132). It is conceivable that whereas a small increase in plasma glucagon stimulates intestinal motor activity, a large one might actually paralyze the gut. This would be consistent with gross jejunal stasis and massive constipation in a patient with an enteroglucagon-producing renal tumor and with disappearance of the motility dysfunction after the tumor had been surgically removed (37).

Large Intestine

In conscious dogs, glucagon ($1.8-90 \times 10^{-9}$ moles/kg) administered by intravenous injection inhibits prostigmin-stimulated motor activity of distal colon (78). In man, motor activity of the rectum stimulated by feeding or morphine is reduced to prestimulation values by glucagon infused at the rate of 8.6×10^{-9} moles/kg-hr (14). However, the question whether endogenous glucagon released from pancreatic or gastrointestinal epithelial tissues may be involved in the regulation of postprandial colonic mass contractions has not been yet tested in more detail. For additional information on the effects of glucagon on gastrointestinal motility, see Chapter 11 by T. M. Lin, pp. 275–305, *this volume.*

Vasoactive Intestinal Polypeptide

It is not known whether, under physiological conditions, VIP interferes with gastrointestinal motility. Three studies have been reported so far on the effect of VIP on alimentary tract motor activity. Piper et al. (84) have demonstrated a relaxant effect of VIP on guinea pig gastric and gallbladder muscles, whereas ileal longitudinal strips were found insensitive to VIP. Jaffer et al. (52) reported that VIP stimulates contractile force of longitudinal muscle of guinea pig duodenum and ileum. And Kachelhoffer et al. (57) obtained shortlasting biphasic responses of the isolated *ex vivo* perfused canine jejunum to intraarterial injection or infusion of the VIP that could be blocked by systemic atropine. This latter phenomenon consisted of brief relaxation and subsequent longer lasting excitation and has been suggested to be involved in aborad bolus propulsion. Due to the limited physiological significance of this type of preparation, however, these effects are most certainly pharmacological. In addition, the above suggestion of propulsive motility was not supported by showing aboral migration of the phenomenon. Nevertheless, considering the possible role of VIP as a peptidergic neurotransmitter substance of the noncholinergic, nonadrenergic inhibitory nervous system (8), the reported events might represent pharmacological counterparts of the physiologically occurring inhibitory-excitatory reflexes along intramural nervous plexuses. For additional information on the effects of VIP on gastrointestinal motility, see Chapter 10 by S. Said, pp. 245–273, *this volume.*

SUMMARY AND CONCLUSIONS

The majority of changes in gastrointestinal motor activity induced by exogenous hormones or candidate hormones of enteric origin is, clearly, unphysiological because of at least one of the following reasons: (a) The threshold dose for eliciting the effect is higher than the dose that induces one-half maximal response (D_{50}) with respect to the identifying action, e.g., on gastric or pancreatic secretions. (b) The rise in the endogenous plasma concentration of a given polypeptide following a meal or during fasting does not coincide with the changes in motor activity occurring in response to the physiological stimulus.

Only the following two actions of gastrointestinal hormones are likely to occur physiologically during the digestive state in dog: (a) retardation of gastric emptying by CCK and (b) stimulation of antral triturating motility by gastrin. Moreover, the following effects of other polypeptides deserve attention since their possible role in gastrointestinal motility cannot be excluded on the basis of recently accumulated knowledge—generation of interdigestive motor complexes (IMCs) in dog and man by motilin, and interruption of the IMC and initiation of digestive motility in the dog by glucagon.

PROJECTIONS FOR THE FUTURE

Within the last decade, research in gastrointestinal motility has been rapidly progressing partly because of a large number of new techniques developed for the study and evaluation of electrical and mechanical motor activity. In recently designed studies, short-time measurements and single-bolus injections of gastrointestinal hormones have been largely replaced by continuous monitoring of their effect over many hours as well as by constant-rate infusion of the peptides reflecting more closely the physiological situation.

Thus, some of the results that have been observed in the past will have to be reevaluated by using physiological dosages, better study designs, and on-line computerized data evaluation. Moreover, the majority of effects of gastrointestinal hormones on digestive tract motility can also be elicited by stimulation of excitatory or inhibitory vagal fibers. Therefore, definite discrimination between and quantitation of nervous and humoral component actions remain a challenge for future research.

Recently, the hypothesis of the duality of actions of gastrointestinal hormones, i.e., of a local "paracrine" and a distant "endocrine" path, has been proposed to explain the multiplicity of effects that this eupeptide system exerts at secretory, muscular, and nervous cells (126). This concept might be particularly helpful in explaining both the local factors that regulate coupling of action potentials with slow waves and the neural control locus that determines the onset and termination of interdigestive and digestive states of motor activity. A variety of enteric hormones or neuroenteric substances have not been considered within the present chapter because of limited knowledge on their effects or relevance in controlling gastrointestinal motor functions. To these belong gastric inhibitory polypeptide, prostaglandins, substance coherin, neurotensin, somatostatin, and the system of endogenous opioid analogues. In designing further experiments on their possibly physiological implications for gastrointestinal motility, it is advisable to take the newly derived concept into sound consideration.

Careful classification and documentation of the endocrine tumor syndromes and of their clinical course and the assay of the total spectrum of neurohormonal substances and peptides related to motor disorders of the gastrointestinal tract are necessary to clarify the pathogenesis of some of the syndromes related to endocrine tumors, the symptomatology of which includes motor disorders of the gastrointestinal tract.

REFERENCES

1. Andersson, K.-E., Andersson, R., and Hedner, P. (1972): Cholecystokinetic effect and concentration of cyclic AMP in gallbladder muscle *in vitro. Acta Physiol. Scand.,* 85:511–516.
2. Bennet, A., Misiewicz, J. J., and Waller, S. L. (1967): Analysis of the motor effects of gastrin and pentagastrin on the human alimentary tract *in vitro. Gut,* 8:470–474.
3. Brown, J. C. (1967): Presence of a gastric motor-stimulating property in duodenal extracts. *Gastroenterology,* 52:225–229.
4. Brown J. C., Cook, M. A., and Dryburgh, J. R. (1972): Motilin, a gastric motor activity-stimulating polypeptide: final purification, amino-acid composition and C-terminal residues. *Gastroenterology,* 62:401–404.
5. Brown, J. C., Cook, M. A., and Dryburgh, J. R. (1973): Motilin, a gastric motor activity stimulating polypeptide: the complete aminoacid sequence. *Can. J. Biochem.,* 51:533–537.
6. Brown, J. C. Mutt, V., and Dryburgh, J. R. (1971): The further purification of motilin, a gastric motor activity stimulating polypeptide from the mucosa of the small intestine of dogs. *Can J. Physiol. Parmacol.,* 49:399–405.
7. Brown, J. C., and Parkes, C. O. (1967): Effect on fundic pouch motor activity of stimulatory fractions separated from pancreozymin. *Gastroenterology,* 53:731–736.
8. Bryant, M. G., Bloom, S. R., Polak, J. M., Albuquerque, R. H., Modlin, I., and Pearse, A. G. E. (1976): Possible dual role for VIP as gastrointestinal hormone and neurotransmitter subtance. *Lancet,* i:991–993.
9. Cameron, A. J., Phillips, S. F., and Summerskill, W. H. J. (1970): Comparison of effects of gastrin, cholecystokinin-pancreozymin, secretin, and glucagon on human stomach muscle *in vitro. Gastroenterology,* 59:539–545.
10. Carlson, G. M., Bedi, B. S., and Code, C. F. (1972): Mechanism of propagation of intestinal interdigestive complex. *Am. J. Physiol.,* 222:1027–1030.
11. Carratu, R., Arcangeli, G., and Pallone, F. (1971): Effects of caerulein on human biliary tract. *Rendic. R. Gastroenterol.,* 3:28–33.
12. Chey, W. Y., Hitanant, S. M., Hendricks, J., and Lorber, S. H. (1970): Effect of secretin

and cholecystokinin on gastric emptying and gastric secretion in man. *Gastroenterology,* 58:820–827.

13. Chey, W. Y., Kosay, S., Hendricks, J., Braverman, S., and Lorber, S. H. (1969): Effect of secretin on motor activity of stomach and Heidenhain pouch in dogs. *Am. J. Physiol.,* 217:848–852.

14. Chowdhary, A. R., and Lorber, S. H. (1977): Effects of glucagon and secretin on food- or morphine-induced motor activity of the distal colon, rectum and anal sphincter. *Am. J. Dig. Dis.,* 22:775–780.

15. Christofides, N. D., Modlin, I., Fitzpatrick, M. L., and Bloom, S. R. (1978): Effect of motilin on gastric emptying of solid meals in man. *Gut,* 19:A436.

16. Chvasta, T. E., and Cook, A. R. (1973): Secretin-gastric emptying and motor activity: natural versus synthetic secretin (36979). *Proc. Soc. Exp. Biol. Med.,* 142:137–142.

17. Code, C. F., and Marlett, J. A. (1975): The interdigestive myoelectric complex of the stomach and small bowel of dogs. *J. Physiol.,* 246:289–309.

18. Connell, A. M., and Logan, C. J. H. (1967): The role of gastrin in gastroileocolic responses. *Am. J. Dig. Dis.,* 12:277–284.

19. Cook, A. R., Chvasta, T. E., and Weisbrodt, N. W. (1972): Effect of pentagastrin on emptying and electrical and motor activity of the dog stomach. *Am. J. Physiol.,* 223:934–938.

20. Debas, H. T., Farooq, O., and Grossman, M. I. (1975): Inhibition of gastric emptying is a physiological action of cholecystokinin. *Gastroenterology,* 68:1211–1217.

21. Debas, H. T., Yamagishi, T., and Dryburgh, J. R. (1977): Motilin enhances gastric emptying of liquids in dogs. *Gastroenterology,* 73:777–780.

22. Dinoso, V., Chey, W. Y., Hendricks, J., and Lorber, S. H. (1969): Intestinal mucosal hormones and motor function of stomach in man. *J. Appl. Physiol.,* 26:326–329.

23. Dinoso, V. P., Meshinpour, H., Lorber, S. H., Gutiérrez, J. G., and Chey, W. Y. (1973): Motor responses of the sigmoid colon and rectum to exogenous cholecystokinin and secretin. *Gastroenterology,* 65:438–444.

24. Dollinger, H. C., Berz, R., Raptis, S., von Uexküll, T., and Goebell, H. (1975): Effects of secretin and cholecystokinin on motor activity of human jejunum. *Digestion,* 12:9–16.

25. Domschke, W. (1977): Motilin: spectrum and mode of gastrointestinal actions. *Am. J. Dig. Dis.,* 22:454–461.

26. Dozois, R. R., and Kelly, K. A. (1971): Effects of gastrin pentapeptide on gastric emptying of liquids. *Am. J. Physiol.,* 221:113–117.

27. Dozois, R. R., Kelly, K. A., and Code, C. F. (1971): Effect of distal antrectomy on gastric emptying of liquids and solids. *Gastroenterology,* 6:675–681.

28. Fara, J. W., and Berkowitz, J. M. (1978): Effects of histamine and gastrointestinal hormones on dog antral smooth muscle *in vitro. Scand. J. Gastroenterol. (Suppl. 49),* 13:60.

29. Fisher, R. S., Lipshutz, W., and Cohen, S. (1973): The hormonal regulation of pyloric sphincter function. *J. Clin. Invest.* 52:1289–1296.

30. Fisher, R. S., Phaosawasdi, K., Boden G., and Kolts, B. (1978): Hormonal effects on the pyloric sphincter in man. *Scand. J. Gastroenterol. (Suppl. 49),* 13:62.

31. Fleckenstein, P., and Oigaard, A. (1977): Effects of cholecystokinin on the motility of the distal duodenum and the proximal jejunum in man. *Scand. J. Gastroenterol.,* 12:375–378.

32. Fleckenstein, P., and Oigaard, A. (1978): Electrical spike activity in human small intestine. A multiple electrode study of fasting diural variation. *Am. J. Dig. Dis.,* 23:776–780.

33. Gerner, T., and Haffner, J. F. W. (1976): Interactions of cholecystokinin (CCK-PZ) and gastrin on motor activity of the isolated guinea pig antrum and fundus. *Scand. J. Gastroenterol.,* 11:823–827.

34. Gerner, T., and Haffner, J. F. W. (1977): The influence of graded distension and carbachol on the motor response to cholecystokinin in the isolated guinea pig antrum and fundus. *Scand. J. Gastroenterol.,* 12:745–749.

35. Gerner, T., and Haffner, J. F. W. (1977): The role of local cholinergic pathways in the motor response to cholecystokinin and gastrin in isolated guinea pig fundus and antrum. *Scand. J. Gastroenterol.,* 12:751–757.

36. Gerner, T. Maehlumshagen, P., and Haffner, J. F. W. (1976): Pressure-responses to cholecystokinin in the fundus and antrum of isolated guinea pig stomachs. *Scand. J. Gastroenterol.,* 11:823–827.

37. Gleeson, M. H., Bloom, S. R., Polak, J. M., Henry, K., and Dowling, R. H. (1971): Endocrine tumor in kidney affecting small bowel structure, motility, and absorptive function. *Gut,* 12:773–782.

38. Green, W. E. R., Ruppin, H., Wingate, D. L., Domschke, W., Wünsch, E., Demling, L., and Ritchie, H. D. (1976): Effects of 13-nle-motilin on the electrical and mechanical activity of the isolated perfused canine stomach and duodenum. *Gut,* 17:362–370.

39. Grossman, M. I. (1977): Physiological effects of gastrointestinal hormones. *Fed. Proc.,* 36:1930–1935.

40. Gutiérrez, J. G., Chey, W. Y., and Dinoso, V. P. (1974): Actions of cholecystokinin and secretin on the motor activity of the small intestine in man. *Gastroenterology,* 67:35–41.

41. Hamilton, S. G., Sheiner, H. J., and Quinlan, M. F. (1976): Continuous monitoring of the effect of pentagastrin on gastric emptying of solid food in man. *Gut,* 17:273–279.

42. Hedner, P., and Rorsman, G. (1972): Acceleration of the barium meal through the small intestine by the C-terminal octapeptide of cholecystokinin. *Am. J. Roentgenol. Rad. Ther. Nucl. Med.,* 116:245–248.

43. Hellemans, J., Vantrappen, G., Janssen, J., and Peters, T. (1978): Effect of feeding and of gastrin on the interdigestive myelectric complex in man. In: *Gastrointestinal Motility in Health and Disease,* edited by H. L. Duthie, pp. 29–31. MTP Press, Lancaster.

44. Hinder, R. A., and Kelly, K. A. (1978): The role of the antral pacesetter potential in canine emptying of solids. In: *Gastrointestinal Motility in Health and Disease,* edited by H. L. Duthie, pp. 459–469. MTP Press, Lancaster.

45. Hunt, J. N., and Ramsbottom, N. (1967): Effect of gastrin II on gastric emptying and secretion during a test meal. *Br. Med. J.,* 4:386–387.

46. Hunt, J. N., and Stubbs, D. F., (1975): The volume and energy content of meals as determinants of gastric

47. Itoh, Z., Honda, R., Hiwatashi, K., Takeuchi, S., Aizawa, I., Takayanagi, R., and Couch, E. F. (1976): Motilin-induced mechanical activity in the canine alimentary tract. *Scand. J. Gastroenterol. (Suppl. 39),* 11:93–110.

48. Itoh, Z., Honda, R., Takeuchi, S., Aizawa, I., Takahashi, I., and Yanaihara, N. (1978): Endogenous release of motilin and gut motor activity in dog and man. *Scand. J. Gastroenterol. (Suppl. 49),* 13:92.

49. Itoh, Z., Takeuchi, S., Aizawa, I., Mori, K., Taminato, T., Seino, Y., Imura, H., and Yanaihara, N. (1978): Changes in plasma motilin concentration and gastrointestinal contractile activity in conscious dogs. *Am. J. Dig. Dis.,* 23:929–935.

50. Itoh, Z., Takeuchi, S., Aizawa, I., and Takayanagi, R. (1977): Effect of synthetic motilin on gastric motor activity in conscious dogs. *Am. J. Dig. Dis.,* 22:813–819.

51. Ivy, A. C., and Goldberg, E. (1928): A hormone mechanism for gallbladder contraction and evacuation. *Am. J. Physiol.,* 86:599–613.

52. Jaffer, S. S., Farrar, J. T., Yau, W. M., and Makhlouf, G. M., (1974): Mode of action and interplay of vasoactive intestinal peptide (VIP), secretin, and octapeptide of cholecystokinin (Octa-CCK) on duodenal and ileal muscle *in vitro. Gastroenterology,* 66:A-62/716.

53. Janson, G., and Martinson, J. (1965): Some quantitative considerations of vagally induced relaxation of the gastric smooth muscle in the cat. *Acta Physiol. Scand.,* 63:351–357.

54. Jennewein, J. M., Hummelt, H., Siewert, R., and Waldeck, F. (1975): The motor-stimulating effect of natural motilin on the lower esophageal fundus, antrum and duodenum in dogs. *Digestion,* 13:246–250.

55. Johnson, L. P., Brown, J. C., and Magee, D. F. (1966): Effect of secretin and cholecystokinin-pancreozymin extracts on gastric motility in man. *Gut,* 7:52–57.

56. Johnson, L. R., Stening, F., and Grossman, M. I. (1970): Effect of sulfation on the gastrointestinal actions of caerulein. *Gastroenterology,* 58:208–216.

57. Kachelhofer, J., Mendel, C., Dauchel, J., Hohmatter, D., and Grenier, J. F. (1976): The effects of VIP on intestinal jejunal loops. *Am. J. Dig. Dis.,* 21:957–962.

58. Kock, N. G., Darle, N., and Dotevall, G. (1967): Inhibition of intestinal motility in man by glucagon given intraportally. *Gastroenterology,* 53:88–92.

59. Lee, K. Y., and Chey, W. Y. (1978): Plasma immunoreactive motilin concentrations during interdigestive and digestive states. *Scand. J. Gastroenterol. (Suppl. 49),* 13:110.

60. Levant, J., Kun, T. L., Jachna, J., Sturdevant, R. A. L., and Isenberg, J. I. (1974): The effects of graded doses of C-terminal octapeptide of cholecystokinin on small intestinal transit time in man. *Am. J. Dig. Dis.,* 19:207–209.

61. Lewis, T. D., Collins, S. M., Fox, J. E., and Daniel, E. E., (1978): Initiation of migrating myoelectric complexes (MMC) by intraduodenal acid. *Gastroenterology,* 74:1055.

62. Lipshutz, W., Tuch, A. F., and Cohen, S. (1971): A comparison of the site of action of gastrin I on lower esophageal sphincter and antral circular smooth muscle. *Gastroenterology,* 61:454–460.
63. Lux, G., Strunz, U., Domschke, S., Femppel, J., Mitznegg, P., Rösch, W., and Domschke, W. (1978): Motilin and interdigestive myoelectric and motor activity of small intestine in man: Lack of causal relationship. *Scand. J. Gastroenterol. (Suppl. 49),* 13:118.
64. Lux, G., Strunz, U., Domschke, S., Femppel, J., Rösch, W., and Domschke, W., (1978): 13-Nle-motilin and interdigestive motor and electrical activity of human small intestine. *Gastroenterology,* 74:1058.
65. MacGregor, I. L., Martin, P., and Meyer, H. J. (1977): Gastric emptying of solid food in normal man and following subtotal gastrectomy and truncal vagotomy with pyloroplasty. *Gastroenterology,* 72:206–211.
66. MacGregor, I. L., Wiley, Z. D., and Martin, P. M. (1978): Effect of pentagastrin infusion on gastric emptying rate of solid food in man. *Am. J. Dig. Dis.,* 23:72–75.
67. Marik, F., and Code, C. F. (1975): Control of the interdigestive myoelectric activity in dogs by the vagus nerves and pentagastrin. *Gastroenterology,* 69:387–395.
68. Matuchansky, C., Huet, P. M., Mary, J. Y., Rambaud, J. C., and Bernier, J. J. (1972): Effects of cholecystokinin and metoclopramide on jejunal movements of water and electrolytes and on transit time of luminal fluid in man. *Eur. J. Clin. Invest.,* 2:169–175.
69. Mayer, C. J., van Breemen, C., and Casteels, R. (1972): The action of lanthanum and D 600 on the calcium exchange in the smooth muscle cells of the guinea pig *taenia coli. Pflügers Arch.,* 337:333–350.
70. Meyer, J. H., MacGregor, I. L., Gueller, R., Martin, P., and Cavalier, R. (1976): ^{99m}Tc-tagged chicken liver as a marker of solid food in the human stomach. *Am. J. Dig. Dis.,* 21:296–304.
71. Mikos, E., and Vane, J. R., (1967): Effects of gastrin and its analogues on isolated smooth muscles. *Nature,* 214:105–107.
72. Misiewicz, J. J., Holdstock, D. J., and Waller, S. L. (1967): Motor responses of the human alimentary tract to near-maximal infusions of pentagastrin. *Gut,* 8:463–469.
73. Mitznegg, P., Bloom, S. R., Domschke, W., Haecki, W. D., Domschke, S., Belohlavek, D., Wünsch, E., and Demling, L. (1977): Effect of secretin on plasma motilin in man. *Gut,* 18:468–471.
74. Morgan, K. G., Schmalz, P. E., Go, V. L. W., and Szurszewski, J. H. (1978): Effects of pentagastrin, G_{17}, and G_{34} on the electrical and mechanical activities of canine antral smooth muscle. *Gastroenterology,* 75:405–412.
75. Mukhopadhyay, A. K., Johnson, L. R., Copeland, E. M., and Weisbrodt, N. W. (1975): Effect of secretin on electrical activity of small intestine. *Am. J. Physiol.,* 229:484–488.
76. Mukhopadhyay, A. K., Thor, P. J., Copeland, E. M., Johnson, L. R., and Weisbrodt, N. W. (1977): Effect of cholecystokinin on myoelectric activity of small bowel of the dog. *Am. J. Physiol.,* 232:E44–E47.
77. Munk, J. F., Gannaway, R. M., Hoare, M., and Johnson, A. G. (1978): Direct measurement of pyloric diameter and tone in man and their response to cholecystokinin. In: *Gastrointestinal Motility in Health and Disease,* edited by H. L. Duthie, pp. 349–359. MTP Press, Lancaster.
78. Necheles, H., Sporn, J., and Walker, L. (1966): Effect of glucagon on gastrointestinal motility. *Am. J. Gastroenterol.,* 45:34–39.
79. Oigaard, A., Dorph, S., Christensen, K. C., and Christiansen L. (1975): The effects of cholecystokinin on electrical spike potentials and intraluminal pressure variations in the human small intestine. *Scand. J. Gastroenterol.,* 10:257–262.
80. Okike, N., and Kelly, K. A., (1977): Vagotomy impairs pentagastrin-induced relaxation of canine gastric fundus. *Am. J. Physiol.,* 232:E504–E509.
81. Ondetti, M. A., Rubin, B., Enel, S. L., Plusec, J., and Sheehan, J. T. (1970): Cholecystokinin-pancreozymin: recent developments. *Am. J. Dig. Dis.,* 15:149–156.
82. Ormsbee III, H. S., and Mir, S. S. (1978): The role of the cholinergic nervous system in the gastrointestinal response to motilin in vivo. In: *Gastrointestinal Motility in Health and Disease,* edited by H. L. Duthie, pp. 113–124. MTP Press, Lancaster.
83. Parker, J. G., and Beneventano, T. C. (1970): Acceleration of small bowel contrast study by cholecystokinin. *Gastroenterology,* 58:679–684.
84. Piper, P. J., Said, S. I., and Vane, J. R., (1970): Effects on smooth muscle preparations of unidentified vasoactive peptides from intestine and lung. *Nature,* 225:1144–1146.

85. Ramirez, M., and Farrar, J. T. (1970): The effect of secretin and cholecystokinin-pancreozymin on the intraluminal pressure of the jejunum in the unanesthetized dog. *Am. J. Dig. Dis.,* 15:539–544.

86. Read, N. W., Smallwood, R. H., Levin, R. J., Holdsworth, C. D., and Brown, B. H. (1977): Relationship between changes in intraluminal pressure and transmural potential difference in the human and canine jejunum in vivo. *Gut,* 18:141–151.

87. Rees, W. D. W., Malagelada, J. R., and Go., V. L. W., (1978): Human interdigestive motor activity: effect of saline and liquid nutrient meals. *Gastroenterology,* 74:1083.

88. Rees, W. D. W., Miller, L. J., Malagelada, J. R., and Go, V. L. W. (1978): Role of gastric acid secretion in the generation of human interdigestive motor activity. *Gut,* 19:A997.

89. Riemer, J., Kölling, K., Ruppin, H., Mayer, C. J., and Wünsch, E., (1977): The effect of 13-norleucine motilin on the electrical activity of rabbit circular duodenal muscle. *Pflügers Arch.,* 368:R24.

90. Rubin, B., Engel, S. L., Drungis, A. M., Dzelzkalns, M., Grigas, E. O., Waugh, M. H., and Yiacas, E. (1969): Cholecystokinin-like activities in guinea pigs and dogs of the C-terminal octapeptide (SQ 19, 844) of cholecystokinin. *J. Pharm. Sci.,* 58:955–959.

91. Ruppin, H., Domschke, S., Domschke, W., Wünsch, E., Jaeger, E., and Demling, L. (1975): Effects of 13-nle-motilin in man—inhibition of gastric evacuation and stimulation of pepsin secretion. *Scand. J. Gastroenterol.,* 10:199–202.

92. Ruppin, H., Mayer, C. J., Domschke, W., Wünsch, E., and Demling, L. (1977): Lack of effect of 13-norleucine motilin on net calcium uptake of isolated rabbit duodenal muscle. *Gastroenterology,* 72:A-100/1123.

93. Ruppin, H., Riemer, J., Mayer, C. J., Kölling, K., Domschke, W., Wünsch, E., and Demling, L. (1977): Ouabain-sensitive contractile response to 13-norleucine motilin of rabbit duodenal muscle. *Gastroenterology,* 72:A-100/1123.

94. Ruppin, H., Soergel, K. H., Dodds, J. W., Wood, C. M., and Domschke, W. (1979): Effects of the interdigestive motor complex (IMC) and 13-norleucine motilin (NLEM) on fasting intestinal flow rate and velocity in man. *Gastroenterology,* 76:1231.

95. Ruppin, H., Sturm, G., Westhoff, D., Domschke, S., Domschke W., Wünsch, E., and Demling, L. (1976): Effect of 13-nle-motilin on small intestinal transit time in healthy subjects. *Scand. J. Gastroenterol. (Suppl. 39),* 11:85–88.

96. Schubert, E., Mitznegg, P., Strunz, U., Domschke, W., Domschke, S., Wünsch, E., Jaeger, E., Demling, L., and Heim, F. (1975): Influence of the hormone analogue 13-nle-motilin and of 1-methyl-3-isobutylxanthine on tone and cyclic 3′, 5′-AMP content of antral and duodenal muscles in the rabbit. *Life Sci.,* 16:263–272.

97. Smith, A. N., and Hogg, D. (1966): Effect of gastrin II on the motility of the gastrointestinal tract. *Lancet,* i:403–404.

98. Snape, W. J., Carlson, G. M., and Cohen, S. (1977): Human colonic myoelectric activity in response to prostigmin and the gastrointestinal hormones. *Am. J. Dig. Dis.,* 22:881–887.

99. Snape, W. J., and Cohen, S. (1978): Stimulation of the isolated cat colon with gastrin or octapeptide of cholecystokinin. *Scand. J. Gastroenterol. (Suppl. 49),* 13:169.

100. Snape, W. J., Matarazzo, S. A., and Cohen, S. (1978): Effect of eating and gastrointestinal hormones on human colonic myoelectrical and motor activity. *Gastroenterology,* 75:373–378.

101. Stemper, T. J., and Cook, A. R. (1976): Effect of a fixed pyloric opening on gastric emptying in the cat and dog. *Am. J. Physiol.,* 230:813–817.

102. Stening, G. F., and Grossman, M. I. (1969): Potentiation of cholecystokinetic action of cholecystokinin (CCK) by secretin. *Clin. Res.,* 17:528.

103. Sterz, P., Guth, P., and Sturdevant, R. (1974): Gastric emptying in man: delay by octapeptide of cholecystokinin and L-tryptophan. *Clin. Res.,* 22:174A.

104. Stewart, J. J., and Burks, T. F., (1977): Actions of cholecystokinin octapeptide on smooth muscle of isolated dog intestine. *Am. J. Physiol.,* 232:E306–E310.

105. Strunz, U., Domschke, W., Mitznegg, P., Domschke, S., Schubert, E., Wünsch, E., Jaeger, E., and Demling, L. (1975): Analysis of the motor effects of 13-norleucine motilin on the rabbit, guinea pig, rat and human alimentary tract *in vitro. Gastroenterology,* 68:1485–1491.

106. Strunz, U. T., and Grossman, M. I., (1977): Antral motility stimulated by gastrin: a physiological action affected by cholinergic activity. In: *Nerves and the Gut,* edited by F. P. Brooks and P. W. Evers, pp. 233–239. Charles B. Slack, Thorofare, New Jersey.

107. Strunz, U. T., and Grossman, M. I. (1978): Effect of intragastric pressure on gastric emptying and secretion. *Am. J. Physiol.,* 235:E552–E555.

108. Strunz, U., Mitznegg, P., Domschke, S., Domschke, W., Wünsch, E., and Demling, L. (1978): VIP antagonizes motilin-induced antral contractions *in vitro.* In: *Gastrointestinal Motility in Health and Disease,* edited by H. L. Duthie, pp. 125–133. MTP Press, Lancaster.

109. Stundevant, R. A. L., Stern, D. H., Resin, H., and Isenberg, J. I. (1973): Effect of graded doses of octapeptide of cholecystokinin on gallbladder size in man. *Gastroenterology,* 64:452–456.

110. Stunkard, A. J., van Itallie, T. B., and Reis, B. B. (1955) The mechanism of satiety: Effect of glucagon on gastric hunger contractions in man. *Proc. Soc. Exp. Biol.,* 89:258–261.

111. Sugawara, K., Isaza, J., Curt, J., and Woodward, E. R., (1969): Effect of secretin and cholecystokinin on gastric motility. *Am. J. Physiol.* 217:1633–1638.

112. Taylor, I., Duthie, H. L., Smallwood, R., and Brown, B. H. (1974): Effect of stimulation on the myoelectrical activity of the rectosigmoid in man. *Gut,* 15:599–607.

113. Toouli, J., and Watts, J. M. (1972): Actions of cholecystokinin-pancreozymin, secretin and gastrin on extra-hepatic biliary tract motility *in vitro. Ann. Surg.,* 175:439–447.

114. Torsoli, A., Ramorino, M. L., and Alessandrini, A. (1970): Motility of the biliary tract. *Rendic. R. Gastroenterol.,* 2:67–80.

115. Vagne, M., and Andre, C. (1971): The effect of secretin on gastric emptying in man. *Gastroenterology,* 60:421–424.

116. Vagne, M., and Grossman, M. I. (1968): Cholecystokinetic potency of gastrointestinal hormones and related peptides. *Am. J. Physiol.,* 215:881–884.

117. Vantrappen, G., Janssen, J., Peeters, T., Bloom, S., Christofides, N. D., and Hellemans, J. (1978): Intraduodenal pH, motilin, and interdigestive migrating motor complex in man. *Scand. J. Gastroenterol. (Suppl. 49),* 13:190.

118. Vantrappen, G., Janssen, J., Peeters, T. L., Bloom, S., van Tongeren, J., and Hellemans, J. (1978): Does motilin have a role in eliciting the interdigestive migrating motor complex (MMC) in man? *Gastroenterology,* 74:1149.

119. Vigna, S. R., and Gorbman, A. (1977): Effects of cholecystokinin, gastrin and related peptides on coho salmon gallbladder contraction *in vitro. Am. J. Physiol.,* 232:E485–E491.

120. Vizi, S. E., Bertaccini, G., Impicciatore, M., and Knoll, J. (1973): Evidence that acetylcholine released by gastrin and related polypeptides contributes to their effect on gastrointestinal motility. *Gastroenterology,* 64:268–277.

121. Weinstein, B., (1968): On the relationship between glucagon and secretin. *Experientia,* 24:404–408.

122. Weisbrodt, N. W., Copeland, E. M., Kearley, R. W., Moore, E. P., and Johnson, L. R. (1974): Effects of pentagastrin on electrical activity of small intestine of the dog. *Am. J. Physiol.,* 227:425–429.

123. Weisbrodt, N. W., Copeland, E. M., Moore, E. P., Kearly, R. W., and Johnson, L. R., (1975): Effect of vagotomy on electrical activity of the small intestine of the dog. *Am. J. Physiol.,* 228:650–655.

124. Wilbur, B. G., and Kelly, K. A. (1973): Effect of proximal gastric, complete gastric, and truncal vagotomy on canine electrical activity, motility, and emptying. *Ann. Surg.,* 178:295–303.

125. Wilbur, B. G., and Kelly, K. A. (1974): Gastrin pentapeptide decreases canine gastric transmural pressure. *Gastroenterology,* 67:1139–1142.

126. Wingate, D. L. (1977): The eupeptide system: A general theory of gastrointestinal hormones. *Lancet,* i:529–532.

127. Wingate, D. L., Pearce, E. A., Hutton, M., Dand, A., Thompson, H. H., and Wünsch, E. (1978): Quantitative comparison of the effects of cholecystokinin, secretin and pentagastrin on gastrointestinal myoelectric activity in the conscious fasted dog. *Gut,* 19:593–601.

128. Wingate, D. L., and Pearce, E. A., (1979): The physiological role of glucagon in the digestive tract. In: *Glucagon in Gastroenterology,* edited by J. Picazo. MTP Press, Lancaster.

129. Wingate, D. L., Pearce, E. A., Thomas, P. A., and Boucher, B. J. (1978): Glucagon stimulates intestinal myoelectric activity. *Gastroenterology,* 74:1152.

130. Wingate, D. L., Ruppin, H., Green, W. E. R., Thompson, H. H., Domschke, W., Wünsch, E., Demling, L., and Ritchie, H. D., (1976): Motilin-induced electrical activity in the canine gastrointestinal tract. *Scand. J. Gastroenterol. (Suppl. 39),* 11:11–118.

131. Wingate, D. L., Thompson, H. H., Pearce, E. A., and Dand, A. (1977): Quantitative analysis of the effects of oral feeding on canine intestinal myoelectric activity. *Gastroenterology,* 72:1151.

132. Wingate, D. L., Thompson, H. H., Pearce, E. A., and Dand, A. (1978): The effects of exogenous cholecystokinin and pentagastrin on myoelectrical activity in the conscious fasted dog. In: *Gastrointestinal Motility in Health and Disease,* edited by H. L. Duthie, pp. 47–60. MTP Press, Lancaster.
133. Yau, W. M., Makhlouf, G. M., Edwards, L. E., and Farrar, J. T. (1973): Mode of action of cholecystokinin and related peptides on gallbladder muscle. *Gastroenterology,* 65:451–456.

Gastrointestinal Hormones, edited by
George B. Jerzy Glass.
Raven Press, New York © 1980.

Chapter 26

Effects of Gut Hormones on Gastrointestinal Sphincters

*Robert S. Fisher and **Sidney Cohen

*Temple University Medical School; and **University of Pennsylvania School of Medicine,
Philadelphia, Pennsylvania 19140*

INTRODUCTION

The role of the gastrointestinal peptide hormones in the physiological control of gastrointestinal sphincters remains unclear. Few subjects in gastroenterology have been of more interest; therefore, much pertinent literature has been generated. This chapter represents an attempt to clarify some of the major issues, and, when possible, emphasizes those studies performed in human subjects. Gastrointestinal hormones may be involved in the regulation of sphincter function by: (a) maintaining resting sphincter pressure; (b) mediating adaptive changes in response to meals and other stimuli; (c) performing a fine-tuning function producing only small changes in sphincter pressure; or (d) playing a permissive role augmenting or potentiating effects mediated by other, nonhormonal pathways.

If the peptide hormones released normally during the digestive process are important in the control of normal sphincter function, then it is possible that some of the symptoms associated with gastrointestinal disorders may be associated with pathophysiological mechanisms of hormone action. There is some evidence to suggest abnormalities of hormone-sphincter interaction in several disorders of the gastrointestinal tract. Each gastrointestinal sphincter is considered individually.

GASTROINTESTINAL HORMONES

The gastrointestinal hormones are a group of polypeptides released from different sites within the gastrointestinal tract following ingestion of a normal meal. They include secretin, gastrin, cholecystokinin (pancreozymin) (CCK), glucagon, vasoactive intestinal polypeptide (VIP), gastric inhibitory polypeptide (GIP), motilin, enterogastrone, villikinin, bulbogastrone, and substance P. All of these polypeptides have not been evaluated for their possible effects on gastrointestinal sphincter function (see Table 1).

There is a structural similarity between some of these hormones, allowing their general subdivision into two major categories: (a) the gastrin-CCK subgroup identified by an identical carboxy-terminal tetrapeptide; and (b) a secretin-glucagon subgroup, characterized by many identical amino acids in sequence. Both VIP and GIP belong to the second group. In general, each sphincter has been demonstrated to respond to all hormones that have been tested. Also, hormone interactions such as addition, potentiation, or antagonism can be shown when combinations are tested. The fact that a hormonal action can be demonstrated does not guarantee its physiological importance. The gastrointestinal hormones are known to have a wide range of biological effects on intestinal

TABLE 1. *Hormonal effects on gastrointestinal sphincters*

Hormone	LES	Pylorus	SO	ICS
Gastrin	↑ (↑)	↓	NT (↓)	↓ (↑)
Secretin	↓ (↓)	↑	↑ (↓)	NT
Cholecystokinin	↓ (↓)	↑ (↑)	↓ (±)	NT
Glucagon	↓ (↓)	↑	NT	NT
Motilin	↑ (↑)	NT	NT	NT

LES, lower esophageal sphincter; SO, sphincter of Oddi; ICS, ileocecal sphincter; NT, not tested; ± responses in both directions depending on species tested; ( ), results of tests in nonhuman species.

absorption, secretion, trophic actions on gastrointestinal organs, insulin release, glycogenolysis, lipolysis, control of appetite, and motor function of the luminal gastrointestinal tract and its sphincters. This latter effect is discussed in depth.

LOWER ESOPHAGEAL SPHINCTER

In 1956, Fyke et al. demonstrated an intraluminal high pressure zone, the lower esophageal sphincter (LES), in the distal aspect of the esophagus (63). In its resting state the LES pressure is 12 to 30 mm Hg above the intraabdominal pressure level. Resting LES pressure is an intrinsic characteristic of the sphincter muscle itself (24–26,108) and is not affected by sphincter location above or below the diaphragm (29,107). Prevention of reflux of gastric contents from a positive pressure cavity, the abdomen (stomach), into a negative pressure cavity, the thorax (esophagus), is the major function of the LES (59). Additionally, it must relax or open appropriately to allow aboral passage of food into the stomach.

Gastrin

Gastrin is a 17-amino acid polypeptide that is released predominantly from the G cells of the gastric antrum and proximal duodenum in man during normal digestion. In the blood it circulates in several forms that may have differing biological activities.

The first evidence suggesting hormonal effects on the LES was provided by Castell and Harris, who demonstrated that inhibition of endogenous gastrin release by exogenous gastric acidification was associated with a marked reduction of LES pressure (20). This observation suggested that resting LES pressure was acid-suppressible and might be dependent on endogenous gastrin. Several groups have demonstrated that changes in intragastric pH are associated with alterations in LES pressure. LES pressure increased during gastric deacidification (6,21,78,110,117) and decreased during gastric acidification (20,21,78) (Fig. 1). Because of the association between gastrin release and intragastric pH (52), it was suggested that the LES pressure changes that occurred in response to altered pH might be mediated by serum concentrations of gastrin. However, when newer techniques of measuring serum concentrations of gastrin were employed, the temporal relationship between intragastric pH and LES pressure was not established (78). LES pressure increases also during the normal course of a protein meal (126). The increment in LES pressure occurs at a time when an increased serum concentration of gastrin has been measured (123,136,151). However, in some studies the correlation between post-meal serum gastrin and LES pressure has been poor (37,43,116,147).

Several investigators demonstrated a LES pressure response to intravenous bolus doses of gastrin and/or pentagastrin (65,108). However, the picture became confused in 1975 when Walker et al. reported that pentagastrin increased LES

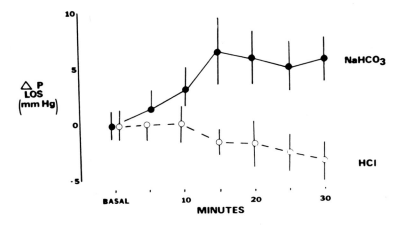

FIG. 1. Mean changes in pressure (ΔP) of lower esophageal sphincter (LES) from the basal level after either gastric alkalinization with sodium bicarbonate (NaHCO₃) or acidification with hydrochloric acid (HCl). *Vertical lines* indicate ± 1 SEM. (From ref. 78, with permission.)

pressure only when infused in pharmacological doses (164). Of interest, Freeland et al. later demonstrated significant increases in LES pressure during infusions of gastrin heptadecapeptide that produced gastrin levels similar to those reported after a meal and at lower doses than those that produced peak gastric acid output (62). Many studies have attempted unsuccessfully to correlate resting LES pressure with resting serum concentrations of gastrin in normal subjects and patients with various disorders (44,49,147,170).

In general, studies performed in other species have confirmed the observations reviewed above. In the opossum it has been demonstrated that passive transfer of graded amounts of rabbit antigastrin antiserum produced a graded diminution of resting LES pressure (Fig. 2) and inhibited the effect of exogenous gastrin on the LES circular muscle (112). A second group employing similar techniques and the same species has not been able to confirm these observations (68). The responses to gastrin of circular smooth muscle strips from the esophagus, LES, fundus, and antrum of the opossum have been studied *in vitro* (Fig. 3) (108). These studies demonstrated the following: (a) LES circular muscle had specific dose-response characteristics to gastrin compared with esophageal, fundic, and antral circular muscle; (b) the threshold concentration of gastrin for LES muscle was 10^{-3} that of circular muscles from adjacent regions; (c) the maximum tension achieved by LES muscle in response to gastrin was twice that of adjacent muscle and was reached at lower concentrations of gastrin; (d) gastrin produced a peak response on LES muscle at a molar concentration 10^7 times less than other pharmacological agents; and (e) the LES muscle response to gastrin was blocked by atropine. Cohen at al. originally postulated that gastrin acted on LES smooth muscle via the local release of acetylcholine

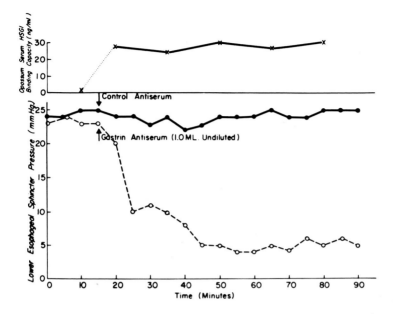

FIG. 2. The effect of 1.0 ml of control serum and 1.0 ml of gastrin antiserum on the resting lower esophageal sphincter pressure of a single animal. Binding capacity of opossum serum from HSGI-1 after the intravenous injection of gastrin antiserum, shown at the **top,** remained unchanged while LES pressure was reduced. (From ref. 112, with permission.)

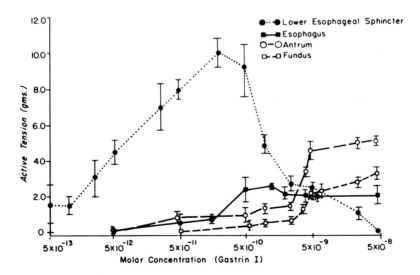

FIG. 3. Dose-response curves for increasing molar concentration of synthetic human gastrin 1, and active tension (g) produced by each muscle. Each point represents the mean $\pm$ 1 SEM of 20 experiments. Sphincter muscle has a lower threshold dose (5×10^{-13}M) and attains a greater increase in active tension. (From ref. 108, with permission.)

(113), but several subsequent studies suggested that gastrin may act directly on the smooth muscle independent of cholinergic pathways (89,172).

Abnormalities in the relationship between serum concentrations of gastrin and LES pressure have been suggested in several gastrointestinal disorders. Although Isenberg et al. reported that there was a correlation between elevated gastrin levels and resting LES pressures in patients with gastrinoma (81), neither they nor other groups have been able to confirm this observation (118,147, 149,171). In patients with pernicious anemia, where serum concentrations of gastrin are also elevated significantly, resting LES pressures were normal or low (51). In these patients the LES pressure responses to both pentagastrin and edrophonium, an inhibitor of acetylcholinesterase, were diminished, suggesting decreased endorgan muscle responsiveness. In patients with achalasia, LES function is characterized by an elevated resting pressure and incomplete post-deglutition relaxation. An exaggerated pressure response of the LES to gastrin has been demonstrated (Fig. 4) (32). The threshold dose of gastrin was lower and the maximal LES pressure response occurred at a lower serum concentration of gastrin. These findings are consistent with denervation supersensitivity of the LES. However, since denervation supersensitivity may be generalized and nonspecific, these findings do not establish that gastrin is an important mediator of resting or adaptive LES pressures under normal conditions.

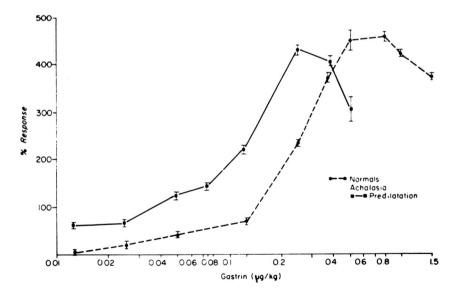

FIG. 4. Dose-response curves of change in LES pressure, expressed as a percentage of initial resting sphincter pressure, against log dose of gastrin 1 in mg/kg. At each point is the mean ± SEM. Data are compiled from responses obtained in 13 normals and 11 patients with untreated achalasia. The LES in patients with achalasia is more sensitive to gastrin 1, but not capable of a greater percentage response. (From ref. 32, with permission.)

Following distal gastric resection, symptomatic gastroesophageal reflux, endoscopic and histological esophagitis, and even stricture formation have been reported (9,33,76,119,169). Since gastrin is produced in and released from the antrum, it has been postulated that abnormal sphincter function may be due to decreased release of gastrin. Interestingly, neither decreased serum concentrations of gastrin nor diminished resting LES pressures have been demonstrated convincingly in these patients (12,99,118,123,147). In patients with LES incompetence with or without hiatal hernia, LES dysfunction appears to be the major cause of reflux (29). Basal sphincter pressure and adaptive pressure responses are decreased. Both decreased basal serum gastrin concentrations (110, 111) and decreased integrated gastrin release (50) have been demonstrated. Furthermore, LES stimulation by synthetic pentagastrin or cholinergic agents has produced subnormal LES pressure responses in patients with LES incompetence (110).

Secretin

Secretin is a 27-amino acid polypeptide that is released from the proximal portion of the duodenum in response to acidification. Although the major function of secretin is thought to be stimulation of pancreatic volume and bicarbonate secretion, its effect on the LES was studied because of its known action at other target organs where gastrin has been shown to act.

When secretin was administered intravenously or released from the duodenal mucosa in human subjects, no change in resting LES pressure was observed (31). In contrast, secretin inhibited significantly the LES pressure response to an intravenous bolus injection of gastrin and shifted the gastrin dose-response curve to higher doses (Fig. 5). When secretin was added to a muscle bath solution *in vitro*, it did not alter muscle responses to other pharmacological agents, but inhibited the muscle response to gastrin (109).

These observations can be summarized as follows: (a) No significant independent effect of secretin on LES pressure has been observed *in vivo*; (b) secretin antagonizes gastrin both *in vitro* and *in vivo*; (c) the antagonism of secretion for gastrin is highly selective; and (d) the interaction between secretin and gastrin at the LES is of the competitive type in its characteristics.

Cholecystokinin

Cholecystokinin (CCK), a 33-amino acid polypeptide, has a C-terminal amino acid sequence identical to gastrin. CCK is released from the proximal part of the small intestine in response to fats, amino acids, and acidification. The primary actions of CCK are gallbladder contraction (cholecystokinetic) and pancreatic enzyme release (pancreozymic).

Both the octapeptide and the whole molecule of CCK have been shown to decrease LES pressure *in vivo* (57,126,127,139,154). When graded doses of CCK

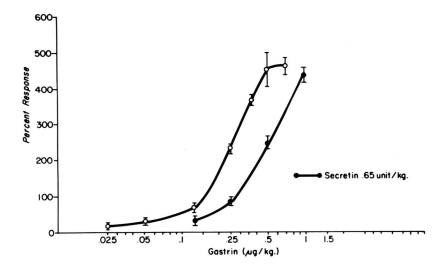

FIG. 5. Dose response curves of lower esophageal sphincter pressure expressed as a percentage of initial resting sphincter pressure against log-dose of gastrin 1 in μg/kg. The curves are those of gastrin 1 give alone to 13 patients and gastrin 1 given against a constant intravenous infusion of secretin at 0.65 U/kg/hr to seven patients. Although the dose-response curve performed during secretin infusion is shifted to higher doses of gastrin, maximal sphincter response is still attained. (From ref. 31, with permission.)

were administered intravenously in either the opossum or man, LES inhibitory dose-response curves were constructed (Fig. 6) (57). CCK decreased LES pressure maximally by 78% in the opossum and 73% in man. Ingestion of fat caused a prompt and sustained decrease of LES pressure (127). Although the mechanism of fat-induced inhibition of LES pressure has not been elucidated clearly, it may be due entirely or in part to the release of CCK from the duodenal mucosa. Studies on CCK effects have been limited because a reliable radioimmunoassay (RIA) for CCK has not been available.

Our knowledge of the effects of CCK on LES muscle, both *in vitro* and *in vivo,* can be summarized as follows: (a) CCK antagonizes the effect of gastrin on LES muscle; (b) it decreases resting LES pressure when administered intravenously, but contracts LES muscle strips *in vitro;* (c) CCK may act on LES muscle by acetylcholine release; and (d) the interaction between CCK and gastrin at the LES is competitive in its characteristics.

Glucagon

There is a strong molecular similarity between glucagon and secretin; 14 amino acids in sequence are identical. Glucagon is released by the pancreatic islet cells and the small intestinal mucosa. Enteroglucagon of small intestinal mucosal origin is released by ingestion of triglycerides or long-chain fatty acids.

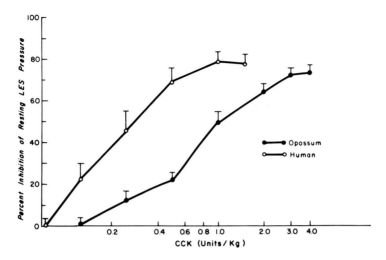

FIG. 6. Log dose-response curves of percentage inhibition of lower esophageal sphincter pressure against dose of intravenous CCK in both opossum and man. For opossums each point represents mean ± SEM for 10 separate experiments. In man each point represents mean ± SEM for 5 separate experiments. (From ref. 57, with permission.)

Exogenous glucagon, administered in large pharmacological doses, has been shown to decrease not only pentagastrin-stimulated LES pressures, but also resting LES pressure (27,85,88). Studies performed on isolated LES muscle strips from dogs were consistent with these findings. Endogenous release of glucagon induced by arginine (28), but not by alanine, infusion (85) has been associated with decreased LES pressure responses to pentagastrin. Hogan et al. reported that resting and pentagastrin-stimulated LES pressures were decreased only at serum concentrations of glucagon above 1,400 pg/ml (79). Recently, a patient with endogenous hyperglucagonemia due to a pancreatic glucagonoma was reported (155). Before surgery, when the fasting serum concentration of endogenous glucagon was 1,200 pg/ml, LES function was normal. However, when pharmacological levels of glucagon were achieved during intravenous infusions of glucagon, LES function was disrupted (Fig. 7).

These observations suggest that endogenous glucagon does not play a role in the regulation of LES function.

Motilin

The observations that acidification of the duodenum inhibited and alkalinization of the duodenum stimulated motility in the transplanted gastric pouch eventually led to the discovery of motilin, a 22-amino acid polypeptide (15). Intravenous infusions of synthetic motilin, 13-norleucine motilin, in dog and man caused dose-dependent increases in LES pressure (45,87,115,120).

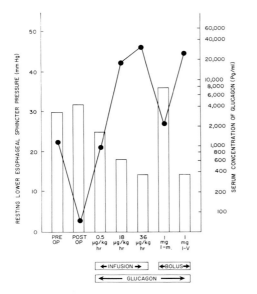

FIG. 7. Resting lower esophageal sphincter pressure (mm Hg) and serum concentration of glucagon (pg/ml) in a patient with a glucagonoma before and after the tumor was removed surgically. Each *bar* represents resting LES pressure determined in a separate study performed pre- and postoperatively and postoperatively during glucagon infusion or after bolus injection. (From ref. 155, with permission.)

Domschke et al. reported that both LES pressure and plasma motilin increased in parallel during duodenal acidification (120), whereas other authors have been unable to document such a correlation (75). In dogs, motilin infusions have reproduced the interdigestive motor activity of the LES (83).

Despite these observations, a physiological role for motilin in the regulation of LES pressure has not been demonstrated convincingly (48).

PYLORUS

The junction of the stomach and duodenum is marked by a confluence of the gastric muscle layers into a prominent muscular ring. Because of the special structure of the thickened circular muscle layer, many early investigators assumed that it was a true sphincter. Thus, it was designated as the pylorus, a term derived from the Greek word meaning gatekeeper. Early studies employing fluoroscopic visualization following ingestion of barium seemed to confirm the sphincteric function of the pylorus (18,93,94). Not only was aboral flow of barium halted abruptly when the pyloric ring closed, but, in addition, retrograde flow of barium from the duodenum into the stomach was seldom observed. When intraluminal pressures were measured at the gastroduodenal junction of man and animals, conflicting results were reported. Most early observers, using various manometric techniques such as the inductograph, balloon sensors, and nonperfused, open-tipped catheters, were unable to demonstrate a consistent zone of high pressure at the gastroduodenal junction (3,5,114,167,168).

In recent years several groups recorded a pyloric high pressure zone in dogs

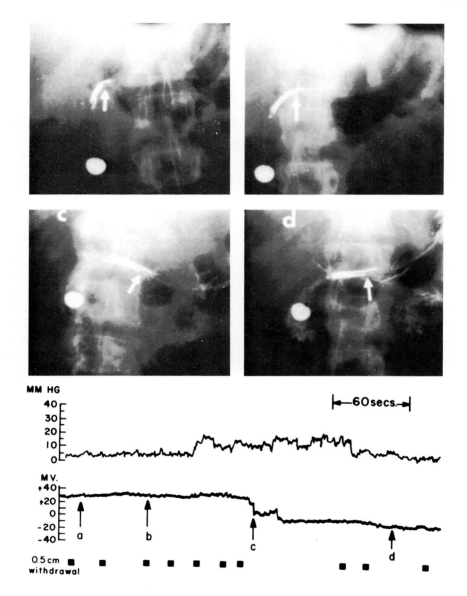

FIG. 8. Simultaneous radiographic, manometric, and potential difference (PD) recordings in a single subject as the tube assembly was withdrawn from duodenum to stomach. X-rays are lettered to correspond to points a,b,c, and d on the recording **(top).** The *arrows* on X-rays mark the position of the mercury-marked middle pressure orifice and the PD electrode. At a and b, the detector is in the duodenum where PD is positive. At c, the PD changes and the pressure tracing shows a zone of elevated pressure (basal pyloric pressure); the X-ray indicates that the recording catheter is within the pyloric channel just proximal to the air-filled duodenal cap. At d, the assembly has been pulled through the pylorus into the stomach with no further change in PD. (From ref. 55, with permission.)

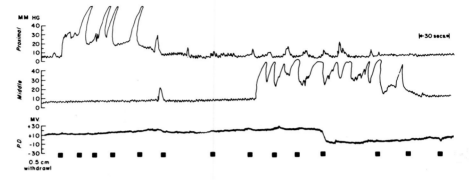

FIG. 9. Pyloric pressure and potential difference (PD) recordings in a single subject during duodenal acidification. Pyloric pressure rose from a resting level of approximately 5 mm Hg, as previously determined, to approximately 25 mm Hg. Duodenal acidification was begun 5 min prior to pull-through and continued throughout the recording. (From ref. 55, with permission.)

using open-tipped catheters with side orifices and/or balloons (14,80). In 1973 Fisher and Cohen were the first to demonstrate a pyloric sphincter high-pressure zone in man (55). They employed infused, open-tipped catheters with side orifices to measure intraluminal pressures. They also measured skin-to-mucosa electrical potential differences during their studies to identify accurately the gastroduodenal junction. They found a resting high-pressure zone at the gastroduodenal junction that measured approximately 2 to 5 mm Hg above the intraduodenal pressure (Fig. 8) and ranged between 5 and 20 mm in length. Whereas resting pyloric pressure was barely detectable, pyloric pressure increased markedly when stimulated by intraduodenal instillation of various agents (Fig. 9). Although Valenzuela et al. confirmed many of these findings in man (160,161), Kaye et al. were unable to detect a pyloric sphincter high-pressure zone (91). The explanation for this discrepancy is not obvious.

Hormonal Responses

Pyloric sphincter pressures have been shown to increase in response to intraduodenal instillation of hydrochloric acid and olive oil in man (55) and dogs (14,80). In addition, duodenal infusion of both hypertonic amino acids and hypertonic glucose increased pyloric pressures in man (Fig. 10) (55). It was postulated that these agents stimulated the release of CCK and/or secretin from the duodenal mucosa, and that pyloric pressures might be increased due to the effects of these hormones. Isenberg et al. had reported previously that the octapeptide of CCK, administered intravenously, increased pyloric sphincter pressure in dogs (80).

Fisher et al. tested the effects of the gastrointestinal hormones—CCK, secretin, and gastrin—on pyloric pressures in man and on strips of pyloric circular muscle obtained from the opossum (58). Both CCK and secretin were found to be

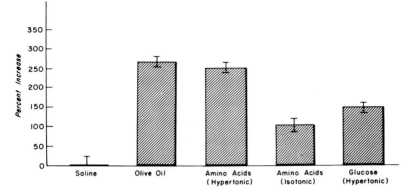

FIG. 10. Pyloric responses to duodenal instillation of various compounds. Data are expressed as percentages of increase in pyloric pressure above basal level. Each bar represents the mean ± SEM. The response to NaCl is not significant. Other responses are significant ($p <$ 0.01). (From ref. 55, with permission.)

agonists, contracting pyloric sphincter muscle (Fig. 11), and gastrin, although it had no effect on resting pyloric pressure, was found to be an antagonist, inhibiting the pyloric sphincter response to intraduodenal hydrochloric acid (Fig. 12). Both endogenously released gastrin and exogenously administered gastrin had similar inhibitory effects (54). Recently, Fisher et al. reported that

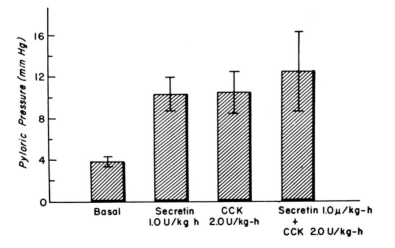

FIG. 11. Human pyloric response to the intravenous administration of secretin and CCK, alone and in combination. Data are expressed in mm Hg above intraabdominal pressure. Each *bar* represents the mean ± SEM of 10 experiments. The human pyloric responses to secretin, CCK, and the combination were significant ($p <$ 0.01). The response to the hormone combination was no greater than the individual hormone maximal responses. (From ref. 58, with permission.)

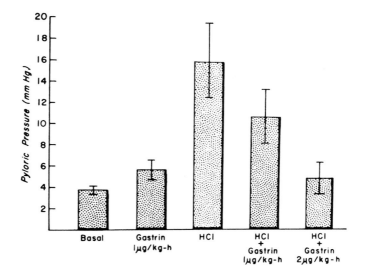

FIG. 12. Human pyloric response to duodenal acidification alone and during intravenous administration of graded doses of gastrin 1. Data are expressed as mm Hg above intraabdominal pressure. Each *bar* represents the mean ± SEM of 10 experiments. Gastrin 1, administered alone, did not significantly alter pyloric pressure ($p < 0.05$). Duodenal acidification by itself significantly increased pyloric pressure to 16.1 ± 3.6 mm Hg ($p < .001$). During gastrin 1 administration at 1 and 2 μg/kg/hr, there was a graded decrease in the response to duodenal acidification. (From ref. 58, with permission.)

pyloric function was not affected by either cholinergic blockade with atropine or direct cholinergic stimulation with bethanechol (135). In addition, cholinergic blockade with atropine did not effect the pyloric pressure responses to exogenous CCK and secretin. Valenzuela had reported previously that atropine decreased the pyloric response to duodenal acidification (160). More recent studies in man have shown that glucagon infusions increase pyloric pressures (134). Interestingly, the serum concentrations of both secretin and glucagon necessary to stimulate the pylorus far exceed those recorded after duodenal acidification or insulin-induced hypoglycemia, respectively (134).

Few other observations in man on pyloric responsiveness to hormones are available for review. Anuras et al. performed studies on opossum pyloric circular muscle and confirmed that CCK was an agonist, but found no effect for secretin (4). Bertaccini et al., studying pyloric function indirectly in the rat by measuring gastric emptying, found that cerulein, an analog of CCK, had a spasmogenic effect (8). Finally, Strunz et al. investigated the effects of 13-nle-motilin and atropine on rabbit pyloric muscle (153). Both 13-nle-motilin and acetylcholine stimulated contraction of isolated pyloric muscle. In addition, 13-nle-motilin caused potentiation of the acetylcholine response.

Reflux of duodenal contents, especially bile, may be an important etiological factor in several gastrointestinal disorders. Contact with bile salts is injurious

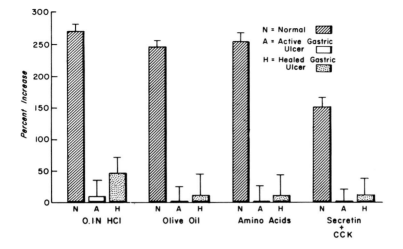

FIG. 13. Pyloric response to intraduodenal stimuli and exogenous hormonal administration in 10 normal subjects and 10 patients with gastric ulcer both before and after healing. Pyloric response is expressed as the percentage increase above the basal pressure. In normal subjects, intraduodenal HCl, olive oil, and amino acids each elevated pyloric pressure significantly; likewise, intravenous secretin and CCK increased pyloric pressure. In patients with gastric ulcer both endogenous and exogenous hormonal stimulation failed to produce a significant rise in pyloric pressure either before or after healing of the ulcer. (From ref. 56, with permission.)

to both gastric and esophageal mucosal surfaces, producing alterations of the mucosal barrier to Na$^+$ and H$^+$ ions as well as histological changes (10,22,38,84). Excessive reflux of bile salts caused by pyloric dysfunction has been suggested as an etiologic factor in the following disorders: gastritis (16,23,41,122), gastric ulcer (11,47,140), alkaline gastritis (7,39,46,162), reflux esophagitis (66,92, 100,152), and gallstone dyspepsia (17,90). Direct studies of pyloric sphincter function have been reported only in patients with gastric ulcer (56,159). Here, the pyloric pressure responses to intraduodenal stimuli and exogenous hormonal administration were suppressed not only while the ulcers were active, but even after the ulcers had healed. (Fig. 13). One group suggested that normal pyloric responsiveness could be restored by acidifying the stomach (53). They postulated that elevated serum concentration of gastrin may inhibit pyloric sphincter function in patients with gastric ulcer.

SPHINCTER OF ODDI

Although some investigators feel that the sphincter of Oddi (SO) may represent an extension of the surrounding duodenal muscle layers (60,61), the majority opinion supports the existence of an anatomical sphincter muscle that functions independently from the contiguous musculature (13,72,77,128). Delmont has suggested that the SO can be divided into five parts (42): (a) the sphincter choledochus proprius; (b) the sphincter pancreaticus proprius, (c) the common papillary sphincter, (d) the infundibulum of the common bile duct, and (e) the pancreatic infundibulum. Of these the common papillary sphincter seems to be the major factor in the control of bile flow into the duodenum.

The major problems in interpreting the available literature are the variations in anatomy and physiology from species to species and the variability in the investigational techniques employed. Toouli and Watts studied the contractile responses of strips of circular muscle from the SO to different stimuli (156,157). Crema et al. also used an *in vitro* preparation in which they isolated the entire lower portion of the common bile duct, leaving the choledochoduodenal junction intact (34,35). Specialized cineradiographic methods have been devised to investigate the region of the SO (158). The majority of manometric studies reported have been indirect, measuring intraluminal pressure within the common bile duct and/or monitoring the bile flow rate across the SO into the duodenum (40,74,133,137,165). Some investigators have measured myoelectrical activity in the region of the SO (82,143,146). The difficulty in interpreting these indirect studies is that they may reflect hepatic secretory pressure, pancreatic secretory pressure, gallbladder contraction, and intraduodenal pressure in addition to SO pressure.

An index of intraluminal pressure at the SO can be obtained directly in man and animals by cannulating the ampulla of Vater with some pressure-recording device (36,73,104,106). A zone of increased pressure has been recorded at the choledochoduodenal junction in most species including cow, pig, cat, dog, opossum, rabbit, and man. The most recent reports in man have determined SO pressures during endoscopic retrograde cannulation of the biliary tract (124,141,163). Unlike the lower esophageal and pyloric sphincters, normal values for resting SO pressure and length have not been established. Normally, the SO has three major functions. First, SO pressure is a determinant of the flow rate of bile and/or pancreatic juice into the duodenum. Second, closure of the SO elevates bile duct pressure above cholecystic pressure, thereby indirectly regulating gallbladder filling. Third, SO pressure may be an important component of the antireflux mechanism at the choledochoduodenal junction.

Hormonal Responses

In 1935, 7 years after CCK was described, it was shown that intestinal extracts containing a cholecystokinetic factor produced relaxation of the SO in the dog (144). Others have confirmed this finding in cat (74,101–103,133), dog (106, 121,144), and man (82,106,124,144). A few investigators have observed increased SO pressures after CCK (106,142,157,166). In the rabbit, CCK elevated SO pressure and decreased biliary flow (145). CCK seems to act directly on the smooth muscle of the SO in that its effect is not blocked by atropine, reserpine, propranolol, phenoxybenzamine, or pentolinium tartrate (74,105). Various family members CCK, including gastrin, pentagastrin, of octapeptide of CCK and cerulein relax the SO (1,105,106). Some authors have reported that gastrin contracts the SO (138), but Lin observed that pressure was decreased at physiological doses and increased at pharmacological doses of gastrin (105).

In the dog, the SO was relaxed by secretin (105,138). Furthermore, the relaxing effect of CCK was potentiated by secretin (106), similarly to the synergism observed in their effect on gallbladder contraction (150) and pancreatic enzyme secretion (70). Nebel et al. reported that secretin increased SO pressure in man during endoscopic cannulation of the ampulla of Vater (125). Next to CCK, the effect of secretin on the SO is the most potent on a molar basis when compared with other peptide hormones (105). Glucagon, like secretin, seems to relax the SO in dogs, but only at doses that are clearly pharmacological (105,106). The effects of the "candidate gastrointestinal hormones" have not been studied.

Disorders in which gallbladder and SO function are disturbed or in which the coordination between gallbladder contraction and SO relaxation may be disrupted may be of clinical importance. Included here would be cholelithiasis, biliary dyskinesia, functional dyspepsia, and papillary stenosis. The role of the gastrointestinal hormones in the pathogenesis of these disorders has not been investigated.

ILEOCECAL SPHINCTER

Because of its relative inaccessibility in man, the ileocecal sphincter has not received continued interest and, consequently, its role in the regulation of colonic function is poorly understood. Whether it functions to regulate aboral flow of ileal contents into the colon or to prevent retrograde movement of cecal contents into the ileum or both has not been determined clearly.

Studies in man that have demonstrated the ileocecal sphincter as an important physiological structure can be summarized as follows. First, the ileocecal junction is characterized by a zone of tonically elevated pressure (19,30). Second, the intraluminal pressure is decreased by proximal and increased by distal distention (19,30). Third, quantitative bacterial counts differ markedly across the ileocecal junction (67). Fourth, removal of the ileocecal junction results in altered bowel function with increased stool frequency and volume (64,98,148).

Studies performed in various animal species have confirmed the above findings (86,95–97). In both cats and dogs the ileocecal junction maintains a tonically elevated high pressure zone. Although the canine ileocecal sphincter is not anatomically distinct, a zone of high pressure, which responds to both proximal and distal distention, can be detected using either nonperfused open-tipped catheter or balloon manometry (95,97). In the cat the ileocecal sphincter is very short and difficult to identify. Therefore, indirect pressure-flow techniques have been employed to provide evidence of an area of resistance that responds both to pharmacological agents and polypeptide hormones (129–132). In most cases, the ileocecal junction pressure response was in the opposite direction of adjacent ileal or colonic muscle. Electrical stimulation of sphincteric nerves increased the junctional resistance to flow, an effect blocked by α- but not by β-adrenegic antagonists (129,130,132). Resistance to transsphincteric flow was increased also by vagal stimulation, a response blocked by atropine sulfate and/or guanethidine (131). Inhibitory responses to electrical stimulation have been reported (86).

A consensus of the existing literature concerning the ileocecal sphincter is difficult to present. It is clear that the ileocecal junction is characterized by a sphincteric high-pressure zone in at least four species (man, monkey, cat and dog). In addition, the magnitude of the intraluminal pressure is affected by neural and hormonal stimulation as well as by intestinal distention.

Hormonal Responses

There have been few studies on hormonal effects on the ileocecal junction pressure (19,95). A single report in man indicated that gastrin decreased ileocecal sphincteric pressure (79). In contrast, studies in dogs demonstrated a slight increase in pressure after feeding (95). Since these observations were made before reliable hormone RIAs were available, they should be repeated.

Clinical importance has been attributed to the ileocecal junction based on postoperative observations. Following operative removal of the ileocecal junction along with the ascending colon, frequent loose bowel movements of increased volume (64,96,98), vitamin B_{12} malabsorption (64), and bacterial colonization of the ileum (67) have been observed. Removal of a comparable segment of left colon failed to produce these effects (98). Finally, removal of the ileocecal junction may accelerate small bowel transit in both man and animals (98).

ARE SPHINCTERIC RESPONSES TO HORMONES "PHYSIOLOGICAL"?

As has been discussed, the resting pressures and adaptive pressure responses of the gastrointestinal sphincters are affected profoundly by the administration of exogenous gastrointestinal hormones. However, the question has been asked, and validly so, as to whether these hormonal effects are of physiological importance. The following criteria for a "physiological" hormonal response have been proposed (69,71,81). First, is the hormonal response in question observed after the release of endogenous hormone during the course of a meal? Second, is the response produced at a dose that is submaximal for the primary known biological action of the hormone? Third, does administration of the hormone, by a continuous intravenous infusion, at a dose that raises the serum concentration to a physiological level, reproduce the event in question? One should ask also whether specific removal of the hormone from the circulation significantly affects sphincter function. Before considering the difficulties encountered in applying these criteria, let us remember that the criteria themselves are somewhat arbitrary and have not been subjected to scientific inquiry.

The techniques that measure gastrointestinal hormones should be sensitive, specific, and quantitative. RIAs have been developed that provide quantitative information about specific hormones. Unfortunately, even the best of these, the RIA for gastrin, has its limitations. Multiple forms of gastrin, including big big gastrin, big gastrin (G-34), hepatadecapeptide gastrin (G-17), and smaller fragments may be present simultaneously within the circulation. The biological actions of each form of circulating gastrin have not been elucidated totally. It is likely that considerable variability may exist. Also, the antisera employed in different RIAs have not been standardized. Some antisera are polyvalent, detecting multiple forms of gastrin; others are univalent, detecting only one form of gastrin. Perhaps in response to some stimuli, one form of gastrin increases while another decreases, resulting in no change in the total serum concentration of gastrin. Until the biological actions of each form of circulating hormone are known, and univalent antisera are available to detect each of these, it will be difficult to correlate confidently serum hormonal concentration and bioactivity. One must also ask whether the actions of synthetic or purified hormones are the same as those of endogenous hormones.

Should the relationship between sphincter pressure and serum concentration of a specific hormone be the same from one individual to another? There might be significant variability in individual dose responsiveness. Likewise, the temporal relationship between hormone release and a change in sphincter pressure must be examined cautiously. It might take time for the concentration of a hormone to reach the threshold necessary for a biological action, or the active substance may be a metabolic product of the parent hormone. Does the serum concentration of a hormone in the peripheral blood actually reflect the concentration at the receptor sites? Some pharmacological agents such as epinephrine are concentrated at their receptors. This would be unusual for a polypeptide, however.

Total elimination of a hormone from the circulation has not been feasible. Most hormones have multiple sites of origin that cannot be removed surgically without distorting the experiment. Another approach would be to develop a specific antiserum to the hormone, which would eliminate the hormone from the circulation. However, how can it be determined that immuno- and bioactivity are identical? In addition, an antiserum that might block one action of a given hormone might have no effect on another of its actions.

In summary, it is difficult to draw conclusions about the "physiological" effects of hormones on gastrointestinal sphincters. More specific RIAs must be made available, and a complete understanding of the actions of each hormone and its various forms must be achieved. We can expect our interpretation of what is physiological to change as our knowledge evolves. Let us remember the histamine-acid secretion story lest we discard prematurely important information about hormone-gastrointestinal sphincter interactions.

SUMMARY AND PROJECTIONS FOR THE FUTURE

The effect of gut hormones on the lower esophageal and pyloric sphincters have been investigated at some length. In contrast, the sphincter of Oddi and especially the ileocecal sphincter have received less attention. The physiological relevance of these hormonal effects has not been established unequivocally for any of the sphincters. As new polypeptide candidate hormones are demonstrated within the gastrointestinal mucosa, their effects must be established. In the future the techniques of molecular biology must be applied to these studies. We must begin to consider not only the distant effects of hormones but also their paracrine and neurocrine effects.

REFERENCES

1. Agosti, A., Mantovani, P., and Mori, L. (1971): Actions of caerulein and related substances on the sphincter of Oddi. *Arch. Pharmacol.,* 208:114–118.
2. Andersson, K. E., Andersson, R., Hedner, P., and Persson, C. G. (1972): Effects of cholecystokinin on the level of cyclic AMP and on mechanical activity in the isolated sphincter of Oddi. *Life Sci.,* 11:723–732.
3. Andersson, S., and Grossman, M. I., (1956): Profile of pH, pressure and potential difference at gastroduodenal junction in man. *Gastroenterology,* 49:364–369.
4. Anuras, S., Cooke, A. R., and Christensen, J. (1974): An inhibitory innervation of the gastroduodenal junction. *J. Clin. Invest.,* 54:529–538.
5. Atkinson, M., Edwards, D. A. W., Honour, A. J., and Rowlands, E. (1957): Comparison of cardiac and pyloric sphincters. *Lancet,* ii:918–924.
6. Bailes, R., Picker, S., and Bremmer, C. G. (1972): The effect of intragastric aluminum hydroxide on lower esophageal sphincter pressures. *S. Afr. Med. J.,* 46:1387–1389.
7. Berardi, R. S., Siroosponi, D., Ruiz, R., Carnes, W., Devaiah, K., Peterson, C., Becknell, W., and Olivencia, J. (1976): Alkaline reflux gastritis. *Am. J. Surg.,* 132:552–559.
8. Bertaccini, G., Impicciatore, M., and DeCaro, G. (1973): Action of caerulein and related substances on the pyloric sphincter of the anaesthesized rat. *Eur. J. Pharmacol.,* 22:320–334.
9. Bingham, J. (1958): Oesophageal strictures after gastric surgery and nasogastric intubation. *Br. Med. J.,* 2:817–819.
10. Black, R. B., Hole, D., and Rhodes, J. (1971): Bile damage to the gastric mucosal barrier; the influence of pH and bile acid concentration. *Gastroenterology,* 61:178–183.
11. Black, R. B., Robert, G., and Rhodes, J. (1971): The effect of healing on bile reflux in gastric ulcer. *Gut,* 12:552–557.
12. Booth, A. D., Rieder, D. D., and Thompson, J. C. (1975): Effect of antrectomy and subsequent vagotomy on the serum gastrin response to food in dogs. *Ann. Surg.,* 181:191–195.
13. Boyden, E. A. (1957): The anatomy of the choledochoduodenal junction in man. *Surg. Gynecol. Obstet.,* 104:641–652.
14. Brink, B. M., Schlegel, J. F., and Code, C. F. (1965): The pressure profile of the gastroduodenal junctional zone in dogs. *Gut,* 6:163–171.
15. Brown, J. C., Cooke, M. A., and Dryburgh, J. R. (1972): A gastric motor activity stimulating polypeptide: Final purification, amino acid composition, and C-terminal residue. *Gastroenterology,* 62:401–404.
16. Butler, B. A., Cheng, J. W. B., Ritchie, W. P., and Delaney, J. (1970): Antral gastritis and parietal cell hyperplasia. *Fed. Proc.,* 29:255–258.
17. Capper, W. M., Butler, T. J., Kilby, J. G., and Gibson, M. J. (1967): Gallstones, gastric secretion and flatulent dyspepsia. *Lancet,* i:413–415.
18. Carson, H. C., Code, C. F., and Nelson, R. A. (1966): Motor action of the canine gastroduodenal junction. *Am. J. Dig. Dis.,* 11:155–162.
19. Castell, D., Cohen, S., and Harris, L. D. (1970): Response of the human ileocecal sphincter to gastrin. *Am. J. Physiol.,* 219:712–715.
20. Castell, D. O., and Harris, L. D. (1970): Hormonal control of gastroesophageal sphincter strength. *N. Engl. J. Med.,* 282:886–890.
21. Castell, D. O., and Levine, S. M. (1971): A new mechanism for treatment of heartburn with antacids: Lower esophageal sphincter response to gastric alkalinization. *Ann. Intern. Med.,* 74:223–227.
22. Chapman, M. L., Rudick, J., and Dyck, W. D. (1969): Electrolyte movements across the

gastric mucosa; the effects of bile on the permeability of the antrum and fundus. *J. Clin. Invest.,* 48:18.

23. Cheng, J., Ritchie, W. P., and Delaney, J. P. (1969): Atrophic gastritis: An experimental model. *Fed. Proc.,* 28:513–515.
24. Christensen, J. J. (1970): Pharmacologic identification of the lower esophageal sphincter. *J. Clin. Invest.,* 49:681–691.
25. Christensen, J. J., Freeman, B. W., and Miller, J. K. (1973): Some physiological characteristics of the esophagogastric junction. *Gastroenterology,* 64:1119–1125.
26. Christensen, J. J., Gomklin, J. L., and Freeman, B. W. (1973): Physiological specialization at esophagogastric junction in three species. *Am. J. Physiol.,* 225:1265–1270.
27. Christiansen, J., and Borgeskov, S. (1974): The effect of glucagon and the combined effect of glucagon and secretin on the lower esophageal sphincter pressure in man. *Scand. J. Gastroenterol.,* 9:615–618.
28. Christiansen, J., Louritzen, K., Moesgard, J., and Holst, J. J. (1977): Effects of endogenous and exogenous glucagon on pentagastrin-stimulated lower esophageal sphincter pressure in man. *Scand. J. Gastroenterol.,* 12:33–36.
29. Cohen, S., and Harris, L. D. (1971): Does hiatus hernia affect competence of the gastroesophageal sphincter? *N. Engl. J. Med.,* 284:1053–1056.
30. Cohen, S., Harris, L. D., and Levitan, R. L. (1968): Manometric characteristics of the human ileocecal junctional zone. *Gastroenterology,* 54:72–75.
31. Cohen, S., and Lipshutz, W. (1971): Hormonal regulation of human lower esophageal sphincter competence: Interaction of gastrin and secretin. *J. Clin. Invest.,* 50:449–454.
32. Cohen, S., Lipshutz, W., and Hughes, W. (1971): Role of gastrin supersensitivity in the pathogenesis of lower esophageal sphincter hypertension in achalasia. *J. Clin. Invest.,* 50:1241–1247.
33. Cox, K. R. (1961): Oesophageal stricture after gastrectomy. *Br. J. Surg.,* 49:307–313.
34. Crema, A., Benzi, G., and Berte, B. M. (1963): The action of some natural substances on the terminal portion of the common bile duct isolated in toto. *Arch. Int. Pharmacodyn. Ther.,* 137:307–317.
35. Crema, A., Benzi, G., Frigo, G. M., and Berte, F. (1965): The responses of the terminal bile duct to morphine and morphine-like drugs. *J. Pharmacol. Exp. Ther.,* 149:373–379.
36. Crispin, J. S., Choi, Y. W., Wisenman, D. G. A., Gillespie, D. J., and Lind, S. F. (1970): A direct manometric study of the canine choledocho-duodenal junction. *Arch. Surg.,* 101:215–218.
37. Csendes, A., Oster, M., and Brandsborg, O. (1978): Gastroesophageal sphincter pressure and serum gastrin studies following food intake before and after vagotomy for duodenal ulcer. *Scand. J. Gastroenterol.,* 13:438–441.
38. Davenport, H. W. (1968): Destruction of the gastric mucosal barrier by detergents and urea. *Gastroenterology,* 54:175–181.
39. Davidson, E. D., and Hersh, T. (1975): Bile reflux gastritis. *Am. J. Surg.,* 130:514–519.
40. Davis, A. E., and Pirola, R. C. (1966): The effects of ethyl alcohol on pancreatic exocrine function. *Med. J. Aust.,* 53:757–760.
41. Delaney, J. P., Butler, B. A., Cheng, J. W. B., Moller, J., Brandsburg, M., and Andrup, E. (1972): Gastritis induced by intestinal juices. *Bull. Soc. Int. Chir.,* 31:176–183.
42. Delmont, J. (1976): An attempt to collate. In: *Proceedings of the Third Gastroenterological Symposium,* edited by J. Delmont. Karger. Nice.
43. Dent, J., and Hansky, J. (1976): Relationship of serum gastrin response to lower esophageal sphincter pressure. *Gut,* 17:144–146.
44. Dodds, W. J., Hogan, W. O., Miller, W. N., Barreras, R. F., Arndorfer, R. C., and Stef, J. J. (1975): Relationship between serum gastrin concentration and lower esophageal sphincter pressure. *Am. J. Dig. Dis.,* 20:201–207.
45. Domschke, W., Lux, G., Mitznegg, P., Rosch, W., Domschke, S., Bloom, S. R., Wunsch, E., and Demling, L. (1976): Relationship of plasma motilin response to lower esophageal pressure in man. *Scand. J. Gastroenterol. (Suppl 39),* 11:81–84.
46. Duplessis, D. J. (1962): Gastric mucosal changes after operations on the stomach. *S. Afr. Med. J.,* 36:471–475.
47. Duplessis, D. J. (1965): Pathogenesis of gastric ulceration. *Lancet,* i:974–977.
48. Eckardt, V., and Grace, N. D. (1976): Lower esophageal sphincter pressure and serum motilin levels. *Am. J. Dig. Dis.,* 21:1008–1011.
49. Eckardt, V. F., Grace, N. D., Osborne, M. P., and Fischer, J. E. (1978): Lower esophageal

sphincter pressure and serum gastrin levels after mapped antrectomy. *Arch. Intern. Med.,* 138:243–245.

50. Farrell, R. L., Castell, D. O., and McGuigan, J. E. (1974): Measurements and comparisons of lower esophageal sphincter pressure and serum gastrin levels in patients with gastroesophageal reflux. *Gastroenterology,* 67:415–422.
51. Farrell, R. L., Nebel, O. T., McGuire, A. T., and Castell, D. O. (1973): The abnormal lower esophageal sphincter in pernicious anaemia. *Gut,* 14:767–772.
52. Feurle, G. E. (1975): Effect of rising intragastric pH induced by several antacids on serum gastrin concentrations in duodenal ulcer patients and in a control group. *Gastroenterology,* 68:1–7.
53. Fisher, R. S., and Boden, G. (1975): Reversibility of pyloric sphincter dysfunction in gastric ulcer. *Gastroenterology,* 69:591–594.
54. Fisher, R. S., and Boden, G. (1976): Gastrin-inhibition of the pyloric sphincter. *Am. J. Dig. Dis.,* 21:468–472.
55. Fisher, R. S., and Cohen, S. (1973): Physiological characteristics of human pyloric sphincter. *Gastroenterology,* 64:67–77.
56. Fisher, R. S., and Cohen, S. (1973): Pyloric sphincter dysfunction in patients with gastric ulcer. *N. Engl. J. Med.,* 288:273–278.
57. Fisher, R. S., DiMarino, A. J., and Cohen, S. (1975): Mechanism of cholecystokinin inhibition of lower esophageal sphincter pressure. *Am. J. Physiol.,* 228:1469–1473.
58. Fisher, R. S., Lipshutz, W., and Cohen, S. (1973): Hormonal regulation of the human pyloric sphincter. *J. Clin. Invest.,* 52:1289–1296.
59. Fisher, R. S., Malmud, L. S., Lobis, I. F., and Roberts, G. (1977): The lower esophageal sphincter as a barrier to gastroesophageal reflux. *Gastroenterology,* 72:19–22.
60. Floguet, J., and Coutin, C. (1975): L' anatomie du sphincter d' Oddi. *Acta Endoscop. Radiocinemat.,* 5:103–108.
61. Floguet, J., Laurent, J., and Plenat, F. (1976): Is the sphincter of Oddi a reality in man? In: *Proceedings of the Third Gastroenterological Symposium,* edited by J. Delmont. S. Karger, Nice.
62. Freeland, G. R., Higgs, R. H., Castell, D. O., and McGuigan, J. E. (1976): Lower esophageal sphincter and gastric acid response to intravenous infusions of synthetic human gastrin I heptadecapeptide. *Gastroenterology,* 71:570–574.
63. Fyke, F. E., Code, C. F., and Schlegel, J. F. (1956): The gastroesophageal sphincter in healthy human beings. *Gastroenterology (Basel),* 86:135–150.
64. Gazet, J., and Kopp, J. (1964): The surgical significance of the ileocecal junction. *Surgery,* 56:565–573.
65. Giles, C. R., Mason, M. C., Humphries, C., and Clark, C. G. (1969): Action of gastrin on the lower esophageal sphincter in man. *Gut,* 10:730–734.
66. Gillison, E. W., Kusakari, K., and Bombeck, C. T. (1972): The importance of bile in reflux esophagitis and the success of its prevention by surgical means. *Br. J. Surg.,* 59:594–599.
67. Gorbach, S., Plaut, A., Malhos, L., and Weinstein, L. (1967): Microorganisms of the small intestine and their relationship to oral and fecal flow. *Gastroenterology,* 53:856–867.
68. Goyal, R. K., and McGuigan, J. E. (1976): Is gastrin a major determinant of basal LES pressure? *J. Clin. Invest.,* 57:291–300.
69. Grossman, M. I. (1968): Physiological role of gastrin. *Fed. Proc.,* 27:1312–1313.
70. Grossman, M. I. (1971): Interaction of gastrointestinal hormones. In: *Structure-Activity Relationships of Protein and Peptide Hormones,* pp. 129–139, edited by W. Creutzfeldt, Schattauer, Stuttgart.
71. Grossman, M. I. (1974): Gastrointestinal hormones: Spectrum of actions and structure-activity relations. In: *Endocrinology of the Gut,* edited by W. Y. Chey and F. P. Brooks, pp. 65–75. Charles B. Slack, Thorofare, New Jersey.
72. Hand, H. B. (1973): Anatomy and function of the extrahepatic biliary system. In: *Clinics in Gastroenterology, Vol. 2,* edited by I. Bonchier, pp. 3–29. Saunders, London.
73. Hauge, C. W., and Mark, J. B. D. (1966): Common bile duct motility and sphincteric mechanism. *Ann. Surg.,* 162:641–652.
74. Hedner, P., and Rorsman, G. (1969): On the mechanism of action for the effect of Cck on the choledochoduodenal junction in the cat. *Acta Physiol. Scand.,* 76:248–254.
75. Hellemans, J., Vantrappen, G., and Bloom, S. R. (1976): Endogenous motilin and the LES pressure. *Scand. J. Gastroenterol. (Suppl. 39),* 11:67–73.

76. Helsinger, N. (1960): Oesophagitis following total gastrectomy. *Acta Clin. Scand.,* 118:190–201.
77. Hendrickson, W. F. (1898): A study of the musculature of the entire extrahepatic biliary system, including that of the duodenal portion of the common bile duct and of the sphincter. *Johns Hopkins Hosp. Bull.,* 9:212–232.
78. Higgs, R. H., Smyth, R. D., and Castell, D. O. (1974): Gastric alkalinization. Effect on lower esophageal sphincter pressure and serum gastrin. *N. Engl. J. Med.,* 291:486–490.
79. Hogan, W. J., Dodds, W. J., Hoke, S. E., Reid, D. P., Kalkhoff, R., and Arndorfer, R. (1975): Effect of glucagon on esophageal motor function. *Gastroenterology,* 69:160–165.
80. Isenberg, J. I., and Csendes, A. (1972): Effect of octapeptide of cholecystokinin on canine pylorus pressure. *Am. J. Physiol.,* 222:420–431.
81. Isenberg, J., Csendes, A., and Walsh, J. H. (1971): Resting and pentagastrin stimulated gastroesophageal sphincter pressure in patients with Zollinger-Ellison syndrome. *Gastroenterology,* 61:655–658.
82. Ishioka, T. (1959): Electromyographic study of the choledochoduodenal junction and duodenal wall muscle. *Tohoku J. Exp. Med.,* 70:73–84.
83. Itoh, Z., Aizawa, I., Honda, R., Hiwatashi, K., and Couch, E. (1978): Control of lower esophageal sphincter contractile activity by motilin in conscious dogs. *Am. J. Dig. Dis.,* 23:341–345.
84. Ivey, K. J., Denbesten, L., and Clifton, J. A. (1970): Effect of bile salts on ionic movement across the human gastric mucosa. *Gastroenterology,* 59:183–186.
85. Jaffer, S. S., Makhlouf, G. M., Schorr, G. A., and Zfass, A. M. (1974): Nature and kinetics of inhibition of lower esophageal sphincter pressure by glucagon. *Gastroenterology,* 67:42–46.
86. Jarrett, R., and Gazet, T. (1966): Studies in vivo of the ileocaeco-colic sphincter in the cat and dog. *Gut,* 7:271–275.
87. Jennewein, H. M., Bauer, R., Hummelt, H., Lepsin, G., Siewart, R., and Waldeck, F., (1976): Motilin effects on gastrointestinal motility and lower esophageal sphincter pressure in dogs. *Scand. J. Gastroenterol. (Suppl. 39),* 11:63–65.
88. Jennewein, H. M., Waldeck, F., Siewert, R., Weiser, F., and Thimm, R. (1973): The interaction of glucagon and pentagastrin on the lower esophageal sphincter in man and dog. *Gut,* 14:861–864.
89. Jensen, D. M., McCallum, R., and Walsh, J. H. (1971): Failure of atropine to inhibit G-17 stimulation of the lower esophageal sphincter in man. *Gastroenterology,* 75:825–827.
90. Johnson, A. G. (1972): Pyloric function and gallstone dyspepsia. *Br. J. Surg.,* 59:449–553.
91. Kaye, M. D., Mehta, S. J., and Showalter, J. P. (1976): Manometric studies on the human pylorus. *Gastroenterology,* 70:477–480.
92. Kaye, M. D., and Showalter, J. P. (1974): Pyloric incompetence in patients with symptomatic gastroesophageal reflux. *J. Lab. Clin. Med.,* 83:198–202.
93. Keet, A. D. (1957): The prepyloric contractions in the normal stomach. *Acta Radiol.,* 48:413–419.
94. Keet, A. D. (1962): Diameter of the pyloric operative in relation to the contraction of the canalis egestorius. *Acta Radiol.,* 59:31–37.
95. Kelley, M., and DeWeese, J. (1969): Effects of eating and intraluminal filling an ileocolonic junctional zone pressures. *Am. J. Physiol.,* 216:1491–1495.
96. Kelley, M., Gordon, E., and DeWeese, J. (1965): Pressure studies of the ileocolonic junctional zone of dogs. *Am. J. Physiol.,* 209:333–339.
97. Kelley, M., Gordon, E., and DeWeese, J. (1966): Pressure response of canine ileocolonic junctional zone to intestinal distention. *Am. J. Physiol.,* 211:614–618.
98. Kolsen, M., Roth, J., Turner, H., and Johnson, T. (1960): Relation of small bowel resection to nutrition in man. *Gastroenterology,* 38:605–615.
99. Korman, M. G., Soveny, C., and Hansky, J. (1972): Extragastric gastrin. *Gut,* 13:346–351.
100. Lambert, R. (1962): Relative importance of biliary and pancreatic secretions in the genesis of esophagitis in rats. *Am. J. Dig. Dis.,* 7:1026–1030.
101. Liedberg, G. (1969): The effect of vagotomy on gallbladder and duodenal pressure during rest and stimulation with cholecystokinin. *Acta Chir. Scand.,* 135:695–699.
102. Liedberg, G., and Halaki, M. (1970): The effect of vagotomy on flow resistance at the choledochoduodenal junction. *Acta Chir. Scand.,* 136:208–215.
103. Liedberg, G., and Persson, C. G. A. (1970): Adrenoreceptors in the cat choledochoduodenal junction studied *in situ. Br. J. Pharmacol.,* 39:619–676.

104. Lin, T. M. (1971): Hepatic, cholecystokinetic and choledochal actions of cholecystokinin, secretin, caerulein and gastrin-like peptides. In: *Proceedings of the International Congress of Physiological Science,* 9:1877.
105. Lin, T. M. (1975): Actions of gastrointestinal hormones and related peptides on the motor function of the biliary tract. *Gastroenterology,* 69:1006–1022.
106. Lin, T. M., and Spray, G. F. (1969): Effect of pentagastrin, cholecystokinin, caerulein, and glucagon on the choledochal resistance and bile flow of the conscious dog. *Gastroenterology,* 56:1178.
107. Lind, J. F., Cotton, D. J., Blanchard, R., Crispin, J., and DiMopolos, G. (1969): Effect of thoracic displacement and vagotomy on the canine gastroesophageal junctional zone. *Gastroenterology,* 56:1078–1085.
108. Lipshutz, W., and Cohen, S. (1971): Physiological determinants of lower esophageal sphincter function. *Gastroenterology,* 61:16–24.
109. Lipshutz, W., and Cohen, S. (1975): Interaction of gastrin I and secretin on gastrointestinal circular muscle. *Am. J. Physiol.,* 222:775–781.
110. Lipshutz, W. H., Gaskins, R. D., Lukash, W. M., and Sode, J. (1973): Pathogenesis of lower esophageal sphincter incompetence. *N. Engl. J. Med.,* 289:182–184.
111. Lipshutz, W. A., Gaskins, R. D., Lukash, W. M., and Sode, J. (1974): Hypogastrinemia in patients with lower esophageal sphincter incompetence. *Gastroenterology,* 67:423–427.
112. Lipshutz, W., Hughes, W., and Cohen, S. (1972): The genesis of lower esophageal sphincter pressure: Its identification through the use of gastrin antiserum. *J. Clin. Invest.,* 51:522–529.
113. Lipshutz, W., Tuch, A. F., and Cohen, S. (1971): A comparison of the site of action of gastrin I on lower esophageal sphincter and antral circular smooth muscle. *Gastroenterology,* 61:454–460.
114. Louckes, H. S., Quigley, J. P., and Hersey, J. (1960): Inductograph method of recording muscle activity especially pyloric sphincter physiology. *Am. J. Physiol.,* 199:301–309.
115. Lux, G., Rosch, W., Domschke, S., Wunsch, E., Jaeger, E., and Demling, L. (1976): Intravenous 13-Nle-motilin increases the human lower esophageal sphincter pressure. *Scand. J. Gastroenterol. (Suppl.* 39) 11:75–79.
116. McCall, I. W., Harvey, R. F., Owen, C. J., and Clendinnen, B. G. (1975): Relationship between changes in plasma gastrin and lower esophageal sphincter pressure after meals. *Br. J. Surg.,* 62:15–18.
117. McCallum, R. W., Kline, M. M., and Sturdevant, R. A. L. (1975): Studies on the mechanism of lower esophageal sphincter pressure response to alkali ingestion. *Clin. Res.,* 23:89.
118. McCallum, R. W., and Walsh, J. H. (1979): Relationship between lower esophageal sphincter pressure and serum gastrin concentration in Zollinger-Ellison syndrome and other clinical settings. *Gastroenterology,* 76:76–81.
119. McKeown, K. (1958): Oesophageal stenosis after partial gastrectomy. *Br. Med. J.,* 2:819–823.
120. Meissner, A. J., Bowes, K. L., Zwick, R. and Daniel, E. (1976): Effect of motilin on the lower esophageal sphincter. *Gut,* 17:925–932.
121. Menguy, R. B., Hallenbeck, G. A., Bollman, J. L., and Grindlay, J. H. (1958): Intraductal pressure and sphincteric resistance in canine pancreatic and biliary ducts after various stimuli. *Surg. Gynecol. Obstet.,* 106:306–312.
122. Menguy, R., and Max, M. A. (1970): Influence of bile on canine gastric antral mucosa. *Am. J. Surg.,* 119:117–124.
123. Morris, D. W., Schoen, H., Brooks, F. P., and Cohen, S. (1974): Relationship of serum gastrin and lower esophageal sphincter pressure in normals and patients with antrectomy. *Gastroenterology,* 66:75.
124. Nebel, O. T. (1975): Manometric evaluation of the papilla of Vater. *Gastroint. Endosc.,* 21:126–128.
125. Nebel, O. T. (1975): Effect of enteric hormones on the human sphincter of Oddi. *Gastroenterology,* 68:962.
126. Nebel, O. T., and Castell, D. O. (1972): Lower esophageal sphincter pressure changes after food ingestion. *Gastroenterology,* 66:778–783.
127. Nebel, O. T., and Castell, D. O. (1973): Inhibition of the lower esophageal sphincter by fat: A mechanism for fatty food intolerance. *Gut,* 14:270–274.
128. Oddi, R. (1887): D'une disposition a sphincter speciale de l'overture canal cholédogue. *Arch. Ital. Biol.,* 8:317–322.

129. Pahlin, P. (1975): Extrinsic nervous control of the ileocecal sphincter in the cat. *Acta Physiol. Scand. (Suppl.),* 426:5–32.
130. Pahlin, P., and Keriventer, J. (1975): Reflexogenic contraction of ileocecal sphincter in the cat following small or large intestinal distension. *Acta Physiol. Scand.,* 95:126–132.
131. Pahlin, P., and Kerwenter J. (1976): The vagal control of the ileocecal sphincter in the cat. *Acta Physiol. Scand.,* 96:433–442.
132. Pahlin, P., and Kerwenter, J. (1976): Sympathetic nervous control of cat ileocecal sphincter. *Am. J. Physiol.,* 231:296–305.
133. Persson, O. A., and Ekman, M. (1972): Effect of morphine, CCK and sympathomimetics on the sphincter of Oddi and intramural pressure of cat duodenum. *Scand. J. Gastroenterol.,* 7:345–351.
134. Phaosawasdi, K., Boden, G., Kolts, B., and Fisher, R. S. (1979): Hormonal effects on pyloric sphincter pressure: are they of physiological importance? *Clin. Res.,* 27:270A.
135. Phaosawasdi, K., Callaghan, M., and Fisher, R. S. (1978): Noncholinergic control of the pylorus. *Clin. Res.,* 26(3):325.
136. Pigott, W. H. (1975): The effect of meat extract stimulation of serum gastrin of patients undergoing proximal gastric vagotomy, alone, and with Finney pyloroplasty. *Br. J. Surg.,* 62:653–655.
137. Pirola, R. C., and Davis, A. E. (1968): Effects of ethyl alcohol on sphincteric resistance at the choledocho-duodenal junction in man. *Gut,* 9:557–560.
138. Raih, T. J., Ashmore, C. S., Wilson, S. D., DeCosse, J. J., Hogan, W. J., Dodds, W. J., and Stef, J. J. (1973): Effect of enteric hormones on the canine choledochal sphincter. *Gastroenterology,* 64:787.
139. Resin, H., Stern, D. H., Sturdevant, R. A. L., and Isenberg, J. I. (1973): Effect of the C-terminal octapeptide of cholecystokinin on lower esophageal sphincter pressure in man. *Gastroenterology,* 64:946–949.
140. Rhodes, J., Barnardo, D. E., Phillips, S. F., Rovelstad, R., and Hofmann, A. (1969): Increased reflux of bile into the stomach in patients with gastric ulcer. *Gastroenterology,* 57:241–248.
141. Rosch, W., Koch, H., and Demling, L. (1976): Manometric studies during ERCP and endoscopic papillotomy. *Endoscopy,* 8:30–33.
142. Sabin, J. O., Siegel, C. I., and Mendeloff, A. I. (1973): Biliary duodenal dynamics in man. *Radiology,* 106:1–15.
143. Salducci, J., Naudy, B., and Pin, F. (1976): Papilla electromyography: Endoluminal recording performed in man by perduodenoscopic cannulation. In: *Proceedings of the Third Gastroenterological Symposium,* edited by J. Delmont. S. Karger, Nice.
144. Sandlom, P., Voegtlin, W. L., and Ivy, A. C. (1935): The effect of Cck on the choledochoduodenal mechanism (sphincter of Oddi). *Am. J. Physiol.,* 93:175–180.
145. Sarles, J. C., Bidart, M. A., Devaux, M. A., Echinard, C., and Castagnini, A. (1976): Action of cholecystokinin and caerulein on the rabbit sphincter of Oddi. *Digestion,* 14:415–423.
146. Sarles, J. C., Midejean, A., and Gayne, F. (1974): Etude electromyographique du sphincter d'Oddi. *Biol. Gastroenterol.,* 7:19–27.
147. Siewert, R., Weiser, H. F., Lepsien, G., Jennewein, H., Waldeck, F., Arnold, R., and Creutzfeldt, W. (1977): The relationship between serum IRG levels and LES pressure under various conditions. *Digestion,* 15:162–170.
148. Singleton, A., Redmond, D., and McMurray, J. (1964): Ileocecal resection and small bowel transit and absorption. *Ann. Surg.,* 159:690–693.
149. Snyder, N., and Hughes, W. (1976): The lower esophageal sphincter pressure in Zollinger-Ellison syndrome. Basal levels and response to calcium infusion. *Clin. Res.,* 24:14.
150. Stening, G. F., and Grossman, M. I. (1969): Potentiation of action of cholecystokinin by secretin. *Clin. Res.,* 17:528.
151. Stern, D. H., and Walsh, J. (1973): Gastrin release in postoperative ulcer patients: evidence for release of duodenal gastrin. *Gastroenterology,* 64:363–369.
152. Stol, D. W., Murphy, G. M., and Collis, J. L. (1974): Duodenogastric reflux and acid secretion in patients with symptomatic hiatal hernia. *Scand. J. Gastroenterol.,* 9:97–104.
153. Strunz, U., Domschke, W., Domschke, S., Mitznegg, P., Wunsch, E., Jaeger, E., and Demling L. (1976): Potentiation between 13-Nle-motilin and acetylcholine on rabbit pyloric muscle *in vitro. Scand. J. Gastroenterol. (Suppl. 39),* 12:29–35.
154. Sturdevant, R. A. L., and Kun, T. (1974): Interaction of pentagastrin and the octapeptide of cholecystokinin on the human lower esophageal sphincter. *Gut,* 15:700–702.

155. Tolin, R. D., Boden, G., and Fisher, R. S. (1979): Effect of endogenous hyperglucagonemia on lower esophageal sphincter pressure and gastric acid secretion. *Am. J. Dig. Dis.*, 24:296–304.

156. Toouli, J., and Watts, J. (1970): The spontaneous motility and the action of cholecystokinin-pancreozymin, secretin and gastrin on the canine extrahepatic biliary tract. *Br. J. Surg.*, 57:858–864.

157. Toouli, J., and Watts, J. (1972): Actions of cholecystokinin-pancreozymin, secretin and gastrin on extra biliary tract motility in vitro. *Ann. Surg.*, 175:439–447.

158. Torsoli, A., Ramorino, W. L., and Carratu, R. (1973): On the use of cholecystokinin in the roentgenological examination of the extrahepatic biliary tract and intestines. *Handbk. Exp. Pharmacol.*, 34:247–258.

159. Valenzuela, S. E., and Defilippi, C. (1976): Pyloric sphincter studies in peptic ulcer patients. *Am. J. Dig. Dis.*, 21:229–332.

160. Valenzuela, J. E., Defilippi, C., and Csendes, A. (1976): Manometric studies on the human pyloric sphincter. Effect of cigarette smoking, metoclopramide and atropine. *Gastroenterology*, 70:481–483.

161. Valenzuela, J. E., Defilippi, C., and Eguiguren, A. L. (1974): Estudio manometrico del esfintes pilorico. *Rev. Med. Chil.*, 102:841–843.

162. Vanheerden, J. A., Phillips, S. F., Adson, M. A., and McIlrath, D. C.: Postoperative reflux gastritis. *Am. J. Surg.*, 129:82–87.

163. Vondrasek, P., Eberhardt, G., and Classen, M. (1974): Endoskopische Halbleitermanometrie. *Inn. Med.*, 3:188–192.

164. Walker, C. O., Frank, S. A., Manton, J., and Fordtran, J. S. (1975): Effect of continuous infusion of pentagastrin on lower esophageal sphincter pressure and gastric acid secretion in normal subjects. *J. Clin. Invest.*, 56:218–225.

165. Walton, B. E., Shapiro, H., and Yenny, T. (1968): Effect of alcohol on pancreatic duct pressure. *Am. J. Surg.*, 31:142–144.

166. Watts, J., and Dunphy, J. E. (1966): The role of the common bile duct in biliary dynamics. *Surg. Gynecol. Obstet.*, 122:1207–1218.

167. Wheelon, H., and Thomas, J. E. (1920): Observations of the motility of the antrum and the relation of rhythmic activity of the pyloric sphincter to that of the antrum. *J. Lab. Clin. Med.*, 6:124–132.

168. Wheelon, H., and Thomas, J. E. (1920–1921): Rhythmicity of the pyloric sphincter. *Am. J. Physiol.*, 54:460–478.

169. Windsor, C. (1964): Gastro-oesophageal reflux after partial gastrectomy. *Br. Med. J.*, 2:1233–1234.

170. Wright, L. F., Slaughter, R. L., Gibson, R. G., and Hirschowitz, B. L. (1975): Correlation of lower esophageal sphincter pressure and serum gastrin level in man. *Am. J. Dig. Dis.*, 20:603–606.

171. Wu, W. C., Hogan, W. J., Whalen, G. E., Hoke, S. E., Go, V. L. W., and Kalkhoff, R. K. (1975): Lower esophageal sphincter responses to enteric hormones in two patients with Zollinger-Ellison syndrome. *Am. J. Dig. Dis.*, 20:716–720.

172. Zwick, R., Bowes, K. L., Daniel, E. E. and Sarnas, K. (1976): Mechanism of action of pentagastrin on the lower esophageal sphincter. *J. Clin. Invest.*, 57:1644–1651.

Gastrointestinal Hormones, edited by
George B. Jerzy Glass.
Raven Press, New York © 1980.

Chapter 27

Effects of Insulin and Glucagon on Secretory and Motor Function of the Gastrointestinal Tract

Tsung-Min Lin

The Lilly Research Laboratories, Indianapolis, Indiana 46285

I. EFFECTS OF INSULIN AND GLUCAGON ON SECRETORY FUNCTION OF THE GASTROINTESTINAL TRACT

EFFECTS OF INSULIN ON GASTROINTESTINAL SECRETION

Gastric Secretion

After the discovery of insulin (6), the action of insulin hypoglycemia on gastric secretion was immediately studied. Before 1930, the studies in which insulins from different sources were used showed conflicting results.

Secretory Responses

Inhibitory effects of insulin on gastric secretion. Ivy and Fisher (96) reported that insulin had no influence on the secretion of gastric juice in the dog. Collazo and Dobreff (28,29,39) found that insulin at the dose of 3 rabbit units per kg of body weight inhibited gastric secretion whereas Fonseca and de Carvalho (56) and Popesco and Dicalesco (178) reported in 1922 that insulin was a strong secretogogue.

Even after 1930 inhibitory actions of insulin on gastric secretion were reported. Karvinen and Karvonen (117) inhibited the histamine-induced secretion from the Heidenhain pouch of the dog and suggested that hypoglycemia was the cause of inhibition that did not occur if hypoglycemia was prevented by administration of glucose. Eisenberg et al. (52) reported that the inhibition of secretion from the Heidenhain pouch by insulin was not dependent on hypoglycemia. Jordan and Quintana (111) found a positive correlation between insulin hypoglycemia and inhibition of gastric secretion that was induced by exogenous and endogenously released gastrin. In fact, this inhibitory action was prevented in the dog by elimination of hypoglycemia, and was believed to be due to interference of insulin with the action of gastrin. Corral-Saleta (32) suggested that insulin had a peripheral and direct inhibitory effect on parietal cells that required no mediation by the vagus. Baron et al. (9) and Eisenberg et al. (51) observed inhibitory action of insulin only when the dose was large and when hypoglycemia was severe. Rouff et al. (186,187) and Burkhole (19) inhibited gastric secretion in the chicken with large doses of insulin.

Biphasic action of insulin hypoglycemia on gastric secretion. Some investigators found that the action of insulin hypoglycemia was biphasic: an initial inhibition was followed by augmentation of gastric secretion in animals (105,168) and man (130).

Stimulation of gastric secretion by insulin. Most investigators who have used adequate methods for studying the problem found that the principal effect of insulin on gastric secretion was stimulatory.

Cascao De Anciaes (21,22) noted that the gastric response to a test meal was increased by insulin. La Barre and De Cespedes (124–127), Kalk and Meyer (113), Necheles et al. (168), Hollander (89,90), Smith et al. (199), Hirschowitz and O'Leary (81,82), Eisenberg et al. (51) Isenberg et al. (95), and Ornsholt et al. (175) all reported that insulin hypoglycemia stimulated gastric secretion in the dog. In man, Okada et al. (173,174), Meyer (160), Roholm (183), Cascao De Anciaes (20,21), Kalk and Meyer (113), Welin and Frisk (232), Hofstein (88), Hollander (89), Glass and Boyd (68), and others (8,33,41,77,94,134,189, 195,202,208) all reported that insulin hypoglycemia increased gastric secretion. In the rat, Lin and Alphin (2,136,137) prepared isolated but vagally innervated total stomach or an innervated gastric fistula with a denervated Heidenhain pouch and found hypoglycemic stimulation of secretion in the vagally innervated stomach or fistula but not in the denervated Heidenhain pouch. Lane et al. also reported insulin stimulation of the gastric secretion in the rat with total gastric fistula (132).

Gastric Components Affected by Insulin Hypoglycemia

The stimulatory effect of insulin is characterized by a moderate increase in secretory volume and by an increase in acidity, mucoprotein, and enzymes in the gastric juice.

Gastric acid. The time course of the acid response to insulin hypoglycemia following a single intravenous dose of insulin in man (64,89,104,160,183,234) and in the dog (113,144) varied under different experimental conditions. When basal secretion was present, Roholm (183) and Meyer (160) found that insulin caused a slight increase in volume in the first one or two 10-min periods, and sometimes a slight decrease in the third 10-min period. This was followed by a sudden rise in both volume and acidity, reaching a maximum in the fourth to sixth 10-min periods. The duration of action could last 1 to 3 hr, depending on the dose. Boldyreff and Stewart (14) found only monophasic stimulation of gastric secretion that was not preceded by inhibition. But Hirschowitz and O'Leary (81,82) reported that a low (0.15 unit/kg) dose produced a single 2-hr secretory response, whereas a larger (> 0.3 unit/kg) dose, a 2-peak response separated by a period of inhibition.

Winkelstein and Hess (234) found that it took 90 to 105 min to show the stimulatory effect of insulin on gastric secretion. But most investigators observed that it did not take more than 15 to 30 min before secretion was stimulated. Glass et al. (69), in a study of nonparietal cell components of gastric secretion in man, reported that insulin caused increases in acidity, mucin, and pepsin secretion without significantly affecting the volume. While the mucoprotein and pepsin secretion rose to peak about 40 min after intravenous administration of 16 to 20 units insulin, the acid output came to a peak about 60 min after the onset of intravenous insulin injection (68,70). Lin et al. (144), by slow intravenous infusion of insulin to dogs under basal conditions, found that volume and acid responses started simultaneously about 45 min after the 1-hr infusion began. The time course of the acid response was monophasic, reaching the maximum 15 min after the 1-hr infusion ended, and the duration of acid secretion lasted an additional 2¾ hr.

Enzymes and mucoprotein. In one of the first studies on this subject, Cascao De Anciaes (20,21) determined the coagulating power of human gastric rennin and found that its activity was increased by insulin. The authors stressed, however, that the stimulation of rennin and increase in acid secretion were unrelated.

Babkin (5) had established rather early that secretion in response to vagus stimulation was rich in pepsin. Boldyreff and Stewart (14) reported that in the dog, gastric secretion stimulated by insulin hypoglycemia had a high pepsin content. Subsequent studies by Welin and Frisk (232), Ihre (93), Saemundsson (189), and Glass et al. (70) in man, by Hirschowitz in the dog (82,86,87), and by Jow et al. in the rat (112), all showed that pepsin secretion was stimulated by insulin hypoglycemia. In patients suffering from schizophrenia, Jacobs et al. (99) observed significant increases of uropepsin excretion after insulin shock.

In addition to pepsin, gastric secretion of mucoprotein was also stimulated by insulin. It was noticed by Babkin (4) and Boldyreff and Stewart (14) that gastric secretion induced by insulin had more visible mucin than that stimulated by histamine and food. Comprehensive studies on the question of mucin secretion were conducted by Glass and associates (64–69), who established the stimulatory effect of insulin on gastric glandular mucoprotein. The increase of mucin and acid secretion actually could occur in the absence of significant changes in the total volume. Glass and Boyd noted a dissociated secretory pattern characterized by a positive mucoprotein and a weak or negative acid response to insulin in the nonoperated patients with atrophy or inflammation of the prepyloric antral area (68) as well as after subtotal gastrectomy (70a). In a study on the three main components of human mucin, they proposed that a test of the response of dissolved mucoprotein and mucoproteose to insulin stimulation might be used for the purpose of evaluating the functional activity of different mucus cells of the gastric mucosa (67). The glandular mucoprotein response to insulin may be used for evaluation of the completeness of vagotomy (70a,89,90), especially when vagotomy was combined with antrectomy or subtotal gastric resection.

Potassium secretion. According to Saemundsson (189), the potassium concentration in the human gastric juice was decreased by insulin. This reduction in potassium concentration was less pronounced after vagotomy than prior to surgery in patients with duodenal ulcer. Jacobson (100) saw an increase in total potassium secretion along with an increase in volume of secretion induced by insulin, but no significant difference in potassium concentration between samples aspirated during basal control and during the postinsulin periods. Hirschowitz and O'Leary (81,82) noticed that insulin at doses greater than 0.3 unit/kg lowered the ratio of potassium concentration in the gastric juice to that in the plasma below 1.0 during the period of inhibition, thereby separating the two peaks of secretion.

Importance of Glucose Level and Gastric Secretory Activity

Since the discovery of the relationship between insulin hypoglycemia and gastric hunger contractions, the importance of blood sugar level in gastric secretory activity has been well recognized. There have been two opposite views of the role of blood sugar on gastric secretion. Some workers hold the view that the effect of insulin hypoglycemia is stimulatory and that this stimulatory effect in man (56,173) and dog (113) could be prevented by administration of glucose. Others believed that insulin hypoglycemia inhibited gastric secretion and that this inhibitory effect could be reversed by elimination of hypoglycemia (111,117).

Most investigators now agree that the primary effect of insulin is stimulatory. Early works of Fonseca and Carvalho (56), Okada et al. (173,174), Meyer (160), Roholm (183), Babkin (5), and La Barre and Cespedes (124–127) all pointed to a positive stimulatory effect of hypoglycemia on gastric secretion. More recent studies by Hollander (89,90), Stein and Meyer (208,209), Winkelstein and Hess (234), Glass and Boyd (68) Glass et al. (70), and Glass and Wolf (70a), Weinstein et al. (228,229), Jemerin (104), Hirschowitz and his associates (78,79,80,82,86), Richardson et al. (181), Isenberg et al. (94) and Chen et al. (23) and Lin et al. (144) all demonstrated a stimulatory effect of insulin on gastric secretion in dog, rat, or man. A dose-response study conducted by Hirschowitz (82) and O'Leary and Eisenberg et al. (51) in the dog and by Isenberg et al. (94,95) and Baron et al. (9) in man established not only optimal doses of insulin for gastric stimulation but also provided an explanation for the inhibitory effect of insulin on gastric secretion.

Okada et al. (173) noticed that the increased gastric secretion induced by insulin was almost completely inhibited by an injection of dextrose, but a profuse secretion again appeared when hypoglycemia recurred. Meyer (160) reported that changes in blood sugar and gastric secretion moved in opposite directions; the maximal gastric response coincided with the maximal lowering of blood sugar curve, and the blood sugar level was the mirror image of the volume curve (160). According to Kalk and Meyer (113), a reduction of blood sugar was not in itself enough to cause gastric secretion, for in diabetes a drastic drop of as much as 200 mg/dl was not enough to elicit acid secretion if this brought the blood sugar only to normoglycemia levels.

This brings our attention to the questions of the adequate dose of insulin and the critical level of hypoglycemia for stimulation of gastric secretion. In the study of Jemerin et al. (104), a correlation between the degree of hypoglycemia and output of acid in the dog was suggested. But Necheles et al. (168), Kneller and Nasset (119), and Eisenberg et al. (51) reported that moderate hypoglycemia (25–50 mg/dl) stimulated gastric secretion, whereas severe (below 25 mg/dl) hypoglycemia caused inhibition of secretion from the stomach of dog and man or even the other digestive glands in the dog (119).

Question of the Adequate Dose

There is little doubt now that for stimulation of gastric secretion there is an optimal insulin dose needed beyond which a smaller response is to be expected. In dose-response studies, Hirschowitz et al. (81,82) found that a low (0.15 unit/kg) dose produced an acid response roughly twice that induced by 0.9 unit/kg. In dogs with Pavlov pouches, Spencer and Grossman (202), over a dose range of 0.06 to 0.5 unit/kg, saw a close relationship between magnitude of peak response and duration of response, both of which were related to the magnitude of fall in plasma glucose. Dozois et al. (41) studied the gastric response of dogs to continuous insulin infusion and found that the degree of hypoglycemia, the dose of insulin up to 0.15 unit/kg, and the gastric secretory response were quantitatively related.

In patients with incomplete vagotomy, Isenberg et al. (94,95) reported that the dose-response to 0.025 to 0.4 unit/kg of insulin was unaltered when compared with that of controls. The optimal dose causing maximal gastric response was 0.2 unit/kg i.v. Baron (8) and Cowley and Baron (33) noted that the peak acid outputs correlated with the lowest concentration of blood glucose and with the rate of fall in any 15-min period. Peak acid outputs were similar after 0.1 to 0.2 unit/kg and were greater than those at either lower or higher doses.

All these studies support the view that: (a) 0.1 to 0.2 unit/kg by single intravenous injection (8,33,81,82,202) or by infusion is the optimal dose for performing pre- and postoperative insulin tests or determining the maximal gastric response, and (b) the gastric secretory response to insulin is not an "all or none" phenomenon (8,202). The results support, instead, the hypothesis that insulin hypoglycemia provides a quantitative glycopenic stimulus producing a quantitative vagal acid response. Severe hypoglycemia consistently inhibited gastric secretion.

Question of Critical Blood Sugar Level

According to Bulatao and Carlson (see Chapter 27II, by T. M. Lin, pp. 667–691, in *this volume*), hunger contractions in the dog started during insulin hypoglycemia when the blood sugar fell to the 70 to 80 mg/dl level. Kalk and Meyer (113) considered the critical level for triggering gastric secretion to be 50 mg/dl. To this value Roholm (183) and many others, especially Hollander (89,90) and Weinstein et al. (229), who made several studies on this subject, agreed. One should bear in mind that the 50 mg/dl value was only a close approximation to which exceptions have been found (81,230) and will be expected to occur in individual situations.

In most, if not all, of the foregoing studies in man or dog, insulin was given as an intravenous bolus. One can argue that the sudden increase in plasma insulin concentration may cause a precipitous fall of blood sugar. Under such circumstances, an accurate estimation of the critical blood sugar level may become difficult. When Lin et al. (144) gave insulin and proinsulin by slow intravenous infusion to the dogs, the first sign of significant increases in volume and acid output, caused by insulin, occurred when hypoglycemia was 42 mg/dl, and that caused by proinsulin occurred when blood sugar level was about 53 mg/dl in the same dogs. The results suggest that even by intravenous infusion of insulin, the fall in blood sugar could have passed the 50 mg/dl mark before signs of gastric stimulation could be noticed. However, the transformation of proinsulin to its active form, insulin, for production of hypoglycemia *in vivo* is a rather slow process (30 min), and the gradual fall of blood sugar to 53 mg/dl at the end of the 1-hr infusion was the point at which slight but significant gastric secretion was first detected. In this sense the existence of a critical blood sugar level set by Hollander, is confirmed (89,90).

Relationship of Blood Sugar Level to the Time Course of the Secretory Curve

In addition to the critical degree of hypoglycemia necessary for initiating gastric secretion, there was discussion about the correlation between the time course of hypoglycemia and the time of gastric response. One view is that the gastric secretory response coincides exactly with the lowering of blood sugar (160). Another view is that there is no relationship between the sugar level and the onset of secretion (183) and that the action of hypoglycemia on gastric secretion is all or none.

Kalk and Meyer (113), in experiments in dog and man, found that the normalization of sugar level coincided with the decrease in the rate of secretion. If glucose were given intravenously, it reduced gastric volume, but the decline in HCl lagged behind. Glass and Boyd (68) noticed that maximal secretion of acid occurred after the blood sugar began to rise from its lowest point, about 60 min after the insulin. Lin et al. (144) showed that the volume and acid secretion continued for an additional 30 to 45 min at the level significantly higher than that of controls after blood sugar was normalized. These findings suggest that (a) the acid and volume responses are not undissociable, (b) once a critical hypoglycemic level is reached and the gastric secretory mechanism is set in motion, this can continue for a while in the absence of obvious hypoglycemia, and (c) the maximal response does not necessarily have to coincide with the lowest blood sugar level.

However, the peak acid output has been shown by Baron (8) and Cowley and Baron (33), Spencer and Grossman (202), and Dozois et al. (41) to coincide with the lowest concentration of blood sugar.

Action of Other Hypoglycemic Agents on Gastric Secretion

That the hypoglycemia itself is responsible for stimulation of gastric secretion is indicated by reports on other agents with hypoglycemic actions. Weiss and Sciales (230) demonstrated that tolbutamide, and Chen et al. (23) showed that hypoglycin A, induced gastric secretion in the dog.

Another aspect of the relationship of sugar metabolism to gastric secretion is the availability of sugar to the vagal centers from which excitatory impulses for gastric stimulation originate. 2-Deoxy-D-glucose (2DG) interferes with the normal metabolism of glucose, which results in an elevation of plasma sugar level and cytoglucopenia. Hirschowitz and Sachs (84) and Duke et al. (45) reported that 2DG was a more powerful stimulus for gastric secretion than insulin, and was superior because of the reliability and reproducibility of response in dog and man. This observation was confirmed in dogs (31,51) and in man (53,175,214). Eisenberg et al. (51) did dose-response studies with insulin and 2DG in dogs with vagally innervated gastric fistula (GF) and denervated Heidenhain pouch (HP). They found that 2DG stimulated secretion from GF and HP. With the GF open, the response to insulin was less than that to 2DG. 2DG *in vitro* inhibited the chloride and acid secretion by the frog gastric mucosa (188).

Importance of the Vagus and the Central Nervous System

Although Weischmann and Gatsweiler observed the antagonistic actions of insulin and atropine on gastric secretion, they interpreted this as evidence of a direct vagotonic effect of insulin (231).

The first indication of the involvement of the parasympathetic mechanism in the stimulation of gastric function was provided by Quigley (179), who showed that insulin-induced gastric motility was inhibited by atropine, adrenaline, vagotomy (216), and glucose. Others (24,27,32,34,36,62,93) who saw an inhibitory effect of atropine on insulin-induced gastric secretion all agreed that the mechanism involved the stimulation of the vagal centers by hypoglycemia. This conclusion was summarized by Hollander (89).

Conclusive evidence of the involvement of the central nervous system (CNS) in gastric secretion induced by insulin hypoglycemia was provided by La Barre and Cespedes (127), who in a cross-circulation experiment between the donor dog and the isolated head of a recipient dog, found that insulin hypoglycemia in the donor caused gastric secretion in the recipient and that this secretion was reversed by injection of glucose (125), inhibited by atropine (126), and abolished by vagotomy. Jogi et al. (105) further demonstrated that the secretory response to insulin remained after decortication but disappeared after decerebration. This indicates that the sites sensitive to hypoglycemia are somewhere below the cerebrum extending to the medulla; the vagi merely serve as a carrier of impulses to the target organs.

The Insulin Test for "Vagality"

In an examination of the vagal innervation of the Pavlov pouch, Jemerin and Hollander (103) found that more than 75% of the vagal fibers were transected in this preparation. A total vagal pouch prepared by Hollander and Jemerin (91) gave uniformly consistent results that enabled them to differentiate vagal from nonvagal pouches (104). But quantitation of the relationship between degree of hypoglycemia and gastric response, at that time, was unsuccessful.

Despite these facts, the validity of insulin hypoglycemia for testing "vagality" of the stomach has been established. Thus according to Hollander (89,90), a positive response to insulin test consisted of a distinct rise in acidity accompanied by hypoglycemia. A negative response was suggestive but not necessarily conclusive proof that all the vagal fibers had been interrupted.

Variation in the anatomy of the peripheral branches of the vagus could be one reason for the variation in the testing results (234). It is thus not surprising that after vagotomy a positive test can still be seen. Weinstein et al. (229) reported that 29% of vagotomized ulcer patients reacted positively to insulin. Ross and Kay (185) found that in 62 of 100 patients, a negative test was found after vagotomy. Smith et al. (200) noticed a negative insulin response immediately after vagotomy but 6 months later negative responses were converted to positive. The conversion was explained on the basis of possible vagal regeneration.

It was reported by Winkelstein and Hess (234) that insulin evoked a significantly higher response in duodenal ulcer patients than in normals. Complete or selective vagotomy has been employed by numerous workers for peptic ulcer therapy during which the insulin test was routinely used (42,43,72,162,172, 191,208,209,220,231).

Hemivagotomy in cats and dogs was reported by Stenning and Isenberg to decrease the peak 15-min and the total 4-hr acid response to insulin by 35 to 50% (210). In man, graded vagotomy was found by Nundy and Baron (171) to produce graded decrease of gastric response to insulin.

Role of the Sympathetic Nervous System

Very little attention has been given to the role of the sympathetic nervous system in gastric function. Quigley and Templeton were the first to mention that the action of insulin and of dextrose on gastric motility in double splanchnicotomized dogs during fasting was slightly greater than that displayed by normal animals. Oberhelman et al. (172) reported that following sympathectomy the gastric secretory response to insulin, food, and histamine all increased and the tolerance to hypoglycemia decreased. This may suggest that under normal conditions the action of the parasympathetic mechanism is balanced by the actions of the sympathetic system.

Pharmacological studies by Quigley (179), Okada et al. (173,174) Kalk and Meyer (113), and others all demonstrated an inhibitory effect of epinephrine on insulin-induced hypersecretion.

Release of Gastrin and Catecholamines by Insulin

Before methods for specific radioimmunoassay (RIA) of gastrin (235) were available, gastrin was measured indirectly by determining the gastric secretory response to methods causing endogenous release of gastrin (54,73), including sham feeding (177,221).

Methods for measuring gastrin have been devised by several groups of workers (62,98,235) and the effect of insulin hypoglycemia on gastrin release has since been studied. The plasma level of gastrin was significantly increased by insulin hypoglycemia (34,62,73,74,203,205,217), feeding (169,224,225), or sham feeding (169,217). Hughes and Green (92) reported that serum gastrin was not clearly related to the blood sugar level, but it was insulin dose-dependent. In duodenal ulcer patients, glucose infusion prevented insulin hypoglycemia and also the increase in plasma gastrin (203).

Walsh et al. assayed gastrin-17 (G-17) in the plasma and found that after complete truncal vagotomy, insulin failed to elicit an acid response from the vagally innervated gastric fistula of the dog, and the rise in plasma gastrin induced by a meal decreased by 50% (224). Atropine inhibited the gastric response to feeding (225) and insulin (34) but not the plasma level of gastrin. In fact, the insulin-induced gastrin release was enhanced by atropine (193). The tonic release of gastrin in patients with anacidity is atropine-resistant; the reduction in gastric acid secretion produced by atropine in acid-secreting subjects serves to blunt the normal inhibitory effect of antral acidification on gastrin release, thereby overcoming any possible atropine blockade of gastrin release in response to feeding (225). The effects of atropine on 2DG-induced gastric acid secretion and gastrin release were the same as those on responses to insulin (175).

According to Tepperman et al. (217), the antrum must be the major site responding to insulin for gastrin release. Denervation of the antral pouch had no effect on the basal plasma gastrin level in the dog, but abolished the plasma gastrin response to sham feeding and insulin hypoglycemia. Stadil and Rehfeld (203) reported that in duodenal ulcer patients, antrectomy abolished insulin-induced gastrin release.

Hansky et al. (74) and Lam and Sircus (130) reported that plasma gastrin levels were increased by insulin in duodenal ulcer patients after incomplete vagotomy, but after complete vagotomy no significant change in gastrin level was seen after insulin. However, Stadil and Rehfeld (205) saw an increase of gastrin before and after truncal vagotomy and believed that release of gastrin by insulin did not depend solely on the vagus.

Insulin releases not only gastrin but also acetylcholine at the vagal nerve endings and epinephrine from the adrenal medulla (204); the former stimulates and the latter inhibits gastric acid secretion. The release of corticoids by insulin (156) has also been reported, but corticoids do not have an immediate stimulatory action on gastric secretion.

Bile Secretion

In 1924, Brugsch and Horster (17,18) found that insulin provoked secretion of bile. This was immediately confirmed (38,60,170,190). Okada et al. (173), who stimulated gastric, pancreatic, and bile secretion with insulin, observed that all these effects were inhibited by atropine, epinephrine, ephedrine, or injection of glucose. They visualized the bile and other secretions induced by insulin as being the result of excitation of the autonomic centers by hypoglycemia, for which the term "humoroneural mechanism" was coined. They also noticed that when both vagi were severed directly above the diaphragm, this regulating mechanism disappeared.

Tanturi and Ivy (215) demonstrated a definite secretory effect on bile secretion in the dog and monkey by stimulation of the vagi peripherally in the neck or centrally by reflex action. Fritz and Brooks (61) showed that in cholecystectomized dogs, bile volume and solids were increased by insulin, diminished by anticholinergics, and abolished by vagotomy. Thornton et al. (219) reported that in the dog, the secretin-induced bile flow was increased by insulin, with bicarbonate concentration remaining unchanged or decreased. There was no greater output of bile salts after insulin than during secretin infusion.

Since insulin hypoglycemia releases gastrin and gastrin is reported to have choleretic action (106,107,237), Nahrwold et al. (165) perfused the antral pouch of the dog with buffered acetylcholine at pH 7, and saw choleresis characterized by increased bicarbonate concentration and output.

The dose-response relationship of insulin and 2DG for biliary and gastric acid secretion was compared in the dog by Jones et al. (108). With appropriate doses of insulin (0.03–2 units/kg) and 2DG (50–400 mg/kg), the maximal choleretic actions of insulin and 2DG were not significantly different. Jones and Brooks (106) believed that the pyloric antrum was the mediator of insulin-induced choleresis. Indeed, Zaterka and Grossman (237) demonstrated that bile secretion was stimulated by gastrin.

The importance of the vagal mechanism on bile secretion during insulin hypoglycemia was evaluated. Evidence showed that an extrahepatic factor, the pylorus (63,106), might be involved in choleresis. In cholecystectomized dogs with pancreatic, gastric, and duodenal fistulae, insulin hypoglycemia increased the bile flow and chloride concentration. Bile flow was not affected by selective hepatic vagotomy but chloride output was decreased (63). Electrical stimulation of the vagus resulted in stimulation of bile secretion in the dog (114). However, in anesthetized rats, the stimulatory action of insulin on bile flow was not suppressed by vagotomy (35).

External Pancreatic Secretion

Conflicting results (30,37,55,57,128,131,222) regarding the effect of insulin hypoglycemia on external pancreatic secretion have been reported. For literature published before 1930, accounts were made by Bachrach[1] and Babkin (5).

In animals, and particularly in human studies, investigation of the action of hypoglycemia is complicated by the inability (a) to obtain pure pancreatic juice and (b) to exclude the gastric juice and bile from entering the duodenum where the release of secretin, CCK, and other hormones can take place. Besides, in the early reports studies were not conducted under steady-state secretory conditions, and thus alteration in secretory response to hypoglycemia was difficult to measure. As will be pointed out later, the action of hypoglycemia is mainly "ecbolic," i.e., enzyme-producing and not "hydrelatic," water-producing. Okada et al. (173) noticed an increase of pancreatic secretion following administration of insulin in man. Frisk and Welin (60) eliminated the possibility of secretin release by aspiration of the gastric juice and found that hypoglycemia increased pancreatic diastase.

Lagerlöf and Welin (129) stated that the volume and bicarbonate secretion from the human pancreas was essentially unaffected by insulin hypoglycemia, but enzyme production was powerfully stimulated. This view has been shared by numerous investigators (59,139,148,149,218).

Thomas and Crider (218) aspirated the gastric juice during induction of pancreatic secretion by continuous infusion of secretin to the dog, and found that enzyme concentration was increased by insulin, whereas volume secretion remained constant. Friedman and Snape (59) came to the same conclusion after

---

[1] A comprehensive and analytical review entitled "The action of insulin hypoglycemia on motor and secretory functions of the digestive tract" was written by W. H. Bachrach in 1953. The treatise, which appeared in *Volume 33* of *Physiological Reviews,* is highly recommended for indepth reading.

studying the effect of hypoglycemia in man. Wang et al. (226) demonstrated that the amylase output remained constant, whereas graded doses of secretin infused produced graded responses in volume secretion. Lin and Grossman (148) and Lin and Ivy (149) showed that in the dog metacholine, which mimics the action of the vagal mechanism, had only enzyme-stimulating action; an increase of amylase activity by hundreds of times was not accompanied by significant change in volume flow.

Several reports indicated negative effect of insulin hypoglycemia on pancreatic secretion in anesthetized animals. La Barre, who reported a stimulatory effect of insulin on gastric secretion in the dog, saw sharp inhibition of pancreatic enzyme production after giving insulin (128). Hebb (75) and Baxter (11) reported that hypoglycemia decreased the output of enzymes from the pancreas of the rabbit through a central action and hyperglycemia increased the output through a peripheral action.

The vagal mechanism is important for the action of insulin hypoglycemia on pancreatic secretion. In man the stimulatory effect of hypoglycemia on volume, bicarbonate, and enzymes was abolished by transthoracic vagotomy (196). After vagisection Dreiling et al. (43,44) found that the response to secretin was unaffected in man, but the enzyme response to insulin hypoglycemia was absent. The role of the vagus for response to hypoglycemia was demonstrated by Lin and Alphin (139) in the chronic pancreatic fistula rat. In a dose range of 0.2 to 2.0 units s.c., insulin increased the volume, bicarbonate and amylase secretion; at the 1 to 2 units doses insulin increased the enzyme output without affecting the volume. This stimulatory action of insulin was abolished by vagotomy. The existence of vagal secretory fibers in the rat was further demonstrated by Alphin and Lin in sham feeding experiments (1).

Vagal stimulation can produce either stimulatory or inhibitory effects on pancreatic secretion, depending on the strength and conditions of stimulation. Hebb (75) maintained that the "trophic" action of vagus stimulation was reversed by hypoglycemia. Lin and Ivy (149) found that weak electrical stimulation of the vagus of the dog during steady-state infusion with secretin caused increase in amylase concentration without significantly affecting volume flow. Strong electrical stimulation of the vagus, however, increased enzyme concentration but decreased drastically volume flow and total amylase output.

Dose-response or kinetic study of the relationship between insulin hypoglycemia and pancreatic secretion has not been done as far as we are aware. But it is reasonable to assume that an optimal dose for hypoglycemic stimulation of pancreatic secretion exists.

Other than vagal excitation as the possible mechanism of action for hypoglycemic stimulation of pancreatic secretion, the release of gastrointestinal hormones by insulin may also play a role in the mechanism of action. The stimulation of pancreatic secretion by gastrin was reported by Gregory and Tracy (71) and the dose-response stimulatory action of the C-terminal peptides of gastrin was reported by Lin et al. (153).

EFFECTS OF GLUCAGON ON GASTROINTESTINAL SECRETION

Gastric Secretion

Secretory Responses

The action of glucagon (15,206), the hyperglycemic-glycogenolytic hormone isolated from the islets of the pancreas on gastric secretion is inhibitory. Early indications of this inhibitory effect were its ability to lower plasma level of pepsinogen (50) and to depress gastric acid secretion in man under fasting conditions (182) or stimulated by a meal in the dog (138).

Effect on meal-induced secretion. In dogs with vagally innervated gastric fistula or Heidenhain pouch, the response to 200 or 400 g of a meat meal was significantly inhibited by glucagon given as a single injection intravenously, subcutaneously, or intramuscularly or by continuous intravenous infusion (121,135, 138,140,143). The effect of a 10 μg/kg dose was seen 15 to 30 min after injection and lasted for 60 to 90 min. By continuous infusion the acid response to a 400-g meal was markedly inhibited by 66 to 99% throughout a 4 ½-hr test.

This inhibitory effect was not due to the hyperglycemic action of glucagon. Glucagon by continuous infusion increased the blood sugar level of the dog for only 1 ½ hr. A hypertonic glucose solution that maintained a blood sugar level higher than that caused by glucagon had no significant effect on the response to the meal (135). In man, glucose solution also failed to influence gastric secretion (201).

This inhibitory action of glucagon was unrelated to the A-V glucose difference, i.e., the tissue utilization of glucose (140). Glucagon caused significant A-V difference only in the initial stage of the intravenous infusion, whereas the inhibition of meal-induced acid secretion lasted for several hours after the A-V difference disappeared (135).

Inhibition of gastrin-induced secretion. The remarkable effectiveness of glucagon for inhibition of meal-induced gastric secretion leads one to believe that glucagon must be effective against gastrin-induced secretion also. Indeed, in the dog the steady-state acid secretion induced by gastrin and its derivatives, the C-terminal penta- and tetrapeptides (140–143,145,150,151,154,223,233), was markedly reduced in the Heidenhain and Pavlov pouches and the gastric fistula when given intravenously, intraportally (223), intramuscularly, or by infusion. Gastrin-induced acid secretion in man (76) and from the gastric fistula of the rat was also very significantly inhibited (151) by glucagon.

Given subcutaneously, the steady-state acid secretion from the Heidenhain pouch was inhibited in a dose-dependent fashion (151). The maximal inhibition was 95% when the dose was 30 μg/kg, and the minimal dose required for inhibition was about 2.5 μg/kg.

Gastric secretory response to endogenous gastrin released by mechanical distention of the stomach (Lin, *unpublished*) was completely abolished by glucagon in the dog. In man gastric secretion stimulated by gastrin pentapeptide was inhibited by endogenously released glucagon (25).

Effect on histamine- and methylxanthin-induced gastric secretion. On histamine-induced gastric secretion glucagon is not as effective as it is on meal- or gastrin-induced secretion (13,26,27,40,138,140,143,152,159) in the dog. Glucagon in a dose range of 20 to 80 μg/kg failed to have any significant inhibitory effect on submaximal or maximal histamine-stimulated secretion. On the other hand, secretion induced by gastrin was reduced by 90% in the same dogs (151).

Published data concerning the effect of glucagon on gastric secretory response to histamine are conflicting. Lin and Alphin (138) at first reported that glucagon was unable to inhibit histamine-induced acid secretion of either the vagally innervated or denervated pouch of the dog stomach. Subsequently transient and modest inhibition was seen in man by Cohen et al. (27). but in other studies in which augmented histamine was used in man (40) or both small and large doses of histamine were employed (26,159), no inhibition was demonstrable. One study showed that glucagon decreased secretory volume without affecting acidity (13).

In order to demonstrate a modest inhibitory effect of glucagon on histamine-induced gastric secretion, the dose ratio of histamine to glucagon must be small. Acid secretion from the Heidenhain pouch induced by a moderate dose (9 μg/kg-hr of the free base) of histamine was significantly inhibited by 25 to 50% whereas comparable secretion induced by gastrin in the same dogs was inhibited by 70 to 90% by the same dose of glucagon (146). In man inhibition of methylxanthine-induced secretion was reported (158).

Inhibition of secretion induced by insulin and sham feeding. The action of sham feeding and insulin hypoglycemia is mainly mediated by the vagal mechanism. Gastric secretion in the dog induced by insulin (140) and sham feeding (143) was completely abolished by glucagon. In ulcer patients glucagon reduced gastric secretion induced by insulin (3).

The inhibition of insulin-induced secretion was mainly, if not entirely, due to the hyperglycemic action of glucagon, which counteracted the effect of hypoglycemia on the vagal centers. The other mechanism that may come into play is the suppression of insulin-induced gastrin release (12), which may also play a part in sham feeding-induced secretion. In addition, sham feeding involves the release of acetylcholine. Glucagon may thus act centrally through hyperglycemic action to reduce vagal tone and peripherally to antagonize the action of acetylcholine. Lin, *(unpublished data)* indicate that glucagon has modest but definite inhibitory action on methacholine-induced secretion.

Characteristics of Inhibition of Gastric Secretion

Since pepsinogen level in the plasma was depressed by glucagon (50), inhibition of pepsin secretion in the gastric juice was also found (182,223). A comparison of the effects of glucagon and secretin on pepsin secretion showed that secretin stimulated the secretion of pepsin whereas glucagon did not (16).

The inhibitory effect of glucagon on gastrin-induced electrolyte secretion in the dog was characterized by decreases in volume and concentration of H^+ and Cl^- and an equimolar increase in Na^+ concentration in the gastric juice (146). On submaximal histamine-induced acid secretion, glucagon caused minimal but significant changes in H^+ and Na^+ concentration in the opposite directions; its major effect was on volume. The K^+ concentration in the gastric juice was not significantly affected. However, in human gastric juice a significant decrease in K^+ concentration was reported (24).

Structure-Function Relationship

The N-terminal histadyl residue of the 29 amino acid polypeptide is important for both hyperglycemic and gastric inhibitory actions of glucagon. Lin et al. (145) infused into dogs the des-histadyl-glucagon, the fragment that was devoid of the histadyl residue, at doses several times of that required for inhibition of gastric secretion by glucagon, and failed to find inhibitory action. In addition to des-histadyl-glucagon, many other fragments of glucagon were tested for inhibition of pentagastrin-induced secretion. The N_{1-27}, N_{1-21}, N_{13-17}, N_{18-29}, and N_{22-29} fragments all failed to inhibit acid secretion (142,145,146). From this it is concluded that all the 29 amino acid residues in the polypeptide are required for gastric inhibitory action.

Question of the Mechanism of Action

The mechanism by which glucagon inhibits gastric acid secretion is unknown. Most probably it is a direct metabolic action of glucagon on the cells of the gastric mucosa, including the acid-producing oxyntic cells. This statement is supported by both direct and indirect evidence.

Lin and Warrick (155) found that the histamine- and pentagastrin-induced acid secretion from the isolated gastric mucosa of *Rana catesbeiana* was significantly inhibited by glucagon *in vitro.*

The indirect evidence comes from studies on gastric mucosal blood flow (MBF). According to Jacobson et al. (101,102), gastric secretory rates are accompanied by directionally corresponding changes in mucosal blood flow. It was found by Lin and Warrick (154) that the gastrin-stimulated steady state clearance of aminopyrine, an indication of MBF, from the Heidenhain pouch and gastric fistula of the dog was significantly decreased by subcutaneous injection of glucagon. This was confirmed (233). Even in the resting fundic pouch, the low rate of MBF was decreased by glucagon (227).

However, the reduction in MBF is unlikely to be the primary factor in the inhibitory action because the ratio of aminopyrine concentration in the gastric juice to that in the plasma was increased by glucagon in both the pouch and the gastric fistula. This indicated that more blood was required for the production of unit quantity of acid, or the efficiency of the oxyntic cells to produce acid was decreased. In this sense the action of glucagon is metabolic (154).

There is no structural analogy between glucagon and histamine on the one hand and glucagon and gastrin on the other. It is unlikely that glucagon acts competitively with either histamine or gastrin at their respective receptor sites. This is especially true for histamine.

The suppression of gastrin release by glucagon (12) is documented and effect of glucagon on the release of other gastrointestinal hormones needs further study.

In some respects the action of glucagon on gastric acid secretion resembles that of the sympathetic system. Lin et al. (147) reported that two β-blocking agents, propranolol and butoxamine, that augmented a steady-state response to pentagastrin, were unable to block the inhibitory action of glucagon. An α-adrenergic blocker, phenoxybenzamine, also failed to prevent the inhibitory action of glucagon.

Hirschowitz (78) and Hirschowitz and Robbin (83) reported a direct inhibitory action of insulin on histamine-stimulated acid secretion in the dog, and on H^+ transport in the guinea pig gastric mucosa *in vitro* (83). This inhibitory effect of insulin in the dog was reversed by slow infusion of potassium chloride (85). But the inhibitory action of glucagon on gastric secretion induced by histamine or gastrin derivatives was neither prevented by prior infusion nor reversed by infusion of KCl following glucagon inhibition (147). This indicates that the inhibitory action of glucagon is not the same as that of insulin.

In addition, glucagon has rather generalized actions on the electrolytes in the body. Its actions on the electrolytes on the small intestine (7), kidney (207), liver, and plasma have been documented. Given subcutaneously in a single injection, glucagon caused instantaneous rise of potassium level in the plasma followed by a gradual fall of both potassium and sodium concentrations in the blood (146). This coincided with diuresis and increased output of electrolytes in the urine. It is very likely that these effects of glucagon are interrelated, since the glucagon fragments that failed to inhibit gastric acid secretion were also devoid of hyperglycemic, diuretic, and hyperkalamic actions.

Question of Physiological Role

Thus far the studies of the inhibition of gastric secretion by glucagon have been pharmacological. Christiansen et al. (25) conducted a dose-response study of the interaction of glucagon and pentagastrin in man and found that the inhibition followed noncompetitive kinetics. Plasma concentrations of pancreatic glucagon in these subjects were comparable with concentrations seen after a protein meal. They infused L-arginine intravenously on a background acid secretion induced by synthetic human gastrin I, and found that arginine increased glucagon concentration to levels seen after a meal and resulted in a significant inhibition of acid secretion. These results favor the view that glucagon may play a physiological role in the regulation of gastric secretion.

External Pancreatic Secretion

In most of the studies *in vivo,* glucagon inhibited pancreatic secretion in the dog (48,97,122,166,167,198,213), cat (122), rat (194), and man (49,58,236). One study (164) showed that glucagon increased the volume and enzyme secretion of a totally isolated canine pancreas stimulated by secretin and CCK. In another study (194) the basal volume, bicarbonate, and protein outputs were all inhibited but the secretion during feeding was increased by glucagon.

The inhibitory effect was first observed by Necheles (167) in nembutalized dogs stimulated by continuous intravenous infusion of secretin, and later, in conscious dogs by Dyck et al. (48), Sweating (213), Nakajima and Magee (166) and others in dogs with chronic pancreatic and gastric fistulae. Studies in man (49,58,236) and in the dog were all conducted under steady-state condition in which pancreatic secretion was stimulated by continuous infusion of secretin or CCK or both, or by constant induction of endogenous secretin release (213).

The inhibitory effect was characterized by reduction of volume, bicarbonate output, and enzyme secretion. Dyck et al. (48) remarked that inhibition of enzyme output was greater than was inhibition of volume and bicarbonate secretion. Nakajima and Magee (166) found dose-related inhibition of pancreatic secretion by glucagon and an inverse relationship between blood sugar level and enzyme output. But the slopes of the dose-response inhibition by glucagon for amylase, lipase, and trypsin were not parallel to each other.

Dose-response inhibition studied by Konturek et al. (122) showed that the inhibition of CCK-induced pancreatic secretion by glucagon was competitive. This remains to be further elucidated. Pancreatic secretion stimulated by endogenous release of secretin or CCK was also inhibited by glucagon. Konturek et al. (122) induced pancreatic secretion in cats with peptone and also by duodenal acidification. Singer et al. (198) did the test with test meal in the dog. In the latter study glucagon inhibited bicarbonate and protein secretion in a dose-dependent manner. Intrajejunal infusion of glucose was found by Dyck (46) to decrease pancreatic volume and bicarbonate outputs; this was probably due to the release of pancreatic glucagon and also glucagon-like substance from the small intestine. However, the effect of glucagon-like substance alone has not been studied.

The mechanism by which glucagon inhibits pancreatic secretion is unknown. On pancreatic slices *in vitro,* glucagon had no effect on the adenylate cyclase (cyclic AMP) activity; nor did it alter the stimulatory effect of VIP or secretin on adenylate cyclase (36,118).

The stimulatory action of gastrin on pancreatic secretion was reported by Gregory and Tracy (71) and that of the C-terminal penta-, tetra-, and tripeptides of gastrin was reported by Lin and co-workers (153). Glucagon was found to suppress basal gastrin level and gastrin release by a meal (12) or bombesin (10). The lack of suppression of secretin release by glucagon was reported (161). It is possible that the suppression of gastrointestinal hormone release may play a role in this inhibitory action. However, in patients with Zollinger-Ellison syndrome, glucagon caused an immediate rise in basal gastrin levels (12).

Glucagon was reported to decrease the mucosal blood flow to the stomach (154) and increase the blood flow to the small intestine (184). What bearing may this increased blood flow to the small intestine have on pancreatic secretion remains to be studied. Necheles (167) mentioned that glucagon initially increased pancreatic secretion in the anesthetized dog. Lin et al. *(unpublished data)* found that small doses (1–5 μg/kg) of glucagon given as single intravenous injection or by infusion over a 10-min period, always increased the volume, bicarbonate, Na, K, Ca, Mg, and protein outputs significantly over and above the steady state secretion induced by secretin and CCK in the first 1 to 5 min after administration. This was followed by the inhibitory phase of secretion. This pattern of secretion was the same as that seen by Necheles. The reason for this observation remains to be studied.

Bile Secretion

The action of glucagon on bile secretion was studied in cholecystectomized dogs with duodenal fistula by Morris et al. (163). Direct collection of bile was made by Jones et al. (109,110) in cholecystectomized dogs with gastric and duodenal fistulae and ligation of the minor pancreatic duct. In the first study glucagon increased bile flow by two- to threefold and augmented the bile salt and electrolyte outputs within 15 min after glucagon administration. In the second study glucagon increased the bile flow and chloride concentration with no effect on bicarbonate concentration; there was a decrease in concentration of the bile salt.

Dyck and Janowitz (47) reported that glucagon augmented the rate of bile flow without altering the composition of hepatic bile in cholecystectomized subjects. Kuska (123) saw brief choleretic action of glucagon in man.

Although in some studies the effect of glucagon was negative, in man (133) or in isolated liver preparation (176), most authors agreed on a choleretic effect of glucagon. In dose-response studies with secretin and glucagon, Jones et al. (109,110) and Kaminski et al. (115,116) found that the calculated maximal responses produced by secretin and glucagon were the same, but the calculated D_{50}s were different. Secretin was about five times as potent as glucagon on a molar basis (109,110). Kinetic studies (115,116) indicated that the inhibition of secretin-induced bile secretion by glucagon was noncompetitive. This suggests that glucagon and secretin do not share the same receptor site for producing bile flow.

Little is known about the mechanism of the choleretic action of glucagon. The stimulatory effect of glucagon on the adenylate cyclase activity is well known (212), and dibutyl cyclic AMP was reported to increase bile flow, bile salts, and electrolyte outputs in the bile of the dog (133). Shoemaker and Van Itallie (197) and Morris et al. (163) showed that the hepatic blood flow was increased by glucagon. The relationship between hepatic blood flow and bile secretion under the influence of glucagon deserves further attention.

REFERENCES

1. Alphin, R. S., and Lin, T.-M. (1959): Effect of sham feeding on pancreatic secretion in the rat. *Am. J. Physiol.,* 197:260–262.
2. Alphin, R. S., and Lin, T.-M. (1959): Preparation of chronic denervated gastric pouches in the rat. *Am. J. Physiol.,* 197:257–259.
3. Ayelett, P. (1962): The effect of glucagon and glucagon-free insulin upon gastric secretion in peptic ulcer patients. *Clin. Sci.,* 22:179–184.
4. Babkin, B. P. (1938): The triple mechanism of the chemical phase of gastric secretion. *Am. J. Dig. Dis.,* 5:467–472.
5. Babkin, B. P. (1944): *Secretory Mechanism of the Digestive Glands.* Paul B. Hoeber, New York.
6. Banting, F. G., Best, C. H., Collip, J. B., Hepburn, J., Macleod, J. J. R., and Noble, E. C. (1922): Physiological effects of insulin. III. Preparation of pancreatic extract containing insulin. *Trans. Roy. Soc. Can.,* 16 (sec V):1–18.
7. Barbezat, G., and Grossman, M. I. (1971): Stimulation of intestinal secretion by peptide hormones. *Science,* 174:422–424.
8. Baron, J. H. (1970): Dose response relationships of insulin hypoglycemia and gastric acid in man. *Gut,* II:826–836.
9. Baron, J. H., Cowley, D. J., Gutierrez, L. V., Iweze, F. I., Spencer, J., and Tinker, J. (1972): Dose-response of gastric acid to insulin in patients with duodenal ulcer. *Gastroenterology,* 62:203–206.
10. Basso, N., Giri, S., Lezoche, E., Materide, A., Materia, A., Melchiorri, P., and Speranza, V. (1976): Effect of secretin, glucagon, and duodenal acidification on bombesin-induced hypergastrinemia in man. *Am. J. Gastroenterol.,* 66(5):448–451.
11. Baxter, S. G.: Blood sugar concentration and pancreatic secretion in the rabbit. *Q. J. Exp. Physiol.,* 21:355–363.
12. Becker, H. D., Reeder, D. D., Lermon, M., and Thompson, J. C. (1973): Effect of glucagon on circulating gastrin. *Gastroenterology,* 65:28–35.
13. Birnbaum, D., Hollander, F., and Weinstein, V. A. (1960): Consistency of gastric acidity with variable secretory rates induced by insulin or glucagon, and histamine. *Proc. Soc. Exp. Biol. Med.,* 105:120–122.
14. Boldyreff, E. B., and Stewart, J. (1932): A study of gastric secretion caused by insulin. *J. Pharmacol. Exp. Ther.,* 46:419–429.
15. Bromer, W. W., Sinn, L. G., and Behrens, O. K. (1957): The amino acid sequence of glucagon. *Diabetes,* 6:234–238.
16. Brooks, A. M., Isenberg, J., and Grossman, M. I. (1969): The effect of secretin, glucagon, and duodenal acidification on pepsin secretion in man. *Gastroenterology,* 57:159–162.
17. Brugsch, T., and Horster, N. (1924): Uber die Leber als Auscheidungsorgan und uber die Wirkung der Cholerectica, insebsondere des Arophans. *Med. Klin.,* 20:661.
18. Brugsch, T., and Horster, H. (1924): A contribution to the physiology of the bile. II. Hyper- and hypo-bile secretion. *Ztschr. Ges. Exp. Med.,* 43:514–538.
19. Burhole, P. G. (1974): Effect of cholecystokinin, secretin, 2-desoxy-D-glucose and insulin on pentagastrin stimulated gastric secretion in fistula chickens. *Scand. J. Gastroenterol.,* 9(1):55–58.
20. Cascao De Anciaes, J. H. (1926): Insulin and gastric functions. *Compt. Rend. Soc. Biol.,* 95:1258–1260.
21. Cascao De Anciaes, J. H. (1928): Insulin und Magenfunktion. *Arch. Verdauungskr.,* 42:377–382.
22. Cascao De Anciaes, J. H. (1931): Insuline, pituitrine et secretion gastrique. *Compt. Rend. Soc. Biol.,* 95:313–315.

23. Chen, K. K., Fleming, W. J., and Lin, T.-M. (1961): Action of hypoglycin A on Blood sugar, gastric secretion and adipose tissue. *Arch. Int. Pharmacodyn. Ther.,* 134:435–446.
24. Christiansen, J., and Hendle, L. (1974): The effect of glucagon on pentagastrin induced gastric secretion of sodium, potassium and calcium in man. *Scand. J. Gastroenterol.,* 9(5):437–440.
25. Christiansen, J., Holst, J. J., and Kalaja, E. (1976): Inhibition of gastric acid secretion in man by exogenous and endogenous pancreatic glucagon. *Gastroenterology,* 70:688–692.
26. Clarke, S. D., Neill, D. W., and Welbourn, R. B. (1960): Effect of glucagon on gastric secretion in the dog. *Gut,* 1:146.
27. Cohen, N., Mazure, P., Dreiling, D. A., and Janowitz, H. D. (1960): Effect of glucagon on histamine stimulated gastric secretion in man. *Gastroenterology,* 39:48–54.
28. Collazo, J. A., and Dobreff, M. (1924): Experimentelle Untersuchungen Über die Wirkung des Insulins auf die aüsere Sekretion der Verdauungsdrüsen. I. Insulinwirkung auf die Sekretion des Magensaftes. *Biochem. Zeitschr.,* 154:349–363.
29. Collazo, J. A., and Dobreff, M. (1924): Insulinwirkung auf die Absonderung der Verdauungssafte. *Klin. Wochenschr.,* 3:1226–1229.
30. Collazo, J. S., and Dobreff, M. (1925): Action of insulin upon the external secretion of the digestive glands. III. Effects upon outer secretion of the pancreas. *Biochem. Zeitschr.,* 165:352–357.
31. Cooke, A. R. (1969): Acid and pepsin secretion in response to endogenous and exogenous cholinergic stimulation and pentapeptide, bethanechol chloride, 2-deoxy-D-glucose in the dog. *Aust. J. Exp. Med. Sci.,* 47:197–202.
32. Corral-Selata, J. M. (1960): Inhibitory action of insulin on the acid secretion of the stomach. *Rev. Espan. Fisiol.,* 16:165–174.
33. Cowley, D. J., and Baron, J. H. (1973): Insulin stimulated gastric acid secretion after vagotomy in man: A dose response study. *Am. J. Dig. Dis.,* 18(7):544–550.
34. Csendes, A., Walsh, J. H., and Grossman, M. I. (1971): Effects of atropine and antral acidification on gastrin release and acid secretion in response to insulin and feeding in dogs. *Gastroenterology,* 60:16–21.
35. Debray, C., De La Tour, J., Roze, C., Souchard, M., and Vaille, C. (1975): Independence from vagal control of biliary secretion in the rat. *Digestion,* 10:413–422.
36. Deschodt-Lankmann, M., Robberecht, P., De Nuf, P., Labbrie, F., and Christophe, J. (1975): *In vitro* interactions of gastrointestinal hormones on cyclic AMP levels and amylase output. *Gastroenterology,* 68:318–325.
37. Deustsch, G., and Drost, E. (1927): Uber Bezieungen zwischen der inneren und aüsseren Sekretion des Pankreas. *Klin. Wochenschr.,* 6:2180–2182.
38. Dobreff, M. (1924): Experimentelle Untersuchungen uber die Wirkung des Insulins auf die aüsere Sekretion der Verdauungsdrüsen: II. Uber den Einfluss des Insulins auf die Gallenabsonderungsfähigheit. *Biochem. Zeitschr.,* 154:364–375.
39. Dobreff, M. (1931): Weitere Untersuchungen uber Insulin und Magensekretion. *Arch. Verdauungskr.,* 1:157–170.
40. Dotevall, G., and Westling, H. (1960): On the effect of glucagon on histamine-induced and spontaneous gastric acid secretion in man. *Scand. J. Clin. Lab. Invest.,* 12:489–492.
41. Dozois, R. R., Carter, D. C., and Kirpatrick, J. R. (1973): Gastric secretory response to continuous insulin infusion in the dog. *Br. J. Surg.,* 60(4):311.
42. Dragstedt, L. R. (1942): Pathogenesis of gastroduodenal ulcer. *Arch. Surg.,* 44:438–451.
43. Dreiling, D. A., Druckerman, L. J., and Hollander, F. (1952): The effect of complete vagisection and vagal stimulation on pancreatic secretion in man. *Gastroenterology,* 20:578–586.
44. Dreiling, D. A., and Hollander, F. (1950): Studies in pancreatic secretion. II. Statistical study of pancreatic secretion following secretion in patients without pancreatic disease. *Gastroenterology,* 15:620–627.
45. Duke, W. W., Hirschowitz, B. I., and Sachs, G. (1965): Vagal stimulation of gastric secretion in man by 2-deoxy-D-glucose. *Lancet,* ii:871–878.
46. Dyck, W. P. (1971): Influence of intra-jejunal glucose on pancreatic exocrine function in man. *Gastroenterology,* 60:864–869.
47. Dyck, W. P., and Janowitz, H. D. (1971): Effect of glucagon on hepatic secretion. *Gastroenterology,* 60:400–404.
48. Dyck, W. P., Rudick, J., Hoexter, B., and Janowitz, H. D. (1969): Influence of glucagon on pancreatic exocrine secretion. *Gastroenterology,* 56:531–537.

49. Dyck, W. P., Texter, E. C., Lasater, J. M., and Hightower, N. C. (1970): Influence of glucagon on pancreatic exocrine secretion in man. *Gastroenterology,* 58:532–539.

50. Earle, A. S., Cahill, G. F., and Hoar, C. S. (1957): Studies on the relationship of glucagon (HGF) to blood pepsinogen concentrations. *Ann. Surg.,* 146:124–130.

51. Eisenberg, M. M., Emas, G. S., and Grossman, M. I. (1966): Comparison of the effect of 2-deoxy-D-glucose and insulin on gastric acid secretion in dogs. *Surgery,* 60:111–117.

52. Eisenberg, M. M., Woodward, E. R., Quintana, R., and Dragstaedt, L. R. (1963): Insulin inhibition of gastric secretion. *J. Surg. Res.,* 3:470–484.

53. Emas, S., and Borg, I. (1972): Stimulation of gastric acid secretion by insulin and 2-deoxy-D-glucose in duodenal ulcer patients. *Digestion,* 7:44–53.

54. Emas, S., Vagne, M., and Grossman, M. I. (1969): Heidenhain pouch response to antral stimulation before and after antral denervation in dogs. *Proc. Soc. Exp. Biol. Med.,* 132:1162–1166.

55. Fonseca, F., and De Carvalho, A. (1926): Action del'insuline sur la secrétion. *Compt. Rend. Soc. Biol.,* 95:1262.

56. Fonseca, F., and De Carvalho, A. (1927): Sur le mecanisme de l'action de l'insuline sur la secretion gastrique. *Compt. Rend. Soc. Biol.,* 96:1327–1328.

57. Fonseca, F., and Trincao, C. (1928): Action de l'insuline sur la secretion du pancreas dans un cas de fistula. *Compt. Rend. Soc. Biol.,* 99:1532–1533.

58. Fontana, G., Costa, P. L., Tassari, R., and Labo, G. (1975): Effect of glucagon on pure human exocrine pancreatic secretion. *Am. J. Gastroenterol.,* 63:490–494.

59. Friedman, M. H. F., and Snape, W. J. (1949): Influence of secretin and insulin on pancreatic secretion in healthy human subjects. *Proc. Soc. Exp. Biol. Med.,* 70:280–282.

60. Frisk, A. R., and Welin, G. (1937): The external pancreatic secretion and the discharge of bile during hypoglycemia following intravenous administration of insulin. *Acta Med. Scand.,* 91:170–182.

61. Fritz, M. E., and Brooks, F. R. (1963): Control of bile flow in the cholecystectomized dog. *Am. J. Physiol.,* 204:825–828.

62. Ganguli, P. C., Hunter, W. M. (1972): Radioimmunoassay of gastrin in human plasma. *J. Physiol.,* 220(2):499–510.

63. Geist, R. E., and Jones, R. S. (1971): Effect of selective and truncal vagotomy on insulin-stimulated bile secretion in dogs. *Gastroenterology,* 60:566–571.

64. Glass, G. B. J. (1949): New physiological and clinical studies on the secretion of mucin in the human stomach. *Rev. Gastroenterol.,* 16:687.

65. Glass, G. B. J., and Boyd, L. J. (1949): The three main components of human gastric mucin; dissolved mucoproteose, dissolved mucoprotein, and mucoid of the gastric mucus. Part I. Differentiation, some physical and chemical characteristics; classification. *Gastroenterology,* 12:821–834.

66. Glass, G. B. J., and Boyd, L. J. (1949): Part II. Method for separation and quantitative determination of each mucous component of the gastric content. *Gastroenterology,* 12:835–848.

67. Glass, G. B. J., and Boyd, L. J. (1949): Part III. Preliminary data on physiological and clinical significance of separate quantitative determination of the dissolved mucoproteose and dissolved mucoprotein in the gastric juice of man. *Gastroenterology,* 12:849–878.

68. Glass, J. B. and Boyd, L. J. (1950): Patterns of response of gastric mucoprotein and acid to insulin: correlation with the underlying disease in the non-operated stomach of man. *Gastroenterology,* 15:438–453.

69. Glass, G. B. J., Boyd, L. J., and Drekter, I. J. (1952): Studies on the non-parietal componenent of gastric secretion in humans. *Gastroenterology,* 20:430–441.

70. Glass, G. B. J., Pugh, B. L., and Wolf, S. (1949–1950): Correlation of acid, pepsin, and mucoprotein secretion by human gastric glands. *Gastroenterology,* 2:571–579.

70a. Glass, G. B. J., and Wolf, S. (1950): Hormonal mechanisms in nervous mechanism of gastric acid secretion in humans. *Proc. Soc. Exp. Biol. Med.,* 73:535–537.

71. Gregory, R. A., and Tracy, H. J. (1964): Constitution and properties of the two gastrins extracted from the hog antral mucosa. *Gut,* 5:103–117.

72. Grimson, K. S., Taylor, H. M., Trent, J. C. et al. (1946): The effect of transthoracic vagotomy upon the function of the stomach and upon the early clinical course of patients with peptic ulcer. *South Med. J.*, 39:460–472.
73. Grossman, M. I. (1967): Neural and new hormonal stimulation of gastric secretion of acid. In: *Handbook of Physiology, sec. 6: Alimentary Canal, Vol. 2.*, Am. Physiol. Soc., pp. 853–863.
74. Hansky, J., Soveny, C., and Korman, M. G. (1972): Role of vagus in insulin-mediated gastrin release. *Gastroenterology*, 63:387–391.
75. Hebb, C. (1936–1937): The effect of insulin administration on the response of the pancreas to parasympathetic stimulation. *Q. J. Exp. Physiol.*, 26:339–354.
76. Handle, L., Jorgensen, S. P., Christiansen, J., and Henriksen, F. W. (1976): Combined effect of glucagon and cholecystokinin on gastric secretion in man. *Scand. J. Gastroenterol. (Suppl.)*, 11:43–46.
77. Hiles, C. H. (1947): Gastric secretory response in hypoglycemia as produced during insulin shock therapy. *Am. J. Med. Sci.*, 214:667–672.
78. Hirschowitz, B. I. (1966): Quantitation of inhibition of gastric electrolyte secretion by insulin in the dog. *Am. J. Dig. Dis.*, 11:173–182.
79. Hirschowitz, B. I. (1966): Characteristics of inhibition of gastric electrolyte secretion by insulin. *Am. J. Dig. Dis.*, 11:182–198.
80. Hirschowitz, B. I. (1967): Continuing gastric secretion after insulin hypoglycemia despite glucose injection. *Am. J. Dig. Dis.*, 12:19–25.
81. Hirschowitz, B. I., and O'Leary, D. K. (1964): Gastric secretion patterns in fistula dogs with varying doses of insulin. *Fed. Proc.*, 22:342 (Abstr.).
82. Hirschowitz, B. I., and O'Leary, D. K. (1964): Dose-response of insulin-stimulated gastric secretion. *Am. J. Dig. Dis.*, 9:379–397.
83. Hirschowitz, B. I., and Robbins, R. C. (1966): Direct inhibition of gastric electrolyte secretion by insulin, independent of hypoglycemia or the vagus. *Am. J. Dig. Dis.*, 11:199–212.
84. Hirschowitz, B. I., and Sachs, G. (1965): Vagal gastric secretory stimulation by 2-deoxy-D-glucose. *Am. J. Physiol.*, 209:452–460.
85. Hirschowitz, B. I., and Sachs, G. (1966): Reversal of insulin inhibition of gastric secretion by intravenous injection of potassium. *Am. J. Dig. Dis.*, 11:217–230.
86. Hirschowitz, B. I., and Sachs, G. (1967): Insulin effects on gastric secretion and blood electrolytes modified by injected potassium. *Am. J. Dig. Dis.*, 12:7–18.
87. Hirschowitz, B. I., and Sachs, G. (1969): Atropine inhibition of insulin, histamine-, and pentagastrin-stimulated electrolyte and pepsin secretion in the dog. *Gastroenterology*, 56:693–702.
88. Hofstein, J. (1933): Action de l'insuline sur la secretion gastrique. Arch. d. Mal. de l'Appar. *Digestif.*, 23:808–826.
89. Hollander, F. (1946): The insulin test for the presence of intact nerve fibers after vagal operations for peptic ulcer. *Gastroenterology*, 7:607–614.
90. Hollander, F. (1948): Laboratory procedure in the study of vagotomy (with particular reference to the insulin test). *Gastroenterology*, 2:419–425.
91. Hollander, F., and Jemerin, E. E. (1938): Preparation of stomach pouch without interruption of vagal supply. *Proc. Soc. Exp. Biol. Med.*, 39:87–90.
92. Hughes, W., and Green, N. (1974): Dose dependence of insulin stimulated gastrin release in the dog. *Gastroenterology*, 66:846 (Abstr.).
93. Ihre, B. (1938): Human gastric secretion: A quantitative study of gastric secretion in normal and pathological conditions. *Acta Med. Scand. (Suppl.)*, 95:1–114.
94. Isenberg, J. I., Stenning, F., Pitcher, J. L., and Brooks, M. (1970): The effect of graded insulin doses on incompletely vagotomized subjects. *Gastroenterology*, 59:698–706.
95. Isenberg, J. I., Stenning, F., Ward, R., and Grossman, M. I. (1969): Relation of gastric secretory response in man to dose of insulin. *Gastroenterology*, 57:395–405.
96. Ivy, A. C., and Fisher, N. F. (1924): The presence of an insulin-like substance in gastric and duodenal mucosa and its relation to gastric secretion. *Am. J. Physiol.*, 157:445–450.
97. Iwatsuki, K., Ono, H., and Hashimoto, K. (1975): Effect of glucagon on pancreatic secretion in the dog. *Jpn. J. Pharmacol. (Suppl.)*, 25:44–45.
98. Jaffe, B. M., McGuigan, J. E., and Newton, W. T. (1970): Immunochemical measurement of vagal release of gastrin. *Surgery*, 68:196–201.
99. Jacobs, J. S. L., Tempereau, C. E., and West, P. M. (1952): The effect of insulin coma on uropepsin secretion. *Science*, 116:86–87.

100. Jacobson, E. D. (1962): The effect of insulin on gastric secretion of potassium. *Am. J. Dig. Dis.*, 7:1061–1065.
101. Jacobson, E. D., Linford, R. H., and Grossman, M. I. (1966): Gastric secretion in relation to mucosal blood flow studied by a clearance technique. *J. Clin. Invest.*, 45:1–13.
102. Jacobson, E. D., Swann, K. G., and Grossman. M. I. (1967): Blood flow and secretion in the stomach. *Gastroenterology,* 52:414–420.
103. Jemerin, E. E., and Hollander, F. (1938): Gastric vagi in the dog. Erroneous assumption of uninterrupted vagal innervation in the Pavlov pouch. *Proc. Soc. Exp. Biol. Med.*, 38:139–146.
104. Jemerin, E. E., Hollander, F., and Weinstein, V. A. (1943): A comparison of insulin and food as stimuli for the differentiation of vagal and nonvagal gastric pouches. *Gastroenterology,* 1:500–512.
105. Jogi, P., Strom, G., and Uvnas, B. (1949): The origin in the CNS of gastric secretory impulses induced by hypoglycemia. *Acta Physiol. Scand.*, 17:212–221.
106. Jones, R. S., and Brooks, F. P. (1965): The pyloric antrum as a mediator of insulin-induced choleresis. *Physiologist,* 8:202 (Abstr.).
107. Jones, R. S., and Brooks, F. P. (1967): Role of pyloric antrum in choleresis after insulin and feeding. *Am. J. Physiol.*, 213:1406–1408.
108. Jones, R. S., Geist, R. E., and Hall, A. D. (1970): Comparison of dose-response relation of insulin and 2-deoxy-D-glucose for biliary and gastric acid secretion in dogs. *Gastroenterology,* 59:665–670.
109. Jones, R. S., Geist, R. E., and Hall, A. D. (1970): Comparison of dose-response of insulin and 2-deoxy-D-glucose for biliary and gastric acid secretion in dogs. *Gastroenterology,* 58:1011 (Abstr.).
110. Jones, R. S., Geist, R. E., and Hall, A. D. (1971): The choleretic effect of glucagon and secretion in the dog. *Gastroenterology,* 60:64–68.
111. Jordan, P. H., and Quintana, R. (1964): Insulin inhibition of gastrin-stimulated gastric secretion. *Gastroenterology,* 47:617–625.
112. Jow, E., Webster, D. R., and Skoryna, S. C. (1960): Effect of glucagon and insulin on gastric secretion in rats. *Gastroenterology,* 38:732–739.
113. Kalk, H., and Meyer, P. F. (1932): Blutzuckerspiegel und Magensekretion. *Zeitschr. Klin. Med.*, 120:692–714.
114. Kaminski, D. L., Dorighi, J., and Jellinek, M. (1974): Effect of electrical vagal stimulation on canine hepatic bile flow. *Am. J. Physiol.*, 227:487–493.
115. Kaminski, D. L., Ruwart, M. J., and Jellinek, M. (1975): Effect of glucagon on secretin stimulated bile flow. *Am. J. Physiol.*, 229:1480–1485.
116. Kaminski, D. L., Ruwart, M. J., and Willman, V. L. (1975): The effect of glucagon on secretin stimulated bile flow. *Fed. Proc.*, 34(3):394 (Abstr.).
117. Karvinen, E., and Karvonen, M. J. (1953): The effect of insulin hypoglycemia on histamine-induced Heidenhain pouch secretion in the dog. *Acta Physiol. Scand.*, 27:350–370.
118. Klaeveman, H. L., Conlon, T. P. and Gardner, J. D. (1974): Effect of gastrointestinal hormones on adenyl cyclase activity in pancreatic exocrine cells. In: *Gastrointestinal Hormones, A Symposium,* edited by J. C. Thompson, pp. 321–344. Univ. of Texas Press, Galveston, Texas.
119. Kneller, A. W., and Nasset, E. S. (1948): Relationship of insulin hypoglycemia to intestinal secretion. *Am. J. Physiol.*, 159:89–93.
120. Konturek, S. J., Demitrescu, T., Radicki, T., Thor, P., and Pucher, A. (1974): Effect of glucagon on gastric and pancreatic secretion and peptic ulcer formation in cats. *Am. J. Dig. Dis.*, 19(6):557–564.
121. Konturek, S. J., Tasler, J., and Obtulowicz, W. (1973): Effect of glucagon on food induced gastrointestinal secretions. *Digestion,* 8(3):220–226.
122. Konturek, S. J., Tasler, V., and Obtulowicz, W. (1974): Characteristics of inhibition of pancreatic secretion by glucagon. *Digestion,* 10(2):138–149.
123. Kuska, J. (1974): Studies of bile secretion in man: Part 3. Influence of sodium dihydrocholate, a diuretic, and glucagon on bile secretion. *Arch. Immunol. Ther. Exp.*, 22(2):207–235.
124. La Barre, J., and De Cespedes, C. (1931): Les variations de la secretion gastrique au cours de L'hypoglycemie insulinique. *Compt. Rend. Soc. Biol.*, 106:480–482.
125. La Barre, J., De Cespedes, C. (1931): Le relevement brusque de la glycemie par injection de dextrose: Supreme-T-U L'exageration postinsulinique de la secretion gastrique? *Compt. Rend. Soc. Biol.*, 106:482–483.

126. La Barre, J., and De Cespedes, C. (1931): Sur L'origine parasympathetique de L'hypersecretion gastrique consecutive a l'administration d'insuline. *Compt. Rend. Soc. Biol.,* 106:484–486.
127. La Barre, J., and De Cespedes, C. (1931): Role of central nervous system in gastric hypersecretion. *Compt. Rend. Soc. Biol.,* 98:1237–1239.
128. La Barre, J., and Destree, P. (1928): Insuline et secretion externe du pancreas. *Compt. Rend. Soc. Biol.,* 98:1237–1239.
129. Lagerlöf H., and Welin, G. (1937): Pancreatic secretion after secretin during insulin hypoglycemia and after graded amounts of secretin. *Acta Med. Scand.,* 91:397–408.
130. Lam, S. K., and Sircus, W. (1977): Cholinergic inhibition and release of gastrin following insulin injection in duodenal ulcer before operation and after complete and incomplete vagotomy. *Am. J. Dig. Dis.,* 22(3):214–222.
131. Lambert, M., and Hermann, H. (1925): Insuline et suc pancreatique. *Compt. Rend. Soc. Biol.,* 92:43–44.
132. Lane, A., Ivy, A. C., and Ivy, E. K. (1957): Vagal gastric secretory nerves in the rat demonstrated with insulin. *Am. J. Physiol.,* 191:262–264.
133. Levin, R. A., and Hall, R. C. (1972): Role of cyclic AMP in bile and pancreatic secretion in man. *Gastroenterology,* 62(4):873, (Abstr.).
134. Levin, E., Kirsner, J. B., and Palmer, W. L. (1948): Preliminary observation on histamine and insulin stimulated gastric secretion during the injection of an enterogastrone concentrate in man. *Gastroenterology,* 10:274–280.
135. Lin, T.-M. (1973): Inhibition of meal-induced gastric acid secretion by glucagon. *Arch. Int. Pharmacodyn. Ther.,* 204:361–367.
136. Lin, T.-M., and Alphin, R. S. (1957): Cephalic phase of gastric secretion in the rat. *Fed. Proc.,* 10:81 (abstr.).
137. Lin, T.-M., and Alphin, R. S. (1958): Cephalic phase of gastric secretion in the rat. *Am. J. Physiol.,* 192:23–26.
138. Lin, T.-M., and Alphin, R. S. (1958): Inhibition of gastric secretion by glucagon and glucose in the dog. *Fed. Proc.,* 17:97 (Abstr.).
139. Lin, T.-M., and Alphin, R. S. (1959): Vagal secretory nerves for pancreatic secretion in the rat. *Am. J. Physiol.,* 197:555–557.
140. Lin, T.-M., and Benslay, D. N. (1962): Action of glucagon on gastrin-, insulin-, histamine-, and meal-stimulated HCl secretion. *Proc. Int. Union Physiologist,* II:383, *XXII International Congress of Physiological Science.* Leiden, Holland.
141. Lin, T.-M., and Benslay, D. N. (1965): Inhibitory effect of glucagon on gastric secretion. *XXIII. International Congress of Physiologic Sciences,* p. 208 (Abstr. 462).
142. Lin, T.-M., Benslay, D. N., and Evans, D. C. (1966): Effect of glucagon and glucagon fragments on gastric HCL secretion. *Fed. Proc.,* 25:513 (Abstr.).
43. Lin, T.-M., Benslay, D. N., and Tust, R. H. (1963): Further study of the effect of glucagon on meal-, histamine-, gastrin-, and sham-feeding induced gastric HCl secretion. *Physiologist,* 6:225.
144. Lin, T.-M., Chance, R. E., and Spray, G. F. (1974): Action of insulin and proinsulin on gastric acid secretion and blood sugar in conscious dogs. *Arch. Int. Pharmacodyn. Ther.,* 211:247–252.
145. Lin, T.-M., Evans, D. C., and Bromer, W. W. (1974): Structure function relation of glucagon for gastric inhibition. *Gastroenterology,* 66:A198/852.
146. Lin, T.-M., Evans, D. C., and Spray, G. F. (1973): Action of glucagon on electrolyte changes in the stomach, kidney, and blood of dogs stimulated by pentagastrin or histamine. *Arch. Int. Pharmacodyn. Ther.,* 202:304–313.
147. Lin, T.-M., Evans, D. C., and Spray, G. F. (1973): Mechanism studies of gastric inhibition by glucagon: Failure of KCl and adrenergic blocking agents to prevent its action. *Arch. Int. Pharmacodyn. Ther.,* 202:314–324.
148. Lin, T.-M., and Grossman, M. I. (1956): Dose response relationship of pancreatic enzyme stimulants: Pancreozymin and methacholine. *Am. J. Physiol.,* 186:52–55.
149. Lin, T.-M., and Ivy, A. C. (1957): Relation of secretin to parasympathetic mechanism for pancreatic secretion. *Am. J. Physiol.,* 189:361–368.
150. Lin, T.-M., and Spray, G. F. (1968): Effect of glucagon on gastric HCl secretion. *Gastroenterology,* 54:1254 (Abstr.).
151. Lin, T.-M., and Spray, G. F. (1971): Inhibitory effect of glucagon on gastric acid secretion

induced by gastrin and its derivatives in dogs and rats. *Arch. Int. Pharmacodyn. Ther.,* 191:88–95.

152. Lin, T.-M., Spray, G. F., and Benslay, D. N. (1970): Action of glucagon on histamine-induced gastric acid secretion in dogs and rats. *Arch. Int. Pharmacodyn. Ther.,* 188:332–340.
153. Lin, T.-M., Spray, G. F., and Evans, °D. C. (1975): Stimulation of gastric and pancreatic secretion by the C-terminal peptides of gastrin. *Physiologist,* 18:292 (Abstr.).
154. Lin, T.-M., and Warrick, M. W. (1971): Effect of glucagon on pentagastrin-induced gastric acid secretion and mucosal blood flow. *Gastroenterology,* 61:328–331.
155. Lin, T.-M., and Warrick, M. W. (1978): Inhibition of histamine and pentagastrin stimulated gastric acid secretion from the isolated stomach of *Rana catesbiana. (unpublished study).*
156. Long, C. N. H., and Fry, F. G. (1945): Effect of epinephrine on adrenal cholesterol and ascorbic acid. *Proc. Soc. Exp. Biol. Med.,* 59:67–70.
157. Lunbosch, J. M., DeGraff, J., and Gerard, A. (1971): Effect of insulin on acid and pepsin secretion in vagotomized and non-vagotomized patients already stimulated by pentagastrin. *Scand. J. Gastroenterol.,* 6(2):183–188.
158. Meiderer, S. E., Deghle, P., and Stadelman, O. (1971): Influence of glucagon and secretin on the gastric secretion of man which is stimulated by methyl xanthine theophylline. *Med. Welt,* 6:209–211.
159. Melrose, A. G. (1960): Effect of glucagon on gastric secretion in man. *Gut,* 1:142–145.
160. Meyer, P. F. (1930): Uber die Wirkung des Insulins auf die Magensekretion. *Klin. Wochenschr.,* 9:1578–1581.
161. Miller, T. A., Watson, L. C., Rayford, P. L., and Thompson, J. C. (1977): The effect of glucagon on pancreatic secretion and plasma secretin in dogs. *USA World J. Surg.,* 1:93–98.
162. Moore, F. D., Chapman, W. P., Schulz, M. D., and Jones, C. M. (1946): Transdiaphragmatic resection of the vagus nerves for peptic ulcer. *N. Engl. J. Med.,* 234:241–251.
163. Morris, T. Q., Sardi, G. F., and Bradley, S. E. (1967): Character of glucagon induced choleresis. *Fed. Proc.,* 26:774 (Abstr.).
164. Murphy, J. J., and McGeeney, K. F. (1974): The effect of glucagon on the exocrine secretion of the perfused canine pancreas. *Irish J. Med. Sci.,* 143:37–41.
165. Nahrwold, D. L., Cooke, A. R., and Grossman, M. I. (1967): Choleresis induced by stimulation of gastric antrum. *Gastroenterology,* 52:18–22.
166. Nakajima, S. D., and Magee, D. F. (1970): Inhibition of exocrine pancreatic secretion by glucagon and D-glucose given intravenously. *Can. J. Physiol. Pharmacol.,* 48:299–305.
167. Necheles, H. (1957): Effect of glucagon on external secretion of the pancreas. *Am. J. Physiol.,* 191:595–597.
168. Necheles, H., Olson, W. H., and Scruggs, W. (1942): Effect of insulin on gastric secretion. *Fed. Proc.,* 1:62 (Abstr.).
169. Nilsson, G., Simon, J., Yalow, R. S. (1972): Plasma gastrin and gastric acid response to sham feeding and feeding in dogs. *Gastroenterology,* 63:51–59.
170. Nitzescu, I. I. (1926): L'insuline et la secretion biliaire. *Compt. Rend. Soc. Biol.,* 95:773.
171. Nundy, S., and Baron, J. H. (1974): Graded vagotomy and gastric secretion. *Am. J. Dig. Dis.,* 19(2):137–142.
172. Oberhelman, H. A., Woodward, E. R., Smith, C. A., and Dragstedt, L. E. (1951): Effect of sympathectomy on gastric secretion in total pouch dogs. *Am. J. Physiol.,* 166:679–685.
173. Okada, S. K., Kuramouchi, T., Tsukahara, T., and Ooinoue, T. (1929): The humoral regulation of the gastric, pancreatic and biliary secretion. *Arch. Int. Med.,* 43:446–471.
174. Okada, S. I., Kuramouchi, T., Tsukahara, T., and Ooinoue, T. (1930): Secretory mechanisms of the digestive juices. *Arch. Int. Med.,* 45:783–813.
175. Ornsholt, J., Brandsborg, O., Brandsborg, M., Lovegreen, A., and Andrup, E. (1977): The influence of atropine on insulin and 2-deoxy-D-glucose-induced acid secretion and gastrin release. *Surg. Res.,* 23(4):246–250.
176. Pessidis, A. C., Bombeck, C. T., Merchant, F., and Nyhus, L. M. (1969): Hormonal regulation of bile secretion: A study in the isolated perfused liver. *Surgery,* 66:1075–1084.
177. Pethein, M., and Schofield, B. (1959): Release of gastrin from the pyloric antrum following vagal stimulation by sham feeding in dogs. *J. Physiol.,* 148:291–305.
178. Popesco, M., and Diculesco, G. (1927): L'action de l'insuline sur la secretion de l'estomac en l'etat normal et pathologique. *Arch. Mal. App. Dig.,* 57:28–43. (from Boldyreff and Stewart.)
179. Quigley, J. P. (1929): Action of insulin on gastric motility of man. *Proc. Soc. Exp. Biol. Med.,* 26:769–770.

180. Quigley, J. P., and Templeton, R. D. (1930): Action of insulin on the motility of the gastrointestinal tract. III a. Action on the pyloric pouch. b. Action on the stomach following double sympathectomy. *Am. J. Physiol.,* 91:482–487.

181. Richardson, C. T., Walsh, J. H., and Cooper, K. A. (1977): Studies on the role of cephalic vagal stimulation in acid secretory response to eating in normal human subjects. *J. Clin. Invest.,* 60(2):435–441.

182. Robinson, R. M., Harris, K., Hlad, C. J., and Eiseman, B. (1957): Effect of glucagon on gastric secretion. *Proc. Soc. Exp. Biol. Med.,* 96:518–520.

183. Roholm, K. (1930): Clinical investigations into effect of intravenous injections of insulin: Gastric secretion in normal individuals. *Acta Med. Scand.,* 73:472–492.

184. Ross, G. (1970): Regional circulatory effects of pancreatic glucagon. *Br. J. Pharmacol.,* 38:735–742.

185. Ross, B., and Kay, A. W. (1964): The insulin test after vagotomy. *Gastroenterology,* 46:379–386.

186. Ruoff, H. J. (1971): The influence of atropine, insulin and 2-deoxy-D-glucose on histamine and pentagastrin stimulated gastric acid secretion in chickens. *Arch. Pharmakol. (Suppl.),* 270:118.

187. Ruoff, H. J., and Sewing, K. F. (1973): Inhibition of gastric acid secretion in chicken by atropine, insulin, and 2-deoxy-D-glucose. *Arch. Pharmakol.,* 273:219–229.

188. Sachs, G., Shoemaker, R., and Hirschowitz, B. I. (1965): Action of 2-deoxy-D-glucose on frog gastric mucosa. *Am. J. Physiol.,* 209:461–466.

189. Saemundsson, J. (1948): Potassium concentration in human gastric juice. *Acta Med. Scand. (Suppl.),* 208:130–139.

190. Sakurai, E. (1926): Experimentelle Untersuchungen uber den Einfluss von Insulin etc., auf die Gallensekretion. *Proc. Imp. Acad.,* 2:185.

191. Schiffrin, M. J., and Ivy, A. C. (1942): Physiology of gastric secretion, particularly as related to the ulcer problem. *Arch. Surg.,* 44:399–414.

192. Schoen, A. M., and Griswold, R. A. (1947): The effect of vagotomy on human gastric function. *Ann. Surg.,* 126:655–663.

193. Schrumpf, E., and Vatn, M. H. (1974): Effect of atropine on insulin stimulated gastrin release and gastric secretion of acid. *Scand. J. Gastroenterology,* 9:665–669.

194. Shaw, H. M., and Heath, T. J. (1973): The effect of glucagon on the formation of pancreatic juice and bile in the rat. *Can. J. Physiol. Pharmacol.,* 51:1–5.

195. Shay, H. (1954): Stress and gastric secretion in man. I. A. study of the mechanism involved in insulin hypoglycemia. *Am. J. Med. Sci.,* 228:630–642.

196. Shingleton, W., Blake, F., and Vitter, J. S. (1950): Pancreatic secretion and response to secretin after vagotomy and sympathectomy. *Fed. Proc.,* 9:315 (Abstr.).

197. Shoemaker, W. C., and Van Itallie, J. (1960): The hepatic response to glucagon in unanesthetized dog. *Endocrinology,* 66:260–268.

198. Singer, M. V., Tiscornia, O. M., De Oliveiro, J. P. M., Demol, O., Levesque, D., and Sarles, H. (1978): Effect of glucagon on canine exocrine pancreatic secretion stimulated by a test meal. *Can. J. Physiol. Pharmacol.,* 56(1):1–6.

199. Smith, C. A., Woodward, E. R., Janes C. W. and Dragstedt, L. R. (1950): The effect of banthine on gastric secretion in man and experimental animals. *Gastroenterology,* 15:718–726.

200. Smith, I. S., Gillespie, G., Elder, J. B., Gillespie, I. E., and Kay, A. W. (1972): Time of conversion of insulin response after vagotomy. *Gastroenterology,* 62:912–917.

201. Solomon, S. P., and Spiro, H. M. (1959): The effect of glucagon and glucose on the human stomach. *Am. J. Dig. Dis.,* 4:775–786.

202. Spencer, J., and Grossman, M. I. (1971): The gastric secretory response to insulin: an "all or none" phenomenon? *Gut,* 12:891–896.

203. Stadil, F., and Rehfeld, J. F. (1972): Hypoglycemic release of gastrin in man. *Scand. J. Gastroenterol.,* 7:509–574.

204. Stadil, F., and Rehfeld, J. F. (1973): Release of gastrin by epinephrine in man. *Gastroenterology,* 65:210–215.

205. Stadil, F., and Rehfeld, J. F. (1974): Gastrin response to insulin after selective, highly selective and truncal vagotomy. *Gastroenterology,* 66:7–15.

206. Staub, A., Sinn, L. G., and Behrens, O. K. (1953): Purification and crystallization of hyperglycemic glycogenolytic factor (HGF). *Science,* 117:628–629.

207. Staub, A., Spring, V., Stoll, F., and Elrick, H. (1957): A renal action of glucagon. *Proc. Soc. Exp. Biol. Med.,* 94:57–60.
208. Stein, I. F. Jr., and Meyer, K. A. (1948): Studies on vagotomy in treatment of peptic ulcer; use of insulin in testing for completeness of vagotomy. *Surg. Gynecol. Obstet.,* 86:473–479.
209. Stein, I. F., and Meyer, K. A. (1948): Vagotomy in the treatment of peptic ulcer. Physiological aspects. *Surg. Gynecol. Obstet.,* 87:188–196.
210. Stenning, F. W., and Isenberg, J. I. (1969): Insulin induced acid secretion after partial vagotomy in dogs. *Am. J. Physiol.,* 217:962–964.
211. Strom, G., and Uvnas, B. (1948): The effect of atropine, scopolamine and some related synthetic drugs on the insulin-induced gastric secretion of the dog. *Acta Physiol. Scand.,* 15:6–9.
212. Sutherland, E. W. (1951): The effect of the hyperglycemic factor and epinephrine on enzyme systems of liver and muscle. *Ann. NY Acad. Sci.,* 54:693–706.
213. Sweeting, J. G. (1968): The effect of glucagon on bile and pancreatic juice. *Gastroenterology,* 54:1276 (Abstr.).
214. Szafran, H., Popiela, T., and Szafran, Z. (1971): The effect of 2-deoxy-D-glucose and insulin stimulation on the secretion of gastric lipase. *Scand. J. Gastroenterol.,* 6:55–58.
215. Tanturi, C. A., and Ivy, A. C. (1938): On the existence of secretory nerves in the vagi for and the reflex excitation and inhibition of bile secretion. *Am. J. Physiol.,* 121:270–283.
216. Templeton, R. D., and Quigley, J. P. (1929–1930): The action of insulin on the motility of the gastrointestinal tract. II. Action on the Heidenhain pouch. *Am. J. Physiol.,* 91:467–474.
217. Tepperman, B. L., Walsh, J. H., and Preshaw, R. M. (1972): Effect of antral denervation on gastrin release by sham feeding and insulin hypoglycemia in dogs. *Gastroenterology,* 63:973–980.
218. Thomas, J. E., and Crider, J. O. (1947): Changes in concentration of enzymes in pancreatic juice after giving insulin. *Proc. Soc. Exp. Biol. Med.,* 64:27–31.
219. Thonton, D. B., Soloway, R. D., Senior, J. R., and Brooks, F. P. (1969): A comparison of choleretic effects of secretin and insulin. *Physiologist,* 12:374 (Abstr.).
220. Thornton, T. F., Storer, E. H., and Dragstedt, L. R. (1946): Supradiaphragmatic section of vagus nerves. *JAMA,* 130:764–771.
221. Uvnas, B., Emas, S., Fyro, B., and Sjodin, L. (1966): The interaction between vagal impulses and gastrin in the control of gastric secretion. *Am. J. Dig. Dis.,* 11:103–112.
222. Villaret, M., and Justin-Besancon, L. (1925): Clinical and physiologic study of pancreatic fistula. *Arch. Mal. App. Dig.,* 15:751–767.
223. Von Heimburg, R. L., and Hollenbeck, G. A. (1964): Inhibition of gastric secretion in dogs by glucagon given intraportally. *Gastroenterology,* 47:531–535.
224. Walsh, J. H., Csendes, A., and Grossman, M. I. (1972): Effect of truncal vagotomy on gastrin release and Heidenhain pouch acid secretion in response to feeding in dogs. *Gastroenterology,* 63:593–600.
225. Walsh, J. H., Yalow, R. S., and Berson, S. A. (1971): The effect of atropine on plasma gastrin response to feeding. *Gastroenterology,* 60:16–21.
226. Wang, C. C., Grossman, M. I., and Ivy, A. C. (1948): Effect of secretin and pancreozymin on amylase and alkaline phosphotase secretion by the pancreas in dogs. *Am. J. Physiol.,* 154:358–368.
227. Warrick, M. W., and Lin, T.-M. (1975): Action of glucagon and atropine on mucosal blood flow of resting fundic pouches of dogs. *Life Sci.,* 17:333–338.
228. Weinstein, V. A., Colp, R. K., Hollander, F., and Jemerin, E. E. (1944): Vagotomy in the therapy of peptic ulcer. *Surg. Gynecol. Obstet.,* 79:297–305.
229. Weinstein, V. A., Hollander, F., Lauber, F. U., and Colp, R. (1950): Correlation of insulin test studies and clinical results in a series of peptic ulcer cases treated by vagotomy. *Gastroenterology,* 14:214–227.
230. Weiss, A., and Sciales, W. J. (1961): The effect of tolbutamide on human gastric secretion. *Ann. Intern. Med.,* 55:406–415.
231. Weischmann, E., and Gatzweiler, W. (1927): Insulin und Magen. Deutsch. *Arch. Klin. Med.,* 157:208–215. (From Boldyreff and Stewart.)
232. Welin, G., and Frisk, A. R. (1936): The amount and acidity of gastric secretion in man and an interpretation of hypoacidity and achylia. *Acta Med. Scand.,* 90:543–570.
233. Wilson, D. E., Ginsberg, B., and Levine, R. A. (1973): Effect of glucagon on histamine- and pentagastrin- stimulated canine gastric acid secretion and mucosal blood flow. *Gastroenterology,* 63:45–50.

234. Winkelstein, A., and Hess, M. (1948): Effect of insulin hypoglycemia on gastric secretion in duodenal ulcer and controls. *Gastroenterology,* 11:326–336.
235. Yalow, R. S., and Berson, S. A. (1970): Radioimmunoassay of gastrin. *Gastroenterology,* 58:1–14.
236. Zajtchuk, R., Amato, J. J., Poloyan, E., and Baker, R. J. (1967): Inhibition of pancreatic exocrine secretion by glucagon. *Surg. Forum,* 18:410–411.
237. Zaterka, S., and Grossman, M. I. (1966): The effect of gastrin and histamine on the secretion of bile. *Gastroenterology,* 50:500–505.

II. EFFECTS OF INSULIN AND GLUCAGON ON MOTOR FUNCTION OF THE GASTROINTESTINAL TRACT

EFFECTS OF INSULIN ON GASTROINTESTINAL MOTILITY

Stomach

In the original study of the relationship between blood sugar and gastric hunger contractions, Bulatao and Carlson (12) found that (a) experimental hyperglycemia produced by intravenous injection of glucose inhibited, whereas hypoglycemia induced by insulin increased, the gastric tonus and hunger contractions in normal dogs; (b) the inhibition of gastric hunger contractions by glucose was not due to the hypertonicity of the injected solution since similar injection of lactose or sodium chloride did not have this effect; (c) the insulin-induced gastric "tetany" that appeared when the blood concentration fell to the 70 to 80 mg/dl level was inhibited by administration of glucose, and (d) insulin produced a preliminary depression of gastric motility followed by excitation during hypoglycemia in diabetic dog. In diabetic dogs, intravenous glucose did not inhibit gastric tonus and hunger contractions except when hypoglycemia and gastric "tetany" were induced by insulin.

The stimulatory action of insulin on gastrointestinal motility was confirmed by Quigley and associates (72–78) and Templeton and Quigley (93), who in addition reported that (a) the essential features of the gastric response were characterized by increase in tone, type A contractions, and prolonged hunger periods; (b) the gastric motility in man was inhibited by introduction of glucose or sucrose into the duodenum, and by subcutaneous injection of atropine or epinephrine (75); (c) in fasting dogs insulin inhibited the motility and depressed the tone of the vagally denervated pyloric and Heidenhain pouches at the same time that the tone and motility of the main stomach was being augmented (77,93); in dogs having vagi sectioned insulin inhibited rather than augmented gastric hunger contractions (78), and (d) in normal or vagotomized dogs intravenous injection of glucose failed to modify gastric motility (74).

The classic observations made by Bulatao and Carlson (12) and by Quigley et al. (72,74,75,77,78) laid the foundation for the elucidation of the mechanism of action of insulin hypoglycemia on gastrointestinal motility. Since both stimulatory (12,72) and inhibitory (12,77,93) effects of insulin on gastric motility were described, subsequent workers were divided in their view about the primary action of insulin. A great majority of investigators reported that the action of insulin hypoglycemia on the stomach was predominantly excitatory in the dog (12,13,44–46,55,56,66,67,73,93,97,100), sheep (33), rat (5), mouse (63), and man (58,72,75). Others saw primarily inhibitory effects of insulin hypoglycemia on the stomach of man (32,84,87) and dog (35,62,65), whereas a few reported that an initial gastric depression was followed by hypermotility in the dog (79), rabbit (70), sheep (2,6,33), and fish (30,31).

In order to clarify the confusion over the pharmacological action of insulin on gastrointestinal motility, the conditions under which the experiments were conducted must be analyzed, and the broad spectrum of physiological effects of insulin must also be taken into consideration before any meaningful interpretation can be given to these apparently contradictory results.

Relationship of Blood Sugar Level to Gastric Motility

Increase of gastric motility by insulin hypoglycemia. Bulatao and Carlson (12) suggested that under ordinary conditions gastric tonus and contraction of the empty stomach increased when tissue glycogen was reduced. This statement appeared to be supported by the evidence that hypoglycemia provoked gastric hypermotility that could be inhibited by intravenous or intraduodenal introduction of glucose (12,72). However, Quigley et al. found that intravenous injection of glucose was without significant effect on the motility or tonus of the Heidenhain pouch (93) or the stomach after vagotomy (78). In addition, the spontaneous motility of the gut could not be modified by intravenous injection of glucose or correlated with spontaneous changes in blood sugar level (62,74).

Most studies support the view that the insulin-induced hypermotility of the stomach was inhibited by glucose administration (12,62,72–76,93,97). In diabetic dogs (12,62) or patients who had high blood glucose level or were resistant to insulin, several times the usual convulsive dose was required to bring about hypoglycemia and gastric hypermotility.

This suggests that the blood sugar level during insulin hypoglycemia must be a critical factor in the initiation of hunger contractions. Bulatao and Carlson (12) found that as blood glucose fell to the 70 to 80 mg/dl level, hunger contractions in the dog started. But others who used different methods to determine blood sugar arrived at some lower figures. Whatever the critical level of hypoglycemia may be, most authors agree that the lowering of blood glucose level was definitely related to increased gastric motility in animals and man (72).

Depression of gastric motility by insulin. A primary depressive action of insulin hypoglycemia on gastric motility was described in man (32,87) and diabetic (12) or normal dogs (65,79). Bulatao and Cárlson found that as the blood sugar fell to convulsion levels, the stomach motor mechanism showed alternate atony and "tetany." In man, Simici et al. (87) saw a period of depression of gastric motility following intravenous injection of 15 units of insulin. Heinz and Palmer (32) noted in 13 patients following subcutaneous injection of 8 to 20 units of insulin, a depression of gastric motility; in one of the patients nearly complete depression lasted for 90 min, during which blood sugar fell to 40 mg/dl. Necheles et al. (65) reported that subcutaneous injection of 0.65 unit/kg of insulin into dogs caused prolonged depression of gastric motility that coincided with low values for blood sugar.

Other studies have shown that insulin had biphasic action on the stomach, a preliminary depression of tonus, and contractions followed by increase in tonus and motility in the dog (79), sheep (2,6,33), and fish (30,31). In the dog the latent increase in gastric motility even passed into a regular type III activity or incomplete tetany (79). The sugar concentration in the blood was not determined in all these studies. Hill (33) found that the initial inhibition and then the increase in activity of the abdomen of the sheep were the direct consequence of the fall in blood sugar. Bowen (6) and Ali et al. (2) reported transitory inhibition of sheep rumen followed by stimulation of motility, and suppression of activity in the reticulum, rumen, and abomasum after insulin hypoglycemia, respectively.

Reversal of insulin hypoglycemia-induced gastric inhibition by glucose. Whereas early studies showed that gastric hypermotility caused by insulin hypoglycemia was inhibited by intravenous injection of insulin (12,72,75,77), several authors reported that the inhibitory effect of insulin hypoglycemia on the stomach was reversed by glucose. Necheles et al. (65), who first inhibited gastric motility with insulin, noticed that "as the blood sugar rose to medium and slightly subnormal value, the typical insulin hypermotility appeared." Subsequently, it was found that the inhibitory effect of insulin hypoglycemia on the reticulum, rumen, and abomasum of the sheep (2), the human colon (39), and the Heidenhain pouch of the dog (56) could all be reversed by intravenous administration of glucose. In anesthetized dogs, the initial gastric relaxation that took place before any marked hypoglycemia ensued was unaffected by glucose infusion, but the second relaxation phase that coincided with insulin hypoglycemia was replaced by gastric activity after glucose was given (35).

Effect of orally or intravenously administered glucose. Quigley (72) demonstrated that the hypermotility of the stomach induced by insulin was inhibited by introduction of dextrose or cane sugar into the duodenum. However, Templeton and Quigley noted that intravenous injection of a 50% solution of dextrose was essentially without effect on the motility of the Heidenhain (93) and pyloric pouches (77), but feeding of dextrose to the animal inhibited the pouch motility. Duodenal activity induced by insulin also was inhibited by oral administration of glucose (76). When intravenous glucose failed to modify the motility in the stomach, ileum, or colon in normal and vagotomized dogs, introduction of glucose, can sugar, or even lactose into the empty stomach succeeded (74). It is of interest to note that lactose given intravenously was without inhibitory effect on hypoglycemia hypermotility (12). This suggests that the mechanism by which lactose or glucose modifies hypoglycemic hypermotility when given orally or intraduodenally must be different from that when given intravenously.

Relationship Between Insulin Hypoglycemia and the Central Nervous System in Hypermotility of the Gut

One of Quigley and Templeton's (77,93) important observations was the fact that the motility of the Heidenhain or pyloric pouch was inhibited, whereas the motility of the vagally innervated main stomach in the same dog was augmented by insulin. In double vagotomized dogs insulin had inhibitory rather than stimulatory effect on hunger contractions, and intravenous injection of glucose was practically without effect on the motility of the vagotomized stomach (78). These observations stimulated the interest of a number of investigators to elucidate the importance of vagal innervation in insulin-induced gastric hypermotility.

Using a carotid-to-carotid cross circulation technique between a donor and a recipient dog, La Barre and Destree (44,45) found that insulin hypoglycemia in the donor caused rhythmic contractions of the stomach in the recipient whose circulation in the head region was supplied solely by the donor. These gastric contractions were relieved by giving glucose to the donor. The gastric motor action of insulin was not influenced by extirpation of the cerebral hemispheres but was abolished by extirpation of the lower autonomic centers. La Barre's conclusion that the action of insulin hypoglycemia was mediated through the vagal centers was in agreement with the findings (77,93) and deductions (78) of Quigley and was confirmed by others.

Thus Mulinos (62) stated that pithed cats maintained by artificial respiration showed no increase in motility of stomach after insulin. Lalich et al. (46) noted that after vagotomy, the stimulation of the dog stomach by insulin was replaced by inhibition that persisted after splanchnicotomy. This led them to believe that the augmenting action of insulin hypoglycemia was on the vagal center. Nga et al. (66) reported that intrathoracic section of left vagus eliminated the motor effect of insulin on the antrum and pylorus. In rabbits gastric hypermotility induced by insulin hypoglycemia was promptly abolished by cervical vagotomy

(70). In vagotomized patients Feldman and Morrison (26) found that insulin decreased gastric tone and delayed gastric emptying beyond the time for emptying after vagotomy. In the sheep the motility of the denervated pouch of the abdomen was unaffected by insulin (33).

Two views are held by those who believe that the primary effect of insulin was the depression of gastric motility. Schapiro and Woodward (84) noted that insulin hypoglycemia inhibited the motor activity of the stomach of 26 subjects but had no effect in 13 vagotomized patients. Jahnberg et al. (35), on the other hand, found that the relaxatory action of insulin was unaffected by vagotomy.

Further evidence of mediation by the vagal mechanism was provided by the action of atropine. Quigley et al. (72,75) were the first to observe the inhibitory effect of atropine on insulin-induced gastric motility in man. This was confirmed by Wilder and Shlutz (97) in the dog and by Hill in the sheep (33). However, Lim and Necheles *(unpublished data)* noted that with viviperfused stomach, the intravenous administration of insulin to the unanesthetized perfuser dog produced an immediate but transient augmentation of the motility in the isolated stomach. Under similar conditions dextrose produced an immediate but transient gastric inhibition. Moreover, Farrel and Ivy (25) reported that intravenous injection of dextrose in the dog inhibited the motility of the autotransplanted gastric pouch, which was also free of innervation.

Only a few studies dealt with the effect of the sympathetic system on hypermotility induced by insulin. Quigley and Templeton (77) noted that the action of insulin and of dextrose on gastric motility in double sympathectomized dogs while fasting was similar to but slightly greater than that displayed by normal animals. This implied that a physiological balance between the sympathetic inhibitory and the vagal excitatory effects existed under normal conditions. Lalich et al. (46) reported that the inhibition of gastric motility on insulin injection after vagotomy persisted after the splanchnics were sectioned, the celiac ganglion and one adrenal gland were removed and the other adrenal gland demedullated. Epinephrine, which mimics the action of sympathetic stimulation, was found to inhibit hypermotility induced by insulin in the hands of most investigators (62,72,75,79,97). However, Ali et al. (2) found that the inhibitory effect of insulin was reversed by epinephrine.

Insulin was found to have no direct effect on the motility of the isolated sheep rumen (35). The gastric relaxation in anesthetized dogs was unrelated to hypokalemia caused by insulin because the effect was unaffected by infusion of potassium chloride (35).

Esophagus

Schapiro and Woodward (84) showed that in 18 subjects the esophageal motility was markedly reduced by insulin. The inhibition occurred in the absence of hypoglycemia and was of short duration.

Small Intestine

Using the double balloon method, Quigley and Solomon (76) found that the duodenal activity in man was increased by subcutaneous injection of insulin and that duodenal hunger contractions could occur in the absence of gastric motility. This stimulatory action of insulin was inhibited by atropine or oral administration of glucose. According to Schapiro and Woodward, insulin primarily had an inhibitory action on the duodenal motility in man (84).

Both stimulatory and inhibitory effects of insulin on the lower part of the small intestine were reported. Krishnan (43) and Gage et al. (28) noted an increase in intestinal motility by giving insulin. Pavel and Milcou (68) saw strong augmentation of amplitude, tonus, and frequency of contraction of rabbit intestine by insulin *in vitro*. According to Bogach et al. insulin increased intestinal motility in the rat (5) and stimulated the tonus and amplitude of contraction and tonus of the jejunum but decreased the activity of the ileum of the dog (4). The interdigestive myoelectric complex (MMC) characteristic of fasting motility patterns in the dog and sheep was replaced by a continuous pattern of activity after injection of insulin. In alloxan diabetic sheep, the recurrence and intensity of MMC were decreased and the normal pattern could be restored by insulin.

The stimulatory effect of insulin on the small intestine was antagonized by atropine *in vitro* (68) and *in vivo* (5) and abolished by double vagotomy in the rat (5) or sheep (11). Ruckelbusch and Fioramonti (82) believed that motility pattern in the sheep after feeding was related to plasma concentration of insulin. This has to be studied further.

It was reported that the activity of the small intestine of the anesthetized guinea pig was inhibited by insulin (61) and that the depression of ileal activity by insulin in the dog was accompanied by hyperglycemia and tachycardia. Kleitsch and Puestow (42) studied the effect of insulin on motility of the isolated intestinal transplants of the dog and noted that physiological saline administered by drip phleboclysis produced a definite increase in rate and strength of peristaltic contractions, whereas insulin caused a progressive diminution of all these parameters.

In isolated intestinal preparations, Winter and Smith (98) first, and then Prasad (71), Abderhalden and Gellhorn (1) and Barlow (3) all saw inhibitory effect of insulin on gut motility.

Colon

Insulin injections produced in dogs an increase in colonic activity that closely paralleled that exhibited by the stomach (66,76). Quigley and Solomon (76) were able to inhibit this effect of insulin by atropine or oral administration of glucose, cane sugar, or lactose. Intrathoracic section of the right vagus was reported to eliminate the stimulatory effect of insulin hypoglycemia on the motility of the proximal colon (66).

In contrast, insulin was found to have an inhibitory effect on the colon of the guinea pig (1,61) and the sigmoid of man (39,57,84). One study showed that the inhibitory action of insulin was unaffected by bilateral vagotomy (84) and another indicated that the activity was increased by intravenous injection of glucagon (39).

GENERAL DISCUSSION

Thus far, three types of actions of insulin hypoglycemia on gastrointestinal motility have been described in the literature: (a) a primary stimulatory, (b) a primary inhibitory, and (c) a biphasic action in which inhibition was followed by excitation. It is noteworthy that in biphasic action seldom was the inhibition preceded by stimulation of gut motility. This was also the case with the gastric secretory response to insulin.

In most of the early studies, only total doses of insulin were recorded; no accurate dosage on unit body weight basis was given. In these studies, the intravenous or subcutaneous dosages of insulin ranged from 0.5 to 5.0 units/ kg in dogs (12,42,46,62,65,73–79,93,97), 0.1 to 0.25 unit/kg in man (32, 39,57,84), and 1.5 to 5 unit/kg in rabbits (70). In some studies stimulatory effect was seen at low doses, whereas inhibitory action was seen as the dosage was increased. Still others found that insulin stimulated motility when given subcutaneously, but depressed the stomach and ileum when injected intravenously (62).

To clarify the contradictions and find explanations for these diversified actions of insulin hypoglycemia, an examination of the purity of insulin itself may bring some relevance. First, "commercial" insulin from different sources was used in different studies. Secondly, advanced technology available today for purification of polypeptides simply did not exist in the 1920s and 1940s. "Crystalline" or "highly purified" insulin does not imply that it is chemically pure. "Monocomponent" insulin was unheard of until a few years ago. To date, we are not aware that any study on motility has ever been done with the synthetic or monocomponent insulin.

But it is of interest to note that as early as 1925 Abderhalden and Gellhorn (1) noted that the inhibitory effect of "commercial" insulin on the small bowel of the rat and colon of the guinea pig was replaced by increased tonus and greater contractions after purification. Indeed, with recent advances in the technology of protein chemistry, more contaminants in "commercial" insulin have been identified and eliminated. Now we understand that the pancreatic islet produces not only insulin from its B cells but also glucagon (7,88) from the A cells, somatostatin from the D cells (21), and pancreatic polypeptide (PP) from the PP cells (14,15,41). Somatostatin in the ovine hypothalamus was not recognized until 1972 and bovine pancreatic polypeptide (BPP) was not known until 1971 (14). Thus before chromatographic methods became available, it was not possible to free insulin completely from glucagon, somatostatin, or PP.

Lately glucagon is well known for its inhibitory effect on gastric motility (89) and secretion (47,80). Somatostatin is one of the most powerful inhibitors of gastric secretion (53,96) and gastrointestinal motility. Minimal doses of somatostatin required for inhibition of antral, duodenal, jejunal, and colonic activity were only 100 to 200 ng/kg (54). In large doses (50–100 μg/kg, i.v.) PP caused vomiting and defecation (50) but in low doses (0.25–1 μg/kg) by slow intravenous infusion, it relaxed the antrum, duodenum, and jejunum (49,54). The relaxing actions of glucagon (16), somatostatin (54), and PP (49) were characterized by an early onset that occurred immediately after administration and short duration of action lasting a few to 30 min depending on the dose. Thirdly, the inhibitory actions of glucagon, somatostatin, and PP are independent of blood sugar level. PP had no effect at all on blood sugar in the dog (52) and somatostatin at doses significantly affecting motility (54) had no effect on insulin and glucagon release or plasma glucose concentration (81).

In view of this some, but not all, of the inhibitory and biphasic actions of insulin may find an explanation, especially when the dosage was large and given as an intravenous bolus *in vivo,* or when the concentration was high *in vitro.*

Equally important is the consideration that insulin hypoglycemia provokes the release of other hormones that have motor effects of their own on the gastrointestinal tract. Soon after method for RIA of gastrin G-17 was established by Yalow and Berson (99), Csendes et al. (19) found that gastrin was released by insulin when the antral pH of the dog stomach was maintained at neutrality. Lin and Chance (50) first reported that feeding and sham-feeding increased the plasma level of PP in the dog. Taylor et al. (90) and Schwartz et al. (85) showed that in man sham-feeding caused a significant rise in PP concentration in the plasma. Subsequently it was found that PP could be released by insulin (27,86) or cholinergics (86,91,92) and the release of PP could be blocked by atropine.

Moreover, insulin hypoglycemia stimulates not only the parasympathetic but also the sympathetic autonomic system. Cannon and associates (13), using the denervated heart as an indicator, obtained evidence for an increased secretion of epinephrine after insulin administration. Houssay et al. (34) demonstrated epinephrine secretion in the recipient dog after injection of insulin by the hyperglycemia appearing in the recipient dog connected to the donor through an adrenal-jugular anastomosis. Drury (20) found that adrenalin release by insulin was caused by lowering of plasma potassium in the rat. Von Euler and Luft (23) reported that in 10 subjects, insulin at 0.1 unit/kg caused a tenfold increase in urinary excretion of epinephrine. A positive relationship between hypoglycemia and secretion of epinephrine was demonstrated by Dunar (22). McCrea et al. (59,60) reported that stimulation of the peripheral end of the sympathetic and vagus nerves was associated respectively with inhibition and initiation of contractions in the stomach. All these results favor the view that exogenous (72,75) and endogenously released epinephrine exerts an inhibitory effect on gastrointestinal motility.

This brings us to the question of the relative effectiveness of intravenously and orally administered glucose for inhibition of insulin-induced hypermotility. First, insulin was reported to inhibit the Heidenhain pouch at the same time that the tone and motility of the main stomach was being stimulated (93). Second, insulin did not have appreciable effect on the motility of the pyloric pouch of the stomach (77). Third, in dogs having the vagi sectioned insulin inhibited rather than augmented the gastric hunger contractions (78).

The lack of stimulatory effect could be explained by the lack of viable vagal innervation in all three preparations. The inhibition could also be due to the presence of inhibitory peptides in the insulin used and excitation of the sympathetic system or the release of inhibitory substances by insulin. But how does one account for the fact that when intravenously administered glucose failed to alter the motility of the Heidenhain pouch or the vagotomized stomach (74), while glucose, cane sugar, or even lactose introduced orally or intraduodenally inhibited these organs (74–78,93)?

Of special interest is lactose that when injected intravenously was unable to inhibit gastric "tetany" during hypoglycemia (12). Yet when given by mouth or intraduodenally, lactose (74) provoked gastric inhibition in both the vagotomized stomach and the Heidenhain pouch. This evidently suggests that the mechanisms by which oral glucose or lactose brings about inhibition of gut motility is not due to hyperglycemia. Recently, new candidate hormones of the gut have been discovered (29). Vasoactive intestinal polypeptide (VIP) (83) was found to inhibit the motility of the smooth muscles of the gut in several species of animals (69). Pure PP showed both stimulatory and inhibitory effects on the stomach, duodenum, and colon of the conscious dog (15,48,50). Pure glucose-dependent-insulinotropic polypeptide (GIP) supplied by Brown (8) was found by Lin et al. (54) to increase the intraluminal pressure in the gastroduodenal junction but lower than in the antrum, descending duodenum, gallbladder, and choledochal sphincter of the conscious dog. "Purified" enteroglucagon prepared by Murphy and associates was also found to relax the stomach and duodenum of the dog (54). All these polypeptides can be released by orally administered glucose (9,27). What role may these hormones play in the regulation of motility when released by oral glucose or insulin?

Besides the vagal release of gastrin, insulin hypoglycemia also releases histamine from the gastric mucosa (17,37). Gastrin was found by Kahlson et al. (37), Johnson and Aureus (36), and Lin and Evans (51) to mobilize histamine from its stores in the gastric mucosa. Whether or not insulin-released histamine has an effect on stomach motility has not been studied. Other mind-gut polypeptides, in particular VIP and somatostatin or paracrine secretions that may be released by vagal excitation should also be taken into consideration whenever insulin hypoglycemia produces an effect on gut motility or secretion. Suffice it to say that what was initially viewed as a simple hypoglycemia-vagal mechanism turns out to be a complicated chain of responses involving the sympathetic autonomic system, other endocrines, and possibly paracrine functions, each of which exerts an effect of its own. The final expression of the effect of insulin hypoglycemia should be considered as the resultant of these forces interacting with each other. Thus, it is not surprising that we find ourselves confused by conflicting results obtained under different experimental conditions.

SUMMARY

Despite the confusion in literature regarding insulin hypoglycemia and gut motility, the current concept of the overall effect of insulin hypoglycemia has not deviated significantly from that conceived originally by Bulatao and Carlson (12) and Quigley et al. (72–78,93). The view that gastric motility is related to reduction of tissue glycogen and enforced energy metabolism of lipids on the part of the smooth muscles (12) is no longer shared by the majority. But the view that the action of insulin-hypermotility is mediated by a vagal mechanism (74–78,93) is well supported.

In essence hypoglycemia is the key that triggers excitation of the vagal centers (44,45,62,78) in the central nervous system, whose messages are carried by the vagi to the targets on the gut. This central excitatory action of insulin hypoglycemia can be reversed or inhibited by giving glucose (12). Peripherally the action is mainly, but not entirely mediated by a cholinergic mechanism, because vagotomy in dogs (26,35,46,66,74–78,93), rabbits (70), sheep (33), rats (5), and man (84) and anticholinergic drugs (33,72,75,97) can block or weaken the response to insulin hypoglycemia.

Insulin hypoglycemia, especially one that is caused by a large dose, stimulates not only the parasympathetic but also the sympathetic mechanism, and the release of gastrointestinal hormones or polypeptides that have effects of their own on gastrointestinal function. Contaminants in "commercial" insulin is no longer a serious problem. But whenever an unexpected effect is seen, the purity of the preparation needs to be examined.

REFERENCES

1. Abderhalden, E., and Gellhorn, E. (1925): Beiträge zur Kenntnis der Wirkung des Insulins. *Pflügers Arch. Physiol.*, 208:135.
2. Ali, T. M., Nicholson, T., and Singleton, A. G. (1976): Stomach motility in insulin-treated sheep. *Q. J. Exp. Physiol.*, 61:321–329.
3. Barlow, O. W. (1931): Effect of insulin on perfused heart and on isolated rabbit intestine. *J. Pharmacol. Exp. Ther.*, 41:217–228.
4. Bogach, P. G., Nga, C. S., and Groisman, S. D. (1973): Effect of insulin hypoglycemia on the motility of the dog jejunum and ileum. *Fiziol Zh. (Kiev)*, 19(4):471–476.
5. Bogach, P. G., Groisman, S. D., and Chan, S. N. (1974): Effect of varying degree of parasympathetic denervation of the stomach, the duodenum and the jejunum on the motor reactions induced by insulin hypoglycemia. *Fiziol. Zh. SSSR. I. M. Sechenova*, 60:1446–1453.
6. Bowen, J. M. (1962): Effects of insulin hypoglycemia on gastrointestinal motility in the sheep. *Am. J. Vet. Res.*, 23:948–954.
7. Bromer, W. W., Sinn, L. G., and Behrens, O. K. (1957): The amino acid sequence of glucagon. *Diabetes*, 6:234.
8. Brown, J. C. (1971): A gastric inhibitory polypeptide. I. The amino acid sequence and tryptic peptides. *Can. J. Biochem.*, 49:255–261.
9. Brown, J. C., Dryburgh, J. R., and Pederson, R. A. (1974): Gastric inhibitory polypeptide

(GIP). In: *Endocrinology of the Gut,* edited by W. Y. Chey and F. P. Brooks, pp. 76–82. Charles B. Slack, Thorofare, New Jersey.

10. Bueno, L. and Ruckelbusch, M. (1975): Effects de l'insuline sur l'activite electrique du jejunum chez le mouton. *Compt. Rend. Sci. Soc. Biol.,* 169:435–439.
11. Bueno, L., and Ruckelbusch, M. (1976): Insulin and jejunal electrical activity in dogs and sheep. *Am. J. Physiol.,* 230:1538–1544.
12. Bulatao, E., and Carlson, A. J. (1924): Influence of experimental changes in blood sugar levels on gastric hunger contraction. *Am. J. Physiol.,* 69:107–115.
13. Cannon, W. B., McEver, M. A., and Bliss, S. W. (1924): A sympathetic adrenal mechanism for mobilizing sugar in hypoglycemia. *Am. J. Physiol.,* 69:46–66.
14. Chance, R. E., and Jones, W. E. (1974): U.S. Patent Office No. 3, 842, 063.
15. Chance, R. E., Lin, T.-M., and Johnson, M. G., et al. (1975): Studies on a new recognized pancreatic hormone with gastrointestinal activities. *Endocrinology (Suppl.),* 96:183, (Abstr. 265).
16. Chernish, S. M., Miller, R. E., Rosenak, B. D., and Schutz, N. E. (1972): Hypotonic duodenography with the use of glucagon. *Gastroenterology,* 63:392–398.
17. Code, C. F. (1956): Histamine and gastric secretion. *Ciba Foundation Symposium: Histamine,* pp. 189–219.
18. Code, C. F., and Marlett, J. A. (1972): The interdigestive myoelectrical complex of the stomach and small bowel of dogs. *J. Physiol.,* 45:1487–1502.
19. Csendes, A., Walsh, J. H., and Grossman, M. I. (1972): Effects of atropine and antral acidification on gastrin release and acid secretion in response to insulin and feeding in dogs. *Gastroenterology,* 63:257–263.
20. Drury, A. (1951): The effect of epinephrine and insulin on the plasma potassium level. *Endocrinology,* 49:663–670.
21. Dubois, M. P. (1975): Immunoreactive somatostatin is present in discrete cells of the endocrine pancreas. *Proc. Natl. Acad. Sci. USA,* 72:1340–1343.
22. Dunar, H. (1953): The influence of the blood glucose level on the secretion of adrenalin and noradrenaline from the suprarenal. *Acta Physiol. Scand. (Suppl.* 102), 28:1–77.
23. Euler, U. S. V., and Luft, R. (1952): Effect of insulin on urinary excretion of adrenaline and noradrenaline. *Metabolism,* 1:528.
24. Farah, A. (1938): Beitrag zur Wirkung des Insulins auf isolierte Abschnitte des Dunndarmes. *Arch. Exp. Pathol. Pharmakol.,* 188:548–554.
25. Farrel, J., and Ivy, A. C. (1926): Studies on the motility of the transplanted gastric pouch. *Am. J. Physiol.,* 76:227–228. (Abstr.).
26. Feldman, M. and Morrison, S. (1948): The effect of insulin on motility of the stomach following bilateral vagotomy. *Am. J. Dig. Dis.,* 15:175 (Abstr.).
27. Floyd, J. C., Jr., Fajans, S. S., Pek, S., and Chance, R. E. (1977): A newly recognized pancreatic polypeptide; plasma levels in health and disease. *Rec. Prog. Horm. Res.,* 23:519–570.
28. Gage, O. M., Ochsner, A., and Cutting, R. A. (1931): The effect of insulin and glucose in normal and obstructed intestine. *Proc. Soc. Exp. Biol. Med.,* 29:264–265.
29. Grossman, M. I. (1974): Candidate hormones of the gut. *Gastroenterology,* 67:730–755.
30. Gzgzyan, D. M., and Kuzina, M. M. (1973): Stomach motor activity in the black sea ray *Daeyatis paetinaca. Zh. Evol. Biochim. Fiziol.,* 9(5):536–539.
31. Gzgzyan, D. M., Kuzina, M., and Tanaschuk, O. F. (1973): The effect of hypophyseal hormones and insulin on motor activity of the stomach in the scorpion fish *Scorpaena porpus. Zh. Evol. Biochim. Fiziol.,* 9(3):301–303.
32. Heinz, T. E., and Palmer, W. L. (1930): A study of the effect of insulin on gastric motility. *Proc. Soc. Exp. Biol. Med.,* 27:1047–1049.
33. Hill, K. J. (1954): Insulin hypoglycemia and gastric motility in the sheep. *Q. J. Exp. Physiol.,* 39:253–260.
34. Houssay, B. A., Lewis, J. T., and Molinelli, E. A. (1924): Accion de la insulina sobre la secrecion de adrenalina. *Compt. Rend. Soc. Biol.,* 91:1011–1013.
35. Jahnberg, T., Abrahamson, H., Jansson, G., and Martinson, J. (1977): Gastric relaxation response to insulin before and after vagotomy. *Scand. J. Gastroenterol.,* 12:229–233.
36. Johnson, L. R., and Aureus, D. (1970): Evidence that histamine is not the mediator of acid secretion in the rat. *Proc. Soc. Biol. Med.,* 134:880–884.
37. Kahlson, G., Rosengten, E., and Svahn, D., and Thunberg, R. (1964): Mobilization and formation of histamine in the gastric mucosa as related to gastric secretion. *J. Physiol.,* 174:400–416.

38. Karef, O., and Mautner, A. (1926): Acceleration of resorption by insulin. *Klin. Wochenchr.,* 5:191.
39. Killenberger, P. G., and Cornwell, G. G. (1964): Effect of insulin hypoglycemia on the human sigmoid colon. *Am. J. Dig. Dis.,* 9:221–228.
40. Kim, K. S., and Shore, P. A. (1963): Mechanism of action of reserpine and insulin on gastric amines and gastric acid secretion and the effect of monoamine oxidase and gastric acid secretion and the effect of monoamine oxidase inhibition. *J. Pharmacol. Exp. Ther.,* 141:321–325.
41. Kimmel, J. R., Hayden, L. J., and Pollack, H. G. (1975): Isolation and characterization of a new pancreatic polypeptide hormone. *J. Biol. Chem.,* 250:9369–9374.
42. Kleitsch, W. P., and Puestow, C. B. (1939): Studies of intestinal motility: The effect of intravenous solutions and of insulin upon peristalsis. *Surgery,* 6:687–696.
43. Krishnan, B. T. (1934): Effect of adrenalin pituitary extract and insulin on the movements of the intestine. *Ind. J. Med. Res.,* 22:161–164.
44. La Barre, J. (1931): Influence of insulin hypoglycemia in the central nervous system on gastric motility. *Compt. Rend. Soc. Biol.,* 107:258–260.
45. La Barre, J., and Destree, P. (1930): Role des centres nerveus superieurs dans l'hypermotilité gastrique consecutive aux états d'hypoglycémie. *Compt. Rend. Soc. Biol.,* 104:112–113.
46. Lalich, J., Youmans, W. B., and Meek, W. J. (1937): Insulin and gastric motility. *Am. J. Physiol.,* 120:554–558.
47. Lin, T.-M., and Alphin, R. S. (1958): Inhibition of gastric secretion by glucagon and glucose. *Fed. Proc.,* 17:97.
48. Lin, T.-M., and Chance, R. E. (1972): Spectrum of gastrointestinal actions of a new bovine pancreatic polypeptide (BPP). *Gastroenterology,* 62:852 (abstract).
49. Lin, T.-M., and Chance, R. E. (1974): Cantidate hormones of the gut: Bovine pancreatic polypeptide (BPP) and avian pancreatic peptide (APP). *Gastroenterology,* 67:737–739.
50. Lin, T.-M., and Chance, R. E. (1974): Gastrointestinal actions of a new bovine pancreatic polypeptide (BPP). In: *Endocrinology of the Gut,* edited by W. Chey and F. P. Brooks., pp. 143–145. Charles B. Slack, Thorofare, New Jersey.
51. Lin, T.-M., and Evans, D. C. (1970): Effect of pentagastrin on gastric HCl secretion and histamine content of the stomach of rats. *Arch. Int. Pharmacodyn. Ther.,* 88:145–155.
52. Lin, T.-M., Evans, D. C., Chance, R. E., and Spray, G. F. (1977): Bovine pancreatic peptide: Action on gastric and pancreatic secretion in dogs. *Am. J. Physiol.,* 1(3):E311–E315.
53. Lin, T.-M., Evans, D. C., Shaar, C., and Crabtree, R. (1976): Action of somatostatin on gastric secretion and mucosal blood flow. Pancreatic output and release of insulin and growth hormone. *Gastroenterology,* 70:A101/959.
54. Lin, T.-M., Spray, G. F., and Bloomquist, W. E. (1978): *Unpublished studies.*
55. Linder, M. M., Bussmann, J. F., and Haselberger, J. (1975): Electric and mechanic gastric activity under insulin. *Chir. Forum Exp. Klin. Forsch.,* 305–308.
56. Lorber, S. H., and Shay, H. (1962): Effect of insulin and glucose on gastric motor activity of dogs. *Gastroenterology,* 43:564–574.
57. Mahler, P. (1930): Der Tonus des menschlichen Magens and Darm in Insulin shock. *Zeit. Ges. Exp. Med.,* 73:817–821.
58. Manville, I. A., and Chuinard, E. G. (1934): Studies on gastric hunger mechanisms. *Am. J. Dig. Dis.,* 1:688–693.
59. McCrea, E. D., and McSwiney, B. A. (1928): The effect on the stomach of stimulation of the peripheral end of the splanchnic nerve. *Q. J. Exp. Physiol.,* 18:301–313.
60. McCrea, E. D., McSwiney, B. A., and Stopford, J. G. (1925): The effect on the stimulation of the peripheral end of the vagus nerve. *Q. J. Exp. Physiol.,* 15:200–233.
61. Meythaler, F., and Graesser, F. (1935): Die Wirkung des Insulins auf den Darm. *Arch. Exp. Pathol. Pharmakol.,* 178:27–35.
62. Mulinos, M. G. (1933): The gastric hunger mechanism. IV. The influence of experimental alterations in blood sugar concentration on the gastric hunger contractions. *Am. J. Physiol.,* 104:371–378.
63. Moniuszko-Jakoniuk, J. (1974): Influence of insulin on the effect of neostigmine in healthy mice and mice with alloxan-induced diabetes mellitus. *Acta Physiol. Pol.,* 25(5); 497–508.
64. Murphy, R. F., Buchanan, K. D., and Elmore, D. T. (1973): Isolation of glucagon-like immunocreativity of gut by affinity chromatography on antiglucagon antibodies coupled to sepharose 4B. *Biochem. Biophys. Acta,* 303:118–127.

65. Necheles, H., Olson, W. H., and Morris, R. (1941): Depression of gastric motility by insulin. *Am. J. Dig. Dis.,* 8:270–273.
66. Nga, C. S., Bogach, P. G., and Groisman, S. D. (1973): Mechanisms of the effect of insulin hypoglycemia on colon motility. *Byull. Eksp. Biol. Med.,* 76:12–15.
67. Okita, O. (1976): Effect of a couple of stimulants on gastric motility. *Jpn. J. Smooth Mus. Res.,* 12(1):37–47.
68. Pavel, I., and Milcou, S. M. (1932): Action de l'insulin sur l'intestin. *Compt. Rend. Soc. Biol.,* 109:776–779.
69. Piper, P, J., Said, S. I., and Vane, J. R. (1970): Effects on smooth muscle preparations of unidentified vasoactive peptides from the intestine and lung. *Nature,* 225:1144–1146.
70. Postlethwaite, R. W., Hill, H. V., and Chittum, J. R. (1948): Effect of vagotomy and of drugs on gastric motility. *Ann. Surg.,* 128:184–194.
71. Prasad, S. (1934): Effect of insulin on the contraction of the intestinal muscle. *Ind. J. Med. Res.,* 21:563–567.
72. Quigley, J. P. (1929): Action of insulin on the gastric motility of man. *Proc. Soc. Exp. Biol. Med.,* 26:769–770.
73. Quigley, J. P., and Barnes, B. D. (1930): Action of insulin on the motility of the gastrointestinal tract. VI. Antagonistic action of posterior pituitary lobe preparations. *Am. J. Physiol.,* 95:7–12.
74. Quigley, J. P., and Hallaran, W. R. (1932): The independence of spontaneous gastrointestinal motility and blood sugar levels. *Am. J. Physiol.,* 100:102–110.
75. Quigley, J. P., Johnson, V., and Solomon, E. I. (1929): Action of insulin on the motility of the gastrointestinal tract. *Am. J. Physiol.,* 90:89–98.
76. Quigley, J. P., and Solomon, E. I. (1930): Action of insulin on the motility of the gastrointestinal tract. V. a. Action on the human duodenum. b. Action on the colon of dogs. *Am. J. Physiol.,* 91:488–495.
77. Quigley, J. P., and Templeton, R. D. (1930): Action of insulin on the motility of the gastrointestinal tract. III. a. Action on the pyloric pouch. b. Action on the stomach following double sympathectomy. *Am. J. Physiol.,* 91:475–481.
78. Quigley, J. P., and Templeton, R. D. (1930): Action of insulin on the motility of the gastrointestinal tract. IV. Action on the stomach following double vagotomy. *Am. J. Physiol.,* 91:482–487.
79. Regan, J. F. (1933): The action of insulin on the motility of the empty stomach. *Am. J. Physiol.,* 104:91–95.
80. Robinson, R. M., Harris, K., Black, C. J., and Eisman, B. (1957): Effect of glucagon on gastric secretion. *Proc. Soc. Exp. Biol. Med.,* 96:518–520.
81. Root, M. A. (1978): Lilly Research Laboratories, *Personal communication.*
82. Ruckebusch, M., and Fioramonti, J. (1975): Insuline-secretion et motricité intestinale. *Compt. Rend. Sci. Soc. Biol.,* 169:435–439.
83. Said, S. I., and Mutt, V. (1973): Isolation from porcine intestinal wall of a vasoactive octapeptide related to secretin and to glucagon. *Eur. J. Biochem.,* 28:199–204.
84. Schapiro, H., and Woodward, E. R. (1959): The action of insulin hypoglycemia on the motility of the human gastrointestinal tract. *Am. J. Dig. Dis.,* 4:787–791.
85. Schwartz, T. W., Grotzinger, U., Schoon, I. M., Stenquist, B., and Olbe, L. (1978): Cephalic-vagal and vago-vagal stimulation of pancreatic polypeptide (PP) secretion in man. *Scand. J. Gastroenterol. (Suppl. 49),* 13:(Abstr. 161).
86. Schwartz, T. W., Holst, J. J., Fahrenkrug, J., Jensen, L., Nelson, O. V., Rehfeld, J. F., Schaffalitzky de Muckadell, O. B., and Stadil, F. (1978): Vagal cholinergic regulation of pancreatic polypeptide secretion. *Clin. Invest.,* 61:781–789.
87. Simici, D., Guires, G., and Dimitriu, C. (1927): L'action de l'insuline sur la motilite et l'evacuation de l'estomac a l'etat normal et pathologique. *Arch. Mal. App. Dig.,* 17:17–18.
88. Staub, A., Sinn, L. G., and Behrens, O. K. (1953): Purification and crystallization of hyperglycemia glycogenolytic factor. *Science,* 117:628–629.
89. Stunkard, S. J., Van Itallie, T. B., and Reis, B. B. (1955): The mechanism of satiety. Effect of glucagon on gastric hunger contraction in man. *Proc. Soc. Exp. Biol. Med.,* 88:258–261.
90. Taylor, I. L., Feldman, M., Richardson, C. G., and Walsh, J. H. (1978): Gastric and cephalic stimulation of human pancreatic polypeptide release. *Gastroenterology,* 75:432–437.
91. Taylor, I. L., Walsh, J. H., Wood, J., Chew, P., and Grossman, M. I. (1977): Bombesin is a potent stimulant of pancreatic polypeptide (PP) release. *Clin. Res.,* 25(4):574A. (Abstr.).

92. Taylor, I. L., Walsh, J. H., Carter, D. C., Wood, J., and Grossman, M. I. (1978): Effect of atropine and bethanechol on release of pancreatic polypeptide and gastrin by bombesin in dog. *Scand. J. Gastroenterol. (Suppl. 49),* 13:(Abstr. 183).
93. Templeton, R. D., and Quigley, J. P. (1929–1930): The action of insulin on the motility of the gastrointestinal tract II. Action on the Heidenhain pouch. *Am. J. Physiol.,* 91:467–474.
94. Unger, R. H., Ohneda, A., Valverde, I., Eisentraut, A. M., and Exton, J. (1969): Characterization of the responses of circulating glucagon-like immunoreactivity to intraduodenal and intravenous administration of glucose. *J. Clin. Invest.,* 47:48–65.
95. Vallenas, G. A. (1956): Effects of glycemic levels on rumen motility in the sheep. *Am. J. Vet. Res.,* 17:79–89.
96. Warrick, M. W., and Lin, T.-M. (1976): Action of somatostatin, metiamide and glucagon on gastric acid secretion from isolated frog gastric mucosa. *Fed. Proc.,* 35:218 (Abstr. 60).
97. Wilder, R. L., and Schultz, F. W. (1932): The action of atropine and adrenaline on gastric tonus and hypermotility induced by insulin hypoglycemia. *Am. J. Physiol.,* 96:54–58.
98. Winter, L. B., and Smith, W. (1924): On the effect of insulin on the isolated intestine of the rabbit. *J. Physiol.,* 58:XII.
99. Yalow, R. S., and Berson, S. A. (1970): Radioimmunoassay of gastrin. *Gastroenterology,* 58:1–14.
100. Yanagisawa, T., Sugaware, K., Kato, M., *et al.* (1976): Studies on factors affecting the motility of the stomach. *Nippon Heikatsukin Gakki Zasshi,* 12:278–279.

EFFECT OF GLUCAGON ON GASTROINTESTINAL MOTILITY

Effect on the Stomach

The inhibitory effect of glucagon on gastric hunger contractions in normal subjects was first described by Stunkard et al. (44). This was associated with decrease in experience of hunger and coincided with a rise in blood glucose levels and an increase in peripheral capillary (A) venous (V) glucose difference. Necheles et al. (35) and Sporn and Necheles (42) demonstrated in conscious dogs a decrease of intraluminal pressure in the stomach and colon following the injection of glucagon and stated that the inhibition was related to the A-V blood sugar difference.

Motility of antrum and pyloric sphincter recorded with pressure transducer strain gauges was suppressed by intramuscular injection of glucagon (25 μg/ kg) in the chronic dog, as shown in Fig. 1. Intraluminal pressure in the stomach was decreased by a low (6.3 μg/kg-hr) but not by a high (25 μg/kg-hr) dose of glucagon, and retardation of gastric emptying in the rat was found to be independent of the presence of thyroid and parathyroid tissue (20).

Studies in man indicated that food intake (39), gastric emptying (4,5,32,33,40), and motility (5,16,20,32,33,37) were reduced by glucagon. Fluoroscopic studies conducted by Chernish et al. (4,5) and Miller et al. (32,33) showed that glucagon stopped the motility of the upper gastrointestinal tract during the intravenous injection of glucagon in a 60-sec period and that the magnitude and duration of inhibition was dose-dependent, lasting for 10 to 30 min. One report showed that gastric and antral motility was inhibited by glucagon after feeding but not in inanition (45,46).

In isolated preparations, glucagon inhibited the activity of the homologous perfused porcine stomach (23) but showed no activity on the human stomach muscle *in vitro* (3).

Effect on the Small Intestines

Conflicting results have been reported on the intestinal effects of glucagon. Inhibition of duodenal (Figs. 1 and 2) and jejunal (13) activity was observed in the conscious dog. Duodenal motility was immediately inhibited by 25 µg/ kg of glucagon given intramuscularly, whereas a large dose (50 µg/kg) often showed biphasic action, an initial stimulation followed by inhibition, as shown in Fig. 3.

In contrast, other investigators found that glucagon stimulated intestinal motility at 10 to 20 µg/kg and inhibited motor and bioelectric activity at 400 to 500 µg/kg doses (36).

Studies in man using radioopaque material (4,5,14,22,32,33,37,38,51) or baloon (8,22) showed that the activity in the duodenum and jejunum was significantly reduced by glucagon. Clinically this relaxing property was applied in hypotonic duodenography (5,32,33) or endoscopic and radiological examination of the gastrointestinal tract in general (21,31,38).

The effect of glucagon on ileal activity was not as distinct as its effect on the stomach, duodenum, or jejunum. Under fasting conditions glucagon might even initiate a few episodes of modest activity immediately after administration (Fig. 3). When gastrointestinal motility was induced by continuous infusion of pentagastrin, glucagon did not suppress the magnitude of ileal contractions but delayed the occurrence of episodes of activity. Glucagon was reported to delay the propulsive movement of the bowel in the small intestine (30,41) and the contractility of the intestinal villi (17).

Effect on the Colon, Rectum, and Anal Sphincter

Motor activities recorded with Quigley's miniature induction coils, pressure transducer strain gages, baloon, or intraluminal catheters were all decreased by glucagon in the dog (26). In man the motility of the colon (6–8,21,22,37) recorded with balloons or intraluminal catheters was also reduced. Glucagon inhibited not only the motility under basal conditions (22,37) but also that stimulated by food, morphine (7,8), prostigmine (6,8), and CCK (6). However, glucagon was reported to cause contraction of the tenia coli *in vitro* (9).

The rectum and the anal sphincter were not as sensitive as the colon to the action of glucagon; the rectum was only slightly inhibited (6,7) and the activity of the anal sphincter was unaffected (6,7).

Effect on the Lower Esophageal, Pyloric, and Ileo-cecal Sphincters

Nearly all the sphincters of the gut are relaxed by glucagon. *In vivo* the lower esophageal sphincter pressure (LESP) was reduced under basal conditions

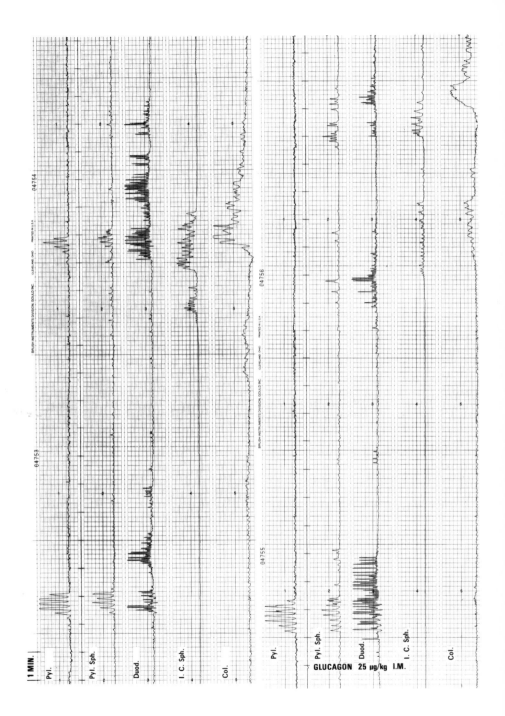

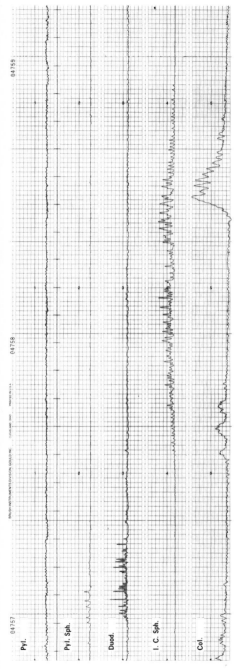

FIG. 1. Effect of glucagon on the motility of the antrum (Pyl), pyloric sphincter (Pyl. Sph.), duodenum (Duod.), ileo-cecal sphincter (I.C. Sph.), and colon (Col.) of the conscious dog under basal conditions. Activity of gut was recorded with pressure transducer strain gages anchored to the serosal wall of the gastrointestinal tract in all the illustrations. Note suppression of rhythmic activities in the antrum, pyloric sphincter, and duodenum.

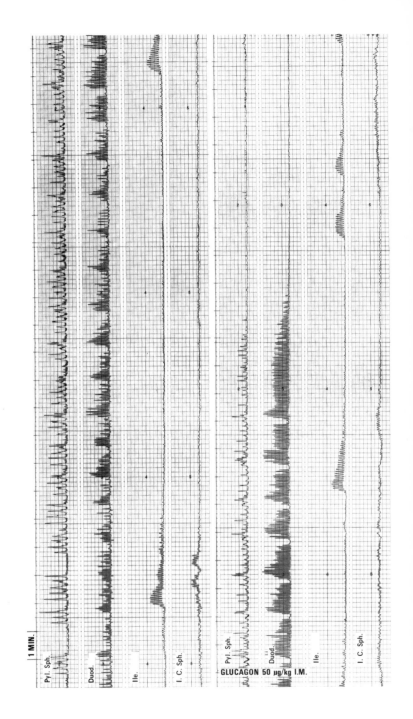

1 MIN.

Pyl. Sph.

Duod.

Ile.

I. C. Sph.

GLUCAGON 50 µg/kg I.M.

Pyl. Sph.

Duod.

Ile.

I. C. Sph.

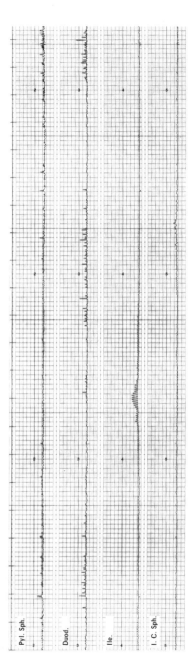

FIG. 2. Effect of a large (50 μg/kg i.m.) dose of glucagon on the motility of the pyloric sphincter, duodenum, ileum (Ile.), and the ileo-cecal sphincter of the conscious dog. Note the initial stimulation of duodenal bulb followed by sustained inhibition.

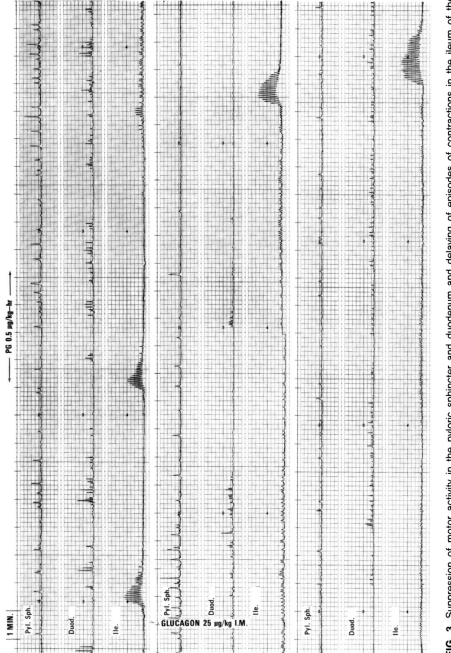

FIG. 3. Suppression of motor activity in the pyloric sphincter and duodenum and delaying of episodes of contractions in the ileum of the conscious dog by glucagon.

(15,19,47), and the stimulatory effect of gastrin on the musculature of LES was diminished by glucagon (19). *In vitro,* glucagon directly counteracted on the action of gastrin on the isolated muscle strips of the LES (19). In the dog, motor activities in the pylorus and ileo-cecal sphincters recorded with pressure transducers were all inhibited under basal conditions or stimulated by pentagastrin, as shown in Figs. 1 and 3.

Effect on Motor Function of the Extrahepatic Biliary Tract

Lin and Spray (24,29) showed that in conscious dogs with gastric, bile, gallbladder, and choledochal fistulae, glucagon increased bile secretion, decreased gastric secretion, and reduced the intraluminal pressure in the gallbladder. The relaxation of the gallbladder was dose-related and the minimal dose was about 2.5 to 5.0 μg/kg i.v. (25). Chernish et al. (5) found that in man glucagon increased the size of the gallbladder when given alone under basal conditions or after a fatty meal. However, this inhibitory effect of glucagon on human gallbladder could not be demonstrated *in vitro* (3).

The action of glucagon on the choledochal sphincter was inhibitory at low doses but became biphasic when the dose was large (25). At high doses glucagon initially increased the resistance of the choledochal sphincter before the final relaxation. The nature of this initial increase in choledochal sphincter tonus in the dog is obscure. It is likely to be related to its initial stimulatory action on the duodenal bulb. The relaxing action of glucagon on the sphincter of Oddi of man was reported recently (34).

Characteristics of the Inhibitory Action of Glucagon

The inhibitory effects of glucagon were characterized by decrease in intraluminal pressure or tonus in the lumen or the sphincters, reduction in amplitude as well as frequency of mechanical contractions, and diminished response to stimulation by gastrin G-17 or insulin (6–8,11,15,22,23,25,26,34,44,49). In addition, the myoelectric activity of the gut was also affected (23).

At very high doses, glucagon in combination with large doses of gastrin caused watery diarrhea in the dog (2). Such an effect of glucagon was mainly due to increased secretion of electrolytes in the jejunum and decreased absorption of electrolytes in the ileum rather than a stimulatory effect of glucagon on the gut muscles.

Possible Mechanism of Action

The mechanism by which glucagon inhibits the activity of the smooth muscles of the gut is poorly understood. One study indicated that the action was mediated through the adrenals (10) because the inhibition of intestinal motility was abolished following the exclusion of the adrenals in the anesthetized cat. In contrast, there is *in vitro* evidence that the inhibitory action was a direct one on the musculature of the gut itself (19). In addition, the effect of glucagon on the musculature of the gallbladder and the choledochal sphincter is probably a direct one also. Glucagon probably increases the intracellular level of cyclic AMP in the choledochal sphincter. Agents such as theophylline and isopreterenol that increase tissue level of cyclicAMP all relax the sphincter *in vitro* (1). In the conscious dog, Lin and Spray (25) failed to prevent the relaxing action of glucagon on the gallbladder and the choledochal sphincter with propranolol, atropine, phenoxybenzamine, or pentolinium tartrate at doses that these drugs showed obvious pharmacological autonomic effects (27,28).

Question of Physiological Role

In all of the studies, so far, the doses required for inhibition of gut motility and relaxation of gallbladder or the sphincters far exceeded those required for glycogenolytic action. The serum level of glucagon caused by infusion of glucagon during inhibition of gut motility was far in excess of that encountered in physiological circumstances (49). This suggests that a physiological role for glucagon in the regulation of the motor activity of the gut and extrahepatic biliary tract is unlikely. This does not, however, rule out conclusively the possibility that glucagon may still have a regulatory role. Further, physiological experiments relating plasma levels of endogenously released glucagon under normal conditions to its biological action on the gut need to be pursued.

Recently glucagon-like immunoreactive substances (entero-glucagon) were extracted from the gut. On purification by gel chromatography, two components were yielded (48,50). The chemical composition of enteroglucagons is still unknown, but it is reasonable to assume that there must be structural analogy to pancreatic glucagon to account for their crossimmunoreactivity with the antibodies to pancreatic glucagon. A good correlation between the log $T_{1/2}$ for gastric emptying and the rate of rise of plasma enteroglucagon after an oral glucose load was reported (40). This observation, of course, could not exclude the involvement of the osmoreceptors in the duodenal bulb or pylorus. Preliminary pharmacological data indicated that the "purified enteroglucagon" prepared by Murphy and Buchanan et al. also inhibited the antral and duodenal motility of the conscious dog at very low doses (26). The conclusive answer to the role of glucagon or enteroglucagon requires more specific and precise assessment of the relation between the plasma levels of pancreatic or enteroglucagon released under physiological conditions and their biologic action on the musculature of the gut.

REFERENCES

1. Anderson, K. E., Anderson, R., Hedner, P., and Persson, C. G. A. (1972): Effect of cholecystokinin on the level of cyclic AMP and on mechanical activity in the isolated sphincter of Oddi. *Life Sci.,* 11:723–732.

2. Barbezat, G. O., Grossman, M. I. (1971): Intestinal secretion: stimulation by peptides. *Science,* 174:422–424.
3. Cameron, A. J., Phillips, S. F., Williams, H. J. and Summerskill, D. M. (1970): Comparison of effects of gastrin, CCK, secretin, and glucagon on human stomach muscle *in vitro. Gastroenterology,* 59:539–545.
4. Chernish, S. M., Miller, R. E., Brunell, R. L., and Rosenak, B. D. (1978): Dose-response to intravenous glucagon as measured by roentgenography. *Radiology,* 127:55–59.
5. Chernish, S. M., Miller, R. E., Rosenak, B. D. and Schulz, N. E. (1972): Hypotonic duodenography with the use of glucagon. *Gastroenterology,* 63:392–398.
6. Chowdhury, A. R., and Lorber, S. H. (1975): Effect of glucagon on cholecystokinin and prostigmine induced motor activity of the distal colon and rectum in humans. *Gastroenterology,* 68:(4), 875. (abstract).
7. Chowdhury, A. R., Lorber, S. H. (1977): Effect of glucagon and secretin on food or morphine-induced motor activity of the distal colon, rectum and anal sphincter. *Am. J. Dig. Dis.,* 22:775–781.
8. Dotevall, G., Koch, N. G. (1963): The effect of glucagon on intestinal motility in man. *Gastroenterology,* 45:364–367.
9. Egbert, E. H., and Johnson, A. G. (1977): The effect of CCK on human *taenia coli. Digestion,* 15(3):217–222.
10. Fasth, S., Hesten, L. (1971): The effect of glucagon on intestinal motility and blood flow. *Acta Physiol. Scand.,* 83:169–173.
11. Ganeshappa, K. P., Walen, G. E., Meade, R. C., and Sorgel, K. H. (1971): The effect of glucagon on jejunal motility, electrolyte and water absorption in man. *Clin. Res.,* 19(3):658.
12. Gerner, T., and Haffner, J. F. (1976): The significance of distension for the effect of glucagon on the fundic and antral motility in isolated guinea pig stomach. *Scand. J. Gastroenterol. (Suppl.),* 10(35):51–53.
13. Granata, L., Leone, D., Paccione, F., and Ruccia, D. (1974): Effect of glucagon on jejunal motility in unanesthetized dog. *Boll. Soc. Ital. Biol. Sper.,* 59(11):780–785.
14. Hicks, T., and Turnberg, L. A. (1974): Influence of glucagon on the human jejunum. *Gastroenterology,* 67:1114–1118.
15. Hogen, W. J., Dodd, W. J., Hoke, S. E. et al. (1975): Effect of glucagon on esophageal motor function. *Gastroenterology,* 69:160–165.
16. Hradsky, M., Stockbruegger, R., and Oestberg, H. (1973): The effect of glucagon on gastric motility, the pylorus and reflux of bile into the stomach during gastroscopic examination. *Scand. J. Gastroenterol.,* 8(20):26.
17. Ih'asz, M., Koiss, I., Nemeth, E. P., Folly, G. and Papp, M. (1976): Action of caerulein, glucagon or prostaglandin E_1 on the motility of the intestinal villi. *Pflüger's Arch. Physiol.,* 364(3):301–304.
18. Jaffer, S. S., Maklouf, G. M., Schorr, B. A., Zfass, A. M. (1974): Nature and kinetics of inhibition of lower esophageal sphincter pressure by glucagon. *Gastroenterology,* 67:42–46.
19. Jennewein, H. M., Waldeck, F., Siewert, R., Weiser, F., Thiman, R. (1973): The interaction of glucagon and pentagastrin on the lower esophageal sphincter in man and dog. *Gut,* 14:861–864.
20. Johansson, H., Segerstrom, A. (1972): Glucagon and gastrointestinal motility in relation to thyroid parathyroid function. *Upps. J. Med. Sci.,* 77(3):183–188.
21. Junsk, K. (1977): Double blind examination of the colon with glucagon. Methods and results. *Roentgenblaetter,* 77(1):8–14.
22. Koch, N. G., Darle, N., Dotevall, G. (1967): Inhibition of intestinal motility in man by glucagon given intraperitoneally. *Gastroenterology,* 53:88–92.
23. Kowalewski, K. O., O'Sullivan, G. O., and Rolodij, A. (1976): Effect of glucagon on myoelectrical and mechanical activity of the isolated homologous perfused porcine stomach. *Pharmacology,* 14(2):115–124.
24. Lin, T.-M. (1974): Action of secretin, glucagon, cholecystokinin and endogenously released secretin and cholecystokinin on gallbladder and bile flow in dogs. *Fed. Proc.,* 33:391. (Abstr.).
25. Lin, T.-M. (1975): Action of gastrointestinal hormones and related peptides on the motor function of the biliary tract. *Gastroenterology,* 69(4): 1006–1022.
26. Lin, T.-M., Bloomquist, W. E., and Warrick, M. W. (1977): *Unpublished studies.*
27. Lin, T.-M., and Evans, D. C. (1973): Effect of propranolol on pentagastrin-induced HCl secretion and mucosal blood flow in dogs. *Gastroenterology,* 64:1126–1129.

28. Lin, T.-M., Evans, D. C., and Spray, G. F. (1973): Mechanism study of gastric inhibition by glucagon: Failure of KCl and adrenergic blocking agents to prevent its action. *Arch. Int. Pharmacodyn. Ther.*, 202:314–324.
29. Lin, T.-M., and Spray, G. F. (1969): Effect of pentagastrin, cholecystokinin, caerulein and glucagon on the choledochal resistance and bile flow of dogs. *Gastroenterology*, 56:1178, (Abstr.).
30. Lish, P. M., Clark, R. B., and Robbins, S. I. (1959): Effect of some physiological substances on gastrointestinal propulsion in the rat. *Am. J. Physiol.*, 197:22–26.
31. Melsom, M., Myren, J., Larson, S., and Moe, A. (1977): Comparison of glucagon and penthidine plus atropine as premedication for peroral endoscopy, A double blind study. *Endoscopy*, 9 (2): 79–82.
32. Miller, R. E., Chernish, S. M., Rosenak, B. D., and Rodda, B. E. (1973): Hypotonic duodenography with glucagon. *Radiology*, 108:35–42.
33. Miller, R. E., Chernish, S. M., Skucas, J., Rosenak, B. D., and Rodda, B. E. (1974): Hypotonic roentgenography with glucagon. *Am. J. Roentg.*, 121:264–274.
34. Nebel, O. T. (1975): Effect of enteric hormones on the human sphincter of Oddi. *Gastroenterology*, 68:(4), 962. (Abstr.).
35. Necheles, H., Sporn, J., and Walker, L. (1966): Effect of glucagon on gastrointestinal motility. *Gastroenterology*, 45:34–39.
36. Nikolov, N. A., and Deleva, Z. I. (1975): Action of glucagon on the motor and bioelectric activity of the small intestine and the stomach in dogs. *Fiziol. Zh. SSSR I. M. Sechenova*, 6(5):774–777.
37. Paul, F. (1974): Quantitative Untersuchungen der Wirkung von Pancreas-Glucagon und Secretin auf der Magen-Darmmotorik mittels electromanometrischer Simultanregistrierungen beim Menschen. *Klin. Wochenschr.*, 52:983–989.
38. Paul, F., and Freyschmidt, J. (1976): The use of glucagon for endoscopic and radiological examination of gastrointestinal tract. *Forschr. Geb. Roentgenstr. Nuklearmed.*, 125(1):310–37.
39. Penick, S. B., and Hinkle, L. E. Jr. (1961): Depression of food intake induced in healthy subjects by glucagon. *N. Engl. J. Med.*, 264:893–897.
40. Ralphe, D. N., Bloom, S. R., Lawden-Smith, C., Thomson, J. (1975): The relationship of human gastric emptying rate and plasma enteroglucagon concentration. *Gut*, 16(5):406.
41. Scott, L. D., and Sommers, R. W. (1974): Effect of glucagon and caerulein on propulsion and motility in the rat small intestine. *Gastroenterology*, 66(4):774. (Abstr.).
42. Sporn, J., and Necheles, H. (1956): Effect of glucagon on gastrointestinal motility. *Am. J. Physiol.*, 187:634. (abstract).
43. Stanciu, C., and Bennett, J. R. (1974): Effect of pancreozymin and glucagon on gastroduodenal motility in normal subjects. *Rev. Med. Chir.*, 78(3):609–613.
44. Stunkard, S. J., Van Itallie, T. B., Reis, B. B. (1955): The mechanism of satiety. Effect of glucagon on gastric hunger contraction in man. *Proc. Soc. Exp. Biol. Med.*, 89:258–261.
45. Takeuchi, S., Aizawa, I., Couch, E. F., and Itoh, Z. (1976): Gastric motor activity-stimulants: Spectrum and chemical architecture of gastrointestinal hormones. In: *Endocrinology of the Gut, Pancreas. Proceedings of International Symposium.* 197–208.
46. Takeuchi, S., Aizawa, I., and Itoh, Z. (1977): Motility of digestive tract and hormones of digestive tract. *Nippon Heikatankin Gakkai Zasshi*, 13(4):199–202.
47. Thomas, P. A., and Earlam, R. J. (1974): The effect of the gastrointestinal polypeptide hormones on the electric activity and pressure of the isolated perfused canine gastro-esophageal sphincter. In: *Proceedings of International Symposium on Gastrointestinal Motility*, 4th:243–250.
48. Unger, R. H., Ohneda, A., Valverde, I., Eisentraut, A. M., and Exton, J. (1968): Characterization of the response of circulating glucagon-like immunoreactivity to intraduodenal and intravenous administration of glucose. *J. Clin. Invest.*, 47:48–65.
49. Valenzuela, J. E. (1976): Effect of intestinal hormones and peptides on intragastric pressure in dogs. *Gastroenterology*, 71:766–769.
50. Valverde, I., Rigopoulou, D., Exton, J., Ohneda, A., Eisentraut, A., and Unger, R. H. (1968): Demonstration and characterization of a second fraction of glucagon-like immunoreactivity in jejunal extracts. *Am. J. Med. Sci.*, 255:415–420.
51. Whalen, G. E., Wu, W. C., Ganeshappa, K. P., Wall, M. J., Kalkhoff, R. K., and Sorgil, K. H. (1973): The effect of endogenous glucagon on human small bowel function. *Gastroenterology*, 64:822.

PROJECTIONS FOR THE FUTURE

In order to understand the true effects of insulin hypoglycemia or glucagon on gastrointestinal secretion and gut motility, one must first of all use the most highly purified materials for investigation. The possible contamination of insulin, glucagon, somatostatin, and pancreatic polypeptide with each other could be the major cause for the confusion reported in literature.

Secondly, both insulin and glucagon are known to influence the release and the plasma level of other hormones or chemical messengers that have actions of their own on either gastrointestinal secretion or motility or both. A clear view of the involvement of the release of these hormones by insulin hypoglycemia and the suppression of their release by glucagon is important for our understanding of the possible mechanisms of action.

Thirdly, the dependence of the action of insulin hypoglycemia on the integrity of the vagal system is well recognized. Evidence at hand suggests that glucagon may have a direct action on the stomach, liver and the smooth muscles of the gallbladder, choledochal sphincter, and the intestine independent of hyperglycemia, vagal innervation, or blood flow. Some of the actions of glucagon are not blocked by anticholinergics, α- or β-adrenergic or autonomic ganglionic blocking agents. The relationship between the effect of glucagon and the activity of second messengers such as the adenyl or guanyl cyclase system remains to be fully explored. This could be the area from which fruitful information about mechanism of action can be obtained.

Both insulin and glucagon can be released under physiological conditions. Their pharmacological actions on secretory and motor activities of the gut have been studied. But the physiological roles of insulin and glucagon, if any, are unknown.

Beside theoretical considerations of mechanisms of action and physiological role, application of insulin and glucagon for diagnostic and even therapeutic use should be expanded. (a) The successful use of glucagon for production of hypotonic duodenography and general relaxation of the bowel for radiographic or endoscopic examination of the gut is rapidly gaining momentum. (b) Because of its effect in increasing the blood flow in the mesenteric arteries, the possibility of using glucagon to improve intestinal blood flow or restore bowel movement soon after abdominal surgery should be considered. (c) Glucagon has been shown to decrease the gastric mucosal blood flow in the dog. The potential for glucagon to reduce gastric bleeding is the other possibility for its clinical use. (d) In view of the general relaxatory action of glucagon on the smooth muscles, clinical trials of glucagon are underway to relax muscles other than those in the gut. Among the latter are the clinical trials of glucagon effects on the ureter and the fallopian tubes, to mention but a few.

Gastrointestinal Hormones, edited by
George B. Jerzy Glass.
Raven Press, New York © 1980.

Chapter 28

Somatostatin and Opiate Peptides: Their Action on Gastrointestinal Secretions

Stanislaw J. Konturek

Institute of Physiology, Medical Academy, Krakow, 31531 Poland

INTRODUCTION

The secretory activity of the digestive glands depends on their intrinsic activity and the interplay of many stimulatory and inhibitory influences arising within the central nervous system (CNS) and alimentary tract. The major systems controlling digestive gland secretion include the autonomic innervation and the gastrointestinal hormones, which show a marked degree of interdependence and interaction. These neurohormonal mechanisms are of two types: the first originates centrally and mediates the anticipatory phase of secretion, and the second originates in the digestive tract itself where both local neural and hormonal mechanisms are activated by the presence of food.

The characteristic feature of the hormone-containing cells of the alimentary tract is their scattered distribution among the exocrine cells of the gastrointestinal mucosa and the pancreas. This provides the anatomical arrangement for the efficient "paracrine" delivery of the hormonal product across the intercellular space directly to the target cells without mediation of circulation (19,71,72).

Some gastrointestinal hormones are also present in the special peripheral neurons within the wall of the gut and in the pancreas, where they may serve as neurotransmitters delivered from the nerve terminals to adjacent tissues by neurocrine path. These peptidergic neurons may be considered as a third division of the autonomic nervous system often referred to as the "purinergic" system (6,11).

It is of interest that some hormonal peptides originally isolated from the digestive tract were then shown to have immunological counterparts in the brain [cholecystokinin (CCK), vasoactive intestinal peptide (VIP), and motilin], and some peptides first isolated from the brain [somatostatin, enkephalin, and thyrotropin releasing hormone (TRH)] were later found to have immunological counterparts in the digestive system.

These rather startling observations were brought together in a unified amine precursor uptake and decarboxylation (APUD) concept formulated by Pearse (71). He observed that neurons and endocrine cells producing peptide hormones share similar ultrastructural characteristics and possess similar cytochemical features such as enzymes capable of producing biogenic amines. On the basis of these findings he postulated that all hormonal peptide-producing cells derive from a neural ectoderm. The discovery of hormonal peptides of dual localization in the brain and the gut is in keeping with this concept.

This chapter presents recent progress in studies on somatostatin and opiate peptides as related to the digestive gland secretion.

SOMATOSTATIN

Somatostatin, a growth hormone-release inhibiting hormone (GH-RIH), was isolated from sheep hypothalami and its amino acid sequence determined in 1973 by Brazeau et al. (10). Subsequently, it was isolated from the hypothalamic tissue of other species and found to have a tetradecapeptide structure, identical to that of ovine peptide (88). The most unexpected finding was the discovery of somatostatin-like immunoreactivity apart from the brain, particularly in the tissues of the digestive system (76). Somatostatin possesses multiple antisecretory actions at both pituitary and extrapituitary sites and is known to affect all basic functions of the digestive system including secretion, motility, absorption, and splanchnic circulation (41).

Structure and Location

Somatostatin originally isolated from ovine and porcine hypothalami is a cyclic tetradecapeptide characterized as the H_2-Ala-Gly-Cys-Lys-Asn-Phe-Phe-

$\quad\quad\quad\quad\quad\quad\quad\quad\quad\quad\quad$ |_____S-S_____

Trp-Lys-Thr-Phe-Thr-Ser-Cys-COOH. Other highly basic forms of somatostatin were also found in extracts of pig hypothalami (89) and shown to have physiochemical properties different from those of somatostatin. These materials are biologically and immunologically active, appear to have several additional amino acids including arginine attached to the NH_2-terminus, and may represent precursor of somatostatin (prosomatostatin). Gel filtration chromatography profiles from the extracts of the stomach, intestine, and pancreas of various species showed at least two peaks, a major peak eluting at the same position as tetradecapeptide somatostatin and a minor peak in the region of the void volume corresponding to "big" somatostatin (17,104). Recent evidence that the latter material can be partially converted by urea treatment to a form eluting in a position identical to tetradecapeptide somatostatin suggests that at least part of big somatostatin may represent an aggregate of somatostatin or somatostatin noncovalently bound to a larger protein (64).

Somatostatin itself is of little therapeutic value because of multiple nonspecific inhibitory actions on the secretory activity of various exocrine and endocrine glands and a short biological half-life of less than 2 min (90a). Recently many somatostatin analogs have been synthesized in an attempt to prolong and increase the biological activity of native peptide (27,87). Some analogs have been thought to be endowed with a dissociated biological action on one or more of the recognized targets of somatostatin. Analogs with such dissociated activities, e.g., [D-Trp⁸]-somatostatin, [D-Trp⁸,D-Cys¹⁴]-somatostatin, and [D-Cys¹⁴]-somatostatin, selectively inhibit growth hormone (GH) and glucagon release more than insulin (65). They are of clinical interest because of their possible usefulness in the treatment of certain endocrinological disorders such as juvenile diabetes, acromegaly, diabetic retinopathy, and other diseases.

Somatostatin originally extracted from the hypothalamus was subsequently demonstrated in even greater amounts in other regions of the brain, particularly in the external zone of the median eminence, the lamina terminalis, and the pineal gland. It was localized by immunocytochemistry (ICC) in nerve cell bodies and in nerve terminals in various hypothalamic nuclei, in the pituitary stalk, and in the posterior pituitary (32). Recent studies (33) on the distribution of immunoreactive somatostatin show that this peptide occurs in neuronal elements in multiple locations in the CNS including the brain cortex and the spinal cord (18). This finding, together with various neurotropic effects of somatostatin, suggests that somatostatin might serve not only as a hypophysiotropic hormone, but also as a neurotransmitter in special neuronal systems in the brain.

Immunoreactive somatostatin has also been demonstrated in various digestive organs such as the stomach, the intestines, the salivary glands, and the pancreas (2,32,33), where it has been localized in the distinctive endocrine cells (D cells) (Fig. 1). In the stomach, D cells were found in the lamina propria, frequently adjacent to the oxyntic and pyloric glands. In the gastric antrum, they predominated in the neighborhood of gastrin-producing cells (76). Many D cells were localized also in the lamina propria of the intestinal mucosa of the entire gut

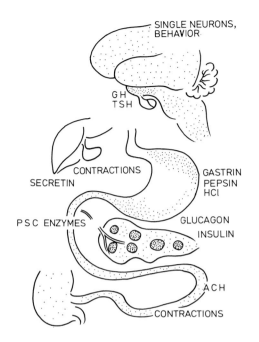

FIG. 1. Multiple locations and multiple effects of somatostatin. (From ref. 27.)

and a few were among the epithelial cells of the Lieberkühn crypts. In the pancreas, the D cells occur in the periphery of the pancreatic islets between A and B cells (32). This particular distribution of D cells, namely, their scattering among the other endocrine and exocrine cells, indicates a possible paracrine (41) rather than an endocrine function.

Somatostatin-like immunoreactivity was also localized to nervous structures of the gut such as the neurons of myenteric plexus (33) and the vagal nerves (101). The accumulation of the somatostatin-like material in the nerve terminals suggests that somatostatin may be released in the digestive tract via neurocrine mechanism by axonal depolarization and serve as an inhibitory neurotransmitter. This assumption has been recently supported by the finding (25) that somatostatin inhibits the release of acetylcholine from the isolated myenteric plexus–longitudinal muscle preparation of the guinea pig ileum, suggesting that this peptide may act as an inhibitory modulator of cholinergic transmission.

Biological Actions

The availability of natural somatostatin and its potent stable analogs as well as sensitive somatostatin radioimmunoassay (RIA) enabled us to determine the full spectrum of biological actions and possible physiological significance of this peptide.

It is now well recognized that somatostatin has many biological effects other than just an inhibition of growth hormone secretion (5). Somatostatin also inhibits the secretion of other pituitary hormones such as thyrotropin (TSH) and prolactin (27,87). A physiological role of somatostatin in the regulation of pituitary hormonal secretion is supported by elegant studies of Arimura et al. (3,4), who showed that passive immunization with somatostatin antiserum increases basal GH concentration, prevents the stress-induced decrease of GH, and increases the TSH response to thyrotropin releasing hormone (TRH). These effects are most likely due to the neutralization of the "tonic" action of endogenous somatostatin, which exhibits an inhibitory control on GH and TSH secretion. The inhibitory effect of somatostatin is more pronounced in the excess of these pituitary hormones regardless of whether their origin is regulatory or autonomous (29).

Pancreatic Somatostatin

At the endocrine pancreas, somatostatin exerts a powerful suppressive effect on the secretion of insulin and glucagon. It inhibits both the acute and chronic phases of insulin and glucagon secretion in response to a variety of stimuli (1,14). It suppresses the release of insulin by glucose, tolbutamide, isoproterenol, gastric inhibitory polypeptide (GIP), glucagon, and secretin. This inhibitory effect is quickly reversible and followed by a rebound of hormone secretion, indicating a short biological action of somatostatin. The decrease in the plasma insulin is associated with a paradoxical decrease in blood glucose level and inhibits release of glucagon (68). In diabetic human subjects somatostatin also causes a marked reduction in blood glucose and in plasma glucagon levels (21). These observations were taken as the first clear-cut evidence that glucagon has an important role in human carbohydrate metabolism and in the hyperglycemia of diabetes. The finding that somatostatin inhibits the secretion of GH, insulin, and glucagon—all involved in the control of carbohydrate metabolism—was considered to have an important therapeutic implication, particularly in the treatment of insulin-dependent diabetes. Recent reports, however, indicate that this is not the case. Somatostatin administered to insulin-deficient diabetics appears to reduce the postprandial hyperglycemia not only by suppressing the excess of glucagon but primarily by delaying the carbohydrate absorption from the gut (21,86,102). Thus the beneficial effects produced by somatostatin in diabetics are not due entirely to inhibition of circulating glucagon. In fact, in patients with maturity-onset diabetes, prolonged administration of somatostatin may even intensify hyperglycemia and hyperketonemia despite the suppression of glucagon secretion. Recently, cases of somatostatinoma, a tumor composed of D cells and producing excessive amounts of somatostatin, have been reported (20,57). Patients with such a tumor developed hypochlorhydria, steatorrhea, and mild diabetes accompanied by hypoglucagonemia and hypoinsulinemia. Removal of the tumor was followed by a remission of hyperglycemia, indicating a causal relationship between hypersomatostatinemia and diabetes in this condition.

Gastrointestinal Somatostatin

Numerous studies in recent years have demonstrated that somatostatin influences a number of gastrointestinal hormones and functions. It was first reported that intravenous somatostatin inhibits markedly the serum gastrin response to feeding in normal subjects and causes a decrease in fasting serum gastrin level in patients with pernicious anemia and with gastrinoma (7). The decrease in basal and postprandial gastrin caused by somatostatin was reported to be similar in normal and hypophysectomized subjects, indicating that the effect is independent of mediation by the GH (79). Since then somatostatin was found to inhibit the release of most gastrointestinal hormones including gastrin (49), secretin (8,51), CCK (51), motilin (66), and pancreatic polypeptide (40).

Somatostatin also inhibits directly the gastrointestinal secretions of electrolytes and enzymes stimulated by a variety of secretagogues, in both man and animals. It is a potent inhibitor of gastric acid secretion induced by exogenous stimulants such as histamine, gastrin, or cholinergic agents acting directly on the oxyntic glands (49). The most sensitive to the inhibitory action of somatostatin appears to be a food-stimulated secretion (Fig. 2), probably because of suppression of the release and action of gastrointestinal hormones involved in the postprandial secretory activities of the oxyntic glands (47,49).

The finding that somatostatin-containing cells and nerves are present in the digestive tract in the close vicinity of endocrine and exocrine cells suggested a possible physiological role of somatostatin as a local hormone, a member of Feyrter's paracrine system (19). Recently, several investigators succeeded, how-

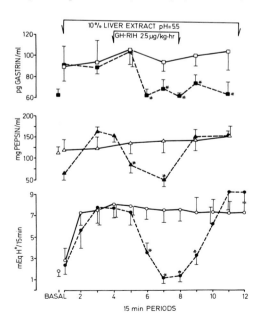

FIG. 2. Effect of somatostatin on meal-induced serum gastrin and gastric acid secretion in six duodenal ulcer patients. (From ref. 47.)

ever, in the development of a sensitive RIA for plasma somatostatin, and Schus-dziarra et al. (90) reported that under basal conditions the concentration of immunoreactive somatostatin in portal blood is significantly higher than in the peripheral venous circulation. This suggests that somatostatin may be released into the blood mainly from the pancreas and the stomach. Pancreatic somatosta-tin can be released by various factors and hormones including high concentration of glucose, arginine, leucine and glucagon (but not insulin), gastrin, secretin, and CCK (35,36). Prompt response of pancreatic somatostatin to various meta-bolic and hormonal stimuli together with a known suppressive effect of somato-statin on glucose intake from the gut and on appetite implies that this peptide may participate in nutrient homeostasis.

The finding that intragastric or intraduodenal administration of HCl solution or acidified peptone meal results in a prompt and marked increase in somatostatin release from the gastric antrum and the duodenum (Fig. 3) suggests that this hormonal peptide may be involved in the antral and duodenal inhibitory mecha-nisms of gastric acid secretion (90). Low pH in the gastric antrum and in the duodenum could suppress gastric acid and gastrin secretion, at least in part, by stimulating the release of somatostatin. Thus somatostatin could explain, at least in part, the well-known feedback suppression of gastrin release and gastric secretion by acidification of the antral and duodenal mucosa.

Duodenal ulcer patients, who were reported to have an abnormality of the mechanisms by which acid inhibits antral gastrin release, were also found to have a failure of somatostatin inhibition of gastrin release due to a relative deficiency of the D cells in their antral mucosa. Polak et al. (77) performed a quantitative immunocytochemical study and showed that in normal human stom-ach tissue there is a preponderance of G cells over D cells (ratio 7:1); in gastric ulcer patients there is a relative decrease in G cells over the D cells, whereas most duodenal ulcer patients show moderate to severe G cell hyperplasia. This remains in agreement with a recent report of Chayvialle et al. (12) that the content of immunoreactive somatostatin in the antral mucosa is significantly lower in duodenal ulcer patients than in healthy subjects. These findings together with the observation of the decreased effect of exogenous somatostatin on acid secretion and gastrin release reported in duodenal ulcer patients (48) emphasize an important role of somatostatin in the pathophysiology of duodenal ulcer disease (Fig. 4).

Somatostatin causes a marked inhibition of pancreatic bicarbonate secretion induced by exogenous secretin and duodenal acidification or feeding (51). The inhibition of secretin-stimulated bicarbonate secretion shows the characteristics of competitive inhibition, suggesting a competition for a common receptor site between somatostatin and secretin (51). This inhibitory effect might be attributed also to some other as yet unknown action of somatostatin including the effect on enzymatic processes involving cyclic AMP or alteration in the transfer of calcium ions (41).

The inhibitory effect of somatostatin on pancreatic response to endogenous

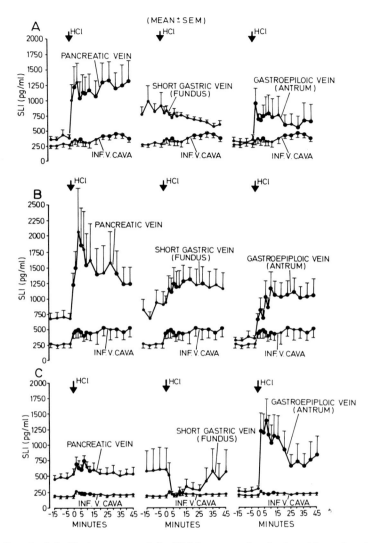

FIG. 3. Somatostatin-like immunoreactivity (SLI) in pancreatic, short gastric, and gastroepiploic vein and in the inferior vena cava in response to intragastric **(A)** and intraduodenal administration of HCl into dogs with a gastric fistula **(C).** ⊙ indicates significant differences ($P < 0.05$) compared to baseline levels. (From ref. 90.)

stimulants such as food or duodenal acidification is usually much stronger than to exogenous secretin (Fig. 5). This finding together with the observation that somatostatin decreases plasma secretin level in tests with duodenal acidification (10) indicates that somatostatin inhibits pancreatic secretion, at least in part, by the suppression of secretin release from the intestinal mucosa.

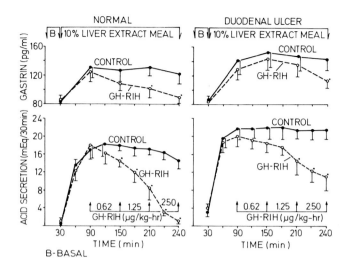

FIG. 4. Effect of graded doses of somatostatin given intravenously and serum gastrin responses to liver extract in healthy subjects and duodenal ulcer patients. Mean ± SEM of six tests on six subjects. *Asterisks* denote significant difference ($P < 0.05$) from control. (From ref. 42a.)

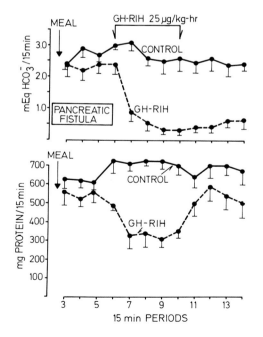

FIG. 5. Effect of somatostatin on meal-induced pancreatic bicarbonate and protein enzyme secretion in pancreatic fistula dogs. (From ref. 51.)

Somatostatin markedly inhibits the secretion of enzymes by the stomach and the pancreas. In fact, this peptide appears to be an even more potent inhibitor of gastric pepsin and pancreatic enzyme secretion than of electrolyte secretion. The potent antisecretory effect of somatostatin on pepsin secretion might explain the prevention by this peptide of the formation of experimental gastroduodenal ulcerations induced by prolonged administration of gastric secretagogues or stress conditions (46). In practical terms somatostatin may be of benefit in the treatment of some forms of peptic ulcerations, e.g., in the preoperative management of duodenal ulcerations in the Zollinger-Ellison syndrome. It has now been applied successfully to patients with bleeding stress ulcers (63), probably due to the reduction of acid-pepsin secretion and prevention of dissolution of thrombi at the site of the bleeding (80). In view of the marked inhibition of pancreatic enzyme secretion, somatostatin has been suggested as a potentially useful therapeutic adjunct to the treatment of acute pancreatitis. This concept is supported by the experimental data indicating that somatostatin reduces the development of acute inflammatory reaction of the pancreas in laboratory animals and by clinical observations that it can prevent pancreatitis-like biochemical disturbances resulting from endoscopic pancreatography (81).

The effect of somatostatin and biliary secretion has not been studied extensively, and the results obtained differ depending on the species examined and the technique of bile collection or peptide administration. Lin et al. (60) observed that it significantly decreases bile flow in the dog, but in other studies performed on man (81) and rats (62) no changes in bile flow or bile composition were noticed.

Somatostatin inhibits intestinal secretion induced by prostaglandin E and theophylline in the rat by a mechanism independent of changes in cyclic AMP in the intestinal mucosa. It also reduces watery diarrhea in a patient with carcinoid syndrome probably due to inhibition of serotonin-induced changes in the intestinal fluid secretion (16a). The changes in the absorption of fat, carbohydrates, and calcium from the gut observed after somatostatin administration might be attributed to changes in the gastrointestinal motility or in the intestinal blood flow (43,102), but they might also be due to the disturbance of the intestinal uptake and transport of absorption products (41).

OPIATE PEPTIDES

The search for opiate-like compounds began after the discovery of opiate receptors in the brain (23). The first of these to be isolated and chemically characterized were two enkephalin pentapeptides (34). Then larger opiate peptides were isolated and designated as endorphins and subdivided into alpha, beta, and gamma, all showing the amino acid sequence contained within the pituitary peptide, beta-lipotropin, which itself has no opiate activity (22,59).

Opiate receptors and enkephalins have been demonstrated recently in the endocrine-like cells and nerves of the digestive tract (78), but their physiological role is completely unknown. This chapter summarizes some of the biological effects of opiate peptides on gastrointestinal secretions.

Structure and Location

The opiate receptors have been identified in the brain by measuring the specific binding of radioactively labeled opiate drugs to cell fragments (75,91). This binding can be specifically blocked by opiate receptor antagonists such as naloxone or naltrexone. Opiate receptors were localized throughout the CNS, particularly in the areas associated with the integration of pain perception and with arousal of emotions (96). The highest concentration of opiate receptors occurs in the first way stations of sensory perception such as substantia gelatinosa of the spinal cord, the trigeminal nuclei, the central thalamus, and the periaqueductal gray matter of the midbrain, which plays a role in drug- and electrically induced analgesia. Opiate receptors are also present in high concentration in the limbic system, especially in amygdala, which are primarily involved with arousal of emotions in man. Vagal nuclei of the brainstem, which participate in visceral reflexes, are also abundant in opiate receptors (5,73,94,96).

Besides the brain, the opiate receptors have also been detected in the digestive tract and found to resemble those in the brain (53–55). Due to the presence of these receptors in the myenteric plexus and the smooth muscle of the gut, opiates specifically inhibit electrically induced contractions of the ileal smooth muscle, and the guinea pig ileum bioassay is now widely used to screen the biological properties of opiate agonists and antagonists.

Opiate-like compounds that have been isolated from the brain or the gut on the basis of this bioassay or displacement of tritiated opiates on synaptosomal preparations, and that have been chemically characterized, are peptides related to a fragment of the C-terminus of the molecule of beta-lipotropin (27), starting at Tyr[61] (where Tyr is tyrosine). Lipotropin is a 91 amino acid pituitary peptide that was discovered by Li et al. (59) and was shown to have some fat-mobilizing activity. In addition to enkephalin pentapeptides, methionine-enkephalin and leucine-enkephalin, which were first isolated and chemically characterized by Hughes et al. (34) in 1975, longer fragments of lipotropin commencing at Tyr[61] were shown to exhibit opiate-like behavior. The most potent of them appears to be beta-endorphin, a fragment containing a 61–91 amino acid sequence of lipotropin. Other fragments such as lipotropin[61-76] (alpha-endorphin) and lipotropin[61-77] (gamma-endorphin) also show considerable affinity to opiate receptors and quite potent contraceptive action (16,22,26,28).

Lipotropin and its major opiate-like fragments are present mainly in the pituitary but they also occur in the brain, although in much lesser concentration (39,56,94). The biological role of lipotropin and its relationship to endorphins and enkephalins is not clear. The observation that lipotropin, which itself has no opiate activity, can generate this activity after incubation with brain extract (58) suggests the presence of specific peptidases in the brain that could cleave lipotropin to endorphins and enkephalins. The suggestion that lipotropin serves as an inactive precursor of opiate peptides seems, however, unlikely because there is good evidence from immunocytochemistry (39) that endorphins exist as such in discrete pituitary cells. In addition, endorphins can be detected in the brain after hypophysectomy, indicating that they are native brain substances rather than cleavage products of lipotropin (13).

The minimum sequence of LPH with opiate activity is enkephalin pentapeptide with Tyr at the N-terminus. It may be defined as the "opioid region" that interacts with the opiate receptor. Removal of C-terminal methionine or leucine from this opioid region strongly reduces the biological activity but does not abolish its binding affinity, whereas the removal of N-terminal tyrosine results in totally inactive tetrapeptide (31,67,100), and this appears to be an important mechanism of inactivation of enkephalin *in vivo* (31). The intact N-terminal tyrosine seems to be essential for binding affinity, but full pharmacological activity requires the presence of C-terminal methionine or leucine. It is of interest that the N-terminus of enkephalin with its benzene ring of tyrosine has some structural feature in common with morphine, suggesting that this portion of the molecule is responsible for binding of both peptides to opiate receptor.

At the present time, a number of enkephalin analogs have been synthesized by replacement of L isomers of amino acids in enkephalin by their D isomer or other alterations of the enkephalin structure that result in the increased binding affinity and biological activity (21,61,74). Some of them such as stable analog FK 33–824 (Sandoz, Switzerland) are many times more potent than morphine in analgesic potency and are active orally (84). They can pass the blood-brain barrier, which prevents natural enkephalin given intravenously from entering the brain. Enkephalins and their stable analogs exhibit cross-tolerance and cross-dependence with morphine and obviously are of clinical interest.

The distribution of enkephalins and endorphins in various tissues can be now conveniently examined by using various techniques such as RIA, ICC, and radiolabeling of opiate peptides. It has been found that the distribution of opiate peptides in the brain is similar to that of opiate receptors (39,53,69,95). In general, the brain areas with a high density of opiate receptors are also rich in enkephalins. Ultrastructurally enkephalins are chiefly confined to nerve fibers and nerve terminals.

Apart from the brain, opiate peptides have been detected also throughout the tissues of the digestive system (Fig. 6). Using two independent methods, RIA and ICC, Polak et al. (78) have demonstrated the presence of enkephalin immunoreactivity both in special endocrine cells of APUD series and in the nerve fibers of the myenteric plexus. The largest concentration of enkephalin was found in the mucosa of antrum and somewhat less in the upper small intestine. Substantial amounts were also detected in the pancreas and in the wall of the gallbladder. Similarly, Sundler et al. (98) reported that enkephalin immunoreactivity occurred in nerve cell bodies and in nerve fibers of the myenteric plexus all along the gut of several species. In some species, except man,

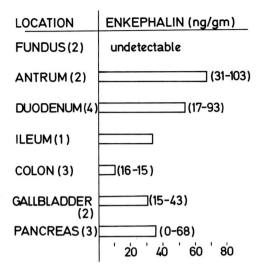

FIG. 6. Distribution of enkephalin in human digestive system. (From ref. 78.)

immunoreactive material was also found in the endocrine cells present mainly in antrum and proximal duodenum. These cells appear to be identical with serotonin-storing enterochromaffin cells, indicating that some endocrine cells may contain both a hormonal peptide and a biogenic amine. The opiate-like peptides occurring in the gut belong to the methionine-enkephalin-type peptides, but in some species also beta-endorphin immunoreactivity was found in the gut.

Biological Actions

The physiological role of opiate peptides is a subject of intensive research carried out in many laboratories. In the brain they appear to play the role of a neurotransmitter or neuromodulator of specific neuronal systems that mediate the integration of sensory information related to pain and emotional behavior. They act as presynaptic or postsynaptic inhibitors and suppress the firing of most neurons tested, particularly those involved in the release of stimulatory neurotransmitters such as acetylcholine or catecholamines (9,15,52,99). They mimic the action of morphine on the brain and result in a great diversity of effects such as limitation of experience of pain, profound tranquilization or analgesia, respiratory depression, changes in the extrapyramidal motor system, and euphoric changes of mood. Other important actions beyond that of pain perception and emotional behavior include the release of pituitary hormones such as prolactin, GH, and antidiuretic hormone (83,105). These effects are prevented by prior administration of naloxone. Beta-endorphin seems to be particularly suitable to control endocrine pituitary functions because it is stored in high concentration in the hypothalamus-pituitary axis and is more resistant to enzymatic degradation than enkephalins.

Effects of Opiate Peptides on Gastric Secretion

Opiates have long been known for the powerful actions on gastrointestinal tract. Morphine and related drugs are known to exhibit pronounced effects on both gastrointestinal motility and secretion (24).

The studies of opiates on the secretory activity of the digestive glands gave conflicting results. Although most pharmacology textbooks describe opiates as inhibitors of gastric secretion, there have been some reports in the past indicating that morphine and related drugs may actually increase gastric secretion (82, 93,106). Our studies (45) on dogs with gastric fistulas and Heidenhain pouches, in which the secretory rate was measured by intrapouch titration of acid, showed that in fasted dogs methionine-enkephalin and its analog increased dose dependently the secretion of acid, reaching a peak of about 17 and 29% of histamine maximum in tests with enkephalin and its stable analogs (FK 33–824) and about 50% in tests with morphine (Fig. 7). This opiate-induced stimulation was not accompanied by any significant change in serum gastrin level, suggesting

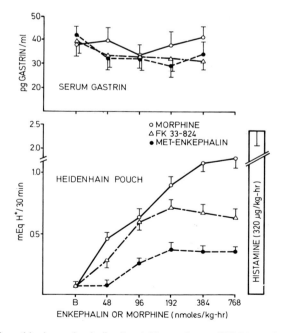

FIG. 7. Effect of methionine-enkephalin, its stable analogue (FK 33–824), and morphine on gastric acid secretion and serum gastrin level in the Heidenhain pouch dog. (From Konturek, *unpublished data*.)

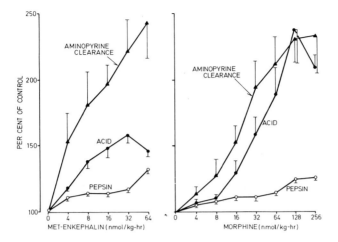

FIG. 8. Effect of methionine-enkephalin and morphine on histamine-induced acid secretion and mucosal blood flow in an *in vivo* canine stomach flap preparation. (From ref. 44.)

that the action of opiates on oxyntic glands is gastrin independent and probably involves direct stimulation of these glands.

When given intravenously during near maximal pentagastrin stimulation, enkephalin augments dose dependently the acid secretory rate, particularly from the denervated portion of the stomach, and this is accompanied by a rise in the gastric mucosal blood flow determined by the aminopyrine clearance technique. Even more pronounced stimulation of gastric secretory rate and substantial increase in the mucosal blood flow (Fig. 8) were observed when enkephalin or morphine was given directly to the artery supplying the flap of the fundic portion of the stomach clamped in the lucite chamber preparation (44). The enhancement of gastrin-stimulated acid secretion by a stable opiate-like peptide analog (FK 33–824) was also observed in rats with perfused stomach preparation (30). The stimulatory effects of opiate peptide in dog and rat can be reversed, at least in part, by the addition of naloxone to enkephalin administration. Naloxone alone (without enkephalin) does not affect basal histamine or pentagastrin-stimulated gastric secretion. This argues against a persisting "tonic" action of endogenous opioid substances but does not exclude such activity under certain conditions such as shock state (85) when enkephalins are produced in large amounts. It should be mentioned, however, that opiate-induced gastric secretion from the innervated and denervated stomach can be easily inhibited not only by naloxone but also by other secretory inhibitors such as anticholinergics or H_2 blockers. This may be explained by the concept of the interaction between binding sites for various parietal cell stimuli including opiate substances. As suggested recently by Soll and Grossman (97), the action of a single agent such as opiate compound may represent, in part, the interaction between this agent and endogenous secretagogues such as histamine or acetylcholine.

The mechanism of opiate-induced stimulation of gastric secretion is unknown, but it is certainly not due to gastrin release. The study with the gastric mucosal blood flow suggests that primary increase in gastric microcirculation and subsequent increased delivery of secretory stimuli to oxyntic glands might be responsible, at least in part, for the observed increase in gastric secretion (45).

The physiological role of opiates as gastric stimulants may be difficult to assess, because neither the mechanism of release nor the amount of enkephalin released from the gut are known. They probably play the role of a local hormone, a member of the paracrine system, because they are quickly removed from the circulation. Our studies with intraportal and systemic administration of enkephalin showed that, unlike morphine, opiate peptides are almost completely inactivated by hepatic transit (45). Thus, because of the marked liver inactivation, the action of natural opiate substances of gastrointestinal origin is probably confined mostly to the digestive system.

Effects of Opiate Peptides on Pancreatic Secretion

The action of opiate peptides on pancreatic secretion has not been studied systematically. The known inhibitory influence of morphine and related drugs has been attributed to pancreatic duct contraction rather than to direct suppression of the secretory activity of the exocrine pancreas. Our recent comparative

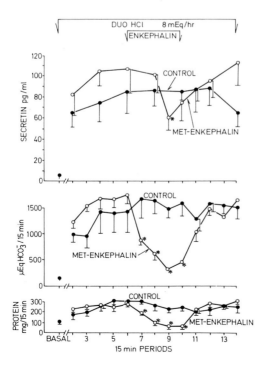

FIG. 9. Effect of methionine-enkephalin on pancreatic bicarbonate and protein secretion and plasma secretin level in response to duodenal acidification in dogs with chronic pancreatic fistulas. (From Konturek, *unpublished data*).

studies (50) showed that both enkephalin and morphine suppress the bicarbonate and protein responses to secretin and CCK and that this suppression possesses the kinetics of competitive inhibition. Opiates were found to be quite effective inhibitors of pancreatic secretion induced by duodenal acidification (Fig. 9). β-endorphin was shown to suppress pancreatic secretion, being a relatively more potent inhibitor than enkephalin.

The most sensitive to opiate-induced inhibition appears to be a meal-induced stimulation of pancreatic secretion. Postprandial stimulation of pancreatic secretion can be almost completely suppressed by opiates. The inhibition of bicarbonate response to a meal is usually accompanied by a marked suppression of plasma secretin level. Naloxone combined with enkephalin or morphine prevents, in part, this inhibition, suggesting that this effect might be mediated, at least in part, by specific opiate receptors. Since naloxone prevents also the suppression of endogenous release of secretin by opiates, it may be assumed that opiate receptors are localized both in secretin-producing cells and in the pancreatic exocrine cells (Fig. 10).

Enkephalin was found to be a potent inhibitor of pancreatic protein secretion, particularly in studies with feeding or duodenal acidification, suggesting that this opiate peptide may suppress the release of CCK from the gut. However, it cannot be determined at this time whether or not opiate peptide affects the release of CCK because, as mentioned before, this peptide also inhibits pancreatic secretory response to exogenous CCK. Direct measurement of plasma CCK

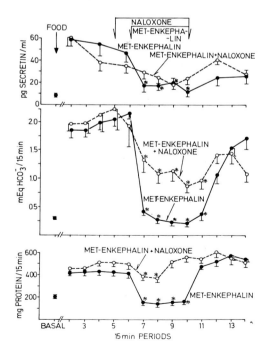

FIG. 10. Effect of methionine-enkephalin alone and in combination with naloxone on meal-induced pancreatic secretion of bicarbonate and protein and plasma secretin level. (From Konturek, *unpublished data*).

level by RIA will clarify a possible role of enkephalin in the release of CCK.

The observation that opiates are potent inhibitors of both bicarbonate and protein secretion from the pancreas suggests that these agents affect the secretory mechanisms common for both parameters of pancreatic secretion. Since opiates are known to suppress the release of acetylcholine in every tissue so far tested (38,70,103), it is possible that enkephalin-induced inhibition of pancreatic secretion could be attributed, at least in part, to removal of the cholinergic background involved in the release and action of intestinal hormones stimulating pancreatic secretion of both bicarbonate and enzyme protein (92).

Opiate peptides are also capable of altering islet cell function (37). They suppress the release of somatostatin-like immunoreactivity and increase the release of insulin and glucagon from the isolated perfused canine pancreas. Since these effects can be reversed by naloxone, it has been suggested that they are mediated by specific opiate receptors. The stimulatory effect of opiates on insulin or glucagon is usually preceded by the suppression of endogenous somatostatin, suggesting that the primary event in opiate action is inhibition of endogenous somatostatin and release of insulin and glucagon from its inhibitory influence.

The physiological role of endogenous opioid substances in the regulation of exocrine and endocrine pancreas is difficult to assess because neither the mechanism of release nor the amount of opiate released is known. The presence of endocrine cells and nerves with enkephalin-like immunoreactivity in the exocrine pancreas and in pancreatic islets raises the possibility that locally secreted opiate substances may influence both exocrine and endocrine secretory activity of the pancreas.

The influence of opiate peptides on biliary and intestinal secretion has not been reported. Opium has been used from antiquity for the relief of diarrhea and dysentery, but this has been attributed to the action of opium alkaloids on gastrointestinal motility (24). Endogenous opiates appear to mimic the action of opium drugs on the motility of the gut as enkephalin was recently shown to inhibit the contractive activity of the gut *in vitro* and to suppress the myoelectric activity of intact intestines *in vivo* (42).

CONCLUSIONS AND PROJECTIONS FOR THE FUTURE

Analysis of the possible physiological functions of somatostatin and opiate peptides is still in an early stage. Most of the information available concerns the pharmacological effects of these peptides, and a great effort has to be made not to indulge in speculation on their physiological role for which the experimental basis is insecure. Highly sensitive RIA of the peptides is now in development, and in the near future we can expect to see whether they are delivered into the circulation by endocrine path as classic gastrointestinal hormones such as gastrin, secretin, or CCK, or whether they are released by paracrine and neurocrine mechanisms and reach their targets by diffusion across the intercellular space. Recent discovery of these peptides in both brain and gut and their location in the latter site in endocrine-type cells and in nerve fibers have revolutionized the concept of the regulation of gastrointestinal secretion. At present it is difficult to conceive, however, how these and a number of other recently discovered hormonal peptides remain in harmonious interplay in the control of gastrointestinal functions. Somatostatin, for example, is capable of suppressing all major digestive functions, and we cannot imagine such a physiological situation in which so many systems would need to be inhibited at once. Exogenous opiate peptides strongly affect both exocrine and endocrine functions of the stomach, pancreas, and gut, yet the blockage of their action by specific opiate receptor antagonists (e.g., naloxone or naltrexone) has little influence on activities of the digestive system. This argues against a persisting "tonic" action of endogenous opiate peptides on the digestive system but does not exclude the possibility of such an action under pathological conditions such as stress states when the opiate peptides are released in large amounts.

Future research should elucidate the mechanism of the release and the spectrum of physiological actions as well as the role of both somatostatin and opiate peptides in the pathophysiology of various diseases of the endocrine and digestive systems. It is possible that these peptides and their potent, long-acting analogs, which have already been prepared, may be useful in the treatment of certain disorders such as acromegaly, diabetes, peptic ulcer, pancreatitis, and other diseases.

REFERENCES

1. Alberti, K. G. M. M., Christensen, S. E., Iversen, J., Seyer-Hansen, A. P., Christensen, N. J., Hansen, A. P., Lundbaek, K., and Orskov, H. (1973): Inhibition of insulin secretion by somatostatin. *Lancet,* 2:1299–2301.
2. Arimura, A., Sato, H., Dupont, A., Nishi, N., and Schally, A. V. (1975): Somatostatin: Abundance of immunoreactive hormone in rat stomach and pancreas. *Science,* 189:1007–1009.
3. Arimura, A., and Schally, A. V. (1976): Increase in basal and thyrotropin-releasing hormone (TRH)-stimulated secretion of thyrotropin (TSH) by passive immunization with antiserum to somatostatin in rats. *Endocrinology,* 98:1069–1072.
4. Arimura, A., Smith, W. D., and Schally, A. V. (1976): Blockade of the stress-induced decrease in blood GH by antisomatostatin serum in rats. *Endocrinology,* 98:540–543.
5. Atweh, S., and Kuhar, M. J. (1977): Autoradiographic localization of opiate receptors in rat brain. I. Spinal cord and lower medulla. *Brain Res.,* 124:53–67.
6. Bishop, A. C., Polak, J. M., Buchman, A. M. J., Bloom, S. R., and Pearce, A. G. E. (1977): Third division of autonomic nervous system. An important element in gut control. *Gut,* 11:A962.
7. Bloom, S. R., Mortimer, C. H., Thorner, M. O., Besser, G. M., Hall, R., Gomez-Pan, A., Roy, V. M., Russell, R. C. G., Coy, D. H., Kastin, A. J., and Schally, A. V. (1974): Inhibition of gastrin and gastric acid secretion by growth-hormone release-inhibiting hormone. *Lancet,* 2:1106–1109.
8. Boden, G., Sivitz, M. C., Owen, O. E., Essa-Koumar, N., and Landor, J. H. (1975): Somatostatin suppresses secretin and pancreatic exocrine secretion. *Science,* 190:163–164.
9. Bradley, P. B., Briggs, I., Gayton, R. J., and Lambert, L. A. (1976): Effects of microiontophoretically applied methionine-enkephalin on single neurons in rat brain stem. *Nature,* 261:425–426.
10. Brazeau, P., Yale, W., Burgus, R., Ling, M., Butcher, J., Rivier, R., and Guillemin, R. (1973): Hypothalamic peptide that inhibits the secretion of immunoreactive pituitary growth hormone. *Science,* 179:77–79.

11. Burnstock, G. (1972): Purinergic nerves. *Pharmacol. Rev.,* 24:509–515.

12. Chayvialle, J. A. P., Descas, F., Bernard, C., Martin, A., Barbe, C., and Partensky, C. (1978): Somatostatin in mucosa of stomach and duodenum in gastrointestinal disease. *Gastroenterology,* 75:13–19.

13. Cheung, A. L., and Goldstein, A. (1976): Failure of hypophysectomy to alter brain content of opioid peptides (endorphins). *Life Sci.,* 19:1005–1008.

14. Chideckel, E. W., Palmer, J., Koerker, D. J., Ensinck, J., Davidson, M. B., and Goodner, C. J. (1975): Somatostatin blockade of acute and chronic stimuli of the endocrine pancreas and the consequences of this blockade on glucose homeostasis. *J. Clin. Invest.,* 55:754–762.

15. Costa, E., Fratta, W., Hong, J. S., Moroni, F., and Yang, H. Y. T. (1978): Interactions between enkephalinergic and other neuronal systems. *Adv. Biochem. Psychopharmacol.,* 217–226.

16. Cox, B. M., Opheim, K. E., Teschemacher, H., and Goldstein, A. (1975): A peptide-like substance from the pituitary that acts like morphine. *Life Sci.,*16:1777–1782.

16a. Dharmsathaphorn, K., Sherwin, R. S., Binder, H. Y., and Dobbins, J. W. (1978): Somatostatin (SRIF) inhibits intestinal fluid secretion. *Clin. Res.,* 26:496A.

17. Dupont, A., and Alvarado-Urbina, G. (1976): Conversion of big pancreatic somatostatin without peptide bond cleavage into somatostatin tetradecapeptide. *Life Sci.,* 19:1431–1434.

18. Epelbaum, J., Brazeau, P., Tsang, D., Brawer, J., and Martin, J. B. (1979): Subcellular distribution of radioimmunoassayable somatostatin in rat brain. *Brain Res. (in press).*

19. Feyter, F. (1953): *Über die peripheren endocrinen (paracrinen) Drüsen des Menschen.* W. Maudrich, Wien.

20. Ganda, O. P., Weir, G. C., Soeldner, J. S., Legg, M. A., Chick, W. L., Patel, Y. C., Ebeid, A. M., Gabbay, K. H., and Reichlin, S. (1977): "Somatostatinoma": A somatostatin-containing tumor of the endocrine pancreas. *N. Engl. J. Med.,* 296:963–967.

21. Gerich, J. E., Lorenzi, M., and Schneider, V. (1974): Effect of somatostatin on plasma glucose and glucagon levels in human diabetes mellitus. *N. Engl. J. Med.,* 291:544–547.

22. Goldstein, A. (1976): Opiate peptides (endorphins) in pituitary and brain. *Science,* 193:1081–1086.

23. Goldstein, A., Lowney, L. I., and Pal, B. K. (1971): Stereospecific and nonspecific interactions of the morphine congener levorphanol in subcellular fractions of the mouse brain. *Proc. Natl. Acad. Sci. U.S.A.,* 68:1742–1747.

24. Goodman, L. S., and Gilman, A. (1965): *The Pharmacological Basis of Therapeutics.* Macmillan New York.

25. Guillemin, R. (1976): Somatostatin inhibits the release of acetylcholine induced electrically in the myenteric plexus. *Endocrinology,* 99:1653–1654.

26. Guillemin, R. (1977): Endorphins, brain peptides that act like opiates. *N. Engl. J. Med.,* 296:226–228.

27. Guillemin, R. (1978): Peptides in the brain. *Science,* 202:390–402.

28. Guillemin, R., Ling, N., and Burgus, R. (1976): Endorphins, peptides d'origine hypothalamique et neurohypophysaire à activité morphinomimetique. Isolement et structure moleculaire de alfa-endorphine. *C. R. Acad. Sci. [D] (Paris),* 282:783–786.

29. Hall, R., Besser, G. M., Schally, A. V., Coy, D. H., Evered, D., Goldie, D. J., Kastin, A. J., McNeilly, A. S., Mortimer, A. S., Phenecos, C. H., Turnbridge, W. M. G., and Weightman, D. (1973): Action of growth hormone-releasing inhibitory hormone in healthy men and in acromegaly. *Lancet,* 2:581–583.

30. Halter, F., and Bublin, E. (1978): Effect of systemic application of a long-acting synthetic methionine enkephalin (FK 33–824) on rat gastric acid secretion. *Scand. J. Gastroenterol.* [Suppl. 49], 13:77.

31. Hambrook, J. M., Morgan, B. A., Rance, M. J., and Smith, C. F. C. (1976): Mode of deactivation of the enkephalins by rat and human plasma and rat brain homogenates. *Nature,* 262:782–783.

32. Hökfelt, T., Efendic, S., and Hellerstrom, C. (1975): Cellular localization of somatostatin in endocrine-like cells and neurons of the rat with special reference to the A_1 cells of the pancreatic islets and the hypothalamus. *Acta Endocrinol.* (Kbh.) [Suppl.], 80:5–40.

33. Hökfelt, T., Schultzberg, M., Johansson, O., Ljungdahl, A., Elfvin, L., Elde, R., Terenius, L., Nilsson, G., Said, S., and Goldstein, M. (1978): Central and peripheral peptide producing neurons. In: *Gut Hormones,* edited by S. R. Bloom, pp. 423–433. Churchill Livingstone, Edinburgh.

34. Hughes, J., Smith, T. W., Kosterlitz, H. W., Forthergill, L. A., Morgan, B. A., and Morris, H. R. (1975): Identification of the two related peptides from the brain with potent opiate agonist activity. *Nature,* 258:577–579.
35. Ipp, E., Dobbs, R. E., Arimura, A., Vale, W., Harris, V., and Unger, R. H. (1977): Release of immunoreactive somatostatin from the pancreas in response to glucose, amino acids, pancreozymin-cholecystokinin and tolbutamide. *J. Clin. Invest.,* 60:760–765.
36. Ipp, E., Dobbs, R. E., Harris, V., Arimura, A., Vale, W., and Unger, R. H. (1977): The effects of gastrin, gastric inhibitory polypeptide, secretin and the octapeptide of cholecystokinin upon immunoreactive somatostatin release by the perfused pancreas. *J. Clin. Invest.,* 60:1216–1219.
37. Ipp, E., Dobbs, R., and Unger, R. H. (1978): Morphine and beta-endorphin influence the secretion of the endocrine pancreas. *Nature,* 276:190–191.
38. Jhamandas, K., Pinksky, C., and Phillis, J. W. (1970): Effect of morphine and its antagonists on release of cerebral acetylcholine. *Nature,* 228:176–177.
39. Johansson, O., Hökfelt, T., Elde, R. P., Schultzberg, M., and Teurenius, L. (1978): Immunochemical distribution of enkephalin neurons. *Adv. Biochem. Psychopharmacol.,* 51–70.
40. Kayasseh, L., Haecki, W. H., Gyr, K., Stadler, G. A., Rittman, W. W., Halter, F., and Girard, J. (1978): The endogenous release of pancreatic polypeptide by acid and meal in dogs. *Scand. J. Gastroenterol.,* 13:385–391.
41. Konturek, S. J. (1977): Somatostatin and the digestive system. *Gastroenterol. Clin. Biol.,* 1:849–854.
42. Konturek, S. J. (1978): Endogenous opiates and the digestive system. *Scand. J. Gastroenterol.,* 13:257–261.
42a. Konturek, S. J. (1978): Somatostatin and gastrointestinal secretion and motility. In: *Gastrointestinal Hormones and Pathology of the Digestive System,* edited by M. Grossman, V. Speranza, N. Basso, and E. Lezoche, pp. 227–234. Plenum Press, New York.
43. Konturek, S. J., Krol, R., Pawlik, W., Tasler, J., Thor, P., Walus, K., and Schally, A. V. (1978): Pharmacology of somatostatin. In: *Gut Hormones,* edited by S. R. Bloom, pp. 457–462. Churchill Livingstone, Edinburgh.
44. Konturek, S. J., Pawlik, W., Walus, K., Coy, D. H., and Schally, A. V. (1978): Methionine-enkephalin stimulates gastric secretion and gastric mucosal blood flow. *Proc. Soc. Expl. Biol. Med.,* 158:156–160.
45. Konturek, S. J., Pawlik, W., Walus, K., Tasler, J., Coy, D. H., and Schally, A. V. (1978): The influence of enkephalin on gastric and pancreatic secretion in dog. *Scand. J. Gastroenterol.* [*Suppl.*], 13:101.
46. Konturek, S. J., Radecki, T., Pucher, A., Coy, D. H., and Schally, A. V. (1977): Effect of somatostatin on gastrointestinal secretions and peptic ulcer production in cats. *Scand. J. Gastroenterol.,* 12:379–381.
47. Konturek, S. J., Swierczek, J., Kwiecien, N., Mikos, E., Oleksy, J., and Wierzbicki, Z. (1978): Effect of somatostatin on meal-induced gastric secretion in duodenal ulcer patients. *Am. J. Dig. Dis.,* 22:981–989.
48. Konturek, S. J., Swierczek, J., Kwiecien, N., and Oleksy, J. (1977): Effect of somatostatin on meal-induced gastric secretion in duodenal ulcer patients. *Gastroenterology,* 72:818.
49. Konturek, S. J., Tasler, J., Cieszkowski, M., Coy, D. H., and Schally, A. V. (1976): Effect of growth hormone release-inhibiting hormone on gastric secretion, mucosal blood flow and serum gastrin. *Gastroenterology,* 70:737–741.
50. Konturek, S. J., Tasler, J., Cieszkowski, M., Jaworek, J., Coy, D. H., and Schally, A. V. (1978): Inhibition of pancreatic secretion by enkephalin and morphine in dogs. *Gastroenterology,* 74:851–855.
51. Konturek, S. J., Tasler, J., Obtulowicz, W., Coy, D. H., and Schally, A. V. (1976): Effect of growth hormone-release inhibiting hormone on hormones stimulating exocrine pancreatic secretion. *J. Clin. Invest.,* 58:1–6.
52. Kosterlitz, H. W., and Hughes, J. (1975): Some thoughts of the significance of enkephalin, the endogenous ligand. *Life Sci.,* 17:91–96.
53. Kosterlitz, H. W., and Hughes, J. (1978): Development of the concepts of opiate receptors and their ligands. *Adv. Biochem. Psychopharmacol.,* 31–44.
54. Kosterlitz, H. W., and Waterfield, A. A. (1975): Opiates and opiate receptors. *Annu. Rev. Pharmacol.,* 15:29–47.
55. Kosterlitz, H. W., and Watt, A. J. (1968): Kinetic parameters of narcotic agonists and antago-

nists with particular reference to N-alkylnoroxymorphone (naloxone). *Br. J. Pharmacol.*, 33:266–276.

56. Krieger, D. T., Liotta, A., Suda, T., Palkvits, M., and Brownstein, M. J. (1977): Presence of immunoassayable β-lipotropin in bovine brain and spinal cord: Lack of concordance with ACTH concentrations. *Biochem. Biophys. Res. Commun.*, 76:930–936.

57. Larsson, L. I., Holst, J. J., Kühl, C., Lundquist, G., Hirsch, M. A., Ingemansson, S., Lindkaer-Jensen, S., Rehfeldt, J. F., and Schwartz, T. W. (1977): Pancreatic somatostatinoma: Clinical features and physiological implications. *Lancet*, 1:666–668.

58. Lazarus, L. H., Ling, N., and Guillemin, R. (1976): β-Lipotropin as a prohormone for the morphinomimetic peptides and endorphins and enkephalins. *Proc. Natl. Acad. Sci. U.S.A.*, 73:2156–2159.

59. Li, C. H., Barnafi, L., Chretien, M., and Chung, D. (1965): Isolation and amino acid sequence of β-LPH from sheep pituitary glands. *Nature*, 208:1093–1094.

60. Lin, T. M., Spray, G. F., and Trust, R. H. (1977): Action of somatostatin (SS) on choledochal sphincter (GS), gallbladder (GB) and bile flow (BF) in dogs. *Fed. Proc.*, 36:557.

61. Ling, N., Minick, S., and Guillemin, R. (1978): Amino-terminal extension analogs of methionine-enkephalin. *Biochem. Biophys. Res. Commun.*, 83:565–570.

62. Linscheer, W. G., and Raheja, K. L. (1978): Effects of somatostatin on gastric acid secretion and on lipid and carbohydrate metabolism in the rat. *Br. J. Pharmacol.*, 64:311–314.

63. Mattes, P., Heil, Th., Raptis, S., Rasche, H., and Scheck, R. (1975): Extended somatostatin treatment of a patient with bleeding ulcer. *Horm. Metab. Res.*, 7:508–511.

64. McIntosh, C., Arnold, R., Bothe, E., Becker, H., Kobberling, J., and Creutzfeldt, W. (1978): Gastrointestinal somatostatin: Extraction and radioimmunoassay in different species. *Gut*, 19:655–663.

65. Meyers, C., Arimura, A., Gordin, A., Fernandez-Durengo, R., Coy, D. H., Schally, A. V., Drouin, J., Ferland, L., Beaulieu, M., and Labrie, F. (1977): Somatostatin analogues which inhibit glucagon and growth hormone more than insulin release. *Biochem. Biophys. Res. Commun.*, 74:630–632.

66. Mitznegg, P., Bloom, S. R., Domschke, W., Domschke, S., Wünsch, E., and Demling, L. (1977): Pharmacokinetics of motilin in man. *Gastroenterology*, 72:413–416.

67. Morgan, B. A., Smith, C. F. C., Waterfield, A. A., Hughes, J., and Kosterlitz, H. W. (1976): Structure-activity relationship of methionine-enkephalin. *J. Pharm. Pharmacol.*, 28:660–661.

68. Mortimer, C. H., Carr, D., Lind, T., Bloom, R. S., Mallinson, C. N., Schally, A. V., Turnbridge, W. M. G., Yeomans, L., Coy, D. H., Kastin, A., Besser, G. M., and Hall, R. (1974): Effects of growth hormone-release inhibiting hormone on circulating glucagon, insulin and growth hormone in normal, diabetic, acromegalic and hypopituitary patients. *Lancet*, 1:697–701.

69. Pasternak, G. W., Simantov, R., and Snyder, S. H. (1976): Characterization of an endogenous morphine-like factor (enkephalin) in mammalian brain. *Mol. Pharmacol.*, 12:504–513.

70. Paton, W. D. M. (1957): The action of morphine and related substances on contraction and on acetylcholine output of coaxially stimulated guinea pig ileum. *Br. J. Pharmacol. Chemother.*, 12:119–127.

71. Pearse, A. G. E. (1977): The diffuse neuroendocrine system and the APUD concept: Related "endocrine" peptides in brain, intestine, pituitary, placenta, and cutaneous glands. *Med. Biol.*, 55:115–125.

72. Pearse, A. G. E., Polak, J., and Bloom, R. S. (1977): The newer gut hormones: Cellular sources, physiology, pathology and clinical aspects. *Gastroenterology*, 22:746–761.

73. Pert, C. B., Kuhar, M. J., and Snyder, S. H. (1976): Opiate receptor: Autoradiographic localization in rat brain. *Proc. Natl. Acad. Sci. U.S.A.*, 73:3729–3733.

74. Pert, C. B., Pert, A., Chang, J. K., and Fong, B. T. W. (1976): [D-Ala²]-Met-Enkephalinamide: A potent, long-lasting synthetic pentapeptide analgesic. *Science*, 194:330–332.

75. Pert, C. B., and Snyder, S. H. (1973): Opiate receptors: Demonstration in nervous tissue. *Science*, 179:1011–1014.

76. Polak, J. M., Bloom, S. R., Sullivan, S. N., Bloom, S. R., and Arimura, A. (1975): Growth-hormone release inhibiting hormone (GH-RIH) in gastrointestinal and pancreatic D cells. *Lancet*, i:1220–1222.

77. Polak, J. M., Grimelius, L., Pearse, A. G. E., Timson, C. M., Arimura, A., and Pearse, A. G. E. (1976): Studies in gastric D cell pathology. *Gut*, 17:400–401.

78. Polak, J. M., Sullivan, S. N., Bloom, S. R., Facer, P., and Pearse, A. G. E. (1977): Enkephalin-like immunoreactivity in the human gastrointestinal tract. *Lancet*, 1:972–974.

79. Raptis, S., Dollinger, H. C., van Berger, L., Schlegel, W., Schröder, K. E., and Pfeiffer, E. F. (1975): Effects of somatostatin on gastric secretion and gastrin release in man. *Digestion*, 13:15–26.

80. Raptis, S., and Rosenthal, J. (1977): Somatostatin—Potential diagnostic and therapeutic value. *Acta Hepatogastroenterol.* (Stuttg.), 24:61–63.

81. Raptis, S., Schlegel, W., and Pfeiffer, E. F. (1978): Effect of somatostatin on gut and pancreas. In: *Gut Hormones*, edited by S. R. Bloom, pp. 446–452. Churchill Livingstone, Edinburgh.

82. Riegel, F. (1900): Ueber den Einfluss des Morphiums auf die Magensaft-secretion. *Z. Klin. Med.*, 40:347–350.

83. Rivier, C., Vale, W., Ling, N., Brown, M., and Guillemin, R. (1977): Stimulation *in vivo* of the secretion of prolactin and growth hormone by β-endorphin. *Endocrinology*, 100:238–240.

84. Roemer, D., Buescher, H. H., Hill, R. C., Pless, J., Bauer, W., Cardineau, F., Closse, A., Hauser, D., and Huguenin, R. (1977): A synthetic enkephalin analogue with prolonged parenteral and oral analgesic activity. *Nature*, 268:547–549.

85. Rossier, J., French, E. D., Rivier, C., Ling, N., Guillemin, R., and Bloom, F. E. (1978): Food-shock induced stress increases β-endorphin levels in blood but not in brain. *Nature*, 270:618–620.

86. Sakurai, H., Dobbs, R. E., and Unger, R. H. (1975): The effect of somatostatin on the response of GH to the intraduodenal administration of glucose, protein and fat. *Diabetologia*, 11:427–430.

87. Schally, A. V. (1978): Aspects of hypothalamic regulation of the pituitary gland. *Science*, 202:18–28.

88. Schally, A. V., Arimura, A., and Kastin, A. J. (1973): Hypothalamic regulatory hormones. *Science*, 179:341–350.

89. Schally, A. V., Dupont, A., Arimura, A., Redding, T. W., Nishi, N., Linthicum, G. L., and Schleisinger, D. H. (1976): Isolation and structure of growth hormone-release inhibiting hormone (somatostatin) from porcine hypothalami. *Biochemistry*, 15:509–514.

90. Schusdziarra, V., Harris, V., Conlon, J. M., Arimura, A., and Unger, R. (1978): Pancreatic and gastric somatostatin release in response to intragastric and intraduodenal nutrients and HCl in the dog. *J. Clin. Invest.*, 62:509–518.

90a. Schusdziarra, V., Harris, V., and Unger, R. H. (1979): Half-life of somatostatin-like immunoreactivity in canine plasma. *Endocrinology*, 104:109–110.

91. Simon, E. J., Hiller, J. M., and Edelman, I. (1973): Sterospecific binding of the potent narcotic analgesic [³H] etorphine to rat-brain homogenate. *Proc. Natl. Acad. Sci. U.S.A.*, 70:1947–1949.

92. Singh, M., and Webster, P. D. (1978): Neurohumoral control of pancreatic secretion. *Gastroenterology*, 74:294–309.

93. Smirnov, A., and Sirokij, V. (1927): Influence of morphine on gastric secretion in fasted dogs (Russian). *J. Expl. Biol. Med.*, 4:694–711.

94. Snyder, S. H. (1975): Opiate receptors in normal and drug altered brain function. *Nature*, 257:185–189.

95. Snyder, S. H. (1977): Opiate receptors in the brain. *N. Engl. J. Med.*, 296:266–271.

96. Snyder, S. H. (1978): Receptors for putative neurotransmitter peptides in the brain. In: *Peptides*, edited by M. Goodman and J. Meienhofer, pp.77–83. Halsted Press Book, New York.

97. Soll, A. H., and Grossman, M. I. (1978): Cellular mechanisms in acid secretion. *Annu. Rev. Med.*, 29:495–507.

98. Sundler, F., Alumets, J., Chang, K. J., and Hakanson, R. (1978): Cellular localization and distribution of leu-immunoreactivity in the gut. *Scand. J. Gastroenterol.* [Suppl. 49], 13:178.

99. Taube, H. D., Borowski, E., Endo, T., and Starke, K. (1976): Enkephalin, a potential modulator of noradrenaline release in rat. *Eur. J. Pharmacol.*, 38:317–380.

100. Terenius, L., Wahlström, A., Lindeberg, G., Karleson, S., and Ragnarsson, U. (1976): Opiate receptor affinity of peptides related to leu-enkephalin. *Biochem. Biophys. Res. Commun.*, 71:175–179.

101. Uvnäs-Wallensten, K., Efendic, S., and Luft, R. (1978): The occurrence of somatostatin-like immunoreactivity in the vagal nerves. *Acta. Physiol. Scand.*, 102:248–250.

102. Wahren, J., and Felig, P. (1976): Influence of somatostatin on carbohydrate disposal and absorption in diabetes mellitus. *Lancet*, 2:1213–1216.

103. Waterfield, A. A., and Kosterlitz, H. W. (1975): Stereospecific increase by narcotic antagonists of evoked acetylcholine output in guinea-pig ileum. *Life Sci.,* 16:1787–1792.
104. Weir, G. C., Goltsos, P. C., Steinberg, E. P., and Patel, Y. C. (1976): High concentration of somatostatin immunoreactivity in chicken pancreas. *Diabetologia,* 12:129–132.
105. Weitzman, R., Fischer, D., Minick, S., Ling, N., and Guillemin, R. (1977): β-Endorphin stimulates secretion of arginine vasopressin *in vivo. Endocrinology,* 101:1643–1646.
106. Yamaguci, I. (1974): A comparative study on the mechanism of action of morphine on gastric acid secretion in dogs. *Jpn. J. Pharmacol.,* 24:779–786.

Gastrointestinal Hormones, edited by
George B. Jerzy Glass.
Raven Press, New York © 1980.

Chapter 29

Bombesin-Like Peptides Activity in the Gastrointestinal Tract of Mammals and Birds

Pietro Melchiorri

Institute of Pharmacology, University of Rome, Rome 0.100, Italy

INTRODUCTION

The numerous publications on peptides of amphibian skin active on the gut have been extensively reviewed in other chapters in this volume by G. Bertaccini (Chapter 13, pp. 315–341) and V. Erspamer (Chapter 14, pp. 343–361).

A finding that emerges from these chapters is that nearly all the peptides found in the amphibian skin have biological and chemical characteristics similar to hormonal peptides already isolated from mammalian tissues.

The bradykinins of the amphibian skin have their duplicate in the mammalian plasma kinins; the tachykinins of the amphibian skin (physalemin, uperolein, phyllomedusin, kassinin) are closely related to substance P of the mammalian brain and gastrointestinal tract; criniaangiotensin II, and endecapeptide found in *Crinia* skin have the same C-terminal pentapeptide as angiotensins II isolated from ox, fowl, and snake plasmas; and, finally, the ceruleins (cerulein, phyllocerulein, Hylambates-cerulein) bear the strictest chemical and biological resemblance to the active portion of the cholecystokinin (CCK) and gastrin molecules (6). In sharp contrast with the above peptide families, the bombesin-like peptides of amphibian skin completely lacked, at the time bombesin was first described, their counterpart in the mammalian organism.

Thus, the question was whether this discrepancy was a real one or whether it simply depended on the fact that bombesin-like peptides had not been sought with suitable methods. The second alternative proved to be correct. Our group has succeeded in demonstrating that the mammalian and avian gut contains one or more peptides endowed with the immunological and biological characteristics similar to those displayed by bombesin and litorin (5,6).

EXTRACTION METHOD AND ASSAYS

Tissue fragments were extracted with 4 parts (w/v) of methanol and, after standing for 24 hr, reextracted with another 4 parts of 80% methanol. Bombesin-like activity was measured by bioassay, gastrin release assay, and radioimmunoassay (RIA).

Bioassay

The rat uterus preparation, pretreated with atropine (0.5–1 μg/ml) and methysergide (0.2 μg/ml), was routinely used in the bioassay of crude extracts and in the follow-up of all extraction, purification, and manipulation procedures. Extracts with sufficiently high bombesin-like activity and semipurified extracts were tested on several *in vitro* and *in vivo* smooth muscle preparations. Rat urinary bladder was used both *in vitro* and *in vivo*, whereas rat colon, guinea pig large intestine and urinary bladder, young cat small intestine, and guinea pig gallbladder were tested *in situ*. (See Chapter 14 by V. Erspamer, pp. 343–362, *this volume*.)

Gastrin Release Assay

The effects of some tissue extracts, semipurified extracts, and chromatographic fractions on gastrin secretion in dogs were measured as previously described (2). The activity of unknown sample was always tested against two doses of bombesin (2 and 5 ng kg^{-1} min^{-1}) in the same dog and the integrated gastrin response was measured for a period of 30 min of intravenous infusion.

Radioimmunoassay

RIA of bombesin-like peptides has been recently described (3), using antibodies obtained by immunization of rabbits with C-terminal nonapeptide of bombesin coupled to bovine albumin. When tissue extracts from animals and man were

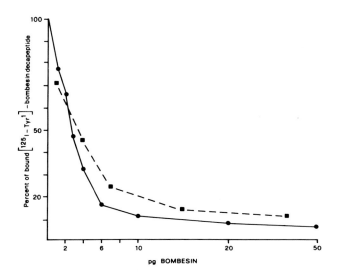

FIG. 1. RIA of bombesin-like peptide in gastric extracts. The curve in the competitive antibody binding assay for the bombesin-like peptides is presented as percent radioactivity of [125]I Tyr[1]-bombesin decapeptide bound to bombesin antibody and plotted against concentrations of cold bombesin or diluitions of gastric extract. *Solid line:* bombesin standards. *Dotted line:* gastric extract dilutions.

diluted and tested by RIA over an eightfold and a fivefold concentration range, respectively, dilution curves could not be distinguished from the standard curves prepared in buffer (Fig. 1).

No cross-reactions were found between the antibody to bombesin and human gastrin I, CCK, cerulein, secretin, glucagon, VIP, GIP, somatostatin, substance P, and eledoisin. However, on a molar basis, the ratio between the dose producing 50% inhibition (ID_{50}) for bombesin and similar peptides was as follows: bombesin 1.0, litorin 0.38, C-terminal tripeptide of bombesin 0.01, BOC-Gln-Trp-Ala-Val-Gly, 0.65.

BOMBESIN-LIKE ACTIVITY OF CRUDE GASTROINTESTINAL EXTRACTS

Table 1 shows bombesin-like activity of different batches of chicken proventriculus and two batches of gizzard mucosa, obtained by bioassay, RIA, and gastrin release assay of methanol extracts.

Bombesin-like activities of crude methanol extracts of gastrointestinal tract of other birds and mammals obtained by bioassay are shown below in ng/g. Values in parentheses were obtained by RIA. No gastrin release assay has been performed on these extracts, since their bombesin-like activity was too low to be detected by this assay. In the case of crude extracts with low concentrations

TABLE 1. *Comparative yields in bombesin-like activity following methanol extraction (ng/g) of chicken proventriculus and gizzard*

Batch	Bioassay	Radio-immunoassay	Gastrin release assay
D Proventriculus	60–80	50	80–90
Gizzard	35–50	35	30–40
G Proventriculus	70–120	80	80–100
Gizzard	40–70	130	30–50
F Proventriculus	100–150	120	—
H Proventriculus	150–170	—	—
I Proventriculus	80–100	—	—
L Proventriculus	110–130	—	—
M Proventriculus	110–120	—	—
N Proventriculus	80–100	—	—
O Proventriculus	60–80	—	—
1977/X Proventriculus	170	102	100–120
1978/A Proventriculus	50	41	30–50

of bombesin-like activity, contaminants interfered heavily also with bioassay, making values of bombesin-like activity below 5 to 10 ng/g unreliable.

Rabbit

Methanol extracts (pool from five animals): Gastric antrum, 25 to 50 (105); gastric fundus, 20 to 30 (42); small intestine, proximal quarter, 6 to 7 (2–4), second quarter, 6 to 7 (<1); third quarter 8 to 10 (<1); distal quarter, 10 (<1); cecum, 8 to 9 (<1), large intestine, 6 to 7 (1); liver, lung, kidney, heart, spleen, and urinary bladder, 5 (<1).

Cat

Methanol extracts (pool from two animals): Gastric antral mucosa, 8 to 10 (3–4); fundic mucosa, 10 to 15; small and large intestine, 5 (<1); gallbladder, pancreas, liver, kidney, heart, lung, spleen, urinary bladder, uterus, ovary, and testicles, 5 (1).

Dog

Methanol extracts (pool from three animals): Gastric fundic mucosa, 15 to 20 (8), antral mucosa 10 to 15, (10–12), mucosa of duodenum, jejunum, and ileum, 5 (<1), mucosa of cecum and large intestine, 5 to 15 (<1), pancreas, 5 (<1).

Rat

Methanol extracts (pools from 10 to 16 animals): Stomach, 30 to 60, 300; small intestine, proximal half, 30 to 40, 200.

Pig

(Minipig, pool from three animals). Methanol extracts: Gastric mucosa, 40 to 70.

Guinea pig

Methanol extracts (pool from five animals): Whole stomach, 40 to 60, small intestine, proximal half, 30 to 40.

Hamster

Methanol extracts (pool from three animals): Whole stomach, 20 to 40.

Man

Methanol extracts (pool of 15 stomachs): Fundic, 20 to 35; antral, 35 to 50; duodenal, 70 to 105; ileal, 8 to 10; and colonic, 7 to 15 mucosae.

Turkey

Pool from five animals: proventriculus, 250 to 400.

Pigeon

Pool from five animals: proventriculus, 500 to 700.

PURIFICATION AND BIOLOGICAL ACTIVITY OF BOMBESIN-LIKE PEPTIDES OF CHICKEN PROVENTRICULUS

Purification of methanol extracts was obtained by the use of alkaline aluminum and Sephadex G25 columns.

Methanol was evaporated and the residue taken up with 90% methanol was loaded on columns containing alkaline alumina in amounts of 100 g per 70 to 100 g tissue. Elution was carried out with ethanol of descending concentration, starting with 90% ethanol, and finally with water. Volumes of the eluates were 100 ml per 100 g alumina.

Table 2 shows the elution profile, from an alumina column, of the bombesin equivalent present in a methanol extract of 470 g of chicken proventriculus. Bombesin-like activity, which was particularly high in this experiment, was estimated by bioassay, RIA, and gastrin release assay. All three methods concordantly showed a major peak of activity in eluates of 60 to 50% ethanol and bioassay and RIA detected a minor peak in eluates of 80% ethanol, which was below the threshold of gastrin release assay.

TABLE 2. *Bombesin-like activity (ng/g) of ethanol eluates from alumina columns loaded with proventricular extracts*

Ethanol eluate	Bioassay	Radio-immunoassay	Gastrin release assay
90_1	—	4	—
90_2	—	4	—
85_1	1	1	—
85_2	1	1	—
80_1	4–5	2	—
80_2	7	2	—
70_1	2	1	—
70_2	—	2	—
60	12	19	—
50	25	45	35–40
40	—	8	—
30	2	4	—
H_2O	2	—	—

Eluates of 60 to 50% ethanol were combined and applied on Sephadex G25 columns. Their elution profiles with 0.1 M formic acid are shown in Fig. 2. Two peaks of bombesin-like activity were obtained with elution volumes of 6% and 69% (expressed as percent of eluted volume from protein peak to salt peak). In each run the minor peak emerged soon after proteins, the major just before bombesin. The bombesin-like activity of pooled fractions of the major peak was 89 ng, as measured by bioassay; 44 ng by RIA; and 55 ng by gastrin release assay per gram fresh tissue, with a yield, referred to the original activity of the crude methanol extract, of 111% by bioassay, 42% by RIA, and 79% by gastrin release assay. Thus, gel filtration increased the specific biological activity as measured by bioassay and gastrin release assay, while it

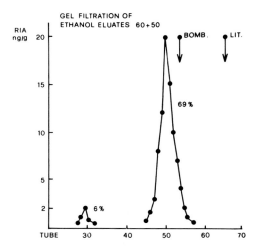

FIG. 2. Elution profile on Sephadex G 25 with 0.1 M formic acid of the bombesin-like activity of chicken proventriculus. This was obtained in the two ethanol eluates from alumina columns, as determined by RIA and expressed in nanograms bombesin per gram fresh tissue. Elution volumes of the bioactivity peaks are expressed as percent of the protein peak (0%) to salt peak. Bomb., bombesin peak; Lit.; litorin peak.

reduced the specific radioimmunoactivity of column eluates. In these two stages of purification, approximately 60% of bombesin-like peptide was lost according to RIA, whereas its biological activity was doubled (bioassay and gastrin release assay).

The biological activity most thoroughly studied was that of the proventricular bombesin-like peptide emerging from Sephadex column loaded with the 60% and 50% ethanol eluate from alumina column. This presented an elution volume very similar to amphibian bombesin and displayed *in vivo* and *in vitro* all the effects characteristic for the amphibian peptide reviewed by V. Erspamer (Chapter 14, pp. 343–362, *this volume*).

It stimulated isolated preparations of rat uterus, large intestine and urinary bladder, guinea pig ileum and urinary bladder, and kitten small intestine; it produced a moderate litorin-like rise of dog pressure; it caused, in the dog, a dose-dependent release of gastrin with ensuing stimulation of gastric acid and pepsin secretion; it contracted the gallbladder of the guinea pig, the cat, and the dog and elicited, in the dog, a profuse secretion of pancreatic enzymes and pancreatic peptide. Finally, it blocked the interdigestive electric complex and the motility of dog stomach and intestine and provoked changes in the pacesetter potentials of the duodenum, similar to those evoked by bombesin. When administered intracisternally in cold-exposed rats, it lowered body temperature by approximately 2°C and blocked the secretion of TSH as compared with untreated controls (3). Since our preliminary communication (5), the occurrence of bombesin-like immunoreactivity in the gastrointestinal tract has been confirmed in the rat by Walsh and Dockray (11), in the man and in the neonatal rabbit by Polak et al. (9), in the frog by Lechago et al. (8), and again in human gut by Polak et al. (10).

BOMBESIN-LIKE PEPTIDES OF THE CENTRAL NERVOUS SYSTEM

Once it was established that the gastrointestinal tract of birds and mammals contained a bombesin-like peptide, it was obvious that this peptide should be sought in the central nervous system (CNS), in analogy to what has been done and is currently being done with other gastrointestinal hormonal peptides (gastrin, CCK, substance P, VIP).

TABLE 3. *Bombesin-like immunoreactivity in the CNS*

Rat (5)	Whole brain	20–45 ng/g
	Hypothalamus	50–100 ng/g
Mini-pigs (3)	Cerebral cortex	5–10 ng/g
	Cerebellum	18–25 ng/g
	Hypothalamus	80–100 ng/g
Rabbit (2)	Cerebral cortex	5–10 ng/g
	Cerebellum	25–50 ng/g
	Hypothalamus	105–130 ng/g

Preliminary experiments carried out in this laboratory (6) have given values of bombesin-like immunoreactivity shown in Table 3. Outside the gastrointestinal tract, bombesin-like peptides have been found in the fetal and neonatal lung (10) and, most important, in the CNS, where they have been described simultaneously by two groups of research workers (2,10).

SUMMARY

The gastrointestinal tract of mammals and birds, especially stomach and upper small intestine, contains bombesin-like peptides. This has been unequivocally demonstrated by RIA and bioassay of these peptides in crude and semipurified gastrointestinal extracts of gastrointestinal tract and by immunohistochemical staining of bombesin-producing cells.

Concentrations of bombesin-like activity may range from a few nanograms to 100–170 ng per gram fresh tissue, depending on tissue sample and animal species. The latter values refer to the chicken proventriculus, which has been the object of a more thorough investigation.

The bombesin-like peptides of the chicken proventriculus showed all the biological effects of bombesin-like peptides of amphibian skin, i.e., stimulation of secretion of gastric acid, pepsin, gastrin, pancreatic enzymes, and pancreatic peptide, and inhibition of gastric and duodenal motility, in dogs.

Bombesin-like peptide isolated from chicken proventriculus elicited a sharp hypothermia and blocked TSH secretion when injected intracisternally to cold (4°C) exposed rats.

Another important extraintestinal localization of bombesin-like peptides in mammals appears to be the CNS, especially the hypothalamus.

CONCLUSIONS AND PROJECTIONS FOR THE FUTURE

The present results demonstrate that, like all other peptide families of the amphibian skin, bombesin-like peptides also have chemical and biological analogs in the mammalian and avian tissues.

Amphibian skin and gut and brain of all examined species of mammals and birds contained one or more peptides that can be classified as belonging to the group of bombesin-like peptides.

At present, it is not possible to answer the question whether the gastrointestinal bombesin-like peptide is chemically identical with one or another of the amphibian bombesins. However, this does not seem to be likely in the chicken, since the main form found in proventricular extracts did not present the same elution pattern from Sephadex G25 columns as bombesin and litorin; nor did the bioassays and RIAs as well as the assays of gastrin release give the same results as those in the amphibian peptides.

Further studies on the avian and mammalian bombesin-like peptides are aimed at elucidation of the chemical structure of these peptides.

ACKNOWLEDGMENT

This work was supported by grants from the Consiglio Nazionale delle Ricerche, Rome, Italy.

REFERENCES

1. Bertaccini, G., Erspamer, V., Melchiorri, P., and Sopranzi, N. (1974): Gastrin release by bombesin in the dog. *Br. J. Pharmacol.,* 52:219–225.
2. Brown, M., Rivier, J., Kobayashi, R., and Vale, W. (1978): Neurotensin-like and bombesinlike peptides: CNS distribution and actions. In: *Gut Hormones,* edited by S. R. Bloom, pp. 550–558. Churchill Livingstone, Edinburgh/London/New York.
3. Erspamer, V., Falconieri-Erspamer, G., Melchiorri, P., and Negri, L. (1979): Occurrence and polymorphism of bombesin-like peptides in G.I. tract of birds and mammals. *Gut (in press).*
4. Erspamer, V., and Melchiorri, P. (1975): Actions of bombesin on secretions and motility of the gastrointestinal tract. In: *Gastrointestinal Hormones,* edited by J. C. Thompson, pp. 575–589. University of Texas Press, Austin and London.
5. Erspamer, V., and Melchiorri, P. (1976): Amphibian skin peptides active on the gut. *J. Endocrinol.,* 70:12P–13P.
6. Erspamer, V., Melchiorri, P., Falconieri-Erspamer, G., and Negri, L. (1978): Polypeptides of the amphibian skin active on the gut and their mammalian counterparts. In: *Gastrointestinal Hormones and Pathology of the Digestive System,* edited by M. Grossman, V. Speranza, N. Basso, and E. Lezoche, pp. 51–64. Plenum Press, New York and London.
7. Greenwood, F. C., Hunter, W. M., and Glover, J. S. (1963): The preparation of I[131] labeled human growth hormone of high specific radioactivity. *Biochem. J.,* 89:114.
8. Lechago, J., Holmquist, A. L., and Walsh, J. H. (1978): Localization of a bombesin-like peptide in frog gastric mucosa by immunofluorescence and RIA. *Gastroenterology,* 74, Part 2:1054.
9. Polak, J. M., Buchnan, A. M. J., Czykowska, W., Solcia, E., Bloom, R. S., and Pearse, A. G. E. (1978): Bombesin in the gut. In: *Gut Hormones,* edited by S. R. Bloom, pp. 541–543. Churchill Livingstone, Edinburgh/London/New York.
10. Polak, J. M., Ghatei, M. A., Wharton, J., Bishop, A. E., Bloom, S. R., Solcia, E., Brown, M. R., and Pearse, A. G. E. (1978): Bombesin-like immunoreactivity in the gastrointestinal tract, lung and central nervous system. *Scand. J. Gastroenterol. (Suppl. 49),* 13:148.
11. Walsh, J. H., and Dockray, H. J. (1978): Localization of bombesin-like immunoreactivity (BLI) in gut and brain of rat. *Gastroenterology,* 74, Part 2:1108.

Gastrointestinal Hormonal Tumors

Gastrointestinal Hormones, edited by
George B. Jerzy Glass.
Raven Press, New York © 1980.

Chapter 30

Gastrinomas

Fl. Stadil

*Department of Surgical Gastroenterology D, Herlev University Hospital,
Copenhagen, Denmark*

HISTORY

In 1955 Zollinger and Ellison (19) described two patients, each of whom was characterized by three features: (a) intractable peptic ulceration so severe that it resisted all medical and surgical treatment short of total gastrectomy, (b) severe hypersecretion of gastric hydrochloric acid, and (c) pancreatic islet cell tumors different from the insulin producing β-cell variety. A few similar cases had been reported earlier, but these papers did not create much interest, and the patients were generally thought to be medical curiosities. Zollinger and Ellison (19), however, proposed that the pancreatic tumors secreted some substance that caused gastric hypersecretion responsible for the ulcer diathesis. This concept of an ulcerogenic tumor syndrome did stimulate a wide interest and caused almost explosive consequences, with publication of additional cases during the following years (2).

A major development was a suggestion by Gregory et al. (4) that the islet cell tumor in the Zollinger-Ellison (Z-E) syndrome was gastrin producing. This suggestion was proved to be correct 4 years later by the same investigators (3). This discovery confirmed the concept suggested by Zollinger and Ellison of the ulcerogenic tumor syndrome. It is now recognized that the severe hypersecretion of gastric hydrochloric acid in patients having the Z-E syndrome is due to the effects of continuous stimulation of the parietal cells by gastrin secreted by the tumors, and that hypergastrinemia over prolonged periods of time, by a trophic action, causes the development of a large parietal cell mass, typical of the Z-E patient.

The concept of a gastric secretagogue secreted by the tumors was exploited diagnostically by the use of various bioassays during the 1960s. Yet, only with the development of radioimmunoassay techniques for gastrin a potent clinical tool became available that changed the diagnostic approach to this disease. The radioimmunoassay (RIA) revealed that more patients suffered from the gastrinoma disease than was suspected previously. In Denmark five to ten patients are diagnosed each year, whereas only two patients were diagnosed before RIAs became available. The true incidence of Z-E syndrome is presumably higher than the present count of one to two cases per million.

The clinical features of the Z-E syndrome can be deduced from the massive and continuous gastric hypersecretion caused by the hypergastrinemia. The acid hyperproduction causes peptic ulcerations with any of its usual complications, such as penetration, perforation, bleeding, or stenosis. It may also lead to diarrhea and steatorrhea due to inactivation of pancreatic lipase at the low pH in the lumen of the upper gut. As the rate of secretion of acid exceeds the neutralizing capacity of the duodenal and upper jejunal secretions, the acid secretion also explains the frequent presence of a multitude of tiny duodenal ulcerations or ectopic chronic peptic ulcers in the post-bulbar or upper jejunal region. The clinical features of the Z-E syndrome were initially presented as a diagnostic triad in the original paper (19). This consisted of the acid hypersecretion, the presence of intractable, fulminating ulcer disease, and the islet cell tumor. Although these features are indeed characteristic of many Z-E patients, none of them had turned out to be necessarily present, as will be shown later.

GASTRINOMAS

The pathology of the gastrinoma tumors may need to be reevaluated, because most of the information contained in the classic papers depended on less sophisticated diagnostic procedures than the ones presently used. Those reports may reflect findings of relatively advanced stages of the disease.

The gastrinoma tumors are found in the pancreas or in the upper duodenum. Only rarely are they found elsewhere, and it is puzzling that an occurrence of the tumor in the antrum seems to be encountered very rarely. Quite often the primary tumors are also difficult to locate in cases when large secondary tumors in lymph nodes, the omentum, or the liver are easily seen. According to the literature the gastrinomas are small, slow growing, and quite often multiple (18).

According to most of the authors, the majority, maybe all, gastrinomas are malignant. This, however, is difficult to judge because of the difficulties in locating tumors, the slow growth of many tumors, and because the histological picture of a gastrinoma often is that of a benign adenoma, when the presence or the later development of metastases proves the tumor to be malignant. In the classic reports about one-half of the patients had metastatic lesions when first diagnosed. This figure may have declined after the introduction of RIA of gastrin in the diagnosis of the Z-E syndrome. The slow growth of many tumors is illustrated by one of the original two patients described by Zollinger and Ellison: At the time of total gastrectomy in 1954 the patient had lymph node metastasis, but she was well 17 years later, having given birth to two children in the meantime (18).

The tumor within the pancreas may be located to a single anatomical area of the gland in approximately one-half of the patients, with a head-body-tail ratio of $4:1:4$ (20). The spread in case of malignancy proceeds by the lymphatic route to paraduodenal, parapancreatic, upper gastric, subpyloric, inferior gastric, or splenic lymph nodes. The local spread is frequently encountered, as are the secondary tumors in the liver. Pulmonary metastases are rarely seen.

Although the tumors are slow growing, it seems that in some patients, or at some stages of the disease, the tumor progresses rapidly in a fashion typical for malignant lesion.

A puzzling feature of the pancreatic endocrine tumors is a frequent occurrence of mixed or multi-hormonal neoplasms (10). Although the clinical tumor syndrome usually is caused by hyperfunction of only one of the cell types found in the tumors, this particular cell type may not necessarily be the dominant tumor cell. Metastases originating from mixed tumors are usually, but not always, composed of the cells responsible for the clinical picture. Consequently, a gastrinoma can only be classified accurately by a combination of clinical, immunocytochemical, and biochemical data (9). It has often been suggested that the Z-E syndrome may be due at times to the islet cell hyperplasia. It is now known that gastrinomas are associated with marked hyperplasia of all endocrine cell types of the pancreatic islets. Hence, a finding of the islet hyperplasia is to be expected in gastrinoma patients, but this hyperplasia does not seem to involve gastrin cells.

The origin of pancreatic gastrinomas may seem obscure, as normal human pancreas does not contain gastrin cells; nor does the pancreas normally produce gastrin. The islets of the pancreas contain at least five well characterized endocrine cells: The A (A_2) (glucagon), B (insulin), D (A_1) (somatostatin), PP (pancreatic polypeptide), and D_1 (bombesin?) cell. In the studies of the ontogeny of the pancreas a transitory phase with pancreatic gastrin cells has been reported in the rat. Such cells are also found in man during the late fetal period. It is likely that the gastrinomas originate from cells related to this category.

GASTRIN

As stated before, the clinical features of the Z-E syndrome are the result of the excessive gastrin production in the tumors. For this reason the knowledge of the physiology and pathology of gastrin is essential for the clinical management of Z-E patients.

Gastrin was originally isolated as a heptadecapeptide (G-17) from hog antral mucosa. Two forms were recognized, one with a sulfated tyrosine residue [G-17 (s) = gastrin II], and one without sulfate [G-17 (ns) = gastrin I]. After development of radioimmunochemical determinations, however, it has become apparent that a number of different gastrins with a common C-terminal structure but different molecular size are found in the blood and tissues. Circulating gastrin in man consists of four main components, which we have named components I–IV (12). Component I has the molecular size of proinsulin. Its structure has not yet been clarified. Components II, III, and IV seem to correspond to gastrin-34 (big gastrin), gastrin-17 (little gastrin), and gastrin-14 (mini-gastrin) found in the mucosa, the identity of which has not yet been finally clarified. A circulating so-called "big big gastrin" with the molecular size of albumin has been also described, but its existence has been seriously questioned.

The biological activity of gastrins is linked to the common C-terminal structure, and it seems that the C-terminal tetrapeptide (gastrin-4) contains all the biological actions of the gastrins. The differences in the molecular size lead to quantitative differences in activity. The most potent gastrins are G-17 and G-14. The bioactivities of gastrins are not influenced by sulfation of the tyrosine residue.

Gastrins are normally produced by the G cells in the stomach and upper intestine. The major source is the antral mucosa, which has a content of about 20 μg gastrin per gram mucosae. Relative to the antrum, the upper duodenum contains 10%, the lower duodenum 1%, and the upper jejunum 0.5% of gastrin per gram mucosae. As in the circulation the main components in the tissues are gastrin-34 and gastrin-17. Normally, these two components seem to constitute 90% of the circulating gastrin, but during stimulation their relative contributions to total gastrin immunoreactivity vary. Gastrin-17 is mainly responsible for the rise in circulating gastrin during the early phase of stimulated gastrin responses. Gastrin-17 is the predominant form of gastrin found in the antrum. In adult man gastrin is not produced in the pancreas.

Gastrin has a number of actions when administered exogenously, most of which can be considered pharmacological in nature. The main physiological actions of gastrin seem to be stimulation of gastric secretion of hydrochloric acid, stimulation of the growth of some of the tissues during long-term hypergastrinemia, and stimulation of the motor activity of the antrum.

The important physiological stimulus for gastrin secretion is the meal. Proteins, peptides, and even amino acids may stimulate gastrin cells directly from the lumen. Cholinergic innervation does not seem to play any significant role in gastrin release in man. Inhibition of stimulated gastrin secretion is mainly due to acid entering the antrum from the upper stomach. The regulation of the function of the unstimulated gastrin cells and of the basal level of circulating gastrin is insufficiently known.

Circulating gastrin can be measured by a number of different RIA techniques that have been developed for gastrin measurements during the last 8 or 9 years. When one relies on gastrin determinations by RIA the knowledge of the specificity of the particular antiserum used in regard to the different gastrins is obligatory. From a clinical point of view, an antiserum that measures all components with equimolar potency is preferable. The mean pattern of gastrin components in serum of patients with Z-E syndrome does not differ from that found in normal subjects or ulcer patients. Occasionally single patients may have unusual patterns, however, with a preponderance of just one or two components (11,12).

CLINICAL FEATURES

Symptoms

Z-E syndrome is diagnosed in all ages. Among the first 260 registered patients, 8% were children.

Some patients may present with dramatic and severe forms of peptic ulcer disease. Of the 30 patients we diagnosed, however, one-third had only episodic symptoms. The clinical spectrum in these patients varied from one single episode of dyspeptic pain lasting a few weeks followed by a symptom-free period of 5 years duration without any treatment, to severe cases with perforated ulcer, hemorrhage, esophagitis, and peptic stricture (14).

One-third of our 30 patients had previously been misdiagnosed and treated by ordinary ulcer surgery. In retrospect, there was little evidence that an aggressive ulcer diathesis was present in most of these patients. On the average it took 5 to 8 years after the onset of symptoms before the first operation was performed. Although the ulcers recurred ultimately, it took from 0.2 to 20 years with a mean of 4.2 years before a second operation was considered necessary. Thus in the majority of our patients the ulcer disease could hardly be described as fulminant. The main symptoms in our patients were dyspeptic pains (in 40%), intermittent or chronic diarrhea (20%), or both (40%). Dysphagia or vomiting was seen occasionally. Compared with the classic descriptions, our patients generally presented less dramatic forms of the disease. Family history of endocrinopathies was obtained in one-third of the patients. In distinguishing these patients from those with ordinary ulcer disease, the most suggestive symptom is probably the chronic diarrhea with or without ulcer pains. A family history of endocrine disorders may also be of value.

Findings

The associated endocrinopathies in Z-E patients or families are usually due to hyperparathyroidism, insulinomas, pituitary tumors, or adrenal cortical adenomas. In a study of the first-degree relatives of 10 Dutch Z-E patients it was found that 30 of 78 family members of 6 of the 10 patients suffered from a total of 50 endocrinopathies (7), one-half of which were newly diagnosed by a simple screening procedure. This illustrates that Z-E frequently is part of a multiple endocrine adenomatosis (MEA, type I—Wermer's syndrome), and that family studies should be carried out whenever possible.

On X-ray films most Z-E patients have a plain-looking single ulcer in the duodenal bulb, and some patients do not have ulcers at all. The presence of multiple ulcers in the stomach and duodenum or ectopic ulcers distal to the duodenal bulb (either in the postbulbar or distal duodenum or in the upper jejunum) is suggestive of a Z-E syndrome. Other regular radiological findings are the giant mucosal folds seen in the gastric body of all patients. At radiological examination of the small intestine a rapid transit is noted, with the contrast scattered throughout most of the small intestine, its torn mucosal pattern suggesting a jejunitis or ileitis. Fluid levels are often apparent due to the increased fluid content of the loops.

At endoscopy chronic ulcers may be seen as in plain duodenal ulcer disease. Characteristic findings are a marked enlargement of the folds in the gastric body and a large volume of juice secreted into the stomach during the examination. A very suggestive finding we have seen in many patients is a marked antral and duodenal irritation, with a multitude of tiny ulcers extending in some cases from the prepyloric region throughout the entire duodenum. In some cases hundreds of such ulcers are seen. This presentation has been mistaken for Crohn's disease of the duodenum.

Patients with Z-E syndrome have massive gastric hypersecretion of acid, and this can be revealed by measurements of the basal and maximally stimulated acid secretion. Such measurements should always be carried out; however, even in gastrinoma patients the basal acid secretion may fluctuate markedly from day to day, and the figures for maximal acid secretion overlap those seen in other conditions. Thus, there is no firm definition of the hypersecretion of acid in Z-E syndrome. The most useful parameter is the basal acid secretion, which normally is below 5 mEq H^+ per hour and much higher in gastrinoma patients. In 30 Z-E patients we found the median basal acid output (BAO) to be between 30 and 40 mEq H^+ per hour. In cases where patients have had earlier gastric operations, the investigator should consider the effects of the previous surgery both on the secretory ability of the stomach and on the correctness of the technique used for the secretory study.

In cases presenting chronic diarrhea, pancreatic secretory studies are sometimes carried out as a part of an investigation of the diarrhea. In such studies an extraordinarily low intraduodenal pH will be found, and this may lead to the diagnosis of the gastrinoma.

All Z-E patients are characterized by hypergastrinemia, which can be demonstrated by analysis of samples of peripheral venous blood, drawn after an overnight fast. As with acid secretion, there will be no clear-cut definition of hypergastrinemia, and there is an extreme individual variability of the levels seen in various patients. In the individual patient the level seem relatively constant, however. In the interpretation of the gastrin determinations it must be remembered that hypergastrinemia may occur as a consequence of other diseases or treatments. Marked hypergastrinemia may be seen in pernicious anemia and in atrophic gastritis. Moderate hypergastrinemia with elevations of one to three times the normal level is seen in many patients with gastric ulcer disease, after vagotomy, after treatment with histamine H_2-receptor antagonists, and possibly in some cases of renal failure. A comparable or more pronounced gastrinemia may also be encountered in ulcer patients suffering from severe gastric stasis due to pyloric stenosis, or after inappropriate Billroth II resections where an antral remnant is retained and excluded from the acid stream. Hypergastrinemia has also been described in cases with hyperplasia of the antral gastrin cells. This condition has not yet been adequately established as a clinical entity, and is probably seen very rarely.

DIAGNOSIS

The diagnosis of Z-E syndrome is made by clinical findings in combination with basal acid hypersecretion and hypergastrinemia. All criteria of acid secretion proposed for the diagnosis of Z-E syndrome yield both false positive and false negative results, and there is no fixed level of acid secretion that permits the correct diagnosis. However, the basal secretion of acid above 20 mEq H^+ per hour is almost diagnostic in the presence of hypergastrinemia. Gastrin measurements are indicated in any ulcer patient with a basal acid secretion above 10 mEq H^+ per hour. Because of the marked day-to-day variations in acid secretion in gastrinoma patients measurements of acid may have to be repeated.

The serum gastrin level, as measured by a proper gastrin antiserum, is a valuable tool in the diagnosis. In our experience, fasting level measured in the morning is the most valuable parameter. In one of 30 patients with a proven gastrinoma, however, gastrin values were at the upper normal range for about 1 year, and were only slightly increased shortly before death from extensive metastatic disease. Markedly elevated gastrin levels (i.e., five times or more the normal range) are diagnostic by themselves when combined with high acid readings. Unfortunately only one-half of the Z-E patients will show this kind of elevation. The magnitude of hypergastrinemia is poorly related to the magnitude of the acid hypersecretion.

Because one-half of the Z-E patients exhibit only moderate hypergastrinemia a number of additional diagnostic tests have been suggested. The ones commonly used have been the secretin, calcium, and meal tests.

Secretin tests are carried out by sampling peripheral venous blood at 5-min intervals for 30 min or longer before and after the intravenous injection of one to three clinical units of secretin per kilogram body weight. In gastrinoma patients gastrin release is acutely and strongly stimulated by secretin, with a mean peak value of about three times the basal level. This response is significantly higher than in duodenal ulcer patients. Originally secretin was believed to lower gastrin concentrations in serum in the duodenal ulcer patients (6). Unfortunately this is not true, and there is an overlap between patients with Z-E syndrome and those with duodenal ulcer disease (16). Due to the unequal incidence of the two diseases, the majority of patients with a positive secretin test in any population will be suffering from duodenal ulcer disease. It follows that in individual cases the diagnostic value of a secretin test may be questionable, and the Z-E syndrome certainly cannot be diagnosed by a particular response to secretin.

The calcium test consists in the measurements of serum gastrin concentration during an infusion of 5 mg Ca^{2+} per hour for 2 to 3 hours. In Z-E syndrome the increase in serum gastrin and acid secretion is higher than in normals and ulcer patients (8). Due to overlapping with ordinary duodenal ulcer patients we found the diagnostic value in the individual cases subjected to the same doubts as listed above (14).

The meal test is based on the autonomous nature of the hypergastrinemia in gastrinoma patients, where only small responses of serum gastrin are seen after stimulation with a protein-rich meal. Its diagnostic value in the individual case is no better than that of the other tests in our experience (16). Meal test may be useful in suggesting antral hyperfunction, also called G cell hyperplasia. In this still inadequately defined entity there may be fasting hypergastrinemia and an exaggerated gastrin response to feeding (17).

These three tests may have clinical interest, but differentiation between patients with duodenal ulcer disease and those with gastrinomas is probably done better by repeated measurements of the basal concentrations of gastrin in serum.

From a practical point of view, Z-E syndrome diagnosis can easily be made in most cases by combining clinical features, acid secretory studies, and gastrin measurements. In a few patients it may be necessary to withhold judgment for a prolonged observation period. One of the main problems is that some cases are bound to be overlooked due to the inadequacy of the screening procedures.

When the diagnosis has been made, efforts should continue to obtain a final proof by locating the tumor(s). Unfortunately, this is often very difficult. Conventional methods such as arteriography, ultrasonic scanning, CT-tomography, peritoneoscopy, and scintigrams are indicated but generally fail. A superior procedure is the simultaneous blood samplings for gastrin assay from pancreatic veins and systemic veins. Portal catheterization procedures with selective catheterization of pancreatic veins and blood sampling can be carried out by percutaneous transhepatic puncture under local anesthesia, as described by Ingemansson et al. (5) and applied to gastrinoma patients by Burcharth et al. (1). The diagnosis can be considered proven by location of the tumor(s) or by the demonstration of hypergastrinemia of pancreatic origin by selective catheterization. It can also be considered proven if hypergastrinemia is unaffected by the total gastrectomy. In theory, the latter could also be due to an intestinal G cell hyperplasia, but such a condition has not yet been described.

TREATMENT

Treatment of Z-E syndrome was formerly by a total gastrectomy, preferably as the first gastric operation. A less extensive surgery would not control the ulcer diathesis, and the other medical alternatives were not effective. On empirical grounds this operation became the treatment of choice, as the survival primarily depended on the prevention of ulcer complications (18).

Between 1972 and 1976 17 Danish Z-E patients were treated by a total gastrectomy, with one operative death. In the remaining patients the symptomatic results were excellent, but some side effects due to biliary reflux, malabsorption, reduced gastric capacity, and dysphagia were seen in some of them. The working capacity was somewhat reduced in most of the patients.

After 1976 total gastrectomy has not been used in any of the Z-E patients in Denmark, due to the development of histamine H_2-receptor antagonist (15). Until now, 17 patients have been treated with continuous administration of Cimetidine in doses from 1 to 3 g/24 hr. In all patients the ulcers disappeared and symptoms were totally relieved after periods ranging from 1 day to 4 weeks. Recurrence of symptoms and ulcers has been seen in four patients during continuous therapy and disappeared after slight adjustment of dosage but the last patient, after 40 months, required a dose increase to 7 g/24 h. Apart from gynecomastia in two patients no biochemical or clinical side effects have become apparent.

In these patients the working stages have been intact. The efficacy and apparent safety of Cimetidine therapy suggest that in the future gastric operations may be superfluous in the majority of Z-E patients but long-term observations are needed. In the group of totally gastrectomized patients, two died after observation periods of 1 and 3 years due to malignant disease. Among the Cimetidine-treated patients, two died from malignant disease after treatment periods of 2 weeks and 6 months.

The control of the ulcer diathesis with Cimetidine treatment can only compete with total gastrectomy if treatment is continuously and carefully controlled by direct and repeated measurements of acid inhibition. Changes in dosage may be needed, and should be promptly carried out if symptomatic relief is not complete. Inadequate treatment can lead to fatal complications. We have found it convenient to centralize the treatment and to educate the patients fully on the nature and the risks of the disease and the nature of the treatment.

The majority of the gastrinomas are malignant, albeit slow growing. As discussed previously the tumor growth may suddenly accelerate, and in our experience the threat posed by malignancy is very real. In one-third of our patients we presently have proof of aggressive invasive disease with widespread secondary tumors. Because of the total symptomatic control of the ulcer diathesis by Cimetidine, as we have previously emphasized, the aim of surgery in Z-E syndrome should be redirected against the cause of the disease if possible, i.e., against the gastrin-producing tumors (15).

In the past radical surgery has rarely been attempted mainly for two reasons. First, pancreatic surgery has been considered to rule out a secondary total gastrectomy, that might be needed in case of failure. This point of view may be unwarranted, since our personal experience with the Whipple operation in two patients earlier treated by total gastrectomy showed that the operations were technically quite possible and that the nutritional and general status of the patients was good. Secondly, the tumors are often difficult to locate and may be multiple. This makes attempts at radical surgery difficult and speaks strongly in our opinion against routine pancreatectomy or blind resections. Pancreatic surgery might be attempted in cases where a single tumor is detected in a location that permits removal by a minor surgery procedure. Major pancreatic surgery should probably be undertaken only if the following two conditions are met: (a) The tumors can be confidently located preoperatively to one particular area of the pancreas; and (b) The presence of tumors in other organs or in the remaining part of the pancreas can be confidently ruled out by preoperative examinations. We have so far operated on five Z-E patients by a Whipple operation, relying on transhepatic portal catheterization with blood sampling for gastrin assay. After an observation time of 1 year or more (this operation appeared to be radical in four patients), who have remained totally well without any other treatment and with serum concentrations of gastrin close to zero. These observations suggest to us that radical surgery may be possible in a substantial number of Z-E patients.

If the tumor growth accelerates and secondary tumors in the liver or elsewhere are diagnosed, cytostatic treatment should be considered. We have used treatment with streptozotocin at 6 to 12 week intervals in cases where secondary tumors became symptomatic (13). Until now we have treated five patients this way, with a marked clinical remission, and a marked fall in the concentrations of circulating gastrin in four. Two patients died after 1 and 3 years, one from age and pulmonary disease, the other from a portal thrombosis. Since the efficiency of cytostatic treatment can be monitored by gastrin measurements, an alternative approach to the one just mentioned would be to treat all patients in which secondary tumors are diagnosed, even if they are not symptomatic. Further experience will be needed to evaluate the benefit from this strategy. If streptozotocin is used, the risks of the serious nephrotoxic actions of the drug should be considered.

REFERENCES

1. Burcharth, F., Stage, J. G., Stadil, F., Jensen, L. I., and Fischerman, K. (1979): Localization of gastrinomas by transhepatic portal catheterization and gastrin assay. *Gastroenterology,* 77:444–450.
2. Ellison, E. H., and Wilson, S. D. (1964): The Zollinger-Ellison syndrome: Reappraisal and evaluation of 260 registered cases. *Ann. Surg.,* 160:512–530.
3. Gregory, R. A., and Tracy, H. J. (1964): A note on the gastrin-like stimulant present in Zollinger-Ellison tumours. *Gut,* 5:115–117.

4. Gregory, R. A., Tracy, H. J., French, J. M., and Sircus, W. (1960): Extraction of a gastrin-like substance from a pancreatic tumour in a case of Zollinger-Ellison syndrome. *Lancet,* i:1045–1048.
5. Ingemansson, S., Larsson, L.-I., Lunderquist, A., and Stadil, F. (1977): Pancreatic vein catheterization with gastrin assay in normal patients and in patients with the Zollinger-Ellison syndrome. *Am. J. Surg.,* 134:558–563.
6. Isenberg, J. I., Walsch, J. H., Passaro, E., Moore, E. W., and Grossman, M. I. (1972): Unusual effect of secretin on serum gastrin, serum calcium and gastric acid secretion in a patient with suspected Z-E-S. *Gastroenterology,* 62:626–631.
7. Lamers, C. B. H., Stadil, F., and van Tongeren, J. H. M. (1978): Prevalence of endocrine abnormalities in patients with the Zollinger-Ellison syndrome and in their families. *Am. J. Med.,* 64:607–612.
8. Lamers, C. B., H., and van Tongeren, J. H. M. (1977): Comparative study of the value of the calcium, secretin and meal stimulated increase in serum gastrin to the diagnosis of Zollinger-Ellison syndrome. *Gut,* 18:128–134.
9. Larsson, L.-I. (1979): Classification of pancreatic endocrine tumours. *Scand. J. Gastroenterol.,* 14, Suppl. 53:15–18.
10. Larsson, L.-I., Grimelius, L., Håkanson, R., Rehfeld, J. F., Stadil, F., Holst, J., Angervall, L., and Sundler, F. (1975): Mixed endocrine pancreatic tumors producing several peptide hormones. *Am. J. Pathol.,* 79:271–284.
11. Rehfeld, J. F., and Stadil, F. (1973): Gel filtration studies on immunoreactive gastrin in serum from Zollinger-Ellison patients. *Gut,* 14:369–373.
12. Rehfeld, J. F., Stadil, F., and Vikelsøe, J. (1974): Immunoreactive gastrin components in human serum. *Gut,* 15:102–111.
13. Stadil, F., Stage, J. G., Rehfeld, J. F., Efsen, F., and Fischerman, K. (1976): Treatment of Zollinger-Ellison syndrome with streptozotocin. *N. Engl. J. Med.,* 294:1440–1442.
14. Stage, J. G., and Stadil, F. (1979): The clinical diagnosis of the Zollinger-Ellison syndrome. *Scand. J. Gastroenterol.,* 14, Suppl. 53:79–91.
15. Stage, J. G., Stadil, F., and Fischerman, K. (1978): New aspects in the treatment of the Zollinger-Ellison syndrome. In: Cimetidine, edited by W. Creutzfeldt, pp. 137–148. Excerpta Medica, Amsterdam and Oxford.
16. Stage, J. G., Stadil, F., Rehfeld, J. F., Fahrenkrug, J., and Schaffalitzky de Muckadell, O. (1978): Secretin and the Zollinger-Ellison syndrome. Reliability of secretin tests and pathogenetic role of secretin. *Scand. J. Gastroenterol.,* 13:501–511.
17. Strauss, E., and Yalow, R. S. (1975): Differential diagnosis of hypergastrinemia. In: *Gastrointestinal Hormones,* edited by J. C. Thompson. University of Texas Press, Austin and London.
18. Zollinger, R. M., and Colemann, D. V. (1974): *Influence of pancreatic tumors in the stomach.* Charles C Thomas, Springfield, Ill.
19. Zollinger, R. M., and Ellison, E. H. (1955): Primary peptic ulcerations of the jejunum associated with islet cell tumours of the pancreas. *Ann. Surg.,* 142:709–723.

Gastrointestinal Hormones, edited by
George B. Jerzy Glass.
Raven Press, New York © 1980.

Chapter 31

Multiple Hormone-Secreting Tumors of the Gastrointestinal Tract

Chung Owyang and Vay Liang Go

Gastroenterology Unit, Mayo Clinic, Rochester, Minnesota 55901

INTRODUCTION

With advances in radioimmunoassay (RIA) and immunohistochemical techniques, the list of endocrine tumors arising from the gut and the pancreas is growing rapidly (Table 1). Until recently, however, the possibility of these endo-

TABLE 1. *Pancreatic endocrine tumors and their associated symptoms*

Cell Type	Tumor type	Clinical state
B	Insulinoma	Hypoglycemia
A	Glucagonoma	Hyperglycemia Migratory dermatitis
D	Somatostatinoma	Hyperglycemia Steatorrhea
G	Gastrinoma	Peptic ulcer Diarrhea
D_1	VIP-oma	Watery diarrhea
D_2	PP-oma	Diarrhea Steatorrhea

crine tumors secreting more than one humoral peptide was not appreciated. Such peptides include gastrin, insulin, glucagon, pancreatic polypeptide (PP), somatostatin, vasoactive intestinal polypeptide (VIP), ACTH, and others. These peptides may be produced in the normal pancreas and gastrointestinal tract, they may occur in these organs only during their developmental stages, or they may be truly ectopic. Currently, nearly all combinations of the above listed hormones have been reported, and as many as six have been found in one tumor. In most cases the tumors are composed of several distinct endocrine cell types, with separate cells being clearly responsible for each secretion. However, it has been shown in a few cases that the same tumor can produce different hormones simultaneously (10). This is not surprising, however, since some normal APUD cells appear to produce more than one substance (23).

MIXED ENDOCRINE PANCREATIC TUMORS: FREQUENCY AND CELL TYPES

The concurrent production of insulin and ACTH by a pancreatic islet cell carcinoma was first reported in 1959 (1), and subsequent similar case reports appeared in 1965 (16) and 1969 (25). The first biochemically proven multiple hormone-producing pancreatic islet cell carcinoma, studied by electron microscopy, was reported by Law et al. (14). They described the case of a 35-year-old black female with metastatic islet cell carcinoma, which was shown to be producing gastrin, ACTH, and MSH. Shortly thereafter, O'Neal et al. (18) reported another case of disseminated islet cell carcinoma that was shown by biochemical assays to produce ACTH, gastrin, MSH, and glucagon; clinical studies also indicated tumor elaboration of parathormone and vasopressin-like substances. Electron microscopic studies demonstrated α type granules within the cytoplasm of the tumor cells. Sircus et al. (24) described two cases of "pancreatic cholera" that featured peptide-secreting adenomatosis of the pancreas. Subsequent bioassay of the tumors and blood by Cleator et al. (4) demonstrated secretin-like and gastrin-like activity. Heitz et al. (9) documented a multicellular, multiple-hormone-producing islet cell tumor that was secreting gastrin and insulin and was associated with amyloid production. Broder and Carter (3), in reviewing 52 cases of pancreatic islet cell carcinoma, found four tumors that secreted two hormones simultaneously (insulin and gastrin in three cases; insulin and glucagon in one case) and one tumor that released three hormones (insulin, gastrin, and glucagon). Two similar cases of multiple-hormone-producing islet cell carcinomas, with detailed morphological and biochemical investigation, were reported by Hammar and Sale (8).

Recently, with improved immunocytochemical techniques, it has become apparent that mixed endocrine tumors of the pancreas are, in fact, much more common than originally postulated. In several reported series (5,11,12,21), the frequency of multiple-hormone producing endocrine tumors, as demonstrated by immunohistology, was as high or greater than 50% (Table 2).

TABLE 2. *Frequency of multiple hormone production in endocrine tumors demonstrated by immunohistology*

	Gastrinomas		Insulinomas		Glucagonomas	
	a	b	a	b	a	b
Insulin	4/18	2/6	3/30	9/9	3/3	1/3
Glucagon	0/18	2/6	0/30	4/9	3/3	3/3
Pancreatic polypeptide	5/18	1/6	1/13	2/9	2/3	0/3
Somatostatin	0/18	2/6	0/30	0/9	2/3	2/3
Gastrin	18/18	6/6	1/30	1/9	0/3	0/3
ACTH	8/14	1/6	—	1/9	—	—
VIP	—	—	—	—	—	1/3

a, Creutzfeldt series (6); b, Larsson series (12).

Polak et al. reported that among the various types of hormone-producing cells in these tumors, there is an extraordinary frequency of PP cells in the tumor tissue (21). In a study of 33 patients with endocrine neoplasms of the pancreas, PP cells were present in 20 of the 33 primary or secondary tumors, and plasma PP levels were markedly elevated in 18 of the 28 patients examined. In the tumor tissue, the immunoreactive PP cells appeared in groups or small clusters, and were located between the cells producing the other hormone. The ratio of PP cells to the number of other hormone-producing cells varied from 10 to 50%. A more recent report from the same group of investigators (28) indicated that PP cells were most frequently observed in glucagonomas (67%), vipomas (50%), and insulinomas (39%), and infrequently in gastrinomas (17%) (Table 3). In patients with pancreatic endocrine tumors, the frequent occurrence of PP cells probably accounts for the observation that plasma concentrations of pancreatic polypeptide are frequently elevated (11,21,28). This has led to the suggestion that a raised plasma PP concentration may be a useful marker for this kind of tumor (28). In contrast with previous reports, Larsson et al. recently reported that, with the exception of WDHA tumors, PP cells occurred no more frequently in mixed tumors than other islet cell types (13) (Table 3). Instead, in most of the patients they found a pronounced hyperplasia of insular and, to a lesser degree, extrainsular PP cells in the pancreas outside the tumor.

TABLE 3. *Frequency of pancreatic polypeptide-containing cells in multiple hormone-producing pancreatic tumors*

	Welbourn Series (18)	Larsson Series (13)
Insulinoma	7/18 (39%)	2/9 (22%)
Glucagonoma	4/6 (67%)	0/3 (0)
Vipoma	10/20 (50%)	3/4 (75%)
Gastrinoma	5/29 (17%)	1/6 (17%)
Corticotrophinoma	1/3 (33%)	—

This observation is especially common in patients with insulinoma, glucagonoma, or WDHA tumors. In contrast, in patients with Zollinger-Ellison syndrome, a different type of hyperplasia was noted, characterized by increases in all demonstrable islet cell types (11). This was thought to be related to the trophic action of gastrin on the islet cell population. This investigator suggested that the hyperplasia of the PP cells surrounding the tumor, rather than an extraordinarily frequent occurrence of PP cells in the tumor proper, is responsible for the elevated level of PP frequently observed in patients with pancreatic endocrine tumors. Further work in tissue morphology is needed to resolve the discrepancy.

More recently, Pearse et al. (20) reported that hyperplasia of pancreatic somatostatin cells (D cells) often occurs in the non-tumorous part of the pancreas that contains an endocrine tumor. In all of the 20 cases investigated, the number of D cells increased fivefold in the uninvolved parts of the pancreas that contained a pancreatic endocrine tumor (insulinoma, glucagonoma, vipoma, or gastrinoma). The most striking increase was found in the normal pancreas that was alongside VIP-producing tumors, and also in the severe watery diarrhea situation that was unassociated with a pancreatic tumor (pseudo-Verner-Morrison syndrome) (22). It was suggested that this phenomenon may represent a hyperplastic and hyperactive response of the somatostatin cells to the high blood concentrations of hormones produced by the tumors. The pathophysiological significance of this observation requires further investigation.

ETIOLOGY AND PATHOGENESIS

The pathogenesis of a multiple-hormone-producing neoplasm of the pancreas is unknown. Until quite recently, the almost universal view was that endocrine cells of the gut and pancreas arose from enterocyte stem cells, or from duct cells. This theory was recently challenged by Like and Orci (15), who studied human fetal tissue, and demonstrated that α, β, and δ cells did not appear to arise from the primitive embryonic duct cells; these investigators failed to identify a primitive precursor cell. An alternative theory was proposed by Pearse (19): Endocrine cells are all derivatives of the neural crest, and thus are both neuroectodermal and, strictly speaking, neuroendocrinal. According to this theory, the cell derivatives of the neural crest possess a common set of cytochemical and ultrastructural characteristics, i.e., amine precursor uptake and decarboxylase, or the so-called APUD system. Members of the APUD cell series are presumed to be capable of polypeptide production and function in many of the endocrine glands. Weichert (27) supported and expanded this concept. He proposed that certain polypeptide-hormone-producing cells of the pancreas, thyroid gland, lung, adrenal gland, parathyroid gland, and gastrointestinal mucosa are derived from neuroectodermal cells, which migrate into the primitive alimentary mucosa, and then are carried passively to their definitive positions where they mature. It is interesting to hypothesize that neoplasia of the primitive stem cells could result in tumors whose cells have the potential to produce a wide variety of polypeptide hormones and vasoactive amines. This would account for the diversity of cell types occurring in these tumors and their corresponding capacity to produce hormones that are not normally present in the adult pancreas. This theory recently received some experimental support when Creutzfeldt (5) demonstrated that there was only one type of cell that occurred in all types of endocrine tumors of the pancreas. These cells contain atypical secretory granules and are argyrophil by the Grimelius procedure. They are similar to the type IV (D_1) cell and may very well be a precursor or stem cell for the endocrine cells (and their tumors) that are derived from the foregut or neurocrest. More recently, this same group of investigators (6) further reported that administration of streptozotocin and nicotinamide to rats for 1 year uniformly produced insulinomas in these animals. Interestingly, by immunohistology, these insulinomas were also found to contain cells that produced somatostatin, glucagon, and pancreatic polypeptide. Ultrastructurally, some cells resembling D cells and cells with small medium electro-dense secretory granules were found in addition to tumor cells containing typical β granules. These findings further support the contention that the mixed endocrine pancreatic tumors originate from precursor or stem cells that have the potential to differentiate into cells capable of producing both pancreatic and extrapancreatic hormones as well as neuronal peptides.

CLINICAL FEATURES

Clinically, the great majority of patients with mixed pancreatic endocrine tumors often present with symptoms characteristic of hypersecretion of only one of the hormones (12). Thus, the potential of these tumors to secrete multihormones is not readily recognized clinically. In a recent review, Larsson (11) reported 25 cases of mixed endocrine tumors of the pancreas. Three of these cases were clinically "silent." The remaining 22 cases presented one of the distinct clinical syndromes characteristic of overproduction of one of the hormonal peptides, despite the fact that the tumors were composed of several distinct endocrine cell types. The reason for this interesting observation is unclear. Possibly, these tumors may secrete only one of the hormones produced, or only one of the hormones released is biologically active. It is also conceivable that various hormones released from the same tumor may have antagonistic physiological actions, and that the subsequent clinical picture may vary according to the cumulative hormonal effect on end organs.

Frequently, it was noted that the secretory products of the predominating tumor cell types could not always explain the most conspicuous clinical picture. This is exemplified in a case reported by Larsson et al. (12) where a 52-year-old man with symptoms of hyperinsulinoma was found at the time of surgery to have a pancreatic mixed endocrine tumor composed of a mixture of glucagon, gastrin, and insulin cells. Immunohistochemical studies revealed that the glucagon cells were most numerous, showing intense immunofluorescence. The gastrin cells were next in frequency, with insulin cells being few in number, and showing only moderate immunofluorescence. Thus, clinical symptoms are not always correlated quantitatively with the most important tumor cell population.

Furthermore, sequential secretion of hormones in patients with pancreatic mixed endocrine tumor has been reported to produce a change in the spectrum of symptoms over a period of years. For example, Broder and Carter (3) reported a case of Zollinger-Ellison syndrome where symptoms of hypergastrinemia developed 3 years prior to the development of hyperinsulinoma. More recently, Hammer and Sale (8) described two additional similar cases, where tumors initially produced symptoms referable to a single hormone, and over a period of years, produced two other endocrine active polypeptides that resulted in a change of clinical symptoms. Morphological investigation of one of the tumors showed no significant ultrastructural changes over a period of 6 years, when a change of symptoms from Zollinger-Ellison syndrome to hyperinsulinoma was noted. Another interesting clinical feature of mixed endocrine pancreatic tumors is that the primary tumor, composed of multiple endocrine cell types, may give rise to metastasis containing only one or two of the cell types (12). Thus, nonradical tumor resection may potentially remove one symptom and substitute another.

TREATMENT

As do gastrinomas, the great majority of mixed endocrine pancreatic tumors have metastasized by the time they are discovered. Thus the treatment is primarily medical. Because of the rarity of this type of tumor, most of the results obtained with pharmacotherapy and/or chemotherapy are, by necessity, anecdotal in nature.

Murray-Lyon et al. (17) first reported the successful use of streptozotocin in the treatment of a case of mixed endocrine pancreatic tumor. The production of insulin as well as gastrin and glucagon by the mixed islet cell carcinoma diminished following streptozotocin administration. This was accompanied by excellent symptomatic relief of hypoglycemia attacks. Similar experiences were shared by Walter et al. (26) when they administered streptozotocin to a patient with a metastatic islet cell carcinoma that was producing insulin and ACTH. The treatment resulted in a significant decline of the insulin and ACTH level, with satisfactory control of hypoglycemic symptoms and regression of signs of Cushing's syndrome. Unfortunately, the use of streptozotocin does not always produce favorable therapeutic responses. Poor responses to streptozotocin were reported by Belchetz et al. (2) in cases of pancreatic islet carcinomas producing ACTH, gastrin, and glucagon. The fulminating hypercorticism was efficiently controlled with metyrapone and aminoglutethimide. Similarly disappointing results were experienced by Hammer and Sale (8) when they treated two cases of multiple-hormone-producing metastatic islet cell carcinoma of the pancreas with streptozotocin. Thus, according to the few scattered reports in the literature, therapeutic responses of this tumor to streptozotocin were about evenly divided between improvement and failure. However, the tremendous variability in the dose, as well as schedule and route of administration of streptozotocin, makes interpretation of the therapeutic response difficult.

CONCLUSIONS

Multihormonal islet cell tumors are more common than is usually appreciated. Clinically, the multi-hormonal potentiality may not be readily apparent, but it is of clinical importance since the spectrum of clinical symptoms may change with time. Thus, ideally, when a pancreatic endocrine tumor is suspected, the patient should be screened for possible hypersecretion of other peptide hormones. Furthermore, since elevated plasma levels of hormones may originate either from the tumor per se or from hyperplasia of the endocrine cells in the non-tumorous part of the pancreas, immunocytochemical studies of the resected tumor should be carried out, along with long term postoperative follow-up that includes the necessary multiple blood hormone determinations.

REFERENCES

1. Balls, K. F., Nicholson, J. T. L., Goodman, H. L., and Touchstone, J. C. (1959): Functional islet cell carcinomas of the pancreas with Cushing's syndrome. *J. Clin. Endocrinol.,* 19:1134–1143.
2. Belchetz, P. E., Brown, C. L., Makin, H. L. J., Trafford, D. J. H., Stuartmason, A., Bloom, S. R., and Ratcliffe, J. C. (1973): ACTH, glucagon and gastrin production by a pancreatic islet cell carcinoma and its treatment. *Clin. Endocrinol.,* 2:307–316.
3. Broder, L. E., and Carter, S. K. (1973): Pancreatic islet cell carcinoma I: Clinical features of 52 patients. *Ann. Intern. Med.,* 79:101–107.
4. Cleator, I. G. M., Thomson, C. G., Sircus, W., and Coombes, M. (1970): Bioassay evidence of abnormal secretin-like and gastrin-like activity in tumor and blood in cases of "cholergic diarrhea". *Gut,* 11:206–211.
5. Creutzfeldt, W.: *Personal communication.*
6. Creutzfeldt, W., Arnold, R., and Frerichs, H. (1978): Insulinomas and gastrinomas. In: *Gut Hormones,* edited by J. R. Bloom, pp. 589–598. Churchill Livingstone, New York.
7. Floyd, J. C., Chance, R. E., Hayashi, M., Moon, N. E., and Fajans, S. S. (1975): Concentrations of a newly recognized pancreatic islet polypeptide in plasma of healthy subjects and in plasma and tumors of patients with insulin-secreting islet cell tumors. *Clin. Res.,* 23:535A.
8. Hammar, S., and Sale, G. (1975): Multiple-hormone-producing islet cell carcinomas of the pancreas. *Hum. Pathol.,* 6:349–362.
9. Heitz, P. H., Steiner, H., Halter, F., Egli, F., and Kapp, J. P. (1971): Multihormonal, amyloid-producing tumor of the islets of Langerhans in a twelve-year-old boy. *Virchows Arch. (Path. Anat.),* 353:312–324.
10. Inglemansson, S., Holst, J. J., Larsson, L.-I., and Lunderquist, A. (1977): Localization of glucagonomas by pancreatic vein catheterization and glucagon assay. *Surg. Gynecol. Obstet.,* 145:509–516.
11. Larsson, L.-I (1978): PP-producing and mixed endocrine pancreatic tumors. In: *Gut Hormones,* edited by S. R. Bloom, pp. 605–610. Churchill Livingstone, New York.
12. Larsson, L.-I., Grimelius, L., Hakanson, R., Rehfeld, J. F., Stadil, F., Holst, J. J., Angervall, L., and Sundler, F. (1975): Mixed endocrine pancreatic tumors producing several peptide hormones. *Am. J. Pathol.,* 79:271–284.
13. Larsson, L.-I., Schwartz, T., Lundqvist, G., Chance, R. E., Sundler, F., Rehfeld, J. F., Crimelius, L., Fahrenkrug, J., Schaffalitzky de Muckadell, D. B., and Moon, N. (1976): Occurrence of

human pancreatic polypeptide in pancreatic endocrine tumors. Possible implication in the watery diarrhea syndrome. *Am. J. Pathol.,* 85:675–684.

14. Law, D. H., Liddle, G. W., Scott, M. W., Jr., and Tauber, S. D. (1965): Ectopic production of multiple hormones (ACTH, MSH and gastrin) by a simple malignant tumor. *N. Engl. J. Med.,* 273:292–296.

15. Like, A. A. and Orci, L. (1972): Embryogenesis of the human pancreatic islets: A light and electron microscopic study. *Diabetes,* (Suppl. 2), 21:511–534.

16. Marks, V., Samols, E., and Bolton, R. (1965): Hyperinsulinism and Cushing's syndrome. *Br. Med. J.,* 1:1419–1420.

17. Murray-Lyon, I. M., Eddleston, A. L., Williams, R., Brown, M., Hoglin, B. M., Bennett, A., Edwards, J. C., and Taylor, K. W. (1968): Treatment of multiple hormone-producing malignant islet cell tumor with streptozotocin. *Lancet,* ii:895–898.

18. O'Neal, L. W., Kipnis, D. M., Luse, S. A., Lacy, P. E., and Garett, L. (1968): Secretion of various endocrine substances by ACTH-secreting tumors—gastrin, melanotropin, norepinephrine, serotonin, parathormone, vasopressin, glucagon. *Cancer,* 21:1219–1232.

19. Pearse, A. G. E. (1969): The cytochemistry and ultrastructure of polypeptide hormone-producing cells of APUD series and the embryologic, physiologic and pathologic implications of the concept. *J. Histochem. Cytochem.,* 17:303–313.

20. Pearse, A. G. E., Polak, J. M., and Bloom, S. R. (1977): The newer gut hormones: Cellular sources, physiology, pathology and clinical aspects. *Gastroenterology,* 72:746–761.

21. Polak, J. M., Bloom, S. R., Adrian, T. E., Heitz, P., Bryant, M. G., and Pearse, A. G. E. (1976): Pancreatic polypeptide insulinomas, gastrinomas, VIPomas and glucagonomas. *Lancet,* i:328–330.

22. Polak, J. M., Bloom, S. R., Arimura, A., and Pearse, A. G. E. (1975): Pancreatic D cells in normal and pathological human pancreas. *Gut,* 16:837.

23. Polak, J. M., Bloom, S. R., Buchan, A. M. T., Bryant, M. G. and Pearse, A. G. E. (1977a): Multiple hormonal APUD cells. *Gut,* 18:A410.

24. Sircus, W., Brunt, P. W., Walker, R. J., Small, C. P., Falconer, C. W. A., and Thomson, C. G. (1970): Two cases of "pancreatic cholera" with features of peptide-secreting adenomatosis of the pancreas. *Gut,* 11:197–205.

25. Vieweg, W. V. R., Graber, A. L., Cerchio, G. M. (1969): Pancreatic islet cell carcinoma with hyperinsulinism and probably ectopic ACTH-MSH secretion. *Arch. Intern. Med.,* 124:731–735.

26. Walter, R. M., Ensinck, J. W., Ricketts, H., Kendall, J. W., and Williams, R. M. (1973): Insulin and ACTH production by a streptozotocin responsive islet cell carcinoma. *Am. J. Med.,* 55:667–670.

27. Weichert, R. F., III. (1970): The neural ectodermal origin of the peptide-secreting endocrine glands. A unifying concept for the etiology of multiple endocrine adenomatosis and the inappropriate secretion of peptide hormones by non-endocrine tumors. *Am. J. Med.,* 49:232–241.

28. Welbourn, R. B., Polak, J. M., Bloom, S. R., Pearse, A. G. E., and Galland, R. B. (1978): Apudomas of the pancreas. In: *Gut Hormones,* edited by S. R. Bloom, pp. 561–569. Churchill Livingstone, New York.

Radioimmunoassays of Gastrointestinal Hormonal Peptides

Gastrointestinal Hormones, edited by
George B. Jerzy Glass.
Raven Press, New York © 1980.

Chapter 32

Problems and Pitfalls in the Radioimmunoassay of Gastrointestinal Hormones

Rosalyn S. Yalow and Eugene Straus

Veterans Administration Hospital, Bronx, New York 10468

INTRODUCTION

Radioimmunoassay (RIA) is a general method employing the reaction of antigen with specific antibody that permits measurement of the concentration of virtually any substance of biologic interest (4,37). The unknown concentration of the antigenic substance in a sample is obtained simply by comparing its inhibitory effect on the binding of radioactively labeled antigen to a limited amount of specific antibody with the inhibitory effect of known standards. There is no requirement in RIA for identity of the labeled and unlabeled antigen or even of the unknown antigen and that used for standard. A necessary, but not sufficient, condition for a properly validated RIA is *immunochemical* identity of unknown and standard antigens. Under these circumstances a dilution curve of the unknown should be superposable along a dilution curve of the standards, preferably over at least a 100-fold range of concentrations. In some instances a RIA procedure may be clinically useful even when it is not properly validated.

A number of factors present problems in the practical application of RIA to measurement of substances in plasma or tissue extracts. These include *nonhormonal* factors such as the lack of sensitivity of the assay system, nonspecific interference in the immune reaction, and damage or destruction of labeled antigen or antibody during incubation and *hormonal* factors such as species specificity of the immune reaction, presence of immunologically related but different hormones, and heterogeneity of hormonal forms.

NONHORMONAL FACTORS

Sensitivity of Assay System

RIA has gained wide acceptance and usage, for it is a method that can make possible detection of substances such as peptide hormones at concentrations of less than 10^{-13} M. In the plasma of normal subjects in the nonstimulated state, these hormones range in concentration from approximately 10^{-12} to 10^{-10} M. Therefore when maximal sensitivity obtains, dilution of the sample in the assay may be sufficient to eliminate most of the effects of artifactual interference in the immune reaction. Furthermore, since extremely small volumes of plasma are usually employed for RIA, multiple sampling as part of stimulatory or suppression tests often permits clinical diagnosis even when the assay *per se* has limited accuracy or precision.

The quantitative aspects of the antigen-antibody reaction and the mathematical considerations that are instructive in optimizing the sensitivity and precision of RIAs have previously been considered in some detail (1,39).

One can gain some insight into the problem from the following highly simplified approach: Consider the RIA reaction to be a bimolecular reaction between an antigen containing a single reactive site (Ag) and a single order of homogeneous combining sites on antibody (Ab) and assume that labeled and unlabeled antigen behave identically. It is obvious that it is inadvisable in a RIA to employ an amount of labeled tracer antigen whose immunochemical concentration is large compared with the concentration of unlabeled antigen in the unknown; e.g., if the tracer concentration is five times the antigen concentration, then a random 5% error in the tracer produces a 25% error in the hormone concentration. It is therefore desirable that the chemical concentration of the tracer be no greater than the minimal concentration of antigen to be determined.

From the mass-action law,

$$[Ag] + [Ab] \underset{k'}{\overset{k}{\rightleftharpoons}} [\overline{AgAb}] \qquad [1]$$
$$F \qquad\quad\ \ B$$

where $F = [Ag]$, the molar concentration of uncomplexed antigen, $B = [\overline{AgAb}]$, the molar concentration of complexed antigen or antibody-combining sites, and [Ab], the molar concentration of uncomplexed antibody. Then

$$B/F = K([Ab^\circ] - B) \qquad [2]$$

where the equilibrium constant for the reaction, $K = k/k'$ and $[Ab°]$ is the total molar concentration of antibody binding sites, i.e., $[Ab°] = [Ab] + [\overline{AgAb}]$.

It is evident from Eq. [2] that when $B \ll [Ab°]$, B/F decreases only slightly for large changes in B; thus if B increases 10-fold from 0.002 $[Ab°]$ to 0.02 $[Ab°]$, the change in B/F is less than 2%. For a sensitive assay, therefore, $[Ab°]$ must be reduced by dilution so that it is not much larger than B; since B, the bound antigen, must be less than the total antigen, it follows that $[Ab°] \cong H$, the minimal hormonal or antigen concentration to be detected.

If we wish to start with $B/F = 1$ in the absence of added unlabeled antigen ("trace" conditions), then from Eq. [2]

$$1 \lesssim K[AB°] \text{ and } [Ab°] \cong H$$

Therefore,

$$H \gtrsim 1/K$$

Thus, there is an inherent sensitivity that can be achieved with any given antiserum. It depends on the equilibrium constant, K, which characterizes the reaction of antigen with the predominant order of antibody binding sites; the higher the value of K, the more sensitive is the assay.

These considerations may need to be modified to take into account the nonidentity of labeled and unlabeled antigen, multiplicity or heterogeneity of antibody binding sites, interaction between binding sites, experimental errors, and so forth. Nonetheless, the more complicated formulations all lead to the same conclusion—in order to achieve a high sensitivity assay, the primary reaction of labeled antigen with antibody must be one of very high energy, that is, having a large equilibrium constant.

Having chosen an antibody with suitable characteristics, it is then necessary to employ as tracer a labeled antigen that does not limit the sensitivity of the assay by its undesirable immunochemical properties or by its inappropriately high concentration. Although in RIA there is no requirement for identity of labeled and unlabeled antigen, chemical alterations that produce a change in the molecular configuration of the labeled antigen may alter its ability to react with specific antibody and somewhat reduce the sensitivity of the assay. For instance, overiodination has been shown to decrease the immunoreactivity of some peptides compared with that of more lightly iodinated preparations (3).

Another type of problem is evident in the choice of tracer for the secretin assay. Secretin is a peptide that contains only an N-terminal histidyl residue and no tyrosyl residue. Substitution of tyrosine in place of phenylalanine in the sixth position simplifies iodination. However, with all antisera we have studied, the use of iodohistidyl secretin as tracer permits a more sensitive RIA than does 6-iodotyrosyl secretin (Fig. 1) (30). We have not had major problems in the iodination of histidyl or sulfated tyrosyl residues. Nonetheless we have demonstrated that, depending on the region of the antigen that reacts with antibody, the presence of both I and SO_3H groups on a tyrosyl residue may result in some steric or charge hindrance to the binding reaction (44).

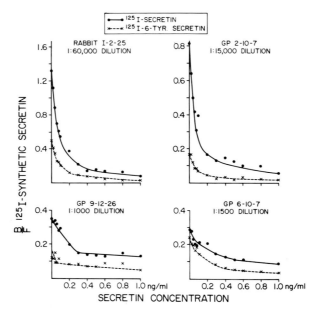

FIG. 1. Standard curves for secretin assay generated using ^{125}I-synthetic secretin and ^{125}I-6-Tyr-secretin as tracers and pure natural secretin for standard. Note that in the three guinea pigs and one rabbit antisera studied there was diminished binding of the labeled preparation to antibody and the standard curve was less sensitive when the ^{125}I-6-Try-secretin was employed. (From ref. 30, with permission.)

Not only is choice of an appropriate labeled antigen necessary to optimize the sensitivity obtainable with any antiserum, but the specific activity of the labeled preparation may also be a limiting factor. It is desirable to employ a tracer that is sufficiently low in concentration so as not to occupy a significant fraction of the high energy antibody-binding sites. Nonetheless the counting rate in the incubation tube must be sufficiently high to assure statistical accuracy. A certain amount of judgment is required to optimize the variables—degree of iodination, chemical amount of tracer, and statistical accuracy—to maximize the sensitivity of an assay procedure.

Perhaps the commonest error is to attribute small, perhaps random, *decreases* in the percent binding of tracer to antibody as due to the presence of hormone. Often in the same assays, there are small *increases* in the percent binding that are ignored since they would then have to be attributed to "negative hormone." Thus the measured basal concentrations often depend on the sensitivity of the assays; with improvements in assay sensitivity the putative fasting levels generally decrease. For instance, in one of the first studies employing the gastrin RIA (19) fasting gastrin levels in 24 patients without recognized gastrointestinal disease were reported to range from 245 to 668 pg/ml. By now, a decade later, there is general agreement that these values are at least 10-fold too high. Another example is an early study of Reeder et al. (24), who reported normal fasting cholecystokinin (CCK) levels to be 5 ng/ml. This was followed by a later paper from the same laboratory (23) in which the levels were reported to average about 700 pg/ml. It is quite likely that even these latter values are too high.

Random or nonrandom nonspecific interference in the immune reaction results in an apparent fasting level that is sensitivity dependent—the better the sensitivity of the RIA the lower is the reported "mean basal concentration."

Chemical Interference in the Immune Reaction

The immune reaction is a chemical reaction and many factors can interfere in this reaction in a nonspecific fashion. Thus the pH, ionic environment, and the introduction of a variety of chemicals may influence the antigen-antibody reaction. If standards and unknowns are in an identical milieu, then the validity of the assay is unaffected, but these effects may reduce the sensitivity of the assay.

The formation of antigen-antibody complexes is usually not pH-dependent in the range 7 to 8.5 but the complexes may dissociate outside this range. The resulting apparent decrease in binding may be falsely interpreted as due to hormone. This must be considered when highly acid or alkaline extracts of tissue are assayed.

High concentrations of salts, even NaCl at the concentration found in a 1:5 dilution of plasma, may inhibit some antigen-antibody reactions (2). The effect of different buffers in altering the standard curves in a typical gastrin assay is shown in Fig. 2. There is clearly a marked lowering of the sensitivity of the

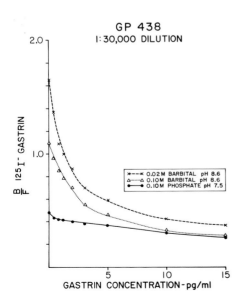

FIG. 2. Standard curves for the radioimmunoassay of gastrin employing different buffers. Higher ionic strength buffers decrease the sensitivity of the assay.

assay when a high ionic strength buffer is employed. The effect of high concentrations of salt may vary among different assay systems and even among different antisera against the same antigen. Nonetheless we have generally obtained assays of better sensitivity when a low ionic strength buffer such as 0.02 M barbital is employed. If, for instance, a high ionic strength buffer is employed to elute a peptide from a Sephadex column, the standards should be prepared in a volume of elution buffer equal to that of the eluates to be assayed. Otherwise the decreases in binding due to the salt may falsely be attributed to the presence of hormone. Serum and tissue proteins may also interfere in the immune reaction. This problem will be considered in the section on heterogeneity of hormonal forms.

Anticoagulants, bacteriostatic agents, and enzyme inhibitors may, in some assays, interfere in the immune reaction. For instance, there is significant, nonspecific interference with the immune reaction in the gastrin RIA in the presence of 40 units heparin per milliliter, an effect not observed at 10 units of heparin per milliliter (43). In the same RIA system, merthiolate, although not sodium azide, was inhibitory at bacteriostatic concentrations (36). Trasylol, a commonly used enzyme inhibitor, is inhibitory in our ACTH RIA (4).

No general conclusions can be drawn concerning which chemicals will inhibit a particular RIA. The unknowns and standards should be in the same milieu. Otherwise, it must be demonstrated that the differences between their milieus do not affect the immune reaction.

Incubation Damage of Labeled Antigen or Antibody

It has long been appreciated that labeled peptides may be damaged by plasma during incubation, an effect that is more marked in concentrated than in highly dilute plasma (5). The peptides damaged during incubation do not bind to specific antibody but may remain in the incubation mixture as small fragments or bind nonspecifically to serum proteins, primarily the α-globulins (5).

Various techniques have been used to evaluate incubation damage of the labeled tracer. One method is to prepare a control mixture containing the labeled antigen and either the unknown sample or the diluent used for the standards, but without antiserum to evaluate differential damage occurring during the incubation period (5,37). When separation of free and antibody bound labeled antigen is effected by adsorption of free labeled antigen to solid-phase material, damaged labeled antigen is considered to be that fraction that fails to be adsorbed. Charcoal, talc, QUSO, and ion-exchange resins are among the specific adsorbents that have been employed. Charcoal, although very widely used, does have some disadvantages. When proteolytic degradation of the labeled peptide is extensive, small fragments and iodotyrosines may be produced that bind to charcoal but that usually do not bind to the other specific adsorbents (31). If the fragment binds to charcoal, the "control" appears to be satisfactory and it is assumed that the tracer is intact. However, the fragments do not bind to specific antibody and the lowered fraction of radioactivity found in the antigen-antibody complexes is often interpreted falsely as due to high hormone concentration. A similar problem obtains with the commonly employed double antibody method, in which the antigen-antibody complexes are precipitated by a second antibody. In this system damaged labeled antigen that does not bind to the first antibody is not precipitated by the second antibody. If this is not appreciated, the effect may be falsely attributed to hormone. Monitoring of the immunologic integrity of the labeled antigen can be performed only by adding excess antibody at the

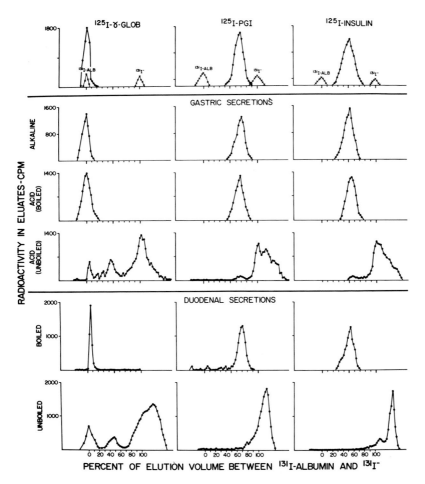

FIG. 3. Sephadex G50 gel chromatography of ^{125}I-human gamma globulin, ^{125}I-PGI, and ^{125}I-human insulin after incubation in standard diluent and in gastric and duodenal secretions. Incubation in unboiled acid gastric juice and unboiled duodenal secretions resulted in altered gel filtration patterns interpretable as due to extensive alterations in each of the labeled substances. (From ref. 31, with permission.)

end of the incubation period, reincubating, and again effecting separation of bound from free labeled hormone. Since this control is wasteful of specific antibody it is generally not employed.

It is evident that if either labeled antigen or specific antibody is altered or destroyed during incubation there is a reduction in the concentration of antigen-antibody complexes and this reduction is likely to be interpreted erroneously as due to high hormonal content. This can be expected to present a major problem, particularly when the fluid to be assayed contains high concentrations of proteolytic enzymes. We have demonstrated (31) that antigen and antibody are destroyed by incubation in unboiled acid gastric juice or unboiled duodenal secretions (Fig. 3). Thus under the usual conditions of sampling, reliable estimates of true hormonal content of these fluids cannot be made because of enzymatic damage to the hormone before assay. It is quite likely that the high values reported by others (17) for gastrin in gastric juice is due to undetected but extensive proteolytic damage to labeled antigen.

HORMONAL FACTORS

Species Specificity

Currently available RIA systems for measurement of many of the gastrointestinal hormones employ antisera raised against the porcine hormone and radioiodine-labeled procine hormone as tracer. The use of a homologous porcine system for study of hormone in species other than the pig requires consideration of the possible species specificity of the immune reaction.

The amino acid sequences of peptides from different species may have diverged during the course of evolution. The divergence has frequently occurred through single base mutations and has generally been conservative, resulting in no significant alteration in the biologic function of the molecule. Species differences are therefore likely to occur in the regions of the molecule that are not directly involved in its biologic action.

The entire secretin molecule appears to be required for its biologic action; there are no reports suggesting that the full spectrum of its biologic activities resides in any fragment of the molecule. It is therefore not surprising that a homologous porcine RIA can be employed to measure secretin not only in the gastrointestinal mucosa of several mammalian species (34) but also in the plasmas of dog and man (32). The situation is quite different for CCK. The COOH-terminal octapeptide (CCK-8) not only has the full spectrum of biologic activities of the intact molecule (CCK-33) but, depending on the bioassay system, has been reported to be as much as 10-fold more bioactive (28). The homologous RIA for porcine CCK-33 (pCCK-33) that we developed did not permit detection of any immunoreactivity in the same monkey and dog extracts in which CCK-like immunoreactivity was measured by a COOH-terminal antiserum with which equimolar amounts of CCK-8 and CCK-33 cross-react identically (33). Our finding of the marked species specificity of antisera directed against the NH_2-terminal of pCCK-33 confirms the earlier work of Go et al. (12), who reported no cross-reactivity of a crude human intestinal extract with an homologous pCCK-33 assay with sufficient sensitivity to detect CCK in pig plasma 60 min after meals. Our findings differ from those of several other laboratories (16,23,48) who have reported the measurement of human plasma CCK with homologous porcine RIAs in which CCK-8 is 20- to 200-fold less immunoreactive than pCCK. We are unable to interpret the findings of Rehfeld (25,26), who employed RIAs using pCCK-33 and CCK-33 labeled through one of its side chains with ^{125}I-hydroxyphenylproprionic acid-succinimide ester. His studies suggested that intact CCK-33 was a very minor component of immunoreactive CCK extracted from porcine or human gut. Mutt and Jorpes (22) purified 6 mg of CCK-33 from the methanol insoluble fraction of the same starting material from which 10 mg of secretin was purified. We interpret these data as indicating that CCK-33 and secretin are to be found in the intestine in approximately the same concentrations. We have found the mean secretin concentration in the pig intestine to average about 3 μg/g wet weight mucosa (34) and the mean CCK-33 concentration to be about 1 μg/g (33). This would be consistent with the extraction data of Mutt and Jorpes (28). If there is as little CCK-33 as reported by Rehfeld, why is so much extractable from the intestine?

Unlike secretin and CCK, which have been purified only from pig gut, the 17 amino acid gastrin peptides have been purified from several mammalian species. Sequence variations among human, porcine, bovine, ovine, canine, and feline gastrins occur only in positions 5, 8, and 10 (see ref. 20 for review). We have been able to use an homologous porcine gastrin RIA to measure immunoreactive gastrin even in the plasma and extracts of the gut of two species of molluscs (29). The guinea pig antiserum used for these studies reacts very poorly with CCK and with C-terminal gastrin fragments consisting of residues 10–17. The finding that molluscan gastrin cross-reacts in our assay system and that the concentrations in pooled blood (40–150 pg/ml) are comparable with those found in the mammalian species suggests very similar molecular configurations and probably homologies among molluscan and mammalian gastrins.

One cannot be certain in predicting for which hormones and in which species there have occurred alterations during the course of evolution. However, it is likely that any such changes have not altered significantly the configuration of the hormonally active site. Thus species differences are apt to be found in regions of the molecule that are not directly involved in its biologic activity. Since antibodies formed in one species against the hormone of another are likely to be directed toward the altered portions of the molecule, it is not surprising that we, and most other groups, have generated anti-pCCK sera against the NH_2 portion of the molecule. Of course if a peptide is treated as a hapten and coupled to a larger protein and there are several sites for coupling, one cannot predict the resulting conformational alterations that contribute to the foreignness of the immunogen.

Immunologically Related but Different Hormones

In RIA, consideration must always be given to the possibility that plasma or tissue extracts contain peptides immunologically (and perhaps biologically) related to the peptide to be assayed. This is of particular concern in assays for the gastrointestinal hormones, many of which can be divided into two families with significant homologies; the secretin-related family consisting of secretin, vasoactive intestinal peptide (VIP), glucagon, and gastroinhibitory peptide (GIP) (see ref. 6 for review) and the gastrin-related family consisting of the gastrins, the CCKs and the ceruleins (see ref. 20 for review), each of which exists in multiple hormonal forms. In general, most antisera developed for assays of the secretin family show little cross-reactivity with other members of the family. However, the cerulein and CCK families share a common C-terminal heptapeptide, and the gastrin family shares a C-terminal pentapeptide with the other two. Therefore an antiserum directed against the C-terminal portion of any member of the family is quite likely to cross-react strongly with other members of the family. For example, we have used an antiserum that reacts more strongly with heptadecapeptide gastrin than with CCK-33 or CCK-8 to measure CCK in brain and gut of several species. This presents no problem, since brain and intestinal gastrin is low or undetectable. However, were such an antiserum used to measure plasma CCK-peptides in normal subjects, the presence of gastrin would have to be taken into account by direct assay of gastrin with an antiserum not sensitive to CCK-peptides and then correcting for the gastrin content in the apparent total immunoreactivity as determined with a CCK-8 antiserum. If the concentrations of the gastrin-like and CCK-like activities are comparable, the determinations are hardly likely to be very precise. Fractionation on Sephadex is also likely to present problems, since 34 amino acid gastrin and 33 amino acid CCK cannot be resolved. Since CCK-33 is a much more basic peptide than G-34, a system that separates on the basis of charge is more likely to provide the required discrimination. Until now there have been no reported assays of plasma CCK using a C-terminal antiserum.

Heterogeneity of Hormonal Forms

Gastrin

It was evident almost from the first application of RIA to the measurement of plasma insulin in man that problems could arise because of differences between the biologic and immunologic potencies of intact hormone and possible metabolic fragments (38). However, the full magnitude of the problem was not appreciated until the many demonstrations during the past decade that generally peptide hormones are found in more than one form in plasma and other tissue extracts. These forms may have partial biologic or immunologic activity. They may represent precursor(s) or metabolic product(s) of the well characterized familiar hormonal form or even be homologous peptides that are independently synthesized or released.

Gastrin, the first gastrointestinal hormone to be measured by RIA, has been shown to be found in plasma and tissue in a bewildering array of hormonal forms. The first evidence for the heterogeneity of gastrin was the demonstration that antral extracts contain two gastrins (I and II) that differ only in the absence or presence, respectively, of an esterified SO_3H on the tyrosyl residue in the 12th position (13,14). These two gastrins appear to behave similarly with respect to all their known biologic properties as well as in virtually all RIA systems. The single exception is a report by Hansky et al. (15) in which porcine gastrin II was shown to be fivefold less immunoreactive than either synthetic human gastrin I or porcine gastrin I.

There is general agreement that the predominant biologically active forms of gastrin in blood and tissue are the heptadecapeptide gastrins (G-17) and the "big" gastrins (G-34). G-34 generally predominates in the plasma of most gastrin hypersecretors (41,42). However, on occasion, G-17 is the predominant form in the plasma of some patients with Zollinger-Ellison syndrome (ZE) (Fig. 4). The hormonal form of gastrin is relevant in determining the clinical significance of its concentration in plasma. Continuous infusion in dogs of equimolar amounts of G-34 and G-17 results in a fivefold higher plasma concentration of G-34 but produces about the same acid response (35). Therefore biologic activity as defined by the traditional dose-response method is different from that defined by plasma concentration-response data. Thus it is necessary to consider the hormonal form in determining the minimal concentration of plasma gastrin that is consistent with ZE. For instance, a plasma concentration of 40 pg G-17/ml would be as potent as 200 pg G-34/ml. G-34 and G-17 cross-react identically on a molar basis with all antisera we use for clinical RIA. The best test for immunochemical identity of G-34 and G-17 is to determine the immunopotency before and after complete tryptic conversion of G-34 to G-17.

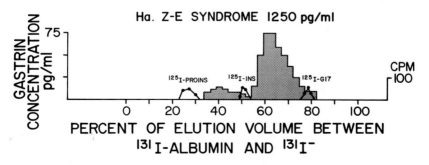

FIG. 4. Sephadex G50 superfine (1 × 200) column gel filtration pattern of plasma from a ZE patient in whom G17 is the predominant form in the circulation. (0.1 M phosphate buffer; 1 ml on column).

There remains some controversy concerning the nature of other hormonal forms of gastrins. We initially demonstrated (45) that in the plasma of ZE patients and in the jejunum of normal subjects there is a minor component of immunoreactivity (generally less than 2%) that elutes in the void volume on Sephadex G50 gel filtration ("big big gastrin," BBG). Furthermore, plasma BBG from ZE patients was shown to be tryptic digestible to G-17 (45). We subsequently further characterized BBG by using void volume fractions from an extract of a ZE tumor (received through the courtesy of Dr. R. Gregory) and showed that it had properties resembling the BBG originally found in ZE plasma (47). Rehfeld et al. (27) has confirmed our finding of the presence of BBG in gastrinomas but concludes "that there are no true macromolecular gastrins in serum or in non-neoplastic gastrointestinal mucosa." Our previous demonstration (45) that the minor BBG component in ZE plasma is tryptic convertible to G-17 confirms that this BBG is a true gastrin molecule, presumably derived from the gastrinoma. What is the nature of BBG in the plasma of those without a gastrinoma?

Some have suggested that BBG might be an artifact introduced by nonspecific

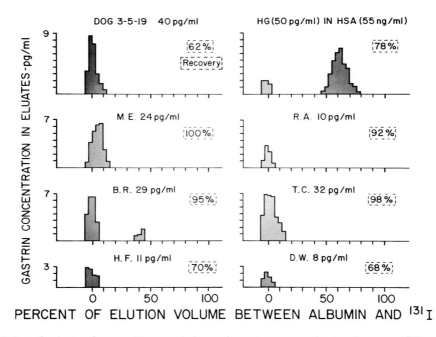

FIG. 5. Sephadex G50 gel filtration of plasma from six antrectomized patients post Billroth II *(6 lower frames),* one dog *(upper left frame),* and of human serum albumin at a concentration of 55 ng/ml fortified with 50 pg HG/ml. One-ml portions were applied to the columns and 1-ml eluates were assayed. The recovery of immunoreactivity from each column is shown in the boxed areas. (From ref. 46, with permission.)

effects of serum proteins (11,27). We have also demonstrated (46) that some BBG does not resemble the BBG identified in plasma and tissue of ZE patients. Sephadex G50 gel filtration patterns of serum albumin (Fig. 5, upper right) or gamma globulin at concentrations comparable with those in plasma and fortified with 50 pg G-17/ml demonstrate that no more than 10% of the added hormone binds to serum proteins. Furthermore, fractionation of the same volumes of dog or human plasma in which the apparent gastrin concentration ranged from 8 to 40 pg/ml demonstrated only "void volume immunoreactivity" (VVI). The amount of such apparent immunoreactivity was not a function of the plasma protein content but was a function of the apparent hormone content as measured at a 1:25 dilution of plasma. Thus in these studies the presence of albumin or gamma globulin did not contribute to the BBG-like activity either by nonspecific interference in the immune reaction or by binding gastrin peptides. However, such experiments leave unanswered the question as to whether all VVI is identical with BBG purified from ZE plasma or tumor. Plasma G-17 and G-34 are not diminished by boiling (40). Furthermore the mucosal and tumor tissues from which BBG was obtained were extracted with boiling water (45,47). It can readily be shown that the apparent hormonal content of some dog and human plasmas can be markedly reduced by boiling for 3 to 10 min at a 1:3 dilution (in normal saline) (46). Thus this cross-reacting material cannot be due to BBG or the smaller gastrins.

In our first report on the RIA for gastrin (40) we recommended boiling a 1:3 dilution of plasma to eliminate nonspecific incubation damage of the tracer that would result in apparently high hormone concentrations. Whether the falsely elevated hormonal content and VVI demonstrable in many fasting plasma samples is due to some such factor has not been fully investigated. However, this method of assuring that the measured immunoreactivity is due to one of the known forms of gastrin is easily effected.

Are there authentic macromolecular gastrins in nongastrinoma plasma or tissue? It seemed easiest to answer this question by employing plasma from an animal species with very high gastrin levels. Many rabbits in our laboratory have fasting gastrin levels considerably higher than those of normal man. A major fraction of the immunoreactivity in these samples elutes in the void volume even though as little as 0.2 ml plasma was applied to 1 × 50 Sephadex G50 columns (Fig. 6). Immunoreactive rabbit plasma gastrin coelutes with albumin on Sepharose 6B gel filtration but remains at the origin on starch block or starch gel electrophoresis *(previously unpublished observations)*. Like G-17, G-34 and authentic BBG the major fraction of immunoreactive gastrin in rabbit plasma is not diminished by boiling. Preliminary experiments confirm that more than 90% of this immunoreactivity is removable from plasma by affinity chromatography *(unpublished observations)*. Thus in rabbit plasma there appears to be an immunoreactive component with some physicochemical properties that would resemble a macromolecular gastrin. The nature of this material has not as yet been fully characterized.

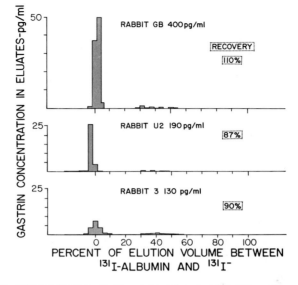

FIG. 6. Sephadex G50 gel filtration of plasma from three rabbits taken after overnight fasting. The same small volume of plasma (0.2 ml) was applied in each case. The apparent void volume immunoreactivity was a function of hormone rather than of protein content.

Secretin

Secretin differs from gastrin in that only a single hormonal form appears to predominate throughout the gastrointestinal tract of all animal species studied including monkey, dog, pig, rabbit, rat, and guinea pig (34). Although it is quite likely that secretin, like other peptide hormones, is synthesized in a larger precursor form we have been unable to detect "big" secretin in the intestinal tissues of any of these species in amounts sufficient for physiocochemical characterization. Our studies fail to confirm the earlier observations of Boden et al. (7) that the major peak of immunoreactive secretin in mucosal tissue has an elution volume on Sephadex between that of insulin and growth hormone.

Vasoactive Intestinal Polypeptide (VIP)

Immunoreactive VIP in gut and brain was shown in some studies to be accounted for by a single component with gel filtration elution patterns indistinguishable from authentic VIP (8,18). More recently, Dimaline and Dockray (9) verified that in pig brain and in muscle from the human colon only a single component of immunoreactive VIP is observed. However, they described four immunoreactive components in human colonic mucosa. Three of these appear to have Sephadex elution volumes identical to that of authentic VIP but are distinguishable from it on the basis of charge. The fourth component elutes later than the other three and could represent a smaller form (9).

Cholecystokinin (CCK)

The nature of plasma CCK has not been described. Several laboratories have reported that the C-terminal fragments including CCK-8 may account for virtually all the recoverable activity in the brain (10,26) or in the gut (26). We have found intact CCK and its C-terminal fragments both in the brain and gut, the apparent relative concentrations depending on the site and extraction technique employed (21,33).

CONCLUSION

This chapter has been concerned primarily with technical problems in RIA and the complications introduced both in bioassay and immunoassay procedures by the existence of heterogeneous forms of most peptide hormones. These problems and pitfalls are common to all assays, whether those in which the reagents are prepared in a research laboratory or those in which commercial sources supply the separate reagents or complete kits. In the latter situation there are additional problems relating to quality control of the kits or other reagents. The manufacturer is responsible for the reliability of the reagents at the time of shipment. However, further problems may be introduced by handling or mishandling of reagents en route to the clinical laboratory. For clinical diagnosis it is generally best wherever possible to use appropriate stimulatory or suppression tests rather than to rely on the absolute accuracy of determinations of hormonal level. Where such testing procedures cannot be employed there is no uniquely satisfactory answer to the general problem of quality control. Use of RIA in a casual manner without insight into its pitfalls can be destructive of its very important role in clinical medicine.

ACKNOWLEDGMENT

These studies were supported by the Medical Research Program of the Veterans Administration.

REFERENCES

1. Berson, S. A., and Yalow, R. S. (1959): Quantitative aspects of reaction between insulin and insulin-binding antibody. *J. Clin. Invest.*, 38:1996–2016.
2. Berson, S. A., and Yalow, R. S. (1968): Radio-immunoassay of ACTH in plasma. *J. Clin. Invest.*, 47:2725–2751.
3. Berson, S. A., and Yalow, R. S. (1969): Recent advances in immunoassay of peptide hormones in plasma. In: *Diabetes,* edited by J. Ostman and R. D. G. Milner, pp. 50–67. Excerpta Medica Foundation, Amsterdam.
4. Berson, S. A., and Yalow, R. S. (1973): General radioimmunoassay. In: *Methods in Investigative and Diagnostic Endocrinology, Part I—General Methodology,* edited by S. A. Berson, and R. S. Yalow, pp. 84–120. North-Holland Publishing Co., Amsterdam.
5. Berson, S. A., Yalow, R. S., Bauman, A., Rothschild, M. A., and Newerly, K. (1956): Insulin-I^{131} metabolism in human subjects: Demonstration of insulin binding globulin in the circulation of insulin-treated subjects. *J. Clin. Invest.*, 35:170–190.

6. Bodansky, M. (1975): The secretin family and evolution. In: *Gastrointestinal Hormones,* edited by J. C. Thompson, pp. 507–518. University of Texas Press, Austin.

7. Boden, G., Murthy, N. S., and Silver, E. (1975): "Big" secretin. *Clin. Res.,* 23:245A.

8. Bryant, M. G., Polak, J. M., Modlin, I., Bloom, S. R., Albuquerque, R. H., and Pearse, A. G. E. (1976): Possible dual role for vasoactive intestinal peptide as gastrointestinal hormone and neurotransmitter substance. *Lancet,* i:991–993.

9. Dimaline, R., and Dockray, G. J. (1978): Multiple immunoreactive forms of vasoactive intestinal peptide in human colonic mucosa. *Gastroenterology,* 75:387–392.

10. Dockray, G. J. (1977): Immunoreactive component resembling cholecystokinin octapeptide in intestine. *Nature,* 270:359–361.

11. Dockray, G. J., Debas, H. T., Walsh, J. H., and Grossman, M. I. (1975): Molecular forms of gastrin in antral mucosa and serum of dogs. *Proc. Soc. Exp. Biol. Med.,* 149:550–553.

12. Go, V. L. W., Ryan, R. J., and Summerskill, W. H. J. (1971): Radioimmunoassay of porcine cholecystokinin-pancreozymin. *J. Lab. Clin. Med.,* 77:684–689.

13. Gregory, R. A., and Tracy, H. J. (1964): The constitution and properties of two gastrins extracted from hog antral mucosa. I. The isolation of two gastrins from hog antral mucosa. *Gut,* 5:103–114.

14. Gregory, R. A., and Tracy, H. J. (1966): Studies on the chemistry of gastrins I and II. In: *Gastrin,* edited by M. I. Grossman, pp. 9–26. University of California, Los Angeles.

15. Hansky, J., Royle, J. P., and Korman, M. G. (1974): Comparison of bioreactive and immunoreactive gastrin. *Aust. J. Exp. Biol. Med. Sci.,* 841–846.

16. Harvey, R. F., Dowsett, L., Hartog, M., and Read, A. E. (1974): Radioimmunoassay of cholecystokinin-pancreozymin. *Gut,* 690–699.

17. Jordan, P. H., Bianca, S. S., and Yip, M. D. (1972): The presence of gastrin in fasting and stimulated gastric juice of man. *Surgery,* 72:352–356.

18. Larsson, L. I., Fahrenkrug, J., Schaffialitsky de Muckadell, O., Sundler, F., Hakanson, R., and Rehfeld, J. F. (1976): Localization of vasoactive intestinal polypeptide (VIP) to central and peripheral neurones. *Proc. Natl. Acad. Sci. USA,* 73:3197–3200.

19. McGuigan, J. E., and Trudeau, W. L. (1968): Immunochemical measurement of elevated levels of gastrin in the serum of patients with pancreatic tumors of the Zollinger-Ellison variety. *N. Engl. J. Med.,* 278:1308–1313.

20. Morley, J. S. (1971): Gastrin and related peptides. In: *Structure-Activity Relations of Protein and Polypeptide Hormones Part I,* edited by M. Margoulies, and F. C. Greenwood, pp. 11–17. Excerpta Medica, Amsterdam.

21. Muller, J. E., Straus, E., and Yalow, R. S. (1977): Cholecystokinin and its C-terminal octapeptide in the pig brain. *Proc. Natl. Acad. Sci. USA,* 74:3035–3037.

22. Mutt, V., and Jorpes, J. E. (1967): Contemporary developments in the biochemistry of the gastrointestinal hormones. *Recent Prog. Horm. Res.,* 23:483–503.

23. Rayford, P. L., Fender, H. R., Ramus, N. I., Reeder, D. D., and Thompson, J. C. (1975): Release and half-life of CCK in man. In: *Gastrointestinal Hormones,* edited by J. C. Thompson, pp. 301–318. University of Texas Press, Austin.

24. Reeder, D. D., Becker, H. D., Smith, N. J., Rayford, P. L., and Thompson, J. C. (1973): Measurement of endogenous release of cholecystokinin by radioimmunoassay. *Ann. Surg.,* 178:304–310.

25. Rehfeld, J. F. (1978): Immunochemical studies on cholecystokinin. I. Development of sequence-specific radioimmunoassays for porcine triacontratriapeptide cholecystokinin. *J. Biol. Chem.,* 253:4016–4021.

26. Rehfeld, J. F. (1978): Immunochemical studies on cholecystokinin. II. Distribution and molecular heterogeneity in the central nervous system and small intestine of man and hog. *J. Biol. Chem.,* 253:4022–4027.

27. Rehfeld, J. F., Schwartz, T. W., and Stadil, F. (1977): Immunochemical studies on macromolecular gastrins: Evidence that "big big gastrins" are artifacts in blood and mucosa, but truly present in some large gastrinomas. *Gastroenterology,* 73:469–477.

28. Rubin, B., and Engel, S. L. (1973): Some biological characteristics of cholecystokinin (CCK-PZ) and synthetic analogues. In: *Frontiers in Gastrointestinal Hormone Research,* edited by S. Andersson, pp. 41–56. Almqvist and Wiksell, Stockholm, Sweden.

29. Straus, E., Gainer, H., and Yalow, R. S. (1975): Molluscan gastrin: Concentration and molecular forms. *Science,* 190:687–689.

30. Straus, E., Urbach, H-J., and Yalow, R. S. (1975): Comparative reactivities of ^{125}I-secretin and ^{125}I-6-tyrosyl secretin with guinea pig and rabbit anti-secretin sera. *Biochem. Biophys. Res. Commun.*, 64:1036–1040.
31. Straus, E., and Yalow, R. S. (1976): Artifacts in the radioimmunoassay of peptide hormones in gastric and duodenal secretions. *J. Lab. Clin. Med.*, 87:292–298.
32. Straus, E., and Yalow, R. S. (1977): Hypersecretinemia associated with marked basal hyperchlorhydria in man and dog. *Gastroenterology*, 72:992–994.
33. Straus, E., and Yalow, R. S. (1978): Species specificity of cholecystokinin in gut and brain of several mammalian species. *Proc. Natl. Acad. Sci. USA*, 75:486–489.
34. Straus, E., and Yalow, R. S. (1978): Immunoreactive secretin in gastrointestinal mucosa of several mammalian species. *Gastroenterology*, 75:401–404.
35. Walsh, J. H., Debas, H. T., and Grossman, M. I. (1974): Pure human big gastrin. Immunochemical properties, disappearance half time, and acid-stimulating action in dogs. *J. Clin. Invest.*, 54:477–485.
36. Yalow, R. S. (1973): Radioimmunoassay: Practices and pitfalls. *Circ. Res.*, 32:I116–I126.
37. Yalow, R. S., and Berson, S. A. (1960): Immunoassay of endogenous plasma insulin in man. *J. Clin. Invest.*, 39:1157–1175.
38. Yalow, R. S., and Berson, S. A. (1961): Immunologic aspects of insulin. *Am. J. Med.*, 31:882–891.
39. Yalow, R. S., and Berson, S. A. (1970): General aspects of radioimmunoassay procedures. In: *"In Vitro" Procedures with Radioisotopes in Medicine*, pp. 455–479. IAEA-SM-124/106, Vienna, Austria.
40. Yalow, R. S., and Berson, S. A. (1970): Radioimmunoassay of gastrin. *Gastroenterology*, 58:1–14.
41. Yalow, R. S., and Berson, S. A. (1970): Size and charge distinctions between endogenous human plasma gastrin in peripheral blood and heptadecapeptide gastrins. *Gastroenterology*, 58:609–615.
42. Yalow, R. S., and Berson, S. A. (1971): Further studies on the nature of immunoreactive gastrin in human plasma. *Gastroenterology*, 60:203–214.
43. Yalow, R. S., and Berson, S. A. (1971): Problems of validation of radioimmunoassays. In: *Principles of Competitive Protein-Binding Assays*, edited by W. D. Odell, and W. H. Daughaday, pp. 374–400. J. B. Lippincott, Philadelphia and Toronto.
44. Yalow, R. S., and Berson, S. A. (1971): Immunochemical specificity of gastrin-antibody reactions. In: *Structure-Activity Relations of Protein and Polypeptide Hormones Part I*, edited by M. Margoulies, and F. C. Greenwood, pp. 48–56. Excerpta Medica, Amsterdam.
45. Yalow, R. S., and Berson, S. A. (1972): And now, "big, big" gastrin. *Biochem. Biophys. Res. Commun.*, 48:391–395.
46. Yalow, R. S., and Straus, E. (1977): Heterogeneity of gastrointestinal hormones. In: *Hormonal Receptors in Digestive Tract Physiology*, edited by S. Bonfils, P. Fromageot, and G. Rosselin, pp. 79–93. Elsevier North Holland Biomedical Press, Amsterdam.
47. Yalow, R. S., and Wu, N. (1973): Additional studies on the nature of big big gastrin. *Gastroenterology*, 65:19–27, 1973.
48. Young, J. D., Lazarus, I., and Chisholm, D. J. (1969): Radioimmunoassay of pancreozymin cholecystokinin in human serum. *J. Nucl. Med.*, 10:743–745.

Gastrointestinal Hormones, edited by
George B. Jerzy Glass.
Raven Press, New York © 1980.

Chapter 33

Radioimmunoassay of Gastrin

*Grace L. Rosenquist and **John H. Walsh

*Department of Animal Physiology, University of California, Davis 95616; and
**Department of Medicine, University of California, Los Angeles, 90024

INTRODUCTION

Other chapters in this volume deal with the cellular origins, structure, and function of the gastrin peptides as well as the molecular heterogeneity of this

---

Abbreviations for peptides: G-17, little gastrin, assumed to be of human origin unless defined by an appropriate abbreviation preceding G as a lower case letter, e.g., pG-17; pG-17, nonsulfated porcine G-17; hG-17, nonsulfated human gastrin; hG-17s, sulfated hG-17; 15-leu-hG-17, hG-17 with leucine substituted in the 15th position; des-G-17, desamido G-17; G-14, minigastrin containing 14 residues; G-34, big gastrin containing 34 residues; G-16, hexadecapeptide of gastrin, the first 16 residues counting from the carboxyl terminus. All gastrin peptides are assumed to be nonsulfated unless "s" is added after the number of the residues.

CCK-8, carboxy terminal octapeptide of cholecystokinin (sulfated); CCK-8ns, non-sulfated CCK-8; CCK-33, cholecystokinin containing 33 residues; CCK-39, cholecystokinin containing 39 resides. All CCK peptides are assumed to be sulfated unless "ns" is added after the number of residues.

family of peptides. It has been pointed out that the major pathological disorder attributed to the secretion of gastrin is caused by excessive gastric acid secretion in the gastrinoma syndrome. Most of the information concerning the physiology and pathophysiology of gastrin has been obtained by use of radioimmunoassay (RIA) techniques. We will review the theoretical and practical considerations in performance of gastrin RIA and present some of the varied approaches in production of antibodies to gastrin, purification of labeled gastrin, and separation of antibody-bound from free labeled gastrin. In addition, we will point out some uses of region-specific antibodies in analysis of the various molecular forms of gastrin.

RADIOIMMUNOASSAY PROCEDURE

Composition of Gastrin and Related Peptides

Gastrin shares a common carboxy-terminal pentapeptide amide with cholecystokinin (CCK) and for this reason must be considered part of the same family of peptides. The presence of both this shared pentapeptide in the biologically active part of the molecule and a sulfated tyrosine supports the concept that gastrin and CCK evolved from a common ancestral gene. Recent evidence indicating a sulfated, CCK-like peptide in intestinal and brain extracts of lamprey, a representative of the oldest group of vertebrates, suggests that CCK peptide may be the more primitive form (28). Intuitively, one might expect a molecule that controls acid release to have evolved later than one that stimulates enzyme release. The structure-activity relationships of these peptides is covered by G. Nilsson in Chapter 6, pp. 127–168, *this volume*. However, the sequences and a short description are included here to aid in understanding the discussions of antibody specificity and gastrin standards. A new system of nomenclature will be used throughout this chapter (16).

Gastrin exists in peptides of differing chain lengths and each molecular size can either exist with the single tyrosine residue sulfated or unsulfated (See Table 1). The well-characterized gastrin peptides range in size from 34 residues down to 14 residues, with the principal activity found in peptides of 17 (G-17) and 34 (G-34) residues. Two larger forms—big, big gastrin (60) and component I (43)—have been identified by immunoreactivity, but have not been purified and sequenced. The sequence differences observed among the mammalian G-34 and G-17 peptides are found in the nonbiologically active part of the molecules and represent single base changes in the DNA.

The CCK peptides found in the intestine include peptides ranging in size from 39 and 33 to 8 residues (11,37,38,41). There is evidence for differences in structure among larger forms of CCK from different species of mammals (51). The octapeptide, which is found in the intestine as well as the brain, is the form with the highest immunoreactivity. Although not nearly as biologically active as the octapeptide, the C-terminal tetrapeptide shared by both gastrin

TABLE 1. Amino acid sequence of gastrin peptides

Residue Number — two numbering systems are shown: superscript [a] = residue numbers using G-34 as the reference peptide (positions 1–34); superscript [b] = numbers using G-17 as the reference peptide (positions 1–17 over residues 18–34).

Metadata and reference sequence (hG-34 is the reference; "—" = residue identical to reference; blank = residue absent):

Name	New Notation	Reference	Source	M.W.
Big gastrin I	hG-34	(25)	Human	3839
	pG-34	(12,25)	Hog	3883
Little gastrin	hG-17	(8)	Human	2098
	pG-17	(22)	Hog	2116
	pG-17	(1)	Cow (Sheep)	2026
		(2)	Dog	2058
		(3)	Cat	2040
Mini gastrin	hG-14	(24)	Human	1647
1-13 NTF[c] of G-17		(23)	Hog	1538
Gastrin fragments and other peptides for evaluating gastrin antibodies				
C[d] term-tetrapeptide	G-4			597
Pentagastrin				769

Residue numbers (G-34): 1[a] 2 3 4 5 6 7 8 9 10 11 12 13 14 15 16 17 | 18 19 20 21 22 23 24 25 26 27 28 29 30 31 32 33 34
Residue numbers (G-17): (— over 1–17) | 1[b] 2 3 4 5 6 7 8 9 10 11 12 13 14 15 16 17

Reference sequence, hG-34:
1 Pca[f], 2 Leu, 3 Gly, 4 Pro, 5 Gln, 6 Gly, 7 (His, 8 Pro, 9 Ser)[g], 10 Leu, 11 Val, 12 Ala, 13 Asp, 14 Pro, 15 Ser, 16 Lys, 17 Lys, 18 Gln, 19 Gly, 20 Pro, 21 Trp, 22 Leu, 23 Glu, 24 Glu, 25 Glu, 26 Glu, 27 Glu, 28 Ala, 29 Tyr[h], 30 Gly, 31 Trp, 32 Met, 33 Asp, 34 Phe-NH2

Differences from reference by peptide:
- pG-34 (Hog): residues 7–9 shown as (His Pro Pro)[g]; residue 22 = Met.
- hG-17 (Human): residue 18 = Pca; C-terminal 17 residues only (18–34).
- pG-17 (Hog): residue 18 = Pca; residue 22 = Met.
- pG-17 (Cow/Sheep): residue 18 = Pca; residue 22 = Met; substitution = Val; substitution = Ala.
- Dog: residue 18 = Pca; substitutions = Ala, Ala.
- Cat: residue 18 = Pca; residue 22 = Met; substitution = Ala.
- hG-14 (Human): C-terminal 14 residues (residues 21–34 / G-17 positions 4–17).
- 1-13 NTF[c] of G-17 (Hog): N-terminal residues 18–30 (G-17 positions 1–13); residue 22 = Met.
- G-4 (C-terminal tetrapeptide): residues 31–34 (Trp-Met-Asp-Phe-NH2).
- Pentagastrin: tBOC[e]-Ala at residue 30 (G-17 position 13), then residues 31–34 (Trp-Met-Asp-Phe-NH2).

[a] Residue numbers using G-34 as the reference peptide.
[b] Numbers using G-17 as the reference peptide.
[c] NTF, N-terminal fragment.
[d] carboxy terminal.
[e] t-Boc, tertiary butyloxycarbonyl.
[f] Pyrrolidone carboxylic acid.
[g] Sequences for residues 7, 8, and 9 for hG-34 and pG-34 are under study (12).
[h] Tyrosine in this position can be sulfated in G-34, G-17, and G-14.
New notation for sulfated peptides—G-34s, G-17s, and G-14s.

TABLE 1A. Amino acid sequences of cholecystokinin and related peptides

Name	Reference	Source	1	2	3	4	5	6	7	8	9	10	11	12	13	14	15	16	17	18	19	20	21	22	23	24	25	26	27	28	29	30	31	32	33	34	35	36	37	38	39
(New notations)																																									
Cholecystokinin -variant (CCK-39)	(37)	hog	Tyr	Ile	Gln	Gln	Ala	Arg	Lys	Ala	Pro	Ser	Gly	Arg	Val	Ser	Met	Ile	Lys	Asn	Leu	Gln	Ser	Leu	Asp	Pro	Ser	His	Arg	Ile	Ser	Asp	Arg	Asp	Tyr^{HSO3}	Met	Gly	Trp	Met	Asp	Phe-NH$_2$
Cholecystokinin (CCK-33)	(38)	hog							—	—	—	—	—	—	—	—	—	—	—	—	—	—	—	—	—	—	—	—	—	—	—	—	—	—	—	—	—	—	—	—	—
Cholecystokinin octapeptide (CCK-8)	(13)																																—	—	—	—	—	—	—	—
Caerulein	(4)	Hyla cerulea																														Pca	Gln	—	—	Thr	—	—	—	—	—

and CCK has been tentatively identified in the intestine (41). Other CCK peptides, now observed only as chromatographic peaks identified by immunoreactivity, still need to be purified, sequenced, and assayed for biological activity (11,41).

Immunization of Animals

Various immunogens have been used to produce gastrin antibodies, including partially purified gastrin (20,44,58) partially purified gastrin conjugated to bovine serum albumin (14,45,62), or synthetic gastrin and gastrin fragments conjugated to bovine serum albumin (34,44). A summary of immunization methods with schedule of injections and proportion of responders is found in Table 2.

On the basis of the results presented in Table 2, as well as our own experience, we would recommend using 50 to 200 μg gastrin conjugated to bovine serum albumin (approximately 75–400 μg) injected into rabbits. The antigen is injected into the back at multiple intradermal sites at intervals of 6 weeks to 3 months. This schedule conserves antigen and usually produces antibodies in 2 to 4 months. For preparation of the immunogen, we conjugate 1 mg of G-17 or G-16. Either gastrin can be used since the linkage occurs either at the free amino of G-16 or through the carboxyl side chains of aspartic or glutamic acids. Use of G-17 has the advantage that some rabbits may develop antibodies specific for the N-terminal sequence of G-17. Such antibodies are useful in distinguishing between the heptadecapeptide and other molecular forms. Gastrin is dissolved in 1 ml 0.05 M ammonium bicarbonate and mixed with 1.5 mg crystalline bovine serum albumin and 10 mg carbodiimide (ECDI, N-ethyl-N' -(3 dimethylaminopropyl) carbodiimide), each in 1.5 ml 0.05 M sodium phosphate, pH 7.0. This mixture is stirred for 4 to 6 hr at room temperature, then dialyzed at 4°C in 0.15 M NaCl, 0.01 M phosphate, pH 7.4 (PBS) for 48 to 72 hr prior to injection. The degree of conjugation of the gastrin and albumin can be estimated by the inclusion of a trace amount of ^{125}I gastrin in the reaction mixture. Efficiency of conjugation also can be estimated by measurement of absorbance at 280 nm of the conjugate before and after dialysis and calculation of the unbound, dialyzable gastrin from the molar extinction coefficient of gastrin.

For immunization, the conjugate is diluted in phosphate buffered saline (PBS) so that the amount to be injected is contained in 1 ml. The antigen is emulsified with an equal amount of Freund's adjuvant and injected into 20 to 40 intradermal sites into the shaved area of a rabbit back. Complete Freund's adjuvant is used for the first and second immunizations. Incomplete Freund's adjuvant can be substituted in later immunizations to decrease the local inflammatory response. Pertussis toxoid also may be injected intramuscularly with the first immunization. The rabbits are bled by the ear artery or vein 4 weeks after the original injection and then checked every 1 to 2 weeks after the original or booster injections for the presence of antibodies. Immunizations are performed every 6 to 12 weeks until antibody is detected. The interval may then be increased until antibody titers have decreased substantially. Antibodies may be detected

TABLE 2. *Immunization methods*

Animal	Antigen	Dose	Adjuvant	Site of injection	Interval between injections/injection schedule	Proportion of responders
Rabbit (34)	hG-16–BSA	8 moles hG-16 per mole BSA, 400μg of gastrin, 2 mg of conjugate	CFA	Footpads	2–3 month interval	3/3
Rabbit (44)	hG-16–BSA	4–8 moles hG-16 per mole BSA, 1 mg as hG-16, 4–7 mg BSA	CFA, then IFA for subsequent injections	Footpads	85 days	10/10 by 6 mos.
Rabbit (44)	hG-17–BSA	4–8 moles hG-17 per mole BSA, 1 mg as hG-17, 4–7 mg BSA	CFA, then IFA for subsequent injections	Footpads	85 days	6/6 by approx. 6 mos.
Rabbit (32)	hG-17–BSA	50 μg hG-17	CFA	Multiple intradermal sites in back	2–3 months	6/6 in 3–4 mos.
Rabbit (19)	Crude porcine gastrin	100–300 μg porcine gastrin	CFA	Sub Q (no location cited)	4 times with 10–14 day intervals, 6 week intervals for 3 months	7/14 in 6 mos.
Guinea pig (58)	Crude porcine gastrin	300 μg porcine gastrin	CFA	Sub Q in inner thigh	2 weeks, 1 month, up to 3 months	1/3 to 1/2 in approx. 4 mos.
Guinea pig (19)	Crude porcine gastrin	100–300 μg porcine gastrin	CFA	Sub Q (no location cited)	4 times with 10–14 day intervals; 6 week intervals for 3 months	6/14 in 6 mos.
Guinea pig (44)	Crude porcine gastrin	Approx. 300 μg porcine gastrin	CFA	Sub Q in inner thigh	30–85 days	1/20 after 4th dose
Guinea pig (46)	Crude porcine gastrin	1mg crude = 130 μg pG-17 by immunoreactivity	CFA	Sub Q in axilla and inguinal areas	5 times in 2.5 months, then monthly	3/9 in 2 mos.
Guinea pig (46)	Crude porcine gastrin conjugated to BSA	Approx. 200 μg pG-17, 2 mg BSA	CFA, then IFA for subsequent injections	Sub Q axilla and inguinal areas	monthly	3/3 in 2–3 mos.

BSA, bovine serum albumin; CFA, complete Freund's adjuvant; IFA, incomplete Freund's adjuvant; Sub Q, subcutaneous

in some rabbits in 1 to 2 months; nearly 100% of the animals respond after 3 months.

Preparation of Labeled Gastrin

Iodination of Gastrin

All iodination methods described in Table 3 are modifications of the chloramine T method of Hunter and Greenwood (30). In our version of the general method, the reagents are added in the following order to a small glass tube: 50 μl of 0.25 M phosphate, pH 7.4, 25 μl of 40 nmoles/ml (or about 2 μg) of hG-17 or pG-17, 10 μl of sodium ^{125}I iodide, 100 mCi/ml (in NaOH) and 10 μl of chloramine T in 0.25 M phosphate, pH 7.4. The reaction is terminated in 15 sec by the addition of 20 μl of sodium metabisulfite, 5 mg/ml in phosphate buffer. This method produces G-17 with a specific activity of greater than 500 mCi/mg. To obtain this specific activity it might be necessary to vary the amount of chloramine T, which is a strong oxidizing agent and changes its potency after prolonged shelf storage. Chloramine T can result in loss of antigenic determinants (33) by oxidizing methionine and tryptophan (5). Although this oxidation is not an apparent problem in gastrin RIA, interesting and potentially useful antibodies that do not react with the oxidized form of these residues may be missed. The use of 15-leu-G-17, which has no methionine in the critical position, may increase the stability of labeled peptide (6).

Purification of Label

Isolation of suitably labeled gastrin has been performed by gel filtration in Sephadex G-10 (34), by starch gel electrophoresis (58), and by ion-exchange chromatography (49). The method of choice is the ion-exchange method, which gives a good separation of mono- and diiodo forms of gastrins with specific activities higher than with the other methods.

In our version of the ion-exchange technique, a preliminary gel filtration step separates gastrin from free iodide and other reactants of smaller molecular size. The gastrins (unlabeled, mono- and diiodinated) are then purified on either amino-ethylcellulose (AE-41, Whatman) (Fig. 1) or DEAE-Sephadex A-25. In the gel filtration, the reaction mixture is diluted with 400 μl 0.25 M phosphate buffer, pH 7.4 and then separated on a 1.0 $\times$ 10 cm column with 0.025 M ammonium bicarbonate containing 0.2 ml plasma protein. The void volume, containing labeled gastrin, is then purified on either AE-41 or DEAE Sephadex columns.

The AE-41 is prepared according to the manufacturer's instructions. The exchanger is cycled four times, alternating between 1 liter of water and 500 ml of 0.5 M NaOH, ending with 1 liter of water (four times). After the pH is adjusted to pH 6.0 with 1 M HCl, the exchanger is washed four more times

TABLE 3. *Preparation and purification of iodinated gastrin*

Purification method	Gastrin type	Isotope	Reactants	Purification of iodinated gastrin	Specific activity	Reference
Sephadex G-10	hG-17 or G-16	[125]I	Buffer system: 0.5 M postassium phosphate pH 7.0 Reaction volume: approx. 110 μl 1–2 μg hormone in 100 μl 0.5 M potassium phosphate pH 7.0 1,000 μCi [125]I 35 μg chloramine T in 10 μl of 0.5 M potassium phosphate pH 7.0 Reaction stopped by addition of 250 μg sodium metabisulfite in 100 μl of 0.5 M potassium phosphate pH 7.0.	Chromatography on Sephadex G-10 column (2.0 × 35 cm) in 0.5 M potassium phosphate pH 7.4	100–325 mCi/mg	(35)
Starch gel electrophoresis	pG-17	[125]I	Buffer system: phosphate buffer pH 7.4 Reaction volume: not stated 20 μl of phosphate buffer, pH 7.4 200–500 μCi of [125]I 0.5–1.0 μg of hormone, 52.2 μg chloramine T in 15 μl buffer Reaction stopped by addition of 96 μg sodium metabisulfite in 20 μl Plasma (20 μl) was added.	Starch gel electrophoresis at a constant voltage, 200–250v or 15–30 mA for 4–6 hr. Fractions (0.5 cm sections) are frozen, then eluted with 1–2 ml of 0.15 M NaCl	Not stated	(58)
AE-cellulose	hG-17	[125]I	Buffer system: 0.05 M phosphate, pH 7.5 Reaction volume: 30 μl 200 μCi of [125]I 5 μg of hormone 5 μg of chloramine T 26 nmoles of sodium metabisulfite in 25 μl Dilute with 500 μl 0.05 M NH₄H CO₃	Chromatography on AE-41 cellulose column (0.9 × 15 cm). Linear gradient from 0.05 to 0.4 M ammonium bicarbonate	350 mCi/mg	(49)
DEAE-Sephadex	hG-17	[125]I	Buffer system: 0.25 M sodium phosphate pH 7.4 Reaction volume: 165 μl 2,500 μCi [125]I 3 μg hormone 30 μg chloramine T Reaction stopped by addition of 100 μg sodium metabisulfite	Chromatography 1st on Sephadex G-10 column equilibrated with 0.05 M imidazole buffer pH 7.5, followed by separation on DEAE-Sephadex column (0.9 cm × 15 cm) equilibrated with imidazole buffer. Elution by linear sodium chloride gradient. (0 to 1.0 M)	Not stated	(10)
DEAE-Sephadex	hG-17	[125]I	Buffer system: 0.25 M sodium phosphate, pH 7.4 Reaction volume: 100 μl 1,000 μCi [125]I 1 μg natural hG-17 20 μg chloramine T Reaction stopped by addition of 100 μg sodium metabisulfite	Chromatography first on Sephadex G-10 column equilibrated with 0.02 M ammonium bicarbonate, followed by separation on DEAE-Sephadex column (1 × 10 cm). Linear gradient from 0.08 to 0.98 M NaCl	> 500 mCi/mg	(32)

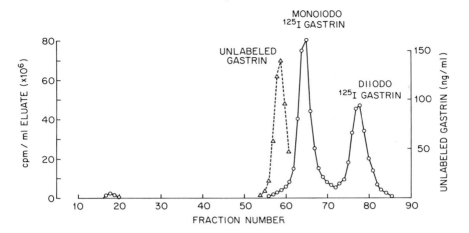

FIG. 1. Elution pattern of labeled gastrin from AE-41 ion exchange column after preliminary purification on Sephadex G-10. Conditions are given in text.

with 1 liter of water and then with 0.5 M ammonium bicarbonate. The material is kept in 0.5 M ammonium bicarbonate at 4°C with a few drops of toluene to prevent contamination. For the fractionation of gastrin, a 1.0×10 cm column is packed and equilibrated with 0.05 M ammonium bicarbonate, pH 8.0. Iodinated gastrin is eluted with a linear gradient from 0.05 to 0.5 M ammonium bicarbonate, and collected in 1-ml aliquots at a flow rate of 8 ml/hr.

Sephadex anion exchanger (DEAE-Sephadex A-25) can be substituted for the AE-41, which is difficult to obtain. The conditions are similar to those used for the AE-41 fractionation except for the following modifications: The Sephadex is suspended and stored in 1.7 M ammonium bicarbonate; the starting buffer is 0.02 M ammonium bicarbonate with 0.08 M NaCl added; after extensive washing with starting buffer, the sample is applied and the gastrins are eluted with a linear gradient by adding 0.02 M ammonium bicarbonate plus 0.98 M NaCl to a 50-ml mixing vessel containing the starting buffer.

Peaks 1 and 2 from both the AE-41 and the DEAE-Sephadex columns are composed of monoiodinated and diiodinated gastrin, respectively (see Fig. 1). The specific activity of fractions from peak 2 should be twice that of fractions from peak 1.

Evaluation of Labeled Gastrin (Label)

Gastrin label should be >80% bound in antibody excess and have nonspecific binding (control) not greater than 10%, preferably less than 5%. Specific activity, a measure of counts per minute (cpm or counts) per unit weight, will affect the sensitivity of the RIA. High specific activity is required for high affinity antibodies.

Nonspecific binding and maximum binding are determined by incubating approximately 2,000 cpm of a fraction containing maximum cpm/ml fraction (peak fraction) of labeled gastrin in triplicate sets of assay tubes. The control tubes contain no antibody; tubes for determining maximum binding contain 10 to 1,000 times more antibody than is necessary to bind 50% of the labeled gastrin. After an overnight incubation, free gastrin is separated from gastrin bound to antibody as described in a later section. Satisfactory binding is greater than 80% in the peak fractions. Suitable fractions are pooled, aliquoted, and frozen so that each aliquot contains enough labeled gastrin for a single assay. Nonspecific binding can be checked with each assay. Maximum binding should be evaluated periodically as an indication of the integrity of the label.

Pure monoiodinated peptide has the same specific activity as the iodide, 15 mCi/μg iodide or 4.16×10^3 dpm/fmole; diiodinated peptide has twice the specific activity, or 8.32×10^3 dpm/fmole. In a gamma counter with 60% efficiency, monoiodinated peptide has a specific activity of 2,500 cpm/fmole and diiodinated peptide has a specific activity of 5,000 cpm/fmole. In the case of gastrin, 1 pg monoiodinated gastrin produces 1,200 cpm, which is equivalent to 900 mCi/mg gastrin.

Specific activity can be estimated empirically by RIA if it can be shown that labeled and unlabeled peptide produce parallel and equivalent displacement of peptide from antibody. For most gastrin antibodies this condition holds true. To determine specific activity by RIA, a dilution of antibody is chosen that produces a bound/free ratio (B/F) of approximately 1.0 with tracer amounts of labeled peptide of approximately 1,000 cpm/2 ml incubation mixture (Fig. 2). B/F is the ratio of cpm associated with labeled gastrin bound to antibody divided by cpm associated with free labeled gastrin. Two types of inhibition curves then are constructed. In one type of curve unlabeled G-17 is added in graded increments to determine the concentration of gastrin that produces 50% inhibition of the initial B/F (ID_{50}). In the other type of curve (Peak 1 and Peak 2), doubling increments of labeled gastrin are added over the range from 1,000 to 32,000 cpm per 2 ml incubation volume. The ID_{50} for labeled gastrin is determined as the cpm/ml that produces 50% inhibition. From these two numbers the specific activity can be calculated simply as the ratio of ID_{50}s for labeled/unlabeled gastrin and expressed as cpm/fmole.

Incubation Procedure

All samples and standards are diluted in 0.02 M veronal or Tris buffers (pH 8.2–8.6) if the assay involves separation with an ion-exchange resin. The buffer should contain 0.02 to 2% albumin, normal rabbit serum, or human serum to minimize absorption of antibody and gastrin peptides to glass.

Standards and serum samples or other unknowns are diluted to contribute

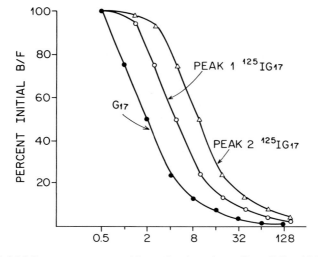

FIG. 2. Autoinhibition curves prepared for estimation of specific activity of labeled gastrin.

a volume of 1 ml to the reaction mixture. Standard curves are prepared first by diluting the standards to contain 1,000, 100, 10 fmoles/ml. Each of these standards is pipetted in amounts of 200 μl, 100 μl, 50 μl, and 20 μl, producing 10 different concentrations with two points of overlap. Buffer is added to bring up the volume to 1 ml. For assays of serum specimens it may be desirable to add gastrin-free serum to the standard samples so as to correct for nonspecific interference by serum protein. Gastrin-free serum can be prepared by affinity chromatography. Aliquots of unknown serum samples, 200 μl and 20 μl, are diluted to 1 ml with standard buffer to give a final concentration of 1/10 and 1/100 in the reaction mixture.

Labeled gastrin and antibody are then added to each tube to give a final 2-ml incubation volume. To each assay tube labeled gastrin is added, approximately 2,000 cpm, plus diluted antibody (predetermined to bind 50% of the labeled gastrin). The non-specific binding controls contain the diluted label and standard buffer instead of antibody. After mixing with a vortex mixer, the tubes are covered and incubated at 4°C for 1 to 3 days. The most reproducible results are obtained when the assays are incubated until equilibrium is reached. Equilibrium is the point at which further incubation does not increase binding of label to antibody.

Premixing of label and antibody before addition to the tube can save some time. However, with some antibodies a portion of the labeled gastrin cannot be displaced even when extreme excesses of unlabeled gastrin are added. With these antibodies, premixing of antibody and labeled gastrin produces an unreliable assay.

Separation of Free Gastrin from Gastrin Bound to Antibody

Several different reagents have been used to separate bound and free gastrin (see Table 4). Of these the following are used: double antibody (20,34); charcoal (26,48); anion exchange resin (58); immune adsorbent (42); polyethylene glycol (42), and ammonium sulfate (40). We routinely use the anion-exchange method of Yalow and Berson (58).

Amberlite IRP-58M (Rohm and Haas) is prepared by mixing 10 g resin with 100 ml standard buffer and stirring gently for 1 hr just prior to the separation procedure. The separation technique requires a similar amount of total protein in each assay tube. Two-tenths ml of resin is transferred to each tube from a container that is continuously stirred to maintain a well-mixed suspension. After the resin has been added the contents of each tube are mixed with a vortex mixer and then centrifuged in a refrigerated centrifuge. After centrifugation, the supernatant fluid is carefully poured into another tube. Both the pellet containing the free gastrin and the supernate containing the antibody-bound gastrin are counted in a scintillation counter.

The advantage of the anion-exchange method is the speed of the operation. Rapid processing is desirable because resin may compete with antibody for free gastrin and prolonged standing (more than 30–45 min) may change the equilibrium. The resin separation technique can be performed on either serum or nonheparanized plasma samples. Since heparin probably competes for resin binding sites and therefore leads to high nonspecific binding, it should not be used in the preparation of plasma samples.

EVALUATION OF RADIOIMMUNOASSAY DATA

Development and Use of the Standard Curve

Counts of labeled gastrin bound to antibody should be corrected for nonspecific binding. B/F ratios or percent labeled gastrin bound are calculated and plotted on the ordinate, with the log concentration of gastrin standards plotted on the abscissa (see Fig. 4). Although the concentration of gastrin is often expressed in pg/ml, a more useful expression is fmoles/ml, which allows easy comparison of concentrations of the various molecular forms.

The amount of gastrin in a sample containing an unknown amount of the hormone is determined by finding the concentration of gastrin standard that produces the same B/F or bound. The sample may need to be diluted so that its B/F falls in the linear portion of the standard curve. The concentration of gastrin in the tube must be corrected for this dilution of the sample to obtain the concentration in the original sample.

The sensitivity of the RIA should be evaluated by determining the detection limit and the ID_{50}. The ID_{50} is the concentration of unlabeled peptide that decreases binding from B/F of 1.0 to 0.5. In antibodies with affinity constants

TABLE 4. *Incubation and separation procedures*

Assay	Description of method	Volume	Buffer	Label	Incubation		Comments and references
					Temperature	Time	
Double antibody	Precipitation of antigen (hormone)—antibody complexes with second antibody. After centrifugation, supernates contain free antigens.	0.5 ml 1st incubation 0.7 ml 2nd incubation	0.01 M Phosphate 0.15 M NaCl, pH 7.4	hG-17	1st-4°C 2nd-4°C	48–72 hr 24 hr	Second antibody is added before the second incubation. Care must be taken to ensure enough globulin (e.g., 10 μg Cohn Fraction II) and second antibody are present to obtain complete precipitation of antigen-antibody complexes. Serum should be heat inactivated; EDTA should be included in reaction mixture (20,31,34,35).
Charcoal[a]	Adsorption of free antigen to charcoal; centrifugation; supernates contain antigen bound to antibody.	1 ml	0.1 M Phosphate, pH 7.5 2 mg BSA/ml	hG-17	4°C	48–72 hr	Uniform protein concentration required in all tubes. No difference in results between coated and uncoated charcoal but coated charcoal easier to handle (21,26,39,48,50).
Resin[b]	Adsorption of free antigen to resin. After centrifugation, supernates contain antigen bound to antibody.	2.0–2.5 ml	0.02 M Veranol, pH 8.4 2.5 mg/ml HSA or 2% Plasmatein[e]	pG-17 hG-17	4°C	2–5 days	Incubation time should be checked with each antibody to ensure equilibrium has been reached. pH optimum of incubation mixture between 8 and 8.5 (50,53,58,36).
Immune adsorbent[c]	Antibody bound to insoluble support; centrifugation; supernates contain free antigen.	2.5 ml	0.02 M Veranol, pH 8.4 2 mg BSA/ml	hG-17	20°C	3 days	Sepharose 4B[c]; Sephadex G-25[c]; or microcrystalline cellulose are supports to which antibody can be bound by cyanogen bromide (9,50).
Polyethylene glycol (PEG)[d]	Precipitation of antigen-antibody complexes with PEG; centrifugation and decantation of precipate; supernates contain free antigen.	2.5 ml	0.02 M Veranol, pH 8.4 2 mg BSA/ml	hG-17	4°C	2 days	Uniform protein concentration required in all tubes (50).
Saturated ammonium sulfate (SAS)	Precipitation of antigen-antibody complexes with SAS; centrifugation and decantation of precipitate; supernates contain free antigen.	1.0 ml	0.02 M Tris, pH 8.4 2.5 mg BSA/ml in 1% normal rabbit serum.	hG-17	4°C	2 days	All tubes should have the same amount of serum or globulin carrier. Tubes are incubated for 30 min at 4°C after addition of 1 ml SAS. SAS is prepared to be saturated at 4°C (40).

[a] Norit A—Neutral Pharmaceutical Grade, Amend Drug and Chemical Co., Irvington, New York.
[b] CG-4B or IRP-58M Amberlite resin from Rohm and Haas, Philadelphia, Pennsylvania; British Drug House, Ltd., Poole, England; Serva, Heidelberg, W. Germany.
[c] Sepharose-4B and G-25 from Pharmacia Fine Chemicals, Piscataway, New York, and micro crystalline cellulose from E. Merck. Ag, Darmstadt, Germany.
[d] Polyethylene glycol—6000 Carbowax from Union Carbide, Norden, AB, Copenhagen, Denmark; Long Beach, California.
[e] Plasmatein from Hyland Laboratories, Costa Mesa, California.

of approximately 10^{11} liters/mole the detection limit is less than 1 pg (0.5 fmole), whereas the ID_{50} for hG-17 is between 2 and 10 pg/ml (1–5 fmoles/ml).

Precision, as expressed as the coefficient of variation of multiple gastrin determinations, should be established both within and between assays (50). The coefficient of variation is equal to the standard deviation divided by the mean gastrin concentration. The accuracy of the assay is determined by the detection of a known amount of gastrin added to serum (recovery).

The semi-log plotting of the assay data results in a nearly linear curve, which allows for linear regression analysis. However, the linearity is extended to include the lower gastrin concentrations (less than 1 fmole/ml) when two other sources of gastrin in the incubation mixture are taken into consideration. The first source is the labeled gastrin added to the incubation. If pure monoiodinated gastrin is employed, 2,500 cpm added to a 2 ml incubation volume is equivalent to approximately 0.5 fmoles/ml gastrin. The second source is gastrin prebound to antibody that is used in the RIA. When high titer antibody is treated with boiling water to liberate prebound gastrin, we have found that many antibodies already have bound up to several hundred ng/ml of endogenous (rabbit) gastrin per milliliter of undiluted serum. If corrections are made for the final dilution of antibody in the RIA, the endogenous prebound gastrin represents a final concentration of 0.1 to 2.0 fmoles/ml. Thus every assay tube contains 0.6 to 2.5 fmoles/ml gastrin before any standard gastrin is added. This probably explains some of the difficulties in constructing sensitive standard curves for concentrations of gastrin less than fmole/ml, even with antibodies with affinity constants as high as 10^{12} M^{-1}.

Standardization

The gastrin RIA should be standardized with gastrin solutions of known concentration and potency. Standards of hG-17s, hG-17, and hG-34 and G-14 are available from the Center for Ulcer Research and Education, Los Angeles, California. Porcine G-17s and hG-17 are available from the Medical Research Council, England. Gastrin peptides are available from the following sources: hG-17 from Boehringer Mannheim, Indianapolis, Indiana; CCK-8ns from Peninsula Laboratories, San Carlos, California; hG-17 and 15-leu-hG-17 from Research Plus, Denville, New Jersey.

Concentrations of the gastrin peptides can be determined by measuring the absorbance at 280 nm and using the appropriate extinction coefficients (see Table 5). Optimally, a measure of biological activity would be sought, but usually immunoreactivity and biological activity correlate quite well. Several standards may be used with each assay to guard against mistakes in dilution or losses of immunologic reactivity of a single standard.

Gastrin peptides should be stored frozen at $-40°C$ or colder. Since gastrin will not stay in solution at low pH, the pH of solutions should be approximately

TABLE 5. *Extinction coefficients and conversion factors*

Peptide	Molecular weight	ϵ^a	Factor $(\mu g/ml)^b$	Factor $(nmoles/ml)^c$
hG-34	3,839	12,261	313	81.6
hG-34s	3,919	10,754	364	93.0
hG-17	2,098	12,261	171	81.6
hG-17s	2,178	10,754	203	93.0
des-hG-17	2,099	12,261	171	81.6
hG-14	1,833	12,261	149	81.6
hG-14s	1,913	10,754	178	93.0
G-4	597	5,377	111	186.0
pCCK-39	4,678	6,884	679	145.3
pCCK-33	3,918	5,377	729	186.0
CCK-8	1,143	5,377	213	186.0
CCK-8ns	1,063	6,884	154	145.3
Caerulein	1,352	5,377	251	186.0

[a] Molar extinction coefficient at 280 nm based on: Trp 5377 molar^{-1} cm^{-1}; Tyr 1507 molar^{-1} cm^{-1}; SO$_3$H-Tyr nil.

[b] Factor $(\mu g/ml) = (M.W./\epsilon) \times 10^3$.

[b,c] Multiply absorbance at 280 nm by factor to get μg/ml or nmoles/ml.

[c] Factor $(nmoles/ml) = 10^6/\epsilon$.

8. We maintain standards from 3 to 10 ng/ml and dilute these for each assay. These standards should be compared with standards not routinely used to check for their stability.

Additionally, for measurement of serum gastrin, the antibody used should have equal reactivity on a molar basis with the major biological forms of gastrin, hG-17, hG-17s, G-34, G-34s, and the slopes of these standard curves should be parallel to those produced by diluted serum from patients with elevated gastrin levels. Additionally, serum gastrin values for normal patients should be compared with values from other laboratories.

Antibody Evaluation

Unlike other reagents which are expected to be homogeneous in the RIA system, antibodies are heterogeneous with respect to affinity, specificity, and concentration. This heterogeneity makes antibody exquisitely versatile, but is also the source of frustration unless the various types of heterogeneity are considered carefully when choosing the ideal antibody for a given RIA. The affinity of the antibody for the peptide to be measured as well as for the label will determine the minimum concentration detectable in the assay. The specificity of the antibody affects whether peptides of similar sequences cross-react with the peptide expected to be measured. The concentration of the highest titer antibody in serum will determine the dilution needed to bind a given label.

Antibody Specificities

Immunochemical studies with peptides of relatively low molecular weight such as gastrin and CCK show that the antigenic determinants (i.e., the sequence recognized by antibody) are generally linear sequences of four to eight amino acids (7). Reports on the specificity of gastrin antibodies suggest there is one main C-terminal antigenic determinant (26,34,44,45,58), a minor N terminal determinant (15), and a third determinant that contains parts of both C and N termini (14).

The high frequency that antibodies are induced to the major antigenic determinant of gastrin (34,45,58,59,61) whose sequence is shared by CCK peptide can create obvious problems in the RIA. However, antibody induced by either conjugated or unconjugated gastrin usually has low cross-reactivity (0.1–5%) with CCK peptides. The left panel of Fig. 3 shows standard curves of antibodies that exhibit increasing cross-reactivity to CCK-8 with respect to hG-17. Antibodies 1611 and 1296 should be used to measure gastrin satisfactorily without undue interference from CCK-8, but these curves do not indicate whether 1296 and 1611 are able to distinguish all forms of gastrin equally well. Figure 4 demonstrated similar affinity of 1296 for various gastrin peptides. Antibody 5135 binds G-17 and CCK-8 equally and measures total gastrin plus CCK without distinguishing between the two. Antibodies with other specificities shown in the right panel of Fig. 3 are defective as all-purpose antibodies but are valuable reagents under certain conditions. Antibody 1295, the antibody directed to the N-terminus of G-17, detects only G-17 and N-terminal fragments of G-17 but does not recognize G-16, CCK-8 or G-34, which is the gastrin that predominates in the circulation (59). Antibody 4, a C-terminal antibody that has high affinity for unsulfated tyrosine (27), detects peptides with sulfated tyrosine poorly. Finally, L6, which is specific for the heptadecapeptide does not detect G-34 or G-14 (or des G-17, G-16 or CCK-8). Nevertheless, this is a valuable antibody for specific measurement of G-17 in a mixture of gastrin molecules.

A specificity profile is a property of a particular antiserum but may change during the course of immunization. Practically, this necessitates checking all bleedings that are used for RIA to be sure the antibody specificity pattern has not changed. Two examples of changing specificities of sera taken from rabbits at various times after the start of immunization are shown in Table 6. Rabbit 5135 at 6 months after immunization was more specific for CCK-8, but at 11 months antibody from the same animal had become more specific for G-17. Antibody 1611 was highly specific for gastrin during early bleedings but developed greater cross-reactivity with CCK peptides after further immunization.

With the wide diversity of antibody specificities available, it might theoretically be possible to analyze serum for all known gastrin-CCK peptide by antibodies alone. Such an analysis would be possible only if antibodies with complete specificity for each molecular form of both peptides were available. A more reasonable approach currently is to make an initial size and/or charge separation by chromatography, then assay the eluted fractions with a smaller, appropriate set of antibodies.

Antibodies of various specificities have been utilized for purposes other than for measuring amounts of serum gastrin-CCK peptides; they have helped to discover errors in published gastrin sequences and helped to identify new gastrin peptides. In the first case, antiserum produced against the natural porcine G-34 recognized the natural peptide, but the synthetic porcine G-34 reacted less than 1/1,000. Since the immunochemical potencies of the synthetic and natural peptide with an antiserum toward G-17 were similar, the differences in sequences between the natural and synthetic big gastrins were thought to be located in the N-terminal end (12). In the second case, the observation that rat gastrin did not react with a specific N-terminal hG-17 antibody (1295) led to the isolation of a peptide that appears to be slightly larger than G-17 *(unpublished observations).*

Unexpected Antibody Specificities

Antibody populations not obvious by RIA, in which only antibodies which bind to label are evaluated, may become apparent when an antiserum is used for immunocytochemistry (12). The concentration of serum usually used in immunocytochemistry is much higher, 10^{-1} to 10^{-2} compared with 10^{-4} to 10^{-6} for RIA. Since binding to a tissue protein is a function of concentration as well as affinity, antibodies of lower affinity, but in higher concentration may bind in tissue sections. In addition, peptides such as gastrin in tissue sections act as multivalent antigens that may increase the effective affinity of the antibody up to 10,000-fold (29). Furthermore, the sensitivity of the flourescent antibody technique in immunochemistry is augmented with the application of a second fluorescent antibody directed to the species immunoglobulin of the first antibody.

Antibodies to the carrier protein such as BSA may create an unexpected problem. A major portion of the total antibody may be to the carrier-peptide junction. These carrier-specific antibodies react with the carrier alone or with the peptide (gastrin) and neighboring amino acid residues of the gastrin carrier. When such antibodies are used to measure gastrin, serum albumin in an unknown sample may bind to the anti-gastrin and may cause a troublesome drop in the binding of the gastrin label. We have found that rabbits immunized with BSA-peptide conjugates produce high titer antibodies to BSA. These antibodies may react with tissue antigens similar to albumin to produce nonspecific immunocyto-chemical staining patterns. In affinity chromatography, when antibodies to gastrin and antibodies to albumin are covalently bound to sepharose beads, the efficiency of gastrin purification may be impaired due to coabsorption of albumin-like molecules from plasma or from tissue extracts.

The reactions described previously are all predictable from the structure of the immunogen, either gastrin or gastrin-protein conjugate. Antibodies cross-

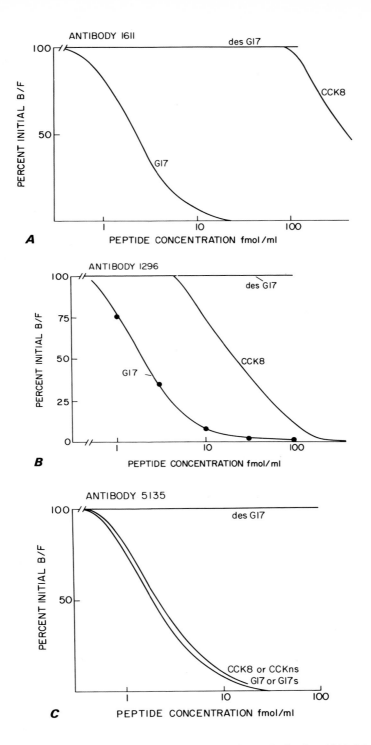

Fig. 3. Specificity patterns of various gastrin antisera. Antibodies 1611 **(a),** 1296 **(b),** and 5135 **(c)** all are specific for the carboxyl-terminal region of gastrin but exhibit increasing affinity for CCK peptides. Antibody L6

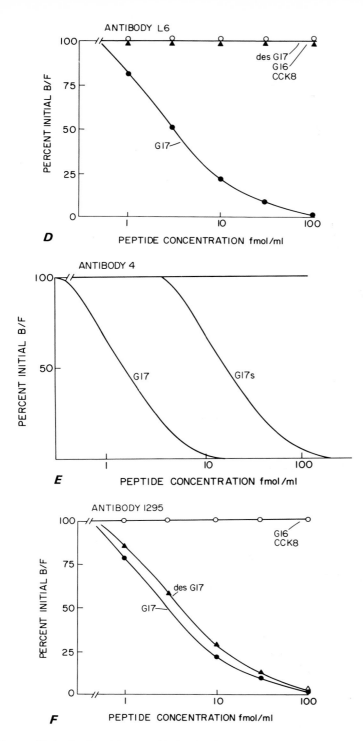

(d) is specific for G-17 and does not bind molecules with slight alterations at either the carboxyl or amino terminus. Antibody 4 **(e)** has higher affinity for nonsulfated than for sulfated gastrin. Antibody 1295 **(f)** is specific for the amino terminal region of G-17 and therefore has high affintiy for desamido G-17 (des-G-17) but no affinity for G-16.

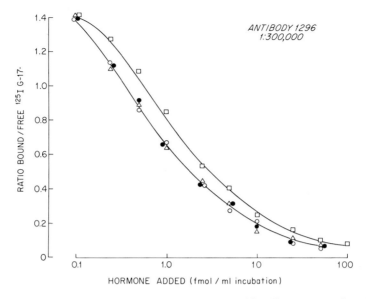

FIG. 4. Specificity of antibody 1296 for various gastrin peptides, illustrating similar affinity for gastrins of different chain lengths containing the same carboxyl-terminal sequence and similar affinity for sulfated and nonsulfated G-17. **Abscissa:** fmoles/ml G-17 or cpm [125]IG-17/ml × 10^{-3}. □, hG-13; ○, hG-17; ●, hG-17s; △, hG-33.

react when there are sequence similarities between the two peptides. In fact specificity refers to the capacity to discriminate between two peptides of similar structure: the greater the difference in binding affinity for two related peptides, the more specific the antibody for the peptide bound with the higher affinity. Sometimes, "cross-reactivities" cannot be explained readily by a comparison of the two molecules under consideration. Perhaps, the antibody-combining site contains residues that form hydrogen bonds, ionic bonds, or bonds involving

TABLE 6. *Change of antibody specificity with time*

Antibody	Time after immunization	ID_{50}[c] G-17	CCK-8	Ratio ID_{50}: G-17/CCK-8
5135[a]	6 months	6.2	5.0	1.24
	11 months	1.4	3.5	0.40
1611[b]	3 months	3.3	1700	0.003
	11 months	1.5	140	0.011

[a] 5135 was immunized with CCK-8-BSA at time 0, 3, and 6 months.

[b] 1611 was immunized with G-17-BSA at time 0, 1.5, 6, and 10 months.

[c] ID_{50}s are expressed in fmoles/ml.

Van der Waal's forces with the cross-reacting substances, although the two substances do not appear to be similar. There are no documented examples of peptides with sequences grossly dissimilar to gastrin binding with gastrin antibody. However, in other systems, such as anti-DNP, structurally dissimilar haptens bind to this antibody (17,47,52). This observation probably is not a unique occurrence and would be expected to happen with gastrin antisera.

INTERPRETATION OF CIRCULATING GASTRIN CONCENTRATIONS

Basal Serum Gastrin Concentrations

Basal serum gastrin concentrations obtained in normal human subjects vary among laboratories that perform this determination (54). The most likely explanations for the reported differences are variations in the nonspecific inhibition of antigen-antibody binding produced by serum proteins and use of standards with varying potency and antibodies with differing specificity for various molecular forms of gastrin. Failure to correct for nonspecific protein effects and use of standard gastrin preparations of less than full potency lead to overestimates of serum gastrin. Use of antibodies that react less avidly with molecular forms of gastrin in the circulation other than the one used as the standard leads to underestimates. For example, some antibodies have lower affinity for sulfated gastrins or for big gastrins than for the nonsulfated G-17 standard. When nonspecific effects are corrected by use of gastrin-free serum and when highly potent standards are used, total serum gastrin concentrations measured with antibodies that have similar affinity for all carboxyl-terminal forms of gastrin average between 10 and 20 fmoles/ml (21–42 pg/ml). Chromatographic studies with serum concentrated by affinity chromatography reveals that approximately two-thirds of this fasting gastrin corresponds to G-34 and most of the remainder corresponds to G-17 (55).

Basal serum gastrin values are increased in certain patients with pathological gastric acid hypersecretion (56). The most common cause of this situation is a gastrin-secreting tumor or gastrinoma that produces the clinical syndrome known as the Zollinger-Ellison syndrome (see Chapter 00). Patients with gastrinomas may have associated hyperparathyroidism or less commonly other endocrine tumors such as pituitary adenomas. The other causes of hypergastrinemia associated with acid hypersecretion are antral gastrin cell hyperfunction and isolated retained antrum.

Increased basal gastrin values are also found in patients with diminished or absent gastric acid secretion and intact antral function (54). The most common cause of this condition is simple atrophic gastritis. In extreme cases this type of gastritis may be associated with pernicious anemia. It also is relatively common in patients with cancer of the stomach. Approximately 20% of patients with advanced renal failure have moderately to markedly increased serum gastrin concentrations. In our experience, most of these patients also are achlorhydric, although some reports in the literature have failed to establish a clear connection between gastric secretion and serum gastrin in patients with renal failure. Surgical vagotomy commonly leads to moderate increases in serum gastrin. This may be due in part to decreased gastric acid secretion and in part to removal of some vagal cholinergic factor that normally inhibits release of gastrin. In general, patients with diminished acid secretion and increased gastrin appear to have increased numbers of antral gastrin cells and increased total antral gastrin content. It is commonly felt that gastrin cell hyperplasia and hyperactivity is due to the removal of an inhibitory effect exerted by luminal acid. However, acute neutralization of gastric contents does not cause a measureable increase in serum gastrin concentration.

Patients with ordinary duodenal ulcer disease have basal gastrin concentrations that fall within the normal range (54). There is limited and conflicting evidence whether or not the proportions of G-17 is increased in the basal serum from these patients. Gastric ulcer patients have an increase in basal gastrin that is due entirely to increased G-34. This hypergastrinemia is not well correlated with gastric acid secretion and does not appear to be accompanied by increased numbers of antral gastrin cells or antral gastrin content.

Serum Gastrin Concentrations after Stimulation

The most potent physiological stimulant of gastric acid secretion and of gastrin release is the presence in the stomach of protein digestion products, peptides and amino acids. A large protein-rich meal produces two- to three-fold increases in serum gastrin consisting of approximately equal increments in gastrin components corresponding to G-34 and G-17. There is some evidence that protein-stimulated gastrin release is increased in patients with duodenal ulcer (36). It is more clearly established that serum gastrin responses to protein are increased in patients with gastric ulcer. In both conditions, the majority of the additional increase is accounted for by G-34 rather than G-17. The most exaggerated increases in gastrin produced by protein meals are found in patients with antral gastrin cell hyperfunction, either associated with gastric acid hypersecretion or with atrophic gastritis. In these patients and in postvagotomy patients, the increased release of gastrin is due to both G-17 and G-34. Unoperated patients with gastrinoma typically show little or no response to a protein meal, although some patients with previous gastrectomy have been found to have considerable responses.

The role of cephalic, vagal, and cholinergic factors in gastrin release is more complicated. Insulin hypoglycemia produces a clear increase in serum gastrin when the gastric contents are maintained at a pH near neutral, but it is not clear that the effects are entirely mediated by the vagus nerve. Sham feeding is a purer cephalic-vagal stimulant but produces very small and often insignificant increases in serum gastrin. However, a magnified response to sham feeding can be produced by prior administration of small doses of atropine, suggesting that there is also a muscarinic, cholinergic factor that inhibits gastrin release (18). This idea is supported by the observation of increased gastrin responses to insulin hypoglycemia, distention of the stomach, and ingestion of a protein meal after pretreatment with low doses of atropine. Very large doses of atropine have been found to inhibit gastrin responses to insulin hypoglycemia and to sham feeding in dogs, but these doses may have been large enough to produce central or nonspecific peripheral effects.

Luminal calcium salts are moderate stimulants of gastrin release in man and are more potent than intravenous calcium, which has a very weak stimulatory effect. The frog peptide bombesin and similar peptides such as litorin are very potent releasers of gastrin when administered intravenously to man or to other mammals. A similar immunoreactive activity has been found in mammalian gut extracts (57). Epinephrine causes gastrin release and may account in part for the increase in gastrin which occurs during insulin hypoglycemia.

Secretin normally is an inhibitor of stimulated gastrin release in man but has a paradoxical stimulatory effect in patients with gastrinoma. An increase in serum gastrin of more than 100 pg/ml and more than 50% above basal values in patients with borderline or increased serum gastrin values within 10 min after rapid intravenous infusion of one or more units of secretin per kilogram body weight seems to be an almost completely specific and reasonably sensitive (85–90%) test for the presence of a gastrin-secreting tumor (54). Gastrinomas also are sensitive to stimulation by intravenous calcium salts. Responses similar to those obtained with intravenous secretin are obtained after infusion of 12 to 15 mg calcium ion per kilogram body weight over a 3-hr period. This test is slightly less specific than secretin infusion because patients without gastrinomas may show moderate gastrin responses to calcium infusion. These tests have been of some value in establishing the diagnosis of gastrinoma in patients with borderline increased serum gastrin values.

SUMMARY AND CONCLUSIONS

The minimum requirements necessary for a reliable RIA are high quality labeled gastrin, unlabeled gastrin standards, high affinity antibody of known specificity, and an easy, but reliable separation technique. The following conclusions may be derived from the previous discussion:

1. *Source of peptide:* High quality peptides can be purchased from a number of places. Peptides for gastrin standards are available through the Center for Ulcer Research and Education, Los Angeles.
2. *Immunization:* The immunization method utilizing gastrin-protein conjugates and complete Freund's adjuvant produces antibodies in close to 100% of

the rabbits immunized. Affinities between 10^{10} and 10^{12} M^{-1} are possible after 4 to 6 months of immunization.

3. *Preparation of labeled gastrin:* Iodinated gastrin produced by the chloramine T method is >90% bindable by antibody and has high specific activity.

4. *Separation technique:* The anion exchange method of separation is the method of choice, because it is reliable and rapid.

5. *Specificity of antibody:* Specificity profiles should be determined by examining binding of antisera to various gastrin peptides and peptides of similar sequences. These profiles should be examined with each bleeding since specificities can change during immunization.

6. *Validation of the RIA:* Validation should include the determining of the assay sensitivity as defined by the detection limit and ID_{50}, assay accuracy by adding known amounts of gastrin peptides to serum, and assay precision as defined by the inter- and intraassay coefficient of variation.

PROJECTION FOR THE FUTURE

The major problem in setting up a gastrin radioimmunoassay is the production of antibody of desired specificity and affinity. Even after a period of 4 to 6 months of immunization, a rabbit may not produce an antibody of the most desirable specificity. During the last few years a method has been developed that may not only shorten the immunization period but also permit selection for desired specificity and affinity. The pioneering work by C. Milstein of Cambridge, England involved forming hybrids of antibody producing cells with tumor cells for the production of specific antibodies. A number of laboratories have expanded on this technique, which involves hybridization, selection of those hybrids that produce the desirable antibody, and then culture of the selected cells. The further refinement of this technique for producing homogenous antibody should encourage the development of a repertoire of antibodies of desired specificities and binding affinities for RIA applications.

REFERENCES

1. Agarwal, K. L., Beacham, J., Bentley, P. H., Gregory, R. A., Kenner, G. W., Sheppard, R. C., and Tracy, H. J. (1968): Isolation, structure and synthesis of ovine and bovine gastrins. *Nature,* 219:614–615.
2. Agarwal, K. L., Kenner, G. W., Sheppard, R. C. (1969): Structure and synthesis of canine gastrin. *Experientia,* 25:346–348.
3. Agarwal, K. L., Kenner, G. W., and Sheppard, R. C. (1969): Feline gastrin. An example of peptide sequence analysis by mass spectrometry. *J. Am. Chem. Soc.,* 91:3096–3097.
4. Anastasi, A., Erspamer, V., and Endean, R. (1968): Isolation and amino acid sequence of caerulein, the active decapeptide of the skin of *Hyla caerulea. Arch. Biochem. Biophys.,* 125:57–68.

Melchers, F., Potter, M., and Warner, N., (Eds.) (1978): *Lymphocyte Hybridomas.* Raven Press, New York.

5. Atassi, M. Z. (1977): Chemical modification and cleavage of proteins and chemical strategy in immunochemical studies of proteins. In: *Immunochemistry of Proteins,* edited by M. Z. Atassi, pp. 1–161. Plenum Press, New York.
6. Baur, S., Bacon, V. C., and Rosenquist, G. L. (1978): Preparation and use of ^{125}I labeled synthetic human (15-leu) gastrin 1-17-I for radioimmunoassay of conventional human gastrins. *Anal. Biochem.* 87:71–76.
7. Benjamini, E., Michaeli, D., and Young, J. D. (1972): Antigenic determinants of proteins of defined sequences. *Curr. Top. Microbiol. Immunol.* 58:85–134.
8. Bentley, P. H., Kenner, G. W., and Sheppard, R. C. (1966): Structures of human gastrins I and II. *Nature,* 209:583–585.
9. Bolton, A. E., and Hunter, W. M. (1973): The use of antisera covalently coupled to agarose, cellulose and sephadex in radioimmunoassay systems for proteins and haptens. *B. B. Acta,* 329:318–330.
10. Brown, T. R., Bagchi, N., Mack, R. E., Booth, E., and Jones, D. P. (1976): Isolation of monoiodinated gastrin using DEAE-sephadex and its characteristics in the gastrin RIA. *Clin. Chem. Acta.,* 67:321–323.
11. Dockray, G. J. (1977): Immunoreactive component resembling cholecystokinin octapeptide in intestine. *Nature,* 270:359–361.
12. Dockray, G. J. (1979): Immunochemistry of gastrin and cholecystokinin: Development and application of region specific antisera. In: *Gastrin and the Vagus,* edited by J. F. Rehfeld. Academic Press, New York.
13. Dockray, G. J., Gregory, R. A., Hutchison, J. B., Harris, J. I., and Runswick, M. J. (1978): Isolation, structure and biological activity of two cholecystokinin octapeptides from sheep brain. *Nature,* 274:711–713.
14. Dockray, G. J., and Taylor, I. L. (1976): Heptadecapeptide gastrin: Measurement in blood by specific radioimmunoassay. *Gastroenterology,* 71:971–977.
15. Dockray, G. J., and Walsh, J. H. (1975): Amino-terminal gastrin fragment in serum of Zollinger-Ellison syndrome patients. *Gastroenterology,* 68:222–230.
16. Dockray, G. J., Walsh, J. H., and Rehfeld, J. F. (1979): Naming gastrin and cholecystokinin. In: *Gastrin and the Vagus,* edited by J. F. Rehfeld. Academic Press, New York.
17. Edmundson, A. B., Ely, K. R., Girling, R. L., Abola, E. E., Schiffer, M., Westholm, F. A., Fausch, M. D., and Deutsch, H. F.: (1974): Binding of 2,4-dinitrophenyl compounds and other small molecules to a crystalline λ-type Bence-Jones dimer. *Biochemistry,* 13:3816–3827.
18. Feldman, M., Richardson, C. T., Taylor, I. L., and Walsh, J. H. (1979): Effect of atropine on vagal gastrin and pancreatic polypeptide release. *J. Clin. Invest.,* 63:294–298.
19. Ganguli, P. C., and Hunter, W. M. (1970): Production of antiserum. In: *Workshop Meeting on Radioimmunoassay Methods,* edited by K. E. Kirkham and W. M. Hunter, pp. 175–176. Churchill Livingstone, Edinburgh.
20. Ganguli, P. C., and Hunter, W. M. (1972): Radioimmunoassay of gastrin in human plasma. *J. Physiol. (Lond.),* 220:499–510.
21. Gedde-Dahl, D. (1974): Relation between gastrin response to food stimulation and pentagastrin-stimulated gastric acid secretion in normal humans. *Scand. J. Gastroenterol.,* 9:447–450.
22. Gregory, H., Hardy, P. M., Jones, D. S., Kenner, G. W., and Sheppard, R. C. (1964): The antral hormone gastrin: The structure of gastrin. *Nature,* 204:931–933.
23. Gregory, R. A. (1974): The gastrointestinal hormones: A review of recent studies. *J. Physiol.,* 241:1–32.
24. Gregory, R. A., and Tracy, H. J. (1974): Isolation of two minigastrins from Zollinger-Ellison tumour tissue. *Gut,* 15:683–685.
25. Gregory, R. A., and Tracy, H. J. (1975): The chemistry of the gastrins: Some recent advances. In: *Gastrointestinal Hormones,* edited by J. C. Thompson, pp. 13–24. University of Texas Press, Austin.
26. Hansky, J., and Cain, M. D. (1969): Radioimmunoassay of gastrin in human serum. *Lancet,* ii:1388–1390.
27. Hansky, J., Soveny, C., and Korman, M. G. (1973): What is immunoreactive gastrin? Studies with two antisera. *Gastroenterology,* 64:740.
28. Holmquist, A. L., Dockray, G. J., Rosenquist, G. L., and Walsh, J. H. (1979): Immunochemical characterization of cholecystokinin peptides in lamprey gut and brain. *Gen. Comp. Endocrinol.,* 37:474–481.

29. Hornick, C. L., and Karush, F. (1972): Antibody affinity III. The role of multivalence. *Immunochemistry,* 9:325–340.
30. Hunter, W. M., and Greenwood, F. C. (1962): Preparation of Iodine-131 labeled human growth hormone of high specific activity. *Nature (Lond.),* 194:495–496.
31. Jackson, B. M., Reeder, D. D., and Thompson, J. C. (1972): Dynamic characteristics of gastrin release. *Am. J. Surg.,* 123:137–142.
32. Jaffe, B. M., and Walsh, J. H. (1979): Gastrin and related peptides. In: *Methods of Hormone Radioimmunoassay,* edited by B. M. Jaffee and H. R. Berman, pp. 455–477. Academic Press, New York.
33. McBurnette, S. K., and Mandy, W. J. (1974): Chemical modification of a rabbit immunoglobulin allotype specificity. *Immunochemistry,* 11:255–260.
34. McGuigan, J. E. (1968): Immunological studies with synthetic human gastrin. *Gastroenterology,* 54:1005–1011.
35. McGuigan, J. E., and Trudeau, W. L. (1970): Studies with antibodies to gastrin: Radioimmunoassay in human serum and physiological studies. *Gastroenterology,* 58:139–150.
36. Mayer, G., Feurle, A. G., Fuchs, K., Ketterer, H., Track, N. S., and Creutzfeldt, W. (1974): Influence of feeding and sham feeding upon serum gastrin and gastric acid secretion in control subjects and duodenal ulcer patients. *Scand. J. Gastroenterol.,* 9:703–710.
37. Mutt, V. (1976): Further investigations on intestinal hormonal polypeptides. *Clin. Endocrinol.* (Suppl.), 5:175s–183s.
38. Mutt, V., and Jorpes, J. E. (1971): Hormonal peptides of the upper intestine. *Biochem. J.,* 125:57p–58p.
39. Nilsson, G. (1975): Increased plasma gastrin levels in connection with inhibition of gastric acid responses to sham feeding following bulbar perfusion with acid in dogs. *Scand. J. Gastroenterol.,* 10:273–277.
40. Patrick, G., and Rosenquist, G. L. (1979): *Unpublished observations.*
41. Rehfeld, J. F. (1978): Immunochemical studies on cholecystokinin II. Distribution and molecular heterogeneity in the central nervous system and small intestine of man and hog. *J. Biol. Chem.,* 253:4022–4030.
42. Rehfeld, J. F., and Stadil, F. (1973): Radioimmunoassay for gastrin employing immunosorbent. *Scand. J. Clin. Lab. Invest.,* 31:459–464.
43. Rehfeld, J. F., and Stadil, F. (1973): Gel filtration studies on immunoreactive gastrin in serum from Zollinger-Ellison patients. *Gut,* 14:369–373.
44. Rehfeld, J. F., Stadil, F., and Rubin, B. (1972): Production and evaluation of antibodies for the radioimmunoassay of gastrin. *Scand. J. Clin. Lab. Invest.,* 30:221–232.
45. Rosenquist, G. L., and Holmquist, A. M. (1974): The specificity of antibodies directed to porcine gastrin. *Immunochemistry,* 11:489–494.
46. Rosenquist, G. L., and Holmquist, A. L. (1979): *Unpublished observations.*
47. Rosenstein, R. W., Musson, R. A., Armstrong, M. Y. K., Konigsberg, W. H., and Richards, F. F. (1972): Contact regions for dinitrophenyl and menadione haptens in an immunoglobulin binding more than one antigen. *Proc. Natl. Acad. Sci. USA,* 69:877–881.
48. Schrumpf, E., and Sand, T. (1972): Radioimmunoassay of gastrin with activated charcoal. *Scand. J. Gastroenterol.,* 7:683–687.
49. Stadil, F., and Rehfeld, J. F. (1972): Preparation of ^{125}I-labelled synthetic human gastrin I for radioimmunoanalysis. *Scand. J. Clin. Lab. Invest.,* 30:361–368.
50. Stadil, F., and Rehfeld, J. F. (1973): Determination of gastrin in serum. An evaluation of reliability of a radioimmunoassay. *Scand. J. Gastroenterol.,* 8:101–112.
51. Strauss, E., and Yalow, R. S. (1978): Species specificity of cholecystokinin in gut and brains of several mammalian species. *Proc. Natl. Acad. Sci. USA,* 75:486–489.
52. Underdown, B. J., and Eisen, H. N. (1971): Cross-reactions between 2,4-dinitrophenyl and 5-acetouracil groups. *J. Immunol.,* 106:1431–1440.
53. Walsh, J. H. (1974): Radioimmunoassay of gastrin. *Nuclear Medicine In Vitro,* edited by B. Rothfeld, p. 231, Lippincott, Philadelphia.
54. Walsh, J. H. (1979): Pathogenetic role of the gastrins. In: *Gastrin and the Vagus,* edited by J. F. Rehfeld. Academic Press, New York.
55. Walsh, J. H. (1979): *Unpublished observations.*
56. Walsh, J. H., and Grossman, M. I. (1975): Gastrin. *N. Engl. J. Med.,* 292:1324–1332 and 1377–1384.

57. Walsh, J. H., Wong, H. C., and Dockray, G. J. (1979): Bombesin-like peptides in mammals. *Fed. Proc.,* 38:2315–2319.
58. Yalow, R. S., and Berson, S. A. (1970): Radioimmunoassay of gastrin. *Gastroenterology,* 58:1–14.
59. Yalow, R. S., and Berson, S. A. (1970): Size and charge distinctions between endogenous human plasma gastrin in peripheral blood and heptadecapeptide gastrin. *Gastroenterology,* 58:609–615.
60. Yalow, R. S., and Berson, S. A. (1972): And now 'big, big gastrin.' *Biochem. Biophys. Res. Commun.,* 48:391–393.
61. Yalow, R. S., and Berson, S. A. (1972): Immunochemical specificity of gastrin-antibody reactions. *Excerpta Medica,* International Congress, Series No. 241, pp. 48–56.
62. Yip, B. S. S. C., and Jordan, P. H., Jr. (1970): Radioimmunoassay of gastrin using antiserum to porcine gastrin. *Proc. Soc. Exp. Biol. Med.,* 134:380–385.

Gastrointestinal Hormones, edited by
George B. Jerzy Glass.
Raven Press, New York © 1980.

Chapter 34

Radioimmunoassay of Secretin, Vasoactive Intestinal Polypeptide, and Motilin

Ta-Min Chang and William Y. Chey

The Isaac Gordon Center for Digestive Diseases and Nutrition, The Genesee Hospital and University of Rochester School of Medicine and Dentistry, Rochester, New York 14642

I. SECRETIN

Secretin was first discovered in 1902 by Bayliss and Starling (1), who demonstrated that acid infusion into a denervated loop of dog jejunum resulted in stimulation of pancreatic secretion and that the extract of the jejunum loop contained a stimulating factor that could be carried by the blood to the pancreas to elicit pancreatic secretory response. The stimulating factor was named secretin, and was the first hormone to be discovered. In 1961, Jorpes and Mutt (13) successfully purified secretin from porcine small intestine as a 27 amino acid polypeptide and soon determined its amino acid sequence (17,18). The structure was then confirmed through chemical synthesis by Bodanszky and co-workers (2,3), and the synthetic peptide was shown to possess the same spectrum of biological activity (16,28).

Despite its being the most potent stimulant of pancreatic bicarbonate and water secretion, the hormonal status of the purified secretin has been questioned, mainly because of frequent failure to observe increase in plasma secretin concentration after a meal correlating well with significant postprandial increase in pancreatic secretion (4,29). Recently, using the improved radioimmunoassay (RIA) methods, a significant rise in the plasma secretin concentration during digestion was observed in man (9,21) and in dogs (15). The important contribution of endogenous secretin to external pancreatic secretion was shown in dogs by the observation that pancreatic bicarbonate secretion could be significantly diminished by intravenous infusion of specific anti-secretin serum (8). In this section the proper method of secretin RIA used in our laboratory that is consistently capable of detecting postprandial increase in plasma secretin concentration in man and dog is discussed.

PRODUCTION OF ANTISERA

High titer anti-secretin sera can be produced in randomly bred New Zealand white rabbit by immunizing the animals with either free secretin or secretin-bovine serum albumin (BSA) conjugate (6,11). However, our experience has shown that immunization with conjugated secretin yields a better chance of obtaining high titer antisera.

Immunization

Before immunization, secretin was conjugated to BSA by mixing 0.6 ml of synthetic porcine secretin (2 mg) in dimethyl foramide with 0.4 ml of 0.05 M potassium phosphate buffer, pH 7.4, 0.4 ml BSA (4 mg) in the same buffer, and then 0.2 ml 1-ethyl-3-(3-diethylaminopropyl)-carbodiimide (EDC) to start the reaction. The reaction mixture was stirred gently for 30 hr at 23°C and then dialyzed at 4°C for 48 hr against 2 liters of 0.01 M potassium phosphate buffer, pH 7.4 containing 0.15 M NaCl. Immunization was then carried out by emulsifying the conjugate with equal volume of complete Freund's adjuvant and injecting 0.4 ml into each rear foot pad of the rabbits. The animals received the same dosage for two additional injections at 4-week intervals. Thereafter, the dose was reduced by using conjugation mixture of 160 μg of secretin with 200 μg of BSA processed with same amount of EDC.

Bleeding was carried out 2 weeks after each injection by venous puncture at the ears and the titer of the antisera determined as the dilution at which 50% of ^{125}I-secretin (approximately 5,000 cpm) was bound after 2-day incubation. Generally, the titer of antisera rose to 1:5 × 10^5 after third immunization in most rabbits and reached to maximum after fifth immunization. The serum with the highest titer (R-1-6) reached to 1:2 × 10^6. It should be mentioned that the above procedure was carried out without monitoring the extent of secretin conjugation to BSA. For less experienced investigators, it is suggested that a small amount of ^{125}I-secretin be added to monitor the extent of conjugation as described by Fahrenkrug et al. (11).

CHARACTERIZATION OF ANTISERUM

Each antiserum should be characterized not only with respect to affinity toward secretin (6) but also to the extent of heterogeneity (14) of antibodies, as done by Fahrenkrug et al. (11). This can be carried out by incubating the antibody, ^{125}I-secretin, and various concentrations of unlabeled secretin (up to 10 ng/ml to ensure saturation) and incubating until equilibrium (usually 4 to 5 days at 4°C). The bound and free counts are then separated and counted. The result is then calculated with correction of the percentage of the tracer bindable with excess antibody according to the following equations:

$$T = \frac{1}{\text{M.W.}} \times \left(\frac{\text{Total counts of tracer}}{\text{Specific radioactivity of tracer}} + \text{unlabeled secretin} \right) \quad [1]$$

$$B = T \times \frac{(B/T)\text{obs}}{\% \text{ Immunoreactive content of tracer}} \quad [2]$$

$$F = (T - B) \times \frac{1{,}000}{V} \quad [3]$$

where T and B are total and bound hormone in pmoles; F, the free hormone concentration in pM; (B/T)obs, the observed bound to total ratio of the tracer counts corrected for blanks; and V, the incubation volume in milliliters. The data are then subjected to a Scatchard plot (19), plot of B/F versus B, yielding the initial slope as effective affinity constant, K_{eff}. This is related to the affinity at the high-energy binding site and hence determines the maximum sensitivity of the assay approachable with the antiserum (10). Whereas the extrapolated intercept at the abscissa measures the total number of binding sites, N, which is used for analyzing the heterogeneity index, α, and average affinity constant, K_0, according to Sip's equation (22) using the graphical analysis of Karush (14) according to equation (4).

$$\log \left(\frac{B}{N - B} \right) = \alpha \log F - \alpha \log K_0 \quad [4]$$

Plot of $\log \left(\frac{B}{N - B} \right)$ versus $\log F$ will obtain α as slope and $\alpha \log K_0$ as intercept at the coordinate. It should be emphasized that these parameters can be accurately measured only if the fraction of tracer bindable by excess antibody is as immunoreactive as the unlabeled peptide. The immunoreactivity of the tracer can be compared with the unlabeled peptide by comparing the Scatchard plot of results of experiments obtained by varying labeled peptide alone with that obtained with tracer amounts of the labeled and varied unlabeled peptide. If the tracer is fully immunoreactive, the two curves should be superimposable.

If correctly measured, antiserum with K_{eff} of $> 10^{11}$ M^{-1} and $\alpha > 0.5$ should be suitable for a sensitive RIA. The antiserum we have used, R-1-6, has the following binding parameters: K_{eff}, 1.0×10^{12} M^{-1}; α, 0.66; K_0, 3.0×10^{11} M^{-1}.

Cross-reactivity of the antibodies with other hormones, particularly the structurally similar vasoactive intestinal peptide (VIP), GIP, and glucagon also should be examined. Our antibodies generally do not cross-react with synthetic GIP, pancreatic glucagon natural porcine cholecystokinin-pancreozymin (CCK-PZ), human gastrin I, pancreatic polypeptide (PP), or motilin at concentrations as high as 10^{-8} M. However, exceptions do exist (6). VIP generally has 0.2 to 0.3% cross-reactivity.

PREPARATION OF RADIOIODINATED SECRETIN

Iodination of secretin can be carried out according to Tai et al. (26), with slight modification. Synthetic porcine secretin (5 μg) in 20 μl of 0.5 M sodium borate buffer, pH 8.0 was mixed with 20 μl of Na [^{125}I] (2 mCi) and immediately followed with 5 μl of 5 mg/ml chloramine T (in 0.05 M borate buffer, pH 8.0). After 2 min at 23°C, the reaction was terminated 2 min later by adding 20 μl of sodium metabisulfite (500 μg) in the 0.05 M borate buffer. The final mixture was diluted with 100 μl of a solution containing 0.5 M sucrose, 0.05 M KI, 1.6% BSA, and 0.02% NaN$_3$, and applied onto a 13 ml column of a mixture of Sephadex G 15/G-50, fine (7/3, w/w) packed in a 10 ml disposable pipet and equilibrated in 0.05 M sodium borate, pH 8.5 containing 0.08 M NaCl, 1% BSA, and 0.02% NaN$_3$. The column was eluted with the same buffer and fractions of 0.4 ml were collected. Radioactivity was monitored by counting 5 μl for 0.2 min. Labeled secretin containing about 15 to 20% of total counts usually peaked at fractions 16–20 and was well separated from high M.W. labeled material (fractions 11–12) and free iodide (fractions 28–36). The ^{125}I-secretin fractions with counts higher than 10^5 (per 5 μl per 0.2 min) were pooled and diluted with 5 volumes of 0.02 M sodium phosphate pH 5.5 containing 1% BSA and 0.02% NaN$_3$, adjusted to pH 5.0, and then chromatographed on a column of SP-Sephadex C25 (10 ml bed) previously equilbrated in the same phosphate buffer containing 0.02 M NaCl (starting buffer). The column was washed with 40 ml of the starting buffer and then eluted with a gradient of 60 ml each of the starting buffer in the mixing reservoir and the diluting buffer containing 0.20 M NaCl in the other. Fractions of 2.1 ml were collected beginning at the time of the sample application. Approximately one-third of the radioactivity was not retained by the column, presumably attributable to the damaged peptide and contaminated free iodide. Whereas immunoreactive ^{125}I-secretin was eluted as a single peak during gradient elution, it was well separated from unlabeled peptide under these conditions, as demonstrated by rechromatography in the presence of the unlabeled secretin (Fig. 1). This procedure is more reproducible than the one reported previously using ammonium

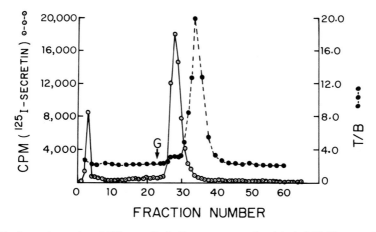

FIG. 1. Rechromatography of ^{125}I-secretin in the presence of unlabeled Mutt's secretin. ^{125}I-secretin (100,000 cpm) was cochromatographed with 1 μg of Mutt's secretin on SP-Sephadex C-25 column as described in the text. The unlabeled peptide was monitored by RIA with a final dilution of 50-fold. The reciprocal of bound to total ratio (T/B) is plotted in the figure to monitor the profile of unlabeled hormone.

bicarbonate buffer (26). The specific radioactivity of the purified tracer after pooling the peak fractions usually ranged between 100 and 200 μCi/μg as measured by the self-displacement method of Stadil and Rehfeld (23). It should be noted that this method is based on the assumption that the labeled and unlabeled peptide are equally immunoreactive and the result is expressed as μCi/μg immunoreactive equivalent of unlabeled peptide. The blank value in RIA with this preparation usually ranges between 6 and 8% and can be reduced to 2 to 4% by rechromatography on SP-Sephadex column. The maximum immunoreactive content of the tracer is also increased from 80 to 83% to 88 to 90% by rechromatography. Since the tracer is stable for 6 weeks when stored at −20°C, we routinely iodinated secretin every 6 weeks and rechromatographed the stored fractions biweekly.

Preparation of tracer from synthetic analog of secretin containing tyrosyl residues also may be satisfactory. However, it should be cautioned that the analog used is as immunoreactive as native secretin. Of known analogs, N^α-(des-Tyr-β-Ala)-secretin (27), N^α-tyrosyl-secretin and tyrosine[1]-secretin (30), appear to be suitable for iodination particularly considering the earlier report of Boden and Chey (5) that the first four amino acid residues from the N-terminal of secretin are not essential for immunoreactivity. The less immunoreactive analog, 6-tyrosyl-secretin (5,30) should not be used.

COLLECTION AND PROCESSING OF PLASMA SAMPLES

Samples of peripheral venous blood were collected into heparinized tubes chilled in an ice bath. Plasma was separated from blood cells by centrifugation at 2,000 × *g* and 4°C for 15 min, divided into 2-ml portions, mixed with Trasylol (500 KIU/ml plasma), and stored at −20°C before assay.

Since plasma samples always contain unidentified interferring substance(s) that nonspecifically inhibit binding of antigen to antibody, it is necessary to remove interferring substance before the assay. Compensation of interference by adding hormone-free plasma is not recommended for two reasons. First, assay in the presence of compensating hormone-free plasma resulted in desensitization of the assay, as demonstrated by comparing the standard curves shown in Fig. 2. Second, the content of interfering substance(s) varies from plasma to plasma (7,25), thus causing assay variation to the extent that is greater than what can be brought about by the postprandial increase of secretin, thereby masking off the observable change. For removing interfering substance from plasma, either the XAD-2 adsorption (25) or the ethanol extraction (20) technique can be used. Recent comparison studies in our laboratory have indicated that the results obtained by both methods are qualitively the same. The simpler and less expensive ethanol extraction procedure is therefore adopted. However, in certain specific experiments in which one wishes to measure the residual plasma secretin level following intravenous infusion of anti-secretin serum (8), the XAD-2 technique (see VIP assay below), should be used, since we found only 35 to 40% of antibody-bound secretin could be removed by ethanol precipitation, whereas all the antibody-bound secretin is separated from free secretin by the XAD-2 resin.

Extraction with ethanol can be carried out by mixing thoroughly 2 ml of the plasma with 2 ml of absolute ethanol and placing it in an ice bath for 20 min before centrifugation at 2,000 × *g* for 25 min to pellet precipitate. An

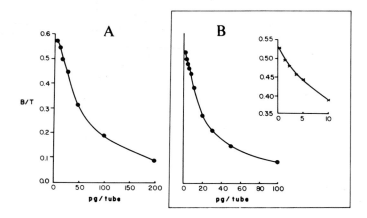

FIG. 2. Comparison of the standard curves of secretin RIA conducted in ethanol extract of hormone-free plasma **(B)** and in hormone-free plasma **(A)**. In the old method **(A)**, 0.2 ml of hormone-free plasma was used in each assay. The standard curve obtained in XAD-2 column extract was equally sensitive as in the ethanol extract.

additional 6 ml of ethanol is then added into the same tube and mixed gently with supernatant without disturbing the pellet, and the mixture is allowed to stay in the ice bath for another 20 min and centrifuged again for 25 min at 2,000 × g. The final clear supernatant is then decanted into another test tube and dried at 40°C under a stream of air, and stored at −20°C before assay. Extract of hormone-free plasma samples in 2 ml alone or containing known amounts of authentic secretin (10,15,25,50, and 100 pg/ml), and a control plasma sample should be included for construction of standard curve, determination of recovery factor, and interassay variation, respectively. Immediately before assay the extract is reconstructed in 1 ml 0.05 M sodium phosphate buffer, pH 7.0 containing 1% BSA and 0.02% NaN$_3$, yielding a semiclear solution that does not require centrifugation before assay.

PREPARATION OF HORMONE-FREE PLASMA

Hormone-free plasma can be prepared by treating pooled plasma from volunteer healthy subjects or experimental animals with dextran-coated charcoal as below. Charcoal (90 mg/ml) is first suspended in a solution of 0.05 M Tris-HCl, pH 7.8 containing 0.1% BSA and 9 mg/ml dextran (M.W. = 86,000) stirred for 2 hr and then pelleted by centrifugation at 2,000 × g for 10 min. After discarding supernatant, the pellet is mixed with pooled plasma at a ratio of 1 ml plasma per ml of the original suspension and then stirred gently for 2 hr at 4°C. The hormone-free plasma is then separated from the bulk of charcoal by centrifugation at 40,000 × g for 20 min, followed by filtration of the supernatant fluid through 5 μm and then 0.2 μm Milipore membranes to remove fine charcoal particles. The 5 μm membrane step can be substituted with 3 steps of filtration through Whatman No. 42 filter paper (20), but the 0.2 μm membrane step should not be omitted. The hormone-free plasma is stored at −20°C after adding Trasylol to final concentration of 500 KIU/ml.

Hormone-free plasma used to coat charcoal for separating bound and free counts is prepared from outdated human plasma by the same treatment after exhaustive dialysis against H$_2$O (five volumes, 6 changes over 48 hr).

ASSAY CONDITIONS

Standard secretin is prepared from natural porcine secretin (GIH) at 5, 10, 15, 25, 50, 100, 150, 250, 500, 1,000, 1,500, and 2,500 pg/ml in 0.05 M sodium phosphate buffer, pH 7.0 containing 1% BSA, 0.02% NaN$_3$, 50 μg/ml protamine-free base and 500 KIU/ml Trasylol (diluting buffer), and stored in 0.5 ml aliquots at −60°C. The standards are thawed only at the time of use and never stored beyond 3 months to ensure reproducibility of the standard curve.

During assay, the unlabeled secretin (i.e., standards or unknown sample) is incubated first with antibody in a final volume of 1.4 ml consisting of 0.4 ml of reconstituted ethanol extract of hormone-free plasma (for standards), recovery standards or of unknown samples; 0.2 ml of standard solution or diluting buffer (for unknowns); 0.8 ml diluted antiserum (1 : 10⁶), in 0.05 M sodium phosphate buffer, pH 7.0 containing 0.1% BSA, 0.02% NaN₃, and 875 KIU/ml Trasylol. After 48 hr at 4°C, 0.2 ml of ¹²⁵I-secretin (approximately 5,000 cpm) diluted in the reconstituting buffer is then added and incubated for another 48 hr. All samples are assayed in duplicate including blanks from each individual subject or experimental animal. Separation of bound and free counts is achieved by adding 0.4 ml dextran- and plasma-coated charcoal suspension and centrifugation and both bound (supernatant) and free (pellet) tracers are counted. The charcoal suspension used is prepared by mixing 1 volume of dialyzed hormone-free human plasma, 1 volume of saline, and 2 volumes of dextran-coated charcoal suspension (90 mg/ml).

CALCULATION OF THE RESULTS

All data are calculated via computer programs loaded to a Monroe model 1860 programmable calculator. All bound to total ratio of tracer counts are corrected for corresponding blank values. A linear standard curve is fitted by the method of unweighted least square plot of the logit transform function of % maximum tracer binding, logit (B/B_0), versus the logarithm of the concentration of added standard secretin (12).

RELIABILITY OF THE ASSAY

The assay sensitivity of the present method is vastly improved over our previous method of compensating interference with hormone-free plasma (15,21),

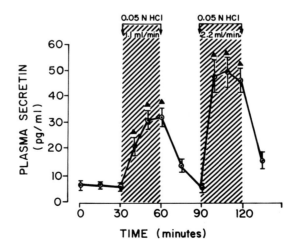

FIG. 3. Plasma secretin concentration in response to duodenal acid infusion at two different rates in five anesthetized dogs. *Triangles* indicate statistical significance of elevation over basal value at $p < 0.05$.

as can be seen by comparing the standard curves shown in Fig. 2. The 95% confident detection limit defined as two standard deviations (2×0.0058, $n = 6$) of the B/T values measured at zero dose divided by the initial slope (0.0176/pg) of the dose response curve (B/T versus dose) (12), is 0.66 pg/tube. The recovery of secretin from ethanol extract was constant over the range concentrations tested (10–100 pg/ml) and was on the average $60.1 \pm 7.1\%$ (mean $\pm$ SD). Correcting the recovery from extraction step, the overall sensitivity of the assay is 1.4 pg/ml (0.46 pM) plasma sample. This sensitivity is slightly improved over the previously reported 2 to 3 pg/ml (9.15), using the XAD-2 adsorption technique mainly due to the use of rechromatographed ^{125}I-secretin and longer preincubation with the antibody. Similar to the XAD-2 adsorption technique (25), the response of plasma secretin concentration to the infusion of a small quantity of HCl into duodenum (Fig. 3) can be consistently observed.

REFERENCES

1. Bayliss, W. M., and Starling, E. H. (1902): Mechanism of pancreatic secretion. *J. Physiol.*, 28:325–353.
2. Bodanszky, M., Levine, S. D., Narayanan, V., Ondetti, M. A., vonSaltza, M., Sheehan, J. T., and Williams, N. J. (1966): Confirmation by synthesis of secretin sequences. In: *Proceedings of the IUPAC International Congress on the Chemistry of Natural Products,* June 26–July 2, Stockholm, Sweden, Section 2C-2.
3. Bodanszky, M., Ondetti, M. A., Levine, S. D., Narayanan, V., vonSaltza, M., Sheehan, J. T., Williams, N. J., and Saba, E. F. (1966): Synthesis of a heptacosapeptide amide with the hormonal activity of secretin. *Chem. Indust.*, 42:1757–1758.
4. Boden, G. (1978): The secretin assay: In: *Gut Hormones,* edited by S. R. Bloom, pp. 169–175. Churchill Livingstone, Edinburgh/London/New York.
5. Boden, G., and Chey, W. Y. (1973): Preparation and specificity of antiserum to synthetic secretin and its use in a radioimmunoassay (RIA). *Endocrinology,* 92:1617–1624.
6. Boehm, M., Lee, Y., and Chey, W. Y. (1974): Radioimmunoassay of Secretin I. Production of secretin antibodies and development of the radioimmunoassay. In: *Endocrinology of the Gut,* edited by W. Y. Chey, and F. Brooks, pp. 310–319. Charles B. Slack, Thorofare, New Jersey.
7. Byrnes, D. J., and Marjason, J. P. (1976): Radioimmunoassay of secretin in plasma. *Horm. Metab. Res.,* 8:361–365.
8. Chey, W. Y., Kim, M. S., Lee, K. Y., and Chang, T. M. (1978): Contribution of endogenous secretin on postprandial pancreatic secretion in dogs. *Scand J. Gastroenterol. (Suppl. 13),* 41:40 (Abstr.).
9. Chey, W. Y., Lee, Y. H., Hendricks, J. G., Rhodes, R. A., and Tai, H. H. (1978): Plasma secretin in fasting and postprandial state in man. *Am. J. Dig. Dis.,* 231:981–988.
10. Ekins, R., and Newman, B. (1970): Theoretical aspects of saturation analysis. *Acta Endocrinol.,* 147:11.
11. Fahrenkrug, J., Schaffalitzky de Muckadell, O. B., and Rehfeld, J. F. (1976): Production and evaluation of antibodies for radioimmunoassay of secretin. *Scand. J. Clin. Lab. Invest.,* 37:281–287.
12. Feldman, H., and Rodbard, D. (1971): Mathematical theory of radioimmunoassay. In: *Principles of Competitive Protein-Binding Assays,* edited by W. D. Odell and W. H. Doughaday, pp. 158–199. J. B. Lippincott, Co., Philadelphia and Toronto.
13. Jorpes, J. E., and Mutt, V. (1961): On the biological activity and amino acid composition of secretin. *Acta Chem. Scand.,* 15:1790–1971.
14. Karush, F. (1962): Immunologic specificity and molecular structure. *Adv. Immunol.,* 2:1–40.
15. Kim, M. S., Lee, K. Y., and Chey, W. Y. (1979): Plasma immunoreactive secretin concentration (IRS) in fasting and postprandial state in dog (Abstr.). *Clin. Res.,* 26:321, 1978; *Am. J. Physiol.,* 236:E539–E544.

16. Konturek, S. J. (1969): Comparison of pancreatic responses to natural and synthetic secretins in conscious cats. *Am. J. Dig. Dis.,* 14:557–565.
17. Mutt, V., and Jorpes, J. E. (1966): Secretin: Isolation and determination of structure (Abstr.). *Proceedings of the IUPAC Fourth International Congress on the Chemistry of Natural Products,* June 26–July 2, Stockholm, Sweden, Section 2C-3.
18. Mutt, V., Magnusson, S., Jorpes, J. E., and Dahl, E. (1965): Structure of porcine secretin. *J. Biochem.,* 4:2358–2362.
19. Scatchard, G. (1949): The attractions of proteins for small molecules and ions. *Ann. NY Acad. Sci.,* 51:660–772.
20. Schaffalitzky de Muckadell, O. B., and Fahrenkrug, J. (1977): Radioimmunoassay of secretin in plasma. *Scand. J. Clin. Lab. Invest.,* 37:155–162.
21. Schaffalitzky de Muckadell, O. B., and Fahrenkrug, J. (1978): Secretion pattern of secretin in man: Regulation of gastric acid. *Gut,* 19:812–818.
22. Sips, P. (1948): On the structure of a catalyst surface. *J. Chem. Phys.,* 15:490–495.
23. Stadil, F., and Rehfeld, J. F. (1972): Preparation of ^{125}I-labeled synthetic human gastrin I for radioimmunoanalysis. *Scand. J. Clin. Lab. Invest.,* 30:361–368.
24. Straus, E., Urbach, H. J., and Yalow, R. S. (1955): Comparative reactivities of ^{125}I-secretin and ^{125}I-6-tyrosyl secretin with guinea pig and rabbit anti-secretin sera. *Biochem. Biophys. Res. Commun.,* 64:1036–1040.
25. Tai, H. H., and Chey, W. Y. (1978): Rapid extraction of secretin from plasma by XAD-2 resin and its application in the radioimmunoassay of secretin. *Anal. Biochem.,* 87:376–385.
26. Tai, H. H., Korsch, B., and Chey, W. Y. (1975): Preparation of ^{125}I-labeled secretin of high specific radioactivity. *Anal. Biochem.,* 69:34–42.
27. Urbach, J. H., Domschke, W., Reib, M., Domschke, S., Rosseliu, G., Wünsch, E., Jaeger, E., Moroder, L., and Demlin, G. L. (1976): Superior immunoreactivity of [125]I-(Des-Tyr-β-Ala)-secretin with rabbit antisera compared to ^{125}I-secretin and ^{125}I-6-tyro-syl secretin. *Horm. Metab. Res.,* 8:459–461.
28. Vagne, M., Stening, G. F., Brooks, F. P., and Grossman, M. I. (1968): Synthetic secretin: Comparison with natural secretin for potency and spectrum of physiological actions. *Gastroenterology,* 55:260–267.
29. Wormsley, K. G. (1973): Is secretin secreted? *Gut,* 14:743–751.
30. Yanaihara, N., Kubota, M., Sakagami, M., Sato, H., Mochizuki, T., Sakura, N., Hashimoto, T., Yanaihara, C., Yamaguchi, K., Zeze, F., and Abe, K. (1977): Synthesis of phenolic group containing analogues of porcine secretin and their immunological properties. *J. Med. Chem.,* 20:648–655.

II. VASOACTIVE INTESTINAL POLYPEPTIDE (VIP)

Vasoactive intestinal polypeptide (VIP), a basic polypeptide of 28 amino residues, was originally isolated from hog small intestine by Said and Mutt (8). Its amino acid sequence has been established (6) and confirmed by chemical synthesis (1). Despite its wide distribution and broad spectrum of biological activity (7), the physiological role of VIP has not been established. However, VIP appears to be of pathophysiological significance since it is hypersecreted into the culture medium of neoplastic cell lines and into plasma of patients with watery diarrhea syndrome (7).

Recently, a sensitive RIA method for VIP has been developed in our laboratory (3). Using this assay we have been able to measure the basal VIP concentration in the plasma of fasting normal human subjects and elevated plasma VIP in patients with Verner-Morrison syndrome, as well as VIP levels in dogs on vagal stimulation (9) and following intestinal ischemia (5). The details of this assay are given below.

PRODUCTION OF ANTI-VIP SERA

Antibody against VIP was prepared by repeated immunization of New Zealand white rabbits with natural porcine VIP conjugated to bovine serum albumin (BSA) by a procedure similiar to that described for secretin (2) and motilin (10). Conjugation of VIP to BSA was carried out by dissolving 0.5 mg of VIP and 1 mg of BSA in 1.2 ml of deionized water and then mixing this with 50 mg of 1-ethyl-3-(3-dimethyl aminopropyl)-carbodiimide in a final volume of 1.4 ml, stirring at 20°C for 20 hr and then dialyzing as described for secretin-BSA (2). Initially, by injection through the foot pad, each rabbit received a whole dose of each conjugated VIP preparation emulsified in an equal volume of Freund's adjuvant in monthly intervals for 2 months, followed by 1/10 of the original dose in the same intervals. Because the animals tended to die from these VIP doses, those animals who survived after the fourth injection and contained a high titer of anti-VIP sera were sacrificed 2 weeks later in order to obtain a large amount of antisera. The final titer usually ranged between

400,000 and 500,000-fold dilution to bind 50% of 10 fmoles of ^{125}I-VIP. The titer of the antibody in a boosted animal did not remain at a high level beyond 4 weeks after the last injection. The antiserum with the highest titer we obtained (1:500,000) had the following binding parameters: effective affinity constant (K_{eff}), 2.9 × 10^{11} M^{-1}; heterogeneity index (α), 0.57; average affinity constant (K_o), 2.4 × 10^{10} M^{-1}, as determined by the methods discussed for secretin assay (2).

PREPARATION OF ^{125}I-VIP

VIP was iodinated by a modified lactoperoxidase method of Thorell and Johansson (11). The initial reaction mixture contained 0.16 M NaOAc, pH 5.6, 2 μg of VIP (0.59 nmoles), 2.7 μg lactoperoxidase (Calbiochem), and 1 mCi of Na [^{125}I] (0.57 nmoles) in a final volume of 51 μl. The reaction was started by the addition of 1 μl H$_2$O$_2$ (0.6 nmoles) and incubated at room temperature. After 30 sec, another aliquot of H$_2$O$_2$ (0.6 nmoles) was allowed to react for another 30 sec before being stopped by the addition of 0.1 ml of a solution containing 100 mM NH$_4$HCO$_3$, 1% BSA, 0.02% NaN$_3$, 60 mM KI, and 0.48 M sucrose, and adjusted to pH 8.5. Iodinated VIP was first separated from lactoperoxidase and free iodide on a 13-ml column of Sephadex G 15/G-50, fine (7/3 w/w) run in 100 mM NH$_4$HCO$_3$ containing 1% BSA, 0.02% NaN$_3$, and 50 μg/ml protamine free base [Sigma as described for secretin (2)]. Approximately 70% of the radioactivity was incorporated into VIP peak. Fractions of

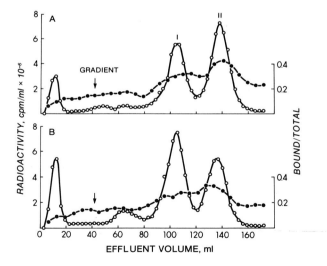

FIG. 1. Purification of ^{125}I-VIP on CM-Sephadex C-25 column. The experimental details are given in the text. **A:** ^{125}I-VIP prepared by lactoperoxidase iodination. **B:** ^{125}I-VIP prepared by chloramine T. *Arrow:* beginning of the gradient. *Open circles,* radioactivity; *filled circles,* immunoreactivity.

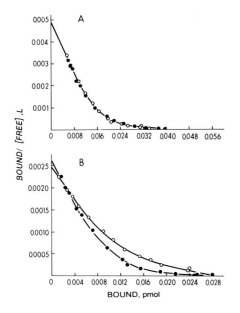

FIG. 2. Scatchard plot of binding of labeled and unlabeled VIP to anti-VIP antibody. **A:** Plot of ^{125}I-VIP peak II compared with plot of native VIP, using peak II as tracer. **B:** Plot of ^{125}I-VIP peak I compared with plot of native VIP, using peak I as tracer. The experimental details and method of data analysis were given in ref. 2.

VIP peaks were then pooled and diluted with equal volumes of a solution containing 0.2 M sucrose, 1% BSA, 0.02% NaN₃, and 50 µg/ml protamine free base, adjusted to pH 6.0, and then applied onto a column of CM-Sephadex C-25 (10 ml bed) previously equilibrated in 50 mM NH₄HCO₃, pH 6.0, containing the same amount of BSA, NaN₃, and protamine. The column was first washed with 20 ml of the equilibrating buffer and then eluted with a gradient of 50 to 250 mM NH₄HCO₃ containing the same amount of BSA and NaN₃ and protamine with 70 ml in each reservoir. The pH of the 250 mM NH₄HCO₃ solution was not adjusted. Fractions of 3 ml were collected starting at the time of sample application and both radioactivity and immunoreactivity were monitored. Two major immunoreactive labeled VIP peaks were resolved during the gradient elution (Fig. 1) and only peak II was fully immunoreactive (Fig. 2). Peak I was unstable and thus not used for RIA. Iodination by Chloramine T method to the same extent of incorporation of [125I] usually yielded less peak II activity and thus is not recommended (Fig. 1). The final specific activity of peak II was 520 ± 100 µCi/nmoles as determined by the self-displacement method. About 88% of the label was bindable to excess antibody and this could be improved to over 90% by rechromatography on CM-Sephadex column. Rechromatography was carried out routinely on a biweekly basis.

COLLECTION AND PROCESSING OF PLASMA SAMPLES

Plasma samples were collected and stored before assay as described for secretin (2). Interference substance(s) was (were) removed by the XAD-2 resin adsorption technique. Each 2-ml aliquot of plasma sample was percolated through a 3-ml bed of XAD-2 resin (packed dry) and recycled once. The column was first washed with 2×2 ml of 50 mM sodium borate buffer, pH 8.5, followed by 2×1.5 ml of H_2O and blown dry with a stream of air. The absorbed VIP was eluted with 2×3.5 ml acid methanol (2 ml of 12 N HCl in 1 liter of methanol), dried at 40°C with a stream of air for 45 to 55 min, and stored at −20°C before assay. For each run, a set of hormone-free plasma [prepared by charcoal treatment as described for secretin (2)], an internal control plasma, and recovery samples (3.9–39 nM in hormone-free plasma), were also processed through XAD-2 column for constructing the standard curve, assessing interassay variation and recovery correction factor, respectively. Immediately before the assay, the dried eluate was redissolved in 0.2 ml 0.01 N HCl and then diluted with 0.8 ml of 50 mM sodium phosphate buffer, pH 7.0, containing 1% BSA, 0.02% NaN_3, and 50 μg/ml protamine (reconstitution buffer).

RADIOIMMUNOASSAY PROCEDURES

Routine RIA was carried out in 13×100 mm glass culture tubes. Added into each tube was 0.4 ml of reconstituted XAD-2 eluate from samples or hormone-free plasma, 0.2 ml of reconstituted buffer containing 0 and 0.89 to 148 fmoles unlabeled VIP standard (prepared fresh by dilution from 5 μg/ml stock solution), and 0.7 ml of diluted anti-VIP serum (1:233,000 in a buffer the same as the reconstituted buffer except that it contained only 0.1% BSA and also 476 KIU/ml Trasylol). The mixture was incubated for 48 hr at 4°C and then mixed with 0.2 ml of ^{125}I-VIP (7–10 fmoles, approximately 5,000 cpm) diluted in the reconstitution buffer and further incubated for another 48 hr before separating bound and free counts by dextran- and plasma-coated charcoal and counted as described for secretin (2). Blank tubes containing XAD-2 eluate of hormone-free plasma (for standard curve) and each individual subject or experimental animal (obtained by pooling excess eluate from each subject and animal) were also incubated to correct for nonspecific binding. Both protamine and BSA were required to keep blank value low.

Calculation of data followed the same procedure as described in the section on secretin RIA.

RELIABILITY OF THE ASSAY

The 95% confidence detection limit was 0.15 pM (0.74 pg/tube) for the present assay. The average recovery of VIP from XAD-2 eluate varied, with batches of XAD-2 resin ranging from 57 to 83%. The mean recovery ± standard deviation from 10 assays was 70.5 ± 5.9% for ^{125}I-VIP and 69.3 ± 9.5% for the unlabeled VIP at 29.6 pM. Recovery from column to column, however, was more constant with coefficient of variation less than 10% and was essentially the same for all the concentrations tested (Table 1). The overall assay sensitivity

TABLE 1. *Comparison of recovery of VIP from XAD-2 column and ethanol extract*

VIP concentration	Recovery from	
	XAD-2 %	Ethanol %
pM		
3.0	55.8 ± 10.0	32.7 ± 4.5
4.4	56.9 ± 6.9	45.3 ± 13.0
7.4	50.5 ± 5.5	57.4 ± 13.6
14.8	57.0 ± 3.4	46.6 ± 2.6
29.6	61.0 ± 2.8	52.8 ± 3.5
73.9	58.5 ± 5.4	50.5 ± 2.5

Natural porcine VIP was added to 2 ml of dog hormone-free plasma to the final concentrations indicated and then processed through XAD-2 column or extract with 66% ethanol. Recovery of VIP in XAD-2 column eluates and ethanol extracts were estimated by RIA as described in ref. 3. Independent standard curves were run by adding corresponding eluates or extracts of hormone-free plasma into assay tubes of standards. The results are presented as mean ± SD from sextuple column eluates or extracts.

with correction of the minimum recovery of 57% was 0.48 pM (1.62 pg/ml plasma). The mean plasma VIP concentration in 78 normal fasting subjects was 5.7 ± 3.4 pM (±SD), with a range of 0 to 15.1 pM, which was comparable to 7.3 pM reported by Fahrenkrug and Schaffalitzky de Muckadell (4), who used ethanol extraction (66% v/v) to reduce interfering substance. We found recovery of VIP by ethanol extraction was slightly lower (Table 1), and the 95% confidence detection limit was reduced to 2.4 pg/tube under the same assay conditions, presumably due to the presence of residual interfering substance in the extract. No significant interference substance remained in the XAD-2

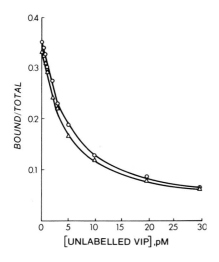

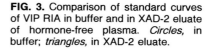

FIG. 3. Comparison of standard curves of VIP RIA in buffer and in XAD-2 eluate of hormone-free plasma. *Circles,* in buffer; *triangles,* in XAD-2 eluate.

eluate as a parallel and almost superimposed standard curves were obtained with XAD-3 eluate and buffer alone (Fig. 3).

REFERENCES

1. Bodanszky, M., Klausner, Y. S., Yand, L. S., Mutt, V., and Said, S. I. (1974): Synthesis of the vasoactive intestinal polypeptide (VIP). *J. Am. Chem. Soc.,* 96:4973–4978.
2. Chang, T.-M., and Chey, W. Y. (1980): Radioimmunoassay of secretin. In: *Gastrointestinal Hormones,* edited by G. B. J. Glass, pp. 797–806. Raven Press, New York.
3. Chang, T.-M., Roth, F., Tai, H. H., and Chey, W. Y. (1979): Radioimmunoassay of vasoactive intestinal polypeptide. *Anal. Biochem.,* 97:286–297.
4. Fahrenkrug, J., and Schaffalitzky de Muckadell, O. B. (1977): Radioimmunoassay of vasoactive intestinal polypeptide (VIP) in plasma. *J. Lab. Clin. Med.,* 89:1379–1388.
5. Modlin, I. M., Mitchell, S. J., and Bloom, S. R. (1978): The systemic release and pharmacokinetics of VIP. In *Gut Hormones,* edited by S. R. Bloom, pp. 470–474. Churchill Livingstone, Edinburgh/London/New York.
6. Mutt, V., and Said, S. I. (1974): Structure of the porcine vasoactive intestinal octacosapeptide. *Eur. J. Biochem.,* 42:581–589.
7. Said, S. I. (1978): VIP: Overview. In *Gut Hormones,* edited by S. R. Bloom, pp. 465–469. Churchill Livingstone, Edinburgh/London/New York.
8. Said, S. I., and Mutt, V. (1970): Polypeptide with broad biological activity: Isolation from small intestine. *Science,* 169:1217–1218.
9. Schaffalitzky de Muckadell, O. B., Fahrenkrug, J., and Holst, J. J. (1977): Release of vasoactive intestinal polypeptide (VIP) by electric stimulation of the vagal nerves. *Gastroenterology,* 72:373–375.
10. Tai, H. H., and Chey, W. Y. (1978): Development of radioimmunoassay for motilin. *Anal. Biochem.,* 87:350–358.
11. Thorell, J. I., and Johansson, B. G. (1971): Enzymatic iodination of polypeptides with ^{125}I to high specific activity. *Biochem. Biophys. Acta,* 251:363.

III. MOTILIN

Motilin, a polypeptide of 22 amino acid residues, was first isolated from duodenal mucosa and subsequently sequenced by Brown and co-workers (1,2,8). Motilin or its analog, norleucine[13]-motilin, has been synthesized and shown to possess a broad spectrum of biological activities (9,11,12). Nevertheless, its physiological role in the gastrointestinal tract still remains to be established. A sensitive RIA of motilin has been developed recently in our laboratory (10) and should be useful for elucidating the physiological role of this peptide.

PRODUCTION OF ANTI-MOTILIN SERA

Motilin antisera were produced by immunization of randomly bred New Zealand white rabbits with synthetic porcine motilin (from Dr. H. Yajima, University of Kyoto, Japan) conjugated to bovine serum albumin (BSA). Motilin (0.5 mg) and BSA (1.0 mg) were dissolved in 1.2 ml of distilled water and then mixed with 0.2 ml of 1-ethyl-3-(3-dimethyl aminopropyl) carbodiimide hydrochloride (5.0 mg) in H_2O. After being stirred for 20 hr at 20°C, the reaction mixture was dialyzed at 4°C against 2 liters of 0.15 M NaCl buffered with 0.01 M potassium phosphate buffer, pH 7.4. The dialyzed conjugate was then emulsified in equal volume of complete Freund's adjuvant and divided into two equal portions and injected into the rear foot pads of each rabbit. After the first three monthly injections of the full dose, the rabbits received 1/10 of the initial dose at monthly intervals until termination of the booster was desired. The animals were bled by venous puncture of the ears 2 weeks after each immunization to obtain antisera. The titer of antibody usually reached a plateau after six immunizations and was maintained by further booster. Our antiserum of highest titer was 1:187,000 to bind 50% of 2.0 fmoles ^{125}I-motilin. The binding parameters determined as described in secretin RIA (3) were: effective affinity constant (K_{eff}), 1.5×10^{12} M^{-1}, heterogeneity index (α), 0.71; and average affinity constant (K_o), 3.4×10^{11} M^{-1}. No cross-reactivity was found for natural porcine secretin, VIP, CCK-PZ, GIP, and human gastrin I (synthetic) at concentrations as high as 10 ng/ml (3.7 nM).

PREPARATION OF ^{125}I-MOTILIN

Motilin contains one tyrosine residue and thus is readily iodinated either by the chloramine T method of Hunter and Greenwood (6) or the lactoperoxidase method of Thorell and Johansson (11). We generally used the former method. Carrier-free Na ^{125}I] (Amersham) (1 mCi) in 10 μl of 0.1 N NaOH was first mixed with 50 μl of motilin (1 μg) in 0.5 M sodium phosphate buffer. After 30 sec at room temperature, the reaction was stopped by adding 50 μl of sodium metabisulfite (250 μg) in the diluted phosphate buffer. The reaction mixture was then diluted with 4 ml of H$_2$O, adjusted to pH 6.0 with 1 N HCl, and immediately loaded onto a CM-Sephadex C-25 column (1 × 20 cm) previously equilibrated with 0.5% BSA in H$_2$O. The column was washed with 20 ml of 0.5% BSA and then eluted with a gradient of 100 ml in each reservoir of 0.5% BSA and 0.3 M ammonium acetate in 0.5% BSA, pH 5.9. Fractions of 2.2 ml were collected and both radioactivity and immunoreactivity were monitered. The major radioactivity peak eluted near the end of gradient contained the most immunoreactive ^{125}I]-motilin and could be stored at −20°C. The product usually has specific radioactivity of 400 to 500 μCi/μg by the self-displacement method and over 90% of the counts were bindable by excess antibody.

COLLECTION AND PROCESSING OF PLASMA SAMPLES

Plasma samples were collected according to the same procedure described in secretin RIA (3) and stored at −20°C in 1 ml aliquots in the presence of Trasylol (500 KIU/ml plasma) until assay. Before the assay, plasma samples were extracted with methanol to remove interfering substances. Briefly, 1 ml of plasma sample was mixed thoroughly with an equal volume of methanol, left in an ice bath for 15 min, and then centrifuged at 2,000 × g and 4°C for 25 min. Without decantating the supernatant, 3 ml of methanol was added to the tube and mixed gently with the supernatant to avoid disturbing the pellet, left in ice for another 20 min, and then centrifuged again. The final supernatant solution was then transfered to another test tube and dried at 40°C under a stream of air. The residue, usually stored at −20°C overnight, was then redissolved in 0.5 ml of 0.05 M Tris HCl, pH 7.8, containing 1% BSA and 0.02% NaN$_3$ and duplicate samples of 0.2 ml were assayed. This two-step extraction method resulted in removal of more protein from plasma than the previously reported one-step extraction (10), and the residue gave a clearer solution on resolution. Samples of hormone-free plasma, recovery standards in hormone-free plasma (50, 100, and 200 pg/ml), and control plasma were also extracted with methanol so as to construct a standard curve and to calculate recovery factor and interassay variation. Hormone-free plasma was prepared as described in the section on secretin RIA (3).

CONDITIONS OF INCUBATIONS

The incubation mixture (1.5 ml) containing 0.2 ml of standard motilin (in reconstitution buffer) or reconstitution buffer alone (samples); 0.2 ml reconstituted methanol extract of hormone-free plasma (for standards) or sample; 0.9 ml diluted antiserum (in 0.05 M Tris-HCl, pH 7.8, containing 0.1% BSA, 0.02% NaN_3), 0.2 ml ^{125}I-motilin (approximately 5,000 cpm, 2.0 fmoles) was incubated at 4° for 48 hr. Bound and free counts were then separated by adding plasma- and dextran-coated charcoal and counted as described for secretin (3).

RELIABILITY OF THE ASSAY

The 95% confidence detection limit defined as 2 SD/m according to Feldman and Rodbard (5) (SD, the standard deviation of measuring bound to total ratio

TABLE 1. *Recovery of motilin from methanol extract*

Concentration (pg/ml)	Recovery %
50	66.1 ± 7.6
100	68.9 ± 7.7
200	66.1 ± 7.6

Native motilin was added to dog hormone-free plasma at indicated concentrations; the plasma was extracted with methanol and assayed as described in the text. The data represent results of eight runs presented as mean ± SE. The overall average ($n = 24$) at all concentrations was 67.9 ± 8.7%.

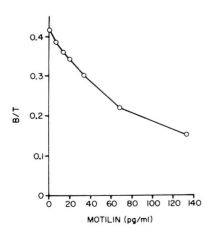

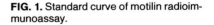

FIG. 1. Standard curve of motilin radioimmunoassay.

at zero dose; m, the initial slope of the dose-response curve as shown in Fig. 1) was 6.8 pg/tube, which was equivalent to 25.0 pg/ml plasma, considering an average recovery of motilin of 67.9% from methanol extract (Table 1). The recovery was consistent for all concentrations tested (Table 1). A human plasma assayed in 5 runs yielded 71.5 ± 10.1 pg/ml (mean ± SD), giving a coefficient of variation of 14%. Thus, the present assay is qualitatively similar to that reported by Dryburgh and Brown (4). Using this assay method, a relationship between cyclic changes in plasma immunoreactive motilin concentration and interdigestive myoelectric activity of the duodenum has been demonstrated (7).

REFERENCES

1. Brown, J. C., Cook, M. A., and Dryburgh, J. R. (1973): Motilin, a gastric motor activity stimulating polypeptide: The complete amino acid sequence. *Can. J. Biochem.,* 51:533–537.
2. Brown, J. C., Mutt, V., and Dryburgh, J. R. (1971): The further purification of motilin, a gastric motor activity stimulating polypeptide from the mucosa of the small intestine of hogs. *Can. J. Physiol. Pharmacol.,* 49:399–405.
3. Chang, T. M., and Chey, W. Y. (1980): Radioimmunoassay of secretin. In: *Gastrointestinal Hormones,* edited by G. B. J. Glass, pp. 797–806. Raven Press, New York.
4. Dryburgh, J. R., and Brown, J. C. (1975): Radioimmunoassay for motilin. *Gastroenterology,* 68:1169–1176.
5. Feldman, H., and Rodbard, D. (1971): Mathematical theory of radioimmunoassay. In: *Principles of Competitive Protein-Binding Assays,* edited by W. D. Odell and W. H. Doughaday, pp. 158–199. J. B. Lippincott, Philadelphia and Toronto.
6. Hunter, W. M., and Greenwood, F. C. (1962): Preparation of iodine-131 labeled human growth hormone of high specific activity. *Nature,* 194:495–496.
7. Lee, K. Y., Chey, W. Y., Tai, H. H., and Yajima, H. (1978): Radioimmunoassay of motilin: Validation and studies on the relationship between plasma motilin and interdigestive myoelectric activity of the duodenum of dog. *Am. J. Dig. Dis.,* 23:789–795.
8. Ruppin, H., and Domschke, W. (1980): Gastrointestinal hormones and motor function of the gastrointestinal tract. In: *Gastrointestinal Hormones,* edited by G. B. J. Glass, pp. 587–612. Raven Press, New York.
9. Schubert, H., and Brown, J. C. (1974): Correction to the amino acid sequence of porcine motilin. *Can. J. Biochem.,* 52:7–8.
10. Tai, H. H., and Chey, W. Y. (1978): Development of radioimmunoassay for motilin. *Anal. Biochem.,* 87:350–358.
11. Thorell, J. I., and Johansson, B. G. (1971): Enzymatic iodination of polypeptides with ^{125}I to high specific activity. *Biochem. Biophys. Acta,* 251:363–369.
12. Wünsch, E., Brown, J. C., Deimer, K. H., Drees, F., Jaeger, E., Muciol, J., Schart, R., Stocker, H., Thamm, P., and Wendleberger, G. (1973): The total synthesis of nor-leucine-13-motilin. *Z. Naturforsch.,* 28:235–240.
13. Yajima, H., Kai, Y., and Kawatani, H. (1975): Synthesis of docosapeptide corresponding to the entire amino acid sequence of porcine motilin. *J. Chem. Soc. Chem. Commun.,* 150–160.

SUMMARY

Sensitive RIA procedures for secretin, VIP, and motilin in plasma have been discussed with respect to production and characterization of antisera, preparation of fully immunoreactive radioiodinated peptides, and elimination of plasma interference factor or factors, as well as the incubation conditions. Specific antibodies against these peptides have been generally produced in rabbits after repeated immunization with peptides conjugated with bovine serum albumin. Characterization of the antibody has been achieved by proper equilibrium binding studies. Radioiodinated secretin and motilin can be successfully prepared by the chloramine T method, whereas VIP should be iodinated by the lactoperoxidase method. Each labeled peptide can be purified by specific purification procedures with gel filtration in conjunction with ion-exchange chromatography. The important effect of plasma interference on the results of these RIA(s) has been determined for each assay. Under the specified assay conditions, the final assay sensitivity of 1.4, 1.62, and 25.0 pg/ml in plasma for secretin, VIP, and motilin, respectively, has been achieved.

PROJECTIONS FOR THE FUTURE

During the past decade, RIA techniques for various gastrointestinal hormones have been reported. The detailed information about specificity and binding affinity of the antibodies, however, has rarely been obtained. Also, the importance of the effect of plasma interference on the results of each assay has been realized only recently. In the past, the failure to deal with plasma interference has led to reports of substantial differences in plasma hormone concentrations among investigators. It is hoped that the methodology discussed in this chapter will be helpful in realization of the importance of these aspects of the RIA. With the present sensitive assay methods, it is now possible to demonstrate a postprandial rise in plasma secretin concentration that correlates with the stimulation of pancreatic flow and bicarbonate secretin.

It is believed that in the near future the roles of secretin in various physiological and pathophysiological states will be more clearly established than in the past. The sensitive RIA for VIP will undoubtedly facilitate exploration in the future of the role of this peptide under normal and pathological conditions. The assay of motilin, although less sensitive than that of secretin and VIP, has enabled us to demonstrate cyclic changes in plasma concentration that may be related to the motor activity of the gastrointestinal tract and, thus, will assist in the exploration of the biological functions of this peptide. It is believed that in the future a higher sensitivity assay of this peptide will be developed through production of antiserum of a higher titer than that presently available.

Gastrointestinal Hormones, edited by
George B. Jerzy Glass.
Raven Press, New York © 1980.

Chapter 35

Radioimmunoassays of Cholecystokinin and Gastric Inhibitory Peptide

* Vay Liang W. Go and ** Chung Owyang

* Mayo Medical School, Gastroenterology Unit, Mayo Clinic, Rochester, Minnesota 55901; and ** Gastroenterology Research Unit, The University of Michigan Medical School, Ann Arbor, Michigan 48109

I. CHOLECYSTOKININ (CCK)

Problem

Although CCK was discovered more than 50 years ago (Ivy and Oldberg, 1928), and the method of radioimmunoassays (RIA) about 30 years ago (Berson and Yalow, 1950) the development of the RIA of CCK has been slow. The several RIAs for CCK that have been published (17,18,22,27,28,39,40) failed to give a reliable value for CCK concentration in human blood. The values are much higher than would be expected from the known biological properties of this hormone. Several factors have contributed to the problem (21). These include: (a) nonavailability of pure human CCK; (b) difficulty in preparing labeled hormone (the only tyrosine residue in porcine CCK is sulfated); (c) instability of labeled and unlabeled hormone in solution; (d) the relatively low immunogenic potency of CCK; (e) high degree of cross-reactivity with gastrin by many antibodies; (f) heterogenicity of CCK (43); and (g) the lack of a reference preparation for use as a working standard. As a result, various laboratories have used different preparations of CCK for labeling, for production of antisera, and for working standards in setting up the assay. This multiplicity of problems has resulted in a lack of agreement among reported values for CCK in the peripheral circulation. Recently Rehfeld developed a sequence-specific RIA for porcine CCK that allows the elucidation of the molecular-heterogeneity of CCK in both brain and gut tissue (44,45).

Radioimmunoassay

In developing a specific RIA of CCK, a highly purified radiolabeled CCK is essential. Recently, a 99% pure preparation of porcine CCK was made available for radiolabeling purposes by Dr. Victor Mutt of the Karolinska Institute, Stockholm, Sweden. In the past, CCK was labeled with ^{125}I or ^{131}I, using the chloramine-T method of Hunter and Greenwood (see ref. 24). However, the specific activities obtained were much lower than those obtained with other gastrointestinal hormones, such as gastrin and glucagon. This was probably due to the fact that the only tyrosine in CCK is sulfated, and this factor renders incorporation of iodine most difficult. To overcome this problem, nonsulfated synthetic analogs or the CCK-39 (containing a nonsulfated tyrosine at the N-terminal) might be used. Radiolabeling of these peptides provides reasonably specific activity; however, they still display such poor immunoreactivity that they cannot be used in any reliable RIA (42). The basic problem is that the CCK molecule and its variant contain three methionyl residues that are so easily sulfoxidized that the radiolabeling procedure may produce subtle damage to the CCK molecule. This leads to a loss of affinity in the labeled antigen for the antibody, since mild oxidates in the conventional iodination procedure (utilizing chloramine-T lactoperoxidase) reduce the immunoreactivity of CCK by 70% to 100% (44).

We recently attempted to overcome this problem (20) by using the modified Bolton and Hunter method (3,20,44), which does not involve any oxidation of the CCK molecule. This technique involves the reaction, under mild conditions, of the peptide hormone with N-hydroxysuccinimide ester of 3-C-4-hydroxyphenyl proprionic acid that has previously been labeled with ^{125}I. The esters react with the free amino groups of the peptides to form amides. This method offers an obvious advantage in that it avoids damage to the peptides, due to direct exposure to ^{125}I, or due to agents or conditions used in the iodination. Using this method, we have obtained stable tracers with high specific activity and immunoreactivity, which are unchanged, from unlabeled CCK-33.

CCK appears to be relatively nonimmunogenic. Using various preparations of porcine CCK (either conjugated to albumin or unconjugated as immunogens), antisera have been obtained in chickens, guinea pigs, and rabbits. These antisera are usually of a low titer. Recently, however, Rehfeld (42) reported CCK-antisera of high quality that were readily produced in guinea pigs, without a previous coupling of CCK to carriers. Another problem with CCK antisera is the frequent cross-reactivity with gastrin. This occurs because both gastrin and CCK share a common biologically active carboxyl terminal pentapeptide sequence (-Gly-

Trp-Met-Asp-Phe-NH$_2$), which is strongly antigenic. To overcome this problem, one may use antisera against a region of the CCK molecule that is specific in this hormone. However, such antisera would recognize the nonbiologically active portion of CCK; therefore, the immunological activity that one measures may not necessarily correlate with the biological activity that one wishes to measure.

Currently, there are no standard reference preparations of gastrointestinal peptide hormones. The crude CCK (20% pure preparation from Karolinska Institute or Boot's preparation) is not satisfactory for repeated use as a standard in the assay system, because of variation in the quoted potency per unit weight, and the different immunological activities that are present in different crude preparations of CCK. The latter observation may explain the discrepancies in values obtained by various published RIA systems. Ideally, therefore, 99% pure porcine CCK with a biological activity of 3,000 Ivy dog units/mg should be used as a reference standard.

Serum Levels

Because of the problems listed above, the reported fasting serum CCK levels vary tremendously. Although the postprandial levels were elevated in all reported studies, the time course and the magnitude differed widely. Rayford et al. (38), using an RIA where 99% pure CCK was employed both as labeled antigen and as a reference standard, reported a mean basal CCK concentration of 731 ± 81 pg/ml. Fifteen minutes after ingestion of a protein meal, CCK levels increased to 912 pg/ml and remained elevated above the basal level until the end of the 240-min test period. Their data differed quite significantly from that of Harvey (27), who reported CCK levels that increased from basal rates of less than 100 pg/ml to levels of 8 to 16 ng/ml within 35 min and declined rapidly to basal values within 45 min postprandially. Recently, using an improved CCK RIA, we reported a mean basal CCK concentration of 150 ± 17 pg/ml (33) that rose rapidly postprandially, reaching a peak between 15 and 30 min, and remained elevated above basal for prolonged periods of time *(unpublished data)*.

No fully documented CCK tumors have yet been described. Rayford et al. (38) found very high fasting serum CCK levels (in the range of 2,000 pg/ml) in postoperative patients with Zollinger-Ellison syndrome. Although gastrin cross-reacted very slightly with their CCK antibody, they found no correlation between high levels of gastrin and high levels of CCK in these patients, suggesting absolute hypercholecystokininemia in patients with Zollinger-Ellison syndrome. Conceivably, the CCK may have originated from a tumor that may have produced both gastrin and CCK. Unfortunately, there were no immunocytochemical studies on the tumors to substantiate this possibility.

It is also interesting to note that Harvey et al. (27) and Low-Beer et al. (33) reported very high fasting levels of CCK (2.9–15 ng/ml) in patients with pancreatic exocrine insufficiency and celiac disease. Many studies have indicated the presence of a feedback system in the secretion of CCK, probably mediated by trypsin. For example, it has been shown that diversion of pancreatic juice from the intestinal tract results in spontaneous pancreatic hypersecretion (23,25). Trypsin inhibitors in the gut similarly evoke increased pancreatic enzyme secretion (26,30). On the other hand, both trypsin and chymotrypsin, when infused into the gut, suppress the excessive pancreatic enzyme secretion in rats with pancreatic fistulae (23). Thus, it seems probable that the elevated fasting levels of CCK in patients with pancreatic exocrine insufficiency may result from the absence of a normal negative feedback of CCK secretion by pancreatic enzymes. Recently, Polak et al. (37) reported that hyperplasia of CCK cells in small intestine mucosa occurred in patients with chronic pancreatitis. This situation is reminiscent of that seen in patients with achlorhydria, who have a hyperplasia of G cells and elevated concentrations of serum gastrin resulting from a failure of feedback inhibition of gastrin secretion by gastric acid. If this observation is confirmed, then measurement of fasting serum CCK level may provide a sensitive test of pancreatic insufficiency. The cause of the unexpected finding of high levels of CCK in patients with celiac disease is currently unknown (33).

Metabolic Fate

Precise studies on the catabolism of CCK have been difficult due to the lack of specific and sensitive assay systems that measure changes in circulating levels of the hormone. Recently Rayford et al. (38) reported the disappearance half-time of porcine CCK from the circulation in man to be 2.44 min. This result is in good agreement with the half-time of 2.59 min for exogenous CCK in dogs as reported by Reeder et al. (41). We (34) recently have determined the metabolic clearance and tissue distribution of CCK in guinea pigs after a pulse injection of ^{125}I CCK [prepared by conjugating 99% pure CCK with the succinimide ester of ^{125}I-P-hydroxyphenyl proprionic acid according to the Bolton-Hunter method (3)]. The half-life of ^{125}I CCK, as determined by measuring the serum immunoprecipitable ^{125}I CCK with CCK antibodies in an RIA system, is 3 min. Tissue distribution studies show a preferential uptake of ^{125}I CCK by the kidneys, liver, stomach, intestine, pancreas, gallbladder, lungs, and the spleen. At 8 min after injection, the kidneys concentrated about half of the total dose of labeled CCK administered. This suggests that the kidneys may play an important role in the catabolism of this hormone. Further studies (32,49) on the fate of CCK in transit through the kidney in dogs demonstrated that the kidney extracted slightly more than one-third of the total CCK presented to it, and that the renal handling of CCK is characterized by high extraction rates and low urinary clearance. More recently, we (33) further demonstrated that the fasting serum CCK concentrations were significantly elevated in patients with renal failure, where serum creatinine was greater than 3 mg/dl and serum concentration of CCK was significantly correlated with the degree of renal insufficiency. The elevated serum CCK is probably responsible for the pancreatic trypsin hypersecretion observed in these patients. The chronic hypercholecystokininemia may also have a trophic influence on the exocrine pancreas, and probably accounts for the greatly enhanced pancreatic exocrine capacity in chronic renal failure.

Heterogeneity

As with gastrin, CCK appears to be heterogenous. Using region-specific RIAs of CCK with antisera specific to region 18–25, 25–30 and 29–33 of CCK-33, Rehfeld (43) recently demonstrated the presence of multiple molecular forms of CCK in the intestine and cerebral cortex of man and pig. The cerebral cortex consists mainly of two small molecular forms, one corresponding to the COOH-terminal octapeptide, and another even smaller COOH-terminal peptide, corresponding to region 30–33 of CCK-33. The intestinal CCK appears to be even more heterogenous. It consists of four main forms, each of which is further heterogenous. However, in both tissue extracts, the predominating CCK-immunoreactive component corresponds to the COOH-terminal octapeptide of CCK. According to these results, it is quite likely that CCK-octapeptide may well be the principal active circulating CCK molecule, and that other larger molecular forms may represent its biosynthetic precursors. An enzyme has now been partially purified from canine and porcine cerebral cortical extracts, by Straus, Malesci, and Yalow, that differs from trypsin that converts CCK to smaller immunoreactive forms of CCK (46). Straus and Yalow recently reported that genetically obese mice with hyperphagia have less immunoreactive CCK in their cerebral cortex than their nonobese littermates. They suggested that the lower amount of CCK in the brain may be causally related to the unrestrained appetite of the obese mice (47). Further studies on the molecular forms of CCK in blood under basal and stimulated states and the biosynthesis of CCK are needed to clarify the role of various CCKs in the gastrointestinal tract.

Summary and Projections for the Future

Due to various problems enumerated earlier, great difficulty has been encountered in the development of sensitive and specific RIAs for CCK. The earlier reported assays have resulted in considerable interlaboratory disagreement on values of CCK in circulation. Over the last few years, with increased experience, some of the major problems have been overcome. This has resulted in a RIA that is quite specific for CCK, with the necessary degree of sensitivity to measure physiological levels of this hormone in animals and in man. However, in view of the problems of heterogenicity, nonequivalence of biological activity and immunoreactivity of the different CCKs, and potential cross-reactivity of gastrin in the assays, CCK RIA will continue to be rather difficult to standardize in the foreseeable future.

II. GASTRIC INHIBITORY POLYPEPTIDE (GIP)

Radioimmunoassay

Shortly following the isolation, purification, and structural determination of porcine GIP, a RIA for GIP was successfully developed by Kuzio et al. (29) in Brown's laboratory. Porcine GIP is used for iodination, and to raise antisera in guinea pigs. The sensitivity range is reported between 25 and 250 pg. Dilution of human serum with either diluent buffer or charcoal-extracted serum that is compared with a standard curve shows parallelism, suggesting a good cross-reactivity between human and porcine GIP. No cross-reactivity could be demonstrated with gastrin, glucagon, secretin, CCK, motilin, and VIP.

Heterogeneity

As with gastrin and CCK, GIP has been shown to circulate in more than one molecular form (6), and the same is true in tissue extracts (13). Column chromatography of postprandial serum of man revealed two peaks of immunoreactive GIP (6). The major component corresponded to ^{125}I-labeled GIP (M. W. of 5,000), and a minor component appeared between the void volume and ^{125}I-labeled polypeptide. Whether these different, but immunologically identical, substances are preferentially released in response to different secretagogues, and whether they have different physiological effects is currently being investigated.

Localization

RIA of tissue extracts and indirect immunofluorescence studies have demonstrated that GIP is localized in the gastrointestinal tract. In man the highest concentrations of GIP were found in the duodenum and jejunum (36). Functional localization of GIP distribution correlated well with anatomical distribution. Using an occluding balloon intestinal perfusion technique and glucose as the stimulus for GIP release, Thomas et al. (46) demonstrated that the GIP secretion was greatest in duodenal perfusion as compared with proximal jejunum perfusion, and secretion decreased markedly as one progressed distally towards the ileum.

Serum Levels

RIA has been applied to the investigation of circulating levels of GIP in man in order to identify a specific secretagogue for its release. Kuzio et al. (29) reported a fasting level of GIP in man of approximately 200 pg/ml. Following a standard breakfast, a biphasic type of response was observed in the circulating GIP levels. The first peak occurred approximately 45 min postprandially, reaching an average circulating level of over 1200 pg/ml. The serum level fell slightly and then remained significantly above normal for more than 4 hr. A somewhat higher fasting level (400 pg/ml) and postprandial peak (3,500 pg/ ml) were later reported from the same laboratory (9), but the time course of the response between the two studies was not grossly different. All three nutrients—fat, glucose, and amino acid mixtures—have been shown to release GIP when ingested or given intraduodenally. Fat is the most potent, followed by glucose and amino acid mixtures (7). The response to glucose and fat is dose-dependent (8,35). The GIP response to oral fat differed significantly from oral glucose, not only in magnitude but also in timing. With glucose the response returned to basal within 180 min and the peak reached was rapid, preceding that of insulin (9). With fat ingestion the peak was reached at 120 to 150 min, but levels did not return to basal within 180 min (9). These differences are probably due to gastric emptying characteristics and the mode of absorption of various nutrients. The intraduodenal instillation of 30 g mixed amino acid solution also stimulated the release of GIP, although to a lesser degree as compared with the other secretagogues (45). In a subsequent study the same group of investigators (47) further demonstrated that the amino acids responsible for the release of GIP are different from the CCK-releasing amino acids as reported by Go et al. (19).

GIP appears to inhibit acid and pepsin secretion in dogs and man (5). The intraduodenal administration of Lipomul demonstrated a 90% inhibition of acid and pepsin output induced by prior pentagastrin injection. This correlated closely with the pattern of increased serum GIP levels during this time interval. In addition, intravenous injection of porcine GIP against a background of 50 to 70% plateau of acid secretion (induced by continuous intravenous administration of pentagastrin) also showed a significant (60%) inhibition of acid and pepsin (5). The serum levels of immunoreactive GIP attained after intraduodenal fat administration are in the range achieved by doses of exogenous porcine GIP capable of inhibiting acid secretion and motility. These observations suggest that GIP might have a physiological role in modulating postprandial gastric secretion and emptying. Furthermore, it has been speculated that an impairment in the release of GIP might be involved in the pathogenesis of gastric acid hypersecretion associated with peptic ulcer disease. However, the mean fasting GIP levels in ulcer patients were not found to be significantly different from healthy controls (7). An exaggerated GIP release following oral glucose (10) or test meal (7) was observed in this group of patients.

Incretin Effects

The incretin effect of GIP is demonstrated by the increased levels of insulin after release of GIP by oral glucose (5). The time course of events is compatible with the concept that GIP is taking part in the physiological regulation of insulin secretion. This, together with the demonstration of release of insulin after intravenous infusion of porcine GIP, further supports the insulinotropic action of GIP first observed by Dupré et al. (15). It is interesting to note that GIP release by oral Lipomul does not increase insulin in man, unless an insulin secretagogue is administered in conjunction with the fat (6). These observations suggest that GIP may be a mediator of the gastrointestinal phase of insulin secretion (enteroinsular axis). Recognition of this possibility prompted several laboratories to study GIP pathophysiology in disorders of carbohydrate metabolism. Subsequent studies revealed that in normal weight individuals with maturity-onset diabetes, the enteroinsular axis is considered to be functional or even overactive. Exaggerated immunoreactive GIP release was observed in non-insulin-dependent chemical diabetics (6), using a 50-g oral glucose tolerance test. A similar exaggeration in the response of obese diabetics was reported by Bloom (2) and Crockett et al. (12). Botha et al. (4) have recorded that fasting immunoreactive GIP rose in acquired pancreatic diabetes and that the response was exaggerated. This observation was confirmed by Ebert et al. (16). Vinik has further demonstrated that insulin treatment of patients with pancreatic diabetes lowered the fasting GIP concentration, but not the response to glucose *(personal communication)*. These observations have led Brown to speculate that the hyperresponse of serum GIP in diabetics to oral glucose or mixed meals may be due to impairment of feedback inhibition by insulin on GIP release, due to attenuated insulin secretion (6). He reported a blunting of serum GIP increases in nondiabetics given an intravenous bolus of insulin after ingestion of fat. Crockett's observation of reduced GIP response to fat ingestion in the face of hyperinsulinemia secondary to intravenous glucose infusion is consistent with a negative feedback role of insulin on GIP (11). However, Anderson et al. (1) reported that hyperinsulinemia concomitant with the clamping of blood glucose in the normal fasting range did not impair GIP increase in response to oral glucose. Since the release of GIP has been shown to be related to the rate and load of glucose absorption (8), the enhanced intestinal absorption of glucose commonly seen in the diabetic state may provide another explanation for the hyperresponse of serum GIP to oral glucose in diabetes. Currently the role of GIP in the pathogenesis of diabetes is uncertain. Whether the pathological secretion of GIP in diabetes is a reflection of the diabetic state or whether GIP is playing a role in the pathogenesis of diabetes mellitus remains to be elucidated.

Excess production of GIP is also seen in other clinical conditions. Enormous elevation of GIP has been reported in juvenile hypoglycemic patients whose postprandial blood sugar decreased to less than 20 mg/100 ml (9). It has been speculated that elevated GIP levels may contribute to the overproduction of insulin by the beta cells of the pancreas. Elevation of serum GIP levels also occurs in patients with dumping symptoms after gastric surgery (48). The overproduction of insulin and decreased intestinal motility, secondary to excess GIP, may be responsible for the symptoms. In addition, patients with chronic renal failure have elevated fasting (30,32) and postprandial (30) serum GIP concentrations. This observation is consistent with the fact that the kidney plays an important role in the metabolism of GIP (30). However, the consequences of this elevated level of GIP on the carbohydrate metabolism in these patients requires further elucidation.

Conclusions and Projections for the Future

A specific and sensitive RIA of GIP is currently available. The use of this assay has revealed some important information on the physiology and pathophysiology in man. The recent demonstration that GIP is heterogenous introduces complications in the quantification of hormonal concentrations and their interpretations, but it also opens new pathways in our understanding of the mechanisms of synthesis and metabolism of this hormone. Obviously, further studies are needed to elucidate the physiological actions, mechanisms, and sites of release of the various molecular forms of GIP. Furthermore, the role of GIP in the enteroinsular axis requires further characterization. This will provide new information regarding the contribution of GIP to the pathogenesis of diabetes mellitus and a number of gastroenterological disorders where abnormalities of the enteroinsular axis (14) have been demonstrated or are reasonably expected to exist.

REFERENCES

1. Anderson, D. K., Brown, J. C., Tobin, T. D., and Andres, R. (1976): Gastric inhibitory polypeptide release after oral glucose and quantification of its normal role in insulin secretion. *Clin. Res.,* 24:455A (Abstr.).
2. Bloom, S. R. (1975): GIP in diabetes. *Diabetologia,* 11:334(A).
3. Bolton, A. E., and Hunter, W. M. (1973): The labelling of proteins and high specific radioactivities by conjugation to a ^{125}I-containing acylating agent. *Biochem. J.,* 122:529–538.
4. Botha, J. L., Vinik, A. I., and Brown, J. C. (1976): Gastric inhibitory polypeptide (GIP) in chronic pancreatitis. *J. Clin. Endocrinol. Metab.,* 42:791–797.
5. Brown, J. C., Dryburgh, J. R., Moccia, P., et al. (1975): The current status of GIP. In: *Gastrointestinal Hormones,* edited by J. C. Thompson, pp. 537–554. University of Texas Press, Austin.
6. Brown, J. C., Dryburgh, J. R., Ross, S. A., and Dupré, J. (1975): Identification and actions of gastric inhibitory polypeptide. *Recent Prog. Horm. Res.,* 31:487–532.
7. Cataland, S. (1978): Physiology of GIP in man. In: *Gut Hormones,* edited by S. R. Bloom, pp. 288–293. Churchill Livingstone, New York.
8. Cataland, S., Crockett, S. E., Brown, J. C., and Mazzaferri, E. L. (1974): Gastric inhibitory polypeptide (GIP) stimulation by oral glucose in man. *J. Clin. Endocrinol. Metab.,* 39:223–228.
9. Cleator, I. G. M., and Gourlay, R. H. (1975): Release of immunoreactive gastric inhibitory polypeptide by oral ingestion of food substances. *Am. J. Surg.,* 130:128–135.
10. Creutzfeldt, W., Ebert, R., Arnold, R., Becker, H. D., Borger, H. W., and Schafmeyer, A. (1977): Serum gastric inhibitory polypeptide (GIP) response in patients with duodenal ulcer (DU), dependence on glucose tolerance. *Gastroenterology,* 72:A-4, 814 (Abstr.).

11. Crockett, S. E., Cataland, S., Falko, J. M., and Mazzaferri, E. L. (1976): The insulinotropic effect of endogenous gastric inhibitory polypeptide in normal subjects. *J. Clin. Endocrinol. Metab.*, 42:1098–1103.

12. Crockett, S. E., Mazzaferri, E. L., and Cataland, S. (1976): Gastric inhibitory polypeptide (GIP) in maturity-onset diabetes mellitus. *Diabetes*, 25:931–935.

13. Dryburgh, J. R. (1976): Thesis: Immunological techniques in the investigation of the physiological functions of gastric inhibitory polypeptide and motilin. University of British Columbia.

14. Dupré, J. (1978): The entero-insular axis. In: *Gut Hormones*, edited by S. R. Bloom, pp. 303–309. Churchill Livingstone, New York.

15. Dupré, J., Ross, S. A., Watson, D., and Brown, J. C. (1973): Stimulation of insulin secretion by gastric inhibitory polypeptide in man. *J. Clin. Endocrinol.*, 37:826.

16. Ebert, R., Creutzfeldt,W., Brown, J. C., Frerichs, H., and Arnold, R. (1976): Response of gastric inhibitory polypeptide to test meal in chronic pancreatitis—relationship to endocrine and exocrine insufficiency. *Diabetologia*, 12:609–612.

17. Englert, E., Jr. (1973): Radioimmunoassay (RIA) of cholecystokinin (CCK). *Clin. Res.*, 21:207 (Abstr.).

18. Go, V. L. W., Cataland, S., and Reilly, W. M. (1974): Radioimmunoassay (RIA) of cholecystokinin-pancreozymin (CCK-PZ) in human serum. *Gastroenterology*, 66:700 (Abstr.).

19. Go, V. L. W., Hofman, A. F., and Summerskill, W. H. J. (1970): Pancreozymin bioassay in man based on pancreatic enzyme secretion. Potency of specific amino acids and other digestive products. *J. Clin. Invest.*, 49:1558–1564.

20. Go, V. L. W., and Owyang, C. (1977): Radioimmunoassay of gastrointestinal hormones. In: *Progress in Gastroenterology, Vol. III*, edited by G. B. J. Glass, pp. 153–178. Grune & Stratton, New York.

21. Go, V. L. W., and Reilly, W. M. (1975): Problems encountered in the development of the cholecystokinin radioimmunoassay. In: *Gastrointestinal Hormones*, edited by J. C. Thompson, pp. 295–299. University of Texas Press, Austin.

22. Go, V. L. W., Ryan, R. J., and Summerskill, W. H. J. (1971): Radioimmunoassay of porcine cholecystokinin-pancreozymin. *J. Lab. Clin. Med.*, 77:684–689.

23. Green, G. M., and Lyman, R. L. (1972): Feedback regulation of pancreatic enzyme secretion as a mechanism for trypsin inhibitor-induced hypersecretion in rats. *Proc. Soc. Exp. Biol. Med.*, 140:6–12.

24. Greenwood, F. C., Hunter, W. M., and Gloven, J. S. (1963): The preparation of ^{131}I-labelled human growth hormone of high specific radioactivity. *Biochem. J.*, 89:114–123.

25. Grossman, M. I. (1958): Pancreatic secretion in the rat. *Am. J. Physiol.*, 194:535–539.

26. Haines, P. L., and Lyman, R. L. (1961): Relationship of pancreatic enzyme secretion by growth inhibition in rats fed soybean trypsin inhibition. *J. Nutrition*, 76:445–452.

27. Harvey, R. F., Dowsett, L., Hartog, M., and Read, A. E. (1973): A radioimmunoassay of cholecystokinin-pancreozymin. *Lancet*, ii:826–828.

28. Harvey, R. F., Dowsett, L., Hartog, M., and Read, A. E. (1974): A radioimmunoassay of cholecystokinin-pancreozymin. *Gut*, 15:690–699.

29. Kuzio, M., Dryburgh, J. R., Malloy, M., and Brown, J. C. (1974): Radioimmunoassay for gastric inhibitory polypeptide. *Gastroenterology*, 6:357–364.

30. Lyman, R. L., Wilcox, S. J., and Monsen, F. R. (1962): Pancreatic enzyme secretion produced in the rat by trypsin inhibitors. *Am. J. Physiol.*, 202:1077–1082.

31. O'Dorisio, T. M., Sirinek, K. R., Mazzaferri, E. L., and Cataland, S. E. (1977): Renal effects on serum gastric inhibitory polypeptide. *Metabolism*, 26:651–656.

32. Owyang, C., Dozois, R. R., and Go, V. L. W. (1976): Metabolism of cholecystokinin (CCK) in dog kidney. *Clin. Res.*, 24:536A.

33. Owyang, C., Go, V. L. W., DiMagno, E. P., Miller, L. J., and Brennan, L. A. (1977): Alteration of serum gastrointestinal hormone levels in renal insufficiency. *Gastroenterology*, 72:1110.

34. Owyang, C., Ng, P., and Go, V. L. W. (1976): Cholecystokinin: Metabolic clearance and tissue distribution. *Gastroenterology*, 70:925 (Abstr.).

35. Pederson, R. A., Schubert, M. E., and Brown, J. C. (1975): Gastric inhibitory polypeptide. Its physiologic release and insulinotropic action in the dog. *Diabetes*, 24:1050–1056.

36. Polak, J. M., Bloom, S. R., Kuzio, M., and Pearse, A. G. E. (1973): Cellular location of gastric inhibitory polypeptide in the duodenum and jejunum. *Gut*, 14:284–288.

37. Polak, J. M., Bloom, S. R., McCrossan, M. V., McCloy, R., South, L. M., Baron, J. H., and

Pearse, A. G. E. (1977): Abnormalities of endocrine cells in patients with duodenal ulceration (D.U.) and with chronic pancreatitis. *Gastroenterology,* 72:822.

38. Rayford, P. L., Fender, H. R., Ramus, N. I., Reeder, D. D., and Thompson, J. C. (1975): Release and half-life of CCK in man. In: *Gastrointestinal Hormones,* edited by J. C. Thompson, pp. 301–318. University of Texas Press, Austin.

39. Reeder, D. D., Becker, H. D., Smith, B. S., Rayford, P. L., and Thompson, J. C. (1972): Radioimmunoassay of cholecystokinin. *Surg. Forum,* 23:361–362.

40. Reeder, D. D., Becker, H. D., Smith, B. S., Rayford, P. L., and Thompson, J. C. (1973): Measurement of endogenous release of cholecystokinin by radioimmunoassay. *Ann. Surg.,* 178:304–310.

41. Reeder, D. D., Villar, H. V., Brandt, E. N., Rayford, P. L., and Thompson, J. C. (1974): Radioimmunoassay measurements of the disappearance half-time exogenous cholecystokinin. *Physiologist,* 17:319 (Abstr.).

42. Rehfeld, J. F. (1978): Problems in the technology of radioimmunoassays for gut hormones. In: *Gut Hormones,* edited by S. R. Bloom, pp. 112–119. Churchill Livingstone, New York.

43. Rehfeld, J. F. (1978): Multiple molecular forms of cholecystokinin. In: *Gut Hormones,* edited by S. R. Bloom, pp. 213–218. Churchill Livingstone, New York.

44. Rehfeld, J. F. (1978): Immunochemical studies on cholecystokinin. I. Development of sequence-specific radioimmunoassay for porcine triacontatriapeptide cholecystokinin. *J. Biol. Chem.,* 253:4016–4021.

45. Rehfeld, J. F. (1978): Immunochemical studies on cholecystokinin. II. Distribution and molecular heterogeneity in the central nervous system and small intestine of man and hog. *J. Biol. Chem.,* 253:4022–4030.

46. Straus, E., Malesci, A., and Yalow, R. S. (1978): Characterization of nontrypsin cholecystokinin converting enzyme in mammalian brain. *Proc. Natl. Acad. Sci. USA,* 75:5711–5714.

47. Straus, E., and Yalow, R. S. (1979): Cholecystokinin in the brains of obese and nonobese mice. *Science,* 203:68–69.

48. Thomas, F. B., Mazzaferri, E. L., Crockett, S. E., Mekhjian, H. S., Gruemer, H. D., and Cataland, S. (1976): Stimulation of secretion of gastric inhibitory polypeptide and insulin by intraduodenal amino acid perfusion. *Gastroenterology,* 70:523–527.

49. Thomas, F. B., Shook, D. F., O'Dorisio, T. M., Cataland, S., Mekhjian, H. S., Caldwell, J. H., and Mazzaferri, E. L. (1977): Localization of gastric inhibitory polypeptide release by intestinal glucose perfusion in man. *Gastroenterology,* 72:49–54.

50. Thomas, F. B., Sinar, D., Mazzaferri, E. L., Cataland, S., Mekhjian, H. S., Caldwell, J. H., and Fromkes, J. J. (1978): Selective release of gastric inhibitory polypeptide by intraduodenal amino acid perfusion in man. *Gastroenterology,* 74:1261–1265.

51. Thomford, N. P., Sirinak, K., Crockett, S., Mazzaferri, E. L., and Cataland, S. (1974): Gastric inhibitory polypeptide response to oral glucose after vagotomy and pyloroplasty. *Arch. Surg.,* 109 (2):177–182.

52. Thompson, J. C., Fender, H. R., Ramus, N. I., Villar, H. V., and Rayford, P. L. (1975): Cholecystokinin metabolism in man and dogs. *Ann. Surg.,* 182:496–504.

53. Young, J. D., Lazarus, L., Chisholm, D. J., and Atkinson, F. F. V. (1970): Radioimmunoassay of pancreozymin cholecystokinin in human serum. *J. Nucl. Med.,* 12:743–745.

Gastrointestinal Hormones, edited by
George B. Jerzy Glass.
Raven Press, New York © 1980.

Chapter 36

Radioimmunoassay of Gut Glucagon-like Immunoreactants

Alister J. Moody and Finn Sundby†

NOVO Research Institute, Novo Allé, DK 2880 Bagsvaerd, Denmark

INTRODUCTION

The discovery of the gut glucagon-like immunoreactants (GLIs), their distribution within the intestine, and their structural relationship to glucagon are described by Sundby and Moody *(this volume).* Gut GLIs are proteins or peptides of enteric origin that are immunochemically distinguishable from glucagon, but that react with many anti-glucagon sera. This chapter reviews the immunochemistry of gut GLIs, the radioimmunoassay (RIA) for gut GLIs, and the results obtained with this method. Readers are referred to Chapter 32 by Yalow and Straus (pp. 751–767, *this volume*) for a discussion of the principles and problems of RIA in general, and to the article by Heding (7) for a description of the methodology of the RIA for gut GLI.

IMMUNOCHEMISTRY

Immunochemistry of Glucagon

Glucagon has two main antigenic sites. One probably consists of the sequence 11–15 (17). This evokes antibodies that react with gut GLIs, mammalian and avian glucagons and that have been called N-terminal specific, cross-reacting, or nonspecific. The other antigenic site is located toward the C-terminal portion of glucagon, and probably consists of glucagon 24–29 (9). This elicits antibodies that react with mammalian glucagons and fragments of glucagon that contain the 24–29 immunoreactant, but that do not react with avian glucagons or gut GLIs. These antibodies are known as specific, glucagon specific, or C-terminal specific. In this chapter anti-glucagon sera that react with mammalian glucagons, avian glucagons, and gut GLIs are termed *anti-glucagon 11–15 sera*. The antisera that react with mammalian glucagons but that do not react with avian glucagons or gut GLIs are termed *anti-glucagon 24–29 sera*. The two types of antisera measure GLI 11–15 and GLI 24–29, respectively. The specificities of the two types of antisera and the sequences of the proposed antigenic sites are shown in Table 1.

Immunochemistry of Gut GLIs

The gut GLIs of a given species are probably formed by a progressive shortening of a common precursor. The porcine gut GLIs, for example, are envisaged as being extended or shortened versions of porcine glicentin, a porcine gut GLI (MW 11,625) with full molar reactivity with anti-glucagon 11–15 sera (25). Glicentin probably consists of a 60-amino acid sequence attached to the N-terminal of a 29 amino acid sequence identical to that of porcine glucagon (13). The C-terminal of the glucagon sequence is attached to a basic octapeptide. Gut GLIs react with anti-glucagon 11–15 sera because they contain a sequence

TABLE 1. *Antigenic sites of glucagon and the specificity of antiglucagon sera*

Antiserum type:	Anti-glucagon 11–15	Anti-glucagon 24–29
Antigenic site:	– 11– 12– 13– 14– 15– –Ser Lys Tyr Leu Asp–	– 24– 25– 26– 27– 28– 29– –Gln Trp Leu Met Asn Thr NH₂–
Reacts with:	Mammalian glucagon, avian glucagon, gut GLI	Mammalian glucagon

homologous with glucagon 11–15. Gut GLIs do not react with anti-glucagon 24–29 sera, despite the probability that they contain a sequence homologous with glucagon 24–29. In the case of glicentin, it has been proposed that the C-terminal octapeptide masks the immunoreactant corresponding to glucagon 24–29 (19). This proposal has been elegantly confirmed by Yanaihara *(personal communication),* who found that synthetic glucagon 17–29 coupled at its carboxyl end to the C-terminal octapeptide of glicentin does not react with an anti-glucagon 24–29 serum.

REAGENTS FOR THE RIA OF GUT GLIs

Standards

Porcine glucagon is the usual standard for the RIA of gut GLIs. If gut GLI is to be measured in whole plasma, the standards should be diluted in plasma that contains aprotinin and has been freed of GLI by treatment with activated charcoal, or by immunoabsorption. Plasma extracts should be dissolved in the same buffer as used for the preparation of the standards.

Samples

Crude gut extracts can be prepared from fresh or freshly frozen intestine either by direct extraction or by extraction of boiled tissues. Acid-alcohol (25) or acetic acid (11) can be used as extraction fluids. Nonspecific effects of the extract on the assay can be minimized by careful neutralization of the extract and adequate dilution of the extract before carrying out the assay. Blood gut GLI should be measured in plasma, prepared by drawing blood into ice-cold tubes containing heparin or EDTA and 500 KIE of aprotinin/ml blood (7). The assay of plasma gut GLI can be carried out on whole plasma or on plasma extracts. If gut GLI is assayed in whole plasma, then the standards must be diluted in plasma as described in the preceding section. The alcohol extraction procedure of Heding (7) has been used for many years in our laboratory. Losses of gut GLI and glucagon during the process are small (about 20%), and the procedure removes plasma proteins that could interfere in the subsequent assay. Acetone extraction, as described by Walters et al. (29), can also be used for the preparation of plasma extracts. Plasma extracts should be reconstituted in the same buffer as is used for the preparation of the standards.

Tracer

The tracer normally used is ^{125}I-labeled glucagon. Porcine glucagon, labeled by a modification of the chloramine-T method and purified by anion-exchange chromatography at 20°C (14), is routinely used in our laboratory.

Antisera

Anti-glucagon 11–15 sera should be selected for use in the RIA of gut GLIs by the following criteria:

(a) their sensitivity to standards and gut GLI;
(b) their relative affinity for the standards and for gut GLI;
(c) the inability of other gut peptides such as GIP, VIP, secretin, and pCCK to inhibit the binding of ^{125}I-glucagon to the antiserum; and
(d) their reactivity with high molecular weight plasma proteins and with the forms of gut GLI in plasma and tissue extracts.

An antiserum should be used for the assay of plasma GLI only if it has the following characteristics: a sensitivity such that the minimum detectable concentration of standard is less than 20 pmoles/liter of standard, an equal affinity for standard and gut GLI so that dilution curves of the standard and gut GLI are superimposable (8), and a negligible reactivity with peptides other than glucagon and gut GLIs.

Separation Procedure

Any procedure that provides satisfactory separation of antibody-bound ^{125}I-glucagon from free ^{125}I-glucagon can be used. In our laboratory the ethanol precipitation technique of Heding (7) has been used successfully for many years.

DESIGN OF THE RIA OF GUT GLIs

An anti-glucagon 11–15 serum can be used in two ways to estimate the gut GLI content of samples. In the first method, the RIA is carried out using the anti-glucagon 11–15 serum only. Anti-glucagon 11–15 sera react with glucagon as well as with gut GLIs, so the sample's content of GLI 11–15 (the total GLI) is the sum of the contributions from gut GLIs and from glucagon. Total GLI is an acceptable measure of gut GLI, provided that the GLI 11–15 attributable to glucagon is low and constant from sample to sample. Total GLI is thus a satisfactory measure of gut GLI in intestinal extracts, and in plasma from the venous drainage of the intestine. When significant amounts of GLI 11–15 are contributed by the A cell of the pancreas, and in particular when the level of secretion may change (e.g., in peripheral plasma after an oral glucose load), it is better to measure gut GLI rather than total GLI. This involves measuring the GLI 11–15 and the GLI 24–29 of the sample with two suitable anti-glucagon sera (7). The GLI 11–15 minus the GLI 24–29 is taken to be a measure of gut GLI, and the GLI 24–29 is taken to be a measure of the pancreatic glucagon in the sample.

Expression of Results

It is preferable to express the results of the RIA for gut GLI in molar equivalents of GLI, rather than in molar concentrations of glucagon, thus underlining that the structure of the material assayed is not known.

Limitations of the RIA for Gut GLI

The RIA for gut GLI has the limitations common to all RIAs in that it does not necessarily measure the biologically active forms of the peptides in plasma, and that plasma proteins inhibit the binding of the label to some antibodies. This latter problem is particularly severe with some anti-glucagon sera (23).

For this reason, if gut GLI is assayed in whole plasma the standards should be prepared in plasma. A more serious limitation is that the assay cannot be used to define the source of the GLIs measured. This problem is common to all RIAs, but it is especially critical in the RIA for gut GLI since the immunoreactivity measured could come from several organs in the body. Even the subtractive technique of Heding (7) does not specifically measure gut GLI. The assay measures GLI 11–15 minus GLI 24–29, and the prefix gut should be used only if there is good reason to assume that the excess GLI 11–15 does indeed come from the intestine. The measurement of gut GLI is very uncertain in fasting plasma, since the basal GLI 11–15 is probably a mixture of gut GLIs, glucagon, and glucagon fragments. After an oral glucose load, when a brisk release of gut GLIs into the mesenteric veins occurs (21), the increase in gut GLI measured by the subtractive technique is a reliable estimate of the peripheral increase in gut GLI.

RIA for Glicentin

This is the first RIA for gut GLI based on an antiserum against a pure gut GLI. Anti-glicentin sera were prepared in rabbits against glicentin coupled to human serum albumin with glutaraldehyde. One of the antisera, R 64, does not react with glucagon, secretin, VIP, PCCK, or GIP and probably reacts with the part of glicentin molecule that is outside the glucagon moiety. A RIA for glicentin using R 64, standards of glicentin, and ^{125}I-glicentin has been developed. The IR glicentin in extracts of porcine intestine was approximately the same as the GLI 11–15 (18). Porcine pancreas was also found to contain IR glicentin (18), confirming the demonstration of IR glicentin in the A cell of the pancreas by immunocytochemistry (20). Fasting levels of IR glicentin in pig plasma were found to be 100 pmoles/liter, and plasma IR glicentin was found to increase two- or threefold after feeding (17). The molecular form of plasma IR glicentin is not yet known.

RESULTS

Tissue Gut GLI

Gut GLI has been measured in the intestinal tracts of many animal species (see ref. 16 for a review). The highest concentrations of gut GLI are found in the lower small intestine and colon, in agreement with the distribution of the L cell in the intestinal mucosa (2). The several forms of gut GLIs found in intestinal extracts are probably native gut GLIs, traces of glucagon (22) and peptide derivatives formed during extraction (26) (Sundby and Moody, *this volume*).

Plasma Levels in Man

This section briefly reviews the values of plasma gut GLI and of plasma total GLI measured by different laboratories. The fasting levels of plasma total GLI and gut GLI in man range from 30 to 433 pmole Eq/liter (see Table 2 for details). This wide range of values is probably a consequence of the differences in the techniques and antisera used by the various laboratories. The levels reported for basal plasma total GLI and gut GLI have fallen during the past few years, and have stabilized between 30 and 90 pmole Eq/liter. Total plasma GLI and gut GLI both increase two- to threefold after an oral glucose load or ingestion of a mixed meal. Maximum plasma total GLI or gut GLI occurs 45 to 60 min after an oral glucose load and 3 hr after a mixed meal. Greater than normal increases in plasma total GLI and gut GLI have been described after oral loads in diabetics, and in subjects whose intestinal function was such that large amounts of unabsorbed nutrients reached the lower small intestine (see Table 3 for details). In all cases where plasma total GLI and gut GLI have been measured in similar patient material, both parameters increased to

TABLE 2. *Fasting and stimulated levels of plasma gut GLI and total GLI in normal man*

Load	Parameter Total/Gut GLI		N	Plasma GLI Fasting	Maximum	Reference
OGTT		Gut GLI	21	109	217 (60)	7
OGTT		Gut GLI	29	138	268 (60)	10
OGTT	Total		18	433	578 (45)	15
OGTT	Total		7	89	126 (45)	28
NIL		Gut GLI	17	37	—	6
OGTT	Total		7	34	40 (60)	5
OGTT		Gut GLI	5	86	115 (60)	4
Meal		Gut GLI	13	28	45 (180)	1

The GLI values are the means, in pmol Eq/liter plasma, of the number of observations given under *N*. The time, in minutes, at which the maximum values were measured, is in parentheses. OGTT, oral glucose load; Meal, mixed meal.

TABLE 3. *Fasting and stimulated levels of plasma gut GLI and total GLI in patients*

Disease[a]	Load	Parameter Total/Gut	GLI	N	Plasma GLI Fasting	Maximum	Reference
C	Meal		Gut GLI	13	97	263 (180)	1
Da	OGTT		Gut GLI	17	176	300 (60)	10
Db	OGTT		Gut GLI	8	242	591 (60)	10
G	OGTT	Total		8	50	312 (60)	3
Gd	OGTT	Total		9	50	598 (60)	3
G	OGTT	Total		5	30	202 (45)	5
G	OGTT		Gut GLI	26	130	300 (30)	24
G	OGTT	Total		7	92	300 (30)	28
G	OGTT	Total		8	490	1590 (30)	15
P	OGTT		Gut GLI	5	86	462 (15–60)	4
S	Meal		Gut GLI	18	45	150 (150)	12
Vt	OGTT	Total		24	28	401 (50)	21
Vs	OGTT	Total		17	39	411 (50)	21

The GLI values are the means, in pmol Eq/liter plasma, of the number of observations given under *N*. The time, in minutes, at which the maximum values were measured, is in parentheses. OGTT, oral glucose load; Meal, mixed meal.

[a] C, Celiac disease; Da, diabetics with IRI response to glucose load; Db, diabetics without IRI response to glucose load; G, gastrectomized subjects; Gd, gastrectomized subjects with dumping syndrome; P, patients with pancreatitis; S, subjects after jejunoileal shunt for obesity; Vs, patients after selective vagotomy; Vt, patients after total vagotomy.

much the same extent after ingestion of the oral load. The increase in total GLI or gut GLI after ingestion of an oral load appears to depend on the degree to which unabsorbed nutrients from the load reach the lower small intestine. Plasma gut GLIs have much the same size distribution as gut GLIs extracted from the intestine (27).

CONCLUSIONS AND PROJECTIONS FOR THE FUTURE

Knowledge of the immunochemistry and partial sequence of glicentin, which was isolated with the aid of the RIA for gut GLI, was crucial in the development of our understanding of the RIA for gut GLI.

It is unlikely that the current RIA, based on anti-glucagon sera, will be able to discriminate between the secretory products of the pancreatic A cell and the intestinal L cell. This pessimistic prognosis is based on growing evidence that an amino acid sequence identical to glucagon's forms part of the gut GLI molecule. It is therefore unlikely that an anti-glucagon serum will react only with gut GLIs (or, indeed, only with glucagon). A RIA specific for gut GLIs can be developed, provided that the antiserum used reacts with the portions of the gut GLI molecule that lie outside the glucagon moiety. An example of such an antiserum was briefly described in a previous section. The subtractive technique of Heding for the assay of plasma gut GLI is an excellent analytical tool, provided that suitable antisera are available. It is to be hoped that the measurement of the plasma levels of gut GLI will replace the measurement of plasma total GLI, since gut GLI is a better measure of the secretion of the L cell than total GLI.

It would be of interest to establish whether the IR glicentin in plasma is glicentin itself, or peptides cleaved from glicentin during or after the secretion of gut GLIs from the L cell. Further investigations with the RIA for glicentin will be of value in establishing the circulating forms of gut GLI and their possible biological role.

REFERENCES

1. Besterman, H. S., Sarson, D. L., Johnston, D. I., Stewart, J. S., Guerin, S., Bloom, S. R., Blackburn, A. M., Patel, H. R., Modigliani, R., and Mallinson, C. N. (1978): Gut-hormone profile in coeliac disease. *Lancet,* i:785–788.
2. Bloom, S. R., and Polak, J. M. (1978): Gut hormone overview. In: *Gut Hormones,* edited by S. R. Bloom, pp. 3–18. Churchill Livingstone, Edinburgh.
3. Bloom, S. R., Royston, C. M. S., and Thompson, J. P. S. (1972): Enteroglucagon release in the dumping syndrome. *Lancet,* ii: 789–791.
4. Botha, J. L., Vinik, A. I., and Brown, J. C. (1976): Gastric inhibitory polypeptide (GIP) in chronic pancreatitis. *J. Clin. Endocrinol. Metabl.,* 42:791–797.
5. Breuer, R. I., Zuckerman, L., Hauch, T. W., Green, W., O'Gara, P., Lawrence, A. M., Foa, P. P., and Matsuyama, T. (1975): Gastric operations and glucose homeostasis. II. Glucagon and secretin. *Gastroenterology,* 69:598–606.
6. Czyzyk, A., Heding, L. G., Malczewski, B., and Miedzinska, E. (1975): The effect of phenformin upon the plasma pancreatic and gut glucagon-like immunoreactivity in diabetics. *Diabetologia,* 11:129–133.
7. Heding, L. G. (1971): Radioimmunological determination of pancreatic and gut glucagon in plasma. *Diabetologia,* 7:10–19.
8. Heding, L. G. (1972): Immunologic properties of pancreatic glucagon, antigenicity and antibody characteristics. In: *Glucagon, Molecular Physiology, Clinical and Therapeutic Implications,* edited by P. J. Lefebvre and R. H. Unger, pp. 187–200. Pergamon Press, Oxford.
9. Heding, L. G., Frandsen, E. K., and Jacobsen, H. (1976): Structure-function relationship: Immunologic. *Metabolism [Suppl. 1],* 25:1327–1329.
10. Heding, L. G., and Munkgaard Rasmussen, S. (1972): Determination of pancreatic and gut glucagon-like immunoreactivity (GLI) in normal and diabetic subjects. *Diabetologia,* 8:408–411.
11. Holst, J. J. (1977): Extraction, gel filtration pattern and receptor binding of porcine gastrointestinal glucagon-like immunoreactivity. *Diabetologia,* 13:159–169.
12. Holst, J. J., Sorensen, T. I. A., Andersen, A. N., Stadil, F., Andersen, B., Lauritsen, K. B., and Klein, H. C. (1979): Plasma enteroglucagon after jejuno-ileal bypass with 3:1 or 1:3 jejunoileo ratio. *Scand. J. Gastroenterol. (in press).*
13. Jacobsen, H., Demandt, A., Moody, A. J., and Sundby, F. S. (1977): Sequence analysis of porcine gut GLI-1. *Biochim. Biophys. Acta,* 493:452–459.
14. Jørgensen, K. H., and Larsen, U. D. (1972): Purification of [125]-I glucagon in anion exchange chromatography. *Horm. Metab. Res.,* 4:223–224.
15. Marco, J., Baroja, I. M., Diaz-Fierros, M., Villanueva, M. L., and Valverde, I. (1972): Relationship between insulin and gut glucagon-like immunoreactivity (GLI) in normal and gastrectomised subjects. *J. Clin. Endocrinol. Metab.,* 34:188–191.
16. Moody, A. J. (1972): Gastrointestinal glucagon-like immunoreactivity. In: *Glucagon, Molecular Physiology, Clinical and Therapeutic Implications,* edited by P. J. Lefebvre and R. H. Unger, pp. 319–341. Pergamon Press, Oxford.
17. Moody, A. J. (1980): Gut GLIs and other enteric glucagon-like peptides. *Br. J. Clin. Pharmacol. (in press).*
18. Moody, A. J., Jacobsen, H., and Sundby, F. (1978): Gastric glucagon and gut glucagon-like

immunoreactants. In: *Gut Hormones,* edited by S. R. Bloom, pp. 369–378. Churchill Livingstone, Edinburgh.

19. Moody, A. J., Jacobsen, H., Sundby F., Frandsen, E. K., Baetens, D., and Orci, L. (1977): In: *Glucagon: Its Role in Physiology and Clinical Medicine,* edited by P. P. Foa, J. S. Bajaj, and N. L. Foa, pp. 129–135. Springer-Verlag, New York.

20. Ravazzola, A., Siperstein, A., Moody, A. J., Sundby, F., Jacobsen, H., and Orci, L. (1979): Glicentin immunoreactive cells, their relationship with glucagon producing cells. *Endocrinology,* 105:499–508.

21. Russell, R. C. G., Thompson, J. P. S., and Bloom, S. R. (1974): The effect of truncal and selective vagotomy on the release of pancreatic glucagon, insulin and enteroglucagon. *Br. J. Surg.,* 61:821–824.

22. Sasaki, H., Rubalcava, B., Baetens, D., Blazquez, E., Srikant, C. B., Orci, L., and Unger, R. H. (1975): Identification of glucagon in the gastrointestinal tract. *J. Clin. Invest.,* 56:135–145.

23. von Schenck, H. (1978): Immunoglobins interfering in the glucagon radioimmunoassay. *Acta Endocrinol.,* 88: (Suppl. 216), 69.

24. Shima, K., Sawazaki, N., Morishita, S., Tarui, S., and Nishikawa, M. (1975): Effect of phenformin on the response of plasma intestinal glucagon-like immunoreactivity to oral glucose in gastrectomised subjects. *Proc. Soc. Exp. Biol. Med.,* 150:232–236.

25. Sundby, F., Jacobsen, H., and Moody, A. J. (1976): Purification and characterization of a protein from porcine gut with glucagon-like immunoreactivity. *Horm. Metab. Res.,* 8:366–371.

26. Unger, R. H., Ohneda, A., Valverde, I., Eisentraut, A. M., and Exton, J. (1968): Characterization of the responses of circulating glucagon-like immunoreactivity to intraduodenal and intravenous administration of glucose. *J. Clin. Invest.,* 47:48–65.

27. Valverde, I., Rigopoulou, D., Marco, J., Faloona, G. R., and Unger, R. H. (1970): Molecular size of extractable glucagon and glucagon-like immunoreactivity (GLI) in plasma. *Diabetes,* 19:624–629.

28. Vance, J. E., Stoll, R. W., Fariss, B. L., and Williams, R. H. (1972): Exaggerated intestinal glucagon and insulin responses in human subjects. *Metabolism,* 21:405–412.

29. Walters, R. M., Dudl, R. J., Palmer, J. P., and Ensinck, J. W. (1974): The effects of adrenergic blockade on glucagon responses to starvation and hypoglycemia in man. *J. Clin. Invest.,* 54:1214–1220.

Gastrointestinal Hormones, edited by
George B. Jerzy Glass.
Raven Press, New York © 1980.

Chapter 37

Radioimmunoassay for Somatostatin in Tissue and Blood

Akira Arimura

Department of Medicine, Tulane University School of Medicine, and Endocrine and Polypeptide Laboratories, Veterans Administration Hospital, New Orleans, Louisiana 70112

INTRODUCTION

Soon after synthetic somatostatin became available, this tetradecapeptide was used to generate a specific antiserum, and using this antiserum investigators established a radioimmunoassay (RIA) method for somatostatin (3,12,17,22,29). With RIA it became possible to determine as small an amount as a femtomole of somatostatin in various biological materials. RIA has now become a most powerful tool for somatostatin research. Because the method of RIA is relatively easy to perform, numerous studies using RIA have been reported. Although much valuable information has been obtained from such studies, there are some data which may have resulted from overlooking pitfalls often encountered during RIA for small peptides such as somatostatin. In this chapter, I have attempted to (a) describe a somatostatin RIA in technical detail so that readers can use this chapter as an experimental manual for the RIA procedure, and (b) discuss a variety of applications and limits of the assay and related problems.

ANTISERUM TO SOMATOSTATIN

Carrier Substances for Somatostatin

Although somatostatin itself can be used as the antigen, its antigenicity is enhanced by conjugating the peptide with a larger carrier molecule. Various carrier substances were described by different investigators, including human α,β-globulin (3), keyhole limpet hemocyanin (14), whelk hemocyanin (17), thyroglobulin (22), human serum albumin (29), and bovine serum albumin (BSA) (12). Chances of success in yielding a good antiserum appear to be affected by the carrier substances used. In our experience, conjugation with human α,β-globulin resulted in an antiserum superior to that obtained with bovine serum albumin. The same result was also observed by another investigator (M. Utsumi, *personal communication*). Keyhole limpet hemocyanin was found by others (14) to be an excellent carrier. Antibodies to the carrier substance may also be generated together with antibodies to somatostatin. With keyhole limpet hemocyanin, which is not present in mammals, the antibody generated against this carrier substance may be quite inert in terms of various reactions that occur during the RIA for somatostatin in mammalian tissue and blood.

Conjugation and Its Effect on the Recognition Site of Antiserum

The antibody to be generated must bind similarly with both somatostatin and the tracer so that they can compete for the limited number of recognition sites on the antibody. Since somatostatin lacks both tyrosine and histidine, which are readily iodinated by conventional methods, Tyr[1]-somatostatin or N-Tyr-somatostatin was synthesized for labeling. However, if the antibody recognizes the N terminus of the somatostatin molecule, it will not bind with ^{125}I-Tyr-somatostatin or ^{125}I-N-Tyr-somatostatin. If either of these tracers is used, it is desirable to use a coupling agent such as glutaraldehyde, which reacts with the free amino group at the N terminus, since the antibody usually recognizes portions of the antigen which are remote from the site of conjugation (4,20). However, it is also possible that glutaraldehyde reacts with the primary amino group of Lys at positions 4 and 9 of the somatostatin molecule. We routinely use this bifunctional coupling agent to conjugate somatostatin with the carrier protein human α,β-globulin.

On the other hand, in order to generate an antibody directed to the N terminus of somatostatin, conjugation should take place at a site distal to the N terminus. In such case, Tyr[11]-somatostatin has been conjugated with a carrier substance by means of bisdiazobenzidine (BDB). The RIA method with antiserum thus generated is carried out using ^{125}I-Tyr[11]-somatostatin as the tracer (29).

In our laboratories, synthetic cyclic somatostatin was coupled with human α,β-globulin by glutaraldehyde. The conjugated peptide was then emulsified with complete Freund's adjuvant and injected into rabbits according to the method described by Vaitukaitis et al. (28). Two out of three rabbits immunized yielded specific antiserum (R101 and R103) with sufficiently high titer. The recognition site of antiserum R101 as tested for cross-reactivity with various synthetic somatostatin analogues, in which amino acids at various positions were replaced by "D" form or other amino acids, was directed to the ring portion of the somatostatin molecule, especially the portion from Asn[5] to Ser[13] (2). Substitution of Lys[4] or Lys[9] with other amino acids resulted in some decrease in binding with antiserum R101.

THE RIA METHOD

Diluent in RIA

Although various diluents are used by different investigators, we have found that 0.25% BSA/0.1% gelatin/0.05 M phosphate buffer/0.08 M NaCl/0.25 M EDTA/0.02% NaN$_3$, pH 7.5, is quite satisfactory and has given consistent results in our RIA.

Standard Preparation

In our laboratory, synthetic cyclic somatostatin (Ayerst No. 24910) has been used as our reference standard preparation. Stock solution, 1 mg/ml 0.1 M acetic acid, can be stored at 4°C for at least 3 months. For working stock solution, it is convenient to prepare 1 ng/μl diluent for RIA from which gelatin is omitted (minus-gelatin diluent). Approximately 200 μl of working stock solution is distributed into a small vial and stored at -50°C without changing activity for 6 months. In our practice, 10 μl of the working stock solution (10 ng somatostatin) is added to 1.94 ml RIA diluent to make the highest standard solution, 512 pg/100 μl, which is serially diluted to 1 pg/100 μl.

Storage of Antiserum

The antiserum is diluted 100 times in the minus-gelatin diluent, a small aliquot is distributed into a small vial and stored at -50°C. This is very stable for at least 1 year. Our antiserum R101 is used at the final dilution of 1:30,000, giving B_0/T of 25 to 45% depending on the specific activity of the tracer, where "B_0" is bound radioactivity without the presence of cold hormone, and "T" represents the total count.

Iodination

For the antiserum directed to the ring portion of somatostatin, either Tyr^1-somatostatin or N-Tyr-somatostatin is labeled with ^{125}I (2). For the antiserum directed to N terminus, Tyr^{11}-somatostatin may be used (29). It is recommended to prepare fresh peptide solution since one of the commonest causes of failure of iodination is old solution. In our laboratories 1 mg/ml 0.1 M acetic acid is prepared.

Although either the chloramine T (16) or the lactoperoxidase method (19) is used for iodination, the latter has given quite satisfactory and consistent results in our experience. It must be kept in mind that with the chloramine T method, sodium metabisulfite should not be used to stop the reaction, since it causes reduction of the disulfide bond of the peptide, leading to loss of binding activity with the antiserum directed to the ring portion of somatostatin.

For purification of labeled products, we have found that ion-exchange chromatography on a carboxymethyl cellulose (CM 22, Whatman) column (0.5 × 17 cm) is quite satisfactory. The method with the CM 22 column is described elsewhere (2).

The tracer thus prepared is quite stable when stored at −50°C. However, when nonspecific binding increases greater than 7%, the tracer should be repurified on the CM column.

RIA Procedure

Sample volume ordinarily used in our laboratory is 100 or 200 μl. First, 300 or 400 μl RIA diluent, 100 or 200 μl sample, and 100 μl diluted antiserum are incubated for 3 to 4 hr at 4°C, and then 100 μl of tracer, approximately 10,000 cpm, is added. After overnight incubation at 4°C, the bound and free hormones are separated by dextran-coated charcoal as described previously (2). The double antibody method can also be used for separation.

Solid-Phase RIA

First, 200 mg cyanogen bromide-activated microcellulose powder is covalently coupled with 50 to 100 μl of the antiserum to somatostatin. Then 200 μg antibody-coupled cellulose is incubated with the tracer and the standard or sample in the buffer, in a capped plastic tube, and rotated gently for 24 hr at 4°C. Next the cellulose powder is washed with cold buffer and counted for radioactivity. The detail of the solid-phase RIA method will be published elsewhere (18). This method has been convenient and simple to perform. It is similar to the other method in sensitivity and accuracy.

Specificity and Sensitivity

With antiserum R101, we have obtained an excellent standard curve in a dose range from 1 to 64 pg/tube. Ten picograms somatostatin replaces 50% of the bound tracer. Sensitivity of the RIA as determined by the amount for the lower limit of 95% confidence limits of the buffer control is 1 pg/tube. Therefore, when 200 μl of the plasma extract is used, the sensitivity is 5 pg/ml.

Antiserum R101 shows no significant cross-reaction with TRH, LHRH, MIF, vasopressin, oxytocin, all pituitary hormones, insulin, glucagon, human pancreatic polypeptide, secretin, VIA, and motilin. The anitserum, however, cross-reacts with synthetic analogues of somatostatin to different extents (2).

DETERMINATION OF SOMATOSTATIN IN TISSUE AND BLOOD BY RIA

Tissue Extracts

When tissue is assayed for somatostatin, it may be homogenized with 1 or 2 N ice cold acetic acid, and the homogenate heated in boiling water for 5 min or heated to boiling point on a hotplate equipped with a magnetic stirrer. The homogenate is then cooled in ice, centrifuged, and the supernatent is lyophilized. The tissue may be placed directly in boiling water and then homogenized, and centrifuged. The supernatant can be assayed immediately by RIA without subjection to further processing. Heating the tissue extracts destroys somatostatin-inactivating enzymes and also denatures proteins, which bind somatostatin and interfere with the RIA. It is recommended to wash the extract with an organic solvent such as ether/ethylacetate mixture (1:3) to remove lipids and other substances. Washing with organic solvents is particularly useful when the affinity of the antibody is relatively low.

When tissue is extracted with acetic acid, lyophilization must be conducted until the acid is completely removed, because the acid remaining in the extracts may suppress the tracer-antibody binding, leading to a falsely high estimate of somatostatin. Immunoreactive somatostatin (IRS) levels in various tissue extracts determined in laboratories using different antisera are in close agreement.

Cerebrospinal Fluid (CSF)

Although somatostatin is relatively stable in CSF (21), it is recommended that CSF be collected in an ice-chilled plastic tube which contains aprotinin

(Trasylol®) (500 KIU/ml), frozen immediately, and stored at −50°C until assayed. CSF can be assayed directly without extraction. However, if the CSF contains considerable concentration of protein, it may interfere with the assay. Although IRS levels in most of the CSF samples show a linear decrease by serial dilutions, those in some CSF samples do not (1). This may indicate that most of the IRS in CSF is immunologically similar, but there is some variation.

Blood

Whole blood or plasma, but not serum, may be used. It is recommended to remove interfering sustances prior to RIA. Whole blood can be collected in chilled 2 N acetic acid, mixed, and stored at −50°C (9). When plasma is used, blood is collected in an ice-chilled tube which contains EDTA (2.5 mg/ml blood) and aprotinin (500 KIU/ml blood) (1,2). Plasma is separated by centrifugation at 4°C and stored at −50°C. At a low pH and temperature, IRS in blood is quite stable (9).

Extraction of IRS in Plasma or Whole Blood

To 0.5 ml EDTA plasma, 50 µl glacial acetic acid is added and mixed, and then 2 ml (4 parts) purified cold acetone is added dropwise while the tube is vortexed. The plasma-acetone mixture is sonicated for 30 sec and centrifuged at 2,000 rpm for 15 min at 4°C. The supernatant is transferred into a gelatin-coated 16 × 100 mm tube. One milliliter of 80% cold acetone is added to the precipitate, mixed by means of a glass rod, and centrifuged. To the pooled supernatant, 0.5 ml water is added to dilute the acetone, and washed with 3 ml of organic solvent (3 parts of ethylacetate and 1 part of anhydrous ether). After vortexing, the mixture may be left on the bench or briefly centrifuged to separate organic and aqueous layers. The upper organic layer is aspirated and the aqueous layer is dried under nitrogen gas flow at 35 to 40°C. The dried residue is stored in a desiccator at 4°C until assayed. Immediately before the RIA, the residue is dissolved in 0.5 ml diluent of RIA and an aliquot is used for RIA. After extraction, the recovery of somatostatin added to plasma in a dose range from 20 to 500 pg/ml averaged 80%.

When the amount of blood to be collected is limited, as with hypophyseal stalk blood, whole blood may be collected in chilled 2 N acetic acid. Four volumes of cold acetone are added to the acid-blood mixture and the extraction is carried out in a method similar to that for plasma extraction. When the volume of pooled acetone extract is too large to wash with organic solvent, the acetone extract may be evaporated to 2 to 3 ml by nitrogen gas and then added with organic solvent. The organic solvent removes lipids and pigments leaving a clear aqueous layer (1,9).

PROBLEMS RELEVANT TO RIA OF PLASMA SOMATOSTATIN

Plasma IRS Levels

In contrast to determination of IRS in tissue extracts, estimates of plasma IRS reported by different investigators vary considerably. Berelowitz et al. (6) determined IRS in unextracted rat serum by RIA using an antiserum specific for somatostatin, and reported the mean levels in the aorta, 304 pg/ml; hepatic portal vein, 495 to 523 pg/ml; hepatic vein, 290 pg/ml; and the hepatic portal vein 5 min after intragastric glucose, 1,550 pg/ml. They reported that IRS in rat serum showed chromatographic similarity with synthetic somatostatin. Pimstone et al. (23) assayed unextracted human serum samples and reported that in 92% of 48 samples, the mean IRS level was 274 $\pm$ 9 (SE) pg/ml, and the remainder showed a level of 1,000 $\pm$ 41 pg/ml. They also reported that oral glucose produced a 15% fall in serum IRS at 120 min and 12% at 150 min. Intravenous intralipid caused a 50% increase in IRS at 60 min and 34% at 120 min. This elevation occurred well after the peak of plasma triglyceride (10 to 30 min). Oxo and arginine produced a downward trend in serum IRS, but these changes were not statistically significant. Schusdziarra et al. (26) measured IRS levels in unextracted plasma obtained from normal and alloxan-diabetic dogs. In normal dogs the mean IRS in peripheral venous plasma was 120 $\pm$ 7.6 pg/ml, and in hepatic portal plasma it was 275 $\pm$ 12.9 pg/ml. In alloxan-diabetic dogs the IRS level in systemic plasma was 285 $\pm$ 22.8 pg/ml during insulin deprivation and 159 $\pm$ 9.9 pg/ml during insulin treatment.

Brazeau et al. (7) added an equal volume of 2 N acetic acid to rat plasma immediately after collection, and neutralized it with NaOH before the RIA. Acid extraction of plasma prevented nonspecific inhibition of the binding of the tracer to the antibody that occurred even when unextracted plasma was incubated with 400 KIU aprotinin. Incubation of ^{125}I-Tyr-somatostatin with rat serum resulted in 60% degradation, as assessed by chromatoelectrophoresis, and a 65% decrease in antibody binding. However, the addition of 0.5 M EDTA to the assay buffer and aprotinin to the serum was associated with incubation damage no greater than that of the buffer controls (10 to 15%). Pimstone et al. (23) reported that IRS levels in systemic plasma obtained from freely moving rats showed three to five intermittent bursts of IRS, rising from undetectable levels ($<$ 96 pg/ml) to peak values of 384 to 2,800 pg/ml. They reported that IRS in the acid extract of plasma was bound to somatostatin antibody immobilized on a Sepharose column, and eluted subsequently with 2 N acetic acid. The total IRS recovered from the Sepharose column using 18 ml of acid-extracted rat plasma from the abdominal aorta corresponded to 360 pg/ml IRS plasma. Gustavsson and Lundqvist (15) extracted pig plasma with acetone followed by washing with anhydrous ether, a method similar to that described in this chapter. IRS levels in the acetone-extracted pig plasma were measured by solid phase RIA (2,18). The mean ($\pm$ SE) IRS level in the pig peripheral plasma was 138 $\pm$ 20 pg/ml, and that in the superior pancreatico-duodenal vein was 256 $\pm$ 60 pg/ml.

IRS levels in acetone-extracted plasma or whole blood of rats, dogs, and humans determined at our laboratory are considerably lower than those reported by others. IRS in normal rat systemic plasma ranged from 5 to 15 pg/ml, and in streptozotocin-treated diabetic rats it ranged from 13 to 41 pg/ml. Basal IRS levels in the hepatic portal vein ranged from 22 to 72 pg/ml. Intravenous injection of secretin (10 μg/100 g body weight) induced an elevation of plasma IRS in the jugular vein to 33 to 89 pg/ml, and in the hepatic portal vein to 126 to 339 pg/ml.

Systemic whole blood of the rat, collected in 2 N acetic acid, was assayed for IRS after acetone extraction (9). The levels, 15.5 to 19.1 pg/ml, were comparable to those in systemic plasma. Hypophyseal portal blood from urethane-anesthetized rats was also measured for IRS. The mean level, 503 $\pm$ 52.9 pg/ml, was significantly greater than those in peripheral blood. IRS levels in hypophyseal portal blood, but not in systemic blood, were affected by the anesthetics used. Higher levels were observed under urethane anesthesia than under pentobarbital (Nembutal®) (113 $\pm$ 18.1 pg/ml) or Althesin[1] (156 $\pm$ 28.4 pg/ml) anesthesia (9). The difference could account in part for the low serum GH levels under urethane anesthesia and higher GH levels under pentobarbital or Althesin (9).

By collecting rat hypophyseal portal blood at 15 to 20 min intervals by means of a specifically devised microfraction collector, it became possible to determine secretion rates of IRS under various experimental conditions. Intracerebroventricular injection of dopamine considerably increased secretion of IRS, whereas norepinephrine moderately did. 5-Hydroxytryptamine did not alter IRS secretion. Acetylcholine did not stimulate IRS release, but prevented gradual decrease in IRS release that spontaneously occurred (10).

Mean IRS level in acetone-extracted dog plasma in the peripheral vein was 7 $\pm$ 1.5 pg/ml; hepatic portal vein, 20 $\pm$ 6.2 pg/ml; v. gastroepiploica dextra, 24 $\pm$ 8.2 pg/ml; v. gastrica brevis, 48 $\pm$ 5.6 pg/ml; and v. pancreatico-duodenalis, 31 $\pm$ 3.7 pg/ml. Intragastric administration of 200 ml 0.1 N HCl or dilatation of the stomach by 500 ml air stimulated IRS release from the body of the stomach, resulting in an increase in IRS in the v. gastrica brevis as high as 4 to 5 pg/ml (in preparation for publication).

We have determined plasma samples from 34 normal men and 26 adult-onset diabetic patients with moderate hyperglycemia, all of whom showed IRS concentration of less than 5 pg/ml. Plasma from three juvenile-type diabetic patients showed slightly higher levels (6.5, 12.5, and 9.5 pg/ml). The reason for such a large discrepancy between our estimates and those of others remains

---

[1]Althesin (Glaxo Laboratories Ltd., Greenford, Middlesex, England) is 0.9% 3α-hydroxy-5α-pregnane-11, 20-dione/0.3% 21-acetoxy-3α-hydroxy-5α-pregnane-11, 20-dione.

to be clarified. Difference in the antiserum alone may not account for the difference in IRS estimates since Schusdziarra et al. (26) also used antiserum R101. Use of extracted and unextracted plasma or different extraction procedures may have caused the discrepancy. Even though plasma is acidified before extraction, our acetone extraction method could precipitate some IRS with plasma macromolecules. It should be noted, however, that the recovery of added synthetic somatostatin after extraction averaged 80%, and that IRS in extracted plasma in the v. gastrica brevis of the dog increased up to 4 to 5 ng/ml after intragastric acid administration.

Characteristics of IRS in Tissue

IRS in extracts of the hypothalamus, stomach, and pancreas shows heterogeneity in chromatographic behavior. IRS in the rat pancreas and stomach (5), as well as in pig hypothalamic extract (25), revealed two and three components by chromatography on Sephadex G-25. The small form migrates in the same zone as tetradecapeptide somatostatin, whereas the big form is eluted with the void volume (13). Both big and small forms have biological activity (13). Part of the big form obtained from rat pancreas extract can be converted into the small form by treatment with 8 M urea, which dissociates noncovalent bonds. This indicates that some of the big form is possibly an aggregate of somatostatin. Spies and Vale (27) extracted and purified pigeon pancreatic tissue by procedures that minimize protein-protein interactions and protease activities. Column gel chromatography on Bio-Gel P-100 yielded a bulk of IRS eluted with the tetradecapeptide somatostatin, and a larger species of IRS which represented 0.5% of the total IRS. This large pancreatic IRS species is dissociated under reducing conditions with thioglycol. Therefore it does not appear to represent a polypeptide with the somatostatin entity linked by a peptide bond. When the same extraction procedure described above was used, a big IRS species with an apparent molecular size of 11,000 to 12,000 daltons was found in rat brain extracts, representing 3 to 5% of the total IRS. The big IRS in rat brain extracts was not changed under reducing conditions with thioglycol. The big species purified from brain and pancreas differed in their immunologic behavior. The RIA was performed with the N-terminally directed antiserum S39 and the centrally directed antiserum S201. The big pancreatic IRS species showed three times more activity in the S39 assay than in the S201 assay. In contrast to these findings, the big brain IRS species is not read by antiserum S39, but only by antiserum S201.

Two larger and more basic IRS species than tetradecapeptide somatostatin were isolated in pure form (2,25) during purification of somatostatin from pig hypothalamic extracts in our laboratory. They completely lacked immunoreactivity in the RIA with S39, but they did show immunoreactivity with antiserum R101 which is directed toward the ring portion of somatostatin. Therefore, these larger IRSs appear to have an extended residue at the N-terminus of somatostatin, and may represent intermediates derived from the prohormone (2).

Pradayrol et al. (24) recently isolated a larger IRS species from acid extracts of porcine upper intestine. Preliminary chemical characterization shows that it has N-terminal serine and that it is composed of somatostatin extended from its N-terminus by an additional peptide.

Characteristics of IRS in Blood

When heparinized rat plasma is chromatographed on a Sephadex G-25 column using 0.03 M ammonium acetate buffer, pH 7.0, one prominent IRS peak is eluted in early fractions with Rf 0.68 to 0.50, corresponding to high peptide concentration as measured by optical density at 278 nm. Synthetic somatostatin is usually eluted at Rf 0.26 to 0.20 after the peak of salts indicated by high electroconductivity. When 20 ng of somatostatin is added to 2 ml plasma and then chromatographed, two IRS peaks are eluted in early fractions and at the somatostatin area, respectively. This suggests that somatostatin added to plasma is bound with large molecular components, probably proteins (2). The binding capacity of plasma appears to vary between individual plasma samples and between species. The binding sites may be saturable, since when a small amount of somatostatin is added to plasma only one IRS peak is eluted in early fractions, whereas with an excess of somatostatin added to IRS, peaks appear in early fractions and at the somatostatin area (2). Conlon et al. (11) reported that at pH 8.8 both endogenous plasma IRS from the pancreatic vein and synthetic somatostatin added to dog plasma or injected *in vivo* were eluted from Sephadex gels in the 150,000 to 200,000 M.W. zone. At pH 2.5, however, both plasma IRS and synthetic somatostatin plasma were eluted in the somatostatin area, 1,600 M.W. zone. These results indicate that somatostatin binds with large molecular components of plasma at pH 8.8, but remains free at pH 2.5. They also reported that ^{125}I-Tyr-somatostatin does not bind with plasma components. Affinity chromatography of plasma samples on columns of immobilized antibodies directed to the central portion of somatostatin removed 95% of both endogenous IRS and somatostatin added to plasma. On the other hand, neither moiety was removed by affinity chromatography with antibodies directed to the N-terminus region of somatostatin. However, in the absence of plasma, somatostatin in buffer or IRS from the pancreas perfused with buffer was bound by both columns of antibodies (11). These data may indicate that the endogenous IRS released by the pancreas is similar in molecular size to somatostatin tetradecapeptide, that both IRS and somatostatin in blood bind to large molecular plasma components, and that the N-terminal region of somatostatin is its probable binding site.

In our recent studies, acetone extracts of dog plasma in the v. gastrica brevis that contained high IRS showed two IRS peaks on chromatography of a Sephadex G-25 column, one being eluted at the somatostatin area and another in more retarded fractions (Arimura et al., *in preparation*). This suggests that one IRS component is of a smaller species than tetradecapeptide somatostatin. The extracts also showed two major peaks on ion-exchange chromatography with CM Sephadex G-25 using ammonium acetate buffer with gradient concentration, pH 4.6. One of the peaks was eluted at the somatostatin area and another in earlier fractions, indicating that the latter is a less basic component. Since these IRSs were assayed by RIA with antiserum R101, which is directed to the ring portion of somatostatin, it is possible that a smaller and less basic IRS species is des [Ala^1, Gly^2]-somatostatin that is biologically fully active (8).

Acetone extracts of whole blood from the rat hypophyseal stalk stump were also subjected to gel filtration and ion-exchange chromatography. In contrast to results in gastric blood, a larger and more basic IRS was observed (9) in addition to the IRS which behaves similarly to somatostatin tetradecapeptide.

SUMMARY AND CONCLUSIONS

A radioimmunoassay method which has been successfully used for many physiological and biochemical studies for the past 4 years in our laboratories has been described in technical detail. Its application and limitation as well as pitfalls have been reported. There is agreement that plasma contains macromolecular components which bind with endogenous and exogenously added somatostatin at neutral and near neutral pH. The presence of such binding components during incubation for RIA is likely to interfere with valid determination of IRS in plasma, leading to false estimates of IRS. To avoid this possible risk, it is recommended to remove those macromolecules of plasma by acidification followed by acetone-organic solvent extraction. Considerable discrepancies in IRS levels in blood reported by us and other investigators may be at least in part interpreted by the use of unextracted and extracted plasma of different extraction methods, rather than different antiserum used. Characteristics of IRS in blood and tissue were determined by various chromatographic analyses. The IRS species appear to be heterogenous, both larger and smaller species being present.

PROJECTIONS FOR THE FUTURE

It is possible to assess the chemical structure of various IRS components in tissue and blood by RIA using antisera with different recognition sites. RIA methods, if properly used, will serve as a powerful tool for studying products during the processes of biosynthesis of somatostatin.

Although recent findings have confirmed that somatostatin is released from the median eminence and that it regulates GH and TSH secretion from the pituitary, it is impossible to monitor the secretory pattern of somatostatin from the median eminence by determining IRS levels in the systemic plasma. Because somatostatin released into the hypophyseal portal vessels may be very small in absolute quantity, quickly diluted by the systemic blood, and rapidly inactivated, it is unlikely that hypothalamic somatostatin constitutes the major portion of circulating IRS. On the other hand, the somatostatin content of the gut and pancreas far exceeds that of the CNS. Gut and pancreatic somatostatin is released into the hepatic portal vessel, wherein high plasma IRS levels, comparable to those in the hypophyseal portal blood, result. However, the total amount of somatostatin released into the hepatic portal vein far exceeds that released into the hypophyseal portal vessel. Although considerable inactivation of somatostatin appears to take place in the liver, gut, and pancreatic somatostatin may still be a major source of circulating IRS.

Significant elevation of IRS in the systemic plasma has been detected in streptozotocin-induced diabetic rats, juvenile-type diabetic patients, and after injection into animals of somatostatin secretagogues such as secretin. These findings suggest that it is possible to determine basal D-cell activities and D-cell reserves by measuring plasma IRS before and after stimulation by an appropriate secretagogue. Although currently available data are limited, parallel changes in D cells in the stomach and the pancreas have been observed; i.e., an increase in IRS content in both stomach and pancreas in streptozotocin-induced diabetic rats which mimics juvenile-type diabetes, and a decrease in ob/ob mice which mimics adult-onset diabetes. Although suppression of glucagon and insulin by somatostatin has been emphasized as an important action of this tetradecapeptide, it is uncertain whether these are the most important physiological effects of endogenous somatostatin. On the other hand, a considerable amount of data suggest an important role for somatostatin in nutrient homeostasis. These include suppression of nutrient uptake by the gut; delay of gastric emptying; possible antagonistic actions on glucagon-induced activation of adenylate cyclase, on accumulation of cAMP, and possibly on glycogenolysis by the liver; and endocrine control of gut and pancreatic exocrine functions, and paracrine regulation of other islet cells. Thus the D-cell reserve test will increase in importance in clinical evaluation of the somatostatin system in various pathological conditions.

ACKNOWLEDGMENTS

Our data were obtained during the studies supported by USPHS grants AM-09094 and AM-07467 and VA grants. The author is greatly indebted to Ms. Alice M. Conradi for her excellent editorial assistance.

REFERENCES

1. Arimura, A. (1979): Radioimmunoassay for somatostatin. In: *Radioassay Systems in Clinical Endocrinology,* edited by G. E. Abraham. Marcel Dekker, New York *(in press).*
2. Arimura, A., Lundqvist, G., Rothman, J., Chang, R., Fernandez-Durango, R., Elde, R., Coy, D. H., Meyers, C., and Schally, A. V. (1978): Radioimmunoassay of somatostatin. *Metabolism* [*Suppl. 1*], 27:1139–1144.

3. Arimura, A., Sato, H., Coy, D. H., and Schally, A. V. (1975): Radioimmunoassay for GH-release inhibiting hormone. *Proc. Soc. Exp. Biol. Med.,* 148:784–789.
4. Arimura, A., Sato, H., Coy, D. H., Worobec, R. B., Schally, A. V., Yanaihara, N., Hashimoto, T., Yanahara, C., and Sukura, N. (1975): The antigenic determinant of the LH-releasing hormone for three different antiserums. *Acta Endocrinol. (Kbh.),* 78:222–231.
5. Arimura, A., Sato, H., Dupont, A., Nishi, N., and Schally, A. V. (1975): Somatostatin: Abundance of immunoreactive hormone in rat stomach and pancreas. *Science,* 189:1007–1009.
6. Berelowitz, M., Kronheim, S., Pimstone, B., and Shapiro, B. (1978): Somatostatin-like immunoreactivity in rat blood. *J. Clin. Invest.,* 61:1410–1414.
7. Brazeau, P., Pelbaum, J., Shaffer Tannenbaum, G., Rorstad, O., and Martin, J. B. (1978): Somatostatin: Isolation, characterization, distribution, and blood determination. *Metabolism [Suppl I],* 27:1133–1137.
8. Brown, M., Rivier, J., Vale, W., and Guillemin, R. (1975): Variability of the duration of inhibition of growth hormone release by N^α-acetylated-des [Ala^1, Gly^2]-H$_2$ somatostatin analogs. *Biochem. Biophys. Res. Commun.,* 65:752–756.
9. Chihara, K., Arimura, A., and Schally, A. V. (1979): Immunoreactive somatostatin (IRS) in rat hypophyseal portal blood: Effect of anesthetics. *Endocrinology,* 104:1434–1441.
10. Chihara, K., Arimura, A., and Schally, A. V. (1979): Effect of intraventricular injection of dopamine, norepinephrine, acetylcholine, and 5-hydroxytryptamine on immunoreactive somatostatin release into rat hypophyseal portal blood. *Endocrinology,* 104:1656–1662.
11. Conlon, J. M., Srikant, C. B., Ipp, E., Schusdziarra, V., and Unger, R. H. (1978): Similarities between circulating pancreatic somatostatin-like immunoreactivity and synthetic somatostatin. *Program of 60th Annual Meeting of the Endocrine Society,* Abstract #240, p. 194.
12. Diel, F., Schneidler, E., and Quabbe, H. (1977): Development of a radioimmunoassay for cyclic somatostatin: Antibody production, comparative radioiodination, and dose response curve. *J. Clin. Chem. Clin. Biochem.,* 15:669–677.
13. Dupont, A., and Alvarado-Urbina, G. (1976): Conversion of big pancreatic somatostatin without peptide bond cleavage into somatostatin tetradecapeptide. *Life Sci.,* 19:1431–1434.
14. Elde, R., Hokfelt, T., Johannson, O., Schultzberg, M., Efendic, S., and Luft, R. (1977): Cellular Localization of Somatostatin. *International Symposium of Somatostatin, Freiburg.*
15. Gustavsson, S., and Lundqvist, G. (1978): Inhibition of pancreatic somatostatin release in response to glucose. *Biochem. Biophys. Res. Commun.,* 82:1229–1235.
16. Hunter, W. M., and Greenwood, F. S. (1962): Preparation of iodine-131 labelled human growth hormone of high specific activity. *Nature,* 194:495–496.
17. Kronheim, S., Berelowita, M., and Pimstone, B. L. (1976): A radioimmunoassay for growth hormone release-inhibiting hormone: Method and quantitative tissue distribution. *Clin. Endocrinol.,* 5:619–630.
18. Lundqvist, G., Gustavsson, S., Elde, R., and Arimura, A. (1979): Solid-phase radioimmunassay for somatostatin. To be published.
19. Miyachi, Y., Vaitukaitis, J. L., Nieschlag, E., and Lipsett, M. B. (1972): Enzymatic radioiodination of gonadotropins. *J. Clin. Endocrinol. Metab.,* 34:23–28.
20. Niswender, G. D., and Midgley, A. R. (1970): Hapten-radioimmunoassay for steroid hormones. In: *Immunological Method in Steriod Determination,* edited by F. G. Peron and B. L. Caldwell, pp. 149–166. Appleton-Century-Crofts, New York.
21. Patel, Y. C., Rao, K., and Reichlin, S. (1977): Somatostatin in human cerebrospinal fluid. *N. Engl. J. Med.,* 29:529–533.
22. Patel, Y. C., Weir, G. C., and Reichlin, S. (1975): Anatomic distribution of somatostatin (SRIF) in brain and pancreatic islets as studied by radioimmunoassay. *Program of the 57th Annual Meeting of the Endocrine Society,* p. 127.
23. Pimstone, B., Berelowitz, M., Kranoid, D., Shapiro, B., and Kronheim, S. (1978): Somatostatin-like immunoreactivity (SRIF-LI) in human and rat serum. *Metabolism [Suppl I],* 27:1145–1149.
24. Pradayrol, L., Chayvialle, J. A., Carliquist, M., and Mutt, V. (1978): Isolation of a porcine intestinal peptide with C-terminal somatostatin. *Biochem. Biophys. Res. Commun.,* 85:701–708.
25. Schally, A. V., Dupont, A., Arimura, A., Redding, T. W., and Linthicum, G. L. (1975): Isolation of porcine GH-release inhibiting hormone (GH-RIH). *Fed. Proc.,* 34:584 (abst. 2065).
26. Schusdziarra, V., Dobbs, R. E., Harris, V., and Unger, R. H. (1977): Immunoreactive somatostatin levels in plasma of normal and alloxan diabetic dogs. *FEBS Lett.,* 81:69–72.

27. Spies, J., and Vale, W. (1978): Investigation of larger forms of somatostatin in pigeon pancreas and rat brain. *Metabolism* [*Suppl. 1*], 27:1175–1178.
28. Vaitukaitis, J., Robbins, J. B., Nieschlag, E., and Ross, G. T. (1971): A method for producing specific antisera with small doses of immunogen. *J. Clin. Endocrinol. Metabol.*, 33:988–991.
29. Vale, W., Ling, N., Rivier, J., Villarreal, J., Rivier, C., Douglas, C., and Brown, M. (1976): Anatomic and phylogenetic distribution of somatostatin. *Metabolism*, 25:1491–1494.

Gastrointestinal Hormones, edited by
George B. Jerzy Glass.
Raven Press, New York © 1980.

Chapter 38

Intraluminal Gastrointestinal Hormones and Their Radioimmunoassay

L. E. Hanssen and J. Myren

Research Laboratory of Gastroenterology, Department of Internal Medicine, Ullevål Hospital, Oslo, Norway

I. SECRETIN

INTRODUCTION

It has been believed that secretin is a hormone that is released by meals and stimulates the pancreas to secrete a copious juice rich in bicarbonate during digestion. It has, however, been difficult to show that secretin determined by radioimmunoassay (RIA) (immunoreactive secretin, IRS) is really released into the blood after a meal in man, probably because of the varying responses in relation to time and pH in the duodenal content.

IRS is released from the duodenal and jejunal mucosa into the blood after infusion of acid into the intestine if the pH is below 3 (2). An intriguing question is whether secretin is really a meal-stimulated hormone. The acid chyme from the stomach may be so well buffered at a pH of 4 to 5 that secretin is not released at all. However, in the interdigestive periods, short-lasting pH spikes down to pH 1 or 2 occur and might cause IRS release (10). Although the acid load delivered to the duodenum in this period is far less than during the digestive period, the importance of secretin for the maintainance of optimal pH in the duodenum should not be denied.

A release of secretin at pH values above 4 from the duodenal and jejunal mucosa has also been looked for. Thus it has been observed that IRS is released into the blood by bile (9) or bile salts (6) at nearly neutral pH. Thus a release of IRS is found at a pH considerably higher than reported when threshold experiments were performed using acid solutions (2). Whether this effect of bile and bile salts is only a facilitating one for the reaction of small amounts of hydrogen ions on the secretin cell (S cell) or is a new release mechanism for IRS has not yet been determined. It has been reported that the highest density of S cells is found in the proximal duodenal mucosa, but the largest S-cell mass is observed in the jejunum, an area of the intestine where HCl from the stomach has been neutralized completely. The bile salts entering the intestine from the papilla of Vater may well be the physiological stimulus for these cells.

Recently it has been suggested that gastrointestinal hormones are released into the secretions entering the gastrointestinal tract at a much higher concentration than that observed in the blood. Thus immunoreactive gastrin has been demonstrated in the gastric juice (12).

EXPERIMENTAL DATA

In the work referred to in this chapter we wanted to investigate whether IRS was present in human duodenal juice. If so, would it be possible to calculate

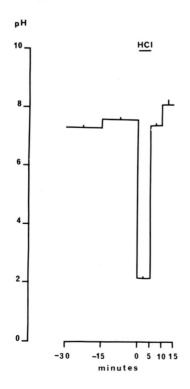

FIG. 1. pH of the duodenal aspirates before and after duodenal acidification with 40 ml 100 mmoles/liter HCl over 5 min. Mean ± SEM, $N = 5$.

the secretin output by continuous aspiration of the duodenal contents? In the blood, secretin concentration of the sample at a given time may be determined if one realizes the short half-life of secretin—2 to 4 min. However, rapid changes might take place in the blood without being noticed if blood samples are drawn every 10 to 15 min.

We have developed and evaluated a method for radioimmunological determination of secretin in duodenal juice of man (5). IRS is extracted into ethanol and the supernatant is evaporated to dryness and resuspended in buffer. Then the secretin RIA (7) is used as for plasma (4).

So that we could examine whether IRS was really present in duodenal juice in man, five healthy young volunteers were fasted overnight and the gastric and duodenal juice collected continuously by means of a Lagerlöf tube. After a control period of 30 min, 40 ml of the 100 mmoles/liter HCl solution was infused over 5 min into the midportion of the duodenum. The aspiration was continued for 15 min. The pH of the aspirates decreased from pH 7 or 8 to pH 2 during the acid infusion (Fig. 1). After cessation of the infusion the pH returned to neutral. The release of IRS into the juice showed a marked increase during acidification (Fig. 2), followed by a rapid return to almost prestimulatory

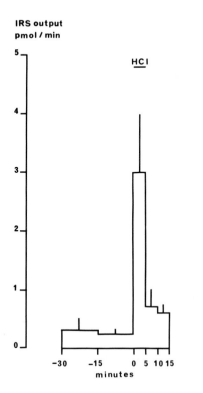

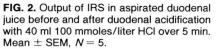

FIG. 2. Output of IRS in aspirated duodenal juice before and after duodenal acidification with 40 ml 100 mmoles/liter HCl over 5 min. Mean ± SEM, $N = 5$.

levels. The simultaneous IRS release into the blood showed a similar pattern (Fig. 3).

We were thus able to show that IRS can really be measured in duodenal juice (5). The control experiments, on the other hand, demonstrated no IRS in gastric juice before and after pentagastrin stimulation, which could be anticipated.

In order to investigate whether IRS was released during a meal, we examined five young volunteers after an overnight fast. A Lavin tube was passed into the proximal duodenum, and the duodenal juice was constantly aspirated throughout the experiment. After a control period of 30 min, the subjects received 250 ml milk fortified with commercial protein powder by mouth.

A high volume of aspirated fluid from the duodenum was obtained during the first hour following the meal (Fig. 4). The amount of IRS in the aspirated duodenal fluid was relatively constant in the control period and during the first digestive hours (Fig. 5). There was, however, a marked increase in IRS output in the late digestive period, while the pH value had returned to neutral (Fig. 6). The IRS output in total aspirates of the duodenal juice did not correlate with the mean pH of the aspirates. The pH spikes down to pH 1 or 2 are short-lived and tend to disappear during digestion. In the interdigestive periods

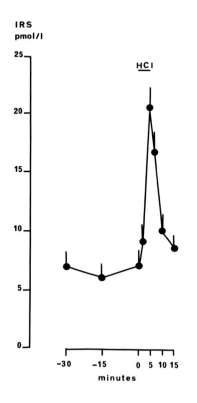

FIG. 3. Plasma IRS before and after duodenal acidification with 40 ml 100 mmoles/liter HCl over 5 min. Mean ± SEM, *N* = 5.

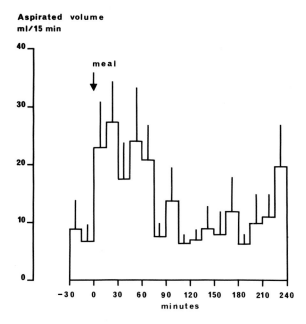

FIG. 4. Volume of duodenal aspirates before and after ingestion of 250 ml milk fortified with protein powder. Mean ± SEM, *N* = 5.

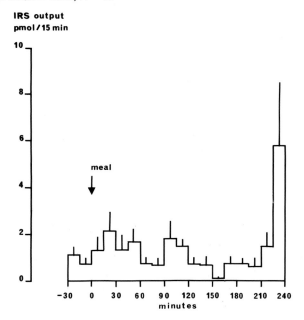

FIG. 5. Output of IRS in aspirated duodenal juice before and after ingestion of 250 ml milk fortified with protein powder. Mean ± SEM, *N* = 5.

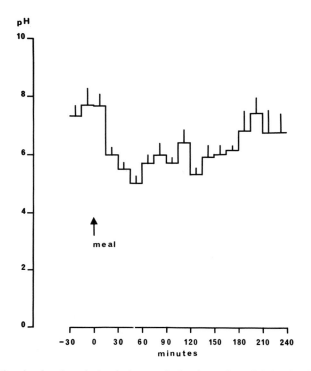

FIG. 6. pH of the duodenal aspirates before and after ingestion of 250 ml milk fortified with protein powder. Mean ± SEM, $N = 5$.

the mean pHs are usually neutral, although rapid pH spikes below pH 3 are seen and may cause IRS release.

The plasma IRS did not change significantly, although there was a tendency to higher mean values towards the end of the experiments. These findings indicate that IRS release into the duodenal juice is more important during the interdigestive period than during a meal.

INTERPRETATIONS

The presence of IRS in the duodenal juice of man may suggest two possible interpretations. The release may be followed by rapid degradation by proteases present in the duodenal juice, which would render the hormone inactive. Furthermore, no reabsorption of the hormone from the duodenal lumen might occur. On the other hand, the release of IRS from the S cells could act as a paracrine secretion that is not supposed to stimulate the pancreas, but might, owing to its high concentration in the duodenum, have a local stimulatory effect on the bicarbonate-producing cells of the duodenal mucosa.

The latter hypothesis is supported by the finding in animal experiments that the duodenal mucosa responds to intravenous secretin injections by an increased secretion of both bicarbonate and fluid. This is shown when both gastric and pancreatic and biliary secretions are diverted (1). A similar response has been elicited by HCl perfusion of a duodenal segment, but not by saline (3,11,13). It has also been shown that only the proximal duodenal mucosa responds with increased bicarbonate secretion to secretin infusion (8). Whether the locally demonstrated released secretin working as a paracrine peptide acts as a physiologic stimulus for this mechanism has not yet been determined.

It is reasonable to believe that the secretin which is released into the duodenum exerts its effect in a paracrine fashion by reaching the target cells at a considerably higher concentration than secretin released into the bloodstream. The relative importance of the duodenal mucosa as compared to that of the pancreas and bile in providing bicarbonate in response to a given stimulus is, however, not adequately known. Nevertheless, the duodenum is able to neutralize acid quicker, if the stimulus, secretin, is secreted in a paracrine manner than if it is secreted into the bloodstream. A direct transport of secretin from the duodenum into the pancreas, e.g., by lymphatic pathway, has not been demonstrated.

SUMMARY AND CONCLUSIONS

It is well established that infusion of HCl into the duodenum is followed by an increase in the blood of the secretin concentration as measured by RIA. It is also observed that the secretin concentration will respond to physiological fluctuations in the pH of the duodenuim, especially the short-lasting pH spikes in the proximal part. During a meal different results have been reported, but in man the mean pH remains above the pH threshold for IRS release. However, a release of IRS has been demonstrated recently after duodenal instillation of bile or bile salts at pH levels 6 to 7.

Recent experiments have shown that in humans the concentration of IRS is much higher in duodenal juice than in the blood after infusion of hydrochloric acid into the duodenum. After a meal a large volume of juice was aspirated from the duodenum without a concomitant increase in IRS output in the juice. However, a marked increase was seen in the late digestive period, when the pH had returned to neutral.

These findings indicate that IRS is released into the duodenal juice of man by acid and after a meal, but that the main importance of secretin in the duodenal juice might be in the late digestive or in the interdigestive period, as a paracrine hormone. The significance of these findings is as yet unknown.

PROJECTIONS FOR THE FUTURE

The presence of a large amount of IRS in the duodenal juice following stimulation may indicate a paracrine type of secretion and the direct effect of the secretin cells' secretion on the duodenal mucosa. Thus the possibility exists that secretin may preferably exert its action on the bicarbonate-producing cells locally. A smaller amount of secretin reaches the pancreas, causing a later response. The problems that require future evaluation include the following: Which role is played by the IRS in the duodenal juice of humans in the neutralization of acid from the stomach? Is this rapid neutralization then disturbed in patients with duodenal ulcer?

Future research should elucidate the significance of the current observations on intraduodenal secretin in the pathogenesis of peptic ulcer.

ACKNOWLEDGMENTS

The technical assistance of Jorunn Bratlie and the inspiring and critical help of Dr. Kristian F. Hanssen and Dr. Johan Haffner are gratefully acknowledged.

REFERENCES

1. Chung, R. S., Johnson, G. M., and DenBesten, L. (1976): The effect of secretin on hydrogen ion transport in the duodenum and jejunum. *J. Surg. Res.,* 20:467–471.
2. Fahrenkrug, J., Schaffalitzky de Muckadell, O. B., and Rune, S. J. (1978): pH threshold for release of secretin in normal subjects and in patients with duodenal ulcer and patients with chronic pancreatitis. *Scand. J. Gastroenterol.,* 13:177–186.
3. Florey, H. W., and Harding, H. E. (1934): Further observations on the secretion of Brunner's glands. *J. Pathol. Bacteriol.,* 39:255–276.
4. Hanssen, L. E. (1980): The effect of atropine on secretin release and bicarbonate secretion after duodenal acidification in man. *Scand. J. Gastroenterol.,* 15 *(in press).*
5. Hanssen, L. E., Hanssen, K. F., and Myren, J. (1977): Immunoreactive secretin is released into the duodenal juice in man. *Acta Hepatogastroenterol.* (Stuttg.), 24:493.
6. Hanssen, L. E., Hotz, J. Hartmann, W., Nehls, W., and Goebell, H. (1980): Immunoreactive secretin (IRS) release following duodenal taurocholate perfusions in the cat. *Scand. J. Gastroenterol.,* 15 *(in press).*
7. Hanssen, L. E., and Torjesen, P. (1977): Radioimmunoassay of secretin in human plasma. *Scand. J. Gastroenterol,* 12:481–488.
8. Himal, H. S., Moqtaderi, F., Kark, A. E., and Rudick, J. (1971): Hormonal regulation of duodenal secretion: Effects of glucagon and secretin. In: *Current Topics in Surgical Research,* edited by D. B. Skinner and P. A. Ebert, pp. 453–463. Academic Press, New York.
9. Osnes, M., Hanssen, L. E., Flaten, O., and Myren, J. (1978): Exocrine pancreatic secretion and immunoreactive secretin (IRS) release after intraduodenal instillation of bile in man. *Gut,* 19:180–184.
10. Schaffalitzky de Muckadell, O. B., Fahrenkrug, J., and Rune, S. J. (1979): Physiological significance of secretin in the pancreatic bicarbonate secretion. *Scand. J. Gastroenterol.,* 14:79–83.
11. Shaffer, R. D., and Winship, D. H. (1972): Acid loss in the human duodenum: Mucosal contribution to neutralization. *Clin. Res.,* 20:466.
12. Uvnäs-Wallensten, K., and Rehfeld, J. F. (1976): Molecular forms of gastrin in antral mucosa, plasma and gastric juice during vagal stimulation of anesthetized cats. *Acta Physiol. Scand.,* 98:217–226.
13. Winship, D., H., and Robinson, J. E. (1974): Acid loss in the human duodenum. *Gastroenterology,* 66:181–188.

Gastrointestinal Hormones, edited by
George B. Jerzy Glass.
Raven Press, New York © 1980.

Chapter 38

Intraluminal Gastrointestinal Hormones and Their Radioimmunoassay

Laurence J. Miller and Vay Liang W. Go

Department of Gastroenterology, Mayo Medical School, Mayo Clinic, Rochester, Minnesota 55901

II. GASTRIN

INTRODUCTION

There has been recent renewed interest in intraluminal gastrointestinal hormones. Evidence for the presence of these hormones in the lumen of the digestive tract is strong, although there are numerous unanswered questions relating to the mechanism of their secretion into the lumen, the regulation of intraluminal versus circulatory release of hormones, and the significance of intraluminal hormones. There are reports of luminal gastrin (9,19,21,22), somatostatin (40), secretin (13), VIP (38), and substance P (38), and we *(unpublished observations)* have recently detected immunoreactivity of cholecystokinin (CCK) gastric inhibitory polypeptide (GIP), and motilin in duodenal secretions. See also the first part of this chapter, I. Secretin, by Hanssen and Myren *(this volume)*.

Since most of the existing literature deals with gastrin, we attempt to review the history of this hormone's demonstration in the lumen, with reference to immunological, biological, and biochemical evidence, the problems in measurement of hormones in digestive luminal contents, and finally the questions raised above.

PRESENCE OF GASTRIN IN THE LUMEN OF THE STOMACH

Nonprotein nitrogen compounds were first observed in the gastric lumen in 1931 by Martin (25). It is interesting that he noted correlations between patients' acid secretory status and the amount of luminal peptide, a concept being actively investigated today. One of these compounds, with an amino acid composition similar to that of gastrin, was examined in the early 1960s by Brummer and co-workers (3,4). The concept of an intact peptide hormone residing in the lumen of the bowel where proteolytic enzymes are present still did not seem tenable until 1964. At that time, Sircus (31) provided evidence of the presence of a nonhistamine gastric acid secretagogue in the gastric lumen of two patients with Zollinger-Ellison syndrome.

Immunological Data

Investigation of intraluminal hormones in healthy man awaited the development of a more sensitive technique—radioimmunoassay (RIA). In 1972 Jordan and Yip (19) used this sensitive and specific technique to demonstrate the presence of large quantities of gastrin in the stomach of healthy man. They reported concentrations of immunoreactive gastrin in fasting gastric juice that ranged from 53 to 584 pg/ml. They showed that betazole promptly stimulated the total output and concentration of immunoreactive gastrin in the lumen, reporting concentrations of hormone in the lumen 400 times that in the circulation. This claim, however, was questioned by two subsequent publications (33,34). In these, the validity of RIA determination of intraluminal peptide concentration was examined, and the conditions necessary for valid determination were defined. See also Chapter 32 by R. S. Yalow and E. Straus, pp. 751–768, *this volume.*

The first problem considers the stability of hormone after entering the luminal milieu. Peptides would be accessible to gastric pepsin, with a pH optimum in the acid range, and pancreatic peptidases, active at neutral pH. Falsely low values for immunoreactive gastrin could be due to degradation of the hormone either *in vivo* in the lumen or after collection of samples. In recovery studies *in vitro*, synthetic human gastrin immunoreactivity disappeared rapidly (less than 1 min) when added to untreated gastric juice (10,33). Addition of aprotinin (Trasylol) did not affect this disappearance (33). Neutralization with NaOH or boiling interrupted this interference with immunoreactivity (33). The gastrin molecule does tolerate boiling at neutral pH for a short time (34). In fact, boiling of gastric juice was shown to be necessary to retain the added gastrin's ability to bind to an anion-exchange resin and to retain its gel filtration (Sephadex

G-50 superfine column) and thin-layer chromatography [butan-1-ol:acetic acid:water (20:3:25) or butan-1-ol:acetic acid:water:pyridine (15:3:12:10) systems] characteristics (34). Similar findings were attained using porcine gastrin I (34). Elution patterns following Sephadex G-50 gel chromatography of this compound were similar after incubation of standard in routine diluent to that attained after incubation in boiled acidic gastric juice, unboiled alkaline gastric juice, and boiled duodenal secretions; however, unboiled acidic gastric juice and unboiled duodenal secretions produced changes in the elution pattern (34).

A second problem considers the validity of the actual RIA determination of hormone concentration in gastric and intestinal juice. RIA measurement of a hormone depends on the competitive inhibition between the unlabeled hormone in the sample and the labeled hormone in the incubation mixture for binding to a specific antibody. This binding is a function of the concentration of hormone in the sample, unlabeled hormone competing with labeled hormone for antibody-binding sites. Antibody-bound hormone is then separated from free hormone. A standard curve is prepared from known standards and the unknown sample values interpolated. Development of a valid RIA therefore depends on (29): (a) the availability of a highly purified hormone for labeling to be used as a reference standard; (b) the stability of this standard under conditions of labeling and of the assay, so as not to interfere with immunoreactivity or biological activity; (c) the availability of antisera with sufficient sensitivity and specificity; and (d) the availability of a valid separation procedure.

In application of this technique to intraluminal samples, conditions (a) and (c) are certainly fulfilled (12). Also, there is much expertise labeling the standard hormone (gastrin) (12). Potential problems arise with the stability of the labeled hormone during incubation with acidic gastric juice and duodenal secretions that contain active proteolytic enzymes. As described above, these conditions, if unaltered, produce damage to the peptide hormone. Also, acidic gastric juice and duodenal secretions have been shown to interfere with binding of gastrin to appropriate antisera (34). These types of problems, degradation of the standard labeled hormone or interference with hormone-antibody binding, would be expected to produce falsely elevated values of immunoreactive gastrin. Straus and Yalow (34) also suggested potential problems with condition (d) by demonstrating that charcoal, the control adsorbent commonly used to assess incubation damage in the gastrin RIA, continued to adsorb labeled gastrin (84%) after the hormone was fragmented by exposure to duodenal secretions. Therefore, the control would have been considered adequate. Amberlite CG-4B resin, a more specific adsorbent, bound only 18% of the labeled peptide under similar circumstances.

The impact of the papers (33,34) criticizing Jordan and Yip's assay techniques was made greater by their reports of only trace amounts of immunoreactive gastrin (33) or less than 40 pg/ml of immunoreactive gastrin (34) in human gastric juice. Since 1976, however, the pendulum has again swung toward believing the presence of gastrin in the lumen of the stomach. One of the authors of these papers, in fact, has reported the presence of gastric luminal gastrin since then (44).

When the above-described technique has been used, immunoreactive gastrin has again been measured in gastric luminal samples in healthy humans by Knight et al. (21) and our group (22,23). This has been primarily true of situations in which acid secretion has been stimulated (21,22). Fasting gastric juice seems to contain little or no immunoreactive gastrin (21,22).

Most data relating to gastric luminal gastrin have been derived from animal or *in vitro* studies. Andersson and Nilsson (1) demonstrated the presence of immunoreactive gastrin in the lumen of antral pouches of dogs. The cat has been a particularly well-studied model, demonstrating luminal immunoreactive gastrin (37,38,40,43,44).

In vitro gastric mucosal preparations have been described that release immunoreactive gastrin from the mucosal (luminal) side of the preparation (2,8,30,49). Schofield et al. (30) showed that acetylcholine stimulated the release of immunoreactive gastrin into the mucosal-side solution when it was applied to either the serosal or mucosal side of the canine preparation. Fiddian-Green et al. (8), using a human antral preparation, found that mucosally applied stimulants (arginine, glycine, acetylcholine) released immunoreactive gastrin only into the mucosal-side compartment, whereas those applied to the serosal side released hormone preferentially into the mucosal solution, but also into the serosal solution.

Biological Data

Combining biological data with the immunological data described above further supports the concept of the presence of intraluminal gastrin. In 1972 Jordan and Yip (20) tested the substance they had identified in human gastric juice to see its secretagogue characteristics in dogs with vagally innervated gastric mucosa and those with vagally denervated Heidenhain pouches. They found that this substance was 79% as active biologically as synthetic human gastrin. Also, it reacted similarly to synthetic human gastrin and differently from histamine in the series of secretory studies. Andersson and Nilsson (1) verified biological activity in the substance they isolated from the dog antral lumen as well. They showed that this substance had the ability to induce secretion in Heidenhain pouch dogs during background stimulation with urecholine. Biological activity has also been demonstrated *in vitro* using a parietal cell preparation (2).

Biochemical Data

The final confirmation of the presence of gastrin in the lumen of the digestive tract is dependent on biochemical verification. Jordan and Yip (20) examined human gastric juice extracts by starch gel electrophoresis, and found the gastrin immunoreactivity at the typical elution zone for heptadecapeptide gastrin.

Knight et al. (21) and our laboratory *(unpublished data)* have also found hepta-decapeptide gastrin to be the predominant form in human gastric juice by chromatographic studies. An *in vitro* human antral preparation also has been shown to release from its mucosal side a biologically active peptide with gastrin immunoreactivity which resembles heptadecapeptide gastrin chromatographically (8,49).

Uvnas-Wallensten and Rehfeld (44) confirmed these data in the cat, demonstrating predominantly heptadecapeptide gastrin in the gastric lumen. This consisted of both sulfated and unsulfated forms.

DUODENAL INTRALUMINAL GASTRIN

Although both the gastric antrum and the duodenum contain gastrin-producing cells (24), and both organs contain approximately equal quantities of this hormone in man (27), most data relating to intraluminal gastrin have been gathered from the level of the stomach. Recently, we (23) quantified the immunoreactive gastrin that arrives at the level of the ligament of Treitz in the distal duodenum in healthy man. Again, samples and the RIA were handled according to the suggestions of Straus and Yalow (34). Immunoreactive gastrin concentrations in basal fasting duodenal samples ranged from 110 to 2,100 pg/ml with an output of 1.6 ± 0.6 ng/min. Intragastric instillation of 400 ml of normal saline stimulated a rapid increase in immunoreactive gastrin arrival at this level of the bowel to approximately five times basal and, despite the diluting volume, hormone concentration increased. These changes were independent of any changes in circulating immunoreactive gastrin. It is of note that large quantities of immunoreactive gastrin were arriving at the ligament of Treitz at a time when gastrin was not detectable in the gastric lumen. This was felt to suggest the duodenal origin of at least a portion of this luminal hormone.

The duodenal contribution to intraluminal gastrin was conclusively demonstrated in the cat by Uvnas-Wallensten et al. (42) using acute duodenal pouches. This release could be stimulated by acetycholine and electrical vagal stimulation, especially during maintenance of intraluminal pH in the neutral or alkaline range.

MECHANISM OF INTRALUMINAL SECRETION OF GASTRIN

Whether the gastrin that appears in the gastric lumen is directly released from the gastrin-producing cells through their villi that project into the lumen, or indirectly arrives in the lumen after release from the granule-containing basal part of the cells is not known (Fig. 1).

The secretory cycle of the gastrin-producing cell has been studied ultrastructurally (11). The hormone-containing granules always seem to be basally located. Normal cells show secretory granules of different electron density, with those from fasting animals containing only dense granules, and with degranulation occurring on refeeding. These observations would tend to support the basal

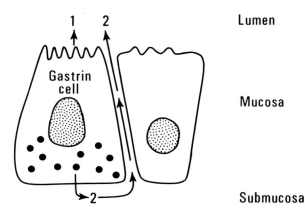

FIG. 1. Gastrin secretion into the gastric lumen may be direct (route 1) or indirect (route 2). These routes are diagrammatically shown here.

release of hormone directly from granules, probably via exocytosis. In this situation the hormone would reach the lumen and the capillaries via diffusion. Forssmann and Orci (11), however, have never seen a granule opening directly into the extracellular space. They postulate, therefore, the intracytoplasmic release of hormone. This could, if present, account for the direct release of hormone from villi into the lumen.

There appears to be a discrepancy between the amount of gastrin released into the lumen and that released into the circulation in different situations. This is actually difficult to interpret because of the large intravascular diluting volume, short circulatory half-life, indeterminate *in vivo* luminal disappearance rate, and possibly different resistances to entry into the blood or lumen. There are certainly some stimuli that release hormone into both the circulation and the lumen [e.g., electrical vagal stimulation in the cat (42)]. This would tend to support the postulated mechanism of indirect arrival in the lumen. There are also, however, times when serum immunoreactive gastrin remains unchanged despite large amounts of hormone released into the lumen [e.g., intraluminal calcium stimulation (22)]. This would tend to support the postulated mechanism of direct release of hormone into the lumen. Uvnas-Wallensten (37) has described the situation in the cat in which 23 times as much gastrin is released into the lumen as is released into the circulation. Perhaps secretion occurs via both routes simultaneously.

Cellular morphology seems to be important in the determination of luminal hormone release. As a rule, the endocrine cells of the gastric fundus are closed cells, lying directly on the basal lamina having no contact with the lumen, whereas the endocrine cells of the antral-pyloric area are open cells, possessing thin cytoplasmic extensions into the lumen (32). It is interesting that no or minute amounts of hormones are released into perfusates of the corpus of the stomach (37,42), whereas hormones are readily released from the antrum (37). This observation is consistent with either theory of hormone secretion into the lumen, direct or indirect. Superficially it might support the direct release theory; however, if hormone were basally released, different resistances to diffusion could explain the same findings. If there were greater resistance to hormone diffusion into the lumen at the level of the corpus than at the level of the antrum, these findings would be consistent with the indirect release theory.

REGULATION OF INTRALUMINAL SECRETION OF GASTRIN

Factors important in the regulation of secretion of gastrin into the lumen of the stomach and duodenum are not clearly defined. The gastrin-producing cell can theoretically be stimulated by way of the lumen, the circulation or nerves. All three routes have been suggested (19,22,36). Human *in vivo* data are quite limited (3,21,23), although an *in vitro* human model is available (8,49). Most information has been systematically collected in the cat by Uvnas-Wallensten and co-workers (36–38,40,43,44). Other animal data are also available (1) (Fig. 2).

Gastric acid secretagogues seem to stimulate the release of immunoreactive gastrin into the gastric lumen. Intragastric instillation of albumin (21) or a calcium solution (22) stimulates hormone release. This secretion into the lumen varies independently from serum gastrin changes (21,22), and the pattern of release into gastric juice can certainly not be inferred from the pattern of release into the circulation (21). It is of note that Knight et al. (21) found significantly greater luminal gastrin release after a stronger stimulus to acid secretion than after a weaker stimulus, albumin versus a saline distension stimulus. Also, human

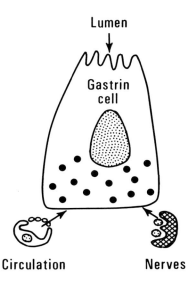

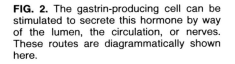

FIG. 2. The gastrin-producing cell can be stimulated to secrete this hormone by way of the lumen, the circulation, or nerves. These routes are diagrammatically shown here.

data (21) support the antral origin of much of this gastrin by showing significantly lesser quantities of immunoreactive gastrin released into the lumen after antrectomy. Parenteral acid secretory stimulants like betazole have also been shown to stimulate the luminal release of gastrin (19).

The cat model has been extensively studied by Uvnas-Wallensten and co-workers (35–40,43,44,46,48). They have previously evaluated the stimulation of acid secretion and the release of gastrin into the circulation by electrical vagal stimulation (35,39,46,48). In 1976 this form of stimulation was shown to release immunoreactive gastrin into the gastric lumen as well (36). This release seems to be noncholinergic since it is not blocked by atropine (43). The ratio of hormone released into the lumen to that released into the circulation in response to this stimulation was rather constant in individual animals, but varied considerably from cat to cat, with ratios ranging from 2 to 23 (mean of approximately 10) (37). Also in this model, the species of gastrin molecules present in the antrum and those released into the circulation and lumen were determined (44). Heptadecapeptide gastrin (component III of Rehfeld) predominated in the antral mucosa, with 5% component II (G34), 1% component I, and traces of component IV (G14). Immediately after stimulation, heptadecapeptide gastrin appeared in the venous effluent and the lumen, with component IV (G14) appearing a few minutes later in the blood. This supports antral release of heptadecapeptide gastrin with subsequent rapid metabolism of this hormone species. The absence of circulating component II (G34) is in contrast with the situation found in man and dog (44).

This group has also added another dimension to the concept of intraluminal gastrin regulation. That is interaction with somatostatin (40,41,43). The gastric somatostatin cells are located in close proximity to the gastrin cells (16). Somatostatin blocks the gastric acid secretion and the gastrin release into the blood, which are stimulated by electrical vagal stimulation (41). Vagal stimulation has been shown to release somatostatin (40), as well as gastrin (36), into the gastric lumen. The somatostatin release, like that of gastrin, is resistant to atropine (43). This release seems to be luminal pH related, with large amounts of somatostatin and small amounts of gastrin released during vagal stimulation and antral perfusion with 0.1 M HCl, and small amounts of somatostatin and large amounts of gastrin released during vagal stimulation and antral perfusion with a slightly alkaline medium (38,40). It has been postulated that the reciprocal occurrence of gastrin and somatostatin in the antral lumen is at least partially due to the local effect of somatostatin on the gastrin-producing cells (40). Apomorphine, a stimulant of dopamine receptors, has been shown in this model to release both gastrin and somatostatin into the antral lumen (43). This release mechanism, like vagal stimulation, is not blocked by atropine, however, it is abolished after vagotomy (43). Thus the effect of vagal stimulation on luminal hormone release might well be an effect of dopaminergic fibers, which travel with the nerve (43).

There is further new information relating to interactions between nerves and hormones (45,47). Heptadecapeptide gastrin has been shown to be present in the vagus (45) and even peripheral nerves (47). Since small amounts of components I and II, putative biosynthetic precursors of the secretory form of gastrin, were also found in nerves, it was suggested that gastrin can be produced there (45). Stimulation of these nerves can be shown to release gastrin (47). The role that this plays in luminal gastrin release is certainly not clear.

SIGNIFICANCE OF INTRALUMINAL GASTRIN

Now that the presence of this hormone in the lumen has been established, investigators are searching for its significance. It would seem to be a great waste to lose a large percentage of gastrin secreted (37) into the lumen if it were just an excretory pathway. Also, however, there continues to be the problem of the coexistence of peptide hormones with active proteolytic enzymes in the bowel lumen. Many of the postulated activities of intraluminal gastrin will await *in vivo* demonstration of delivery of biologically active hormone to the mid and distal gut—thus far, its presence has been demonstrated only as far distally as the ligament of Treitz (23).

The most exciting potential activity of luminal gastrin is its trophic activity for the mucosa of the gastrointestinal tract. Gastrin has been shown to stimulate RNA, DNA, and protein synthesis in mucosa along the entire length of the bowel, except for the esophagus and antrum (5,6,17). Because a number of observations related to growth of gastrointestinal mucosa cannot be explained by a systemic factor, but require a mechanism with a gradient having greatest effects proximally and lesser effects distally, a trophic component of chyme must be postulated. Johnson et al. (18) have recently shown that gastrin can exert its trophic effect on the bowel mucosa when administered intraluminally. They showed that this effect was not mediated by absorption and subsequent recirculation of the hormone (18), in spite of the observation that pentagastrin can be absorbed intact from the bowel and stimulate acid secretion (26). The effect, also, was not a nonspecific effect of the amino acid content since control animals were perfused with 1,000 times more amino acids than would result from the total hydrolysis of the dose of gastrin used.

Recent *in vitro* work has demonstrated the presence of specific gastrin receptor sites on parietal cells, with access both from the serosal and mucosal sides of the tissue (14,15). This suggests that luminal hormone might play a role in regulation of acid secretion. In fact, exogenous heptadecapeptide gastrin instilled into the stomach of healthy subjects has been shown to stimulate acid secretion, concurrently with its disappearance from the lumen, but with no measurable increase in serum concentrations (9). This stimulation of acid secretion was dose related (9).

Other roles have been proposed for luminal gastrin. Quinn and Fiddian-Green (7,28) suggested duodenal or gastrinoma gastrin release into the circulation. Uvnäs-Wallensten and Rehfeld (44) suggested that it could affect gastrointestinal motility since concentrations similar to those which occur in the gastric lumen cause contraction of smooth muscle preparations and antagonize the CCK-induced contraction of the pyloric sphincter.

SUMMARY AND CONCLUSIONS

The presence of intraluminal gastrin in the stomach and duodenum has been well established by immunological, biological, and biochemical techniques. Demonstration of its presence requires unique handling of luminal contents because of pH, osmolar, and enzymatic characteristics that could interfere with RIA and provide artifactual results. Investigation into the mechanism of its secretion into the lumen, the regulation of its appearance in the lumen, and the significance of its presence in the lumen is currently in progress.

PROJECTIONS FOR THE FUTURE

In the future, the mechanism of gastrin secretion into the lumen, its regulation, and significance should all be well defined. Along with this, the same questions will have to be answered for the other gastrointestinal peptide hormones. This should change our concept of the lumen of the digestive tract, adding new significance to this already complex and important organ.

REFERENCES

1. Andersson, S., and Nilsson, G. (1974): Appearance of gastrin in perfusates from the isolated gastric antrum of dogs. *Scand. J. Gastroenterol.,* 9:619–621.
2. Askew, A. R., Vinik, A. I., Grant, B. J., Terblanche, J., and Louw, J. H. (1977): Evidence for biological activity of immunoreactive gastrin released by the mucosal surface of the human antrum. *S. Afr. J. Surg.,* 15:126 (abst.).
3. Brummer, P., and Kulonen, M. (1960): Chromatographic pattern of ninhydrin-staining compounds in gastric juice and its relation to acid gastric secretion. *Acta Med. Scand.,* 167:61–64.
4. Brummer, P., Seppala, P., and Kulonen, M. (1961): Chromatographic pattern of ninhydrin-staining compounds in gastric juice. Polypeptide residues of pepsinogen. *Acta Med. Scand.,* 170:187–189.
5. Enochs, M. R., and Johnson, L. R. (1977): Trophic effects of gastrointestinal hormones: Physiological implications. *Fed. Proc.,* 36:1942–1947.
6. Enochs, M. R., and Johnson, L. R. (1977): Hormonal regulation of gastrointestinal tract growth; Biochemical and physiologic aspects. In: *Progress in Gastroenterology, Vol. 3,* edited by George B. Jerzy-Glass. Grune & Stratton, New York.
7. Fiddian-Green, R. G. (1977): Is peptic ulceration a hormonal disease? *Lancet,* 1:74–76.
8. Fiddian-Green, R. G., Aitchison, J. M., and Vinik, A. I. (1976): *In vitro* release of gastrin from oriented sheets of human antral mucosa II. *Gastroenterology,* 70:961 (abst.).
9. Fiddian-Green, R. G., Farrell, J., Havlichek, D., Jr., Kothary, P., and Pittenger, G. (1978): A physiological role for luminal gastrin? *Surgery,* 83:663–668.
10. Fiddian-Green, R. G., Knight, N., and Vinik, A. I. (1977): Regulation of gastrin release into human gastric juice. *Gastroenterology,* 72:1159 (abst.).
11. Forssmann, W. G. and Orci, L. (1969): Ultrastructure and secretory cycle of the gastrin-producing cell. *Z. Zellforsch. Mikrosk. Anat.,* 101:419–432.
12. Go, V. L. W., and Owyang, C. (1977): Radioimmunoassay of gastrointestinal hormones. In:

Progress in Gastroenterology, Vol. 3, edited by George B. Jerzy-Glass, pp. 153–178. Grune & Stratton, New York.

13. Hanssen, L. E., Hanssen, K. F., and Myren, J. (1978): Immunoreactive secretin is released into the duodenal juice. *Scand. J. Gastroenterol. [Suppl. 49]*, 13:79 (abst.).
14. Hedenbro, J. L., Fink, A. S., and Fiddian-Green, R. G. (1978): Binding of luminal gastrin to canine parietal mucosa *in vitro. Gastroenterology,* 74:1045 (abst.).
15. Hedenbro, J. L., Fink, A. S., and Fiddian-Green, R. G. (1978): Directions of access to gastrin receptor sites in canine parietal mucosa. *Scand. J. Gastroenterol. [Suppl. 49]*, 13:84 (abst.).
16. Hökfelt, T., Efendić, S., Hellerström, C., Johansson, O., Luft, R., and Arimura, A. (1975): Cellular localization of somatostatin in endocrine-like cells and neurons of the rat with special references to the A_1-cells of the pancreatic islets and to the hypothalamus. *Acta Endocrinol. (Kbh.) [Suppl.]*, 200:1–41.
17. Johnson, L. R. (1977): New aspects of the trophic action of gastrointestinal hormones. *Gastroenterology,* 72:788–792.
18. Johnson, L. R., Copeland, E. M., and Dudrick, S. J. (1978): Luminal gastrin stimulates growth of distal rat intestine. *Scand. J. Gastroenterol. [Suppl. 49]*, 13:95 (abst.).
19. Jordan, P. H., Jr., and Yip, B. S. S. C. (1972): The presence of gastrin in fasting and stimulated gastric juice of man. *Surgery,* 72:352–356.
20. Jordan, P. H., Jr., and Yip, B. S. S. C. (1972): The canine secretory response to gastrin extracted from gastric juice of man. *Surgery,* 72:624–629.
21. Knight, N. F., Fiddian-Green, R. G., and Vinik, A. I. (1978): *In vivo* release of gastrin into human gastric juice. *Br. J. Surg.,* 65:118–120.
22. Krawisz, B. R. (1978): Gastric luminal gastrin release in man: Effects of calcium and pH. *Gastroenterology,* 74:1173 (abst.).
23. Krawisz, B. R., Miller, L. J., and Go, V. L. W. (1978): Quantification of luminal immunoreactive gastrin (iG) secretion in man. *Scand. J. Gastroenterol. [Suppl. 49]* 13:105 (abst.).
24. Larsson, L. I., Hakanson, R., Sjoberg, N. O., and Sundler, F. (1975): Fluorescence histochemistry of the gastrin cell in fetal and adult man. *Gastroenterology,* 68:1152–1159.
25. Martin, L. (1931): Total nitrogen and nonprotein nitrogen partition of gastric juice obtained after histamine stimulation. *Johns Hopkins Med. J.,* 49:286–301.
26. Morrell, M. J., and Keynes, W. M. (1975): Absorption of pentagastrin from gastrointestinal tract in man. *Lancet,* 2:712.
27. Nilsson, G., Yalow, R. S., and Berson, S. A. (1970): Distribution of gastrin in the gastrointestinal tract of human, dog, cat and hog. *Sixteenth Nobel Symposium: Frontiers in Gastrointestinal Hormone Research,* Stockholm.
28. Quinn, T. J., and Fiddian-Green, R. G. (1977): Luminal gastrin and gastrin release. *Lancet,* 2:307–308.
29. Rodbard, D., Rayford, P. L., Cooper, J. A., and Ross, G. T. (1968): Statistical quality control of radioimmunoassays, *J. Clin. Endocrinol. Metab.,* 28:1412–1418.
30. Schofield, B., Tepperman, B. L., Kende, E. M., and Tepperman, F. S. (1976): *In vitro* release of gastrin by a morphologically-oriented canine antral mucosa preparation. *Gastroenterology,* 70:935 (abst.).
31. Sircus, W. (1964): Evidence for a gastric secretagogue in the circulation and gastric juice of patients with the Zollinger-Ellison syndrome. *Lancet,* 2:671–672.
32. Solcia, E., Capella, C., Vassallo, G., and Buffa, R. (1975): Endocrine cells of the gastric mucosa. *Int. Rev. Cytol.,* 42:223–286.
33. Stadil, F., Malmstrom, J., Miyata, M., and Rehfeld, J. F. (1975): Effect of histamine on immunoreactive gastrin in gastric juice and in serum. *Surgery,* 77:345–350.
34. Straus, E., and Yalow, R. S. (1976): Artifacts in the radioimmunoassay of peptide hormones in gastric and duodenal secretions. *J. Lab. Clin. Med.,* 87:292–298.
35. Uvnas, B., Uvnas-Wallensten, K., and Nilsson, G. (1975): Release of gastrin on vagal stimulation in the cat. *Acta Physiol. Scand.,* 94:167–176.
36. Uvnas-Wallensten, K. (1976): Gastrin release and HCl secretion induced by electrical vagal stimulation in the cat. *Acta Physiol. Scand. [Suppl.]*, 438:1–39.
37. Uvnas-Wallensten, K. (1977): Occurrence of gastrin in gastric juice, in antral secretion, and in antral perfusates of cats. *Gastroenterology,* 73:487–491.
38. Uvnas-Wallensten, K. (1978): Vagal release of antral hormones. In: *Gut Hormones,* edited by S. R. Bloom, pp. 389–393. Churchill Livingstone, Edinburgh.

39. Uvnas-Wallensten, K., and Andersson, H. (1977): Effect of atropine and methiamide on vagally induced gastric acid secretion and gastrin release in anesthetized cats. *Acta Physiol. Scand.,* 99:496–502.
40. Uvnas-Wallensten, K., Efendić, S., and Luft, R. (1977): Vagal release of somatostatin into the antral lumen of cats. *Acta Physiol. Scand.,* 99:126–128.
41. Uvnas-Wallensten, K., Efendić, S., and Luft, R. (1977): Inhibition of vagally induced gastrin release by somatostatin in cats. *Horm. Metab. Res.,* 9:120–123.
42. Uvnas-Wallensten, K., Efendić, S., and Luft, R. (1978): Release of gastrointestinal hormones into the duodenal lumen of cats. *Horm. Metab. Res.,* 10:173.
43. Uvnas-Wallensten, K., Lundberg, J. M., and Efendić, S. (1978): Dopaminergic control of antral gastrin and somatostatin release. *Acta Physiol. Scand.,* 103:343–345.
44. Uvnas-Wallensten, K., and Rehfeld, J. F. (1976): Molecular forms of gastrin in antral mucosa, plasma and gastric juice during vagal stimulation of anesthetized cats. *Acta Physiol. Scand.,* 98:217–226.
45. Uvnas-Wallensten, K., Rehfeld, J. F., Larsson, L.-I., and Uvnas, B. (1977): Heptadecapeptide gastrin in the vagal nerve. *Proc. Natl. Acad. Sci. U.S.A.,* 74:5707–5710.
46. Uvnas-Wallensten, K., and Uvnas, B. (1976): Gastric clearance of gastrin during acid secretory responses to vagal activation and its effect on peripheral gastrin levels. A study on anesthetized cats. *Acta Physiol. Scand.,* 97:349–356.
47. Uvnas-Wallensten, K., and Uvnas, B. (1978): Release of gastrin on stimulation of the sciatic and brachial nerves of the cat. *Acta Physiol. Scand.,* 103:349–351.
48. Uvnas-Wallensten, K., Uvnas, B., and Nilsson, G. (1976): Quantitative aspects of the vagal control of gastrin release in cats. *Acta Physiol. Scand.,* 96:19–28.
49. Vinik, A. I. (1978): Regulation of gastrin release from oriented sheets of human antral mucosa *in vitro.* In: *Gut Hormones,* edited by S. R. Bloom, pp. 156–157. Churchill Livingstone, Edinburgh.

Candidate Peptide Hormones and Chalons

Gastrointestinal Hormones, edited by
George B. Jerzy Glass.
Raven Press, New York © 1980.

Chapter 39

Intestinal Phase Hormone That Stimulates Gastric Acid Secretion

Marshall J. Orloff, Paul V. B. Hyde, Louis D. Kosta, Roger
C. L. Guillemin, and Richard H. Bell, Jr.

*Department of Surgery, University of California Medical Center, San Diego,
San Diego, California 92103*

Although stimulation of gastric acid secretion by food in the intestine was identified early in this century (38,53,78), and humoral mediation of this phenomenon was suggested over three decades ago (25,61,87), it has been recognized only recently that the intestinal phase of gastric secretion plays an important role in acid production during digestion. Moreover, it is only within the last decade that research has provided convincing physiologic evidence that the stimulatory intestinal phase is mediated by one or more hormones.

The term "intestinal phase of gastric secretion," as used generally and in this chapter, refers to *stimulation* of gastric acid production by food in the intestine. It should not be confused with inhibition of acid secretion arising in the small bowel, which is known to be caused by certain foods, particularly fats, hyperosmolar sugar solutions, and acid. Undoubtedly, the gastric secretory response to food in the gut reflects the net effect resulting from these stimulatory and inhibitory mechanisms.

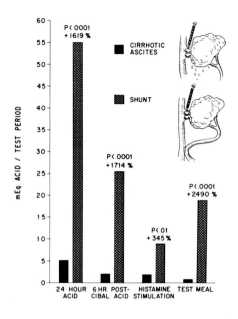

FIG. 1. Effect of portacaval shunt on Heidenhain pouch acid secretion in dogs with liver disease, portal hypertension and ascites. The data represent the mean results in 4 dogs. PCS produced marked acid hypersecretion in all tests. (From ref. 74, with permission.)

PORTACAVAL SHUNT-RELATED GASTRIC HYPERSECRETION

The consistent observation of profound gastric acid hypersecretion in dogs with a portacaval shunt (PCS) was largely responsible for recent interest in the intestinal phase of gastric secretion (13,19,23,42,52,74,85) (Fig. 1). Numerous studies have shown that PCS-related hypersecretion is most marked following ingestion of protein (13,81,85), and that it is not related to the cephalic or antral phases of gastric acid secretion, since it is not abolished by truncal vagotomy (42) or antrectomy (13,42,56,62,73,77). It has been shown to occur following systemic shunting of venous blood draining the small intestine, but not after hepatic bypass of venous blood from the stomach, proximal duodenum, pancreas, and spleen (11,12,30,54). Substantial evidence suggests that the striking acid hypersecretion associated with PCS is due to unmasking of the intestinal phase of gastric secretion by hepatic bypass of a gastric secretory stimulant in portal blood that normally is inactivated to a considerable extent by the liver.

In 1966, we began a series of experiments in dogs directed at answering the question of humoral mediation of PCS-related acid hypersecretion and of the intestinal phase of gastric secretion. The first of these studies involved measurements in antrectomized dogs of the Heidenhain pouch secretory response to an intestinal meal during isovolemic autotransfusion of blood from the portal vein to the thoracic aorta, to simulate an acute PCS (4). Combination of an intestinal meal with portal-systemic autotransfusion resulted in significantly greater gastric acid secretion than an intestinal meal alone or portal-systemic

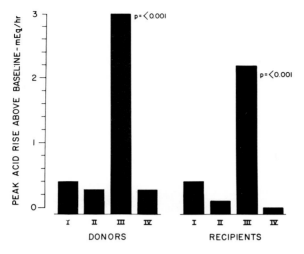

FIG. 2. Mean peak elevations of Heidenhain pouch acid secretion during cross-transfusion in four experimental groups of dogs as follows: I, Cross-transfusion alone from intact donors (8 pairs); II, Cross-transfusion from intact donors receiving intestinal meal (8 pairs); III, Cross-transfusion from donor with PCS receiving intestinal meal (10 pairs); IV, Cross-transfusion from donor with PCS in absence of meal (8 pairs). The recipients in all experiments had a Heidenhain pouch but otherwise were intact. (From ref. 73, with permission.)

autotransfusion alone. These results suggested that a humoral agent in portal blood was responsible for PCS-related gastric hypersecretion.

To further examine the question of humoral mediation, we conducted studies using the classic physiologic technique of controlled, isovolemic cross-transfusion (73). Heidenhain pouch acid output was measured during cross-transfusion of systemic blood between an antrectomized "donor" dog with a PCS and an intact "recipient" dog, in the presence and absence of food in the donor's intestine. The intestinal meal in the donor dog with a PCS stimulated marked acid secretion, not only in the donor, but also in the intact recipient that received the donor's blood by cross-tranfusion (Fig. 2). No significant rise in recipient acid output was produced by cross-transfusion alone, by donor feeding in the absence of a PCS, or by a donor PCS in the absence of an intestinal meal. These results provided direct evidence for humoral mediation of PCS-related gastric hypersecretion.

We next sought to determine whether the humoral mediator of PCS-related hypersecretion was a secretagogue absorbed from food or a hormone of endogenous origin. To this end, we compared the Heidenhain pouch secretory response to an intestinal meal with the response to balloon distention at physiologic pressures 20 cm distal to the duodenal-jejunal junction before and after PCS (92). Intestinal distention stimulated gastric hypersecretion in shunted animals to the same extent as an intestinal meal (Fig. 3). Moreover, a single 20-min period of intestinal distention stimulated as much acid secretion as repeated

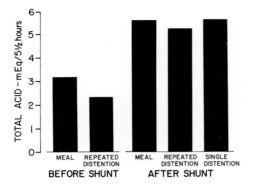

FIG. 3. Heidenhain pouch acid secretion for 5½ hr in response to an intestinal meal, a single 20-min period of balloon distention of the jejunum at physiologic pressures, and repeated balloon distention of the jejunum for 20 of each 30 min. Data represent mean results in 16 dogs. Intestinal distention stimulated as much acid secretion as an intestinal meal.

balloon distention or as an intestinal meal. These results suggested that the humoral agent was a hormone that originated in the intestine.

To determine the site of origin of the hormone responsible for PCS-related hypersecretion, our next experiments examined the gastric secretory responses of a Heidenhain pouch to the introduction of food into isolated segments of jejunum, ileum, and colon before and after PCS (72). Food in the isolated jejunum produced substantial gastric acid secretion before PCS, and sustained acid hypersecretion after PCS (Fig. 4). Food in the isolated ileum stimulated modest gastric secretion in unshunted dogs, but PCS did not enhance acid output, and food in the colon failed to produce a gastric secretory response. It was concluded that the jejunum was the major source of the humoral agent responsible for PCS-related acid hypersecretion.

The applicability of the striking findings of dog experiments to humans with PCS was unknown as of 1969. Indeed, up to that time a number of studies of basal and histamine stimulated gastric secretion in patients with PCS had not shown an increase in acid production (9,20,76,83,84,88,96). However, all of

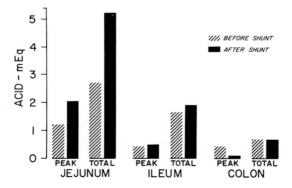

FIG. 4. Comparison of mean Heidenhain pouch acid responses to food in isolated segments of jejunum, ileum and colon before and after PCS. Each *bar* represents 16 studies in 8 dogs. Acid secretion was stimulated only by food in the jejunum. (From ref. 72, with permission.)

these clinical studies suffered from failure to examine the intestinal phase of gastric secretion. Accordingly, we undertook a study of the gastric secretory response to instillation of a liquid meal directly into the upper jejunum in 10 normal subjects, 20 ambulatory patients with compensated cirrhosis, and 15 ambulatory, compensated cirrhotic patients who had undergone PCS (67). The PCS group was subsequently expanded to 52 patients, and 11 patients were studied both before and after PCS. As other workers had reported, patients with PCS were found to have normal levels of basal- and histamine-stimulated gastric acid secretion. However, each of the 52 shunted cirrhotic patients responded to an intestinal meal with a marked, prolonged, and highly significant hypersecretion of acid that, at its peak, averaged 709% above the basal level (Fig. 5). Food in the intestine of normal subjects and unshunted cirrhotics failed to stimulate gastric secretion. It was concluded that hepatic bypass of portal blood unmasked the intestinal phase of gastric secretion in humans, just as it did in dogs.

As we had done in dog experiments, our next study in humans compared the gastric secretory response to balloon distention of the upper jejunum for 20 min at physiologic pressures with the response to an intestinal meal (65). Studies were performed in normal subjects, unshunted cirrhotic patients, and cirrhotic patients with PCS. Balloon distention of the jejunum did not stimulate acid secretion in normal subjects and unshunted cirrhotic patients, but produced a highly significant output of acid in every cirrhotic patient with a PCS, similar in magnitude to the secretory response to an intestinal meal (Fig. 6). These results suggested that PCS-related hypersecretion in humans, as in dogs, was mediated by an endogenous hormone rather than by a substance absorbed from food.

Our final study in humans was directed at localizing the intestinal site from which the intestinal phase hormone (IPH) originates. For this purpose we compared the gastric secretory responses to the instillation of food directly into the jejunum (just beyond the ligament of Treitz) and into the ileum (2½–3

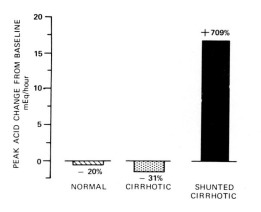

FIG. 5. Mean peak gastric acid response to an intestinal meal in 10 normal subjects, 20 patients with cirrhosis, and 15 cirrhotic patients with a PCS. (From ref. 67, with permission.)

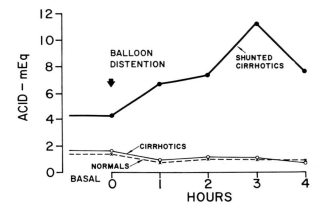

FIG. 6. Mean hourly gastric acid secretion after balloon distention of the jejunum for 20 min in 5 normal subjects, 10 patients with cirrhosis, and 10 cirrhotic patients with a PCS. (From ref. 65, with permission.)

feet proximal to the ileocecal valve) in cirrhotic patients with and without PCS (1,66). In the patients with PCS, food in the ileum did not stimulate acid secretion but food in the jejunum produced a marked and highly significant hypersecretion of gastric acid (Fig. 7). These results suggested that the stimulatory IPH in humans originated mainly in the jejunum, just as it did in dogs.

The nature of the gastric secretory stimulant in portal blood has been the subject of much speculation and considerable study. Early considerations focused on histamine (absorbed from proteins in the gut) as a result of two reports of increased levels of peripheral arterial blood histamine following a protein meal

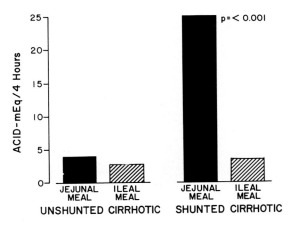

FIG. 7. Comparison of mean 4-hr total gastric acid response to a jejunal meal and an ileal meal in 5 unshunted cirrhotic patients and 10 cirrhotic patients with PCS.

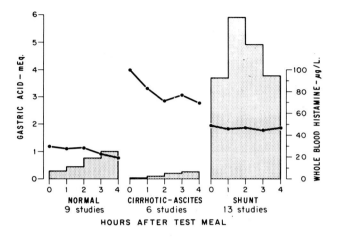

FIG. 8. Mean arterial whole blood histamine levels and Heidenhain pouch acid secretion in response to a meat meal in four normal dogs, six dogs with congestive cirrhosis and ascites, and the same cirrhotic-ascitic dogs after PCS.

in dogs with a PCS (82,86), and several reports of increased histamine levels in urine and gastric mucosa in rats with a PCS (16,21,22,79). However, there is substantial evidence against the proposal that histamine is the mediator of PCS-related acid hypersecretion. As we (75,98) and others (28,31,59,60) have shown, measurements in dogs of arterial whole blood and plasma histamine by modern techniques, and of urinary histamine (81) have shown no significant changes in response to eating before and after PCS, and no significant differences in comparisons between nonshunted and shunted dogs, despite enormous PCS-induced acid hypersecretion (Fig. 8). Acid hypersecretion has been observed with foods other than proteins and, as we have shown, occurs with balloon distention of the jejunum. Intestinal antibiotics have been shown to eliminate histamine formation in the gut (35,97), but not to influence PCS-related acid hypersecretion (13). Studies in dogs have failed to demonstrate a significant amount of histidine decarboxylase in gastric mucosa or an increase in gastric mucosal histamine following PCS (62,90). Finally, recent studies in shunted rats (50) showed no increases in gastrointestinal synthesis or urinary excretion of histamine, contrary to previously reported findings.

Another candidate that has been proposed as the stimulant responsible for PCS-related gastric hypersecretion is gastrin (6,18,30,39,90,95). However, antrectomy does not prevent the gastric hypersecretion associated with PCS (13,42, 56,62,77), and gastrin levels in peripheral blood and gastrointestinal tissues in dogs (14) and rats (80) have shown a decline after PCS rather than a rise. Furthermore, a major argument against the involvement of gastrin is evidence that gastrin is not inactivated (2,3,10,24,64), or is only slightly inactivated (30,91) by the liver, whereas the portal blood stimulant clearly undergoes marked hepatic inactivation. If the agent is gastrin, it must exist in a form different from that detected by current radioimmunoassays (RIAs).

In addition to histamine and gastrin, it has been suggested that the gastric secretory stimulant is some other type of secretagogue absorbed from food, and considerations have included proteins or protein derivatives, amino acids, and ammonia (13,28). The occurrence of PCS-related gastric hypersecretion during fasting, during balloon distention of the intestine, in the absence of protein, and after intestinal antibiotics argue against the likelihood that the agent is a secretagogue absorbed from protein-containing food.

PHYSIOLOGIC EVIDENCE FOR AN INTESTINAL PHASE HORMONE

In addition to the early work that established the existence of a stimulatory intestinal phase of gastric secretion, and the studies of PCS-related gastric hypersecretion that demonstrated humoral mediation of the intestinal phase, a number of recent studies in dogs and humans have provided important physiologic evidence for the existence of a unique IPH. Studies in both dogs (15,17,39–41,43, 44,47,63,94) and humans (5,34,36,37,63,93) have consistently shown that instillation of proteins, peptides, or amino acids into the duodenum or jejunum stimulates substantial acid secretion from the innervated and denervated stomach. Under some circumstances in dogs, instillation of proteins or protein products into the duodenum has provoked release of antral and duodenal gastrin (55), and elevation of peripheral serum gastrin concentration (43,44,47). However, in studies that demonstrated marked stimulation of acid secretion from a denervated gastric pouch by an intestinal meal, no increase in peripheral serum gastrin levels was detected by Debas et al. (17) in dogs with an intact antrum, or by Way et al. (94) in antrectomized dogs. Moreover, in four separate studies in humans, intraduodenal instillation of liver extract, peptone or amino acids provoked substantial gastric acid secretion without an increase in serum gastrin concentration (34,36,45,46).

Most important, substantial recent evidence has shown that food in the intestine potentiates the cephalic and gastric phases of gastric acid secretion, and augments the maximal secretory response to the known gastric stimulatory hormones. Studies from six laboratories have shown that an intestinal meal of protein in dogs with a denervated and/or innervated stomach significantly augments the maximal acid secretory response to pentagastrin (17,39,40,43,93,94), endogenous gastrin (15,17,39,40,43,94), histamine (17,39,40,94), vagal stimulation (39,40), cholecystokinin (CCK) (94), and bethanechol (94). In addition, it has been demonstrated recently in humans that instillation of liver extract into the duodenum augments the maximal secretory response to pentagastrin (45). In each of these studies, the investigators have concluded that the augmentation must be due to release of an intestinal hormone that is distinct from gastrin. Grossman (29) has proposed the name "entero-oxyntin" for this intestinal phase hormone.

TABLE 1. *Physiologic characteristics of the intestinal phase hormone (IPH) compared with the established physiologic characteristics of the known gastric stimulatory agents*

	IPH	Gastrin	CCK	Bombesin	Histamine
Augments maximal response to pentagastrin and gastrin	+	0	0	0	+
Increases serum gastrin level	0	+	0	+	0
Is substantially inactivated by liver	+	0	0	0	+
Antrectomy markedly diminishes effect of endogenous release	0	+	0	+	0
Augments maximal response to histamine	+	+	+	+	0
Increases blood histamine level	0	0	0	0	+
Characteristics different from IPH		4/6	2/6	4/6	2/6

The characteristics of the IPH that set it apart from the known gastric stimulatory hormones are summarized in Table 1. IPH is not gastrin because an intestinal meal consistently augments the maximal response to exogenously administered pentagastrin and endogenously released gastrin. No known form of gastrin produces such augmentation. Furthermore, most studies in dogs and all studies in humans have shown that serum gastrin concentration does not increase during the acid secretory response to an intestinal meal. Additionally, unlike IPH, gastrin is not substantially inactivated by the liver.

IPH is not CCK because CCK competitively inhibits pentagastrin- and gastrin-stimulated acid secretion. In addition, an intestinal meal has been shown to augment the maximal acid secretory response to CCK. Moreover, unlike IPH, CCK is not metabolized by the liver. Finally, CCK is a relatively weak agonist, and IPH produces substantially greater stimulation of acid secretion than CCK.

IPH is not bombesin because it is well-established that: (a) bombesin acts by releasing gastrin, (b) the response to bombesin is associated with a rise in serum gastrin levels, (c) antrectomy greatly reduces the response to bombesin, and (d) bombesin is not substantially metabolized by the liver. All of these characteristics are distinctly different from those of IPH.

Evidence that IPH is not histamine is the finding that an intestinal meal augments the maximal response to histamine. Furthermore, distention of the intestine by a balloon (in the absence of food containing histamine or histamine precursors) stimulates acid secretion, and intestinal antibiotics that eliminate histamine formation in the gut do not alter the intestinal phase. Additionally, repeated studies using modern assay techniques have failed to demonstrate an increase in histamine levels in whole blood, plasma, or urine during the gastric secretory response to a meal.

On the basis of several recent studies, the suggestion has been made that amino acids absorbed from the intestine stimulate gastric acid secretion by a direct action on the oxyntic cells, and are responsible for part or all of the intestinal phase of gastric secretion. It is well established that amino acids are capable of directly stimulating the parietal cell (49). Systemic intravenous administration of amino acids in dogs and humans has been shown to stimulate acid secretion from the innervated and denervated stomach to the same extent as instillation of amino acids in the duodenum or jejunum (37,45,47,48,51,57, 58,63), and to produce no changes in serum gastrin concentration (37,45,47,48). Administration of amino acids by the portal venous route in dogs has been observed to have little or no gastric stimulatory effect, in contrast with systemic administration (47,57). Interestingly, intraduodenal administration of amino acids in dogs and humans has been found, predictably, to result in a much lower level of amino nitrogen in peripheral blood than systemic administration, but to stimulate gastric acid secretion to the same degree (37,45,47). One study in dogs (57), which requires confirmation, was reported to show augmentation by systemic intravenous amino acid administration of the maximal acid secretory response to pentagastrin and histamine, whereas a similar study in humans (45) failed to show augmentation of the maximal pentagastrin response. Although absorption of amino acids could account for some of the gastric secretory response to food in the intestine, this phenomenon cannot explain the gastric secretory response to balloon distention of the intestines that has been conclusively demonstrated in dogs and humans (61,65,87,92). Moreover, amino acids in the gut must be absorbed into the portal venous system before reaching the systemic circulation; yet intraportal administration of amino acids had little or no gastric stimulatory effect. Most important, the fact that instillation of amino acids into the intestine produced much lower levels of amino nitrogen in peripheral blood than systemic administration, yet caused as much acid secretion (37,45,47), suggests that the intestinal amino acid meal stimulated the oxyntic cells by a different mechanism from that involved in the stimulatory response to systemic infusion.

WORK ON ISOLATION OF THE INTESTINAL PHASE HORMONE FROM HOG INTESTINAL MUCOSA

On the basis of the many studies that provided strong physiologic evidence for hormonal mediation of the intestinal phase of gastric secretion, we undertook a program directed at extracting a gastric stimulatory hormone from the small intestinal mucosa of hogs (7,8,68–70). Based on existing knowledge of the structure-activity relationships of the known gastrointestinal hormones that stimulate or inhibit gastric secretion, the assumption was made that IPH was likely to be an acidic peptide of low molecular weight. Accordingly, the classic method of Gregory and Tracy (26,27) for extracting small acidic peptides was used. Briefly, it consisted of heating fresh intestinal mucosa from 3,000 hogs to precipitate proteins and large molecular weight peptides, absorption of the supernatant

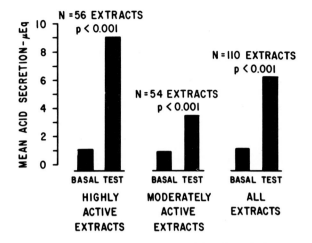

FIG. 9. Gastric secretory response to 110 batches of hog intestinal mucosa extract (HIME) in rats with acute gastric fistula. (From ref. 70, with permission).

on DEAE cellulose, alkali elution of the material attached to the cellulose, acid precipitation of the eluate, and extraction of the precipitate into isopropanol.

Gastric Stimulatory Activity of HIME *In Vivo*

Each hog intestinal mucosa extract (HIME) from 110 separate batches of intestinal mucosa was tested for stimulatory activity in a group of 12 rats with acute gastric fistulas (7,8,68–70). A dosage standard was adopted for all studies such that one standard dose of HIME contained 2 mg protein. One standard dose of HIME was administered intravenously over a 30-min period to the rats, and gastric acid secretion was measured for 2 hr. The batches of HIME were classified as highly active, moderately active, or inactive according to stringent criteria. All 110 batches of HIME were active in the rats with acute gastric fistulas, and 56 were highly active (Fig. 9).

Twenty batches of HIME that were highly active in the rats were tested subsequently in dogs with Heidenhain pouches. One standard dose (2 mg protein) was given intravenously over a 30-min period and pouch acid secretion was measured for 3 hr. Figure 10 shows the secretory response to 12 batches of HIME that were tolerated without adverse reaction. All batches of HIME were highly stimulatory, producing a mean 22-fold increase in acid production above the basal level, and a mean 12-fold greater acid output than the control infusion of diluent.

The gastrin content of 73 batches of HIME was measured by RIA in two separate laboratories. The gastrin content ranged from 0 to 48.9 ng per standard

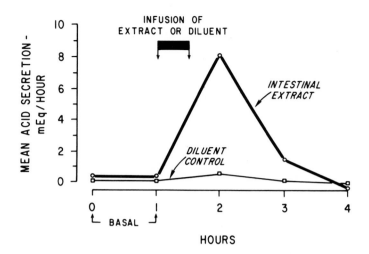

FIG. 10. Response of Heidenhain pouch to intravenous infusion of one standard dose of HIME in dogs (mean of 12 batches of HIME). (From ref. 70, with permission.)

dose of HIME, and averaged 5.80 ng. The minimal stimulating dose of hog gastrin in the acute gastric fistula rat was found to be 2,000 ng, which was approximately 350 times greater than the mean gastrin content of HIME. No batch of HIME contained sufficient gastrin to produce an acid secretory response.

Figure 11 shows the gastric secretory responses to increasing doses of HIME and, for comparison, the dose-response curve of pentagastrin in rats with an

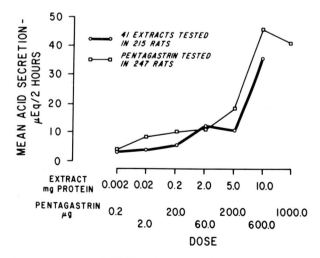

FIG. 11. Dose-response curves of HIME and pentagastrin in rats with acute gastric fistula. (From ref. 70, with permission.)

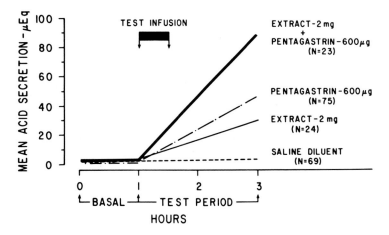

FIG. 12. Augmentation of maximal pentagastrin secretion by HIME in rats with acute gastric fistula. (From ref. 70, with permission.)

acute gastric fistula. As the dose of HIME was increased, there was an increase in the secretory response in a linear dose-response relationship. The minimal stimulating dose of HIME was 0.2 mg protein. The largest dose of HIME tested, 10 mg protein, stimulated almost as much acid output as did the maximal stimulating dose of pentagastrin.

The capacity of HIME to augment the maximal secretory response to pentagastrin was tested in acute gastric fistula rats, using four separate batches of HIME. The gastric secretory response was significantly greater following simultaneous administration of one standard dose of HIME plus a maximally stimulating dose of pentagastrin than following administration of either agent separately. Figure 12 summarizes the experiments showing significant augmentation of maximal pentagastrin secretion by HIME.

Hepatic metabolism of HIME was investigated by comparing the gastric secretory responses to portal vein and inferior vena cava infusions of extract in acute gastric fistula rats. Systemic infusion of one standard dose produced a mean 2-hr acid output of 9.56 ± 1.11 μEq, whereas portal venous infusion produced a mean secretion of only 2.48 ± 0.66 μEq, reflecting substantial inactivation of HIME by the liver (Fig. 13). As has been demonstrated previously in other species, there was marked inactivation of pentagastrin by the liver, but no hepatic inactivation of hog gastrin.

To summarize these *in vivo* studies, HIME was found to contain a potent stimulant of gastric acid secretion that acted in a regular dose-response relationship on both the innervated and denervated stomach, was not gastrin in any of its immunoassayable forms, significantly augmented the maximal secretory response to pentagastrin, and was substantially inactivated by the liver. HIME was found to have all of the known physiologic properties of IPH.

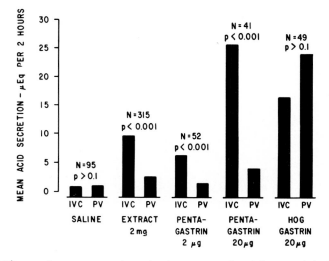

FIG. 13. Gastric secretory responses to systemic venous and portal venous infusions of HIME, pentagastrin, and hog gastrin in rats with acute gastric fistula. (From ref. 70, with permission.)

Stimulatory Activity of HIME In The Frog Isolated Gastric Mucosa

The isolated gastric mucosa of the frog *Rana pipiens* has been used in our laboratory for over a decade in studies of gastric secretion, and we have found it to be a highly sensitive and reliable bioassay model. The secretory response of the frog isolated gastric mucosa to increasing doses of HIME is shown in Fig. 14, which also shows the dose-response curves for pentagastrin and leucine-

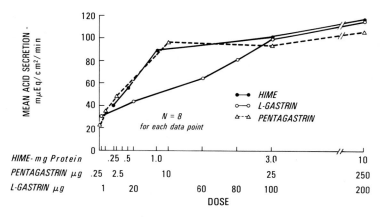

FIG. 14. Dose-response curves of HIME, pentagastrin and l-gastrin in frog isolated gastric mucosa. Each data point is the mean of eight mucosa experiments.

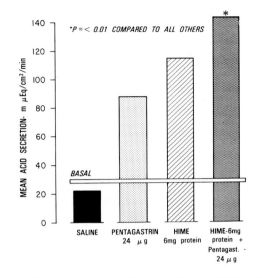

FIG. 15. Augmentation of maximal pentagastrin secretion by HIME in frog isolated gastric mucosa. Each bar represents the mean of eight mucosa experiments.

gastrin. Increasing doses of HIME stimulated increasing acid secretion in a linear dose-response relationship. The largest does of HIME tested, 20 mg protein (10 standard doses), stimulated as much acid output as the maximal stimulating doses of pentagastrin and 1-gastrin.

The capacity of HIME to augment the maximal secretory response to pentagastrin is shown in Fig. 15. HIME and pentagastrin together stimulated significantly more acid secretion than either agent separately. In separate experiments, HIME similarly augmented the maximal response to 1-gastrin (33,71).

We also studied the capacity of HIME to augment the acid secretory response to other gastrointestinal hormones in the frog isolated gastric mucosa. The results of studies with CCK are shown in Table 2. The maximal stimulatory dose of CCK was found to be 100 ng. The combination of HIME and CCK stimulated significantly more acid secretion than a maximally stimulating dose of CCK alone. As expected, no secretory response to bombesin, the gastrin-releasing hormone, was detected in studies using the frog isolated gastric mucosa.

Table 3 shows the results of studies of augmentation of the secretory response to histamine by HIME (32). In separate experiments, the maximal stimulating dose of histamine phosphate was found to be 10 μg and the minimal stimulating dose was found to be 1.0 μg. HIME produced significant augmentation of the maximal response to histamine.

Although the extraction procedure of Gregory and Tracy is reported to produce histamine-free extracts, studies were performed to determine the histamine content of HIME using a highly sensitive enzymatic radioisotopic microassay

TABLE 2. *Studies of augmentation of the maximal secretory response to CCK by hog intestinal mucosa extract (HIME) in the frog isolated gastric mucosa*

Test substance and dose	Number of mucosae	Adjusted mean acid $m\mu$ Eq/cm²/min
Saline	8	22.5
CCK (100 ng)	8	77.0
HIME (10 standard doses)	8	96.3
CCK (100 ng) plus HIME (10 standard doses)	8	98.2[a]
Pentagastrin (24 μg)	8	87.9

One standard dose of HIME contains 2 mg protein.
Adjusted mean acid was obtained by subtracting basal acid secretion.
Data were analyzed by the multiple comparison test of D. B. Duncan (*Biometrics*, 2:1, 1955.) and the one-side multiple comparison test of C. W. Dunnett (*Am. Statistical Assoc. J.* 50:1096, 1955.)
  [a] $p < 0.05$ compared with CCK alone.

of histamine (89). The mean histamine content of six batches of HIME averaged 0.22 μg per standard dose of extract. Since the minimal stimulatory dose of histamine was found to be 1.0 μg, the histamine content of HIME was below the level required to stimulate acid secretion in the frog isolated gastric mucosa. Furthermore, when HIME was passed through a carboxymethyl cellulose column that removed all assayable histamine, the histamine-free HIME retained all of its gastric stimulatory activity.

In summary, the studies of HIME in the frog isolated gastric mucosa confirmed and extended the findings of studies in the rat and dog. HIME was found to contain a potent agent that stimulated acid secretion in a linear dose-response pattern and augmented the maximal secretory responses to pentagastrin, 1-gas-

TABLE 3. *Studies of augmentation of the maximal secretory response to histamine by hog intestinal mucosa extract (HIME) in the frog isolated gastric mucosa*

Test substance and dose	Number of mucosae	Adjusted mean acid $m\mu$ Eq/cm²/min
Saline	8	16.8
Histamine phosphate (10 μg)	8	76.7
HIME (3 standard doses)	8	80.8
HIME (3 standard doses) plus Histamine phosphate (10 μg)	8	104.0[a]
Pentagastrin (24 μg)	8	91.4

One standard dose of HIME contains 2 mg protein.
Adjusted mean acid was obtained by subtracting basal acid secretion.
Data were analyzed by the multiple comparison test of Duncan and the one-sided multiple comparison test of Dunnett.
  [a] $p < 0.05$ compared with either agent alone.

trin, CCK and histamine, indicating that its effect was not due to the presence of any of these well-recognized stimulatory substances.

Work In Progress On Characterization Of HIME

Initial experiments were conducted to provide information on the size, stability, and chemical nature of the active agent(s) in HIME. It was found that the gastric stimulatory activity of HIME in the acute gastric fistula rat persisted after incubation for 48 hr at room temperature in pH 7.0 buffer, and was diminished significantly by dialysis tubing with a M.W. cutoff of 3,500 daltons. Hydrolysis in 6 N HCl under vacuum for 20 hr destroyed the stimulatory acitvity. Amino acid analysis of HIME showed it to be 46% protein, and to contain a large number of acidic amino acids. These properties are consistent with those of a low molecular weight peptidic compound.

Fractionation of HIME on a G-25 Sephadex gel filtration column yielded four distinct pools, one of which, corresponding to an approximate M. W. of 300 to 1,500 daltons, had significant acid stimulatory activity in the frog isolated gastric mucosa. Fractionation of HIME on a G-10 Sephadex gel filtration column yielded seven distinct pools, two of which were highly active. Ion exchange chromatography of these active pools with DEAE cellulose and SP-Sephadex suggested that the active material was a cation. When the intestinal mucosal slurry was placed directly on a G-25 Sephadex gel filtration column, three highly stimulatory zones were obtained: a protein zone corresponding to a M. W. of 5,000 to 3,000, a protein zone corresponding to a M. W. of 2,000 to 1,000, and a salt zone. The activity of the most stimulatory protein zone was significantly diminished by acid hydrolysis.

SUMMARY

The existence of a stimulatory intestinal phase of gastric acid secretion has been suspected, but largely ignored, for many years. Recently, however, it has become clear that the intestinal phase plays an important role in acid production during digestion. The intestinal phase is of additional interest in relation to the profound gastric acid hypersecretion associated with portacaval shunt (PCS). Substantial evidence indicates that PCS-related gastric hypersecretion is due to unmasking of the intestinal phase by hepatic bypass of a humoral stimulant in portal blood that is normally degraded to a considerable extent by the liver. Studies in our laboratory during the past 12 years have provided strong physiologic evidence for humoral mediation of both the intestinal phase of gastric secretion and of PCS-related hypersecretion by a hormone that arises in the small intestine, particularly in the jejunum. Furthermore, our studies have demonstrated that this intestinal phase hormone (IPH) exists in humans as well as in dogs, rats, and pigs. Additionally, recent work by a number of investigators as well as our group has provided convincing evidence that IPH is different from any of the known gastric stimulatory hormones.

With these physiologic observations as a background, we have used a classic method for extracting acidic peptides to prepare a hog intestinal mucosa extract (HIME) that has all of the known physiologic properties of an IPH. Specifically, HIME contains a potent stimulant of gastric acid secretion that acts according to a linear dose-response relationship, that is not gastrin in any of its immunoassayable forms, that significantly augments the maximal acid secretory responses to pentagastrin, gastrin, CCK and histamine, and that is substantially degraded by the liver, in contrast with gastrin and CCK. Efforts at isolating the gastric stimulatory substance in HIME suggest that it is a peptide of low molecular weight.

PROJECTIONS FOR THE FUTURE

Work directed at isolating IPH from HIME continues to be a major endeavor of our laboratory. Thus far, studies indicate that IPH is a peptide. Future efforts will be directed at further purification and eventual isolation of IPH from HIME, establishing proof of homogeneity, determination of the primary sequence and, finally, total synthesis. Once IPH has been isolated and synthesized, efforts will be undertaken to develop a RIA and to determine cross-reactivity with the known digestive hormones. Availability of synthetic IPH will make it possible to conduct a wide range of physiologic studies on the actions and metabolism of the hormone. Ultimately, it will be important to demonstrate IPH in humans, and to determine its role in normal digestion and in digestive disease.

ACKNOWLEDGMENTS

This work was supported in part by Grants No. AM-12281 and AM-19875 from the National Institutes of Health, and Grant No. 77243 from the John A. Hartford Foundation, Inc.

The authors gratefully acknowledge the important help of many colleagues, students, and technical personnel who contributed to the studies described in this review during the past 12 years.

REFERENCES

1. Abbott, A. G., Rosen, H., and Orloff, M. J. (1970): Site of origin of the hormone responsible for gastric hypersecretion in humans with portacaval shunts. *Surg. Forum,* 21:340–343.
2. Amure, B. O., and Ginsburg, M. (1964): Inhibitors of histamine catabolism and the action of gastrin in the rat. *Br. J. Pharmacol.,* 23:476–485.
3. Bridgwater, A. B., Kuroyanagi, Y., Geisel, T., and Necheles, H. (1963): Pancreozymin-cholecystokinin injected by portal and systemic routes. *Proc. Soc. Exp. Biol. Med.,* 112:1056–1058.
4. Brown, G. E., Faustina, G. E., and Orloff, M. J. (1967): Humoral mediation of the intestinal phase of gastric secretion. *Surg. Forum,* 18:298–300.
5. Buxton, B., Wasunna, A. E. O., Bedi, B. S., and Gillespie, I. E. (1972): Role of the jejunum and the ileum in the acid response of dogs to a meal. *Gastroenterology,* 63:270–272.

6. Castaneda, A., Griffen, W. O., Jr., Nicoloff, D., Leonard, A. S., and Wagensteen, O. H. (1960): Antral hyperfunction following portacaval shunt. *Surg. Forum,* 11:349–351.
7. Chandler, J. G., Rosen, H., Kester, K. C., and Orloff, M. J. (1972): Isolation of the hormone responsible for intestinal phase of gastric secretion from pig intestinal mucosa. *Surg. Forum,* 23:382–384.
8. Chandler, J. G., Rosen, H., Kester, R. C., and Orloff, M. J. (1973): Extraction of the hormone responsible for the intestinal phase of gastric secretion from the intestinal mucosa of the pig. *Gastroenterology,* 64:707.
9. Clarke, J. S., Costarella, R., and Ward, S. (1958): Gastric secretion in the fasting state and after antral stimulation in patients with cirrhosis and with portacaval shunts. *Surg. Forum,* 9:417–420.
10. Clarke, J. S., Hall, R., Devor, D., and Rizer, J. (1967): Failure of gastrin inactivation. In: *Gastric Secretion. Mechanism and Control,* edited by T. K. Shnitka, J. A. L., Gilbert, and R. C. Harrison, p. 357. Pergamon Press, Toronto.
11. Clarke, J. S., McKissock, P. K., and Cruze, K. (1959): Studies on the site of origin of the agent causing hypersecretion in dogs with portacaval shunt. *Surgery,* 46:48–55.
12. Clarke, J. S., Miller, I., and McKissock, P. K. (1966): Increased acid secretion from Heidenhain pouches by shunting colonic venous blood around the liver. *Arch. Surg.,* 92:653–656.
13. Clarke, J. S., Ozeran, R. S., Hart, J. C., Cruze, K., and Crevling, V. (1958): Peptic ulcer following portacaval shunt. *Ann. Surg.,* 148:551–566.
14. Clendinnen, B. G., Reeder, D. D., Jackson, B. M., Miller, J. H., and Thompson, J. C. (1970): Effect of portacaval shunting on postprandial serum gastrin levels in dogs. *Surg. Forum,* 21:339–40.
15. Curt, J. R. N., Isaza, J., Woodward, E. R., and Dragstedt, L. R. (1971): Potentiation between intestinal and gastric phases of acid secretion in Heidenhain pouches. *Arch. Surg.,* 103:709–712.
16. Day, S. B., Skoryna, S. C., Webster, D. R., and MacLean, L. D. (1963): Gastric hypersecretion and histamine levels in liver, stomach, duodenum, and blood following portacaval shunt in rats. *Surgery,* 54:764–770.
17. Debas, H. T., Slaff, G. F., and Grossman, M. I. (1975): Intestinal phase of gastric secretion: Augmentation of maximal response of Heidenhain pouch to gastrin and histamine. *Gastroenterology,* 69:691–698.
18. Dragstedt, L. R. (1957): The physiology of the gastric antrum. *Arch. Surg.,* 75:552–557.
19. Dubuque, T. J., Jr., Mulligan, L. V., and Neville, E. C. (1957): Gastric secretion and peptic ulceration in the dog with portal obstruction and portacaval anastomosis. *Surg. Forum,* 8:208–211.
20. Ferrarese, S., Ronzini, V. (1966): Gastric secretion in cirrhotics after portasystemic shunts. *Gaz. Int. Med. Chir.,* 71:882–889.
21. Fischer, J. E., and Snyder, S. H. (1965): Histamine synthesis and gastric secretion after portacaval shunt. *Science,* 150:1034–1035.
22. Fisher, J. E., and Snyder, S. H. (1965): Increased histamine snythesis: a possible final common pathway in gastric acid hypersecretion. *Surg. Forum,* 16:331–332.
23. Gerez, L., and Weiss, A. (1936): Uber die Magensaftsekretion bei Eckscher Fistel. *Ztschr. ges. Exp. Med.,* 100:281–288.
24. Gillespie, I. E., Grossman, M. I. (1962): Gastric secretion of acid in response to portal and systemic venous injection of gastrin. *Gastroenterology,* 43:189–192.
25. Gregory, R. A., and Ivy, A. C. (1941): The humoral stimulation of gastric secretion. *Q. J. Exp. Physiol.,* 31:111–128.
26. Gregory, R. A., and Tracy, H. J. (1961): The preparation and properties of gastrin. *J. Physiol. (Lond.),* 156:523–543.
27. Gregory, R. A., and Tracy, H. J. (1964): The constitution and properties of two gastrins extracted from hog antral mucosa. *Gut,* 5:103–114.
28. Griffen, W. O., Slesh, M. Z., and Mooney, C. S. (1969): Gastric secretagogues following portacaval shunt. *Surgery,* 66:111–117.
29. Grossman, M. I. (1974): Entero-oxyntin. In: Candidate hormones of the gut. *Gastroenterology,* edited by M. I. Grossman. 67:730–755.
30. Hayashi, K., Rheault, M. J., Semb, L. S., and Nyhus, L. M. (1968): The effect of splenocaval shunt on gastric secretion and liver function as compared with other shunting procedures in the dog. *Surgery,* 64:1084–1091.
31. Hubens, A. (1966, 1967): Contribution a l'étude de l'hypersécrétion acide de l'estomac apres

transposition porto-cave, chez le chien. *Acta Gastroenterol. (Belg.) (2 parts),* 29:1009–1037, and 30:7–55.

32. Hyde, P. V. B., and Orloff, M. J. (1979): Augmentation of histamine-stimulated gastric secretion by the intestinal phase hormone. *Surg. Forum,* 30: 360–362.

33. Hyde, P. V. B., Skivolocki, W. P., Guillemin, R. C. L., Sayers, H. J., and Orloff, M. J. (1978): Augmentation of pentagastrin and gastrin stimulated acid secretion by the intestinal phase hormone. *Surg. Forum,* 29:392–394.

34. Ippoliti, A. F., Maxwell, V., and Isenberg, J. I. (1976): Demonstration of the intestinal phase of gastric acid secretion in man. *Gastroenterology,* 70:896.

35. Irvine, W. T., Duthie, H. L., Ritchie, H. D., and Waton, N. G. (1959): The liver's role in histamine absorption from the alimentary tract. Its possible importance in cirrhosis. *Lancet,* i:1064–1068.

36. Isenberg, J. I., Ippoliti, A. F., and Maxwell, V. L. (1977): Perfusion of the proximal small intestine with peptone stimulates gastric acid secretion in man. *Gastroenterology,* 73:746–752.

37. Isenberg, J. I., and Maxwell, V. (1978): Intravenous infusion of amino acids stimulates gastric acid secretion in man. *N. Engl. J. Med.,* 298:27–29.

38. Ivy, A. C., Lim, R. K. S., and McCarthy, J. E. (1925): Contributions to the physiology of gastric secretion. II. The intestinal phase of gastric secretion. *Q. J. Exp. Physiol.,* 15:55–68.

39. Jordan, P. J., Jr. (1967): Relationship between stimulating mechanisms of gastric acid secretion in dogs. *JAMA,* 199:149–155.

40. Jordan, P. J., Jr., and de la Rosa, C. (1964): The regulatory effect of the pyloric gland area of the stomach on the intestinal phase of gastric secretion. *Surgery,* 56:121–134.

41. Kelly, K. A., Nyhus, L. M., and Harkins, H. N. (1965): A reappraisal of the intestinal phase of gastric secretion. *Am. J. Surg.,* 109:1–6.

42. Kohatsu, S., Gwaltney, J. A., Nagano, K., and Dragstedt, L. R. (1959): Mechanism of gastric hypersecretion following portacaval transposition. *Am. J. Physiol.,* 196:841–843.

43. Konturek, S. J., Kaess, H., Kwiecien, N., Radecki, T., Dorner, M., and Teckentrupp, U. (1976): Characteristics of intestinal phase of gastric secretion. *Am. J. Physiol.,* 230:335–340.

44. Konturek, S. J., Kwiecien, N., Fckina, A., Radecki, T., and Mikos, E. (1978): Role of antral gastrin in gastric and intestinal phases of gastric secretion. *Scand. J. Gastroenterol. (Suppl.),* 13, 49:99.

45. Konturek, S. J., Kwiecien, N., Obtulowicz, W., Mikos, E., Sito, E., and Olesky, J. (1978): Comparison of intraduodenal and intravenous administration of amino acids on gastric secretion in healthy subjects and patients with duodenal ulcer. *Gut,* 19:859–864.

46. Konturek, S. J., Kwiecien, N., Obtulowicz, N., Sito, E., and Olesky, J. (1978): Intestinal phase of gastric secretion in patients with duodenal ulcer. *Gut,* 19:321–326.

47. Konturek, S. J., Radecki, T., and Kwiecien, N. (1978): Stimuli for intestinal phase of gastric secretion in dogs. *Am. J. Physiol.,* 234:E–64–69.

48. Konturek, S. J., Tasler, J., Cieszkowski, M., and Jaworek, J. (1978): Comparison of intravenous amino acids in the stimulation of gastric secretion. *Gastroenterology,* 75:817–824.

49. Konturek, S. J., Tasler, J., Obtulowicz, W., and Cieszkowski, M. (1976): Comparison of amino acids bathing the oxyntic gland area in the stimulation of gastric secretion. *Gastroenterology,* 70:66–69.

50. Kowalewski, K., Russell, J. C., and Koheil, A. (1971): Excretion of ^{3}H-histamine in urine of rats with portacaval shunts. *Proc. Soc. Exp. Biol. Med.,* 136:760–764.

51. Landor, J. H., and Ipapo, V. S. (1977): Gastric secretory effect of amino acids given enterally and parenterally. *Gastroenterology,* 73:781–784.

52. Lebedinskaja, S. I. (1933): Uber die Magensekretion μ Eckschen Fistulhunden. *Ztschr. Ges. Exp. Med.,* 88:264–270.

53. Leconte, P. (1900): Fonctions gastro-intestinales. *Cellule,* 17:285–318.

54. Leger, L., Cachin, M., and Pergola, F. (1960): Ulcères gastro-duodénaux après anastomose porto-cave. A propos de quelques documents personnels. *Presse Méd.,* 68:63–66.

55. Llanos, O. L., Villar, H. V., Konturek, S. J., Rayford, P. L., and Thompson, J. C. (1977): Release of antral and duodenal gastrin in response to an intestinal meal. *Ann. Surg.,* 186:614–618.

56. Macpherson, W. A., Miller, I., Nishikawa, W. Y., McKissock, P. K., and Clarke, J. S. (1962): The importance of the antrum in gastric hypersecretion after shunt. *Surg. Forum,* 13:271–273.

57. Mariano, E. C., Beloni, A., and Landor, J. H. (1978): Some properties shared by amino acids and entero-oxyntin. *Ann. Surg.,* 188:181–185.

58. Mariano, E. C., and Landor, J. H. (1978): Gastric secretory response to intravenous amino acids in eviscerated dogs. *Arch. Surg.,* 113:611–614.

59. McPhedran, N. T., Bett, H. D., Stone, R. M., and Goldberg, M. (1967): The nature and source of a gastric secretagogue. *Arch. Surg.,* 95:606–608.

60. McPhedran, N. T., Bett, H. D., Stone, R. M., and Goldberg, M. (1968): Some observations on the cause of the gastric hypersecretion following portacaval shunt. *Bull. Soc. Int. Chir.,* 27:286–290.

61. Nagano, K., Johnson, A. N., Jr., Cobo, A., and Oberhelman, H. A., Jr. (1959): Effects of distention of the duodenum on gastric secretion. *Surg. Forum,* 10:152–155.

62. Newman, P. H., Reeder, D. D., Davidson, W. D., Schneider, E., Miller, J. H., and Thompson, J. C. (1969): Acid secretion following portacaval shunting: role of vagus, gastrin, intestinal phase and histamine. *Arch. Surg.,* 99:369–375.

63. Okada, S., Kuromochi, K., Tsukahara, T., and Ooinoue, T. (1930): Pancreatic function. V. The secretory mechanism of digestive juices. *Arch. Intern. Med.,* 45:783–813.

64. Olbe, L. (1960): Influence of portacaval transposition on gastric secretion in dogs. *Acta Physiol. Scand. (Suppl.),* 175:110–111.

65. Orloff, M. J., Abbott, A. G., and Rosen, H. (1970): Nature of the humoral agent responsible for portacaval shunt-related gastric hypersecretion in man. *Am. J. Surg.,* 120:237–243.

66. Orloff, M. J., Abbott, A. G., and Rosen, H. (1971): Jejunal origin of the hormone responsible for the intestinal phase of gastric secretion and portacaval shunt-related hypersecretion in man. *Gastroenterology,* 60:703.

67. Orloff, M. J., Chandler, J. G., Alderman, S. J., Keiter, J. E., and Rosen, H. (1969): Gastric secretion and peptic ulcer following portacaval shunt in man. *Ann. Surg.,* 170:515–527.

68. Orloff, M. J., Charters, A. C., and Knox, D. G. (1975): Hepatic metabolism of the intestinal phase hormone. *Gastroenterology,* 68:964.

69. Orloff, M. J., Charters, A. C., and Nakaji, N. T. (1976): Isolation of the hormone responsible for the intestinal phase of gastric secretion. *Gastroenterology,* 70:990.

70. Orloff, M. J., Charters, A. C., Ill, and Nakaji, N. T. (1976): Further evidence for an intestinal phase hormone that stimulates gastric acid secretion. *Surgery,* 80:145–154.

71. Orloff, M. J., Skivolocki, W. P., Guillemin, R. C. L., and Sayers, H. J. (1978): Augmentation of pentagastrin and gastrin stimulated acid secretion by the intestinal phase hormone. *Gastroenterology,* 74:1139.

72. Orloff, M. J., Villar-Valdes, H., Abbott, A. G., Williams, R. J., and Rosen, H. (1970): Site of origin of the hormone responsible for gastric hypersecretion associated with portacaval shunt. *Surgery,* 68:202–208.

73. Orloff, M. J., Villar-Valdes, H., Rosen, H., Thompson, A. G., and Chandler, J. G. (1969): Humoral mediation of the intestinal phase of gastric secretion and of acid hypersecretion associated with portacaval shunts. *Surgery,* 66:118–130.

74. Orloff, M. J., and Windsor, C. W. O. (1966): Effect of portacaval shunt on gastric acid secretion in dogs with liver disease, portal hypertension and massive ascites. *Ann. Surg.,* 164:69–80.

75. Orloff, M. J., Windsor, C. W. O., Thompson, J. C., and Goodhead, B. (1966): Studies of blood histamine in relation to the gastric hypersecretion associated with portacaval shunts. *Gastroenterology,* 50:861.

76. Ostrow, J. D., Timmerman, R. J., and Gray, S. J. (1960): Gastric secretion in human hepatic cirrhosis. *Gastroenterology,* 38:303–313.

77. O'Sullivan, W. D., Cantlin, M. L., Sweeney, R. D., Rosteing, H. M., and Foster, W. C. (1960): Role of residual stomach in hypersecretion of Heidenhain pouch after portacaval transposition. *Surg. Forum,* 11:347–348.

78. Pavlov, I. P.: Translated by Thompson, W. H. (1902): *The Work of the Digestive Glands, 1st edition.* Charles Griffin & Company, London.

79. Reichle, F. A., Brigham, M. P., Tyson, R., and Rosemond, G. P. (1968): Histidine metabolism after portacaval shunt in the rat. *J. S. Res.,* 8:320–325.

80. Reichle, F. A., Reeder, D. D., Reichle, R. M., and Thompson, J. C. (1974): Serum gastrin, gastrointestinal tissue gastrin, and gastric hypersecretion after portacaval shunt in rats. *Surg. Forum,* 25:418–420.

81. Rex, J. C., Code, C. F., and ReMine, W. H. (1964): Gastric secretion of acid and urinary excretion of histamine in dogs with portacaval transposition. *Ann. Surg.,* 160:193–201.

82. Rutherford, R. B., Mehlman, B., and Brickman, R. D. (1966): Regional contributions to portal blood histamine in the dog. *Surgery,* 60:159–170.

83. Schriefers, K. H., Schreiber, H. W., and Esser, G. (1963): Zur Frage der Magensaftsekretion

und des Magen-Duodenalulcus beim Pfortaderhochdruck der Lebercirrhose und nach portocava-len Shunt-Operationen. *Arch. Klin. Chir.,* 302:702–715.

84. Scobie, B. A., and Summerskill, W. H. J. (1964): Reduced gastric acid output in cirrhosis: quantitation and relationships. *Gut,* 5:422–428.
85. Silen, W., and Eiseman, B. (1959): The nature and cause of gastric hypersecretion following portacaval shunts. *Surgery,* 46:38–47.
86. Silen, W., and Eiseman, B. (1961): Evidence for histamine as the agent responsible for hypersecretion after portacaval shunts. *Surgery,* 50:213–219.
87. Sircus, W. (1953): The intestinal phase of gastric secretion. *Q. J. Exp. Physiol.,* 38:91–100.
88. Tabaqchali, S., and Dawson, A. M. (1964): Peptic ulcer and gastric secretion in patients with liver disease. *Gut,* 5:417–421.
89. Taylor, K. M., and Snyder, S. H. (1972): Isotopic microassay of histamine, histidine, histidine decarboxylase and histamine methyltransferase in brain tissue. *J. Neurochem.* 19:1343–1358.
90. Thompson, J. C. (1969): Alterations in gastric secretion after portacaval shunting. *Am. J. Surg.,* 117:854–865.
91. Thompson, J. C., Reeder, D. D., Davidson, W. D., Charters, A. C., Bruckner, W. L., Lemmi, C. A. E., and Miller, J. H. (1969): Effect of hepatic transit of gastrin, pentagastrin and histamine measured by gastric secretion and by assay of hepatic vein blood. *Ann. Surg.,* 170:493–505.
92. Villar-Valdes, H., Thompson, A. G., Chandler, J. G., and Orloff, M. J. (1969): Endogenous origin of the humoral agent responsible for gastric hypersecretion associated with portacaval shunt. *Surg. Forum,* 20:360–362.
93. Wasunna, A. E. O., Buxton, B. F., and Bedi, B. S., and Gillespie, I. E. (1971): Acid responses of denervated fundic (Heidenhain) pouches to meals compared with those to histamine and pentagastrin. *Scand. J. Gastroenterol.,* 6:407–410.
94. Way, L. W., Cairns, D. W., and Deveney, C. W. (1975): The intestinal phase of gastric secretion: A pharmacological profile of entero-oxyntin. *Surgery,* 77:841–850.
95. Wilken, B. J., Hunt, D., Lowe, C. E., Billups, W. A., and Hardy, J. D. (1969): Gastrin inhibition of gastric secretion before and after portacaval shunt. *Surg. Gynecol. Obstet.,* 129:22–26.
96. Wilkinson, F. O. W., and Riddell, A. G. (1965): Studies on gastric secretion before and after portacaval anastomosis. *Br. J. Surg.,* 52:530–535.
97. Wilson, C. W. M. (1954): The metabolism of histamine as reflected by changes in its urinary excretion in the rat. *J. Physiol.,* 125:534–545.
98. Windsor, C. W. O., Thompson, J. C., and Orloff, M. J. (1965): Effects of experimental liver disease and portacaval shunts on gastric acid secretion and blood histamine. *Surg. Forum,* 16:322–324.

Gastrointestinal Hormones, edited by
George B. Jerzy Glass.
Raven Press, New York © 1980.

Chapter 40

Villikinin: Characterization and Function

* Eszter Kokas, ** John J. Pisano, and * Benny Crepps

* *Department of Physiology, University of North Carolina School of Medicine, Chapel Hill, North Carolina 27514; and ** Section on Physiological Chemistry, Laboratory of Chemistry, National Heart, Lung and Blood Institute, Bethesda, Maryland 20205*

INTRODUCTION

The earliest experiments on the control of villous motility dealt with the local effects of mechanical and chemical stimuli (3,7,8,46). Prevailing thought was strongly influenced by those experiments, so when it was later shown that villous activity was much higher in fed dogs compared with fasted animals, it was proposed that the stimulation was caused by the local mechanical and chemical action of chyme (19). However, it was then demonstrated that feeding greatly stimulated villous motility in an isolated jejunal loop prepared by connecting the mesenteric artery and vein with the carotid-jugular circulation (20). To account for this new observation it was proposed that chyme, in addition to a local action, caused the release of a factor in the duodenum that entered the bloodstream and stimulated motility. This experiment marked a conceptual turning point. Emphasis was now directed away from local effects of mechanical and chemical stimuli to the possible occurrence of a physiologically significant intrinsic factor that controls villous motility. The theory was supported by additional experiments, and the intrinsic motility factor was named villikinin (24).

VILLOUS MOTILITY

Intestinal villi are a characteristic feature of mammalian small intestine mucosa and they are readily observed in an exteriorized jejunal loop of a pentobarbital-anesthetized animal. Viewed through a stereomicroscope, 40 × magnification, two forms of villi are observed—finger-like and leaf-like. The former occur in carnivores and the latter both in herbivores and omnivores (9,10, Table 1). Finger-like villi exhibit three types of movements: (a) contraction followed by relaxation; (b) pendular movements, i.e., swaying to and fro without shortening; and (c) tonic or sustained contraction. Contractions, followed by a return to the original length, are described also as pumping movements and are herein referred to as villous motility (41, 46, 47; Fig. 1). Each villus moves independently of its neighbors and of peristalsis. The pendular villous movements occur when the mucosal surface comes into contact with liquid. They are of relatively short duration and appear to be propulsive in nature (46). Tonic villous contractions are seen in agonal or preagonal states and are thought to be a pathological rather than a physiological feature (47). Leaf-like villi never show pumping movements, but are compressed by the circular contractions of the muscularis mucosae (9).

PHYSIOLOGICAL SIGNIFICANCE OF VILLOUS MOTILITY

It seems reasonable to assume that lymph flow is promoted by the pumping action of the villi. As far back as 1851 it was postulated that the central lacteals of the villi empty during contraction and fill during relaxation (1). Histological

TABLE 1. *Villous form in relation to diet*

Dietary class	Villous form	
	Finger-like	Leaf-like
Herbivorous	Chicken	Gopher
	Pigeon	Guinea pig
		Hamster
		Rabbit
		Squirrel
Carnivorous	Cat	
	Dog	
	Eagle	
	Fox	
Omnivorous	Man	Opossum
	Monkey	Pig
		Rat

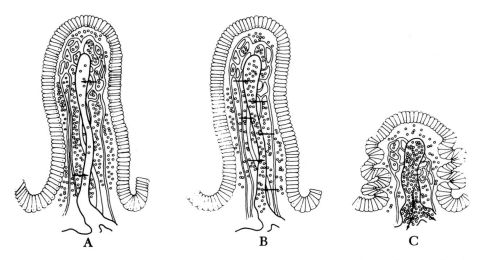

FIG. 1. Variations in height, volume, and shape of a finger-like villus as it goes from a relaxed state (**A** and **B**) to a contracted state (**C**). *Arrows* show the postulated movement of particles from interstitial tissue into the central lacteal when the villus is relaxed (**A** and **B**) and their subsequent ejection when the villus contracts (**C**). (From ref. 41.)

studies have shown that during fat absorption the central lacteals are empty in contracted villi and full with fat droplets in relaxed villi (39). It also has been observed that villous stimulants increase lymph flow from the thoracic duct of anesthetized dogs (12). However, the villous-pump theory of absorption was not supported in a study that involved the use of a special absorption chamber. It was reported that the central lacteals do not empty when the villi shorten (48). More research is needed in this area.

Another effect of the pumping action of villi is to agitate the chyme. This may be observed in fed dogs where one is especially impressed with enormously active villi stirring and mixing chyme. The probable consequence of this activity is to present fresh material to the absorptive surface. Substances that stimulate villi enhance absorption (14,22,31,38,40) and those that inhibit motility decrease absorption (18,30).

HORMONAL CONTROL OF VILLOUS MOTILITY

Villous motility in the small intestine is affected by: (a) local mechanical and chemical stimuli (19,46,47); (b) parasympathetic and sympathetic nerve stimulation (7,36,47); and (c) extracts of small intestine mucosa (21). We will review published and unpublished experiments on the hormone-like activity of the active principle in mucosal extracts, villikinin, as well as present new data on its chemical characteristics.

Several observations support the theory that intestinal villous motility is controlled by a unique gastrointestinal hormone. They include: (a) Villous motility is much higher in fed than in fasted dogs. Although there are individual variations in the number of contractions, typically one observes, in a mm² circumscribed field containing approximately 30 villi, approximately 200 contractions per minute in fed dogs, but only approximately 60 contractions per minute in fasted dogs. In fasted animals the basal count is remarkably constant for several hours (17). (b) Intraduodenal administration of 0.1 N HCl markedly stimulates the villi in an isolated jejunal loop transplanted into the carotid-jugular circulation (20,21). (c) Perfusion of an isolated intestinal loop of a fasted dog via the carotid-jugular circulation of a fed dog markedly stimulates the villi of the fasted dog (26). (d) In cross-circulation experiments involving carotid-jugular anastomosis of two animals, introduodenal administration of 0.1 N HCl into one animal substantially increased the villous motility of both animals. Saline and bicarbonate, on the other hand, are without effect (2,28). (e) A substance can be extracted from the mucosa that stimulates villous motility by intravenous injection (21). Thus, it appears that acid chyme releases a substance that can enter the bloodstream and stimulate villi. All the evidence indicating a hormonal mechanism for the control of villous motility has been obtained in dogs; other animal species should be tested. One laboratory has reported that it was unable to obtain evidence for a hormonal mechanism in pigeons (4).

VILLIKININ ACTIVITY

Activity is expressed as the contraction index CI, (16):

$$CI = \frac{\text{experimental count} - \text{basal count}}{\text{basal count}}$$

Units of villikinin are determined by intravenous assay. Ten units in a 10-kg dog causes a 50% increase in the number of contractions. From the equation it is apparent that a 50% increase is equivalent to a CI of 0.5. A typical dose-response curve, plotted on a semi-log scale, is depicted in Fig. 2. The response increases with increasing doses up to 8 units/kg. The threshold dose is 0.25 units/kg. Occasionally, large doses of crude HCl mucosal extracts cause an initial inhibition of villous motility, followed by an increase above the basal count, suggesting the presence of an inhibitory factor, antivillikinin (17). The active and inhibitory principles in these HCl extracts can be separated easily by dialysis; villikinin passes through the membrane whereas antivillikinin is retained (17,24).

Villous motility is stimulated by villikinin when administered topically, intravenously, or intraarterially. The characteristic actions of the hormone after intravenous injection are: (a) the rate of contracting villi increases 1 to 3 min after injection; (b) the maximal effect is reached in 5 to 8 min, and (c) the rate of contractions returns to the basal level within 15 min (Fig. 3). There is no effect on the tunica muscularis, no change in peristaltic activity or blood

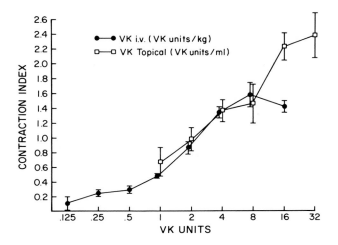

FIG. 2. Dose-response curve (semi-logarithmic) of porcine villikinin extracted from mucosa by the trichloroacetic acid-Dowex 50 method (see text). *Vertical lines* indicate standard error of the mean.

pressure (although there is a slight vasodilation in the villi), no tachyphylaxis, and no increase in mucus formation on the exposed mucosal surface (6). Villikinin does not alter pancreatic exocrine secretion nor does it cause the gallbladder to contract (24). It does not affect the rabbit duodenum or guinea pig *in vitro* (16). Villikinin does not appear to have a direct effect on villous smooth muscle. Its action is blocked by hexamethonium and other ganglionic blockers (35). Isoproterenol, a β-agonist, applied topically, stimulates villous motility and norepinephrine, an α-agonist, is inhibitory. Their actions are blocked by propranolol and phentolamine, respectively (15). Acetylcholine initially stimulates

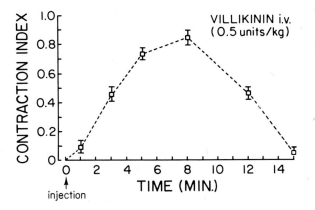

FIG. 3. Typical action curve of canine villikinin prepared by the trichloroacetic acid-Dowex 50 method (see text). *Vertical lines* indicate SEM.

villous motility but this is followed by a state of relaxation (15). Atropine blocks acetylcholine but not villikinin; the effect of adrenergic receptor antagonists on villikinin has not been tested.

DISTRIBUTION OF VILLIKININS

Crude extracts of villikinin were first prepared from canine mucosa obtained by scraping the small intestine. The mucosa was ground with sand, boiled in 0.1 N HCl, neutralized with NaOH, centrifuged, and treated with charcoal to remove histamine and other known gastrointestinal hormones (21). Villikinin was found only in mucosa of the small intestine, with the highest concentration occurring in the duodenal mucosa (33). Active preparations have been obtained from the mucosa of different mammalian species including man (23,27,34). The effect was not related to the presence of histamine, choline (24), secretin, cholecystokinin (CCK), or adenosine in the samples (25). Villikinin enters the circulation (29) and has been found in human, canine, and bovine plasma (plasmavillikinin), (5,43) as well as in human and canine lymph (44). Active preparations also have been extracted from human and canine urine (urovillikinin) (5,37, 42,45), suggesting that villikinin is cleared by the kidney. Although there are differences in the potencies of villikinin preparations from various animals and tissues, villikinin from all sources produces similar responses (5), and the hormone is not species-specific (23). Villikinin increases in human urine after a meal and after intraduodenal HCl administration (37).

ACTIVITY OF OTHER SUBSTANCES

A number of gastrointestinal hormones and other active substances, most of them present in the intestinal mucosa, have been compared with villikinin (Tables 2a, 2b; ref. 6). Although some stimulate motility in doses as small as 1.0 ng/kg, they also have other effects such as causing mucus secretion, cyanosis or anemia in the villi, and altering blood pressure and peristalsis. Not shown in table 2 are unpublished preliminary observations on the pancreatic secretion and gallbladder contraction. Many of the hormones studied have significant effects on these organs. It is noteworthy that even when administered in high doses, villikinin has the distinctive feature of stimulating the villi without causing other effects. Methionine-enkephalin and α-endorphin come close to resembling villikinin (Table 2b) since they stimulate motility and have only minor effects on other parameters. However, another opiate peptide, leucine-enkephalin, administered intravenously inhibited motility, stimulated mucus secretion, and caused anemia (Table 2b). Naloxone blocked the action of the opioid peptides on the villi but naloxone was without effect on villikinin.

Bombesin is another peptide with a rather specific action on villi (Table 2b). Infused in the minute dose of 1 ng/kg/hr it has a weak stimulant action but

TABLE 2a. *Summary of the effect of gastrointestinal hormones*

Substance	Route of administration	V.M.	M.S.	Anemia or cyanosis	Peri	B.P.
Cholecystokinin-pancreozymin	Intravenous	+--	+	0	-	↓
	Topical	--	+	0	-	
	Intraarterial	+-				
Enterogastrone	Intravenous	-	+	++	+	↑
	Topical	-	+	+	0	
Human gastrin	Intravenous	-+	0	0	0	↓
	Topical	+	0	0	0	
Pentagastrin	Intravenous	-	+	0	0	0
	Topical	-	+	0	0	
Gastric inhibitory peptide	Intravenous	-	+	+	0	0
	Topical	-	0	0	0	
Glucagon	Intravenous	---	0	+	---	0
	Topical	---	+	+	---	
	Intraarterial	---	0	++	---	
Secretin	Intravenous	-0	0	0	0	↓
	Topical	0	0	0	+	
	Intraarterial	+-	0	0	0	
Villikinin	Intravenous	+++	0	0	0	0
	Topical	+++	0	0	0	
	Intraarterial	+++	0	0	0	

+, Stimulation; -, inhibition; 0, no effect; +, slight; ++, moderate; +++, strong stimulation; -, slight; --, moderate; ---, strong inhibition; ↑, Increase; ↓, decrease; V.M., villous motility; M.S., mucus secretion; B.P., arterial blood pressure; Peri., peristalsis; + -, stimulation followed by inhibition; - +, inhibition followed by stimulation.

this lasts less than 5 min and is followed by slight inhibition. At 10 or 100 ng/kg/hr bombesin consistently inhibits motility.

The effects of other gastrointestinal hormones and vasoactive substances are listed in Tables 2a and 2b.

NEW PREPARATIONS OF VILLIKININ

Recent studies have centered on the preparation of suitable quantities of villikinin for its chemical characterization. Extracts of dog mucosa prepared by the HCl-charcoal method were desalted and further purified by hanging curtain continuous flow paper electrophoresis at pH 8.6. One major peak of activity was found (13,16,45). It was associated with a ninhydrin-positive peak on the anodal side of the curtain. Pepsin and trypsin treatment did not alter the activity of purified canine villikinin (16). The substance also resists heating up to 100° in dilute acid, passed through a dialysis membrane and could not be separated

TABLE 2b. *Summary of the effect of vasoactive substances*

Substance	Route of administration	V.M.	M.S.	Anemia or cyanosis	Peri	B.P.
Eledoisin	Intravenous	−+	+	+	↓	
	Topical	+	+			
	Intraarterial	+	0			
Cerulein	Intravenous	−	+	+	↑	↓
	Topical	−−	+	+		
	Intraarterial	+−	+			
Ranatensin	Intravenous	−−−	+	+	↑	↑
	Topical	−−	0			
Substance P	Intravenous	+−	+++		↑	↓
	Topical	−−	++			
Bradykinin	Intravenous	+	0		↓	↓
	Topical	0	0	+	↓	
	Intraarterial	++	0		↓	
Histamine	Intravenous	++	+			↓
	Topical	+−	+			
	Intraarterial	+−	++			
Kallidin	Intraarterial	++	0	+	↓	
Serotonin	Intravenous	+−	+		↑	↑
	Topical	−	+	+	↑	
	Intraarterial	−	0	+	↑	
Neurotensin	Intravenous	−	+	+	0	↓
	Topical	−	+	++	0	
Bombesin	Intravenous	+−	0	0	0	0
	Topical	+	0	0	0	
Prostaglandin E₁	Intravenous	−−	+	+	0	0
	Topical	−−	+			
	Intraarterial	−−	+	+	0	
Opiate Peptides Met-enkephalin	Intravenous	++	0	0	↑	0
	Topical	++	+	0		
Leu-enkephalin	Intravenous	−	+	+	0	0
	Topical	+−				
α-endorphin	Intravenous	+	+	0	0	0
	Topical	+	+	0	0	
β-endorphin	Intravenous	0	0	0	0	0
	Topical	0				
γ-endorphin	Intravenous	0	0	0	0	0
	Topical	0	0	0	0	0

+, Stimulation; −, inhibition; 0, no effect; +, slight; ++, moderate; +++, strong stimulation; −, slight; −−, moderate; −−−, strong inhibition; ↑, Increase, ↓, decrease; V.M., villous motility; M.S., mucus secretion; B.P., arterial blood pressure; Peri., peristalsis; + −, stimulation followed by inhibition; − +, inhibition followed by stimulation.

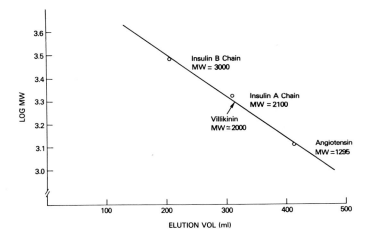

FIG. 4. Peak of villikinin activity *(arrow)* observed when porcine villikinin was filtered through Bio-Gel calibrated with known peptides.

from salt on a Sephadex G-25 column that has an exclusion limit of 5,000 (16).

Working on the assumption that villikinin is a polypeptide, a new extraction procedure has been developed which avoids heating, HCl and charcoal. Mucosa was homogenized in a trichloroacetic acid solution and the clear supernatant solution obtained after centrifugation was passed over a Dowex 50 column. Trichloroacetic acid passes through the column and the adsorbed villikinin was eluted with 0.2 M pyridine. It appears just after elution of the bulk of adsorbed substances. The eluate was freeze-dried and bioassayed.

Seven thousand and 5,400 units of villikinin were isolated from the small intestine of 75 pigs and 100 dogs, respectively. One unit of porcine villikinin weighed 5 μg. This material was still quite crude but it was 100 times more potent than a typical HCl-charcoal extract used previously. One peak of villikinin activity (tested by intravenous injection) was observed when porcine villikinin was filtered through Bio-Gel P-4. Its apparent M. W. was 2,000 (Fig. 4) and the peak accounted for 35% of the applied activity. The M. W. of canine villikinin estimated on a Bio-Gel P-10 column with the use of several markers was 2,500. As previously observed with cruder preparations, the peak fractions strongly stimulated the villi and had no other effects.

Pronase, Nagarse (subtilisin BPN'), and papain, but not trypsin or pepsin, inactivated villikinin (Table 3). The exopeptidases, leucine aminopeptidase and carboxypeptidase A also inactivate but carboxypeptidase B is without effect. Chymotrypsin partially inactivated villikinin, suggesting that the digest contained a less potent fragment. Enough porcine villikinin was recovered from gel filtration for testing with leucine aminopeptidase. The enzyme completely inactivated

TABLE 3. *Actions of proteases on villikinin[a]*

Enzyme	Action
Pronase	Inactivation
Papain	Inactivation
Subtilisin BPN'	Inactivation
Leucine aminopeptidase	Inactivation
Carboxypeptidase A	Inactivation
Chymotrypsin	Partial inactivation
Carboxypeptidase B	No effect
Trypsin	No effect
Pepsin	No effect

[a] Canine, porcine, and bovine villikinins were tested.

the sample as expected. The enzyme studies indicate that villikinin is a polypeptide with free amino- and carboxy-termini.

CONCLUSIONS

Although dog intestinal villi respond to a number of physiologically active substances, the majority are inhibitory. Those that are stimulatory (as well as the inhibitors) also produce other effects, including: (a) increase mucus secretion, (b) cause anemia or cyanosis, (c) alter peristalsis, and (d) alter blood pressure. Villikinin, even in very high doses, shows a characteristic long-lasting stimulant action and none of these side effects. The other agents also may be affected by specific blocking agents such as atropine, antihistamine, or naloxone. Ganglionic blockers are the only agents so far tested that block villikinin.

Substitution of the original HCl-charcoal purification by the trichloroacetic acid-Dowex 50 procedure has given a product that is at least 100 times more potent. When porcine villikinin obtained by the later procedure was gel-filtered, 35% of the activity was recovered in a single peak with an apparent M. W. of 2,000. Canine villikinin similarly treated gave a single peak with a M. W. of 2,500. The porcine and canine preparations were similarly inactivated by proteases. Thus, villikinin appears to be polypeptide.

PROJECTIONS FOR THE FUTURE

The proof of the hypothesis that villikinin is a single hormonal polypeptide awaits further experimentation. Our efforts are now directed to the isolation, purification, and complete characterization of villikinin.

REFERENCES

1. Brücke E. (1851): *Sitzung. Kaiser. Akad. der Wissensch. Wien.,* 6:214.
2. Brunson, W. D., and Kokas, E. (1967): Presence of villikinin, secretin and cholecystokinin in the duodenal content. *Physiologist,* 10:136.

3. Hambleton, B. F. (1914): Note upon the movements of the intestinal villi. *Am. J. Physiol.*, 34:446–447.
4. Hooper, P. A., and Schneider, A. (1970): Evidence against the existence of hormonal control of small intestinal villous movement in the pigeon. *Life Sci.*, 9:1269–1273.
5. Johnston, C. L., Kokas, E., and Barrow, E. (1967): Plasma Villikinin. *Proc. Soc. Exp. Biol. Med.*, 125:281–284.
6. Joyner, W. L., and Kokas, E. (1973): Effect of various gastrointestinal hormones and vasoactive substances on villous motility. *Comp. Biochem. Physiol.*, 46A:171–181.
7. King, C. E., and Arnold, L. (1922): The activities of the intestinal mucosal motor mechanism. *Am. J. Physiol.*, 59:97–121.
8. King, C. E., Arnold, L., and Church, J. G. (1922): The physiological role of the intestinal mucosal movements. *Am. J. Physiol.*, 65:80–92.
9. Kokas, E. (1930): Vergleichendphysiologische Untersuchungen über die Bewegung der Darmzotten. *Pflüger's Arch. Ges. Physiol.*, 225:416–420.
10. Kokas, E. (1932): Vergleichendphysiologische Untersuchungen über die Bewegung der Darmzotten II. *Pflüger's Arch. Ges. Physiol.*, 229:486–491.
11. Kokas, E. (1948): Die Bewegung der Darmzotten und ihre hormonale Regelung. *Ztschr. Vitamin-Hormon-Fermentforsch.*, 2:98–112.
12. Kokas, E., Crepps, B., and Karika, J. (1973): The effect of some intestinal hormones on lymph-flow. *(Unpublished data)*.
13. Kokas, E., Davis, J. L., and Brunson, W. D. (1971): Separation of villikininlike substance from intestinal mucosal extract. *Arch. Int. Pharmacodyn. Ther.*, 191:310–317.
14. Kokas, E., and Gál, G. (1929): Resorptionsbeschleunigung durch Hefeextrakt. *Biochemische Ztschr.*, 205:380–387.
15. Kokas, E., and Gordon, H. A. (1970): Adrenergic and cholinergic receptors of intestinal villi in dogs. *J. Pharmacol. Exp. Ther.*, 180:56–51.
16. Kokas, E., and Johnston, C. L. (1965): Influence of refined villikinin on motility of intestinal villi. *Am. J. Physiol.*, 208:1196–1202.
17. Kokas, E., and Johnston, C. L. (1966): Evidence for an intestinal inhibitor of villous motility. *Arch. Int. Pharmacodyn. Ther.*, 160:211–222.
18. Kokas, E., and Kokas, F. (1948): Über die Wirkung von Ephedrin auf die Zottenbewegung und die Resorption von Glucose aus dem Darm. *Arch. Int. Pharmacodyn. Ther.*, 76:457–462.
19. Kokas, E., and Ludány, G. (1930): Weitere Untersuchungen über die Bewegung der Darmzotten. *Pflüger's Arch. Ges. Physiol.*, 225:421–428.
20. Kokas, E., and Ludány, G. (1932): Die Beobachtung der Zottenbewegung am überlebenden Darm. *Pflüger's Arch. Ges. Physiol.*, 231:20–23.
21. Kokas, E., and Ludány, G. (1933): Die hormonale Regelung der Darmzottenbewegung. I. *Pflüger's Arch. Ges. Physiol.*, 232:293–298.
22. Kokas, E., and Ludány, G. (1933): Die Wirkung der Gewürzmittel auf die Bewegung der Darmzotten und die Glycoseresorption. *Arch. Exp. Pathol. Pharmakol.*, 169:140–145.
23. Kokas, E., and Ludány, G. (1933): L'hormone excitant les mouvements des villosités intestinale (villikinine) est elle spécifique? *C. R. Soc. Biol.*, 113:1447–1449.
24. Kokas, E., and Ludány, G. (1934): Hormonale Regelung der Darmzottenbewegung II. *Pflüger's Arch. Ges. Physiol.*, 234:182–186.
25. Kokas, E., and Ludány, G. (1934): Über das Villikinin. *Pflüger's Arch. Ges. Physiol.*, 234:589–593.
26. Kokas, E., and Ludány, G. (1934): Nouvelles recherches sur la régulation hormonal des mouvements des villosités intestinales. *C. R. Soc. Biol.*, 117:972–973.
27. Kokas, E., and Ludány, G. (1934): Vergleichendphysiologische Untersuchungen über das Villikinin. *Arb. Ung. Biol. Forschungsinstitut*, 7:263–266.
28. Kokas, E., and Ludány, G. (1935): Über Aktivierung des Villikinins. *Pflüger's Arch. Ges. Physiol.*, 236:166–174.
29. Kokas, E., and Ludány, G. (1936): Résorption de la villikinine par l'intestin. *C. R. Soc. Biol.*, 122:413–415.
30. Kokas, E. and Ludány, G. (1937): Die Wirkung des Cocains auf die Glykoseresorption aus dem Darm. *Arch. Int. Pharmacodyn. Ther.*, 56:180–184.
31. Kokas, E., and Ludány, G. (1938): Relation between the "villikinin" and the absorption of glucose from the intestine. *O. J. Exp. Physiol.*, 28:15–22.

32. Ludány, G. (1933): Présence, dans l'intestin du foetus, d'une hormone excitant les mouvements des villosités intestinales (villikinine). *C. R. Soc. Biol.,* 113:1449–1450.
33. Ludány, G. (1935): Teneur en villikinine des differentes parties du tube gastrointestinale. *C. R. Soc. Biol.,* 117:974–976.
34. Ludány, G. (1935): Villikinin im menschlichen Darme. *Klin. Wochenschr.,* 141:123–124.
35. Ludány, G., Gáti, T., Rausch, J., and Hideg, J. (1960): Ganglionblocker und Darmzottenbewegung. *Arch. Int. Pharmacodyn. Ther.,* 127:402–409.
36. Ludány, G., and Jourdan, F. (1935): Influence du pneumogastrique et du sympathique sur la motricité des villosités intestinales. *C. R. Soc. Biol.,* 119:1189–1190.
37. Ludány, G., Svatoš, A., Gàti, T., and Gelencsér, F. (1962): Die Darmzottenbewegung fördernde Wirkung des Harns. (Urovillikinin) nach Nahrungsaufnamhme und Duodenumsäuerung. *Arch. Int. Pharmacodyn. Ther.,* 140:138–142.
38. Magee, H. E., and Reid, E. (1931): The absorption of glucose from the alimentary canal. *J. Physiol.,* 73:163–183.
39. Mahler, P., and Nonnebruch, W. (1932): Arbeiten über die Physiologie und Pathologie des Dünndarms. V. Die Fettresorption im gereizten Darm. *Ztschr. Ges. Exp. Med.,* 85:112–114.
40. Mahler, P., Nonnenbruch, W., and Weiser, J. (1932): Arbeiten über die Physiologie und Pathologie des Dünndarms II. Über Änderungen der Resorptionsgeschwindigkeit (Versuche mit Schleimstoffen, Adsorbentien, Gewürzen und entzundungserregenden Agenzien). *Ztschr. Ges. Exp. Med.,* 85:82–94.
41. Sessions, J. T., Viegas de Andrade, S. R., and Kokas, E. (1968): Intestinal villi: Form and Motility in Relation to Function. *In: Progress in Gastroenterology,* Vol. I, edited by G. B. J. Glass, pp. 248–260. Grune & Stratton, New York.
42. Svatoš, A. (1959): Über villikininartige Wirkung des Harns. *Experientia,* 15:479.
43. Svatoš, A., and Bartos, V. (1967): Villikinin activity of the blood serum in young and aged men. *Sbornik. Ved. Fak. KU. Hradci Kralove,* 10:245–250.
44. Svatoš, A., Brzek, V., and Bartos, V. (1964): Influence de l'application intraveineuse de la lymphe humaine et du sérum sanguin sur l'activité motrice de la musculature lisse de l'appareil digestif du chien. *J. Physiol. (Paris),* 56:659.
45. Svatoš, A., Quisnerová, M., and Gáti, T. (1960): Vergleichende elektrophoretische Untersuchungen der Zottenbewegung stimulierenden Substanzen in der Duodenal-schleimhaut und im Harn. *Arch. Int. Pharmacodyn. Ther.,* 126:315–320.
46. Verzár, F., and Kokas, E. (1927): Die Rolle der Darmzotten bei der Resorption. *Pflüger's Arch. Ges Physiol.,* 217:397–412.
47. Verzár, F., and McDougall, E. J. (1936): *Absorption from the Intestine,* pp. 53–70. Longmans, Green and Co., London.
48. Wells, H. S., and Johnson, R. G. (1934): The intestinal villi and their circulation in relation to absorption and secretion of fluid. *Am. J. Physiol.,* 109:387–402.

Gastrointestinal Hormones, edited by
George B. Jerzy Glass.
Raven Press, New York © 1980.

Chapter 41

Bulbogastrone: Physiological Evidence for Its Significance

Göran Nilsson

Department of Physiology, Faculty of Veterinarian Medicine, Swedish University of Agricultural Sciences, Uppsala, Sweden; and Department of Experimental Surgery, Serafimerlasarettet, Stockholm, Sweden

INTRODUCTION

The observation that high levels of acidity in the stomach or in the duodenum cause a reduction of gastric acid secretion early (40) indicated the existence of mechanisms exerting inhibitory influences on the acid-secreting glands of the stomach. According to Babkin (8), Sokolov working in Pavlov's laboratory was the first to demonstrate that acid in contact with the duodenal mucosa induces inhibition of gastric secretion. Subsequent studies performed by different groups confirmed the observation by Sokolov. Pincus et al. (42,43) made the observation that the luminal pH of the duodenum had to be below 2.5 before inhibition appeared. Such low pHs had not been frequently found in the duode-num, and the physiological significance of the inhibitory mechanism was therefore questioned.

However, experimental evidence from studies in which the acid gastric content was prevented from reaching the duodenal mucosa strongly suggested that the duodenum must be involved in the control of gastric acid secretion. Thus surgical resection (9,23,46) or translocation (9) of the duodenum increased the acid responses from vagally denervated pouches of Heidenhain type in dogs. Similarly, elimination of the acid influence on the duodenum by removing the parietal cell-bearing mucosa of the stomach (26) significantly increased the acid responses in Heidenhain pouch dogs.

The related observations led Andersson and Uvnäs (7) to postulate the existence of a pH gradient within the duodenum with low pHs in the upper duodenum and higher pHs more distally. If so, it could be possible to evoke inhibition from the most proximal portion of the duodenum. To substantiate their hypothesis they constructed in dogs pouches of the first 3 to 4 cm of the duodenum corresponding to the duodenal bulb. When the bulbar pouches were perfused with acid, a considerable reduction of test meal-induced acid secretion from the gastric fundic pouches was noted (7).

In other studies it was shown that inhibition did not occur (5) or was insignificant (24) if pouches constructed of the distal portion of the duodenum were acidified (Figs. 1 and 2).

These results compared favorably with observations in studies where the intraluminal pH of the antrum-duodenum region was registered (2) (see Fig. 3). There it was noted that pH in the lumen of the human duodenal bulb was better correlated to the pH of the gastric antrum than to the pH of the remaining portion of the duodenum. Thus when the antral pH was low (1 to 2) also the bulbar pH was low (1 to 3), whereas the pH distal to the entrance of the bile and pancreatic ducts was higher and constantly around 6.5 to 7.5. Similar results were later obtained in studies on dogs (10). After the demonstration that conditions for a pH-sensitive inhibitory mechanism exist exclusively in the bulbar

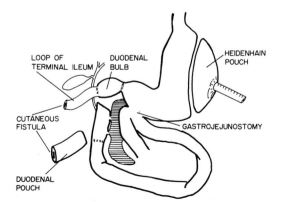

FIG. 1. Surgical preparations in dogs used in studies of acid-induced duodenal inhibition of gastric secretion. From Andersson et al. (5).

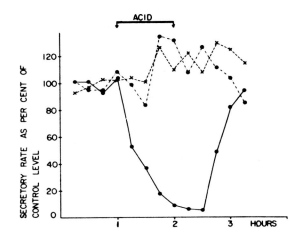

FIG. 2. Inhibition and lack of inhibition following acid perfusion of isolated pouches of the duodenal bulb (●--●), distal duodenum (●---●), or terminal ileum (x---x). Acid secretion induced by the intravenous infusion of exogenous gastrin. From Nilsson (29).

portion of the duodenum and that inhibition does not occur when pouches from lower duodenum are acidified, subsequent work has been designed to study the characteristics of the inhibition originating from the duodenal bulb.

SECRETORY STIMULANTS COUNTERACTED BY THE BULBAR MECHANISM

In a series of investigations acid secretion was induced by different means and isolated bulbar pouches were perfused with 0.1 M hydrochloric acid causing a persistent pH of 1.1 to 1.3 in the effluent perfusates. Bulbar acidification effectively reduced acid responses to stimulants that release gastrin since acid responses to test meal stimulation (6,7,35), sham feeding (6,31,34), or insulin hypoglycemia (6,30) were inhibited.

Also when acid secretion is induced by exogenous gastrin, inhibition is evident (3,5,33,36). The inhibition seems to be competitive since acid responses to low doses of gastrin are more suppressed than responses induced by higher doses (3). Such a dose-related inhibition is illustrated in Fig. 4. The competitive nature of the mechanism is also indicated in studies where stimulation of the HCl glands has been induced by the intravenous infusion of the same amount of gastrin in each experiment and the bulbar mechanism activated at different degrees by perfusing bulbar pouches with solutions of varying pHs (3). Reduction of secretory inhibition resulting from elevation of the intrabulbar pH is depicted in Fig. 5.

The related results demonstrating inhibition of acid responses to exogenous

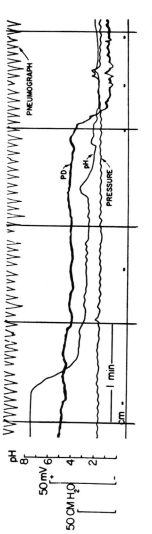

FIG. 3. Recording of pH, PD, and pressure from the gastroduodenal junction in man. The intraduodenal pH gradient is illustrated by the decrease in pH 2 cm distal to the pylorus. The pylorus is recognized by the fall in PD in the right section of the figure. From Andersson and Grossman (2).

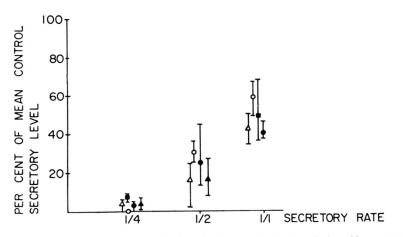

FIG. 4. Percent inhibition of acid secretion from fundic pouches in dogs induced by exogenous gastrin following reduction of the intrabulbar pH to 1.1–1.3. From Nilsson (29).

gastrin indicate that the bulbar mechanism interferes with gastrin at the parietal cell level rather than by suppressing the release of gastrin from the antrum.

As a matter of fact, later investigations (34) have indicated that no reduction of gastrin release occurs at acidification of the bulbar mucosa (Fig. 6).

It is well established that gastrin together with vagal excitation will cause the HCl glands to secrete optimally. Thus if gastrin-releasing tissues are removed,

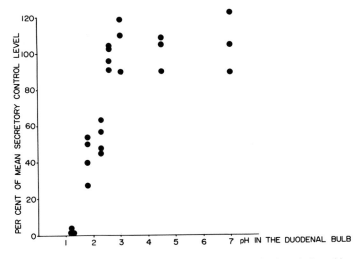

FIG. 5. Percent inhibition of acid secretion from fundic pouches in dogs induced by exogenous gastrin (approximately ¼–⅓ of maximal secretory rate) following bulbar perfusion with buffer solutions of different pHs. From Andersson and Nilsson (3).

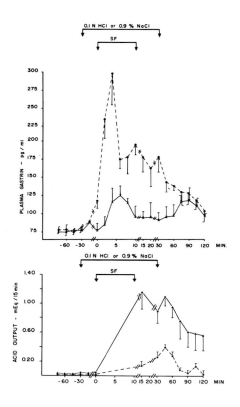

FIG. 6. Acid responses and plasma concentration of gastrin-like immunoreactivity in a dog at 10 min of sham feeding at perfusion of bulbar pouches with acid or saline. Symbols represent mean of 4 experiments. Vertical bars indicate the SD. From Nilsson (34).

acid responses to stimulation by short periods of sham feeding (45,49) or to low doses of insulin (39) may be abolished. However, if sham feeding is prolonged (45,49) or higher doses of insulin (39,41) are administered, the HCl glands may secrete significant amounts of acid also in absence of gastrin. When acid secretion is stimulated by prolonged sham feeding or by higher doses of insulin, inhibition becomes less efficient as stimulation is increased (Fig. 7).

These results were taken as evidence that the bulbar mechanism lacks efficiency in interfering with the vagal excitation of the HCl glands (32). This concept has been supported also by results from subsequent studies. Intravenous infusion of the stable choline ester betanechol in dogs activates acid secretion without causing release of gastrin. This indicates that cholinergic excitation may stimulate the parietal cells more or less independently of gastrin (52). When betanechol is used for stimulation of acid secretion in bulbar acidification experiments, no or little inhibition is found (37).

Also, basal acid secretion in dogs is suppressed when the pH in the duodenal bulb becomes acid (38) (Fig. 8). The true nature of basal acid secretion is not known and may perhaps be of different origin on different occasions. It is not, however, unreasonable to assume that under certain basal conditions nervous activation may arise that releases gastrin and excites the HCl glands which

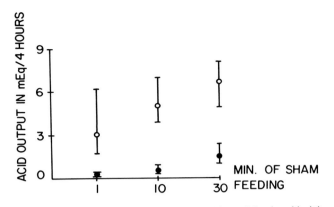

FIG. 7. Acid responses following sham feeding for 1, 10, or 30 min with (●) or without (○) acid perfusion of bulbar pouches. From Nilsson (31).

may result in secretion of acid gastric juice. If so, bulbar inhibition of basal acid secretion also may be due to an interference with gastrin at the oxyntic gland level.

Whereas gastrin-induced acid secretion is profoundly inhibited, acid responses to histamine are not reduced by acid perfusion of bulbar pouches in dogs (5). The interpretation of these results is complicated by the insufficient knowledge about the role that histamine plays in activation of acid secretion. It is well established from experiments in the rat that gastrin activates the histidine decar-

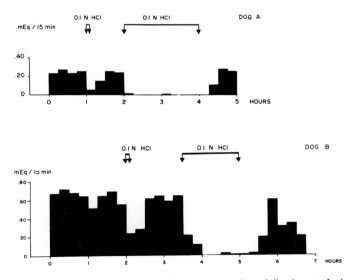

FIG. 8. Inhibition of basal acid secretion in Pavlov pouch dogs following perfusion of bulbar pouches with 0.1 M HCl for varying periods of time. From Nilsson (38).

boxylase of the gastric mucosa that in turn converts histidine to histamine. Whether the formed histamine indeed contributes to the activation of the HCl glands is still the matter of an animated discussion. If histamine is physiologically involved in the stimulation of the parietal cells, the bulbar mechanism might hypothetically act by interfering with the stimulatory effect that gastrin exerts on the activation of the enzyme histidine decarboxylase and thus inhibiting the formation of histamine. Experiments supporting or disqualifying this hypothesis are lacking.

pH-DEPENDENCE OF THE BULBAR MECHANISM

Using the preparation with isolated pouches of the duodenal bulb pH of bulbar perfusates may easily be maintained at a certain level over long periods of time. If moderate doses of gastrin are given to induce acid secretion corresponding to one-fourth to one-third of the maximal secretory rate inhibition is evident when pH of the bulbar perfusate is decreased below 2.5 (3) (see Fig. 5). If, however, smaller amounts of gastrin are used for stimulation, significant inhibition of acid secretion is apparent at even higher pHs (Fig. 9). Thus already a reduction of the intrabulbar pH below pH 5 significantly suppresses acid secretion (3). A similar activation of the bulbar mechanism at higher pHs has been seen (31) when sham feeding for 10 min has been used as secretory stimulus (Fig. 10). The related results indicate that a relatively

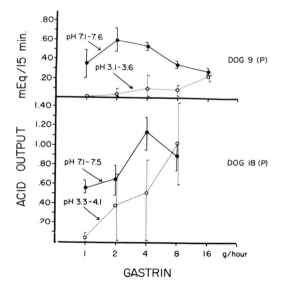

FIG. 9. Dose-response curves to gastrin at perfusion of bulbar pouches with buffer solutions of different pHs. Symbols represent the mean of 3 experiments in a dog. Vertical bars indicate the range. From Andersson and Nilsson (3).

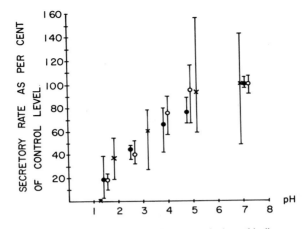

FIG. 10. Acid responses to 10 min of sham feeding at perfusion of bulbar pouches with buffer solutions of different pHs. Symbols represent the mean of 3 experiments in a dog. Vertical bars indicate the range. From Nilsson (31).

moderate increase of the acidity within the duodenal bulb is sufficient to activate the pH-sensitive inhibitory mechanism there, and that the mechanism may operate under the pH conditions normally existing in the duodenal bulb of the dog (10).

NATURE OF THE BULBAR INHIBITORY MECHANISM

The acidification of bulbar pouches effectively reduces acid secretion from both vagally innervated (3,5,6,7,30,31,33–37) and vagally denervated (3,5) gastric pouches indicating that inhibition is not mediated by vagovagal pathways. Results also suggest that inhibition is not mediated by intramural reflex activity arising from the bulbar mucosa and acting on the HCl glands since acid responses in Heidenhain pouches (3,5) are profoundly inhibited. The finding that intramural reflexes do not mediate the bulbar inhibition is supported also by studies of Andersson and Sjödin (6), who found that transection of the pylorus did not abolish the inhibition of acid secretion stimulated by different means.

In another study (33) bulbar inhibition of acid secretion by gastrin was studied in the same dogs before and after transection of the pylorus and following transplantation of the bulbar pouches to the abdominal wall (Fig. 11). Transection of the pylorus or complete denervation of the bulbar pouches did not significantly reduce the inhibition or change the inhibitory pattern which proves that bulbar inhibition is indeed mediated by a humoral agent. The name bulbogastrone has been given to this hypothetical factor (4).

The nature of this factor has been the matter of some speculation. Secretin or cholecystokinin-pancreozymin has been suggested to be the humoral factor mediating inhibition. However, when isolated bulbar pouches are perfused with

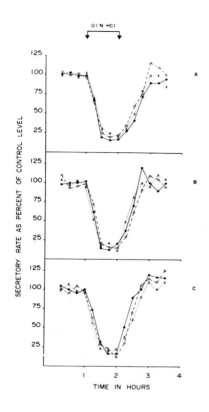

FIG. 11. Inhibition of acid responses to exogenous gastrin following acidification of bulbar pouches before **(A)** and after **(B)** transection of the pylorus and transplantation **(C)** of the bulbar pouch. Each curve illustrates one experiment. All experiments performed in the same dog. From Nilsson (33).

acid in dogs provided with both a gastric pouch and a pancreatic fistula, inhibition of acid secretion occurs but no stimulation of either bicarbonate or enzyme secretion is present (4). Considering that bulbar acidification does not induce pancreatic secretion and that relatively large doses of secretin and cholecystokinin-pancreozymin have to be given to cause inhibition, neither of these two hormones is likely to be the humoral factor mediating bulbar inhibition. Instead, a hypothetical factor named bulbogastrone has been suggested (4). Attempts to isolate this factor from the duodenal mucosa of pigs have given extracts with inhibitory properties from the proximal portion of the duodenum, whereas inhibition by extracts from distal duodenum has been insignificant (4). The bulbogastrone principle is therefore probably not identical with the previously suggested enterogastrone released by digested fat in contact with the mucosa of the upper small intestine (24). All studies performed so far support the idea that the bulbogastrone principle interferes with gastrin when inhibiting acid secretion and that this inhibition is exerted at the parietal cells rather than by preventing gastrin release (3,5,33,34,36). Interestingly, sham feeding in combination with bulbar acidification causes a considerably greater increase in concentration of gastrin-like immunoreactivity than does sham feeding alone (Fig. 6).

The great gastrin-like responses at bulbar acidification in these experiments may mean that the humoral factor released from the bulbar mucosa at bulbar acidification is a gastrin-like peptide cross-reacting with the antigastrin antibodies used. If this is true, a gastrin-like bulbogastrone may act at the parietal cells by binding to the same receptors as gastrin. The intrinsic activity of the bulbogastrone-gastrin receptor complex may be very low or lacking, which may result in a competitive inhibition of gastrin-induced excitation of the HCl glands.

INFLUENCE OF BULBAR ACIDIFICATION ON OTHER FUNCTIONS OF THE STOMACH

Bulbar acidification does not only reduce the secretion of hydrochloric acid from the stomach. Also, the output of pepsin is significantly reduced following stimulation by a test meal (35) (Table I).

In a study that was never completed, Andersson (1) perfused isolated bulbar pouches with acid and registered the motor activity in isolated fundic pouches of Heidenhain type. Bulbar acidification in such experiments almost abolished the spontaneous motor acitivity present in the vagally denervated gastric pouch.

Whether the inhibition of pepsin secretion and gastric motility mentioned above can be ascribed to the previously mentioned bulbogastrone principle, to some other not identified humoral factor, or to impulses mediated by intrinsic or extrinsic nerves, respectively, remains to be clarified.

INHIBITION IN SPECIES OTHER THAN THE DOG

The most extensive investigations on duodenal inhibition induced by acid have been performed in dogs. However, results are available from experiments also in other species.

TABLE 1. *Acid secretion (mEq/hr), pepsin concentration (PU Hb/10^{-4}), and pepsin output (PU Hb/10^{-4}) in Pavlov pouch dogs following test meal stimulation with or without bulbar acidification*

Experimental procedure	Secretion registered	Hours following start of feeding		
		1	2	3
Test meal	Acid secretion	4.73	4.61	3.40
	Pepsin conc.	215	141	150
	Pepsin output	3,204	1,975	1,465
Test meal and 0.1 M HCl in the duodenal bulb	Acid secretion	*1.98*	2.47	3.23
	Pepsin conc.	*151*	139	136
	Pepsin output	*1,139*	1,140	1,243

Acid perfusion of the duodenal bulb was performed during the first hour after feeding was started and is indicated by figures in italics. Figures represent average values from 25 controls and 19 inhibitory experiments in 5 dogs. From Nilsson (35).

Studies in cats have given contradictory results inasmuch as some authors
(22) have noted profound inhibition of acid secretion whereas others have failed
to demonstrate secretory inhibition (14,54). In our own experiments *(unpublished
observations)* in which isolated pouches of the upper duodenum were perfused
with 0.1 N HCl and acid secretion induced by pentagastrin, minute inhibition
was observed. However, this inhibition was considerably less pronounced than
inhibition in dogs elicited at a similar bulbar pH (1.1 to 1.3) and at a similar
rate of acid secretion from the stomach (approximately 50% of maximal secretory
rate in the cat). Considering the results related above, there is reason to believe
that the inhibitory mechanism is present also in cats although its quantitative
importance may be of little significance. In another study using ligation technique, Lundberg and Andersson (27) obtained results that were taken as evidence
for the existence of a pH-sensitive inhibitory mechanism also in the upper duodenum of the rat.

In man convincing results exist demonstrating that adequate conditions are
present in the proximal portion of the duodenum for a pH-sensitive inhibitory
mechanism to operate (6). Several studies show that the instillation of hydrochloric acid into the duodenum elicits profound inhibition of acid secretion
(17–19,48). As for dogs it has been claimed that a humoral factor may be
responsible for the inhibition present in man. Blood transfused from a person
with acidified duodenum may cause inhibition of gastric secretion in the receiver
of the transfused blood (19).

QUANTITATIVE IMPORTANCE OF THE BULBAR MECHANISM

In the studies reported in this chapter the bulbar mechanism has been studied
by a technique that not only permits the intrabulbar pH to remain constant
over a longer period of time. Perfusions have also been performed at a slight
overpressure (5 to 10 cm H_2O), which ensures a close contact between the
perfusion solution and the mucosal cells. Thanks to this experimental procedure,
high reproducibility of the experiments in dogs has been present and quantitative
estimations can be done. From the related studies the bulbar mechanism appears
as an extraordinarily potent inhibitory mechanism with the ability to abolish
also considerable acid responses.

In the intact gastrointestinal tract the stomach empties its acid content inter-
mittently into the duodenum. It is reasonable to assume that the bulbar mechanism under such conditions exerts a more moderate inhibitory influence on
acid secretion than in the experimental situation with isolated bulbar pouches
distended with acid solutions. The quantitative importance of the bulbar inhibitory mechanism in regulating acid secretion is not known. Possibly, experiments
in which acid secretion is determined before and after surgical resection of
the upper duodenum or experiments in which acid is prevented from reaching
the bulbar mucosa may offer a better estimation of the quantitative importance
of the bulbar mechanisms.

For example, Konturek and Grossman (23) found that acid responses to gastrin were increased by approximately 40% when the segment corresponding to the duodenal bulb was surgically removed.

DO FACTORS OTHER THAN ACID ACTIVATE THE BULBAR MECHANISM?

A number of studies exist indicating that hypertonic solutions of proteins, carbohydrates, and salts may induce inhibition of gastric acid secretion from the duodenum. On the other hand, several authors have failed to demonstrate such inhibition [for references, see Nilsson (36)]. The effect of bulbar perfusion with hypertonic solutions (40%) of peptone, glucose, or sodium chloride on acid responses induced by peptavlon has been studied. No significant inhibition of acid secretion was noted in these experiments, indicating that the bulbar mechanism is not activated by high osmolarity (36).

It is well established that digestion products of fats when present in duodenum and the jejunum induce inhibition of the gastric secretion (25). Only a few single experiments have been done to study whether the bulbar mechanism is activated by this stimulus. According to the experiments performed (S. Andersson, *personal communication*), digested fat evokes no inhibition when perfused through bulbar pouches.

In an attempt to determine whether cholinergic excitation of the bulbar region induces inhibition of gastric secretion, investigators have perfused bulbar pouches with acetylcholine solutions of low concentrations (36). Interestingly enough, such perfusions initiate some inhibition of gastric secretion evoked by peptavlon. The results may be taken as evidence for the existence of a cholinergic release mechanism for bulbogastrone. Further support that vagal (cholinergic) mechanisms may cause release of an inhibitory agent from the upper gastrointestinal tract has been obtained also from other sorts of experiments in dogs. Truncal transection of vagi has given rise to increased acid secretion from Heidenhain pouches (13,15,47). A similar effect has been demonstrated also following selective extragastric abdominal vagotomy (53). Furthermore, it has been shown that vagal excitation induced by insulin hypoglycemia (11,16,20,21,28,53) or by sham feeding (45,50) evokes inhibition of acid secretion initiated by different means. Following surgical removal of the pyloric antrum and the duodenal bulb, vagal excitation by sham feeding no longer suppresses acid responses to exogenous gastrin in Heidenhain pouch dogs (51).

DEFECTIVE DUODENAL INHIBITION OF GASTRIC SECRETION: AN ETIOLOGIC FACTOR IN ULCER DISEASE?

Shay et al. (48) have propounded the hypothesis that hypersecretion of acid gastric juice in duodenal ulcer disease may be due to a less effective duodenal inhibitory mechanism. Later findings by Johnston and Duthie (17) have supported this concept.

Investigations of duodenal inhibition in man are complicated by certain difficulties. The number of experiments is in general small. Difficulties exist to repeat experiments in the same individual. The position of the tubes in the duodenum cannot be exactly controlled which may cause a less adequate duodenal acidification. In addition, experiments on duodenal ulcer patients have often been performed during an active period of the disease. The portion of the upper duodenum responsive to reduction of the intraluminal pH may under such conditions be too ulcerated or edematous to respond normally to instillation of hydrochloric acid. Duodenal ulcer patients having indications of a defective duodenal inhibitory mechanism should therefore be persuaded to participate in additional inhibitory tests when the ulcerated area has healed and become normalized. Until such studies have been performed under adequate experimental conditions and in sufficient number, the defective duodenal inhibition of gastric secretion as an etiological factor in duodenal ulcer disease remains only an exciting hypothesis. Duodenal inhibition of gastric secretion may, however, be defective also in other respects in duodenal ulcer disease.

Experiments in dogs indicate that the bulbar mechanism interferes with the stimulatory action of gastrin at the parietal cells but does not counteract cholinergic stimulation of these glands. Dragstedt (12) has suggested that vagal hyperactivity may be present in patients having duodenal ulcer disease. If such stimulation of cholinergic nature predominates in this disease, inhibitory influences arising on acidification of the duodenal mucosa may be less effective in reducing acid secretion in the duodenal ulcer patient than in normal man. Under such circumstances reduced inhibition would be due not to a defective inhibitory mechanism in the duodenum but to the inability of this mechanism to interfere with a pathological stimulus acting on the HCl glands (37).

PITFALLS IN THE STUDIES OF BULBAR INHIBITION

As in most experimental studies, conflicting results have been reported from investigations of the mechanism by which acid in the duodenum inhibits gastric secretion.

Some methodological aspects of crucial importance will be mentioned here. Control experiments should be carried out to determine the secretory capacity of the gastric pouch. On the basis of such experiments the stimulant should be adjusted to induce a submaximal rate of acid secretion from the fundic pouch Control experiments have to be performed to avoid normal fluctuations in secretion of gastric juice during intravenous infusions of histamine or gastrin being interpreted as inhibition. Perfusion of isolated pouches of the duodenum has to be done under a slight overpressure (5 to 10 cm H_2O) to enable the solution to come in contact also with the deepest portions of the duodenal pouches. pH of the effluent perfusate from duodenal pouches should be repeatedly controlled.

Dogs having isolated pouches of the duodenal bulb should be regularly used in experiments with bulbar acidification. Too long periods before experiments are started or between experiments may lead to failure to demonstrate bulbar inhibition. If so, the inhibitory mechanism may be reactivated by daily perfusions of bulbar pouches with acid solutions for a 1 or 2 weeks (G. Nilsson, *unpublished observations*).

SUMMARY AND CONCLUSIONS

A mechanism responsive to reduction of the pH inhibiting gastric acid secretion has been demonstrated to exist in the duodenum of dog, man, cat, and rat. The mechanism seems to be located exclusively at the duodenal bulb where the pH conditions exist permitting such a mechanism to operate. The mechanism seems to suppress acid secretion by interfering with the stimulatory action of gastrin at the oxyntic glands. The mechanism is mediated by a humoral principle, so far not isolated but named bulbogastrone. The inhibitory mechanism is supposed to get into operation when the gastric acid content after a meal becomes high and the acid is emptied into the duodenum. Since basal acid secretion is inhibited, the mechanism may in addition contribute to the suppression of acid secretion between meals.

ACKNOWLEDGMENTS

The author's studies referred to in this paper have been supported by research grants from the Swedish Medical Research Council. The secretarial assistance of Mrs. Ewa Kallerman is gratefully acknowledged.

REFERENCES

1. Andersson, S. (1975): Bulbogastrone. In: *Symposium on Gastrointestinal Hormones*, pp. 555–562. University of Texas Press, Austin.
2. Andersson, S., and Grossman, M. I. (1965): Profile of pH, pressure and potential difference at the gastroduodenal junction in man. *Gastroenterology*, 49:364–371.
3. Andersson, S., and Nilsson, G. (1969): pH-dependence of the mechanism in the duodenal bulb inhibiting gastric acid responses to exogenous gastrin. *Acta Physiol. Scand.*, 76:182–190.
4. Andersson, S., Nilsson, G., Sjödin, L., and Uvnäs, B. (1973): Mechanism of duodenal inhibition of gastric acid secretion. In: *Nobel Symposium XVI. Frontiers in Gastrointestinal Hormone Research*, pp. 223–238. Almquist & Wiksell, Stockholm.
5. Andersson, S., Nilsson, G., and Uvnäs, B. (1967): Effect of acid in proximal and distal duodenal pouches on gastric secretory responses to gastrin and histamine. *Acta Physiol. Scand.*, 71:368–378.
6. Andersson, S., and Sjödin, L. (1972): Inhibition of gastric secretion by acidification of the duodenal bulb before and after transection of the pylorus. *Scand. J. Gastroenterol.*, 7:151–156.
7. Andersson, S., and Uvnäs, B. (1961): Inhibition of postprandial gastric secretion in Pavlov

pouches by instillation of hydrochloric acid into the duodenal bulb. *Gastroenterology*, 41:486–490.

8. Babkin, B. P. (1950): *Secretory Mechanism of the Digestive Glands*. Paul B. Hoeber, New York.
9. Brackney, E., Thal, A. P., and Wangensteen, O. H. (1955): Role of duodenum in the control of gastric secretion. *Proc. Soc. Exp. Biol. Med.*, 88:302–306.
10. Brooks, A. M., and Grossman, M. I. (1970): Postprandial pH and neutralizing capacity of the proximal duodenum in dogs. *Gastroenterology*, 59:85–89.
11. Burstall, P. A., and Schofield, B. (1951): An inhibitory component in the gastric response to insulin hypoglycemia in Heidenhain pouches in dogs. *J. Physiol.*, 115:19,20P.
12. Dragstedt, L. R. (1942): Pathogenesis of gastroduodenal ulcer. *Arch. Surg.*, 44:438–450.
13. Emås, S., and Grossman, M. I. (1969): Response of Heidenhain pouch to histamine, gastrin and feeding before and after truncal vagotomy in dogs. *Scand. J. Gastroenterol.*, 4:449–457.
14. Emås, S., Svensson, S. O., and Borg, I. (1971): Effect of duodenal acidification or exogenous secretin on acid gastric secretion stimulated by histamine, pentagastrin or human gastrin I in conscious cats. *Digestion*, 5:17–30.
15. Evans, S. O., Zubiran, J. M., McCarthy, J. D., Ragins, H., Woodward, E. R., and Dragstedt, L. R. (1953): Stimulating effect of vagotomy on gastric secretion in Heidenhain pouch dogs. *Am. J. Physiol.*, 174:219–225.
16. Jemerin, E. E., Hollander, F., and Weinstein, V. A. (1943): A comparison of insulin and food as stimuli for the differentiation of vagal and non-vagal gastric pouches. *Gastroenterology*, 1:500–512.
17. Johnston, D., and Duthie, H. L. (1964): Effect of acid in the duodenum on histamine-stimulated gastric secretion in man. *Gut*, 5:573–580.
18. Johnston, D., and Duthie, H. L. (1965): Inhibition of gastric secretion in the human stomach. *Lancet*, 2:1032–1036.
19. Johnston, D., and Duthie, H. L. (1966): Inhibition of histamine-stimulated gastric secretion by acid in the duodenum in man. *Gut*, 7:58–68.
20. Jordan, P. H., Jr., and Quintana, R. (1964): Insulin inhibition of gastrin-stimulated gastric secretion. *Gastroenterology*, 47:617–625.
21. Karvinen, E., and Karvonen, M. J. (1953): The effect of insulin hypoglycemia on histamine-induced Heidenhain pouch secretion in the dog. *Acta Physiol. Scand.*, 27:350–370.
22. Konturek, S., Dubiel, J., and Gabrys, B. (1969): Effect of acid infusion into various levels of the intestine on gastric and pancreatic secretion in the cat. *Gut*, 10:749–753.
23. Konturek, S., and Grossman, M. I. (1965): Localization of the mechanism for inhibition of gastric secretion by acid in intestine. *Gastroenterology*, 49:74–78.
24. Konturek, S., and Grossman, M. I. (1965): Effect of perfusion of intestinal loops with acid, fat or dextrose on gastric secretion. *Gastroenterology*, 49:481–489.
25. Kosaka, T., and Lim, R. K. S. (1930): Demonstration of the humoral agent in fat inhibition of gastric secretion. *Proc. Soc. Exp. Biol. Med.*, 27:890–891.
26. Landor, J. H., Ross, J. L., and Gay, G. R. (1962): The importance of acid inhibition in the regulation of gastric secretion. *Arch. Surg.*, 85:695–700.
27. Lundberg, B., and Andersson, S. (1974): The role of the upper duodenum in controlling gastric acid secretion in the rat. *Scand. J. Gastroenterol.*, 9:623–627.
28. Necheles, H., Olsson, W. H., and Scruggs, W. (1942): Effect of insulin on gastric secretion. *Fed. Proc.*, 1:62.
29. Nilsson, G. (1968): Studies on the bulbar inhibitory mechanism, p. 384. In: *The Physiology of Gastric Secretion*. Universitetsförlaget, Oslo.
30. Nilsson, G. (1969): Effect of acid in the duodenal bulb on gastric secretory responses to insulin hypoglycemia. *Acta Physiol. Scand.*, 75:476–483.
31. Nilsson, G. (1969): Effect of acid in the duodenal bulb on gastric secretory responses to sham feeding. *Acta Physiol. Scand.*, 77:308–315.
32. Nilsson, G. (1969): Studies on the mechanism by which acid in the duodenal bulb inhibits gastric acid secretion. Dissertation, Stockholm.
33. Nilsson, G. (1974): Effect of acidification of totally denervated pouches of the duodenal bulb on gastric acid secretion in dog. *Acta Physiol. Scand.*, 92:569–571.
34. Nilsson, G. (1975): Increased plasma gastrin levels in connection with inhibition of gastric acid responses to sham feeding following bulbar perfusion with acid in dogs. *Scand. J. Gastroenterol.*, 10:273–278.

35. Nilsson, G. (1975): Effect of acid in the duodenal bulb on acid and pepsin responses to test meal in dog. *Scand. J. Gastroenterol.,* 10:279–282.
36. Nilsson, G. (1975): Effect of bulbar perfusion with acid, hypertonic solutions and acetylcholine on gastric acid secretion in dogs. *Scand. J. Gastroenterol.,* 10:283–287.
37. Nilsson, G. (1975): Effect of bulbar acidification on gastric acid responses to urecholine in Pavlov pouch dogs. *Acta Physiol. Scand.,* 95:258–262.
38. Nilsson, G. (1975): Effect of bulbar acidification on basal secretion of acid and gastrin in dog. *Acta Physiol. Scand.,* 95:477–481.
39. Olbe, L. (1964): Effect of resection of gastrin releasing regions on acid response to sham feeding and insulin hypoglycemia in Pavlov pouch dogs. *Acta Physiol. Scand.,* 62:169–175.
40. Pavlov, I. P. (1910): *The Work of the Digestive Glands, Ed. 2,* translated by W. H. Thompson. Griffin, London.
41. Pevsner, L., and Grossman, M. I. (1955): The mechanism of vagal stimulation of gastric acid secretion. *Gastroenterology,* 28:493–499.
42. Pincus, I. J., Friedman, M. H. F., Thomas, J. E., and Rehfuss, M. E. (1944): A quantitative study of the inhibitory effect of acid in the intestine on gastric secretion. *Am. J. Dig. Dis.,* 11:205–208.
43. Pincus, I. J., Thomas, J. E., and Rehfuss, M. E. (1942): A study of gastric secretion as influenced by changes in duodenal activity. *Proc. Soc. Exp. Biol. Med.,* 51:367–368.
44. Preshaw, R. M. (1973): Inhibition of pentagastrin stimulated gastric acid output by sham feeding. *Fed. Proc.,* 32:1067 (abst.).
45. Preshaw, R. M., and Webster, D. R. (1967): A comparison of sham feeding and teasing as stimuli for gastric acid secretion in the dog. *Q. J. Exp. Physiol.,* 52:37–43.
46. Quintana, R., Kohatzu, S., Woodward, E. R., and Dragstedt, L. R. (1964): Mechanism of duodenal inhibition of gastric secretion. *Arch. Surg.,* 89:585–591.
47. Schmitz, E. J., Kanar, E. A., Storer, E. H., Sauvage, L. R., and Harkins, H. N. (1952): The effect of vagotomy of the main stomach on Heidenhain pouch secretion. *Surg. Forum,* 3:17–22.
48. Shay, H., Gershon-Cohen, J., and Fels, S. S. (1942): A self regulatory duodenal mechanism for gastric acid control and an explanation for the pathologic gastric physiology in uncomplicated duodenal ulcer. *Am. J. Dig. Dis.,* 9:124–128.
49. Sjödin, L. (1972): Potentiation of the gastric secretory responses to sham feeding in dogs by infusions of gastrin and pentagastrin. *Acta Physiol. Scand.,* 85:24–32.
50. Sjödin, L. (1975): Inhibition of gastrin-stimulated canine acid secretion by sham feeding. *Scand. J. Gastroenterol.,* 10:73–80.
51. Sjödin, L., and Andersson, S. (1977): Effect of resection of antrum and duodenal bulb on sham feeding induced inhibition of canine gastric secretion. *Scand. J. Gastroenterol.,* 12:43–47.
52. Sjödin, L., and Nilsson, G. (1974): Plasma gastrin levels and gastric acid secretion in dogs during administration of urecholine. *Scand. J. Gastroenterol.,* 9:747–750.
53. Stening, G., and Grossman, M. I. (1970): Gastric acid response to pentagastrin and histamine after extra-gastric vagotomy in dogs. *Gastroenterology,* 59:364–371.
54. Stening, G. F., Johnson, L. R., and Grossman, M. I. (1969): Effect of secretin on acid and pepsin secretion in cat and dog. *Gastroenterology,* 56:468–475.
55. Sun, D. C. H., and Shay, H. (1960): Mechanism of action of insulin hypoglycemia on gastric secretion in man. *J. Appl. Physiol.,* 15:697–703.

Gastrointestinal Hormones, edited by
George B. Jerzy Glass.
Raven Press, New York © 1980.

Chapter 42

Antral Chalone and Gastrones

George B. Jerzy Glass

Gastroenterology Research Laboratory, Department of Medicine, New York Medical College, New York, New York 10029

The topics of this chapter include two closely related subjects. One of these, "antral chalone," is a purely hypothetical hormone and is said to be formed in the gastric mucosa on acidification of the antrum to pH 1.5 to 2.0. Its existence has never been proven beyond doubt, and its isolation has never been attempted. The other, called "gastrone," appears to be a mixture of two chemically different materials, called "gastrone A" and "gastrone B," which are united by their biological ability to inhibit gastric acid secretion. Most remarkably, from the time when both names, "antral chalone" and "gastrone," had been coined (1957 and 1958), the pathways of the studies dealing with them practically have never crossed; nor did they meet in the preceding 20 years during which their existence had been suspected. Although the work on "antral chalone" has remained in the sphere of strictly physiological research and hypothetical argumentation, reaching a "dead end," that on "gastrone" forged slowly ahead in the direction of its chemical and physical fractionation, biological assays for its quantitation, and immunological tracing.

Accordingly, the section on "antral chalone" describes the physiological arguments supporting and refuting its hypothetical existence, whereas the more extensive section on "gastrone" deals with the evolution of our knowledge and the current status of information available on gastrone(s).

I. Antral Chalone

HISTORICAL BACKGROUND

Seventy-five years ago in Pavlov's laboratory Sokolov (29,29a) reported that exogenous acidification of the gastric mucosa reduced secretory response of the stomach to a meal. His thesis and his findings were acknowledged and expanded by workers in Babkin's laboratory (4,6).

This inhibitory effect, reported in 1935, was confirmed and demonstrated to be proportional to the concentration of acid in the stomach by Wilhelmj and collaborators (41). This was the first clear-cut evidence for an inhibitory feedback mechanism related to secretion of acid in the stomach.

The extension of this original line of research on the inhibitory effect on gastric acidity of acid in the stomach was carried on in 1952 and 1954 in the work by Oberhelman et al. (24) and Woodward et al. (43) and then continued by Longhi et al. (20), Dragstedt et al. (7), Gillespie (9), Woodward and Dragstedt (42), and Gillespie and Grossman (10), who showed that acidification of the antrum resulted in suppression of gastrin release and inhibition of gastric secretion. This was consistent with the earlier clinical observations by Ogilvie (25) in 1938 of a high incidence of recurrence of peptic ulcer in patients who had undergone the Finsterer type of surgery comprising exclusion of the antrum. Ogilvie explained this finding by the elimination, in this type of operation, of the antral inhibitory feedback mechanism produced in man by the acidification of the antrum and depressing the acid secretion.

MECHANISM OF ANTRAL INHIBITION OF GASTRIC ACID SECRETION

Interpretation of the mechanism of antral inhibition of the gastric acid secretion by acidification of gastric antrum includes several possibilities, which have been recently reviewed by Wheeler (40).

The first mechanism consists of reduction of the release of gastrin from the antrum by lowering the antral pH to about 1.5. The role of the acidification of antral mucosa in the inhibition of gastrin release has been well established (see Grossman, 11). It is supported by reduction of the gastrin response to antral distension (20), reduction of gastrin release in response to acetylcholine (10), and loss of continually released gastrin from nonstimulated antral pouch on acidification of the antrum (3). Gillespie (9) perfused the antra of three two-stage gastrectomized patients with diluted acid and observed inhibition of histamine-stimulated acid secretion when the pH of the antrum was lowered to 1.5, which was then expanded by the work of Gillespie and Grossman (10), quoted above, with gastrin response to acetylcholine. This was also noted in vagotomized and nonvagotomized patients during surgery for duodenal ulcer, which suggested a humoral pathway of this inhibition (19), and was also supported by the subsequent work of Anderson and Grossman (2,3), and more directly by Yalow and Berson (45), who showed that the lowering of the pH in the antrum causes a fall in the serum gastrin. The possibility of a direct action of the acid in the antrum on gastrin-producing cells was also considered (1).

The second plausible mechanism of the antral inhibition of the acid secretion was thought to be the possible existence of an intramural reflex from the antrum. Since it has been demonstrated, however, that the application of a local anesthetic to the antral mucosa did not prevent the inhibition of acid secretion on acidification of the antrum, the intramural inhibitory reflex causing antral inhibition became improbable (26).

The third possible mechanism of the inhibitory effect of the lowering of the antral pH on the HCl output in the stomach could be the stimulation of the formation of an antral inhibitor that would depress gastric acid secretion. This was considered by Harrison et al. in 1956 (13). The concept of an antral inhibitory hormone, antral chalone, was introduced by Jordan and Sand (16,17) in 1957 on the basis of physiological considerations.

PHYSIOLOGICAL SUPPORT FOR THE EXISTENCE OF GASTRIC CHALONE

The concept of the antral chalone was developed in the early 1960s by Thompson and his group (31–38). The experimental work in that laboratory, based on cross-transfusion studies (38) and on transplanted gastric pouches (34), provided an initial support for the presence of an inhibitory antral hormone; the antrum left in continuity seemed to offer protection against jejunal or marginal ulcers. An inhibitor has been shown to be transferred from the portal blood of animals when the antrum was acidified. The acidification of the isolated vagally denervated host antrum inhibited acid secretion from host and transplanted fundic pouches in response to acetylcholine perfusion of a transplanted antral pouch. This evidence had not been abolished by subsequent studies (22). Anderson and Grossman (2,3) performed antrectomy on Heidenhain pouch dogs and observed a marked augmentation of the submaximal response to gastrin. Although the antrectomy did not also increase the responsiveness of the dog secretion to histamine (33), as should be expected following the loss of the antral chalone, the augmentation of the response to gastrin after antrectomy was interpreted as a support for the hypothesis of antral chalone.

The concept that the innervated antrum suppresses gastric secretion has been used by Holle (14) to support the rationale of the proximal selective vagotomy for treatment of duodenal ulcer. Although many authors concluded that vagus also contains fibers that inhibit gastric secretion (8,18,30,39), yet, as noted by Thompson (33), this vagal inhibition of gastric secretion was effective only against gastrin and not histamine, and acted only on the vagally denervated (Heidenhain) pouches and not on vagally innervated stomachs. Accordingly, the characteristics assigned to the antral chalone differed in some aspects from those proposed for vagogastrone (33), a hormone-like substance, presumably secreted by vagus and inhibitory to gastric acid secretion (12).

DOUBTS CONCERNING ACTIVITY OF CHALONE

The other physiological studies on this problem have either not supported the existence of antral chalone (5,23,27,28) or, if inhibition was demonstrated, could alternatively explain this by changes in gastrin release, by duodenal inhibitory mechanism, or by inhibitory reflexes (27,28).

Most of the subsequent findings were also very complex, interpretated ambiguously, and difficult to duplicate. This was true, e.g., for the experiments on resection of the proximal half of the antrum in Heidenhain pouch dogs that had a transplant of the distal half of the antrum to the transverse colon, and where a significant rise of acid output was observed. This was also true for the suppression of gastrin- and histamine-stimulated acid secretion in dogs by the irrigation of the antrum with acid (35); here the inhibition was obtained only at a fast rate of irrigation, but not at a slow rate (9), or could not be duplicated at all (27). The results of the cross-circulation studies in anesthetized and conscious dogs (35), and the experiments on homo-transplantations of antral and fundic pouches in dogs with denervated antral and fundic pouches made from their own stomachs (34) spoke for the existence of the antral hormone. Yet, the experiments with the divided antral pouches produced evidence both for and against the existence of a humoral antral inhibitor.

The complexity of the relationship between the antral chalone and other endogenous inhibitors of acid secretion has been augmented by different meanings that have been assigned to chalone-like features of the inhibitors and by the antimitotic activity of the chalones (21). Also, whereas originally the physiological significance of a chalone was identified with that of the inhibitory secretory hormone, the later investigators had noted that many hormones existed whose actions were inhibitory either on the secretory function only or on the motor function only of gastrointestinal organs. Moreover, their endocrine action could have included inhibitory effects on one of the functions and a stimulatory one on the other. Furthermore, the inhibitory activity that initially was considered to be due to the activity of the chalone itself could be also explained, as commented by Wormsley (44), by the inhibitory action of other factors. These could exert their action on the nerve terminals near the cell surface, by the interaction with receptors on the cell surface, by the inhibition of the synthesis of cell proteins, or by the production or release of the stimulatory antagonistic hormones. Some additional complexity has been added by the existence of the biphasic inhibition-rebound pattern, which, e.g., is instrumental in the acidification of the duodenum (40).

Because of all these considerations, the possible mechanisms of the inhibitory activity of the antrum on gastric secretion could be very complex and the inhibition of the gastrin release could be only one of its components. Thompson, who in the early 1960s championed the concept of antral chalone (31,36,37,38) and in 1964 reviewed the evidence for and against antral chalone at the Gastrin Conference in Los Angeles (32), in a 1966 postscript to his 1964 presentation wrote that "it is yet not possible to make a definite statement on antral chalone. The majority of evidence at this time is against its existence. If there is an antral chalone, its physiological significance is obviously questionable" (32). In his most recent review on this subject in 1974 (33) Thompson maintains his former conclusions without reservation.

CONCLUSIONS

In view of the increasing scope of positive information on the existence of antral gastrone (gastrone B) described in Part II, the physiological arguments against its existence cited above are becoming increasingly irrelevant, as is the disappointment in antral chalone reiterated in 1974 by Thompson, whose exclusively physiological work on antral chalone had ended in 1966.

It is obvious that further progress in gastrone investigations will also include antral chalone, after work in this area had to stop because of inadequate approaches used for its exploration. The current proliferation of our knowledge on gastrointestinal peptide hormones justifies the change of approach to antral chalone in expectation of new sources of information on this subject, especially in regard to its identity with gastrone A. It is of interest in this context that Chang et al. found in the dog antral juice an inhibitory material to gastric secretion that highly resembles in its characteristics and activity gastrone A from human gastric juice (see Part II of this chapter).

REFERENCES

1. Andersson, S. (1969): Physiologic mechanisms inhibiting gastric secretion of acid. *Am. J. Surg.,* 117:831–840.
2. Andersson, S., and Grossman, M. I. (1965): Effect of antrectomy on gastric secretion of acid and pepsin in response to histamine and gastrin in dogs. *Gastroenterology,* 49:246–255.
3. Andersson, S., and Grossman, M. I. (1966): Effect of denervation and subsequent resection of antral pouches on secretion from Heidenhain pouches in response to gastrin and histamine. *Gastroenterology,* 51:4–9.
4. Babkin, B. P. (1950): *Secretory Mechanism of the Digestive Glands.* Paul B. Hoeber, New York.
5. Blair, E. L. (1967): The effects of tissue extracts on the stomach. In: *Gastric Secretion: Mechanisms and Control,* edited by J. K. Shnitka, J. A. L. Gilbert, and R. C. Harrison, pp. 263–281. *Proceedings of the Symposium on Gastric Secretion,* University of Alberta, Edmonton. Pergamon Press, Oxford.
6. Day, J. J., and Webster, D. R. (1935): The autoregulation of the gastric secretion. *Am. J. Dig. Dis. Nutr.,* 2:527.

7. Dragstedt, L. R., Kohatsu, S., Gwaltney, J., Nagano, K., and Greenlee, H. B. (1959): Further studies on the question of an inhibitory hormone from the gastric antrum. *Arch. Surg.,* 79:10–21.

8. Emås, S., and Grossman, M. I. (1969): Response of Heidenhain pouch to histamine, gastrin, and feeding before and after truncal vagotomy in dogs. *Scand. J. Gastroenterol.,* 4:497–503.

9. Gillespie, I. E. (1959): Influence of antral pH on gastric acid secretion in man. *Gastroenterology,* 37:164–168.

10. Gillespie, I. E., and Grossman, M. I. (1962): Effect of acid in pyloric pouch on response of fundic pouch to injected gastrin. *Am. J. Physiol.,* 203:557–559.

11. Grossman, M. I. (1968): Antral gastric inhibitory mechanisms. In: *The Physiology of Gastric Secretion,* edited by L. S. Semb and J. Myren, pp. 352–355. *Proceedings of the NATO Advanced Study Institute,* Lysebu, Oslo, May 1967, Universitetsforlaget, Oslo.

12. Grossman, M. I. (1974): Vagogastrone. In: Candidate hormones of the gut. *Gastroenterology,* 67:754–755.

13. Harrison, R. C., Lakey, W. H., and Hyde, H. A. (1956): The production of an acid inhibitor by the gastric antrum. *Ann. Surg.,* 144:441–449.

14. Holle, F. (1970): Surgery of gastroduodenal ulcer based on form and function. Importance, reasoning, technique and results in 580 cases, 300 of them postexamined. *Chir. Orthop.* 54:1.

15. Johnson, Jr., A. N. (1964): Acid inhibition by the gastric antrum. *Am. J. Physiol.,* 203:557.

16. Jordan, Jr., P. H., and Sand, B. F. (1957): Antral inhibition of gastric secretion. *Proc. Soc. Exp. Biol. Med.,* 94:471–474.

17. Jordan, Jr., P. H., and Sand, B. F. (1957): A study of the gastric antrum as an inhibitor of gastric juice production. *Surgery,* 42:40–49.

18. Kaynan, A., Ben-Ari, G., Kark, A. E., and Rudick, J. (1973): Effects of parietal cell vagotomy on acid and pepsin secretion in gastric fistula dogs. *Ann. Surg.,* 178:204–208.

19. Koster, K. H., and Rune, S. J. (1963): Antral control of gastric acid secretion. *Lancet* ii:1183–1188.

20. Longhi, E. H., Greenlee, H. B., Bravo, J. L., Guerrero, J. D., and Dragstedt, L. R. (1957): Questions of an inhibitory hormone from the gastric antrum. *Am. J. Physiol.,* 191:64–70.

21. Maugh, T. H. (1972): Chalones: Chemical regulation of cell division. *Science,* 176:1407–1408.

22. Monetti, G. (1973): The antral control of gastric secretion. *Chir. Gastroenterol.,* 7:191–229.

23. Nyhus, L. M., Rheault, M. J., and Semb, L. S. (1965): The effect of antral acidification on the intestinal phase of gastric secretion in the Heidenhain pouch dog. *Acta Physiol. Scand.,* 65:11–19.

24. Oberhelman, Jr., H. A., Woodward, E. R., and Zubiran, J. M. (1952): Physiology of the gastric antrum. *Am. J. Physiol.,* 169:738–748.

25. Ogilvie, W. H. (1938): The approach to gastric surgery. *Lancet,* ii:295–299.

26. Redford, M. and Schofield, B. (1965): The effect of local anesthesia of the pyloric antral mucosa on acid inhibition of gastrin-mediated acid secretion. *J. Physiol. (Lond.),* 180:304–320.

27. Rheault, M. J., Semb. L. S., Harkins, H. N., and Nyhus, L. M. (1965): Acidification of the gastric antrum and inhibition of gastric secretion. *Ann. Surg.,* 161:587–591.

28. Semb, L. S. (1969): Studies on inhibition of gastric secretion; with special reference to acidification of the gastric antrum and the inhibitory substance in gastrice juice. Thesis, Oslo, Universitatsverlaget, 1–41.

29. Sokolov, A. P. (1904): Analysis of the secretory work of the stomach in the dog. Thesis. Vaisberg & Gershunim, St. Petersburg (in Russian).

29a. Sokolov, A. P. (1904): Zur Analyse der Abscheidungsarbeit des Magens bei Hunden. *Jahresber Forstchr Thier-Chem.,* 34:369–40 (Abstr.).

30. Stening, G. F., and Grossman, M. I. (1970): Gastric acid response to pentagastrin and histamine after extragastric vagotomy in dogs. *Gastroenterology,* 59:364–371.

31. Thompson, J. C. (1962): The inhibition of gastric secretion by the duodenum and by the gastric antrum: A review. *J. Surg. Res.,* 2:181–196.

32. Thompson, J. C. (1966): The question of an antral chalone. In: *Gastrin,* edited by M. I. Grossman, pp. 193–228. UCLS Forum in Medical Sciences, No. 5, Los Angeles, University of California Press.

33. Thompson, J. C. (1974): Antral chalone. In: *Candidate Hormones of the Gut,* edited by M. I. Grossman. *Gastroenterology,* 67:752–753.

34. Thompson, J. C., Daves, I. A., Davidson, E. D., and Miller, J. H. (1965): Studies on the

humoral control of gastric secretion in dogs with autogenous and homotransplanted antral and fundic pouches. *Surgery,* 58:84–109.

35. Thompson, J. C., Davidson, E. D., Miller, J. H., and Davies, R. E. (1964): Suppression of gastrin-stimulated gastric secretion by the antral chalone. *Surgery,* 56:861–867.

36. Thompson, J. C., Lerner, H. J., and Tramontana, J. A. (1962): Inhibition of cephalic and antral phases of gastric secretion by antral chalone. *Am. J. Physiol.,* 202:716–720.

37. Thompson, J. C., Lerner, H. J., and Tramontana, J. A. (1962): Action of antral inhibitory hormone (antrogastrone) on gastric secretion stimulated by vagus, gastric antrum or histamine. In: *Second World Congress of Gastroenterology,* Munich, pp. 72–74.

38. Thompson, J. C., Tramontana, J. A., Lerner, H. J., and Stallings, M. O. (1952): Physiologic scope of the antral inhibitory hormone. *Ann. Surg.,* 156:550–569.

39. Walsh, J. H., Csendes, A., and Grossman, M. I. (1972): Effect of truncal vagotomy on gastrin release and Heidenhain pouch acid secretion in response to feeding in dogs. *Gastroenterology,* 63:593–600.

40. Wheeler, M. H. (1974): Inhibition of gastric secretion by the pyloric antrum. *Gut,* 15:420–432.

41. Wilhelmj, C. M., O'Brien, F. T., and Hill, F. C. (1936): The inhibitory influence of the acidity of the gastric contents on the secretion of acid by the stomach. *Am. J. Physiol.,* 115:429–440.

42. Woodward, E. R. and Dragstedt, L. W. (1960): Role of the pyloric antrum in regulation of gastric secretion. *Physiol. Rev.,* 40:490–504.

43. Woodward, E. R., Lyon, E. S., and Landor, J. (1954): The physiology of the gastric antrum: Experimental studies on isolated antrum pouches in dogs. *Gastroenterology,* 27:766–785.

44. Wormsley, K. G. (1970): Inhibition of gastrointestinal secretion. *Gut,* 11:883–887.

45. Yalow, R. S., and Berson, S. A. (1970): Radioimmunoassay of gastrin. *Gastroenterology,* 58:1–14.

II. Gastrones

HISTORICAL BACKGROUND

In the early 1940s considerable evidence had already accumulated for the possible existence of a secretory depressant in the achlorhydric human gastric juice, which exerted a depressor effect on gastric acid secretion. This concept was derived from the work on dogs with gastric pouches by Brunschwig and associates (19–23,98) who, in a series of publications dating from 1939 to 1943, reported the presence of a secretory depressant in the anacid human gastric juice of patients with gastric cancer or pernicious anemia. Shortly thereafter, these findings were confirmed by Kirsner et al. (65) and then significantly expanded by Code and his group (9,10,25–29,59,72). In a series of experimental studies on dogs with Heidenhain pouches dating from 1948 to 1953, Code et al. delivered much information on this subject and partly clarified the origin of this inhibitory material. In 1953, Hood and associates (59) in Code's laboratory concluded that antral mucosa was the most probable source of this secretory depressor.

Brunschwig's group (22) had also recognized that acidic juices from dog stomach produced inhibition of gastric secretion as well, but to a degree about four to ten times less than the achlorhydric human gastric juices. Smith et al. (108), using six dogs with Heidenhain pouches, found that normal human gastric juice collected after feedings, and then pooled, dialyzed, lyophilized, and injected intravenously to dogs at doses of 0.5 to 1.0 mg/kg body weight caused 59% inhibition of acid secretion, on the average, in 80% of the 35 tests. This inhibition was associated with reduction of the volume of gastric juice, but not of the pepsin output.

In the discussion of this work at the National Meeting of the American Gastroenterological Association in 1958, Code coined the name "gastrone" for this inhibitory material (26). He considered the possibility that this material in question could have a chalone-like activity, i.e., that of an inhibitory hormone to gastric secretion.

It is rather remarkable that the pathways of the investigations on "antral chalone" and on "gastrone" have not really crossed thereafter. This is unusual in view of the fact that both of these putative factors appear to originate in the antrum or at least to be derived from it in great part, and that an inhibitory activity on gastric secretion has been attributed to both. While the investigations on "antral chalone," similar to that on "bulbogastrone," (see Chapter 41, pp. 929–969, *this volume*) have remained strictly in the area of physiological experimentation, the work on "gastrone" centered mainly on biochemical purification of this material, its biological assay, and on its possible hormonal nature.

In the early 1960s, the interest in gastric inhibitory factor has increased and since that time, several authors in the United States (7,11,13,32,63,71,79–81,87) and abroad (31,68,82–86,88–91,95,99–104,111,113) studied the inhibitory effect of gastric juice and some of its fractions on gastric acid secretion. Its chemical and physiological nature remained, however, unexplored, which in 1963 incited this author to participate in a joint research project with C. F. Code from Mayo Clinic to attempt to better clarify the nature of gastrone and to develop better methods for its fractionation and purification. This work was carried on for 5 years, and continued in successive collaboration with K. Kubo and R. Fiasse (33–35,54,55,67), W. S. Rosenthal and J. T. Balanzo (1–3,52,56,92–94), J. D. Lopes (73–75), A. Gindzienski and S. Yano (38,38a, 57), and most recently with V. Murty, K. Kojima, and B. L. Slomiany (86a).

METHODS OF ASSAY

The assays on gastrone were done initially on dogs with innervated and with Heidenhain pouches (19–23,27–29,31,32), and later on rats with pyloric ligation (33,35,63,67,80–84,86,88,90,91,99,102) by the Shay et al. technique (105). Subsequent attempts to use frog gastric mucosa (87a) or separated parietal cells from the normal rat gastric mucosa for the gastrone assays (68,84,111) were inadequate. The assays of inhibitory gastrone activity on rats with chronic gastric fistula (1,3,38,38a,57,73), and Ghosh-Lai stomach preparations (2,86a) showed substantial merits and have been used in our later studies more extensively.

Bioassay on dogs with total or innervated gastric pouches using meat feedings were developed initially by Brunschwig et al. (21). Assays on dogs with dener-vated (Heidenhain) pouches replaced the former in the 1950s and were standard-ized by Code and his associates (see 27,53) (Fig. 1). The most accurate assay (28) was obtained in a pouch secreting at 50% or more of the maximal rate obtainable with histamine stimulation by calculating the inhibitory activity of gastrone from the dose-response curve at three different doses as the amount of inhibitor required to produce 50% inhibition of acid secretion. The disadvan-tages were: (a) large quantities and cost of materials to be tested; (b) difficulties in the preparation and maintenance of the Heidenhain pouches; and (c) pyroge-nicity of several of the gastrone containing materials in dogs, a species known to be especially sensitive to pyrogens. This could have disturbed the interpretation of the test and caused elimination of the assays showing elevation of $t°$ of more than 0.8 C° (4,12,14,16) (see pp. 954–956).

Bioassay on rats with pyloric ligation was introduced into the study of gastrone by Menguy and Smith (80,81) with the use of the Shay et al. (105) method, and was improved by Brodie and Knapp (15). This was adopted also in Code's laboratory and used in our early joint research (33–35,53–55). The inhibitory material was given intravenously, its effect on gastric secretion determined 4 hr later, the results compared with those on the control animals, and the gastrone activity calculated as ID_{50} from the intercept of the dose response line at the 50% inhibition level (Fig. 2). The advantages of this test were a lower dose

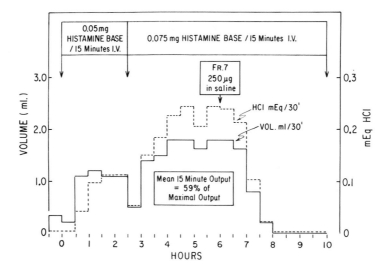

FIG. 1. Gastrone assay on a dog Heidenhain pouch, stimulated by a constant infusion of histamine. (From ref. 53.)

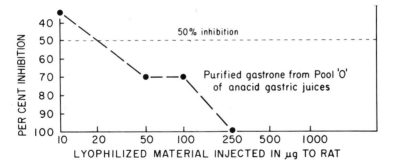

FIG. 2. Rat assay of gastrone activity. The purified gastrone is represented by peak 7 obtained from the Sephadex G-100 column as described by Fiasse, Code, and Glass, ref. 33. This is assayed at four concentrations to form a dose-response curve, the intersection of which with the line at 50% inhibition corresponds to the dose of 20 μg. This dose is here accepted as the measure of the degree of activity of the material tested. (Modified from ref. 53.)

of material, the lesser cost of animals needed for the assay, and resistance of rats to pyrogenic action of gastrone. The applicability of this method to gastrone assay was described in detail in publications listed in this chapter. The shortcomings of this method included a large number of rats necessary for each of the assays. A similar technique was used by Huff et al. (60) in the assay of urogastrone.

Bioassay on rats with chronic gastric fistula, introduced by Komarov et al.

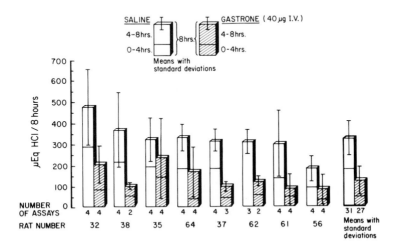

FIG. 3. Hydrochloric acid output in eight rats with chronic gastric fistula following intravenous administration of saline and gastrone. The first columns represent the secretion in saline controls, the second ones, the secretions after 40 μg gastrone injected intravenously to the same rat. Each column represents a mean of several assays in the same rat, serving as its own control. (From ref. 3.)

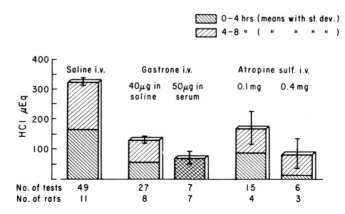

FIG. 4. Effect of gastrone and atropine on hydrochloric acid output in chronic gastric fistula rats. The number of tests and rats used for each of the means is listed in the graph. The inhibitory activity of gastrone at the dose of 50 μg/200 g rat was greater than that of 0.4 mg atropine sulfate i.v. (From ref. 3.)

(66) and improved by Brodie and associates (17,18), has been successfully used for the study of the effects of various stimulants and inhibitors of gastric secretion (70). It was applied to the assay of gastrone by Balanzo and Glass (3,38,38a,73). Its important advantage was reutilization of the same rat serving as its own control for several weeks. The results of this method obtained with gastrone preparations are exemplified in Figs. 3,4, and 5.

The modification of bioassay on Ghosh-Lai preparations of the rat stomach

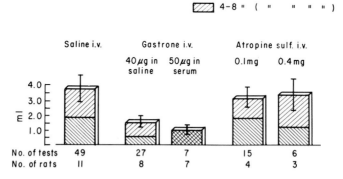

FIG. 5. Effect of gastrone and atropine on volume of gastric secretion in chronic gastric fistula rats. The graph is arranged similarly to Fig. 4. It shows that the effect of atropine given at a dose of 0.4 mg i.v. was exerted only on the concentration of gastrone and not on its output in the gastric juice, and that the effect of gastrone given at doses of 40 and 50 μg i.v. in saline or in serum was more pronounced on the volume of gastric secretion than that of 0.4 mg of atropine. (From ref. 3.)

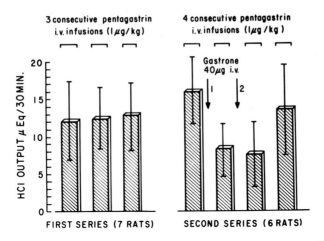

FIG. 6. Effect of gastrone (40 μg) on pentagastrin-stimulated HCl secretion in Ghosh-Lai rats. Each of the two 40 μg gastrone (fraction 7) intravenous injections caused about 50% inhibition of pentagastrin-stimulated acid secretion in the ½ hr collections of the perfusate. (From ref. 2)

(37,69) has been successfully utilized in our laboratory for the assay of the HCl outputs in the rat stomach, following maximal stimulatory dose of pentagastrin or histamine, and the gastrone assay (2). Its main advantage is the isolation of the stomach, which permits the total collection of rat gastric juice without the necessity of accounting for losses through the pylorus. Examples of these assays are shown in Figs. 6 and 7.

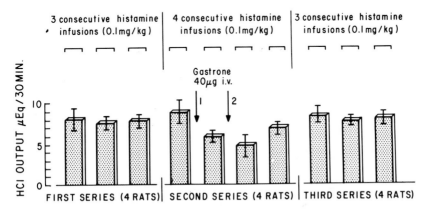

FIG. 7. Effect of gastrone (40 μg) on histamine-stimulated HCl secretion in Ghosh-Lai rats. Series I and III represent the controls, whereas in series II, 40 μg gastrone was injected twice intravenously prior to histamine infusions. Each of these gastrone doses caused reduction of the HCl output by about 30 to 40%, as compared with controls. (From ref. 2.)

SOURCES OF GASTRONE

The best source of gastrone are anacid gastric juices obtained from humans with histamine fast anacidity, which obviously is a very limited source. Other studies have been done using as a source material acid human gastric juices, human gastric mucosa, dog gastric juice from the fundus and the antrum, dog gastric mucosa, and hog gastric mucin.

Anacid Human Gastric Juice

In the original work of Brunschwig et al. (19–23), the gastric juice from achlorhydric patients with gastric cancer or pernicious anemia was mostly used. Kirsner et al. injected 25 mg of alcoholic precipitate of achlorhydric gastric juice from otherwise healthy persons and inhibited acid secretion by 70% (65). Anacidity produced by X-irradiation of the stomach of originally hyperacid patients was not associated with the formation of secretory depressant in the gastric human secretions (65).

Code and associates (27) and Blackburn et al. from Code's group (10) injected 10 to 25 mg alcoholic precipitate of the achlorhydric gastric juice to dogs and obtained 70 to 75% inhibition. The precipitate of human gastric juice from pernicious anemia patients produced the greatest inhibition. Some Japanese workers dialyzed and lyophilized gastric juices from achlorhydric noncancer and non-pernicious anemia patients and obtained inhibition of gastric secretion in rats by 79%, on the average, and if gastric juice was derived from cancer patients, this inhibition reached almost 100% (86). In our laboratory, using rats with pyloric ligation, we obtained 50% inhibition of gastric secretion at doses of 1.8 to 3.2 mg of dialyzed and lyophilized pooled achlorhydric gastric juice from patients with histamine fast anacidity, gastric cancer, and pernicious anemia (34,54,67).

Normal Acid Human Gastric Juice

It was early recognized that acid gastric juice with or without alcohol precipitation produced much less inhibition of gastric secretion than the anacid juice, so that 100 mg of such precipitate from acidic gastric juice of healthy individuals produced a mean inhibition of only 22% in dogs with Heidenhain pouches (27). When rats with pyloric ligation were used in which doses of 2 to 6 mg of normal human dialyzed and lyophilized gastric juice per 200 g rat were injected, a mean inhibition of about 80 to 85% was obtained in two series (80,81), and of 58 to 87% of doses of 1 to 4 mg, respectively (87a). The 30 min boiling, trypsin digestion, and charcoal treatment as well as precipitation with 66% acetone or 66% ammonium sulfate did not destroy the inhibitory activity (87a).

Achlorhydria of the gastric juice is not a condition *sine qua non* of its inhibitory activity, since Japanese authors gave 4-mg dialyzed and lyophilized acid gastric juice from patients with and without gastric cancer to rats and obtained 59 to 65% inhibition (82–84). It is not clear why the normal acid gastric juice exerted some inhibitory activity in rats with pyloric ligation, while this effect in dogs with Heidenhain pouches was much less pronounced (19–22). It is most probable, we believe, that the presence of gastrone A resistant to acid-peptic digestion (see below) is responsible for the inhibitory activity of the normal acid gastric juice observed.

Pepsin secretion was not inhibited in these experiments, although the volume of gastric juice and its acidity declined markedly. With some exceptions, similar lack of gastrone effect on pepsin was also observed by Semb (99–101,103). Miyoshi et al. (84) and Moriga (86) have observed development of atrophic lesions in rats on prolonged parenteral administration of dialyzed and lyophilized normal human gastric juice or that from patients with anacidity, which they related to prolonged effects of gastrone. In an extensive work (75) with Lopes and Ito from our laboratory *(in preparation for publication)*, on rats injected for prolonged time with gastrone B material processed from human gastric juices, no development of atrophic lesions was observed. Most probably, the effects observed by Japanese authors pertained not to the effects of gastrone, but either to the presence of gastric auto-antibodies in those materials or development of these antibodies in rats as result of administration of various antigens-containing gastric juice, as described by Smith et al. (106–109), Wolf et al. (112), and Hennes et al. (58) in dogs and by our group in rats (see ref. 51).

Dog Gastric Juice

The Mayo group found rather early that the inhibitory factor was also present in canine gastric juice, especially when obtained from Pavlov pouches after cholinergic stimulation (72). It was also present, but at a lesser concentration, in denervated Pavlov pouches and Heidenhain pouches after histamine injection or after metacholin (27), but absent from Heidenhain pouch secretion (108).

Hood et al. (59) from the same group demonstrated that whereas 100 mg of the alcoholic precipitate of fundic gastric juice of dog after urecholin stimulation produced only 8% inhibition, that derived from antral mucosa under similar conditions caused 56% inhibition of acid output in the dog.

Menguy (76) much later reconfirmed this finding in rats with pyloric ligation. The dialyzed and lyophilized juice from antral pouches of dogs at the dose of 6 mg per 200 g weight caused 86% inhibition on the average, whereas no effect was obtained with gastric juice from denervated or innervated fundic pouches. Also Semb (100) observed that the dialyzed and lyophilized juices secreted by vagally denervated dog antral pouches contained a gastric secretory inhibitory substance (GIS) that inhibited basal secretion and that was stimulated by gastrin. These materials, returned to the dog from which the antral juice was obtained, inhibited secretion of acid from the vagally denervated pouch on stimulation with histamine, gastrin or the feeding. Some of these extracts produced elevation of body temperature, however, but the fever, according to Semb, did not correlate with the inhibition of acid secretion (see p. 954).

Human Gastric Mucosa

Whereas 19% of the acid extracts from gastric mucosa of normal humans and patients with gastric carcinoma given to dogs after neutralization produced inhibition of gastric secretion, those of PA patients produced inhibition in one-half of them at a relatively low dosage (21). Yet, in rats Kubo et al (68) obtained a mean inhibition of gastric acid secretion by 97 and 77.5%, respectively, using extracts of human gastric mucosa from normals and patients with cancer of the stomach.

Hog Gastric Mucosa

Code et al. (29) and Blackburn et al. (9) obtained a good correlation between the dose of the fresh hog gastric mucus injected intravenously and the percent inhibition of gastric secretion in dogs with Heidenhain pouches. Most potent materials were obtained when extraction was performed at pH 8.5, which gave the mean inhibition of 43 to 98%. In most instances there was a definite pyrogenic effect with rise in temperature of 2 to 3 degrees, which made the results questionable. When the extraction was performed at pH 4, however, there was no increase in body temperature and 30 mg of this extract intravenously caused inhibition of acid secretion by 45 to 71%.

Saliva studied initially on dogs by Code's group (29) produced inhibitory activity on gastric acid secretion that was less than that of hog gastric mucin. This was confirmed by Smith et al. (108). Alcohol precipitates of human saliva at a 50 mg dose caused 55% inhibition in one series (29), but in another series at a double dose only 24 to 26% inhibition (27). Menguy and Berlinski (77) confirmed the presence of inhibitory activity in saliva on rats with pyloric ligation. This amounted to more than 50% at times, when as little as 6 mg of dialyzed and lyophilized saliva was used. The highest inhibition was obtained (78) with saliva of patients with gastric ulcer and gastric carcinoma, whereas that of duodenal ulcer patients was the lowest and that of healthy individuals, intermediate. This generated some speculation in its interpretation. The dialyzed and lyophilized parotid saliva exerted practically no inhibitory activity at the dose of 6 mg (77), whereas the submaxillary and still more sublingual saliva, at the same doses, showed most marked inhibitory activity ranging from 60 to 82%. The authors (77) proposed the name of "sialogastrone" to distinguish salivary material from other gastrone preparations.

Baume et al. (5) suggested the derivation of the inhibitory gastric material in saliva from bacterial contamination of gastric lumen with *Neisseria catarrhalis*. When growth of bacteria was prevented in saliva no inhibitory effect was obtained

(6). More recently, Baume et al. (6) purified and concentrated human saliva 30-fold by extraction of proteins with phenol, and digestion with proteolytic enzymes, followed by dialysis. The inhibitory material obtained was of polysaccharide or mucopolysaccharide nature, had an estimated M. W. of over 100,000 daltons on Sephadex G-100 column, and appeared, we believe, to be related to the material recovered from human gastric juice, referred to as "gastrone A" (53). This should be clearly differentiated from gastrone B that is derived from pyloric antrum in man and dog and from the antrum and crypt cells of the duodenal bulb in dogs (see p. 947). Neither of these two gastric materials has any relationship to the bacterial contaminants and is present in the gastric contents after removing bacterial contamination by incubation with antibiotics (Glass and Lopes *unpublished*). Lymph from thoracic duct of fasting dogs was reported by Rudick et al. (96,97) to contain inhibitory material to rat gastric secretion, after it was extracted by chloroform/methanol, and after removal of serum proteins by isoelectric precipitation at pH 5. This material was further fractionated by Rosenthal and Rudick (94) in our laboratory with filtration on Sephadex G-100 and called "chylogastrone." It has a more than 100-fold potency as compared with previous lymph material, so that inhibition occurred in rats at the dose of 100 μg per 100 g body weight.

Other Sources

Other materials from the oral cavity, stomach, gastric juice and mucosa, blood serum, and ovarian cysts were also studied. The neutral and mucopolysaccharides from hog gastric mucosa (9,40,41), blood group substance A from hog gastric mucosa (63), and glycoproteins from ovarian cysts (108) were either inactive or produced very low inhibitory activity. Also pneumococcus polysaccharide (27), synovial fluid (108), heparin (27,110a), gonadotropic hormone (27), pepsin (76), hog intrinsic factor concentrate (63), chondroitin sulfate (36,76), orosomucoid of canine origin (76), serum albumin (108), normal human serum (63), and bovine corpus vitreum (108) were either inert or exhibited a low inhibitory activity on acid secretion in various bioassays. All these assays were done, however, with various doses of materials tested, and were not well controlled.

ATTEMPTS TO PURIFY GASTRONE FROM HUMAN GASTRIC JUICE

Fractionation by Cohn's method 10

Fractionation by Cohn's method 10 was performed on pools of acid and anacid human gastric juices by N. Ibanez in our laboratory using ethanol sulfate precipitations in the cold (see ref. 54). Inhibitory activity was found in the supernatants of fraction 2, which produced 70% inhibition of gastric secretion at a dose of 5 mg i.v. without causing pyrogenicity in dogs with Heidenhain pouches. The yield and activity of this material were small, however, so that further fractionation was not deemed promising.

Continuous Electrophoresis on Paper Curtain

Anacid gastric juices were filtered and centrifuged, the supernatants were pooled, dialyzed and lyophilized, and submitted to continuous electrophoresis in the refrigerated Spinco apparatus on paper curtain in borate buffer of pH 9 and 0.06 ionic strength (41,67). The total of 157 fractions was collected from the curtains, pooled according to the location on the curtain, dialyzed, lyophilized, identified by paper electrophoresis in borate buffer of pH 9 and ionic strength of 0.24 (39), and assayed for inhibitory activity on acid secretion in C. F. Code's laboratory on dogs with Heidenhain pouches stimulated by continuous intravenous administration of histamine (28). The inhibitory activity was concentrated at the anodic end of the partition corresponding to the area of mucous substances staining with PAS and only slightly with amido black, and in a cathodic fraction staining wtih amido black only and corresponding in location to that of γ-globulin mobility (54). Because of the low inhibitory activity in the dog assay and polydispersity of the inhibitory material on the electrophoretic partition this technique as used alone was inadequate. Yet, it could not be followed by further fractionations by other means because of the shortage of the source material.

Fractionation on IRC-50 (XE-64) Column

This technique was applied to the initial fractionation of gastrone in association with K. Kubo, N. J. Ibanez, and Z. E. Castro-Curel (41,67). Seventy-five to 100 ml of lyophilized anacid gastric juice were applied to the column, eluted first with 0.2 M citrate buffer of pH 3.2, then with 0.2 M phosphate buffer, pH 4.6, and finally with 1.0 M phosphate buffer, pH 5.2. Only very small amounts of trailing material from the second and third elution showed a definite but inconsistent inhibitory activity, which was not adequate for further concentration.

Fractionation of Gastric Mucous Substances

Japanese workers (Miyoshi et al., 82–85; Kubo et al., 68; and Wakisaka et al., 111), all belonging to the same group, fractionated gastric mucin by the method developed in our laboratory (see ref. 43). This consists of consecutive precipitation of gastric juice with trichloracetic acid and acetone, followed by isoelectric precipitation of the supernatant with dilute HCl. They found that the so-called "mucoproteose fraction" (see ref. 43) from anacid gastric juice that contains the bulk of mucus glycoproteins dissolved in gastric juice was very active, which could indicate that gastrone activity was here confined mostly to gastric glycoproteins (gastrone A?). It also caused cytoplasmic atrophy, karyo-pycuosis, and degeneration of mitochondria of parietal cells.

Mucoproteose was fractionated further on Sephadex G-75 column, where it dissociated into a higher molecular weight fraction (above 40,000), staining strongly with PAS on paper electrophoresis in borate buffer, pH 9.0 (39), and containing much carbohydrates (54). It was inactive on dog bioassay. The second fraction of lower molecular weight was retarded on Sephadex G-75 and caused reduction of gastric acid secretion by about 33% at a dose of 5 mg in dogs (54,55). This material on paper electrophoresis moved to the cathode by endosmosis and stained strongly with amido black, but not with PAS stain (gastrone B?)

Fractionation on Sephadex G-100 Column

A few years later, Fiasse et al. (33) fractionated gastrone on Sephadex G-100 column, which yielded two major fractions: (a) a weakly active carbohydrate-containing high molecular weight glycoprotein material, later called gastrone A (53); this was resistant to peptic digestion and obviously was the source of inhibitory activity of the acid gastric juice of humans and dogs. Some of the preliminary data pertaining to its composition have been described (33,46,48,53). (b) The other inhibitory material, later called gastrone B (53) or "fraction 7" (33), was a glycopeptide (Fig. 8). This had an inhibitory activity on HCl output in rats with pyloric ligation at an intravenous dose ranging from 10 to 15 μg per 100 g body weight. It had electrophoretic mobility and staining properties of γ-globulin, but on immunoelectrophoresis behaved differently than IgA or IgG. Its protein content by Lowry method was 17.1% only. It contained also 3.2% carbohydrates as determined by orcinol method (Fig. 9), and its molecular weight was estimated as below 12,000 (Fig. 10). On refractionation (Fig. 11) it resolved into three bands located close to each other, of which one was major, and two minor. This suggested that gastrone B could be further purified. Heating at 100°C for 15 min at acid, neutral, or alkaline pH caused marked decrease or abolition of the inhibitory activity and change of its electrophoretic pattern.

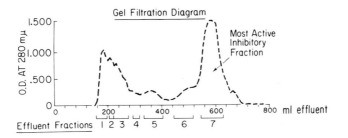

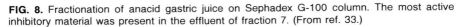

FIG. 8. Fractionation of anacid gastric juice on Sephadex G-100 column. The most active inhibitory material was present in the effluent of fraction 7. (From ref. 33.)

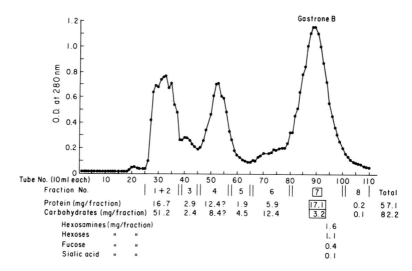

Tube No. (10ml each)	10	20	30	40	50	60	70	80	90	100	110	
Fraction No.			1+2	3	4	5	6		7		8	Total
Protein (mg/fraction)			16.7	2.9	12.4?	1.9	5.9		17.1		0.2	57.1
Carbohydrates (mg/fraction)			51.2	2.4	8.4?	4.5	12.4		3.2		0.1	82.2
Hexosamines (mg/fraction)									1.6			
Hexoses " "									1.1			
Fucose " "									0.4			
Sialic acid " "									0.1			

FIG. 9. Fractionation of gastrone B (fraction "7") on Sephadex G-100 column. The fractionation pattern was drawn using Gaussian curves technic. It showed seven fractions, of which the seventh contained the highest amount of gastrone B, and highest inhibitory activity in gastric secretion. Each of these seven fractions was analyzed for proteins and total carbohydrate content, and fraction 7 in addition for individual sugars. Results are shown at the bottom of the figure. The total protein content was 41% and carbohydrate content 59% in the material applied to the column. (From ref. 56.)

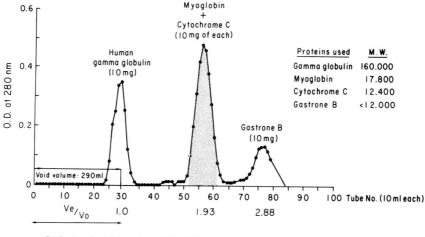

Proteins used	M.W.
Gamma globulin	160.000
Myoglobin	17.800
Cytochrome C	12.400
Gastrone B	<12.000

Sephadex G-100 in saline. LKB 3 X 90 cm column
Ascending flow 30 ml/hr

FIG. 10. Fractionation of gastrone B on Sephadex G-100 column with the use of markers. Estimated mol. wt. of gastrone B was lower than that of the mixture of myoglobulin and cytochrome C, i.e. below 12,000. The calculation of the estimated molecular weight from the position of markers as read from Ve/Vo shown on the graph, places its molecular weight below 9,000 daltons. (From ref. 56.)

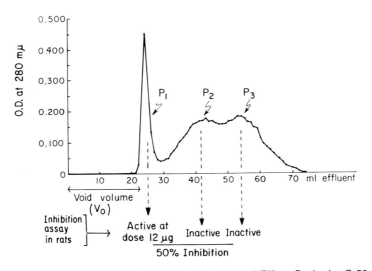

FIG. 11. Refractionation of fraction 7 from anacid gastric juice ("R") on Sephadex G-50 (coarse) column. Of the three fractions obtained, only the first peak corresponding to the first fraction eluted caused maximal inhibitory gastrone activity at dose of 12 μg/rat weight. (From ref. 33.)

Gastrone B was sensitive to pepsin digestion, which resulted in marked reduction of its inhibitory activity after incubation with pepsin at pH 2.0 and obliteration of peak 7 (Fig. 12). This explains its absence or its low activity in acid gastric juices (Fig. 13), and its presence in the *in vivo* neutralized normal acid gastric juice (53). The existence of two similar materials in anacid gastric juice has also been detected and confirmed by Rheault and colleagues (88–91).

A few years later in association with J. D. Lopes (73,74), we attempted to fractionate "fraction 7" further, to which aim serveral chromatographic tech-

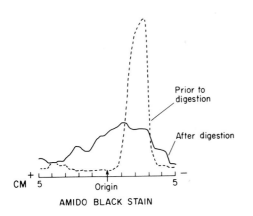

FIG. 12. Paper electrophoretic tracings of fraction 7 from anacid gastric juice ("S") prior to and after pepsin digestion. The active inhibitory material showed slightly cathodic mobility, typical for fraction 7. After digestion by pepsin, this peak underwent obliteration of its tracing, which corresponded to the loss of its inhibitory activity. (From ref. 33.)

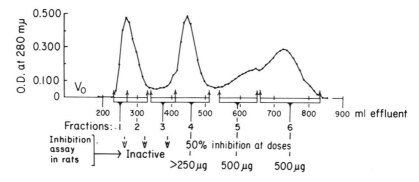

FIG. 13. Fractionation of the acid gastric juice ("Q") on Sephadex G-100 column. Of the several peaks obtained, the first was inactive, the second caused 50% inhibition only at a dose above 250 μg/rat, and peaks 5 and 6 were active at the doses of 500 μg/rat, indicative of very weak inhibitory activity of the acid gastric juice. (From ref. 33.)

niques were used, of which some were promising. One of these consisted of sequential use of two Biogel columns, P-30 and P-6, which were used in sequence. This yielded three subfractions, the first of which was a glycoprotein of M. W. at least 30,000 and inactive on rat bioassay. The second, of M. W. close to or below 9,000, was active on rats with chronic gastric fistula at a dose below 11 μg/100 g, at which it reduced the 4-hr volume of gastric juice and HCl output by 50–60% without any pyrogenic effect. The third subfraction, of a lowest M. W. (about 2,000), could not be assayed because of its low yield (see refs. 48, 56).

FRACTIONATION OF GASTRONE FROM CANINE ANTRAL MUCOSA

In order to obtain larger supply of the source material for purification of gastrone, we used canine antral mucosae, which were known from previous work of other authors to contain and elaborate antral gastrone (27,59,91,99–101). In collaboration with A. Gindzienski and S. Yano (38,38a,57), the inhibitor of the HCl secretion was extracted from the mucosal scrapings of the commercially available frozen canine antra.

Thirteen batches of frozen dog stomachs, each containing five to six frozen samples, were thawed, opened along the greater curvature, and washed under a stream of cold water and saline. The pyloric antra were carefully dissected from the adjacent duodena and fundal portions of the stomachs, the antral mucosae were gently peeled off the submucosae, and scraped with glass slides. The scrapings were suspended in bisulfite buffer (64), which dissolved even poorly soluble mucus, and thoroughly homogenized in a slow rotating Virtis homogenizer. They were then centrifuged at 30,000 $\times$ g for 1 hr in the refrigerated centrifuge, the supernatant was removed by filtration and dialyzed in the Hollow

Fiber Osmolizer, using a Biofiber "80" system at 160 cm H_2O pressure, with elution volume of 14 liters water. The soluble material was then concentrated in vacuum at 35°C in a Rotar vaporizer, transferred to Biofiber "50" system, and again eluted with 14 liters of water. The material remaining in the beaker "50" was now desalted on Biogel P-2 column, concentrated by evaporation, lyophilized, redissolved in saline, and refractionated on Biogel P-10 and by preparative acrylamide disc electrophoresis.

The second peak, obtained on Biogel P-10 (the first peak after the breakthrough fraction), was desalted by gel filtration on Biogel P-2. The inhibitory activity was concentrated exclusively in this fraction, which also formed a single peak on preparative acrylamide disc electrophoresis. The active inhibitory materials on gas-liquid chromatography had a carbohydrate content of 8.9%, with a molar ratio of galactosamine to glucosamine, to galactose, to glucose, to fucose, to mannose, to sialic acid equal to $3:3:3:3:2:1:1/3$. The inhibitor was probably a glycopeptide of a M. W. estimated to be between that of glucagon and insulin (4,000–6,000), which were used as markers of this fractionation (38,38a,57).

In more than 40 fasting rats with chronic gastric fistula the intravenous dose of 15 μg of this gastrone material inhibited nonstimulated HCl output in rats with chronic gastric fistula by 40 to 69%, as compared with saline injected to the same rat as control. This difference was statistically significant, with a p value between 0.05 and 0.01 during the first 2 hr of inhibition (Fig. 14).

The inhibitory activity of this material was not associated with pyrogenicity as determined by the thermocouple rectal measurements during the 6 hr bioassay in rats, which did not show any rise in temperature. Rats producing highest HCl output under basal conditions also had the highest inhibition of the acid output following intravenous administration of this gastrone preparation.

The effect of the three batches of the inhibitor prepared by this method on pentagastrin-stimulated HCl secretion at the dose of 6 μg/kg S. C. was tested on 30 rats with chronic gastric fistula at a dose of 15 μg/200 g body weight i.v. (57). The results obtained were compared with saline controls. The three batches of material injected to those rats reduced the HCl output by 34%, 51%, and 60%, respectively, on the average. This reduction was statistically significant at a p value below 0.05 to 0.01. The inhibition of pentagastrin-stimulated gastric secretion lasted 3 hr (Fig. 15).

Most recently the initial steps of gastrone fractionation were changed in order to improve the yield of active material (V. Murty, K. Kojima, B. L. Slomiany, and G. B. J. Glass, 86a). About 20 g of scrapings obtained from commercially available freeze-dried dog antra were suspended in 100 ml bisulfite buffer, pH 8.6, and left overnight at 4°C with continuous stirring. The homogenate was centrifuged for 1 hr at 30,000 × g, the supernatant was filtered, and the pellet remaining on the filter was resolubilized with 60 ml bisulfite buffer. The process was repeated. The supernatant, in the total volume of 210 ml, was fractionated through a series of tubular cellulose Spectra/Por membranes, 40 to 50 mm in

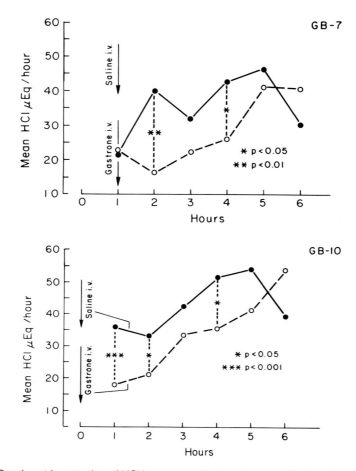

FIG. 14. Basal gastric secretion of HCl in ten rats with chronic gastric fistula after intravenous administration of gastrone (15 μg per 200 g weight) or saline. Gastrone B was obtained from pool 10 of dog antral mucosa. Note inhibition of gastric HCl secretion that started within the first hour after gastrone administration and lasted for 5 hr. The statistical significance of these differences as compared with controls is shown by asterisk. No increase in t° was recorded throughout the duration of the test in any of the rats. (Unpublished, ref. 38.)

length and 25 to 30 mm in diameter, having a well determined cutoff ranges of M. W. 12,000, 8,000, 3,500, and 2,000 daltons. The dialyzates obtained by dialysis against disulfite buffer at 4°C, totaling 14 liters, were changed over a period of 3 days. Each of the pooled dialyzates was concentrated under low pressure at 25°C and in each case the desalting was performed prior to use of the next cutoff membrane of the lowermost molecular weight. Several fractions obtained, of different molecular weights, were freeze dried and tested for their inhibitory activity on gastric acid secretion in Ghosh-Lai rats.

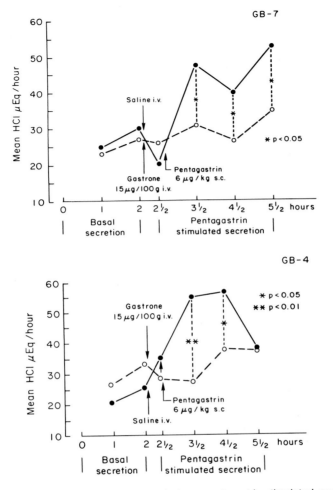

FIG. 15. Effect of gastrone (15μg/200 g wt. i.v.) on pentagastrin-stimulated gastric acid se-cretion in ten rats with chronic gastric fistula. Note reduction of the gastrone output that started within ½ hr after administration of gastrone and ended 3½ hr later. The statistical significance of the inhibition is shown by asterisks for each of the sets of data. No increase in t° was recorded in any of the rats throughout the duration of the tests. (Unpublished, ref. 38.)

Most of the inhibitory activity was found in the gastrone preparation nondia-lyzable through Spectra/Por membrane of 2,000 daltons; this was retained in the sac, and dialyzable through the Spectra/Por membrane of 3,500 M. W. cutoff. This "2,000–3,500 gastrone fraction" was fractionated further by gel filtration on Biogel P-10 column with 0.1 M sodium acetate of pH 4.0 as eluant.

A sharp and tall peak 1 in the area of the void volume, and a short, wider and somewhat delayed peak 2 were detected at 280 nm optical density. Peak

1 contained most of the inhibitory activity of this fraction, as shown by testing in the Ghosh-Lai isolated rat stomach preparation on 200 to 250 g Sprague-Dawley rats. This preparation was continually perfused with 0.9% NaCl solution buffered with 0.1 M sodium bicarbonate to pH 7. Gastric acid stimulation was maintained at a constant level by intravenous pentagastrin infusion at the rate of 0.5 g (25% maximal capacity) per kg/hr. Gastrone preparation was administered as a 0.5 ml bolus into the femoral vein at doses ranging from 12.5 to 50 μg per 200 g rat body wt. Collections were obtained for 3 hr, every 30 min. Gastric juice volumes were measured and titrated electrometrically. An average 30 to 40% inhibition was obtained and maintained for 2 hr following intravenous administration of 50 μg gastrone bolus, without any pyrogenicity.

Another gastrone fraction of somewhat less inhibitory activity was processed from peak 1 of the P-10 column fractionation of the "3,500 to 8,000 gastrone fraction." This inhibited gastric secretion by 50% for 2 to 2 ½ hr after intravenous administration of this material at a dose of 100 μg/100 g rat body weight, again without any temperature increase.

Further fractionation and purification of these materials on ion-exchange columns and by other techniques is now in progress.

QUESTION OF PYROGENICITY OF GASTRONE-CONTAINING MATERIAL

A question raised by gastrone activity is whether its inhibitory action on acid secretion is not due to a presence of contaminating pyrogens.

In dogs, injected with a non-fractionated anacid gastric juice, a non-infrequent elevation of the temperature was observed at the onset of Brunschwig research about 40 years ago. It was discussed extensively by C. F. Code at the Symposium on Gastric Secretion at the University of Alberta in 1965 (27). Although it was observed by other investigators about that time, the increase in temperature was by no means consistent, even in dogs susceptible to pyrogen reactions. According to Semb (101) and Code (27), who studied this problem in detail, pyrexia could not be considered the basic responsible factor in the production of the gastric acid inhibition following intravenous administration of gastrone to dogs.

More recently, Cowley (31) revived this problem by intravenously injecting to three pouch dogs "fraction 7" purified by Fiasse et al. in our laboratory (33). He obtained a significant correlation in the regression curves of temperature rise and the acid inhibition; yet this was not absolute, and no pyrexia developed in some of the Cowley's dogs injected with low gastrone doses, despite an outstanding (40–75%) inhibition of HCl output (see Glass, 45). Similar observations, as mentioned above, were made before on dogs with Heidenhain pouches in Code's (27) and Semb's (100,101) laboratories.

The possibility of endotoxin playing a role in causing inhibition of acid secretion in dogs after gastrone injection was raised by Cowley (31), echoed by

Thompson (110), and subjected to doubt by this writer (45,46) because of the following considerations:

(a) Whereas gastrone B is a glycopolypeptide containing large peptide moiety and no lipids, as shown by negative staining with sudan black on electrophoresis and very low carbohydrate content in biochemical analysis (J. D. Lopes and J. Badurski, see 48,56), endotoxin is a glycolipopolypeptide (8). (b) Whereas endotoxin molecular weight ranges from 15,000 to several hundred thousand daltons (8), that of gastrone B is at the most in the neighborhood of about 9,000 or below, as shown by Lopes (73,74) in our laboratory with the use of Sephadex filtration and protein markers (see 48,56). Moreover, inhibitory activity has been recently demonstrated in gastrone-like material of molecular weight between that of glucagon and insulin (4,000 to 6,000) (57). (c) Whereas endotoxin is derived from bacteria that may contaminate saliva and grow in the anacid stomach, gastrone B is entirely absent from saliva, in which only a weak inhibitor of a high molecular weight (gastrone A) is present. (d) The cellular source of gastrone B in man appears to be pyloric glands and surface epithelium of the antrum and crypt epithelium of the duodenal bulb in the dog, as shown by immunofluorescent indirect Coons' test (30) with rabbit anti-gastrone serum (52). (e) Endotoxin acts on gastric secretion in dogs through its pyrogenic effect (12,16), whereas small doses of gastrone B may inhibit gastric secretion in the dog and especially in the rat without raising temperature at all (27,53).

Blickenstaff and Grossman (12), after injections of bacterial pyrogens to dogs, found that the maximal inhibition of gastric secretion occurred after the maximal change in rectal t° had taken place. The analysis of the data by Semb (100) obtained on dogs with antral and Heidenhain pouches and injected with gastrone demonstrated that the relationship between body temperature and inhibition of gastric secretion was probably different from that encountered by others utilizing bacterial pyrogens.

The complete removal of endotoxin from gastric juice is technically impossible, as communicated to the present writer in frequent discussions with various specialists in this area. We attempted, therefore, to reduce the bacterial invasion of the human stomach prior to collection of the anacid gastric juices in two volunteers by oral administration of tetracycline or ampicillin for 1 week and reducing in this way contaminating pyrogens. This did not reduce, however, the inhibitory activity of the "fraction 7" (gastrone B) which was processed from the gastric juices of these men after administration of antibiotics (unpublished data).

Furthermore, we sent to a private research laboratory which was doing Limulus assay [Amebocyte (E-toxate) (Sigma)] for the endotoxin, an active gastrone B material processed on Sephadex G-100. We obtained ambiguous report on the presence of endotoxin in material sent [no gel formation, with some increases in viscosity, opacity, and starchy granules (unpublished data)].

In our studies in rats, no correlation was observed between the pyrogenic reaction and the inhibition of gastric secretion. Menguy et al. (79–81) and Semb (100,101), who used rats for the bioassay of the inhibitory activity of gastrone, also found, at that time, that rats only rarely responded with a pyrogenic reaction to intravenous administration of gastrone-containing materials, and that this did not correlate at all with the inhibition of gastric acid secretion following gastrone. The time pattern of gastrone's inhibitory effect on rat gastric secretion also does not follow the time pattern observed in those rats in which gastric secretion was inhibited by injections of pyrogen (57,99).

According to Brodie and Kundrats (16) the inhibition of gastric secretion in pylorus-ligated rats occurred only when body temperature were raised $0.8°$ C or more. All our rats had, therefore, lately an electronic control of rectal $t°$ for the duration of 5 hr following intravenous administration of active gastrone preparation. No increase in the rectal $t°$ above $0.5°C$ was noted in almost all of these rats (38,38a,57).

Thus, our recent data do not corroborate the role of pyrexia due to bacterial contamination in the inhibition of gastric secretion in rats injected with gastrone B-containing material. (See note in proof, p. 970.)

QUESTION OF INTRALUMINAL SECRETION OF GASTRONE

One of the important issues of the gastrone research is whether gastrone is secreted into the gastric lumen from gastric mucosa and whether it has inhibitory activity on gastric secretion also from the lumen, and not only when it is adminis-tered intravenously.

J. D. Lopes in our laboratory (73) administered gastrone B contained in "fraction 7" at a single dose of 300 μg intragastrically by a gastric tube to each of the seven male Sprague-Dawley rats provided with chronic gastric fistula. This dose was derived from 3 mg lyophilized human anacid gastric juice, obtained by fractionation on Sephadex G-100 column. The gastric contents were continu-ally aspirated before and after gastrone administration and the volume of gastric secretion and its HCl content were measured for the duration of 5 to 6 hr. In six out of seven rats used for this experiment, a highly significant (p below 0.001) decrease of gastric volume and HCl content were observed (see 48 and 56) (Fig. 16).

It was not clear, however, whether the effects of intragastrically administered gastrone were due to its passage into circulation after absorption in the small intestine, or whether they were due to its topical action on the glandular cells of the gastric fundus. Since gastrone-like material has been detected in the fasting dog lymph after its oral administration to the fasting dog (94,96,97), this observation may speak for the intestinal absorption of gastrone. Yet, in line with the current concepts of the existence of the paracrine gastrointestinal secretion of various peptide hormones (Chapter 23, pp. 529–564) one cannot rule out the possibility that gastrone may belong to the group of peptides, the secretion of which affects gastric mucosa by a paracrine effect. The increasing

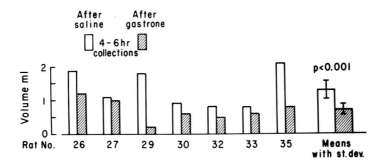

FIG. 16. Effect of intragastric administration of gastrone B (150 μg per 100 g wt.) on the juice volume in seven rats with chronic gastric fistula. Six of the seven rats are the same as the ones in the previous figure. Collections were obtained for 4 hr in each of the rats. Note the significant reduction of the mean juice output after intragastric administration of gastrone. No increase in $t°$ was recorded in any of the rats during the entire duration of the experiment. (From ref. 56.)

amount of information on the possible existence of a paracrine topical inhibitory effect on gastric secretion, that is exerted by some of the gastrointestinal hormones and peptides (such as somatostatin and others; see Chapters 15, 23, pp.363,529, *this volume*) make this mechanism of the inhibitory effect of gastrone on secretion of gastric acid rather plausible.

ANTIBODY TO GASTRONE B

Antibody to gastrone B was raised in our laboratory by Rosenthal et al. (92,93) in rabbits by repeated injections of gastrone B obtained from pooled anacid human gastric juices by fractionation on Sephadex G-100 column and emulsified in Freund's adjuvant. On immunoelectrophoresis this anti-gastrone antibody could be classified as belonging to the class of IgG globulins. On double immunodiffusion tests on Ouchterlony plates this antibody formed a single precipitant arc against the "fraction 7" from Sephadex G-100 fractionation (gastrone B), at concentrations of 0.25 to 0.5 mg/ml. Fractions containing gastrone A-like material that were obtained from saliva, and were devoid of gastrone B, did not react with this antibody. A single precipitant arc was also formed when three pooled unfractionated anacid human gastric juices were tested against four various rabbit anti-gastrone B sera. No precipitant lines were obtained with three normal acid human gastric juices, one of which was neutralized *in vivo* (Fig. 17) (93).

The precipitating nature and possible biological activity of anti-gastrone antibody have been demonstrated by the removal of the biological inhibitory activity of gastrone B from gastrone B solution by the rabbit anti-gastrone B serum, as demonstrated in 15 bioassays on 4 rats (93). The control experiments performed with the supernatants from mixtures of normal rabbit serum and gastrone

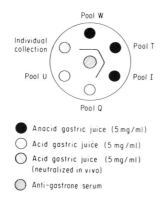

FIG. 17. Double diffusion in agar gel of pools of fractionated gastric juice set against anti-gastrone serum. Note precipitation lines between the anti-gastrone serum and the three pools W, T, and I of the anacid gastric juices, suggesting the presence of the immunoreactive gastrone in these three pools. Note absence of the precipitation line between the anti-gastrone serum and the acid gastric juice (pool U) and the neutralized *in vivo* acid gastric juice. The latter suggests that the absence of gastrone from the assay pool of acid juices is not exclusively due to the digestion by the acid but also probably to the low or absent gastrone content in the acid secreting stomach. (From ref. 93.)

B revealed persistence of inhibitory activity similar to that obtainable with gastrone B alone. No gastrone B antibody was present in normal rabbit sera, and the antibody to gastrone B did not demonstrate any cross-reactivity with other nondialyzable materials in the human gastric juice (93).

The presence of only one antigenic determinant for precipitating antibody formation and absence of cross-reactivity with gastrone A-like and other components of gastric juice suggests that gastrone B preparation may be more specific for the immunological purposes than we have thought initially. The homogenity of the gastrone preparations, used as antigen, supports the possibility that this antibody can be used for further exploration of the role of gastrone in gastrointestinal physiology and pathology. Nevertheless, it is obvious at this point that further purification of gastrone B, if successful, may permit development of new and more sensitive and specific anti-gastrone immune sera. This, in turn, may open the road to the radioimmunoassays of gastrone.

CELLULAR DERIVATION OF GASTRONE

The immunofluorescent technic has been very rewarding in determining the cellular derivation of various biologically significant components of the gastrointestinal mucosa in man and other species. This was true, e.g., for the successful tracing of microsomal antigens in parietal cells of various species (see 47,51) and of intrinsic factor in parietal cells of man (62) and peptic cells of the rat (51). More recently, the immunocytochemistry has played a crucial role in the detection of the cellular derivation and localization of gastrointestinal hormones (see Chapters 1–3, pp. 1–70, *this volume*).

FIG. 18. Normal human antral mucosa exposed in indirect Coons' test to anti-gastrone B rabbit serum and fluoresceinated goat anti-rabbit IgG. Note fluorescence of surface epithelium and pyloric glands; (A) ×100; (B) ×250. (From ref. 52.)

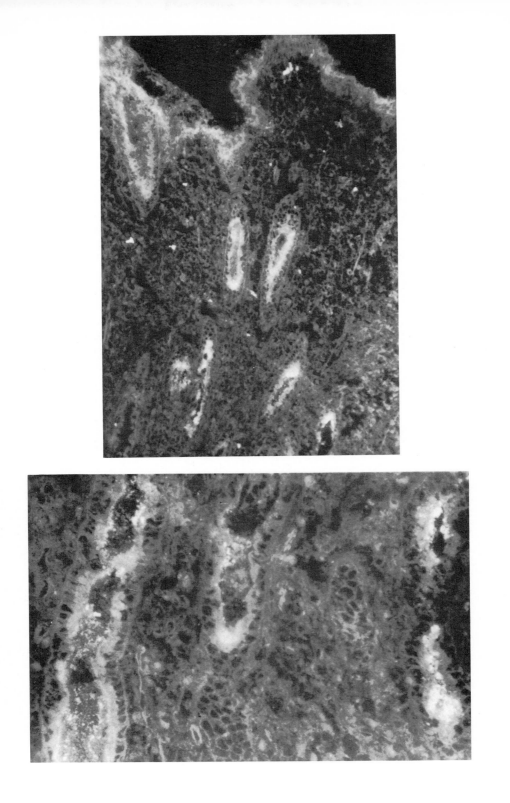

The pyloric glands and pyloric surface epithelium of man and the dog and of the duodenal bulb crypts of the dog were exposed to immunofluorescent Coons' test (30), using the antibody to human and dog gastrone raised in rabbits (92,93). We obtained immunofluorescence of these structures when rabbit sera containing antibodies to these materials were used (52). No immunofluorescence was obtained with various other control tissues or normal rabbit sera (52). These findings suggested the derivation of gastrone B from the surface epithelium and pyloric glands of the antrum in man (Fig. 18) and the dog (Fig. 19) and from the crypts (Fig. 20) and the villous epithelium (Fig. 21) of the duodenal bulb in the dog. The fundic glands in humans and in dogs did not show any fluorescence, however, with anti-gastrone antibody (52). Only a nonspecific staining has been obtained at times with surface epithelium of the fundus of man and dog stomach, when exposed to anti-gastrone serum. This staining was similar in intensity to that obtained with normal rabbit serum. It could be easily differentiated from the true immunofluorescence obtained with gastrone-containing materials (52).

In one patient with atrophic gastritis and pyloric metaplasia, a striking immunofluorescence of the surface epithelium of the fundic mucosa was obtained. If verified on a larger material of cases it could indicate the formation of gastrone B in the metaplastic fundal mucosa of patients with atrophic gastritis and gastric anacidity.

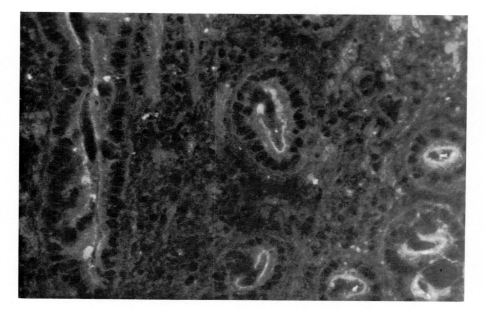

FIG. 19. Dog pyloric mucosa exposed in indirect Coons' test to anti-gastrone B rabbit serum and fluoresceinated goat anti-rabbit IgG. Note fluorescence of pyloric glands. ×250. (From ref. 52.)

The localization of gastrone B by immunofluorescence in the human and dog antral and duodenal bulb dog mucosa is in accord with the presence of gastrone activity in the extracts from these areas obtained in the 1950s and 1960s by Hood et al. (59), Livermore and Code (72), Menguy (76), and Semb (99,100,102).

Thus, these findings (52) have narrowed the site of gastrone B production in man to the surface epithelium of the antrum and to pyloric glands, and in the dog to the antral mucosa and that of duodenal bulb. A material inhibitory to gastric secretion and localized in the duodenal bulb, called bulbogastrone, had been stipulated to exist on the basis of physiological evidence by Andersson et al. in 1969 (see Chapter 41 by R. Nilsson, pp. 911–928, *this volume*). It has to be determined whether "bulbogastrone," postulated to be derived from duodenal bulb and not yet chemically and immunologically studied, is related to or identical with gastrone B in dogs, which produces the immunofluorescence in Coons' test with crypts and villi of the duodenal bulb (Figs. 20 and 21).

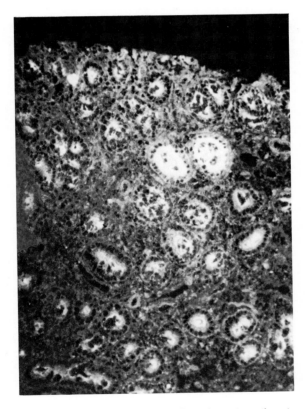

FIG. 20. Dog duodenal mucosa exposed in indirect Coons' test to anti-gastrone B rabbit IgG. Note striking fluorescence of the crypts and its epithelium. ×100. (From ref. 52.)

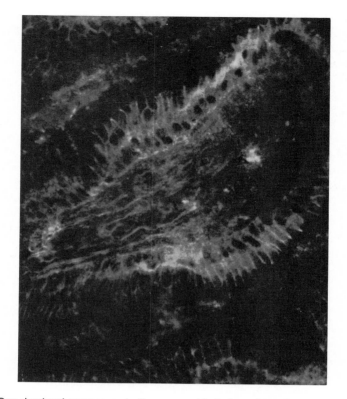

FIG. 21. Dog duodenal mucosa and villus exposed in indirect Coons' test to anti-gastrone B rabbit serum and fluoresceinated goat anti-rabbit IgG. Note fluorescence in a few areas of the apical portion of the villous epithelium and at the basal membrane. ×250. (From ref. 52.)

It is striking, of course, that the cellular derivation of gastrone B is not from single cells scattered through the gastric mucosa, as is the case with the hormonal peptides of the gastrointestinal tract, discussed at length in this volume. A relatively large mass of the epithelial cells from the antrum and pyloric glands in man and also from the crypts and villous epithelium of the duodenal bulb in the dog gives the fluorescence, in our system, with antibody to gastrone B. This would fit well with the finding that gastrone B represents as much as 8 to 10% of the total dry weight of nondialyzable materials of the anacid gastric juice (33). Furthermore, it is consistent with a relatively low biological inhibitory activity of gastrone B. This is much weaker per unit of weight than that of peptide hormones derived from single cells of the gastro-pancreatico-intestinal endocrine system of the body.

Nothing known at present about the inhibitory gastrointestinal peptide hormones detectable in the gastric antrum would make one believe that one or more of these peptides is the cause of the inhibition of acid secretion attributable to gastrone. Those detectable in the antrum, such as somatostatin, GLIs, or VIP have different time patterns of inhibitory activity on acid secretion, different sensitivity to high temperature and peptic digestion, and much higher inhibitory activity on gastric secretion per unit of weight than gastrone. All this speaks in favor of a paracrine mechanism of the gastrone effect on acid secretion. Yet, there is no information available as yet to which extent this activity, if any, plays any role in the physiological control of gastric acid secretion.

SUMMARY AND CONCLUSIONS

Because of inadequate purification of gastrone, its identification and quantitation by radioimmunoassays is not yet available; hence no advanced exploration has been made possible of its distribution in the body, its mechanism of action and its role, if any, in influencing the levels of gastric acid secretion. The only methods available so far for its detection and quantification in body fluids have been, until now, only its bioassays. Although initially they were done on dogs with Heidenhain pouches, for the last 20 years the assays on rats with pyloric ligation, chronic gastric fistulae or Ghosh-Lai 'isolated' *in vivo* rat stomachs have replaced the former.

The work on purification of gastrone, which until recently was based on live sources of this material in form of anacid human gastric juices or dog secretions from antral pouches, has been most recently extended to frozen dog antral mucosae, available commercially.

The more recent methods of fractionation of gastrone were based on molecular sieving on Sephadex or Biogel columns. These demonstrated the presence of two major components of different chemical nature, different physicochemical characteristics, and different biological activity in gastrone material. The first, called "gastrone A," represents material of high molecular weight, mostly polysaccharide in nature, resistant to peptic digestion, present both in acid and anacid gastric juices, endowed with a moderate inhibitory activity on gastric acid secretion at a dose of 100 to 200 μg/200 g/rat body weight on intravenous administration, and resembling or identical with another inhibitor of gastric acid secretion present in saliva called "sialogastrone." The other material, called "gastrone B," is probably a mixture of two or more glycopeptides of molecular weight ranging from about 8,000 to 9,000 daltons, to 2,000 to 3,500 daltons, depending on source material and method of fractionation. It still contains some impurities, is sensitive to peptic digestion and depending on source material and the method of purification, shows more or less inhibitory activity on intravenous administration on acid secretion in the dog and rat, at doses about 15 to 20 μg/per 200 g rat body weight. Further purification of this material on Biogel column somewhat improved the activity of this material, but the attempts to purify it further on ionic exchange columns met with difficulty due to its poor solubility above pH 4.0.

The more recent attempts at purification of gastrone from scrapings of dog antral mucosa were made by: (a) the consecutive use of Biofiber "80" and "50" systems, followed by refractionation on Biogel P-10 and desalting on P-2; this yielded material of an estimated M. W. between 4,000 and 6,000 daltons as estimated by the use of column markers and which had inhibitory activity on gastric acid secretion in rats with chronic gastric fistula, at doses of about 25 μg/200 g body weight; and (b) the dialysis of the extracts from antral mucosal scrapings, through the standardized Spectro/Por membranes of 2,000 to 3,500 daltons permeability, which inhibited gastric acid secretion at doses of 12.5 to 25 μg/200 g rat body weight.

No pyrogenicity was found in the bioassays on rats as controlled by thermocouple measurements of rectal t°. The Limulus assay for endotoxin in the gastrone containing material gave ambiguous results. The prolonged oral administration of antibiotics to two volunteer patients prior to collection of their gastric juices to be used for recovery of gastrone did not affect their inhibitory activity.

The intraluminal discharge of gastrone B from antral surface epithelium and glandular epithelium is probable, especially because of its showing inhibitory effect on acid secretion in the rats on oral administration. Since this effect appears to be somewhat delayed it cannot be ruled out that some part, at least, of gastrone becomes absorbed in the small intestine, from which it may pass in circulation and act on parietal cells. Another very probable alternative is the paracrine mode of inhibitory action of gastrone on parietal cells, directly from its source of origin, or as a result of its topical action from the lumen.

An antibody to gastrone B was raised in rabbits. This yielded a single precipitant arc with gastrone B and gastrone B-containing human anacid gastric juices from PA patients or those with advanced atrophic gastritis and anacidity. The addition of the anti-gastrone B caused a precipitate and removal of inhibitory acitivity of gastric juice on acid secretion in the rats, not observed in controls. The antibody to gastrone B did not cross-react with gastric juice fractions containing gastrone A only.

The exposure in an indirect Coons' test of histological sections of various parts of the stomach and duodenal mucosa from man and dog to immune rabbit serum against gastrone B and fluresceinated anti-γ-globulin produced a striking immunofluorescence with the antral and pyloric glands epithelium in man and dog, and the crypts and villous epithelium of dog duodenal bulb. No immunofluorescence with fundic glands and fundic surface epithelium or with parietal and peptic cells, was obtained under these conditions.

The mutual ratio of gastrones A and B in gastric juices may vary markedly, depending on the degree of peptic digestion to which gastrone B had been exposed, the pH of the gastric juice presence of pepsin, the degree of the contamination of the gastric juice with saliva, and the technique used for collection and preservation of gastric juice fractions. This explains the divergent data on gastrone in the literature.

Several materials with inhibitory activity on gastric acid secretion found in various body fluids have been called gastrones, with appropriate adjectives or prefixes. These are: salivary gastrone (sialogastrone), gastrone from duodenal bulb (bulbogastrone), gastrone from lymph (chylogastrone), gastrone from dog antral juice (antrogastrone), and gastrone from the urine (urogastrone). Some of these materials, such as sialogastrone and antrogastrone, are most probably related to gastrone A, and others, such as bulbogastrone and chylogastrone, to gastrone B. Urogastrone has no relation whatsoever to materials discussed in this chapter.

PROJECTIONS FOR THE FUTURE

The further exploration of gastrones requires clarification of several basic and still unanswered problems:

(a) The determination of whether the acidification of the antrum, followed by inhibition of gastric acid secretion, is associated with intraluminal, endocrine, or paracrine discharge of gastrone.

(b) Exploration of the mode of action of gastrone A and B in the human and animal stomach.

(c) Continuation and expansion of attempts at better fractionation and purification of gastrone A and B by more complex techniques, including extraction, delipidation, dialysis through Spectro/Por membranes, followed by molecular sieving on Biogel columns with markers, ion-exchange chromatography, and acrylamide gel electrophoresis. These investigations will have to be preceded by accumulation of a large stock of source materials (dog antral gastric mucosa, neutralized juice from dog antral pouches, sublingual saliva, etc.) needed to obtain large amounts of active materials to be studied. These should be screened by controlled bioassays of the inhibitory activity of fractions obtained on rats with chronic gastric fistula or Ghosh-Lai preparations of isolated stomach.

(d) Continuation of the attempts at removal of occasional pyrogenicity from some of the source materials, and use of bioassays on species not sensitive to pyrogens.

(e) Obtaining more specific antisera for each of the highly active gastrone materials, with the aim of ultimate development of radioimmunoassays that would allow for better quantification and identification of active gastrone fractions.

ACKNOWLEDGMENT

These studies were supported by Research Grant-in-Aid AM-00068–27 from the NIAMDD, National Institues of Health, Bethesda, Maryland.

REFERENCES

1. Balanzo, J. T., and Glass, G. B. J. (1972): Removal of the gastric inhibitory activity from gastrone solutions by anti-gastrone antibodies. *Fed. Proc.*, 31:354. (Abstr.).
2. Balanzo, J. T., and Glass, G. B. J. (1975): Secretion of hydrochloric acid in Ghosh-Lai rat preparation following stimulation with histamine and pentagastrin and inhibition by gastrone and atropine. *Digestion*, 13:291–303.

3. Balanzo, J. T., and Glass, G. B. J. (1975): Bioassay of inhibitory activity of gastrone on basal HCl secretion in rats with chronic gastric fistula. *Digestion,* 13:334–343.
4. Bandes, J., Hollander, F., and Bierman, W. (1948): The effect of physically induced pyrexia on gastric acidity. *Gastroenterology,* 10:697–707.
5. Baume, P. E., Baxter, C. H., and Nicholls, A. (1967): Concentration and partial characterization of human salivary gastrone. *Am. J. Dig. Dis.,* 12:965–972.
6. Baume, P. E., Baxter, C. H., and Nicholls, A. (1968): The source of a gastric secretory inhibitor from human saliva. *Aust. Ann. Med.,* 17:42–48.
7. Baume, P. E., and Law, D. H. (1966): Investigation of the possible mode of action of gastrone as endogenous inhibitor of gastric secretion. *Am. J. Dig. Dis.,* 11:951–957.
8. Bennet, I. L., and Cluff, L. E. (1957): Bacterial pyrogens. *Pharmacol. Rev.,* 9:427–475.
9. Blackburn, C. M., and Code, C. F. (1949): The inhibition of gastric secretion in dogs by human gastric juice and gastric mucin. *J. Natl. Cancer Inst.,* 10:337–338.
10. Blackburn, C. M., Code, C. F., Chance, D. P., and Gambill, E. E. (1950): Confirmation of the presence of a gastric secretory depressant in gastric juice of humans. *Proc. Soc. Exp. Biol. Med.,* 74:233–236.
11. Blair, E. L. (1967): The effects of tissue extracts on the stomach. In: *Gastric Secretion: Mechanisms and Control,* edited by T. K. Shnitka, J. A. L. Gilbert, and R. C. Harrison, pp. 263–281. *Proceedings of the Symposium on Gastric Secretion,* University of Alberta, Edmonton, 1965. Pergamon Press, Oxford.
12. Blickenstaff, D., and Grossman, M. I. (1950): A quantitative study of the reduction of gastric acid secretion associated with pyrexia. *Am. J. Physiol.,* 160:567–571.
13. Britton, B. H., Jr., and Wolf, S. (1959): An *in vitro* test for a hydrochloric acid inhibitor in human gastric content. *Clin. Res.,* 7:152 (Abstr.).
14. Brodie, D. A. (1970): Drug-induced inhibition of gastric secretion. In: *Progress in Gastroenterology, Vol. II,* edited by G. B. J. Glass, pp. 92–110. Grune & Stratton, New York.
15. Brodie, D. A., and Knapp, P. G. (1966): The mechanism of the inhibition of gastric secretion produced by ligation in the pylorus-ligated rats. *Gastroenterology,* 50:787–795.
16. Brodie, D. A., and Kundrats, S. K. (1964): The effect of pyrexia on gastric secretion. *Gastroenterology,* 47:171–178.
17. Brodie, D. A., Marshall, R. W., and Moreno, O. M. (1962): The effect of ulcerogenic drugs on gastric acidity in the rat with chronic gastric fistula. *Gastroenterology,* 43:675–679.
18. Brodie, D. A., Marshall, R. W., and Moreno, O. M. (1962): Effect of restraint on gastric acidity in the rat. *Am. J. Physiol.,* 202:812–814.
19. Brunschwig, A., Clarke, T. H., van Prohaska, J., and Schmitz, R. L. (1940): A secretory depressant in the achlorhydric juice of patients with carcinoma of the stomach. *Surg. Gynecol. Obstet.,* 70:25–30.
20. Brunschwig, A., Clarke, T. H., van Prohaska, J., and Schmitz, R. L. (1941): A gastric secretory depressant in extracts of achlorhydric carcinomatous stomachs. *Ann. Surg.,* 113:41–46.
21. Brunschwig, A., van Prohaska, J., Clarke, T. H., and Kandel, E. (1939): A secretory depressant in gastric juice of patients with pernicious anemia. *J. Clin. Invest.,* 18:415–422.
22. Brunschwig, A., Rasmussen, R. A., Camp, E. J., and Moe, R. (1942): Gastric secretory depressant in gastric juice. *Surgery,* 12:887–891.
23. Brunschwig, A., Schmitz, R. L., and Rasmussen, R. A. (1941): Experimental observations of achlorhydria of gastric cancer. *J. Natl. Cancer Inst.,* 1:481–488.
24. Chang, F. M., Pathak, S. R., and Law, D. H. (1969): Studies of gastric inhibitory substance (G.I.S.). *Clin. Res.,* 299 (Abstr.).
25. Code, C. F. (1952): Physiological gastric secretory inhibition. *Univ. Manitoba Med. J.,* 86–89.
26. Code, C. F. (1958): Discussion. *Gastroenterology,* 34:210.
27. Code, C. F. (1967): The recognition and assay of gastrone. In: *Gastric Secretion: Mechanisms and Control* edited by T. K. Shnitka, J. A. L. Gilbert, and R. C. Harrison, pp. 377–404. Pergamon Press, Oxford. *Proceedings of the Symposium on Gastric Secretion,* University of Alberta, Edmonton, 1965.
28. Code, C. F., Blackburn, C. M., Livermore, G. R., Jr., and Ratke, H. V. (1949): A method for the quantitative determination of gastric secretory inhibition. *Gastroenterology,* 13:573–587.
29. Code, C. F., Ratke, H. V., Livermore, Jr., G. R., and Lundberg, W. (1949): Occurrence of gastric secretory inhibitor activity in fresh gastric and salivary mucin. *Fed. Proc.,* 8:26 (Abstr.).

30. Coons, A. H., and Kaplan, M. H. (1950): Localization of antigen in tissue cells. II. Improvements in a method for the detection of antigen by means of fluorescent antibody. *J. Exp. Med.*, 91:1–13.
31. Cowley, J. F. (1973): Effect of partly purified gastrone on acid secretion, body temperature and leukocyte count in the dog. *Gastroenterology*, 65:43–53.
32. Cowley, J. F., Code, C. F., and Fiasse, R. (1969): Gastric mucosal blood flow during secretory inhibition by gastrin pentapeptide and gastrone. *Gastroenterology*, 56:659–665.
33. Fiasse, R., Code, C. F., and Glass, G. B. J. (1968): Fractionation and partial purification of gastrone. *Gastroenterology*, 54:1018–1031.
34. Fiasse, R., Code, C. F., and Glass, G. B. J. (1968): Gastrone and its partial purification. In: *The Physiology of Gastric Secretion*, edited by L. S. Semb and J. Myren, pp. 356–361. *Proceedings of the NATO Advanced Study Institute*, Lysebu, Oslo, May, 1967, Universitetsforlaget, Oslo.
35. Fiasse, R., Kubo, K., Code, C. F., and Glass, G. B. J. (1966): Purification of gastrone, endogenous inhibitor of gastric secretion. *Gastroenterology*, 50:842 (Abstr.).
36. Gerard, A., DeGraef, J., Lev, R., and Glass, G. B. J. (1967): Secretion of a chondroitin sulfate-like substance by the chief cells of the dog gastric mucosa. *Proc. Soc. Exp. Biol. Med.*, 124:1070–1073.
37. Ghosh, M. N., and Schild, H. O. (1958): Continuous recording of acid gastric secretion in the rat. *Br. J. Pharmacol. Chemother.*, 13:54–61.
38. Gindzienski, A., Yano, S., and Glass, G. B. J. (1976): Partial purification of gastrone from canine antral mucosa. The bioassay of its inhibitory activity on HCl secretion in rats with chronic gastric fistula. *Gastroenterology*, 70:A-29/997 (Abstr.).
38a. Gindzienski, A., Yano, S., and Glass, G. B. J. (1976): Gastrone purification from canine antral mucosa. Its bioassay on rats with chronic gastric fistula. In: *Tenth International Congress of Gastroenterology*, Budapest, Hungary, June 1976, 780, p. 688 (Abstr.).
39. Glass, G. B. J. (1961): Paper electrophoresis of gastric juice in health and disease. *Am. J. Dig. Dis.*, 6:1131–1192.
40. Glass, G. B. J. (1962): Biologically active materials related to gastric mucus in the normal and diseased stomach of man. *Gastroenterology*, 43:310–325.
41. Glass, G. B. J. (1963): Mucosubstances of gastric secretion in man and their biological activity. *Ann. NY Acad. Sci.*, 106:775–793.
42. Glass, G. B. J. (1965): The natural history of gastric atrophy. A review of immunologic aspects and possible links to endogenous inhibitors of gastric secretion. *Am. J. Dig. Dis.*, 10:376–398.
43. Glass, G. B. J. (1967): Current status of the "glandular mucoprotein" and "mucoproteose" fractions of the gastric mucin: A review of 15 years' progress in this area. *Ann. NY Acad. Sci.*, 140:804–834.
44. Glass, G. B. J. (1974): Gastrone, endogenous inhibitor of gastric secretion. In: *Satellite Symposium on Gastrointestinal Hormones, XXVI International Congress of Physiological Sciences*, Krakow, Poland. *Rendiconti di Gastroenterologia*, 6:76 (Abstr.).
45. Glass, G. B. J. (1974): Is the inhibitory effect of gastrone on gastric acid secretion due to contamination with pyrogen (endotoxin)? *Gastroenterology*, 66:1099–1103.
46. Glass, G. B. J. (1974): Gastrone. In: Candidate hormones of the gut. *Gastroenterology*, 67:740–742.
47. Glass, G. B. J. (1974): *Gastric Intrinsic Factor and Other Vitamin B_{12} Binders. Biochemistry, Physiology, Pathology and Relation to Vitamin B_{12} Metabolism.* Georg Thieme Publishers, Stuttgart.
48. Glass, G. B. J. (1975): Endogenous inhibitors of gastric secretion. In: *Proceedings of the J. Earl Thomas. Memorial Symposium on Functions of the Stomach and Intestine*, edited by M. H. F. Friedman, pp. 423–446. Thomas Jefferson University, Nov. 1973. University Park Press, Baltimore/London/Tokyo.
49. Glass, G. B. J. (1975): Endogenous inhibitors of gastric secretion. *Biol. Gastroenterol. (Paris)* (Suppl. 3), 8:245–261; *Arch. Fr. Mal. Dig.*, 64:5, Juillet-Aout.
50. Glass, G. B. J. (1977): Gastrone, endogenous inhibitor of gastric secretion. In: *Satellite Symposium on Gastrointestinal Hormones. XXVI International Congress of Physiological Sciences*, Krakow, 1974. *Materia Medica Polona*, 9:118–123.
51. Glass, G. B. J. (1977): Immunology of atrophic gastritis. *NY State J. Med.*, 77:1697–1705.
52. Glass, G. B. J., Balanzo, J. T., and Rosenthal, W. S. (1973): Cellular localization of gastrone in gastroduodenal mucosa by immunofluorescence. *Am. J. Dig. Dis.*, 18:270–288.

53. Glass, G. B. J., and Code, C. F. (1968): Gastrone, endogenous inhibitor of gastric secretion. In: *Progress in Gastroenterology,* Vol. I, edited by G. B. J. Glass, pp. 221–247. Grune & Stratton, New York.

54. Glass, G. B. J., Code, C. F., Kubo, K., and Fiasse, R. (1967): Fractionation of endogenous inhibitor of gastric secretion (gastrone) by physicochemical means. In: *Gastric Secretion: Mechanisms and Control,* edited by T. K. Shnitka et al, pp. 405–425, *Proceedings of the Symposium on Gastric Secretion.* University of Alberta, Edmonton. Pergamon Press, Oxford.

55. Glass, G. B. J., Kubo, K., Castro-Curel, Z., Fiasse, R., and Code, C. F. (1965): Partial purification of gastric acid inhibitor (gastrone) from human gastric juice. *Fed. Proc.,* 24:407 (Abstr.).

56. Glass, G. B. J., and Rosenthal, W. S. (1974): Gastrone today. In: *Endocrinology of the Gut,* edited by W. Chey and F. P. Brooks, pp. 126–142. Charles B. Slack, Thorofare, New Jersey.

57. Glass, G. B. J., Yano, S., and Gindzienski, A. (1976): Inhibition by gastrone of the pentagastrin stimulated secretion of HCl in rats with chronic gastric fistula. In: *First International Symposium on Gastrointestinal Hormones,* edited by M. I. Grossman. Asilomar, California, Abstr. 051.

58. Hennes, A. R., Sevelius, H., Lewellyn, T., Joel, W., Words, A. H., and Wolf, S. (1962): Atrophic gastritis in dogs. Production by intradermal injection of gastric juice in Freund's adjuvant. *Arch. Pathol.,* 73:281–287.

59. Hood, R. T. Jr., Code, C. F., and Grindlay, J. H. (1953): Source of a possible gastric secretory inhibitor in canine gastric juice and effect of vagotomy on its production. *Am. J. Physiol.,* 173:270–274.

60. Huff, J. W., Risley, E. A., and Barnes, R. H. (1950): Preparation and properties of a purified antisecretory substance, urogastrone. *Arch. Biochem.,* 25:133–140.

61. Jacob, E., and Glass, G. B. J. (1969): The participation of complement in the parietal cell antigen—antibody reaction in pernicious anemia and atrophic gastritis. *Clin. Exp. Immunol.,* 5:141–153.

62. Jacob, E., and Glass, G. B. J. (1971): Localization of intrinsic factor and complement fixing intrinsic factor—intrinsic factor antibody complex in parietal cell of man. *Clin. Exp. Immunol.,* 8:512–527.

63. Katzka, I., and Riss, L. (1962): A gastric secretory inhibitor in normal and pernicious anemia. *Gastroenterology,* 43:71–74.

64. Kim, Y. S., and Horowitz, M. I. (1971): Solubilization and chemical and immunochemical characterization of sparingly soluble canine gastric mucins. *Biochim. Biophys. Acta,* 236:686–701.

65. Kirsner, J. B., Nutter, P. B., and Palmer, W. L. (1940): Studies on anacidity: The hydrogen-ion concentration of the gastric secretion, the gastroscopic appearance of the gastric mucosa, and the presence of a gastric secretory depressant in patients with anacidity. *J. Clin. Invest.,* 19:619–625.

66. Komarov, S. A., Bralow, S. P., and Boyd, E. (1963): A permanent rat gastric fistula. *Proc. Soc. Exp. Biol. Med.,* 112:451–453.

67. Kubo, K., Castro-Curel, Z., Ibanez, N., Glass, G. B. J., and Code, C. F. (1964): Fractionation of gastrone, inhibitor of gastric secretion. *Gastroenterology,* 46:758 (Abstr.).

68. Kubo, K., Nishi, S., Miyake, T., Yoshizaki, R., and Miyoshi, A. (1962): Assay of gastric secretion inhibitor *in vivo* and *in vitro* with special reference to gastric juice of patients with carcinoma of the stomach. *Jpn. Arch. Intern. Med.,* 9:494.

69. Lai, K. S. (1964): Studies on gastrin. I. A method of biological assay of gastrin. *Gut,* 5:327–333.

70. Lambert, R. (1968): Use of the rat in the exploration of experimental peptic ulcer and sequellae of gastrectomy. In: *Progress in Gastroenterology Vol. I,* edited by G. B. J. Glass, pp. 40–66. Grune & Stratton, New York.

71. Law, D. H., and Baume, P. E. (1965): Two possible modes of action of gastrone. *Clin. Res.,* 13:256 (Abstr.).

72. Livermore, Jr., G. R., and Code, C. F. (1952): A possible gastric secretory inhibitor in canine gastric juice. *Am. J. Physiol.,* 168:605–611.

73. Lopes, J. D., and Glass, G. B. J. (1975): Purification of gastrone, endogenous inhibitor of gastric acid secretion and its bioassay on rats with chronic gastric fistula. *Clin. Res.,* 23:439A (Abstr.).

74. Lopes, J. D., and Glass, G. B. J. (1975): L'inhibiteur de la sécrétion gastrique et son bioassay sur les rats arec une fistule gastrique chronique. *Forum International Francophone de Recherches en Gastroenterologie,* Sherbrook, June 16–17, Abstr. 72.

75. Lopes, J. D., Ito, H., and Glass, G. B. J. (1979): Prolonged i.v. administration of gastrone B to rats. *(In preparation for publication).*
76. Menguy, R. (1967): Gastric inhibitory substance. In: *The Stomach, Including Related Areas in the Esophagus and Duodenum,* edited by C. Thompson, D. Berkowitz, E. Polish, and J. H. Moyer, pp. 145–157. *The 13th Hahnemann Symposium,* Grune & Stratton, New York.
77. Menguy, R., and Berlinski, M. (1967): Source of sialogastrone, a gastric inhibitory substance in human saliva. *Am. J. Dig. Dis.,* 12:1–6.
78. Menguy, R., Masters, Y. F., and Gryboski, W. (1964): Content of gastric inhibitory substance in saliva of patients with various gastric disorders. *Gastroenterology,* 46:32–35.
79. Menguy, R., Masters, Y. F., and Gryboski, W. (1965): Studies on the origin of the gastric inhibitory substance in the gastric juice. *Surgery,* 58:535–539.
80. Menguy, R., and Smith, W. O. (1959): Inhibition of gastric secretion in the rat by normal human gastric juice. *Proc. Soc. Exp. Biol. Med.,* 102:665–667.
81. Menguy, R., and Smith, W. L. (1960): Inhibition of gastric secretion in the rat by normal and abnormal human gastric juice. *Proc. Soc. Exp. Biol. Med.,* 105:238–239.
82. Miyoshi, A. (1962): Development of gastric anacidity: Its clinical and pathological study. *Annual Meeting of Japanese Gastroenterological Association. Jpn. Arch. Gastroenterol.,* 118–122.
83. Miyoshi, A., Inouye, T., Miyake, T., Okuda, Y., Kubo, K., Nakamura, T., Hatano, M., Nishi, S., Kanematsu, Y., and Yoshizaki, R. (1961): Inhibition of rat gastric secretion by human gastric juice (so-called gastrone activity). *Nippon Rinsho,* 9:2167–2175.
84. Miyoshi, A., Miyake, T., Kubo, K., Nishi, S., and Yoshizaki, R. (1962): Assay of gastric secretion inhibitor *in vivo* and *in vitro.* In: *Proceedings of the World Congress of Gastroenterology,* Munich 2:67–71. S. Karger, Basel.
85. Miyoshi, A., Moriga, M., and Suyama, T. (1968): A gastric secretion inhibitory substance in human saliva. In: *Proceedings of the VII International Congress of Gastroenterology,* July 7–13, Prague, edited by O. Gregor and O. Riedl, pp. 213–218. Schattauer, Stuttgart, New York.
86. Moriga, M. (1968): Studies on "gastric secretory inhibitor" and "gastric atrophy producing factor." *Jpn. Arch. Intern. Med.,* 15:175.
86a. Murty, V., Kojima, K., Slomiany. B. L., and Glass, G. B. J. Further attempts at fractionation of antral gastrone and its assays on Ghosh-Lai rat stomach. *(In preparation for publication).*
87. Olson, W. H., Walker, L., and Necheles, H. (1954): Depression of gastric secretion without elevation of temperature following injection of pyrogens. *Am. J. Physiol.,* 116:393.
87a. Peissner, L., and Tang, J. (1960): Preliminary studies of the inhibitory factor in human gastric juice. *Physiologist,* 176:393–395.
88. Rheault, M. J., Deschenes, J., and Tetreault, L. (1970): Demonstration chez le rat d'un facteur gastrique inhibiteur de la secretion gastrique. *Can. J. Surg.,* 13:288–294.
89. Rheault, M. J., Rouse, D., and Tetreault, L. (1975): Influence de diverses voies d'administration sur l'efficacite pharmacologique du facteur inhibiteur gastrique chez le rat. *Union Med. Can.,* 104:970–976.
90. Rheault, M. J., and Tetreault, L. (1972): Proprietés inhibitrices du suc gastrique humain sur la secretion gastrique du rat. Différence quantitative d'inhibition selon cinq états physiopathologiques. *Can. J. Surg.,* 15:374–383.
91. Rheault, M. J., and Tetreault, L. (1976): La gastrone. *Union Med. Can.,* 105:1141–1146.
92. Rosenthal, W. S., Balanzo, J. T., and Glass, G. B. J. (1972): Antibody to gastrone, endogenous inhibitor of gastric secretion and use in detection of gastrone's cellular origin. *Gastroenterology,* 62:801 (Abstr.).
93. Rosenthal, W. S., Balanzo, J. T., and Glass, G. B. J. (1973): Antibody to gastrone—endogenous inhibitor of gastric secretion. *Am. J. Dig. Dis.,* 13:349–359.
94. Rosenthal, W. S., and Rudick, J. (1971): Chylogastrone: Gastric secretory inhibitor in thoracic duct lymph of man and dog. *Am. J. Physiol.,* 220:452–456.
95. Rowe, P. B., Fenton, B. H., and Beeston, D. (1964): Further observations on the gastric secretory depressant in human gastric juice. *Gastroenterology,* 46:748 (Abstr.).
96. Rudick, J., Gajewski, A. K., Pitts, C. L., Semb, L. S., Fletcher, T. L., Harkins, H. N., and Nyhus, L. M. (1965): Gastric inhibitors in fasting canine thoracic duct lymph. *Proc. Soc. Exp. Biol. Med.,* 120:119–121.
97. Rudick, J., Gajewski, A. K., Pitts, C. L., Semb, L. S., Fletcher, T. L., Harkins, H. N., and Nyhus, L. M. (1966): Inhibition of gastric secretion by fractionated lymph. Elaboration of gastrone-like substance during digestive phases in dogs. *Am. Surg.,* 32:513–520.

98. Scott, V. B., Moe, R., and Brunschwig, A. (1943): Further studies on properties of the gastric secretory depressant in gastric juice. *Proc. Soc. Exp. Biol. Med.,* 52:45–46.
99. Semb, L. S. (1966): The effects of a gastric inhibitory substance on gastric secretion in the pylorus ligated rat. *Acta Physiol. Scand.,* 66:374–382.
100. Semb, L. S. (1966): Studies on a gastric inhibitory substance isolated from juice of the gastric antrum in the dog. The effect of intravenous injection of isologous extracts of antral juice on the gastric secretion of acid and pepsin in Heidenhain pouch dogs stimulated by histamine, gastrin and feeding. *Scand. J. Gastroenterol.,* 1:253–267.
101. Semb, L. S. (1969): Studies on inhibition of gastric secretion; with special reference to acidification of the gastric antrum and the inhibitory substance in gastric juice. Thesis, Oslo, Universitatsverlaget 1–41.
102. Semb, L. S. (1969): Effects of gastric and jejunal juice extracts on gastric secretion. *Acta Physiol. Scand.,* 77:385–395.
103. Semb, L. S. (1972): Effect of human and canine gastric juice extracts on gastric secretion and aminopyrine clearance in Heidenhain pouch in dogs. *Acta Hepatogastroenterol.,* 19:264–271.
104. Semb, L. S., Gjone, E., and Rosenthal, W. S. (1970): Bioassay for gastric secretory inhibitor in extract of pancreatic tumor from patient with WDHS-syndrome. *Scand. J. Gastroenterol.,* 5:409–414.
105. Shay, H., Sun, D. C. H., and Gruenstein, M. A. (1954): A quantitative method for measuring gastric secretion in the rat. *Gastroenterology,* 26:906–913.
105a. Sigma (1973): Technical Bulletin 210.
106. Smith, W. O., Duval, M. K., Joel, W., Honska, W. L., and Wolf, S. (1960): Gastric atrophy in dogs induced by administration of normal human gastric juice. *Gastroenterology,* 39:55–61.
107. Smith, W. O., Duval, M. K., Joel, W., and Wolf, S. (1959): The experimental production of atrophic gastritis using a preparation of human gastric juice. *Surgery,* 46:76.
108. Smith, W. O., Hoke, R., Landy, F., Caputto, R., and Wolf, S. (1958): The nature of the inhibitory effect of normal human gastric juice on Heidenhain pouch dogs. *Gastroenterology,* 34:181–187.
109. Smith, W. O., Joel, W., and Wolf, S. (1958): Experimental atrophic gastritis associated with inhibition of parietal cells. *Trans. Assoc. Am. Physicians,* 71:306.
110. Thompson, J. C. (1974): Antral chalone. In: *Candidate Hormones of the Gut,* edited by M. I. Grossman. *Gastroenterology,* 67:752–753.
110a. Thompson, J. C., Vakil, H. C., and Miller, J. H. (1964): Mast cell degranulation and gastric secretion: Inhibitory role of heparin. *Fed. Proc.,* 22:214 (Abstr.).
111. Wakisaka, G., Miyoshi, A., Miyake, T., Kubo, K., Nishi, S., Okuda, Y., Kanematsu, Y., Okawa, S., Yoshizaki, R., and Inouye, T. (1962): Studies on the effect of the gastrone. *In vitro* experiment with special reference to fundamental study. In: *Annual Meeting of the Japanese Gastroenterological Association (Personal communication).*
112. Wolf, S., Smith, W. O., Caputto, R., Trucco, R., and Johnson, P. C. (1957): The biological activities of the large macromolecular components of human gastric content. *Trans. Am. Clin. Climatol. Assoc.,* 69:147–153.
113. Yamagata, S., and Ueno, K. (1962): The experimental studies of gastric secretory inhibitor in human gastric juice. *Jpn. J. Gastroenterol, Proceedings of the 48th Annual Meeting,* p. 94 (Abstr.).

Note Added in Proof: Most recently, through the courtesy of Dr. M. I. Grossman, which is gratefully acknowledged, 150 μg gastrone B from canine antral mucosa was assayed in the Los Angeles V.A. Hospital, Lipid Research Laboratory, for the content of β-hydroxy myristic acid, one of the constituents of bacterial endotoxin (Luderitz et al., *J. Infect. Dis.,* 128:S17–S29, 1973). This was found to be 1.4%. In the same laboratory, a human urinary gastric inhibitor (HUGI) was found to contain 3½ times more of this acid than gastrone B (5%), HUGI, as well as an equivalent in terms of myristic acid, amount of *E. coli* endotoxin caused depression of the gastrin G-17 stimulated cat gastric acid secretion by 64% and a rise in t° by 1.4°C, both for 90 min. (M. I. Grossman and D. Rachmilewitz, *personal communication).* To what extent this valuable information applies to gastrone B activity cannot be stated at this time. The duration of gastrone effect on acid secretion extends up to 5 hr or more (see 4 graphs on pp. 952–953), but the difference may be the function of the dose. The contents of the β-hydroxy myristic acid in various gastrone preparations has not yet been determined, and this fatty acid is not the only pyrogen in endotoxin. Further work on these aspects of the problem will be helpful.

Gastrointestinal Hormones, edited by
George B. Jerzy Glass.
Raven Press, New York © 1980.

Chapter 43

Work in Progress on Some of the Candidate Hormones

Viktor Mutt

Karolinska Institute, S-10401 Stockholm, 60 Sweden

In addition to the recognized gastrointestinal hormones, there are a number of "candidate hormones" (1,2). (see Chapters 39–42 of this volume, pp. 877–970) Some of these have been identified chemically, but not enough physiological studies have been carried out to show whether or not they are hormones in the original sense of this term. Others are still physiological principles, known by their actions only.

This chapter does not review the whole field of candidate hormones. It is confined to a brief description of work in progress in a group of collaborating laboratories, with the object of isolating from intestinal and gastric tissue hormonal peptides, which on immunochemical grounds have been claimed to be present in the particular tissue but have not yet been isolated from it. These laboratories are also studying some previously unrecognized peptides which have now been identified either by a purely chemical method or by physiological studies.

It is becoming increasingly evident that the peptide pattern of the gastrointestinal tissue is far more complex than previously believed, and that much more work will have to be done before a coherent picture of the chemistry and physiology of these peptides will emerge.

REFERENCE

1. Grossman, M. I. (1974): Candidate hormones of the gut. *Gastroenterology*, 67:730–755.
2. Grossman, M. I. (1975): Additional candidate hormones of the gut. *Gastroenterology*, 69:570–571.

I. PURIFICATION OF A PEPTIDE WITH BOMBESIN-LIKE PROPERTIES FROM PORCINE GASTRIC AND INTESTINAL TISSUE

T. J. McDonald

Department of Biochemistry II, Karolinska Institute, S-104 01 Stockholm 60, Sweden

During a systematic investigation of porcine nonantral gastric tissue extracts, certain fractions were noted to cause acid and pepsin secretion in chronic gastric fistula cats despite the presence in these fractions of such inhibitors of acid secretion as the vasoactive intestinal polypeptide (VIP) and immunoreactive somatostatin. Further investigation demonstrated that intravenous (i.v.) administration of these impure extracts to conscious dogs resulted in a significant elevation of plasma immunoreactive gastrin (IRGa) which was dose responsive and at least partially resistant to prior atropinization or beta blockade. It was markedly reduced, however, by prior removal of the gastric antrum and abolished by prior treatment of the extracts with alpha-chymotrypsin (6). Investigation of a similar porcine intestinal extract fraction revealed similar bioactivity (7), and all information to date suggests that the active peptide present in both the intestinal and gastric extracts is identical. This section briefly outlines the properties, so far known, of highly purified preparations of the gastric and intestinal peptide and discusses its possible relationship to bombesin, a tetradeca-peptide isolated from frog skin (1), which also has potent gastrin-releasing properties (3). Radioimmunological and immunohistochemical evidence of the presence in the mammalian gut of a peptide similar to amphibian bombesin has been reported (3,10,15).

PURIFICATION PROCEDURE

Details of tissue extraction (6,9), purification procedures (6,8), radioimmunological assays (RIAs) and chemical techniques (6,8,12), and the *in vivo* biological assays for plasma IRGa-elevating activity (6), gastric acid and pepsin secretion in chronic gastric fistula cats (13,14), antral motility in conscious cats (2), gall-bladder contraction in the anesthetized guinea pig (5), and pancreatic protein output in the anesthetized cat (4) have been described. The starting material for the purification of the gastric peptide has been described (6), whereas that for the intestinal peptide was a side fraction from the purification of intestinal VIP (11).

The criterion for increase in purity of the active fractions was an increase in the potency of plasma IRGa-elevating activity, but increases in potency of gallbladder contraction and pancreatic protein-stimulating activities occurred during the purification of both peptides. Intravenous infusion of the active gastric and intestinal fractions into cats with chronic gastric fistulas resulted in significant increases in acid and pepsin secretion. Intravenous administration of these active fractions into conscious cats decreased the frequency of high-amplitude antral contraction peaks (greater than 30 cm H_2O) and increased those of low amplitude (between 3 and 10 cm H_2O), an effect similar to that seen with pentagastrin administration (2).

PROPERTIES OF THE PURIFIED PEPTIDE

After a final carboxymethyl cellulose (CMC) chromatography, the highly purified intestinal peptide on bolus i.v. injection into conscious dogs at a dose of 150 ng-kg^{-1} resulted in a rapid fivefold increase in plasma IRGa. Isotachophoretic analysis of the highly purified gastric and intestinal peptide preparations (both after a final CMC chromatography) indicated that both preparations were dominated by one component. On silica gel thin-layer chromatography, both peptides exhibited a discrete ninhydrin-positive spot with an identical R^f value that was midway between that of standard porcine secretin and synthetic bombesin. N-terminal analysis of both these highly purified preparations revealed a dominant alanine residue, but the presence of a blocked N terminus has not yet been completely excluded. Analysis for C-terminal amide structures revealed, in both peptides, the presence of a C-terminus methionine alpha-amide residue, and preliminary evidence indicates that the penultimate residue is leucine. Reverse phase high-pressure liquid chromatography of the highly purified gastric and intestinal preparations revealed, in each case, a sharply defined dominant protein elution peak with identical retention times. The plasma IRGa-elevating and gallbladder-contracting activity was confined to the dominant peak and was not found in the small residual contaminant peaks. Assay of fractions, generated during the preparation of the intestinal peptide, for immunoreactive bombesin (IRB) showed that the peak IRB consistently coincided with the peak gastrin-releasing activity (7,8).

SUMMARY

An apparently identical peptide from the porcine nonantral gastric and intestinal tissue has been found to possess potent gastrin-releasing activity. The concomitant activities of increase of acid and pepsin secretion and changes in antral motility are at least partially consistent with the release of gastrin. Both peptides exhibit the ability to increase protein output from the pancreas and to contract the gallbladder—activities which are consistent with the release of cholecystokinin-pancreozymin—but the possibility of a direct effect on target organs has not been excluded. The mammalian peptide exhibits cross-reactivity in a RIA system based on amphibian bombesin, but this reactivity may not be complete (6), perhaps due to structural differences between the two molecules. The immunological cross-reactivity and the similar spectrum of bioactivities suggest that the peptide purified from porcine gut is the mammalian counterpart to amphibian bombesin. The peptide has been highly purified and preliminary chemical evidence suggests that the C-terminus is composed of leucyl-methionine amide. Complete structural characterization of the mammalian peptide is essential to determine the similarities and dissimilarities between the mammalian and amphibian peptides with bombesin-like properties.

REFERENCES

1. Anastasi, A., Erspamer, V., and Bucci, M. (1971): Isolation and structure of bombesin and alytesin, two analogous active peptides from the skin of the European amphibians Bombina and Alytes. *Experientia, 27*:166–167.
2. Desvigne, C., Vagne, M., Faivre, M., and Desvigne, A. (1977): Action de proglumide sur la secretion acide et la motricité gastrique stimulées par la pentagastrine chez le chat. *Gastroenterol. Clin. Biol., 1*:447–454.
3. Erspamer, V., and Melchiorri, P. (1975): Actions of bombesin on secretions and motility of the gastrointestinal tract. In: *Gastrointestinal Hormones: A Symposium,* edited by J. C. Thompson, pp. 575–589. University of Texas Press, Austin.
4. Jorpes, E., and Mutt, V. (1966): Cholecystokinin and pancreozymin, one single hormone? *Acta Physiol. Scand., 66*:196–202.
5. Ljungberg, S. (1964): Biologisk styrkebestämning av cholecystokinin. *Sven. Farm. Tidskr., 68*:351–354.
6. McDonald, T. J., Nilsson, G., Vagne, M., Ghatei, M., Bloom, S. R., and Mutt, V. (1978): A gastrin releasing peptide from the porcine nonantral gastric tissue. *Gut, 19*:767–774.
7. McDonald, T. J., Nilsson, G., Vagne, M., Ghatei, M., Bloom, S. R., and Mutt, V. (1978): Purification of a porcine intestinal peptide with bombesin-like properties. *Scand. J. Gastroenterol.* [*Suppl. 49*], 13:149 (abst.).
8. McDonald, T. J., Nilsson, G., Vagne, M., Ghatei, M., Bloom, S. R., and Mutt, V. (1979): Purification of a peptide with bombesin-like properties from porcine gastric and intestinal tissue. *In preparation.*
9. Mutt, V. (1959): Preparation of highly purified secretin. *Ark. Kemi., 15*:69–74.
10. Polak, J. M., Bloom, S. R., Hobbs, S., Solcia, E., and Pearse, A. G. E. (1976): Distribution of a bombesin-like peptide in human gastrointestinal tract. *Lancet, 1*:1109–1110.
11. Said, S. I., and Mutt, V. (1972): Isolation from porcine intestinal wall of a vasoactive octacosapeptide related to secretin and glucagon. *Eur. J. Biochem., 28*:199–204.
12. Tatemoto, K., and Mutt, V. (1978): Chemical determination of polypeptide hormones. *Proc. Natl. Acad. Sci. USA, 75*:4115–4119.
13. Vagne, M., and Perret, G. (1976): Effect of duodenal acidification on gastric mucus and acid secretion in conscious cats. *Digestion, 14*:332–341.
14. Vagne, M., Perrett, D. S., and Desvigne, A. (1974): Dosage de l'activité protéolytique du suc gastrique par une méthode automatique. *Path. Biol. (Paris), 22*:359–364
15. Walsh, J. H., and Holmquist, A. L. (1976): Radioimmunoassay of bombesin peptides: Identification of bombesin-like immunoreactivity in vertebrate gut extracts. *Gastroenterology, 70*:948 (abst.).

II. CHEMICAL ASSAY FOR NATURAL PEPTIDES: APPLICATION TO THE ISOLATION OF CANDIDATE HORMONES

Kazuhiko Tatemoto

Department of Biochemistry II, Medical Nobel Institute, Karolinska Institute, S-104 01 Stockholm 60, Sweden

We have been systematically isolating some naturally occurring polypeptides from extracts of porcine intestinal tissue using a chemical assay system based on characteristic chemical structures, rather than a bioassay system based on biological functions, to follow the purification.

ASSAY SYSTEM BASED ON CHARACTERISTIC CHEMICAL STRUCTURES

The characteristic chemical structures used in these studies are the C-terminal alpha-amide structures of polypeptides which occur often in many hormonal peptides, as for example, oxytocin, gonadoliberin, calcitonin, tyroliberin, gastrin, cholecystokinin, secretin, substance P, α-melanotropin, pancreatic polypeptide, vasoactive intestinal peptide (VIP), vasopressin, and many others (2,3). The alpha-amide bond of a naturally occurring polypeptide may be formed from its precursor as the result of specific enzyme reactions. This was demonstrated by Suchanek and Kreil (5) in the formation of C-terminal -Gln-NH$_2$ of melittin from C-terminal -Gln -Gly-OH of the precursor molecule. Since the common degradation reactions of polypeptides do not produce the C-terminal alpha-amide structures, it may be worthwhile to first isolate peptides containing such structures and then examine them for possible biological activities. The presence of such peptides can be demonstrated directly in tissue extracts by using a chemical assay system described previously (6), in which peptide fragments having the C-terminal alpha-amides are released enzymatically, and then selectively isolated and identified by thin-layer chromatography. By use of this technique. it was found that a large number of hitherto unknown polypeptides containing C-terminal alpha-amides were present in porcine intestinal extracts in addition to the known polypeptide amides, secretin, cholecystokinin, and vasoactive intestinal peptide (6).

CHEMICAL STRUCTURES AND BIOLOGICAL PROPERTIES OF THREE RECENTLY ISOLATED PEPTIDES

The following section describes preliminary data on the chemical structures and biological properties of some of those previously unknown polypeptides recently isolated in this laboratory.

PHI Peptide: A New Porcine Peptide

One of these newly discovered polypeptides, PHI, containing isoleucine amide at its C terminus, was isolated from porcine intestinal extracts by purification being followed solely by the chemical assay method described. The terminal analysis of the pure peptide preparation indicates that this peptide has N-terminal histidine and C-terminal isoleucine amide.

Since the biological properties of this newly isolated peptide are not yet known, a chemical name was given to it based on its species origin (porcine, *P*), its N-terminal amino acid (histidine, *H*), and its C-terminal amino acid (isoleucine, *I*).

Partial sequence analysis suggests that PHI has structural similarities to members of the secretin-glucagon family, although its structure is distinct from that of secretin, VIP, or any other known peptide.

Bataille et al. (1) have examined the binding of PHI to various known receptor and immunological systems. It was found that PHI effectively inhibited the binding of ^{125}I-vasoactive intestinal peptide to the receptors in various rat tissue membranes and activated adenyl cyclase in the same membrane systems. In contrast, it did not cross-react with the VIP antibodies.

A preliminary report suggests that PHI releases glucagon and insulin in an isolated rat pancreas (J. T. Szecowka, *personal communication*). It is probable that further physiological investigations will reveal yet unknown biological properties of this peptide.

Secretin II: A Secretin-Like Peptide

During the chemical assay studies it was noted that there might be a peptide other than secretin with C-terminal valine amide (6). A new peptide of secretin-like molecular structure has now been isolated from porcine intestinal extracts using the chemical assay, instead of bioassay, to follow the purification of this peptide. The thin-layer chromatography of the tryptic fragments of this peptide revealed that four of the five tryptic fragments were identical to those of secretin, but the N-terminal fragment was different. The biological and chemical nature of this secretin-like peptide is under investigation.

CCK III: A Cholecystokinin-Like Peptide

Detailed chromatographic studies during the purification of cholecystokinin revealed the presence of three distinct molecular forms which exhibited cholecystokinin bioactivities *(unpublished)*. When the chemical assay and the bioassay methods were used, another cholecystokinin molecule, more basic than the two known cholecystokinin molecules (CCK-33 and CCK-39) (4), was isolated from porcine intestinal extracts. A preliminary study indicates that the biological properties of this peptide are similar to those of the known cholecystokinin molecules. Preliminary chemical analysis, however, indicates that the N-terminal amino acid of the CCK-like peptide is arginine, instead of lysine (CCK-33) or tyrosine (CCK-39), whereas the C-terminal amino acid is phenylalanine amide which is the same for the other CCK molecules. Further studies on chemical structure of this peptide are underway.

REFERENCES

1. Bataille, D., Laburthe, M., Dupont, C., Tatemoto, K., Vauclin, N., Rosselin, G., and Mutt, V. (1978): VIP-like effects of a newly isolated intestinal peptide (PIHIA). *Scand. J. Gastroenterol.* [*Suppl. 49*], 13:13.
2. Dayhoff, M. O. (1972): Hormones, active peptides and toxins. In: *Atlas of Protein Sequence and Structure, Vol. 5,* edited by M. O. Dayhoff, pp. D173–D227. National Biomedical Research Foundation, Silver Springs, Md.
3. Hunt, L. T., and Dayhoff, M. O. (1976): Hormones and active peptides. In: *Atlas of Protein Sequence and Structure, Vol. 5,* edited by M. O. Dayhoff, Suppl. II, pp. 113–145. National Biomedical Research Foundation, Silver Springs, Md.
4. Mutt, V. (1976): Further investigations on intestinal hormonal polypeptides. *Clin. Endocrinol.* [*Suppl.*], 5:175s–183s.
5. Suchanek, G., and Kreil, G. (1977): Translation of melittin messenger RNA *in vitro* yields a product terminating with glutaminylglycine rather than glutaminamide. *Proc. Natl. Acad. Sci. USA,* 74:975–978.
6. Tatemoto, K., and Mutt, V. (1978): Chemical determination of polypeptide hormones. *Proc. Natl. Acad. Sci. USA,* 75:4115–4119.

III. GASTROZYMIN

Monique Vagne

INSERM U 45, Hôpital Edouard-Herriot, 69374 Lyon, Cedex 2, France

Gastrozymin was discovered by Blair et al. (1) who described a pepsin secretion-stimulating principle occurring in extracts of intestinal and gastric tissues. But as yet the isolation of gastrozymin has not been realized. The problem is complicated because stimulation of pepsin secretion may be obtained by hormones such as gastrin (2) and secretin (5).

We have previously described (6) separation of a peptide fraction from porcine intestinal mucosa which has a pepsin secretion-stimulating action, and, which because of its chemical and physiological properties should be different from secretin.

This fraction was obtained from the chromatography of the concentrate of thermostable intestinal peptides (CTIPs) (3) on Sephadex G-25 equilibrated and eluted with 0.2 N acetic acid. The major stimulation of pepsin was obtained with the 39–42 fraction, which elutes before the 51–66 fraction that is the starting material of the hitherto isolated intestinal hormones (secretin, cholecystokinin, VIP, motilin, etc). On extraction of the 39–42 fraction with methanol, the active material was found to be soluble in methanol at pH 4 but insoluble at pH 7.5. This insoluble fraction was further purified on carboxymethyl cellulose and the active material was eluted with 0.04 M ammonium bicarbonate and then chromatographed on Sephadex G-50. This fraction purified further was 120 times more potent than the starting material and was effective at a dose of 10 μg·kg^{-1}. The activity was abolished by trypsin and chymotrypsin proteolysis.

The pepsin-stimulating effect was obtained with secretions of both the innervated and denervated stomach preparations of conscious cats, in a gastric fistula conscious dog, and in gastric fistula anesthetized rats. The same fraction showed a stimulating effect on bile secretion in anesthetized guinea pigs (4) with bile duct canulations, cystic duct ligations, and gastric fistulas. A stimulation of pancreatic juice and bicarbonate output was obtained in anesthetized cats with pancreatic duct canulations and gastric fistulas.

As all these actions qualitatively resemble those of secretin, a systematic comparison with secretin was made. This showed that the dose-response curves, for all these activities, had significantly different slopes. Furthermore, the comparison of the doses of secretin and gastrozymin fractions needed for different actions showed that gastrozymin was relatively more potent than secretin on pepsin secretion and more potent on bile secretion than on pancreatic secretion (six to eight times).

Gastrozymin also differs from secretin in several chemical characteristics:

1. It is eluted before secretin on Sephadex G-25 and G-50, even in the presence of 8 M urea, and therefore probably has a higher molecular weight.
2. It is eluted with a higher concentration of ammonium bicarbonate on carboxymethyl cellulose, and therefore probably is more basic in nature.
3. It has solubility differences with secretin, in that it is insoluble in methanol at pH 7.5 whereas secretin is soluble, is insoluble in 80% ethanol at −30°C whereas secretin is soluble, and is not extracted into butanol from 0.1 M ammonium bicarbonate whereas secretin is extracted.

Further purification will show whether all the effects are produced by one or several peptides still present in our fraction and whether or not there is any structural relation between gastrozymin and secretin or its precursor(s).

REFERENCES

1. Blair, E. L., Harper, A. A., and Lake, H. J. (1953): The pepsin stimulating effect of gastric and intestinal extracts in cats. *J. Physiol. (Lond.),* 121:20–21 P.
2. Gregory, R. A., and Tracy, H. J. (1974): The constitution and properties of two gastrins extracted from hog antral mucosa. *Gut,* 5:103–107.
3. Mutt, V. (1978): Hormone isolation. In: *Gut Hormones,* edited by S. R. Bloom and M. I. Grossman, pp. 21–27. Churchill Livingstone, Edinburgh.
4. Perret, G., Gelin, M. L., Vagne, M. et al. (1978): Technique de recueil de la bile chez le cobaye. Etude de l'action de la sécrétine et de la gastrozymine. *Gastroenterol. Clin. Biol.,* 2:817–824.
5. Pratt, C. L. G. (1940): The influence of secretin on gastric secretion. *J. Physiol. (Lond.),* 98:1P.
6. Vagne, M., Mutt, V., Perret, G., and Lemaitre, R. (1976): A fraction isolated from porcine upper small intestine stimulating pepsin secretion in the cat. *Digestion,* 14:89–93.

IV. ENTERO-OXYNTIN

Monique Vagne

INSERM U. 45, Hôpital Edouard-Herriot, F-69374, Lyon, Cedex 2, France

The intestinal phase of gastric secretion has been shown to be humorally mediated (2,3,7), and Grossman (4) has named this humoral factor entero-oxyntin (4). One group obtained a gastrin-free preparation from hog intestine capable of stimulating acid secretion (1,6), but no complete isolation has been reported. Way et al. (9) determined the pharmacological profile of the humoral factor of the intestinal phase as a substance released by the intestine that acts on a receptor of the parietal cell different from that of gastrin, stimulates basal acid secretion, and increases maximal acid secretion induced by all known stimulants of gastric acid secretion.

SEARCH FOR POSSIBLE OCCURRENCE OF ENTERO-OXYNTOCIN IN PORCINE INTESTINAL TISSUE

We began to investigate the possible occurrence of entero-oxyntin in porcine intestinal tissue extracts by systematically testing all the side fractions obtained during the isolation of secretin and cholecystokinin for the ability to increase maximal acid secretion stimulated by pentagastrin in conscious cats equipped with a denervated pouch and a gastric fistula. We found such activity in the concentrate of thermostable intestinal peptides (CTIPs) (5), which on Sephadex G-25 chromatography was eluted in the 49–50 fraction, which is just before the fraction containing all the hitherto isolated intestinal hormones (secretin, cholecystokinin, VIP, motilin, etc).

SEPARATION AND TESTING OF THE ACTIVE FRACTION

A methanol extraction of the 49–50 fraction left the activity in the insoluble material which was further purified by chromatography on diethylaminoethyl

(DEAE) cellulose. The testing of this DEAE fraction was done in the following ways:

1. Given alone, the DEAE fraction produced at a dose of 1,200 $\mu g \cdot kg^{-1}hr^{-1}$ an increase in both volume and acid output, by 28 and 25%, respectively, of the maximal response obtained in cats with pentagastrin (peak values per 15 min).
2. Given during intravenous infusion of pentagastrin which induced a maximal acid response (32 $\mu g \cdot kg^{-1}hr^{-1}$), this fraction induced an increase by 25% of the maximal acid output.

An increase of pepsin output was also obtained in both types of experiments.

Adjusting the pH of the DEAE fraction to 7.8 resulted in the formation of a precipitate which gave an increase of pentagastrin maximally stimulated acid output of 39% at a dose of 500 $\mu g \cdot kg^{-1}hr^{-1}$. Although high doses were required to give a large increase in acid output, the threshold dose was less than 40 μg. Our fraction is still very complex, and therefore purification of the active material may be expected to give a great increase in specific activity.

The CCK content of this fraction cannot be implicated in the increase of maximally stimulated acid secretion since we have confirmed the finding of Way (8) that, in the cat, CCK and pentagastrin are full agonists.

SUMMARY AND CONCLUSIONS

These data indicate that our active fraction is consistent so far with the previously defined profile of the mediator of the intestinal phase of gastric secretion named entero-oxyntin, in that it stimulates basal and maximal acid secretion to the same extent and therefore acts on a different receptor from that of gastrin on the parietal cell.

REFERENCES

1. Chandler, J. G., Kester, R. C., and Orloff, M. J. (1972): Isolation of the hormone responsible for intestinal phase of gastric acid secretion from pig intestinal mucosa. *Surg. Forum.* 23:382.
2. Debas, H. T., Slaff, G. F., and Grossman, M. I. (1975): Intestinal phase of gastric acid secretion: Augmentation of maximal response of Heidenhain pouch to gastrin and to histamine. *Gastroenterology,* 69:691–698.
3. Gregory, R. A., and Tracy, H. J. (1960): Secretory responses of denervated gastric pouches. *Am. J. Dig. Dis.,* 4:308–323.
4. Grossman, M. I. (1974): Candidate hormones of the gut. *Gastroenterology,* 67:730–757.
5. Mutt, V. (1978): Hormone isolation. In: *Gut Hormones,* edited by S. R. Bloom, pp. 21–27. Churchill Livingstone, Edinburgh.
6. Orloff, M. J., Guillemin, R. C. L., and Nakaji, N. T. (1977): Isolation of the hormone for the intestinal phase of gastric secretion. *Gastroenterology,* 72:A10/820.
7. Sircus, W. (1953): The intestinal phase of gastric secretion. *Q. J. Exp. Physiol.,* 38:91–100.
8. Way, L. W. (1971): Effect of cholecystokinin and caerulein on gastric secretion in cats. *Gastroenterology,* 60:560–565.
9. Way, L. W., Cairns, D. W., and Deveney, C. W. (1975): The intestinal phase of gastric secretion: A pharmacological profile of entero-oxyntin. *Surgery,* 77:841–860.

V. FRACTION PURIFIED FROM PORCINE UPPER SMALL INTESTINE WHICH INDUCES THE ABSORPTION OF WATER AND SODIUM IN THE DUODENUM OF RAT

Danielle Pansu

Ecole Pratique des Hautes Études and INSERM U 45, Hôpital Eduoard-Herriot, 69374, Lyon, Cedex 2, France

During the studies on the effect of gastrozymin (5) on intestinal secretion, we found that certain gastrozymin-containing fractions induced an increase in duodenal water and sodium absorption in rats (4), whereas the gastrozymin fractions obtained at a next step of purification did not modify the duodenal absorption. Recognizing that a fraction different from gastrozymin could be involved with duodenal absorption, we reinvestigated the early fractions obtained from a concentrate of intestinal peptides (CTIP) (3) chromatographed on Sephadex G-25. We found that the most active fraction on duodenal absorption was the fraction 43–46, whereas the most active fraction for gastrozymin-like activity was 39–42.

The activity on duodenal absorption was determined in Wistar rats, in which duodenal loops were made *in situ*. These were filled with a solution containing 0.138 M NaCl and $^{14}CPEG$ and ^{22}Na as markers; the final content was collected after 1 hr, and the movement of water and sodium was measured.

The fraction 43–46 was found to be methanol soluble at pH 4 but insoluble at pH 7.5. This insoluble fraction was chromatographed on carboxymethyl cellulose and eluted with 0.04 M ammonium bicarbonate. With a sixfold increase of activity from the starting material, this fraction at a dose of 250 μg/100 g body weight produced a water absorption of 0.37 $\pm$ 0.04 ml/hr. Incubation of this fraction with chymotrypsin suppressed the activity on duodenal absorption, indicating a peptidic nature of the active principle.

In contrast with this active fraction, secretin, cholecystokinin, and somatostatin induced a duodenal secretion of water and sodium. Pentagastrin induced a duodenal absorption but decreased the ileal absorption, whereas our fraction, which did not contain immunoreactive gastrin, induced a duodenal absorption without changing the ileal absorption. Both prolactin (2) and angiotensin (1) have been previously demonstrated to increase intestinal absorption, but radioimmunoassays have eliminated the presence of both peptides in our fraction. It seems probable that the activity described is due to a peptide which has not yet been characterized.

REFERENCES

1. Bolton, J. E., Munday, K. A., Parsons, B. J., and Poat, J. A. (1974): Effect of angiotensin on fluid transport by rat jejunum in vivo. *J. Physiol.,* 241:33–34 P.
2. Mainoya, J. R. (1975): Further studies on the action of prolactin in fluid and ion absorption by the rat jejunum. *Endocrinology,* 96:1158–1164.
3. Mutt, V. (1978): Hormone isolation. In: *Gut Hormones,* edited by S. R. Bloom, pp. 21–27. Churchill Livingstone, Edinburgh.
4. Pansu, D., Bosshard, A., Vagne, M., and Mutt, V. (1978): A fraction isolated from upper small intestine inducing the absorption of water and sodium in duodenum of rats. *Scand. J. Gastroenterol.* [*Suppl. 49*], 13:139.
5. Vagne, M., Mutt, V., Perret, G., and Lemaitre, R. (1976): A fraction isolated from upper small intestine stimulating pepsin secretion in the cat. *Digestion,* 14:89–93.

VI. PORCINE INTESTINAL PEPTIDE WITH C-TERMINAL SOMATOSTATIN: ISOLATION AND CHARACTERIZATION

Lucien Pradayrol, J. Chayvialle, and A. Ribet

INSERM U. 151 C.H.U. Rangueil, F-31052 Toulouse, Cedex, France

In order to investigate the intestinal modulation of pancreatic secretion, we have been interested in naturally occurring peptides able to inhibit pancreatic secretion. At least two approaches to this problem were possible. First, we could have chosen a physiological model to follow and purify previously uncharacterized peptides showing such an inhibitory activity. Second, we could have investigated the possible occurrence in the intestinal tissue of known substances with this property but which had not previously been isolated from intestinal tissue. We started with the latter approach, and somatostatin, a tetradecapeptide isolated from ovine hypothalamus and chemically characterized by Brazeau et al. (2), appeared to be the best candidate. An identical peptide has been also isolated and characterized by Schally et al. (16) from porcine hypothalamus. Somatostatin-like immunoreactivity (SLI) and bioactivity have been shown to be widely distributed in the central nervous system and digestive tract tissues (1,3,6,19), and somatostatin or somatostatin-like material has been localized immunohistochemically in the pancreatic cell islets (9) and subsequently in the gastrointestinal mucosa (12). Radioimmunoassay in conjunction with physiological tests allowed us to investigate the porcine intestinal peptides.

During our isolation work, higher molecular weight immunoreactive forms of growth hormone–release inhibiting factor (GH-RIF) have been reported in extracts of ovine hypothalamus (10,19), rat pancreas and stomach (1), human serum (7), and human pancreatic somatostatinoma (8), but no final characterization of these peptides has been reported.

PURIFICATION

The radioimmunological determination (4) of the SLI content of the porcine intestinal peptide concentrate (11) and of the material obtained from the peptide concentrate showed that the immunoreactive material was purified, although in low yield, jointly with secretin, up to the step of carboxymethyl cellulose chromatography. At this step, SLI material was eluted after the secretin fraction. The purification of the post-secretin fraction has been carried out with a chromatography on carboxymethyl cellulose sandwiched between two chromatographies on Sephadex G-25.

The final purification of the material eluted from the second chromatography on Sephadex has been processed by high-performance liquid chromatography (HPLC), using a reverse-phase column (15). The peptide eluted in the main peak exhibited biological and radioimmunological activities.

COMPARATIVE STUDIES OF THE INTESTINAL PEPTIDE AND GH-RIF

We first reported (14) differences in the chromatographic behavior of the partially purified intestinal SLI peptide and GH-RIF. The intestinal peptide appeared less hydrophobic on phenyl-Sepharose column and did not migrate on countercurrent distribution in a n butanol/0.1 M NH_4HCO_3 (v/v) system.

The purified material was well differentiated from GH-RIF during isotachoelectrophoresis (13). The intestinal molecule gave a plateau with lower light absorbance at 254 nm and a mobility different from that of GH-RIF.

CHARACTERIZATION OF THE INTESTINAL PEPTIDE

Degradation with trypsin and analysis of the tryptic peptides (13) suggest that the C-terminal tetradecapeptide of the intestinal peptide is identical to hypothalamic somatostatin. As to the N-terminal part of the molecule, preliminary results seemed to indicate that the somatostatin sequence was preceded by heptapeptide (13), but more recent results indicate that this extension is longer (H. Jörnvall, *personal communication*).

ACTIVITY OF THE INTESTINAL PEPTIDE

A preliminary report (17) showed that in conscious dogs provided with gastric and pancreatic fistulas, the intestinal SLI peptide had inhibitory properties on slightly stimulated enzymatic pancreatic exocrine secretions similar to the ones of GH-RIF. In contrast with GH-RIF, it does not exhibit appreciable inhibitory activity on gastric secretion.

SUMMARY AND CONCLUSIONS

A porcine intestinal peptide belonging to the somatostatin family of peptides has been isolated from porcine upper small intestine. This peptide, immunologically identical to GH-RIF, was found to differ from it in several biological and chemical properties.

The preliminary chemical analysis of this peptide suggests that it is a higher molecular weight form of somatostatin. The existence of a trypsin-cleavable bond between the N-terminal alanine of GH-RIF and the first basic residue of the extension might mean that this peptide is a prohormonal form of GH-RIF. Work has been undertaken in our laboratory to study enzymatic conversion products of this molecule.

According to preliminary biological observations and because of rather large quantities of this peptide found in extracts from the upper small intestine, it is not improbable that it has a role in modulating pancreatic secretion.

PROJECTIONS FOR THE FUTURE

During the isolation procedure, we have not localized the tetradecapeptide isolated from the hypothalamus. Further work will show whether this has been due to loss of it during the preparation of the peptide concentrate or whether only the larger form is present in the intestinal tissue.

REFERENCES

1. Arimura, A., Sato, H., Dupont, A., Nishi, N., and Schally, A. V. (1975): Somatostatin: Abundance of immunoreactive hormone in rat stomach and pancreas. *Science,* 189:1007–1009.
2. Brazeau, P., Vale, W., Burgus, R., Ling, N., Butcher, M., Rivier, J., and Guillemin, R. (1973): Hypothalamic polypeptide that inhibits the secretion of immunoreactive pituitary growth hormone. *Science,* 179:77–79.
3. Brownstein, M., Arimura, A., Sato, H., Schally, A. V., and Kizer, J. S. (1975): The regional distribution of somatostatin in the rat brain. *Endocrinology,* 96:1456–1461.
4. Chayvialle, J. A. P., Descos, F., Bernard, C., Martin, A., Barre, C., and Partensky, C. (1978): Somatostatin in mucosa of stomach and duodenum in gastroduodenal disease. *Gastroenterology,* 75:13–19.
5. Hartley, B. S. (1970): Strategy and tactics in protein chemistry. *Biochem. J.,* 119:805–822.
6. Kronheim, S., Berelowitz, M., and Pimstone, B. L. (1976): A radioimmunoassay for growth hormone release-inhibiting hormone: Method and quantitative tissue distribution. *Clin. Endocrinol.,* 5:619–630.
7. Kronheim, S., Berelowitz, M., and Pimstone, B. L. (1978): The characterization of somatostatin-like immunoreactivity in human serum. *Diabetes,* 27:523–529.
8. Larsson, L.-I., Hirsch, M. A., Holst, J. J., Ingemansson, S., Kühl, C., Jensen, S. L., Lundqvist, G., Rehfeld, J. F., and Schwartz, T. W. (1977): Pancreatic somatostatinoma. Clinical features and physiological implications. *Lancet,* 1:666–668.
9. Luft, R., Efendic, S., Hökfelt, T., Johansson, O., and Arimura, A. (1974): Immunohistochemical evidence for the localization of somatostatin-like immunoreactivity in a cell population of the pancreatic islets. *Med. Biol.,* 52:428–430.
10. Millar, R. P. (1978): Somatostatin immunoreactive peptides of higher molecular weight in ovine hypothalamic extracts. *J. Endocrinol.,* 77:429–430.
11. Mutt, V. (1976): Further investigations on intestinal hormonal polypeptides. *Clin. Endocrinol.* [*Suppl.*], 5:175s–183s.

12. Polak, J. M., Pearse, A. G. E., Grimelius, L., Bloom, S. R., and Arimura, A. (1975): Growth-hormone release-inhibiting hormone in gastrointestinal and pancreatic D cells. *Lancet,* 1:1220–1222.
13. Pradayrol, L., Chayvialle, J. A., Carlquist, M., and Mutt, V. (1978): Isolation of a porcine intestinal peptide with C-terminal somatostatin. *Biochem. Biophys. Res. Commun.,* 85:701–708.
14. Pradayrol, L., Chayvialle, J., and Mutt, V. (1978): Pig duodenal somatostatin: Extraction and purification. *Metabolism [Suppl. 1],* 27:1197–1200.
15. Rivier, J. E. (1978): Use of trialkyl ammonium phosphate (TAAP) buffers in reverse phase HPLC for high resolution and high recovery of peptides and proteins. *J. Liquid Chromatoge.,* 1:343–366.
16. Schally, A. V., Dupont, A., Arimura, A., Redding, T. W., Nishi, N., Linthicum, G. L., and Schlesinger, D. H. (1976): Isolation and structure of somatostatin from porcine hypothalami. *Biochemistry,* 15:509–514.
17. Susini, C., Vaysse, N., Bommelaer, G., Esteve, J. P., and Ribet, A. (1979): Abstract submitted to A.G.A. meeting, New Orleans.
18. Vale, W., Brazeau, P., Rivier, C., Brown, M., Boss, B., Rivier, J., Burgus, R., Ling, N., and Guillemin, R. (1975): Somatostatin. *Recent Prog. Horm. Res.,* 31:365–397.
19. Vale, W., Ling, N., Rivier, J., Villarreal, J., Rivier, C., Douglas, C., and Brown, M. (1976): Somatostatin. Anatomic and phylogenetic distribution of somatostatin. *Metabolism [Suppl. 1],* 25:1491–1494.
20. Woods, K. R., and Wang, K.-T. (1967): Separation of dansyl-amino acids by polyamide layer chromatography. *Biochim. Biophys. Acta,* 133:369–370.

Subject Index